FOUNDATIONS OF ORIENTATION AND MOBILITY

SECOND EDITION

Bruce B. Blasch,
William R. Wiener,
and Richard L. Welsh
Editors

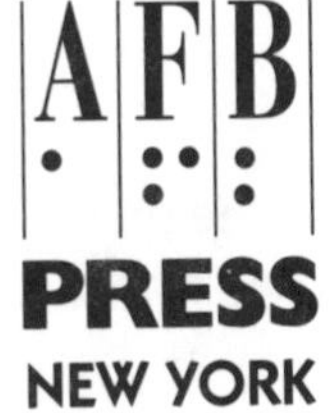

NEW YORK

Printed in the United States of America

Library of Congress Cataloging-in-Publication Data

Foundations of orientation and mobility / Bruce B. Blasch, William R. Wiener, Richard L. Welsh, editors — 2nd ed.
p. cm.
Includes bibliographical references and index.
ISBN 0-89128-946-1
1. Visually handicapped—Rehabilitation. 2. Visually handicapped—Orientation and mobility. 3. Blind—rehabilitation. 4. Blind—perception. I. Blasch, Bruce B. II. Wiener, William R. III. Welsh, Richard L.
HV1626.F68 1997
362.4'18—dc21 97-27613
CIP

The development of this publication was sponsored in part by the U.S. Department of Veterans Affairs, VA Rehabilitation Research and Development Service, Washington, DC (Administrative Project to Atlanta VA Medical Center, Rehabilitation Research and Development Center).

The mission of the American Foundation for the Blind (AFB) is to enable persons who are blind or visually impaired to achieve equality of access and opportunity that will ensure freedom of choice in their lives.

It is the policy of the American Foundation for the Blind to use in the first printing of its books acid-free paper that meets the ANSI Z39.48 Standard. The infinity symbol that appears above indicates that the paper in this printing meets that standard.

This book is dedicated to Donald Blasch and Everett "Butch" Hill, whose commitment and leadership were significant in the development of the profession of orientation and mobility. Both men were contributors to the first edition of this text, and both passed away in the early days of the preparation of this second edition.

CONTENTS

FOREWORD

The first edition of *Foundations of Orientation and Mobility* was published by the American Foundation for the Blind in 1980. The appearance of this text was a milestone in the development of a key discipline in the rehabilitation and education of persons who are blind or visually impaired. It was also a milestone in the delivery of services in the field of blindness and visual impairment, for the ability to travel safely and on one's own is an essential skill for individuals who wish to live independently. A text that disseminated information and in that way advanced the practice of orientation and mobility (O&M) therefore had a profound impact on both the profession of O&M and the people who benefitted from improved instruction.

The first edition of this book made a memorable contribution by assembling together for the first time in one place diverse and technical information from a variety of sources. This second edition builds on the essential foundation laid down by its predecessor. In the chapters that follow, students and practitioners of O&M will find material that elaborates on the theoretical background of their discipline and carries it into areas such as low vision, technology, and the international sphere that have seen notable activity and growth over the last decade. They will find reflected here the broad panorama of what now constitutes the discipline of O&M as we approach the next century.

The editors and authors contributing to this text have provided a vital service to the field of blindness and visual impairment by enriching the knowledge available to us all. By supporting and collaborating with them, we at the American Foundation for the Blind have been pleased to play the critical role that the foundation always strives to fill—improving the quality of life of persons who are blind or visually impaired.

Carl R. Augusto
President
American Foundation for the Blind

PREFACE

As I paged through the chapters of the first edition of *Foundations of Orientation and Mobility* a decade ago, I was persuaded to the conviction that what I was reading was what years of professional practice had instructed me is the vital substance of rehabilitation medicine. The chapters comprised a compilation of the scientific and ethical foundations common to many branches of the practice of human rehabilitation.

Rehabilitation was properly presented as a process whereby a person, once impaired by loss of structural integrity or functional use, achieves optimal levels of performance compatible with his or her current abilities. It allows the person once again to participate in personally chosen life pathways and to enjoy the satisfying qualities that life offers.

Rehabilitation requires an interdisciplinary contribution by many care-related practitioners to assist the disabled person to seek and to gain his or her goals. It employs not only interventions of a medical, surgical, and nursing design, but also personal assistance, physiological reconditioning, retraining, reeducation, and environmental modification. Corrective, adaptive, and substitute technologies were seen as therapeutic applications for accomplishing physical, psychological, spiritual, social, vocational, and recreational wholeness for a disabled person. It adds the dimension of concern for function into the care equation, a concern which is often left to rest in negative balance for the person after preventive and curative measures are undertaken.

Now in the second edition of this preeminent textbook for the orientation and mobility specialist, the luster of heritage of the profession has been burnished even brighter by close interlocking of the sciences contributing to understanding of sight and seeing and orientation and mobility with the functional goals of rehabilitation and special education practices for people who are blind or have low vision. Contributing authors with a wide range of clinical study and research experience have made complex subject topics accessible from the physical, biological, and psychosocial sciences. Since information about the world around each person is acquired through a rich complex of sensory channels, the importance of addressing multiple perceptual losses has been more fully explored in this new edition. Emphasis is placed on the related effects of loss of sensation in one body system as it affects others, such as where one has both visual and physical impairment. The primacy of the visual experience is evident in consideration of principles guiding each person's ability to experience the dimensions of self, the place of self in the personal space of his or her perceived universe, and the societal interactions empowered by improved orientation and mobility. For the instructor, the guide, the mentor, and the friend, the importance of recognizing the unique personhood of each visually impaired person becomes clear in this edition's topical subject presentations. Thus every effort in the process of rehabilitation and special education becomes exclusively individualized.

With demobilization of veterans of military service following World War II, the rehabilitation movement was begun in America. Many returnees to civilian life had sustained permanent impairment and disability through vital loss of structure and function. There were the amputees. There were the blinded. There were the head and spinal injured. There were the burned, and many more. Rehabilitation grew out of this overwhelming need for assistance and continues to serve with cessation of each military conflict and national emergency. Pioneers banded together to make a life better for people who are disabled from whatever cause or diagnosis in military or civilian life. The heroes of the rehabilitation movement were many. Rusk, Krusen, Covalt, and Switzer in physical and vocational rehabilitation. Hoover, Williams, Carroll, Bledsoe, and Blasch in orientation and mobility. There were many agencies that banded together, including the Military Services, the Veterans Service Organizations, the Veterans Administration, other Federal agencies, and the American Foundation for the Blind. It is especially impressive to note that some of these early heroes and pioneers—Bledsoe, Whitstock and Farmer—who contributed to the first edition of this book have also contributed to this second edition.

But that is what this book is about. So read and study. Become a professional with knowledge, skill, and a guiding ethic. If you use this text as a student, then you will benefit in your student life. If you use this book as a basis for your professional dedication, then many will benefit.

John W. Goldschmidt, MD
Director
Rehabilitation Research and Development Service
U.S. Department of Veterans Affairs

ACKNOWLEDGMENTS

Many years ago, two naive instructors in training programs for mobility specialists began the task of "correcting a deficiency." This deficiency was the lack of a comprehensive textbook for orientation and mobility (O&M) specialists. After numerous hours preparing the first edition, a sudden insight prompted the statement, "The past five years have helped us to understand why such a book was not attempted by wiser individuals." As with many experiences, however, only the positive aspects have been remembered, particularly the feedback about the value of the textbook and the interaction with and assistance of many people who contributed to the production of "Big Red." Forgotten were the missed football games, hunting trips, times away from young families, and long weekends devoted only to manuscript preparation, review, and editing.

With a twinge of guilt about outdated materials, fading memories, a fresh dose of enthusiasm from Bill Wiener, and support from the U.S. Department of Veterans Affairs and the American Foundation for the Blind (AFB), the task of bringing "Big Red" into the twenty-first century was begun.

As with any task of this magnitude, many individuals have provided us with sustaining support. Most significant, have been our wives (Barb, Peg, and Dee respectively), who provided us with nourishment, cheerful work environments, advice, and loving encouragement. Our young adult children, with the fresh perspective of their own university experiences, offered a pride and respect in the task their fathers were undertaking. These sources of support maintained our desire to complete the task.

The breadth of the subject matter covered in this text necessitated a close collaboration with many of the outstanding professionals in the field. We owe them a special thank-you not only for their efforts in completing their chapters, but also for the knowledge they shared with us.

The support from our employers—the U.S. Department of Veterans Affairs, Rehabilitation Research and Development Service; Western Michigan University; and Pittsburgh Vision Services—have continued to encourage our efforts. We would like to also express our appreciation to AFB and Carl Augusto for continuing to support professionalism in our field through textbooks such as "Big Red." Also, for helping with many of the processing details we want to thank Erica Wyse, Lou Ann Grossberg, and Mike Williams at the Atlanta Veterans Affairs Medical Center, Rehab R&D Center.

Readers of this text will find that it is dedicated to Donald Blasch and Everett ("Butch") Hill and that a description of their accomplishments is included later in these pages. In addition to what we have summarized about their memorable accomplishments, we would also like to add something here about their equally memorable personalities. In the case of Donald Blasch, his distinguished career and especially his concern for students were facilitated and enhanced by his wife, Virginia. His support, wisdom, and willingness to listen are missed by many. Everett Hill, who had a limited supply of suits and ties (if any) and an abundance of "Rock 'n' Roll" records, was noted for his dedication to family and basketball as well as to the profession of O&M. In all of his endeavors, he acknowledged the support of his closest colleague and wife, Mary Maureen Snook Hill. He was a true friend who would give of himself freely.

The project has demonstrated again that teaching and learning are inseparable processes. Our debt to both our teachers and our students is clear to us, even though it has been difficult to distinguish when we were teaching and when we were being taught.

Finally, our colleagues across the world, other mobility specialists, have inspired us by their commitment to their profession, their commitment to their mobility students, their interest in this project, and their willingness to share their knowledge any place, any time.

Bruce B. Blasch
William R. Wiener
Richard L. Welsh

THE CONTRIBUTORS

Bruce B. Blasch, Ph.D., is Senior Health Scientist at the Veterans Affairs Medical Center in Atlanta and the Rehabilitation Research and Development Center in Decatur, Georgia. He is also Clinical Associate Professor, Department of Rehabilitation Medicine, at Emory University School of Medicine in Atlanta, Georgia.

William R. Wiener, Ph.D., is Chairperson and Professor, Department of Blind Rehabilitation and Co-coordinator, Rehabilitation Counseling/Teaching Program, Departments of Blind Rehabilitation and Counselor Education/Counseling Psychology, at Western Michigan University in Kalamazoo, Michigan.

Richard L. Welsh, Ph.D., is Vice President of Pittsburgh Vision Services in Pittsburgh, Pennsylvania.

Chapter Authors

Billie Louise Bentzen, Ph.D., is Director of Research at the Carroll Center for the Blind in Newton, Massachusetts; Adjunct Professor, Department of Psychology, at Boston College in Chestnut Hill, Massachusetts; and President of Accessible Design for the Blind in Berlin, Massachusetts.

Michael J. Bina, Ed.D., is Superintendent of the Indiana School for the Blind.

C. Warren Bledsoe is Board Member (Emeritus) of the Maryland School for the Blind in Baltimore, Maryland, and was Consultant to the U.S. Department of Health, Education, and Welfare, Social and Rehabilitation Services Administration, Office for the Blind and Visually Handicapped.

Robert H. Bradley, Ph.D., is Professor, Center for Research on Teaching and Learning, at the University of Arkansas at Little Rock.

Harvey C. Clark, M.Ed., is Blind Rehabilitation Specialist, O&M Section, Southeastern Blind Rehabilitation Center, at the Veterans Affairs Medical Center in Birmingham, Alabama.

John E. Crews, Ph.D., is Executive Director of the Governor's Council on Developmental Disabilities in Atlanta, Georgia; Adjunct Senior Associate in Rehabilitation Medicine at Emory University School of Medicine in Atlanta, Georgia; and Clinical Professor, Department of Mental Health and Human Services, at Georgia State University in Atlanta.

Robert J. Crouse, Ed.D., is Executive Director of the Blind and Low Vision Services of North Georgia, Inc., in Smyrna, Georgia.

William R. De l'Aune, Ph.D., is Research Psychologist, Rehabilitation Research and Development Center, at the U.S. Department of Veterans Affairs in Decatur, Georgia; Clinical Assistant Professor,

Rehabilitation Medicine, at Emory University School of Medicine in Atlanta, Georgia; Clinical Professor, Department of Mental Health and Human Services, at Georgia State University in Atlanta; and Associate Professor, Vision Rehabilitation Program, at the Pennsylvania College of Optometry in Philadelphia.

Paul Ehresman, M.Ed., is an Orientation and Mobility Instructor at the Missouri School for the Blind in St. Louis, Missouri.

Leicester W. Farmer, Sr., M.A., was, at the time of writing, Technology Transfer Specialist and Director of the Electronic Travel Aids (ETAs) Section of the Veterans Affairs Blind Rehabilitation Center in Hines, Illinois.

Lukas Franck, M.A., is Supervisor of Community Instruction at Seeing Eye, Inc. in Morristown, New Jersey.

Duane Geruschat, Ph.D., is Director of Educational Support at the Maryland School for the Blind in Baltimore and Research Associate in Ophthalmology at the Johns Hopkins School of Medicine in Baltimore, Maryland.

David A. Guth, Ph.D., is Professor, Department of Blind Rehabilitation, at Western Michigan University in Kalamazoo, Michigan.

Rodney Haneline, M.A., is Director of Admissions and Graduate Services at Leader Dogs for the Blind in Rochester, Michigan.

Everett W. Hill, Ph.D., now deceased, was Professor, Department of Special Education, at George Peabody College for Teachers at Vanderbilt University in Nashville, Tennessee.

William H. Jacobson, Ed.D., is Professor, Department of Rehabilitation, at the University of Arkansas at Little Rock.

Elga Joffee, M.Ed., M.P.S., is Director of the Information Center at the American Foundation for the Blind in New York.

Steven J. LaGrow, Ed.D., is Professor and Head, Department of Rehabilitation Studies, at Massey University in New Zealand.

Gary D. Lawson, Ph.D., is Associate Professor, Department of Speech Pathology and Audiology, at Western Michigan University in Kalamazoo, Michigan.

Dennis Lolli is an Orientation and Mobility and Low Vision Education Consultant at the Perkins Outreach Service and Educational Consultant for the Hilton/Perkins Program in Watertown, Massachusetts.

Richard G. Long, Ph.D., is an Orientation and Mobility Specialist and Teacher in Clayton County, Georgia Public Schools, and Clinical Assistant Professor, Department of Rehabilitation Medicine, at Emory University School of Medicine in Atlanta, Georgia.

Nurit Neustadt-Noy, Ph.D., is Rehabilitation Consultant and Director, International Training Program, at the Carroll Center for the Blind in Newton, Massachusetts and Professor at Tel Aviv Teachers' College in Israel.

Lydia Peterson, M.S., is an Orientation and Mobility Specialist at the Saint Paul Public Schools in Minnesota.

John J. Rieser, Ph.D., is Professor and Chair, Department of Psychology and Human Development, at George Peabody College for Teachers at Vanderbilt University in Nashville, Tennessee.

Christine A. Roman, Ph.D., is Clinical Instructor, Vision Studies Program, Department of Instruction and Learning, at the University of Pittsburgh in Pennsylvania; Coordinator, Project CRIB, at Western Pennsylvania School for Blind Children; and Infant Development Specialist at the Western Pennsylvania Hospital.

Sandra Rosen, Ph.D., is Associate Professor and Coordinator, Programs in Visual Impairment, at the San Francisco State University in California.

Deborah Rower, MPA, M.S. Special Education, was, at the time of writing, Mobility Supervisor at the Lighthouse, Inc., Hudson Valley Region, in New York.

Dona Sauerburger, M.A., is an orientation and mobility specialist in Baltimore, Maryland.

Annette C. Skellenger, Ed.D., is Assistant Professor, Programs in Special Education, Department of Educational Psychology, University of South Carolina in Columbia.

Eileen Siffermann, M.A., M.Ed., is an orientation and mobility specialist in Tucson, Arizona.

Audrey J. Smith, Ph.D., is Executive Director, Institute for the Visually Impaired, and Associate Professor, Department of Graduate Studies in Vision Impairment, at the Pennsylvania College of Optometry in Philadelphia.

Daniel L. Smith, M.A., is an Orientation and Mobility Specialist at the Central Blind Rehabilitation Center in Hines, Illinois.

Robert H. Whitstock, J.D., was, at the time of writing, Vice President, Programs, at the Seeing Eye, Inc. in Morristown, New Jersey.

George J. Zimmerman, Ph.D., is Associate Professor and Associate Chair, Department of Instruction and Learning and Coordinator, Vision Studies Program in Special Education, at the University of Pittsburgh in Pennsylvania.

IN MEMORIAM

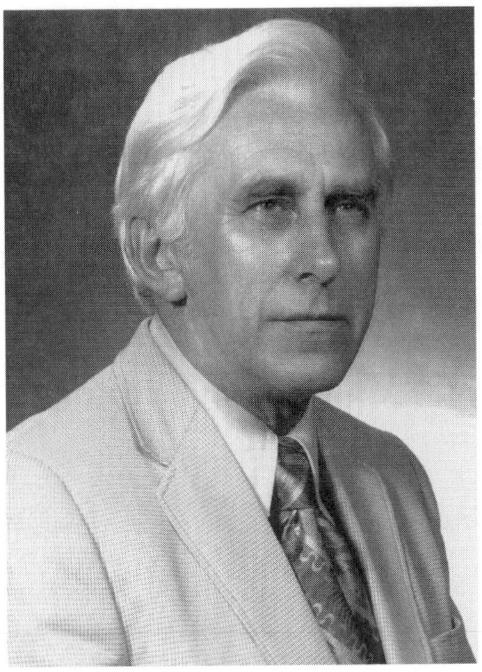

Donald Blasch was cast in many roles during his distinguished career: counselor to many veterans, teacher to many students, mentor, leader, pioneer, role model, uncle, and friend. He entered the blindness field in 1951, as a counselor at the Hines VA Medical Center where his responsibilities were to assist blinded veterans, particularly those from the Korean War. Toward the end of the 1950's, he spearheaded a pilot program that applied the Hines approach to mobility instruction to children with a visual impairment. In 1961, he became the first director of Western Michigan University's orientation and mobility program. Under his leadership the program became an institute in 1967 and achieved departmental status in 1972. Don was instrumental in establishing the AAWB Interest Group IX and the AEVH orientation and mobility group. He was the first chair of the AEVH O&M group and served on numerous committees at all levels in both professional organizations. He also began the first professional rehabilitation teacher training program. In recognition of his professional contributions, Don was the recipient of many awards, including: Buddy Award, The Seeing Eye (1966); Lawrence E. Blaha, AAWB (1977); Migel Award, AFB (1977); Alfred Allen Memorial Award, AAWB (1979); Ambrose B. Shotwell Award, AAWB (1981); and the WMU Distinguished Service Award (1982).

IN MEMORIAM

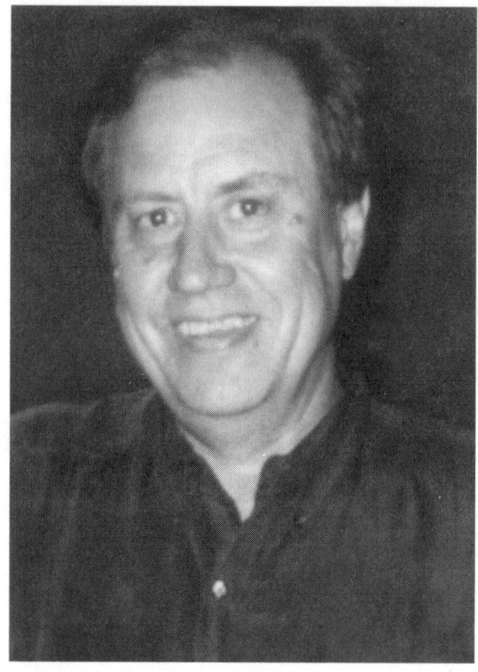

Everett Hill was a man with dedication and energy for a wide variety of interests and the profession of orientation and mobility. He accepted a job teaching mobility at the Minneapolis Society for the Blind (MSB) in 1966. Recognizing the complexity of this "simple task of mobility," he pursued his formal education in O&M at Western Michigan University. After graduation, he returned to MSB and then to the Missouri School for the Blind. In 1970, he accepted a position at Florida State University (FSU) as a faculty member. While at FSU, he collaborated on the first book of O&M techniques.

In 1974, Butch returned to Western Michigan University to complete a Masters degree in special education and a Doctorate in education. His first major research effort, the Hill Test of Selected Positional Concepts, became the first norm-referenced assessment tool in O&M. In 1979 he joined the faculty at Peabody College, where he continued to teach and inspire students who have gone on to further develop the profession of O&M. He authored more than 40 papers, and contributed chapters to various textbooks. He is especially noted for his significant research and publications in the areas of spatial orientation, infancy, and early childhood. From 1988 to 1990 he served as the chair of Division Nine. Because of his significant contributions to Division Nine, the Newcomer-Hill Award was established in 1992 to honor an individual at each International AER Conference in recognition of major contributions made to Division Nine during the previous two years. At this same conference, he was awarded the highest honor in O&M, the Lawrence E. Blaha Award. Through his behavior he has inspired a generation of practitioners.

Introduction

Bruce B. Blasch, William R. Wiener, and Richard L. Welsh

The ability to move independently, safely, and purposefully through the environment plays an important role in human development. The infant who learns to crawl, the toddler who takes her first steps, and the child who negotiates stairs by herself are each recognized as having accomplished an important developmental task. When a young child is first allowed to cross a street, run an errand to the neighborhood store, or travel back and forth to school on his own, he is generally considered to have passed other developmental milestones. When an adolescent receives permission to travel alone in a complex downtown area or to drive a car, it is recognition of the fact that her skill and judgment in moving independently through the community have developed even further. Each of these accomplishments increases the status of the individual in the eyes of others and has a positive impact on his own self-concept.

The exhilaration associated with achieving these developmental milestones should serve as a predictor of the intensity of the frustration that accompanies a person's loss of the ability to move independently through the community. This occurs when people with visual impairments, especially older people, are no longer able to drive a car. A lack of mobility among people with severe visual impairment or other disabilities also seems to contribute to the depression that some people with disabilities feel early on in their experience with a disability.

Geruschat and Smith in Chapter 3 of this text eloquently describe the contribution of vision to mobility:

> There is no other sense that can gather and process the same volume and richness of information as quickly as sight. In addition to the *speed* and *volume* of information obtained through sight is the *distance* from which the information can be obtained. In a mobility context, distance means anticipation, the ability to preview the travel path, which provides the individual with the ability to be proactive through the avoidance of obstacles and the identification of a curb or stairs before arriving at them. (p. 60)

The significance of mobility accomplishments perhaps should have been seen as a predictor of the strong desire to learn to be independently mobile that characterized the young men and women who lost their vision during World War II and who were gathered at Valley Forge Army Hospital in 1945 for rehabilitation services. The energy that resulted from this urgent desire to be mobile fueled the development of the profession of orientation and mobility (O&M).

As the first O&M specialists faced the challenge of helping people who are blind or visually impaired learn how to safely travel, they recognized the need for a broad base of understanding about human functioning and the impact of blindness. When the training of O&M specialists shifted from the U.S. Veterans Administration (VA) to universities across this country, the curricula that were developed drew from a wide range of professions and disciplines in order to provide the new O&M specialists the information they needed.

THE KNOWLEDGE BASE OF ORIENTATION AND MOBILITY INSTRUCTION

The professional specialty of O&M instruction for persons with visual impairments emerged in recognition of the importance of independent movement in human functioning. Whether a person's visual impairment is congenital and evident at birth or whether it occurs later in life, it can have a major negative impact on a person's functional mobility and, therefore, on the quality of his or her life (Lowenfeld, 1964; Carroll, 1961). Fortunately, this kind of negative impact can be lessened or overcome through instruction.

Although formal instruction of children who are blind generally preceded formal rehabilitation programs for adults who lost their vision later in life, school programs did not introduce formalized instruction in O&M (Bledsoe, 1980). With the exception of the early work of Francis Campbell in the United States and the work of schools for blind children in Germany (Allen, 1969), there is little evidence of formal instruction in mobility being provided for children. The development of the Seeing Eye program represented the first systematic instruction in O&M in the United States. This was followed by the development of the long-cane method of travel in the army's rehabilitation program following World War II and the refinement of this approach in the Veterans Administration facilities in the 1950s (Bledsoe, 1980).

It was not until the training of O&M specialists moved to universities in the 1960s that an effort was made to define the body of knowledge that mobility specialists needed to carry out their responsibility to help people learn how to travel independently without vision or with severely reduced vision. Those who were charged with the responsibility for developing the first university programs divided the content of their training programs into three general areas. First, they had to teach those who would be instructors the actual techniques and methods that visually impaired people use to achieve independent O&M. Second, they knew that O&M specialists would need a solid understanding of the basic human systems through which people receive, interpret, and act on information about the environment, especially in the absence of visual information. Finally, they needed supervised practice as teachers so that they could develop and refine their ability to actually teach people who are blind or visually impaired successfully and to modify the basic teaching as needed when confronted by students who had other impairments or limitations in addition to vision loss.

In the early days of the university training programs for O&M specialists, faculty members selected courses from other departments in the university through which the future instructors could learn about audiology, kinesiology, psychology, and other areas of information that were considered important for an instructor to know. Multiple textbooks were required to cover all of the necessary information and relevant articles from various disciplines were shared with the students.

The first edition of *Foundations of Orientation and Mobility,* which was published in 1980, pulled together for the first time in a single text much of the diverse background knowledge needed by O&M specialists. This information was intended to provide O&M specialists with enough information about the physiology and functioning of human perceptual and motor systems to understand why the mobility techniques would be successful, how to improve them further, and how to modify them for students or clients with special needs in addition to their loss of vision. It was not intended to be a book of techniques or teaching methods. Other texts cover that information (Hill & Ponder, 1976; Jacobson, 1993; LaGrow & Weessies, 1994).

Although many of the chapter authors in the first edition of *Foundations of Orientation and Mobility* were themselves O&M specialists, some chapters were authored by specialists in the various disciplines represented in the text. They tried to make their work relevant to the needs of O&M specialists, but sometimes did not succeed. Sixteen years later the editors, while preparing this updated version of the text, have been impressed by the number of O&M specialists who have become experts in the related disciplines represented in this volume. Every chapter but one has been authored or coauthored by a person who was trained as an O&M specialist and who has spent time practicing that profession.

Even more impressive, throughout the text there are numerous references to research studies which have been designed and implemented by O&M specialists. These studies have further advanced the O&M profession and the quality of services which are provided to people who are blind and others who experience functional limitations in mobility and require systematic instruction in order to learn how to overcome these limitations.

REVIEW OF THE TEXT

The text is divided into four sections: human systems; mobility systems; the learner; and the progression of the profession.

Human Systems

In the first section, six primary human systems are presented and the significance of each for O&M is discussed. The section leads off with a unique overview of perception as it relates to the control of locomotion without vision. Central to the role of the O&M specialist is the ability to understand how people receive and interpret information about the environment, especially when vision, the primary channel for receiving such information, is blocked or deficient in some way. Perception is a complex topic and most attempts to present an overview of it tend to oversimplify it or make it difficult to understand. Guth and Rieser in Chapter 1 present the basic concepts of perception using examples from O&M situations only. Although the chapter requires careful reading, the time spent is a good investment. The basic concepts of perception are found throughout all of the following chapters and the issue of what a client is perceiving in any given situation is the most frequently recurring question in the O&M specialist's practice.

Although the act of perceiving the information represented by sensory stimuli is a critical building block, the resulting conceptualization of space and how a client uses such concepts are of central importance to independent travel. Long and Hill in Chapter 2 present one of the more extensive treatments of spatial orientation found in the mobility literature to date. They have captured the best thinking of the field on this topic and packaged for the entering professional in such a way that this information can be effectively used with students much sooner than was possible in the past. This chapter also updates some of the standard terminology in the mobility field regarding spatial orientation. The editors expect that these improved terms will introduce greater conceptual clarity and consistency in future discussions of spatial orientation.

One of the more important and fastest growing areas of knowledge for the O&M specialist relates to the topic of low vision. Since the publication of the first edition of this text in 1980, the role of the O&M specialist in working with clients who have low vision has continued to expand. Geruschat and Smith in Chapter 3 provide the beginning instructor with sufficient information to understand how various types of low vision affect mobility. They also address how the O&M specialist can assess the functional mobility limitations of the low vision student and how best to provide instruction designed to increase the low vision student's safe and independent travel.

In Chapter 4, Wiener and Lawson present

solid and comprehensive information about hearing, an extremely important sense for people with visual impairments. The O&M specialist needs to know how hearing is assessed, how to interpret audiograms for specific clients, and how hearing can be improved. All of this basic information is provided. This chapter also reviews research that is relevant to the O&M specialist's ability to understand and use hearing. This research ranges from the classical studies done at Cornell University many decades ago to the most current studies being done and shared in this textbook for the first time.

In Chapter 5, Rosen provides the basic information that the O&M specialist needs to understand the mechanics of bodily movement as well as the awareness of movement. The kinesthetic sense provides a great deal of important information to people, especially when vision is absent or significantly impaired. The O&M specialist helps his students understand how to attend to and interpret this information.

In Chapter 6, Welsh reviews information relevant to the psychological and social functioning of people with visual impairments, especially in mobility situations. Psychosocial factors play a prominent role in a person's success as a visually impaired traveler when other systems are functioning normally and when they are not. An understanding of psychosocial factors is recommended for the O&M specialist in order to structure mobility learning experiences that result in success and confidence building.

Mobility Systems

The second section of the text addresses the tools, materials, and features of the environment that the O&M specialist and his students use to facilitate independent travel without vision or with severely impaired vision. Farmer and Smith in Chapter 7 briefly review the standard long cane, the development of which launched the O&M revolution. They then review and explore the various efforts to develop and disseminate electronic travel aids and close with a review of adaptive mobility devices. It is recommended that the O&M specialist understand all of these tools and have a conceptual basis for evaluating each next generation of technology that will emerge.

In Chapter 8, Whitstock, Franck, and Haneline review the history and the principles underlying the use of specially trained dogs as a mobility system that is of value to many visually impaired travelers. Most O&M specialists will not work directly in the process of helping a person who is blind or visually impaired learn how to use a dog for mobility purposes. Increasingly, dog guide training programs depend on O&M specialists to provide basic O&M instruction for people who will go on to use dog guides. O&M specialists also assist dog guide users with orientation to new areas. For all of these reasons, O&M specialists need to understand how dog guides work, how they are trained, and how handlers are taught to use their dogs.

Bentzen, in Chapters 9 and 10, adds other tools and information to the O&M specialist's repertoire. In her comprehensive presentation of orientation aids, Bentzen provides the information that an instructor needs to develop aids which permit a blind traveler to understand spatial layouts and store such information for future reference. Electronics and computers are quickly changing this area of information as new orientation aid products arrive in this rapidly expanding market.

The environments themselves that orientation aids try to depict are also changing rapidly. Many of these changes are fueled by legislation and public policy which require that public environments be made accessible. Others are caused by changes in traffic control aids that facilitate movement through the environment for vehicles while creating serious new challenges for the pedestrian who is blind or visually impaired. It is recommended that O&M specialists be informed about such changes and help their students understand them and how to negotiate safely through these changing environments. In Chapter 10, Bentzen reviews the emerging changes in the built environment and provides suggestions for how visually impaired travelers can continue to move independently in a rapidly changing world.

The Learner

The third major section of the text focuses on the various kinds of people who require instruction from O&M specialists. Although all students can use the human systems described in Part One, and they all use one or all of the mobility systems discussed in Part Two, the approaches that O&M specialists use for different kinds of students will change from one student to another.

All instruction is directed by the basic information that is encompassed by the term "learning theory." Jacobson and Bradley in Chapter 11 review various theories about how learning occurs and how it can best be facilitated by teachers. The examples that illustrate the theories of learning are taken primarily from mobility situations. In this way the student can more readily understand how these theories apply to mobility instruction and how instruction can be modified to respond to the special needs of individual clients.

In Chapter 12, Zimmerman and Roman present the standard approach to teaching children and adults who are visually impaired how to travel, while the remaining chapters in this section address the special characteristics of many learners whose age, other disabilities, or health conditions require variations in the standard approach. The basic principles of program design that Zimmerman and Roman articulate apply across all settings. For learners of all kinds, it is important that O&M specialists work closely with the student, parents, and other family members when appropriate in understanding what they want to accomplish and selecting the goals and approaches that will be used. It is also important that O&M specialists work closely with parents and family members of mobility students and other team members to make certain that they understand what is being taught and what can be expected of the visually impaired person following mobility training. This is especially important as O&M specialists find themselves teaching students with more complex patterns of multiple impairments and working in various kinds of multidisciplinary or transdisciplinary teams in which the responsibility for the students' learning is shared among team members.

Chapters 13 and 14 provide O&M specialists with the theoretical and practical information they need to modify their approaches to instruction appropriately for preschool-aged learners as well as for older adults. Both groups have particular needs related to their ages that may require specific consideration from the O&M specialist.

The final five chapters of this section further illustrate the need for O&M specialists to modify approaches to instruction for various types of learners whose needs and styles of learning are affected by the presence of other impairments. For many years newly trained O&M specialists have felt that they needed more information about how best to serve people whose visual impairment was complicated by hearing loss, cognitive impairments, the effects of stroke, and other multiple disabilities. Information in this area has been expanded to the point where graduating O&M specialists should feel more comfortable as they begin to serve the more complex needs of these students. However, real comfort in this area of service will only result from appropriately supervised experience in teaching these learners.

The final chapter of this section also provides a bridge to the final section of the textbook, which will address the progression of the profession. Chapter 19 addresses the expanding concept of providing mobility instruction to people with various functional limitations but who are not visually impaired. Although this concept has been discussed by O&M specialists for at least 25 years and was included as a chapter in the first edition of this text, it is still an underrecognized opportunity to develop and expand the O&M profession. Blasch, LaGrow, and Peterson provide a rationale for this development, along with many practical suggestions for how to approach the mobility needs of people with functional limitations but without visual impairment.

Progression of the Profession

In the fourth and final section of the book, the progression of the O&M profession is reviewed. Wiener and Siffermann trace the movement of O&M toward increasing professionalism while highlighting the issues that face the profession both now and in the future. This development has been built on the work of those who were responsible for launching the profession in the army and VA programs following World War II. Bledsoe, in Chapter 21, has chronicled in a very personal way the steps that were taken to formalize, preserve, and further advance the insights that he, Richard Hoover, and Russell Williams had developed with the help of hundreds of visually impaired people.

In Chapter 22 Neustadt-Noy and LaGrow offer the first comprehensive analysis of how formal O&M instruction has spread around the globe. Although the manner of training instructors and delivering the services varies from country to country, this chapter provides strong evidence of the recognition of the importance of formal mobility instruction. It also foresees an even stronger demand for mobility instruction in the future.

In the final two chapters of the text, the focus is on the future of the profession. In Chapter 23 Crouse and Bina discuss the methods used to organize and manage formal O&M services from the administrative point of view. Regardless of the soundness of the theory underlying the practice of O&M, unless the financial resources are available and the legal and procedural requirements are met, mobility services will not be available and will not continue to expand.

Finally, in Chapter 24, De l'Aune provides the information and encouragement that O&M specialists need if they are going to contribute scientifically to the further growth and development of their profession. If this textbook is successful, O&M specialists will have sufficient background and information to draw upon the theories of many different disciplines in developing and testing new approaches for helping people with visual impairments and functional mobility limitations be independently mobile.

LOOKING FORWARD

This brief preview of the content and layout of this text brings us full circle to the starting point for this revised edition. It is the intention of this work to help prepare beginning O&M specialists in such a way that they will have the breadth and depth of information and the professional commitment that will enable them to be effective instructors and encourage their participation in the continuing growth of the knowledge base of the mobility profession. If this book fulfills its goals, there will soon be a need for a third edition, and, more important, there will be greater numbers of people with visual impairments who will have been helped to become or remain independently mobile.

PART ONE

Human Systems

CHAPTER 1

Perception and the Control of Locomotion by Blind and Visually Impaired Pedestrians

David A. Guth and John J. Rieser

As a result of congenital glaucoma, John has a visual field of 10 degrees and a visual acuity of 20/100. John exercises by walking several miles a day, usually along highly familiar routes. While out walking, he finds it difficult to remain oriented to distant places in his surroundings. John has found, for example, that when he attempts to devise a shortcut back home, he sometimes walks in the wrong direction. Jane has albinism, a full visual field, and a visual acuity of 20/400. Although she, like John, is "legally blind," she has little difficulty remaining oriented to places that are out of view, even while walking long and complex routes. What accounts for this difference in John's and Jane's spatial orientation?

Jill was recently blinded in an automobile accident and has begun working with an orientation and mobility (O&M) instructor. During O&M lessons, Jill frequently misjudges things as she is exploring them with her long cane. On today's lesson, for example, she mistook a crack in the sidewalk for a curb. Jack is also totally blind, but he has been traveling with a long cane for many years and rarely makes such misjudgments. What is it about Jack's experience that makes him a better perceiver than Jill?

Waverly is a sighted student in the first semester of her university's O&M program. She describes herself as a "human pinball" as she bounces from wall to wall while blindfolded and walking down a hallway with her long cane. How is it, she wonders, that her friends who are blind are able to walk straight down the center of the same hallway?

This chapter deals with questions such as these about the role of perception in the everyday pedestrian travel of people who are blind and visually impaired. Although the scientific study of perception has flourished since the 1800s, the profession of O&M became well established only in the 1960s (Wiener & Welsh, 1980). In large part the rapid expansion of O&M since then has been due to the effectiveness of tools and techniques that enable perception, most notably the long cane and the associated touch-technique promoted by Hoover (1946, 1950).

This chapter emphasizes the ecological approach to perception pioneered by James Gibson (1966, 1979; see also Neisser, 1976; Pick, 1980a, 1980b; von Hofsten, 1985). Earlier approaches to the study of perception emphasized situations in which both the perceiver and the surround-

We thank Daniel Ashmead, Emerson Foulke, Lukas Franck, Robert LaDuke, Joe Lappin, Jack Loomis, Herbert L. Pick, Jr., and Paul E. Ponchillia for many helpful conversations about the ideas in this chapter, and the late Everett Hill for years of comradeship in this enterprise.

ings were stationary. These approaches were often difficult to apply to the skillful perception of moving observers, and they ignored the possibility that movement itself contributed useful information. Gibson recognized the ubiquity of object motion as well as self motion and the central role of this movement in perception. He also stressed the importance of exploratory movements for perceiving the surroundings and controlling locomotion.

One of Gibson's major contributions was his idea that perception and action are a cycle: People act in order to learn about their surroundings and they use what they learn to guide their actions. From this perspective, the critical defining features of *perception* include the exploratory actions of the perceiver and the knowledge of the surroundings gained while engaged in looking, listening, touching, walking, and other forms of direct observation. Following Gibson's lead, this chapter is selectively focused on perceivers' exploratory actions and the resulting knowledge that is used for orientation and mobility (O&M). *Orientation* means knowledge of one's distance and direction relative to things observed or remembered in the surroundings and keeping track of these "self-to-object" spatial relationships as they change during locomotion (Hill & Ponder, 1976; Howard & Templeton, 1966; Rieser & Garing, 1994). *Mobility* means moving safely, gracefully, and comfortably (Foulke, 1971; Suterko, 1973). Mobility depends in large part on perceiving the properties of the immediate surroundings.

SOURCES OF PERCEPTUAL INPUT

Looking

Looking involves movements of the eyes, head, and body that control what appears in the visual field. People with normal vision can see about 180 degrees of their surroundings at a glance; they can see things small and large; they can see things near and far; and they can see the self-to-object and the object-to-object spatial relationships among things.

There is substantial variability in what can be seen by persons with low vision. Two general categories of low vision are distinguished in this chapter that have different functional implications for O&M: impairment of the size and shape of the visual field and impairment of visual acuity and contrast sensitivity.

Impaired Visual Fields

Many individuals with impaired vision see only portions of the visual field (see Chapter 3). For some, a fairly well-defined "tunnel" restricts central vision to a small visual angle. This angle is often in the range of 2 to 20 degrees (as a rule of thumb, when holding one's fist at arm's length, the fist subtends about 5 degrees of visual angle). Others see little when looking straight ahead but have normal peripheral vision. And still others see normally at locations scattered throughout the visual field.

Being able to see the broad visual field makes it relatively easy to perceive the shapes of large objects such as buildings and to perceive the spatial layout (i.e., the object-to-object relationships) of the things in the immediate surroundings (Millar, 1994). Accomplishing the same tasks with a small visual field depends to a much greater extent on scanning the surroundings and integrating what has been seen. Even the identification of a familiar building can be tedious and time consuming when the building can be seen only one piece at a time.

Impaired Acuity and Contrast Sensitivity

Acuity is defined as the ability to resolve small details. Visual acuity is typically assessed under good lighting conditions with a chart that displays progressively smaller black letters or numbers on a white background (see Chapter 3). Visual acuity depends on visual contrast—a difference in the amount of light reflected from one region of space to the next. Much smaller details are more visible in high-contrast situations than in low-contrast situations, a fact understood by every sighted person who has attempted to read in the diminishing light of evening. Contrast sensitivity and acuity are related but they are not the same. It is common for older persons to have corrected acuities that are near normal (assessed in high-contrast situations) and yet to be functionally blind when attempting to walk at twilight or in other low-contrast situations.

Listening

People often identify and locate things by listening to the sounds that the things themselves emit or the sounds that result when listeners interact with them. Many things emit sounds that enable them to be easily identified—people (their voices, their footsteps), automobiles (their engines, tire noise) and other machines, and environmental sounds (dripping water, wind blowing through trees). Other things do not themselves emit sounds but nevertheless are easily identifiable because they modulate the sounds created by human exploratory actions—for example, grass and gravel and concrete surfaces are identifiable by listening to footfalls or the striking and sliding of a long cane; and water, oil, and cereal can be distinguished by listening to them being poured into containers. Gaver (1993) investigated sounds caused by exploratory actions in order to understand how they specify properties of explored things and suggested that different exploratory actions are best suited to identifying different properties. He distinguished "scraping sounds" (like those caused by sliding a cane across the ground), which are useful for detecting a surface's texture from "impact sounds" (like those caused by striking the walking surface with a cane), which are useful for detecting a surface's hardness.

Safe and graceful walking often depend on knowing the location of or "localizing" objects and surfaces in the immediate surroundings. The localization of a sound source requires information about both its direction and its distance (for reviews, see Grantham, 1995, and Chapter 4). The time of arrival of sounds as well as sound intensity at the two ears vary with the location of a sound source, and these are important cues for judging sound-source direction. A cue used to judge the distance to a sound source is *familiar intensity*—knowing the loudness of a particular sound source and knowing how this varies with distance. People are poor at judging their distance to stationary, unfamiliar sound sources. In situations in which a sound source and a listener are moving relative to one another, lawful acoustic changes provide information about sound-source distance. For example, Ashmead, Davis, and Northington (1995) demonstrated that the pattern of change in sound intensity that can be observed when walking toward an unfamiliar sound source is a useful cue for perceiving its distance.

Also in dynamic situations, the reflection and attenuation of sounds by environmental features can help to localize those features. Waverly, the pinballing O&M student mentioned in this chapter's introduction, learned that her friends who were blind could walk much straighter than she could because they could use reflected sounds to hear their distance from the hallway's walls and could therefore use the walls as guidelines (see Strelow & Brabyn, 1982). Sound attenuation resulting from the presence of an object between a pedestrian and a sound source often makes it easy to localize the object. For example, blind pedestrians can readily localize bus shelters and other large objects that occur between themselves and busy streets by the "sound shadows" they cast.

Touching

Touching is used to discover the properties of the immediate surroundings. Touching involves the *cutaneous sense*—feelings of pressure, vibration, temperature, and pain, for example, resulting from the stimulation of neural end-organs embedded within the skin and the tissues below the skin (see Heller & Schiff, 1991). As Loomis and Lederman (1986) have pointed out, however, touching also involves detecting the relative positions and movements of the parts of the body. For example, while manually exploring a cold metal object, knowledge of the positions of the fingers and hands relative to each other and changes in these positions during exploration make it easy to tell that the object is a mailbox and not a parking meter. This type of perception is sometimes called *proprioception* (e.g., Pick, 1980a; Chapter 5) and sometimes *kinesthesis* (e.g., Loomis & Lederman, 1986). The neural end-organs involved in proprioception are receptors in and around the muscles, tendons, and joints.

Perception often involves a *proximal* or near stimulus and a *distal* or far stimulus (Aslin & Smith, 1988; Gibson, 1962). The distal stimulus is the object or event that is perceived, whereas the proximal stimulus is the pattern of sensation at the receptor organs. In the case of touching, the proximal stimulus is the stream of cutaneous and proprioceptive input, and the distal stimulus is whatever object or environmental feature is being explored. This chapter focuses squarely on distal stimuli and on the exploratory methods used by skillful perceivers to obtain information about them.

With a long cane, pedestrians who are blind can extend their touching well beyond arm's length. Long canes are powerful perceptual tools with which skillful users can, for example, perceive the material, slope, and elevation of the upcoming walking surface; and the location and dimensions of the obstacles and openings along their paths. In the case of exploring an obstacle with the long cane, the proximal stimulus is the pattern of pressure and deformation that occurs where the hand is gripping the cane, but the distal stimulus is the obstacle itself. The later sections "What Pedestrians Need to Know and How They Find It Out" and "Perceiving during Three Everyday Activities," examine several everyday perceptual feats that are accomplished with a long cane.

Walking

Walking is both an action and itself an important source of perceptual input (so too are other means of human locomotion such as crawling and propelling a wheelchair). Walking involves sequences of motor control commands to the muscles (*efference*) and feedback from the body about the movements resulting from those commands (*afference*). Efferent commands and afferent feedback are each assumed to play a role in keeping track of one's path of locomotion (Klatzky et al., 1990).

Some afferent feedback is proprioceptive and some is vestibular. The vestibular system of the inner ear is sensitive to the rotary and linear acceleration of the head as well as to its tilt. As the head turns, hairs in one or more of the three semicircular canals of the vestibular system are bent in a way that signals the direction and extent of the turn. Straight line movements and tilts of the head are signaled by the bending of hairs in another part of the vestibular system, the *utricle* (see Pick, 1980a; Chapter 5).

Another type of feedback resulting from walking is information about environmental flow. *Environmental flow* refers to the lawful changes in a pedestrian's distances and directions to things in the surroundings that occur while walking. Maintaining orientation is a matter of keeping track of environmental flow. Consider the basic geometry of this flow: When a pedestrian merely turns in place, self-to-object directions all change by the same amount and the distances remain the same. However, when a pedestrian walks straight ahead, the distances and directions change at different rates depending on their distance and direction from the pedestrian and the pedestrian's direction of locomotion. For example, imagine that you are walking along a sidewalk and that there is a bench 10 feet straight ahead of you, a tree 10 feet away from you and 45 degrees to your left, a parked car 20 feet away and 45 degrees to your left, and a flower bed 10 feet away and 90 degrees to your left. While you walk toward the bench, its direction would remain a constant straight ahead, the direction of the flower bed would change at a faster rate than the direction of the tree, and the direction of the tree would change at a faster rate than the direction of the car. Upon your arrival at the bench, your distance to it would be zero, your distances to the tree and the car would be smaller than their original distances of 10 feet and 20 feet, and your distance to the flowers would be greater than their original 10 feet. Environmental flow is three-dimensional, occurring in the vertical as well as the horizontal plane. Kennedy (1993), for example, found that people who were congenitally blind understood that as you approach a building, accurate pointing at the building's roof requires that you point steeper and steeper as you get closer and closer.

The environmental flow created by walking can readily be perceived by looking and listening. While walking, people with normal vision are continuously exposed to this flow; their broad visual fields enable them to observe how their movements affect their spatial relationships to large numbers of the objects and features of their surroundings (see Gibson, 1966; Lee, 1980). Environmental flow is also available acoustically when people walk in the vicinity of sound-making objects and notice how their locomotion affects their spatial relationships to the objects. In addition, some environmental flow may be perceptible as people walk in the presence of directionally specific sources of heat and odor. It is argued later (in the section "Perceiving During Three Everyday Activities," below) that experiences such as seeing and hearing environmental flow are crucial to the development of skillful spatial orientation.

Wind, Temperature, and Odors

Other useful sources of perceptual input include feeling the wind, feeling changes in temperature, and smelling odors. In areas crowded with tall buildings, wind flow perpendicular to the line of travel is often a cue that a street is being approached or that an alley or some other break in a row of buildings is being passed. In open areas, the wind's direction can sometimes be used to identify one's general facing direction. Feeling the wind involves direct mechanical stimulation of the skin by the wind as well as stimulation resulting from the movements of body hair and clothing.

Information about one's location and facing direction can also be obtained via temperature changes such as those felt when walking into the shade in familiar surroundings and when walking past the open door of an air-conditioned bus. The "hot spot" felt when the sun is shining on the face can be used to determine facing direction if the sun's direction is known. A variety of cutaneous receptors respond to changes in temperature, including "warm" and "cold" receptors, and *nociceptors* that respond to noxious temperature (see Stevens, 1991, for a review).

Odors usually indicate that one is in the general vicinity of their source, for example, a fast-food restaurant or a leather-goods store. Odors carried by the wind may also provide some directional information if the wind's direction is known. To be smelled, a substance must give off vapors and those vapors must be fat-soluble since the nose's sensory receptors are surrounded by fatlike material (see Sekuler & Blake, 1994).

BASIC CONCEPTS AND DEFINITIONS

Perceptual Learning

Most of the O&M tasks discussed in this chapter involve perceptual learning, and an important role of the O&M instructor is to provide opportunities for perceptual learning to occur. *Perceptual learning* can be thought of as the education of attention (Gibson, 1969)—with practice and experience, perceivers come to notice the features of situations that are relevant to their goals and not to notice the irrelevant features. Three general principles of perceptual learning seem particularly applicable to O&M. The first is that unskillful perceiving requires much concentration and attention, whereas skillful perceiving requires less attention and is more easily combined with other tasks. The second is that unskillful perceiving involves noticing both the relevant and irrelevant features of sensory stimulation without understanding their meaning, whereas skillful perceiving involves narrowing ones focus to relevant features and understanding the situations they specify. The third principle is that unskillful perceiving often involves attention to the proximal stimulus, whereas skillful perceiving involves attention to the distal stimulus.

Consider how these three principles apply to the task of learning to use the long cane. First, novice long-cane users sometimes have difficulty dividing their attention between the mobility-related information provided by their canes and the information they use to maintain spatial orientation. With practice, the twin tasks of mobility and maintaining orientation become more smoothly coordinated. Second, novices pay attention to both the relevant and the irrelevant vibrations and sounds of their canes, but more experienced users selectively attend to those which specify functionally important conditions such as drop-offs and obstacles. Third, although novices may attend to the proximal forces at the hand that accompany such events as the dropping or stopping of the cane tip, experienced cane users "feel" the distal drop-off or obstacle.

Motor Learning

Motor learning is often distinguished from perceptual learning and refers to the acquisition—through practice and experience—of specific and often highly complex patterns of movement. The patterns most obviously relevant to O&M are those of long-cane techniques such as the touch and constant-contact techniques that involve coordinated movements of the hands and feet (see LaGrow & Weessies, 1994).

Two topics discussed in the motor-learning literature seem especially relevant to O&M: the "degrees-of-freedom problem" (Rosenbaum, 1991) and the development of automaticity. As discussed in the previous section for perceptual learning, the learning of long-cane skills will be used to illustrate these concepts. A degree of freedom is a dimension in which movement is free to vary. Rosenbaum pointed out that the joints of the arm have seven degrees of freedom: the shoulder has three since it can move up and down, from side to side, and can twist; the elbow has two since it can bend and twist; and the wrist has two since it can move up and down and turn from side to side. With all of these degrees of freedom, there are a large number of ways that the cane tip can be moved from side to side. For many motor skills, including moving the long cane, an important goal is to minimize the energy required for performance (Schmidt, 1991). Another goal is to perform consistently—for example, to consistently place the cane's tip in the same place relative to the body. To assist their novice students to achieve these goals, O&M instructors typically encourage students to "lock up" degrees of freedom; that is, to keep their shoulder and elbow joints in a fixed position and to move only the wrist. Initial instruction may involve locking up all but one degree of freedom—the side to side movement of the wrist—and then later "unlocking" a second degree of freedom—the up and down movement of the wrist necessary to perform the touch technique. Motor learning research (e.g., McDonald, vanEmmerik, & Newell, 1989) suggests that for many skills, novice learners often use a strategy of locking up degrees of freedom, which they gradually unlock as skill is acquired.

Automaticity relates to the attention required to perform a motor skill—the less attention required, the more automatic the skill is said to be. A key feature of attention is its limited capacity: It is possible to take in only a limited amount of information, and attending to some things interferes with attending to other things. Learning long-cane techniques is attentionally demanding, requiring that learners concentrate on their hands, feet, and cane tips in order to judge whether they are moving in the proper synchrony. These attentional demands of motor learning can compete with the attentional demands of perceptual learning described in the preceding section. Consequently, many O&M instructors try to avoid overloading their students' attentional capacity during early lessons with the long cane by working in open, obstacle-free areas. This enables students to focus on developing automaticity in their manipulation of the long cane before shifting their attention to its use as a perceptual tool.

Perceptual-Motor Coordination

Pedestrians coordinate the forces and directions of their actions with the perceived sizes, distances, and directions of the objects in their surroundings (Rieser, Pick, Ashmead, & Garing, 1995). Mobility depends on skill at coordinating actions with the properties of the immediate path. For example, the path taken around an obstacle must fit the obstacle's size and its distance and direction from a pedestrian. To negotiate a curb gracefully, a pedestrian's step height must fit the curb's height. Similarly, maintaining orientation depends on coordinating one's actions with the properties of the further-ranging surroundings. For example, when walking in familiar neighborhoods and rooms, skillful travelers keep track of how their walking affects their distances and directions to objects remembered in the surroundings, and they use this information to help guide their walking path.

Perceptual-motor coordination is learned. All experienced O&M instructors have observed novice cane users clumsily negotiating curbs due to misjudging their distance from the curb or stepping too high or too low to surmount it. The learning of perceptual-motor coordination occurs during the many opportunities that pedestrians who are blind have to explore curbs of various heights with their long canes and to notice which step distances and heights fit safely with which perceived curb distances and heights.

In some situations the coordination of actions with the perceived surroundings is continuously guided by feedback while in other situations actions are preplanned and executed without external feedback. Examples of the former include walking parallel to a nearby wall or parallel to a street, using the sounds reflected by the wall or emitted by traffic to maintain the line of travel. Examples of the latter are stepping over a gutter after judging its width with the long cane and stepping up a curb after judging its height with the cane.

Perception and Knowledge

Perception is influenced by what a person knows, and it is useful to distinguish three types of knowledge that are relevant to O&M: procedural knowledge, episodic knowledge, and conceptual knowledge (Anderson, 1995; Tulving, 1983). *Procedural knowledge* refers to knowledge of how to do things and where to do them. For pedestrians who are blind, an important kind of procedural knowledge is knowledge of motor procedures. Familiar examples include knowing how to make 90- and 180-degree turns, knowing how to react to the movements of a dog guide, and knowing various long-cane techniques. Knowing the situations in which a particular motor procedure will yield a particular kind of information is especially useful for O&M. For example, knowing to use the touch-and-drag technique to locate the seam along the edge of a parking lot can enable a blind pedestrian to avoid veering into the lot.

Episodic knowledge refers to knowledge of particular places and events, that is, of particular episodes of experience. Orientation and mobility each rely heavily on episodic knowledge. For orientation, knowledge of the places within a neighborhood and knowledge of efficient routes between those places is useful episodic knowledge. For mobility, knowledge of particular environmental hazards and their locations is useful—even knowing that a neighborhood has an area of broken pavement without knowing its location can help by increasing one's vigilance for it. The contribution of episodic knowledge to O&M is evident from the increasing speed and efficiency with which pedestrians who are blind travel as they acquire familiarity with an area.

Finally, *conceptual knowledge* (sometimes referred to as *semantic knowledge*) refers to knowledge of general patterns, not of specific instances of a pattern. The profession of O&M has traditionally emphasized the development of conceptual knowledge such as the layout and traffic patterns of typical intersections, cardinal directions, street and avenue numbering systems, the street–curb–grass–sidewalk–yard arrangement of some neighborhoods, and changes in the sun's direction with time of day and season. Such general concepts can be applied to familiar and unfamiliar environments, and play a particularly important role in exploring and learning about unfamiliar neighborhoods.

Perceptual Error

This section describes two common types of perceptual error of concern to O&M instructors and visually impaired pedestrians: *detection errors* (when the presence or absence of an important environmental feature or event is misjudged) and *localization errors* (when the distance or direction to an environmental feature or event is misjudged).

Detection Errors, Curb Ramps, and Risk

Safe travel depends on detecting critical environmental features such as stairways and curb ramps and events such as traffic movements. *Signal detection theory,* originally developed for the analysis of electronic communication systems, has become the conventional framework used to characterize the errors that people can make during detection judgments (see Green & Swets, 1966; Macmillan & Creelman, 1991). The essentials of signal detection theory are summarized in Table 1.1.

Table 1.1. Essentials of Signal Detection Theory

Is It Really There?	Think It's There?	
	Yes	**No**
Yes	True positive (Hit)	False negative (miss)
No	False positive	True negative

Sensitivity: One's ability to discriminate among alternative environmental features (e.g., curb cut vs. sidewalk) and events (e.g., turning vs. nonturning vehicles), measured as a discrepancy between the hit rate and the false positive rate. Sensitivity is influenced by the sensory input given by the environmental feature or event (which may be reduced by a sensory impairment), the differences in this input among the alternatives, and the normal variability in this input for each of the alternatives.

Criterion: The amount of evidence one requires in order to decide if something is or is not present, measured as the degree to which "yes" or "no" responses dominate. In addition to the specific evidence obtained in a particular instance, this is affected by the perceiver's belief about the probability of the thing being present, by the potential benefits and costs associated with being right or wrong, and by the perceiver's general goals (e.g., maximize safety, maximize travel speed).

Consider, for example, a pedestrian who is blind who is traveling with a long cane along a level sidewalk and is approaching a downward-sloping curb ramp. Each sweep of the cane affords the possibility of detecting the curb ramp. In the vocabulary of signal detection theory, a "negative" result occurs each time the pedestrian does not detect a curb ramp and a "positive" result occurs whenever the pedestrian does detect one. Given that both positive and negative judgments can be right or wrong, signal detection theory provides a straightforward way to think about the four resulting possibilities: namely, true positives or "hits" (the curb ramp was there and it was detected); false positives (the curb ramp was not there but the pedestrian thought that it was); true negatives (the curb ramp was not there and the pedestrian did not think it was present); and false negatives or "misses" (the curb ramp was actually there but the pedestrian did not detect it).

Signal detection theory distinguishes two general sources of detection error. One is a lack of perceptual *sensitivity.* This would be the case if a pedestrian were insensitive to the change in slope encountered at a curb ramp, perhaps because the change was very slight (e.g., a 2-degree downward slope) or because the pedestrian had diabetes-related neuropathy of the feet and legs (Kozel, 1995; Ponchillia, 1993). Sensitivity is measured as a discrepancy between the hit rate and the false positive rate.

The second general source of detection error is a perceiver's detection *criterion,* that is, how much evidence is needed to decide that a particular environmental feature or event is or is not present. People choose their own criteria, and their choices can serve to minimize some types of error at the expense of others. Continuing with the curb-ramp example, suppose a pedestrian's cane sweeps over a piece of sidewalk that slopes downward toward the street and which may or may not be a curb ramp. Variations in the slopes of sidewalks due to factors such as erosion and tree roots commonly mislead people into the false positive identification of a sloped section of sidewalk as a curb ramp. In such situations, however, there is a low cost associated with a cautious criterion that leads to a false positive (i.e., when a curb ramp is not there but the pedestrian thinks it is). But because of the risk associated with walking into a street without knowing it, there may be a high cost associated with a more relaxed criterion that leads to a miss (i.e., when a curb ramp is there but the pedestrian fails to detect it).

An individual's choice of a criterion usually involves a safety–efficiency trade-off. Criteria that increase travel safety usually decrease travel efficiency and vice versa. Considering the curb ramp example again, pedestrians are probably wise to try to minimize the miss rate even though this will increase the false positive rate. For example, when approaching a street and detecting what *may* be a curb ramp, a pedestrian could stop and explore further before continuing on. O&M instructors emphasize safety at the cost of efficiency (e.g., see Bennett, 1991) but skilled pedestrians who are blind vary in their willingness to make this trade-off. Brabyn and Foulke (1988; unpublished transcripts) observed highly skilled blind travelers in a large city and interviewed the travelers about the choices they made. One participant, whose detection error caused him to cross against a traffic light, commented, "There was an element of danger there. We're always dealing with a probability of getting hurt which is higher than for other people. . . . We are gambling more," and "How close to the brink do we always exist? It drives mobility instructors crazy. They're seeking a form of perfection that I think doesn't exist." At present, the ability of O&M instructors to provide objective information about risk-taking behaviors is severely limited by the fact that little is known about the probability of injury associated with various decision criteria.

Localization Errors

The second category of perceptual error is localization error, which is error measured relative to the distance or direction of something's actual location. There are two types of localization error. One is *constant error* which occurs when people consistently misjudge an object's location—for example, by consistently underestimating how far it is to busy streets heard in the distance or consistently judging the opposite corner of an intersection to be to the left of its actual location (see Participant 1 in Figure 1.1).

The second type of localization error is *variable error,* which occurs when people are uncertain of a thing's exact location and therefore vary in their judgments of its distance or direction. They may, for example, sometimes overestimate and sometimes underestimate in their judgments of the distance to busy streets. Or they may sometimes judge the opposite corner to be to the left of its true location and sometimes judge it to be to the right.

WHAT PEDESTRIANS NEED TO KNOW AND HOW THEY FIND IT OUT

The previous two sections presented general concepts that are relevant to a wide range of O&M situations. The next two sections focus more narrowly and selectively on specific types of information that are used to guide locomotion (this section) and on specific O&M tasks ("Perceiving During Three Everyday Activities," section, below).

This section introduces two broad classes of information whose perception is necessary for skillful pedestrian travel, and it discusses some of the ways that people who are visually impaired go about getting this information. The focus is first on pedestrians' need for information about the characteristics of the walking surface and

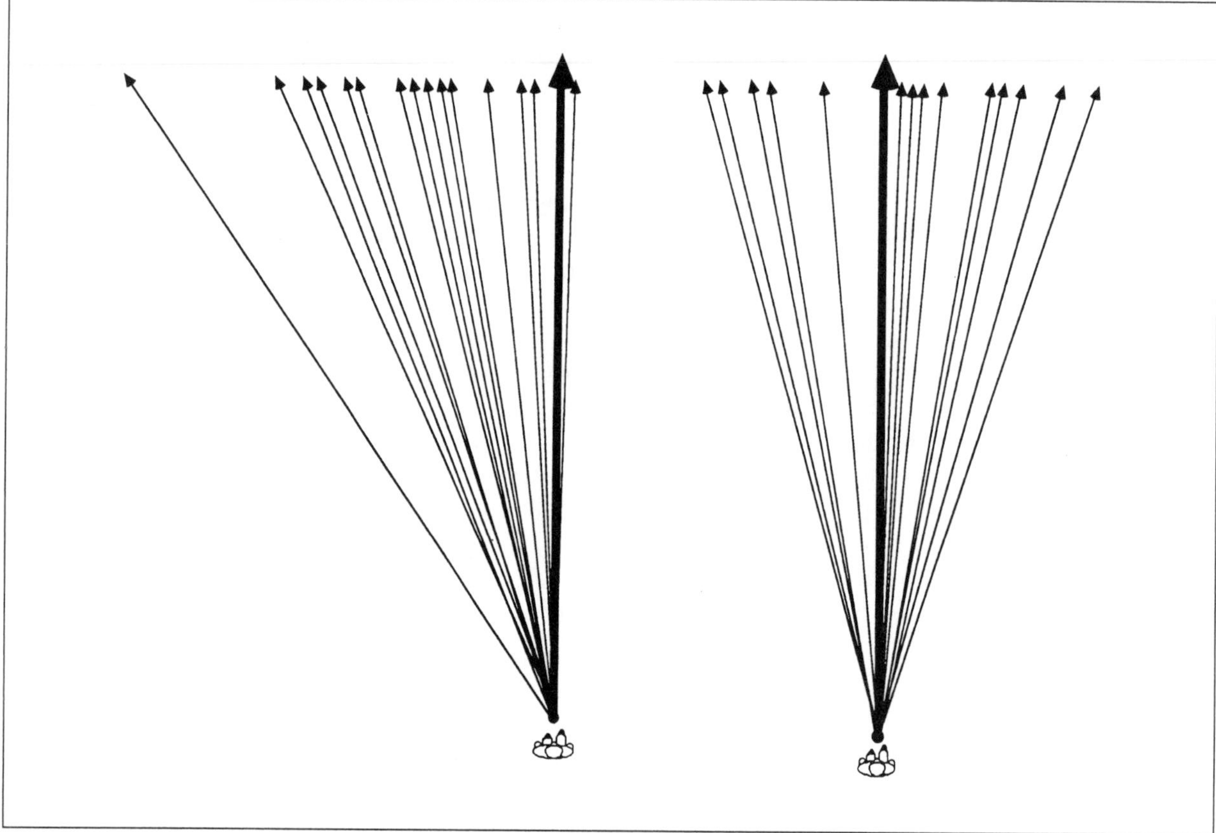

Figure 1.1. Response directions of two participants who are blind in the 15 trials of a street-crossing alignment experiment. The heavier arrow shows the direction the participants were attempting to face. While the two participants exhibited similar variable error, only Participant 1 exhibited a sizable constant error.

second on pedestrians' need for information about spatial relationships. This is not intended to be a comprehensive review of everything a pedestrian needs to know—for additional relevant discussion and examples, the reader should see Foulke (1971, 1983, 1985), Jannson (1990), Strelow (1985), Gibson (1958), Hill and Ponder (1976), Jacobson (1993), and LaGrow and Weessies (1994).

Information about Walking Surfaces

Material and Texture

Successful O&M requires knowledge of the surface being walked upon and the surface being walked toward. Travel would be difficult if pedestrians were unable to distinguish between concrete and grass or between tile and carpet. Textural changes in surfaces of the same material—for example, a change from smooth to bumpy concrete—can be used as landmarks and are increasingly being used to warn of upcoming hazards (see Chapter 10). Perception of the upcoming walking surface enables the motor preplanning that is necessary to maintain safety. For example, adjustments of posture and gait can be made in anticipation of slippery, soft, or springy surfaces, and surfaces that cannot support a pedestrian's weight can be avoided.

Pedestrians with Low Vision. Consider the wintertime problem of judging whether the walking surface just ahead is a puddle of water or a patch of ice. To judge this, pedestrians with unimpaired vision may take into account the surface's visible texture, reflectance, and opacity. The judgment is often easy to make, and pedestrians can then plan efficient detours to avoid puddles or can make the kinetic adjustments necessary to maintain their balance while walking on ice. Persons with low vision, on the other hand, cite walking in icy conditions as a major mobility problem regardless of the level of outdoor illumination (Smith, De l'Aune, & Geruschat, 1992). It may be the case that this is a greater problem for persons with impaired acuity than for persons with impaired fields and good scanning skills, because impaired acuity reduces the distance from which details such as the spectral highlights of the walking surface can be seen. Pedestrians with low vision who have particular difficulty under such conditions may wish to consider using a long cane to augment their visual preview of the walking surface.

Pedestrians Who Are Blind. Pedestrians who are blind usually inspect the walking surface with the cane or the foot. Relevant to this type of exploratory action is the research of Lederman and Klatzky (1987; Klatzky & Lederman, 1987), which documents the ways in which people go about discovering specific properties of objects when exploring them with the hand. To discover surface texture, for example, the most common exploratory procedure is *lateral motion*—rubbing the hand back and forth across a surface. Deformations of the skin as well as vibrations felt while rubbing across the elements of a surface appear to be important bases of perceiving texture by touch (Pick, 1980b; Taylor & Lederman, 1975) and the lateral motion of the hand is well suited to maximizing these. A comparable example of exploring via the foot is the practice of some dog-guide users of rubbing a foot back and forth along the ground in order to detect the change in pavement texture that occurs at the juncture of a concrete sidewalk and an asphalt road.

Another of Lederman and Klatzky's exploratory procedures that can readily be generalized to perception via foot or cane is the *pressure* procedure whereby people poke or squeeze a surface to determine its hardness. Consider, for example, the practice during winter travel of poking the nearby snow with the tip of the long cane in order to locate the hard-packed walking path. Similarly, consider the poking of the cane into fallen leaves in order to determine whether the sidewalk is beneath.

Long cane techniques appear to vary in the properties of the walking surface about which they are most informative. Consider the touch technique (Jacobson, 1993): The sounds heard and the vibrations felt as the cane strikes the walking surface would each appear to be useful for perceiving its hardness. The striking of the cane creates *impact sounds* (Gaver, 1993) that vary according to the hardness of a surface. It also creates an extended version of the pressure exploratory procedure described above, which should be well suited to detecting surface hardness.

Seemingly better suited to identifying the texture of the walking surface is the constant-contact technique. This technique is identical to the touch technique except that it involves sliding the cane back and forth across the walking surface (Fisk, 1986; LaGrow & Weessies, 1994). Like the touch technique, the constant-contact technique simultaneously creates felt vibrations and sounds. The back-and-forth sliding of the cane is essentially an extended version of the lateral-motion exploratory procedure described above. The constant contact technique also produces *scraping sounds* (Gaver, 1993), which vary according to the material being scraped, its texture, and the speed with which the cane is moved.

Changes in Elevation: Ramps and Drop-Offs

Changes in the elevation of the walking surface occur regularly in many travel environments. These may be the gradual change of a ramp or the abrupt change of a drop-off. Commonly experienced ramps and drop-offs are those at curbs and curb ramps, along sidewalks in disrepair, at stairways, and at the edges of rapid-rail platforms. Detection errors at ramps and drop-offs can result in stumbles and falls as well as in missing useful information about one's location.

Pedestrians with Low Vision. Peceiving changes in the elevation of the walking surface is a well-documented difficulty of pedestrians with low vision (Genesky, Berry, Bikson, & Bikson, 1979; Kalloniatis & Johnston, 1994; Long, Rieser, & Hill, 1990; Smith, De l'Aune, & Geruschat, 1992). Impaired acuity results in reduced perceptual sensitivity to many of the depth cues that normally specify changes in height. For example, a sudden change in the visible texture of the walking surface often indicates a drop-off, but a person with impaired acuity may be unable to resolve enough textural detail to see the change. Similarly, the inability to resolve small details can make it difficult to discriminate a drop-off from a shadow or from a change in the color or shading of the walking surface, especially in low contrast situations. The source of difficulty is probably different for persons with severely impaired visual fields. Unless they are traveling with a long cane, these persons should visually scan the walking surface ahead of themselves to be certain of detecting any ramps or drop-offs in their way.

A visual cue for detecting the height of an impending drop-off is the rate at which the surface whose view is blocked (occluded) by the drop-off comes into view as one is walking toward it. The general importance of dynamic visual changes at occluding edges was emphasized by Gibson (1979). The usefulness of attending to these changes as a curb is being approached by a visually impaired pedestrian was noted by Brady (1988; see also O'Donnell & Smith, 1994). Frank Brady, who had lost vision in one eye, recommended that: "As you approach the street, keep your eye on the edge of the curb so you can observe its relative movement against the background of the street's surface. The higher the curb, the faster will this relative motion occur and the more street paving will come into view" (p. 54).

Because the visual perception of changes in the elevation of the walking surface is sometimes problematic for persons with low vision, O&M instructors may encourage their clients to look for the visible features of the environment that are associated with such changes. Railings are associated with stairs, for example, and street signs are associated with curbs and curb ramps. Also helpful are contrast and color cues such as crosswalk lines and differences in the color or shade of the sidewalk and street (see O'Donnell & Smith, 1994; and Geruschat & Smith, this volume, for reviews). The usefulness of such environmental regularities for detecting drop-offs and ramps is another illustration of the value of conceptual knowledge.

Pedestrians Who Are Blind. Pedestrians who are blind who travel with long canes are usually informed of the presence of drop-offs such as curbs, steps, and holes by the sudden drop of their cane's tip over the edge of the drop-off. When using the touch technique, pedestrians may also hear the cane strike the walking surface later than it normally would have (or not hear it strike at all). Novice long-cane users sometimes miss drop-offs, and Murakami and Shimuzu's (1990) account of 120 falls from rapid-rail platforms suggests that even experienced long-cane users sometimes fail to perceive drop-offs in time to react safely. LaGrow and Weessies (1994) noted that well-defined curbs are becoming increasingly scarce at street corners as communities replace curbs with curb ramps. Because blind pedestrians no longer experience a drop-off at the end of every block, they have fewer incidental opportunities for learning and practicing the skillful detection of drop-offs.

Curb ramps are probably the most frequently experienced instance of downward slopes, and they are a dominant nonvisual cue for identifying the location of streets. How well can they be detected? On the one hand, Cratty (1965) reported that over 78 percent of a sample of 30 adults who were blind could detect ramps that had 1-degree slopes. On the other hand, Bentzen and Barlow (1995) reported that blind pedestrians who were traveling in unfamiliar areas often failed to detect streets that were entered via curb ramps. Of Bentzen and Barlow's 80 blind participants, 75 percent were good-to-excellent travelers according to self-reports and the reports of O&M instructors, and 66 percent reported traveling independently at least five times per week. These persons' detection performance increased as slope increased: they stopped before entering a street on 49 percent, 70 percent, and 89 percent of trials where the curb ramps were ≤4 degrees, 5 degrees, and \$6 degrees, respectively. Of the 80 street-entry points studied by Bentzen and Barlow, only 14 were detected by all participants, and 12 of these had curb ramps with slopes of 5 degrees or more.

What may account for the superior performance of Cratty's participants? Under Cratty's indoor conditions, the slope of the specially constructed walkway changed every 8 feet, alternating between level sections and sections that were sloped upward or downward. Because the participants were guided along the path, they were free to devote their full attention to the task. In contrast, Bentzen and Barlow's participants guided themselves along unfamiliar city blocks and searched for any cues that could help them detect their arrival at a street. Because the blocks varied in length, conceptual knowledge of the length of typical blocks was of limited value. In addition, the participants' attention was divided among a variety of tasks including cane manipulation, staying on path, and seeking information about the presence of a street. It is therefore not surprising that people are less sensitive to the presence of underfoot ramps during everyday travel than they are in laboratory tests designed to assess performance under ideal conditions.

Information about Spatial Relationships

Successful O&M logically requires knowledge of object-to-object and self-to-object spatial relationships (Rieser, Guth, & Hill, 1982). To get to their destinations, pedestrians need information about the arrangement or *layout* of the objects in their surroundings—that is, the distances and directions that relate the objects to one another. Without this knowledge of object-to-object relationships, pedestrians can proceed to their destinations only by a trial and error search, by using systematic exploration techniques, or by soliciting assistance. When pedestrians do solicit assistance, they often seek information about object-to-object relationships such as the direction of their destination from the nearest intersection (LaGrow & Mulder, 1989).

However, even sophisticated knowledge of the relative locations of places is useless unless pedestrians can keep track of where they stand and which way they are facing relative to those places. Maintaining orientation involves keeping up to date on the continuous changes in these self-to-object relationships that occur during locomotion. Knowledge of self-to-object relationships is likewise essential for mobility, since safe travel relies on coordinating locomotion with the locations of the objects, openings, and hazards in the immediate surroundings. It is the latter type of self-to-object relationship and the related perceptual-motor coordination which are emphasized in the section below, while self-to-object relationships involving more distant objects are considered in the section "Perceiving during Three Everyday Activities" and Chapter 2.

Self-to-Object Relationships

The moment-to-moment safety and efficiency of pedestrian travel often relies on perceiving one's direction and distance to the obstacles and openings in the immediate surroundings. To get to their destinations, pedestrians must steer around the obstacles and through the openings that lie along their paths. Obstacles and openings are perceptual as well as functional opposites. Gibson (1979) pointed out that for visual perception, an obstacle is something that blocks out increasingly greater amounts of the visible background as it is approached. The rate of this change increases as one's distance from the obstacle decreases and is greatest just before collision. Conversely, an opening reveals increasingly greater amounts of the visible background as it is approached. As a person walks toward an open doorway, for example, increasingly greater amounts of whatever is on the other side of the doorway come into view (see also Strelow, 1985). Gibson's insight for vision is quite general and applies to other senses as well. For example, obstacles that occur between a pedestrian and a sound source block out increasingly greater amounts of sound as they are approached while openings "reveal" increasingly greater amounts of sound as they are approached.

Pedestrians with Low Vision. Detecting the presence and location of objects in the immediate surroundings is a problem for many persons with low vision (Kalloniatis & Johnston, 1994; Smith, De l'Aune, & Geruschat, 1992), with small obstacles that occur in only one region of space reported to be the most troublesome. For example, Genesky et al. (1979) found that fewer adults with low vision reported problems with obstacles such as trees, lamp posts, and parking meters than reported problems with unexpected small objects at head, foot, or chest level. Objects at eye level were more frequently reported to be a problem by persons with severe field impairments than by those with lesser field impairments or with impaired acuity only. This may be because pedestrians with severe field impairments tend to monitor the walking surface ahead of themselves more than the space directly in front of the head (Long, Rieser, & Hill, 1990).

The finding that *unexpected* small obstacles are more difficult for persons with low vision provides another illustration of the role of knowledge in perceiving. Whether or not an obstacle is detected is determined in part by the type and severity of the visual impairment, the size of the obstacle, the visual contrast of the obstacle with its surroundings, and the pedestrian's distance from the obstacle. But it is also influenced by a pedestrian's knowing what to look for and where to look for it—that is, by the pedestrian's episodic and conceptual knowledge. For example, a pedestrian who knows the location of an obstacle such as a low-hanging tree branch knows when and where to look for it and is therefore more likely to detect it. Similarly, a pedestrian with the conceptual knowledge that guy wires occur near utility poles is more likely to be looking for—and therefore to detect—these wires when walking in the vicinity of utility poles.

Pedestrians Who Are Blind. For many pedestrians who are blind, the long cane is the primary means of detecting and locating the obstacles and openings in the immediate surroundings. Obstacles are located when the cane collides with them during locomotion and openings are located when an obstacle gives way to open space.

Listening also provides useful information for detecting and locating stationary objects that emit or reflect sound. For example, Ashmead, Hill, and Talor (1989) had children who were congenitally blind (ages 5–12 years) travel a 27-foot (8.2-meter) route along a sidewalk that was sometimes clear and sometimes contained a "roadblock"—a masonite box to be detected and steered around. The children traveled without canes; the size of the box and its location along the route were varied; and potential cues from wind, light, shadows, and the texture of the walking surface were minimized. The children readily used reflected sounds to perceive their self-to-box spatial relationship and to steer around the box. That six of the ten children had not received formal O&M instruction suggests that this kind of perceptual-motor coordination can develop in the absence of systematic training.

Moving Objects. In contrast to situations that require localizing a stationary object are those in which an object such as a vehicle or another pedestrian is moving. Athletes on the soccer field and goal-ball court alike can perceive an approaching ball's trajectory and move to intercept it. For mobility, pedestrians need to anticipate the trajectories of moving objects in order to avoid collisions. Street crossing is one task that depends on perceiving the trajectory and timing of oncoming vehicles. Research shows that even young children with normal vision can visually perceive an approaching automobile's *time-to-arrival*—the time until the automobile will pass them by (Lee, Young, & McLaughlin, 1984). They judge the timing accurately, well before they can act on it by crossing streets safely.

Two types of visual information seem particularly useful for perceiving object motion. One is intrinsic to the object's visual image. For the situation in which a vehicle is coming head-on toward an observer, the vehicle's time-to-arrival is specified by the ratio of the size of the vehicle's visual image and the instantaneous rate of the image's expansion (Lee, 1980). This can be generalized to situations in which a pedestrian on a sidewalk is watching a car approach and judging the time until the vehicle will pass by. The other type of information depends on being able to see the moving object relative to a stable frame of reference. In studies in which people are asked to judge whether or not a visible stimulus is moving, they can detect much slower movements when the movement is framed within stable visible surroundings than when it is presented against a totally dark background.

There has apparently been no research to date about the skill with which persons with low vision perceive the trajectories and timing of moving objects such as motor vehicles. However, it seems reasonable to assume that under high contrast conditions the skill of individuals with impaired acuity or contrast sensitivity but with normal visual fields could be quite good. This makes sense, first, because detection of the vehicle's image size and changes in image size depend on being able to see the vehicle's large contours, not its specific details. Second, with a large visual field it is usually possible to see both the vehicle and its surroundings.

Conversely, it seems reasonable to expect that persons with small visual fields would be less skillful at perceiving vehicle motion. This makes sense because a field restriction can limit the ability to see an object's large contours (especially a nearby large object) as well as the object's surroundings.

Another reason that a person with a small visual field may have difficulty perceiving the trajectory of a moving object is that trajectory judgments depend on keeping an object in view (i.e., tracking it) over part of its path. Although individuals with large fields can easily track a visible object as it moves across the peripheral field (the peripheral retina is highly sensitive to object motion), individuals with small fields must work hard to keep the object within the visual field. This is a perceptual "Catch 22" for persons with small fields because perceiving trajectories depends upon visual tracking and visual tracking depends upon perceiving trajectories.

Listening also provides information about the trajectories of moving objects. The perceptual-motor skill of blind athletes diving to block goal balls moving at 30–35 miles per hour attests to the usefulness of listening for this purpose. This general topic is considered further in the discussion of street crossing alignment in the section "Perceiving During Three Everyday Activities."

Object-to-Object Relationships

Because the visual perception of object-to-object relationships was addressed in the section "Sources of Perceptual Input," this section focuses on the nonvisual perception of these relationships. A pedestrian who is blind can scan with the hand(s) or the long cane in order to perceive the object-to-object relationships of nearby things. Listening can also provide information about object-to-object relationships such as the relationship of two cars on a street. Walking, however, is the principal nonvisual means of learning object-to-object relationships. How this is accomplished is considered in the remainder of this section as well as in the section "Perceiving During Three Everyday Activities."

Several studies have examined the methods by which people learn object-to-object relationships while walking without vision. Tellevik (1992) had blindfolded sighted persons learn an unfamiliar layout of objects in an unfamiliar room and an unfamiliar layout of objects in a room that had been previously explored. His findings suggested that knowledge of the general configuration of the room provided a spatial framework within which learning object-to-object relationships was more efficient and effective.

Extending Tellevik's work, Hill et al. (1993) asked 65 people who were totally blind to explore a small room-sized space in order to discover the

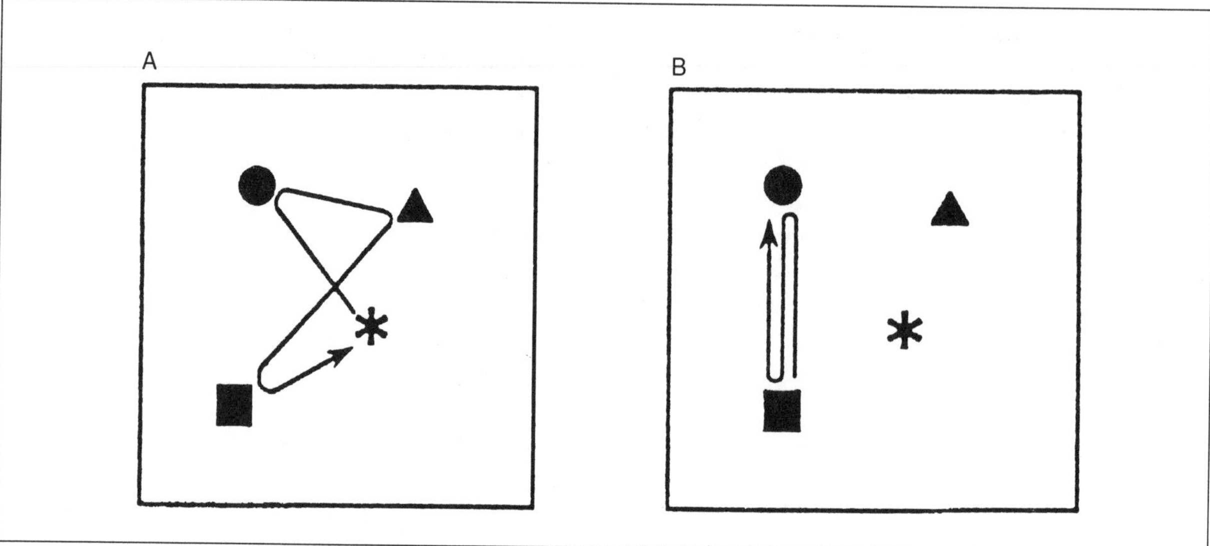

Figure 1.2. Schematic representation of the experimental layout and examples of exploratory patterns. *Panel A:* Exploratory cycles (cyclic patterns). *Panel B:* Back-and-forth exploration.

Source: Reprinted, by permission, from F. Gaunet and C. Thinus-Blanc, "Exploratory Patterns and Reactions to Spatial Change: The Role of Early Visual Experience." In B. G. Bardy, R. J. Bootsma, & Y. Guiard (Eds.), *Studies in Perception and Action III*. Mahwah, NJ: Lawrence Erlbaum.

five objects there and to learn their object-to-object relationships. After 7 minutes of independent exploration, object-to-object learning was assessed by asking a participant to judge the direction from each object to every other object. Participants were videotaped as they explored the space and were also asked to describe how they attempted to learn the object-to-object relationships. The 15 most accurate participants were found to have performed significantly more straight-line linking movements than the 15 who were least accurate; that is, the most accurate participants strategically walked directly from the objects to the perimeter of the space and from one object to another much more often than the other participants. Some of the best performers also used their canes to establish links by repeatedly sweeping them among the objects and from the perimeter of the space to the objects.

In a similar study, Gaunet and Thinus-Blanc (1995) found that pedestrians who were blind who used a predominately back-and-forth exploratory strategy for learning an unfamiliar layout acquired more accurate object-to-object knowledge than those who used a cyclic strategy (see Figure 1.2).

Pedestrians who are blind have a much greater need to remember object-to-object relationships than do pedestrians with vision. For example, a normally sighted traveler need not learn and remember where the turnstiles of a frequently used subway station are in relation to the subway's escalators or where the escalators are in relation to the tracks; these spatial relationships can be easily spotted on each trip.

PERCEIVING DURING THREE EVERYDAY ACTIVITIES

This section examines the role of perception in three of the everyday activities of pedestrians who are blind or visually impaired, namely (1) using a long cane to perceive surfaces and objects; (2) crossing streets at traffic-signal controlled intersections; and (3) learning the spatial layout of an unfamiliar place while walking within the place. For the first two activities nonvisual perception only is considered, third activity similarities and differences among persons with varying degrees of vision and visual experience are considered.

Perceiving with a Long Cane

What do a screwdriver and a long cane have in common? Each is a tool used to extend touch and which enables the user to perceive the world beyond its tip. The carpenter perceives the movements of the screw (Gibson, 1966; von Bekesy, 1967) just as the pedestrian who is blind perceives the objects and features of the immediate surroundings.

Instruments that extend touch are common in the natural world. For example, Burton (1993) described the nocturnal jerboa's use of its whiskers to preview the walking surface. While walking, the jerboa places the tip of its whiskers where it plans to place its foot on the next step (Sokolov & Kulikov, 1987). This biological adaptation to traveling in the dark is similar to Hoover's (1950) description of the touch technique: "The distal cane tip . . . always touches in front of the foot which is in arrears (the one about to be brought forward) making sure this foot will have a safe and unobstructed spot upon which to be placed" (p. 362). The long cane affords preview of the walking surface and the lower portion of the space in front of a pedestrian (Barth & Foulke, 1979). Although this preview is limited to the reach of the cane, it has been sufficient to provide a generally safe alternative to the use of human guides and dog guides.

This section is focused on information about the immediate surroundings that is relayed via the sounds, felt vibrations, and locations of the cane. The important complementary issue of the likelihood of protection against various kinds of obstacles and holes in the walking surface when different canes, techniques, styles of grasping, and patterns of cane–foot coordination are used is not discussed.

Identifying Surfaces and Materials

How well can people detect the properties and identities of surfaces while exploring them with tools like long canes? Schenkman (1986) performed an early systematic study of this. In two similar experiments, four common walking surfaces (concrete, asphalt, sand, and linoleum) were tapped with various long canes. In the first experiment ("sound only"), the participants listened and guessed which of the surfaces was being tapped by the experimenter. They were told whether their guesses were right or wrong, but were not given the correct answer when their guesses were wrong. In the second experiment ("touch only"), the participants did the tapping themselves but were outfitted with a sound system so that they could not hear the sounds they were producing.

In the sound-only experiment, participants' judgments averaged 67 percent correct overall, with judgments of the individual items ranging from 43 percent correct for asphalt to 93 percent correct for sand. Performance was not as good in the touch-only experiment, averaging 55 percent correct overall and ranging from 38 percent correct for asphalt to 96 percent correct for sand.

Schenkman's experiments demonstrated that people could identify surfaces with a long cane, by sound as well as touch. But although their performance was much better than chance, the participants erred much of the time, confusing some of the test surfaces with others. These confusions were not random—for example, while sand was rarely confused with any of the other possibilities, concrete and linoleum were often mistaken for each other.

Errors reflect that participants confused a particular surface's sound or feel with the sound or feel of another surface. Because the stimuli were presented one modality at a time, Schenkman's experiments did not examine the extent to which combining the modalities—as they are combined during everyday experience—would help. Consider two reasons that two modes may be better than one. First, it might be the case that the acoustic characteristics of the sounds resulting from tapping some surfaces are highly similar (Schenkman demonstrated this to be the case for concrete and linoleum) and therefore difficult to discriminate whereas the tactual feel is less similar (or vice versa). In this case, participants who had access to both sound and touch should make fewer errors than those who had access to only one modality of input. Second, it might be the case that sounds and touch vibrations are similarly difficult to discriminate on their own, but that when presented together one modality can be used to help disambiguate the other.

Guth, Rieser, and Yen (1995) extended Schenkman's single-mode experiments to investigate the potential advantages of multimodal perception. Their participants used a 30-centimeter wooden rod to explore 30 everyday surfaces and materials. Participants attempted to identify the stimuli under conditions in which they could be (1) felt with the rod and heard, (2) felt with the rod but not heard, and (3) heard but not felt. Among the stimuli most relevant to O&M were concrete, gravel, ceramic tile, steel, wood, glass, carpet, water, and plastic. Participants were allowed to tap, scrape, and stir these things except in the listening-only condition in which they directed an experimenter's manipulation of the rod.

Five of the 30 stimuli (e.g., thin steel) were easy to identify in the listening-only condition but relatively difficult in the touching-only condition; the opposite was true for 8 stimuli (e.g., concrete); and for 12 of the stimuli (e.g., wood) there was an advantage of the combined listening and touching condition over either of the single-mode conditions.

The auditory and tactile input from tools like long canes is often a sufficient basis for identification, as indicated by the rate of 28 percent correct identifications over all 30 of Guth, Rieser, and Yen's items. But participants erred on two-thirds of the identifications, even when they could listen to as well as feel the results of their explorations. This low rate can be accounted for in part by the perceptual similarity of many of the stimuli, such as the similar feel of smooth ceramic tile and glass, and the similar sounds of gravel and plastic beads. It is important to note that in the conditions described above, the participants did not know what kinds of surfaces and materials to expect. In most everyday situations, however, people have rich knowledge of what to expect. When exploring familiar places, they have episodic knowledge of the place from their earlier visits, and in unfamiliar places they usually have conceptual knowledge of some of the likely contents of the place. To assess the role of knowledge, Guth, Rieser, and Yen asked participants to identify the same stimuli on a second set of trials. But before doing so, the participants were told the names of all 30 items. They therefore knew what to expect and, accordingly, they doubled their success rate, correctly identifying 64 percent of the stimuli.

A final issue about identifying surfaces and materials with tools like long canes is the extent to which perception is affected by the perceptual tool. Schenkman (1986) found that among 32 cane–tip combinations, some worked much better than others. For example, in his sound-only experiment, 54 percent of participants' judgments were correct when using the Swedish laser cane with a nylon tip and 83 percent were correct when using a British cane with a nylon tip. It seems sensible that such assessment of the information-gathering characteristics of canes should play an important role in their evaluation. It would be useful to know, for example, how identification of the walking surface is affected by long-cane features such as rotating tips designed to reduce snagging.

Perceiving the Dimensions of Obstacles and Openings

Pedestrians who are blind use their long canes to judge the dimensions of the objects and openings they encounter. Consider the geometry of such skills: Begin by imagining that you are traveling with a cane that is 4 feet (1.2 meters) long and that your cane collides with an object. To discover the dimensions of the object, you move the tip of your cane first from the right side of the object to the left and then from the object's bottom to its top. You use the information you pick up during this exploration to decide whether to walk around the object or to step over it. Now imagine the same situation, except that you are traveling with a cane that is 8 feet (2.4 meters) long.

What is different about these two scenarios? A principal difference is that to move the cane tip the same distance from side to side or top to bottom, a 4-foot cane requires twice as much angular displacement of the wrist, hand, and arm as an 8-foot cane. That is, the movements of the wrist, hand, and arm that occur while exploring an object with a long cane vary not only as a function of the object's actual dimensions, but also as a function of cane length. Consequently, to accurately perceive an object's dimensions, the perceiver must take into account the length of his or her cane.

For explorations with the tip of the cane, one might suppose that accurate perception requires that a pedestrian have extensive experience with a cane of a single length. Through perceptual learning, a pedestrian who is blind could learn the one-to-one correspondence between the particular cane's various movements and the information specified by those movements. But what would happen if this hypothetical pedestrian were to travel with a cane that was markedly shorter or longer than his or her customary cane? Would perception be inaccurate and locomotion suffer? What about blind children whose canes "grow" with them? Does each new cane require a lengthy new round of perceptual learning? That this may not be the case is suggested by Burton's (1994) study of blindfolded sighted adults, who used probes similar to aluminum canes to help them cross holes in the floor of up to 35 inches (0.9 meters) across. The probes used by Burton's inexperienced participants varied in length from 48 to 60 inches (1.22 to 1.52 meters), and this variation was not found to affect performance.

Another variable that may affect a cane user's perception of the dimensions of an opening is his or her distance from the opening. Although the boundaries of an opening sometimes make contact with the tip of a pedestrian's cane, this contact will be higher on the shaft of the cane when the pedestrian is nearer to the opening. In a relevant study, Barac-Cikoja and Turvey (1991) had sighted persons use a wooden rod to estimate the width of unseen openings between two posts. As shown in Figure 1.3, a participant made the estimate by using his or her free hand to adjust the opening between an identical pair of posts. For openings that were actually the same width, judgments were strongly influenced by the opening's distance from a participant's hand. That is, the participants consistently judged the nearer openings to be wider than the farther ones. This suggests that perception was misled by the greater angles through which the rod had to be moved to explore the nearer openings. It seems likely that novice cane users would be similarly influenced and, assuming that the location of shaft contact can be accurately perceived, that perceptual learning would be reflected in more accurate perception among experienced cane users.

The Barac-Cikoja and Turvey research also raises new questions about the perceptual effects of variations in the physical characteristics of long canes other than length. For example, in two of their experiments, a cylinder of lead was inserted into the hollowed-out end of one rod, and this rod was sometimes held at its heavy end and sometimes at its light end. When the rod was held at its heavy end, participants consistently perceived the openings to be wider than they perceived the same openings to be when the rod was held at its lighter end. These perceptual differences can be related to differences in the forces present at the hand that are unrelated to either the length of the rod or the angle through which the wrist moves. It remains to be seen whether perception is similarly affected by variations such as those in the weight of long-cane tips and the uniformity of long-cane shafts.

Crossing Streets without Vision

This section considers four of the central tasks involved in crossing streets at traffic-signal controlled intersections. The tasks are according to their temporal sequence: detecting the street (a detection task), aligning the body (a localization task), initiating the crossing (a detection task), and walking a straight path across the street (a localization task). The selective emphasis of this section is the pedestrian who relies solely on nonvisual information and who uses a long cane. Related information about pedestrians who travel with dog guides can be found in Chapter 8 of this volume.

The perceptual demands of street crossing have increased dramatically since the early days of professional O&M in the 1940s and 50s. Some of the factors responsible for this are the replace

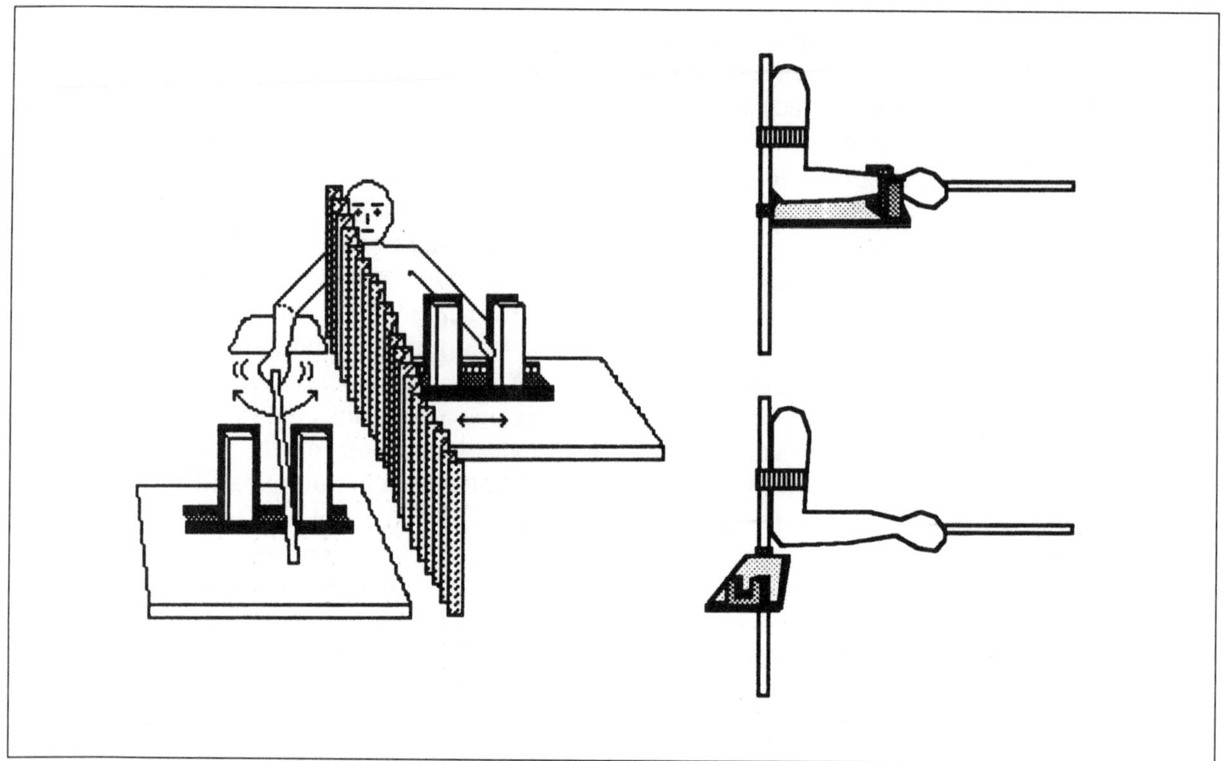

Figure 1.3. A diagram of test situation used to assess discrimination of gap widths explored with a rod that was manipulated without vision.

Source: Reprinted, with permission from APA and the authors, from D. Barac-Ci Koja and M. T. Turvey, "Haptically Perceiving Size at a Distance," *Journal of Experimental Psychology: General,* 122 (1993) 349.

ment of curbs with curb ramps, an increase in the complexity of intersection layout, the evolution of quieter motor vehicles (see Chapter 4), the widespread enactment of right- and left-turn-on-red laws, and the increased use of traffic signals whose timing varies according to the volume and location of traffic (Institute of Transportation Engineers, 1989, 1995).

Street Detection

A street should be detected before it is crossed. Bentzen and Barlow's (1995; Barlow & Bentzen, 1995) 80 participants who were blind reported using 22 different cues to detect streets they approached via curb ramps. Of these, the predominant cues were ramp slope and the presence of traffic in the to-be-crossed street (the "perpendicular" street). However, neither of these cues may be present at an intersection: Sidewalks and streets are sometimes level and even with each other (Hapeman, 1993; Wardell, 1980), and streets sometimes continue the upward or downward slope of a hilly terrain. Traffic waxes and wanes according to the time of the day and the day of the week, and some streets controlled by traffic signals rarely carry much traffic (Hall, Rabelle, & Zabihaylo, 1994).

Nor are the other cues reported by Bentzen and Barlow's participants reliably available. These include, for example, the upward camber of a street as it extends away from a sidewalk, curbs encountered to the side of a curb ramp, the stop-and-go pattern of traffic in the parallel street, other pedestrians, textural differences between a sidewalk and a street, the seam at the base of a curb ramp, and the end of a line of buildings (the latter detected via a disappearing sound shadow, the absence of reflected sounds, changes in air flow or temperature, and/or cane contact). At intersections where reliable cues for street detection are not available, it makes sense to consider installing a standardized cue such as underfoot warning tiles.

Episodic and conceptual knowledge each play important roles in street detection. Episodic knowledge such as knowing about a change from a pebbly sidewalk to an asphalt street at a particular corner makes it easy to detect the street. Conceptual knowledge such as knowing the typical relationship of the end of a building line to a street is useful for predicting when to expect a street. However, environmental variability sometimes limits the usefulness of such conceptual knowledge. Of Bentzen and Barlow's ten most difficult-to-detect streets, for example, five either had no building line on their approach path or had a building line whose distance from the street varied from the others along the route.

Alignment

Before crossing a street that has been detected, pedestrians who are blind often need to adjust their facing direction so that they are aligned with the opposite street corner. The physical features of a familiar environment can sometimes be used to establish this alignment. For example, an edge of a sidewalk that leads to a street and *is known* to be perpendicular to it can be a useful guide for alignment when accessed with the long cane or the foot, or both (see Hill & Ponder, 1976). Idiosyncratic environmental features such as the bars of sewer grates and the sides of mailboxes are also sometimes used when their spatial relationship to the direction of correct alignment is known.

Traffic sounds are another important source of information for alignment, and at some intersections they may be the only source. Traffic sounds enable pedestrians who are blind to align themselves in relation to the trajectory of traffic (e.g., to be facing parallel to the trajectory of parallel-street traffic). Chew (1986) and Guth, Hill, and Rieser (1989) assessed the skill with which experienced blind pedestrians aligned themselves parallel to and perpendicular to traffic that ranged from a single car to heavy traffic. These experiments revealed a wide range of individual differences, with some participants exhibiting substantially more performance variability (i.e., variable error) than others and some participants exhibiting a consistent response bias (i.e., constant error) such as facing away from parallel street traffic. Even those participants with the least variable error exhibited sufficient trial-to-trial variability that they would have occasionally walked into the intersection instead of across the street had they maintained their initial alignment direction while crossing. The acoustic basis of the use of traffic sounds for alignment is unclear and requires further investigation. Although blind pedestrians are able to use distant vehicles as directional beacons, they also appear to derive useful information while passing vehicles are close to them (Guth, Hill, & Rieser, 1989).

Audible traffic signals (ATS) can also provide useful information for alignment. Stevens (1993) assessed the alignment skill of 18 persons who were totally blind. They aligned themselves at a complex offset intersection using a traditional ATS system, which simultaneously emits sounds from both sides of a street, and an alternating ATS system, which alternates the sounds from one side of a street to the other. Participants were substantially more accurate with the alternating ATS than with the traditional ATS (average error = 6 degrees versus 28 degrees, respectively). The perceptual advantage of the alternating ATS system apparently is that the speaker on the opposite side of the street can serve as an auditory beacon because its sounds are not masked by the sounds of the speaker on the pedestrian's side. Notably, *average* performance with the alternating ATS was comparable to the performance of the *best* subjects in the studies of the use of traffic sounds for alignment.

Initiating the Crossing

Once properly positioned and aligned, a pedestrian must determine when to start out across a street. The usual signal to initiate a crossing is the parallel-street surge; that is, a pedestrian should begin crossing "when parallel traffic accelerates from a stopped position" (Hill & Ponder, 1976, p. 75). However, this can be a difficult detection task at modern intersections. It may be difficult, for example, to differentiate the many surging traffic movements at a complex intersection: With a leading turn arrow, the first surge of parallel-street traffic may be traffic turning into a pedestrian's intended path. Turn arrows on the perpendicular street can sometimes lead to surges in perpendicular-street traffic that "sound like" a parallel-street surge, especially if a pedestrian is misaligned. And parallel-street traffic making right or left turns on red can be mistaken for the appropriate surge. The perceiver's task is to sort through these possibilities and detect the appropriate surge from among the potential false positives. The likelihood and ease of doing so is undoubtedly increased at familiar intersections at which the cycle and timing of traffic movements are known and predictable.

Other sources of difficulty are the growing number of cars which are difficult to hear under the best of acoustic conditions (Chapter 4) and the near absence of parallel-street surges at some intersections (Hall, Rabelle, & Zabihaylo, 1994; Chapter 10). Contributing to the absence of the traditional surge is the rapidly increasing use of traffic-actuated signal systems. These systems maximize traffic flow and thereby minimize the occurrence of surges and even eliminate phases of the traffic-light cycle (e.g., turn arrows) when there is not enough traffic to warrant them (Institute of Transportation Engineers, 1995). (A corollary problem associated with actuated systems is variability in the time available to cross a street. Following a surge, there may not be sufficient time to get across the street before the light on the perpendicular street turns back to green. This problem is typically overcome with a pedestrian-activated traffic-signal cycle. This solution may require some adaptation for pedestrians who are blind, however, in order that the pedestrian control be easy to find, and the onset of the appropriate pedestrian cycle be identified [see Chapter 10]).

Maintaining a Straight Path across the Street

Once a properly aligned pedestrian has stepped into the street, it is important that he or she walk a reasonably straight path across it. There is sometimes information available for continuous guidance—for example, the sounds of a steady stream of parallel-street traffic can be used to maintain a constant distance from that street. At some geometrically complex intersections, tactual guidestrips, accessed with the long cane, provide a means of continuous guidance (see Taraya, 1995). Stevens (1993) has demonstrated the usefulness of alternating ATS systems for street-crossing guidance (in addition to their previously described usefulness for alignment): with minimal practice, her participants were able to stay within a 10-foot (3-meter) crosswalk while crossing a six-lane street.

On some occasions, however, there is little or no information available for guidance. A large body of evidence documents the inability of pedestrians who are blind or are sighted and blindfolded to maintain a straight path (i.e., to "veer") in the absence of external guidance (e.g., Rouse & Worchel, 1955; Cratty & Williams, 1966; Guth & LaDuke, 1995; see Guth & LaDuke, 1994, for a review). Over repeated attempts to maintain a straight-line trajectory, some people exhibit constant error—an overall tendency to veer in a particular direction. However, whether or not they exhibit constant error, even highly experienced blind pedestrians exhibit variable error sufficient to result in veering into the parallel street when crossing at intersections. The implications of this are that performance variability should be expected by blind pedestrians and O&M instructors alike, and that O&M instructors should emphasize the quick application of recovery procedures when such to-be-expected errors are detected (see Hill & Ponder, 1976; Jacobson, 1993; LaGrow & Weessies, 1994).

In an unpublished training experiment, Guth and LaDuke sought to reduce the veering tendency of five persons who were blind who exhibited a severe and directionally consistent veering tendency. The training procedure involved *bandwidth feedback* (Schmidt, 1991; Sherwood, 1988), whereby feedback was given only when performance deviated beyond set limits. During each of the 20 trials of a training session (12–20 training sessions per participant) a participant started with his or her back to a wall, walked away from the wall, and then attempted to stay within a 6.6-foot (2-meter) wide, 66-foot (20-meter) long path defined by two parallel infrared beams. If either beam was crossed, a signal heard through the participant's earphones identified the direction of error and the trial ended. The participant was also informed of the distance that he or she had traveled before the beam was broken.

The training was effective for all five participants, with veering after walking 82 feet (25 meters) reduced from an average of about 26 feet (8 meters) to the left or right of the intended path to an average of about 5 feet (1.5 meters). None of the participants could articulate what had been learned. Instead, they reported that they had "found the groove" or that they had learned what it "felt like" to walk straight. The training apparently enabled the participants to learn the motor commands and/or to recognize the motor feedback (kinesthetic, vestibular) associated with walking a straight-line path.

Path Integration, Cognitive Mapping, and Spatial Orientation

To plan a route through a familiar area, pedestrians who are blind or visually impaired need to think about the spatial layout of the objects and paths in the area. To travel successfully through the area, they first must know their starting place and facing direction and then must keep track of where they are within the remembered spatial layout. While traveling through an unfamiliar area, pedestrians often have the additional goals of discovering what objects are there and of learning their object-to-object relationships.

Learning object-to-object relationships (*cognitive mapping*) and keeping track of self-to-object relationships can each be accomplished in different ways, some relying primarily on information from self-movement (e.g., walking) and some relying on the use of external reference information and landmarks (see Chapter 2). In this section the information available from walking and present instructional and cognitive strategies that may improve the skill of maintaining orientation while walking are presented.

There is a long line of research about the use of information about self-movement to keep track of self-to-object relationships. This skill has variously been called "path integration," "spatial updating," "dead reckoning," and "inertial navigation" (Rieser & Garing, 1994; Schone, 1984). The latter two terms, originally applied to the piloting of vehicles such as ships, refer to measuring the distance and direction of each leg of a trip and using this information to compute the current distance and direction from a reference location. Darwin (1873) noted a similar ability in animals and humans that could not be explained on the basis of external reference information, and there has since been an abundance of research about the path integration abilities of animals (e.g. Muller & Wehner, 1988), of adults and children with normal vision (Klatzky et al., 1990; Rider & Rieser, 1988), and of people with visual impairments (Loomis et al., 1993; Rieser, Guth, & Hill, 1986; Worchel, 1951).

For a pedestrian who is totally blind, path integration is responsible for much of his or her knowledge of object-to-object relationships. Consider the following example of how this works: If a pedestrian leaves Object A and, while walking, is able to keep track of her self-to-Object A relationship, then when she encounters Object B she should know the Object A-to-Object B relationship. Likewise, if the pedestrian encounters Object C after leaving Object B, she will then know the Object B-to-Object C relationship. Research has shown that in such situations, people can learn both the directly experienced relationships (e.g., A to B, B to C) and those which can be logically inferred (e.g., A to C) (Book & Garling, 1981; Rieser, Guth, & Hill, 1982, 1986).

To assess the path integration skill of pedestrians who are blind, Hill et al. (1993) asked 60 individuals to walk paths varying in length and complexity. At the end of these walks, a pedestrian's judgment of the direction of the path's starting point was measured by having the pedestrian turn to face it. The pedestrian's judgment of the distance back to the starting point was then measured by having the pedestrian attempt to walk to it. The paths ranged in length from 20 to 66 feet (6 to 20 meters) and included one to seven turns ranging from 40 to 120 degrees. All 60 subjects judged directions and distances with better-than-chance levels of accuracy, but substantial individual differences were evident, especially on the longer, more complex routes. For example, even on the seven-turn routes, the most accurate subject averaged only 15 degrees and 1.6 feet (0.5 meters) of error while the least accurate subject averaged 100 degrees and 13 feet (4 meters) of error.

Similar findings have been obtained in studies in which the task was to maintain orientation to multiple objects. For example, Rieser, Guth, and Hill (1986) used sighted-guide techniques to show individuals who were blind the locations of five objects in an unfamiliar room. Participants were then led along a J-shaped route from one of the objects to a new place in the room and were asked to judge the direction of each of the objects. Overall, the participants averaged 30 degrees of error, but again there was a wide range of individual differences, with averaged individual errors ranging from 10 to 120 degrees.

Consider two of the possible causes of individual differences in path integration skill: One hinges on differences in the learning of how locomotion affects self-to-object relationships. How is it that people learn how a nearly infinite set of locomotor movements affects their spatial relationships to a nearly infinite set of possible object locations in their surroundings? The other hinges on differences in cognitive encoding strategies—individuals may differ in the degree to which they create a frame of reference and use that frame of reference to help keep track of their location within a place. Each of these is discussed below.

The Learning of Perceptual-Motor Coordination

In order to relate self-movement to knowledge of the locations of objects in the surroundings, one needs to know the geometry of how locomotion affects self-to-object relationships. The general characteristics of this geometry were described in the discussion of walking in the section, "Sources of Perceptual Input." It is easy to think about how people with unimpaired vision learn the geometry of their self-movements, since the rich environmental flow of changing self-to-object relations can be observed during locomotion (Rieser et al., 1995). Blindfolded sighted adults and adults who were blinded after early childhood performed similarly well on path integration tasks, suggesting that persons with late-onset blindness are able to maintain their knowledge of the effects of self-movement throughout years of blindness. Individuals who were blinded early in life are capable as well. Although they have been found to perform more poorly than individuals with late-onset blindness and sighted individuals on average (e.g., Rieser, Guth, & Hill, 1986), some congenitally blind persons perform with the same skill as the most accurate blindfolded sighted persons and persons with late-onset blindness.

This leads to two related questions. First, what accounts for the skill of some persons who are congenitally blind, given that they did not have the visual input with which to observe the complex changes in self-to-object relationships that result from locomotion? Second, how might the learning of perceptual-motor coordination be used to assist poor performers to sharpen their performance?

The geometry of self-movement would suggest that path integration difficulty probably lies more with straight-line movements (translations) than with turns (rotations). Because any rotation changes all self-to-object relationships by the same amount, attending to the direction of a single sound source while turning would be logically sufficient for learning the effects of turning movements on self-to-object relationships. However, as described in "Sources of Perceptual Input," earlier in this chapter, the geometry is more complex for translations. The high levels of skill of some persons who are congenitally blind might result from their attention to how their movements affect their spatial relationships to familiar sound-making objects, and we suggest that teaching take the same approach. That is, O&M instructors could direct their clients' attention to the relationship of their locomotion and the corresponding audible changes in self-to-object distances and directions. (Note that it is difficult to localize unfamiliar sound-making objects, so using familiar ones is potentially important.) Instructors attempting to enhance path integration skills could also attempt to systematically increase the number of sound sources being attended to. If multiple sources can be attended to, then the effects of translation on multiple self-to-object relationships can be observed. It may be helpful to begin practice by directing attention to a single auditory landmark, then to two, then to three, and so forth. A potential problem with this scheme is that the sound sources will mask each other, making localization difficult or inaccurate. A potential solution is to alternate the sound sources in a manner similar to that described earlier for alternating audible traffic signals. Talor (1993) suggested this approach to training and found that persons who initially experienced difficulty isolating three distinctive sound sources in a room reported that this difficulty disappeared as they became more familiar with the sound sources.

A perceptual learning hypothesis has been proposed here to account for differences in the path integration skills of persons who are totally blind. A similar hypothesis may apply to persons with low vision. Rieser, Hill, Talor, Bradfield, and Rosen (1992) assessed knowledge of the object-to-object relationships among landmarks in a familiar area of their towns of persons whose low vision varied in type and age at onset. Those persons whose visual fields were severely impaired from an early age (birth–3 years) performed significantly worse on average than those with an early- or late-onset acuity impairment or a late-onset field loss. It may be that an early-onset field loss has the same effect on the development of path integration skill as does early-onset total blindness. That is, persons with severely restricted fields have little access to environmental flow while walking. This is not the case for persons with impaired acuity and broad fields because under high contrast conditions even persons with acuities below 20/1000 experience compelling environmental flow while walking (Long, Rieser, & Hill, 1990).

Real and Imagined Spatial Frameworks

The strategies with which people attempt to acquire and use information influence their success as travelers. Textbooks of O&M techniques are replete with "recovery" strategies with which to reestablish orientation once a traveler is disoriented. However, fewer strategies are presented for becoming familiar with a novel environment or for maintaining orientation. This section describes promising strategies involving perceiving self-movement in relation to a spatial framework. The discussion begins with an anecdote in support of these strategies that is followed with less direct empirical evidence.

The anecdote concerns Everett Hill, our research collaborator. Hill prided himself on never becoming lost when blindfolded. With one exception, we could never get him lost, even when outfitting him with a sound system that made it impossible to use sound cues and then guiding him along tortuously circuitous routes that were explicitly designed to ensure that anyone would become lost. We believe the one exception is deeply informative. On that occasion we were discussing O&M and walking around an empty gymnasium, trying to design better tests of spatial orientation. Hill was being pilot tested on path-integration tests—being guided along circuitous routes and asked to point back at his starting point. Hill failed, missing by more than 100 degrees. He knew he performed poorly and it made him angry. He tried again, and was lost again. Then he realized the problem, tried again and forever after localized his starting point to within 10 degrees, even after walking routes with 30 turns, which varied from gradual to abrupt and from about 20 degrees to 720 degrees.

Hill's explanation was that while talking he lost track of his location within the gymnasium. Knowing this, he tried on the next trial to keep track of his starting place as he walked but found it difficult to keep up with all of the turns. Puzzled by this unaccustomed difficulty, he realized that he had forgotten to use his backup strategy for maintaining orientation—imagining himself standing within a framework. He said that sometimes in this situation he imagined himself inside a large grid and perceived his changing positions and the objects encountered along the way relative to this imaginary grid. At other times, like on this occasion, he merely supposed that he was at a particular place within the actual space, even though he knew that he was probably imagining himself in the wrong place. But doing so gave him a spatial framework within which it was easy for him to maintain his orientation to his starting point and to the things he encountered as well as to learn the object-to-object relationships of those things.

In familiar places, it is possible to call to mind one's knowledge of the framework of the place and the objects within it and then to perceive self-movement relative to that knowledge. It may be the case that skillful travelers do this more consistently than unskillful ones. This seems like a teachable skill. In unfamiliar places, however, travelers may be in a strategic dilemma: On the one hand they are attempting to learn the arrangement of objects and the framework of the new place via their self-movement, and on the other hand this knowledge would help them perceive their self-movement.

If Hill's example is generally applicable, then imagining *any* spatial framework would help. Hill understood that he was in a large gymnasium and he knew its dimensions, so he imagined occupying it from an arbitrary observation point. Hill was a talented individual with exceptional spatial imagery, so it may be the case that such real or imagined spatial-framework strategies would be of limited use to less talented individuals. There are indications, however, that this may not be the case. Rieser and Frymire (1995; see also Rieser, Garing, & Young, 1994) tested six blindfolded sighted young adults' skill at using a spatial-framework strategy to keep track of their starting place as they walked along irregular 33- to 66-foot (10 to 20-meter) routes in an open field. In the No-Knowledge Condition the participants didn't know where in the field they were actually starting and were simply asked to try to keep track of the starting location while they were walking. In the Imagined-Surroundings Condition participants were asked to imagine being in a familiar open area that they knew well and which had several landmarks to help them track their position. The imagined surroundings were usually a front or back yard. Judgments were more accurate in the Imagined Surroundings Condition than in the No-Knowledge Condition.

The use of an imagined framework strategy would seem to be particularly useful to pedestrians who are blind in very large open areas that contained object-to-object relationships of importance, but whose perimeters were distant from the relevant objects and irrelevant to the pedestrian's travel goals. Consider, for example, a typical atrium lobby of a large hotel. The interior of such a lobby may cover an acre or more, containing several "open-air" restaurants and lounges, food carts, seating areas, elevators and escalators, fountains and objects of art, and so forth. A guest who is blind may be interested in learning only particular object-to-object relationships—for example, the relationships among the elevators, concierge desk, front door, a breakfast stand, and a particular restaurant. Using an imagined framework strategy while traveling among these locations with a sighted guide may be an efficient and effective way to obtain the desired knowledge.

But pedestrians who are blind are able to use

an imagined framework strategy? Using such a strategy requires two things: One is that people are able to generate an image of a spatial framework, imagining that they are there, and the other is that once they have generated this image, they are able to perceive their locomotion relative to the imagined framework. We have already discussed the evidence showing that blind pedestrians are able to perceive their locomotion relative to the places that they actually occupy. It seems likely that the same path integration would occur within an imagined place. Although less is known about the ability to generate an image of a spatial framework, we summarize below the conclusions of two lines of research that seem relevant.

First, evidence suggests that individuals who are congenitally blind are capable of generating and manipulating spatial images (de Beni & Cornoldi, 1988; Hollins, 1985; Kerr, 1983; Lehtinen-Railo & Juurmaa, 1994; Marmor, 1977). The research leaves open the question of whether persons with congenital blindness may be slower to generate images or less precise in the images they generate, but it is clear that they are able to process images and decide about the properties of imagined things in the same ways as blindfolded sighted individuals.

Second is evidence suggesting the ability to call to mind knowledge of familiar rooms while standing in other rooms. Rieser, Halpin, and Hill (unpublished study) asked 40 individuals whose onset of blindness occurred before the age of 1 year and 20 individuals whose onset of blindness occurred after the age of 4 years to explore a 15- by 15-foot (4.6- by 4.6-meter) room occupied by five common objects and to learn the relative positions of the objects. After this learning phase they traveled to another building. They were then asked to imagine standing in a given spot in the recently learned room and to turn to face the targets as if they were actually occupying that spot. Both groups were successful at this: the individuals with late-onset blindness averaged 30 degrees of error, which was significantly better than the 55-degree average of those with early-onset blindness. Within each group, however, individuals ranged from lows of under 15 degrees of error to highs exceeding 100 degrees. The sources of these errors are not known. It may be that the participants differed in how accurately they learned the space, how accurate an image of the space they were able to call to mind, or some combination of these.

CONCLUSION

Pedestrians on the move guide their locomotion in relation to the objects and events in their surroundings. Doing so requires information about the characteristics, identity, and location of those objects and events. Perceiving is defined as obtaining that information by looking, listening, touching, and other forms of active, direct observation.

Even the most experienced pedestrians (those who are normally sighted, visually impaired, and blind alike) make errors. They stumble over objects they failed to detect; they barely escape collisions when crossing streets; and they lose their way when exploring new places. Such errors occur for a variety of reasons including situations where the information is impoverished, a lack of perceptual and motor skill, inattention, and a willingness to take risks. O&M instructors often work with persons who are novices at traveling independently under the conditions of their visual impairments and/or who are novices at traveling under the conditions of the environments they wish to master. During O&M lessons instructors have the chance to observe many perceptual errors that reflect a lack of perceptual and motor skill. In order to assist, they provide instruction focused on perceptual and perceptual-motor strategies used to acquire and act on environmental information that is useful for O&M. They also arrange situations where the strategies can be practiced safely in the sometimes risky contexts where they are needed. Assisting blind and visually impaired persons in becoming more skillful perceivers is a central role of O&M instructors. This chapter has been an attempt to assist them in becoming more effective in this role.

Suggestions/Implications for O&M Specialists

1. To guide their locomotion, people need information about the characteristics, identity, and location of the objects and events in their surroundings. Perception is defined as obtaining that information by looking, listening, touching, and other forms of active, direct observation.
2. Motion of the self, the motion of objects, and exploratory activities are essential sources of information for perceiving one's surroundings and guiding locomotion.
3. Impairment of the size and shape of the visual field and impairment of visual acuity and contrast sensitivity have different functional implications for O&M.
4. Objects and surfaces can be identified by the sounds they make, sounds they reflect, and sounds produced from their interaction with travelers' footsteps, and long canes.
5. Touching, used to discover the properties of the immediate surroundings, involves both the cutaneous sense and proprioception. Long canes are tools used to extend touching.
6. Walking involves efference (motor control commands to the muscles) and afference (feedback from the body about the movements resulting from those commands). Both are believed to play a role in keeping track of one's path of locomotion.
7. The vestibular system of the inner ear detects the rotary and linear movements of the head as well as its tilt. It too plays an important role in keeping track of one's path of locomotion.
8. Environmental flow refers to the continuous lawful changes in one's directions and distances to things in the surroundings that occur during locomotion. Maintaining orientation can be thought of as keeping track of environmental flow. The complex geometry of environmental flow may help explain why some persons have difficulty maintaining spatial orientation.
9. Pedestrian safety depends on proficiently adjusting one's movements in relation to the perceived characteristics of the immediate path. This is an important type of perceptual-motor coordination.
10. Perception and knowledge are interrelated in functionally important ways. Especially relevant to O&M are procedural knowledge, episodic knowledge, and conceptual knowledge.
11. The concepts of "sensitivity" and "criterion," borrowed from signal detection theory, provide useful ways for O&M instructors to think about the perceptual errors that pedestrians make in detecting the presence of environmental features and events.
12. Long cane techniques such as the touch and constant-contact techniques vary in the properties of the walking surface about which they are most informative. This is due to differences in the felt vibrations, sounds, and forces arising from the various techniques.
13. Successful O&M requires information about the layout (object-to-object relationships) of the objects in one's surroundings. Even sophisticated knowledge of the relative locations of objects is useless, however, unless pedestrians know where they stand and which way they are facing relative to those objects.

(*continued on next page*)

Suggestions/Implications for O&M Specialists (continued)

14. The movements of the wrist, hand, and/or arm that occur while exploring an object with a long cane vary not only as a function of the object's dimensions, but also as a function of cane length. Therefore to perceive an object's dimensions, one must somehow take into account the length of his or her cane.
15. The perceptual demands of nonvisual street crossing have increased dramatically in recent years. Among the responsible factors are the replacement of curbs with gently sloped curb ramps, an increase in the complexity of intersection layout, the design of quieter motor vehicles, right- and left-turn-on-red laws, and traffic-actuated traffic signals.
16. The physical features of the environment encountered at an intersection are useful for street-crossing alignment only to the extent that their spatial relationship to the direction of correct alignment is known.
17. Path integration is responsible for much of a totally blind person's knowledge of object-to-object relationships. Path integration makes it possible to learn relationships that are directly experienced as well as those which can be logically inferred from the experienced relationships.
18. A person who had an early onset of blindness or an early onset of a severe restriction of his or her visual field may have difficulty acquiring path integration skills. This may be due to difficulty in observing the complex changes in self-to-object relationships that occur during locomotion.

ACTIVITIES FOR REVIEW

1. Develop an activity with which you can demonstrate to others the environmental flow that occurs when a pedestrian walks a straight-line path. Your activity should illustrate the geometric complexity of the environmental flow as described in this chapter. Explain why maintaining orientation means the same thing as keeping track of environmental flow.
2. Observe an O&M lesson. Analyze the lesson in terms of the extent to which the instructor emphasized procedural, episodic, and conceptual knowledge.
3. Pedestrian travel can be a risky business. Using everyday language and practical examples, write a script in which you explain to a client how the choice of a criterion involves a safety/efficiency trade-off.
4. Visit several traffic-signal controlled intersections that vary in complexity and traffic volume. For one crossing at each intersection, list all of the sources of information available to pedestrians who are blind and visually impaired for (1) street detection, (2) alignment, (3) initiating the crossing, and (4) walking a straight path across the street. For each source of information, distinguish whether it is always present and whether it depends on the pedestrian's familiarity with the intersection in order to be useful.

5. Explain how a difference in the learning of perceptual-motor coordination may account for the difference in John and Jane's spatial orientation that is described in the first paragraph of this chapter.
6. List three reasons that the detection of curbs and ramps can be problematic for pedestrians with low vision.
7. With the assistance of a partner, use nonvisual path integration to learn the object-to-object relationships among several objects in a large room. While you are outside of the room, have your partner arrange the objects in a layout that is unfamiliar to you. Then, using your partner as a sighted guide, use a path integration strategy to learn the layout. Devise a simple test of your path integration skill and use it to test your knowledge of the arrangement of the objects.

CHAPTER 2

Establishing and Maintaining Orientation for Mobility

Richard G. Long and Everett W. Hill

This chapter is about spatial orientation of individuals who are blind or visually impaired. It focuses on spatial problems they must solve to move efficiently from place to place and the strategies or tools they use to solve them. The problems can be illustrated by questions visually impaired travelers often must answer, such as "How far and in which direction is my destination? How will I keep track of my location along a route as I travel? Which way do I turn next to continue traveling toward my destination? If I become disoriented, how will I relocate the travel path? Where is my destination in relation to other places I want to go, and what are the shortest and safest routes that lead from place to place?" To answer questions like these, blind or visually impaired travelers use a variety of problem-solving strategies. These strategies include the use of landmarks and information points for orientation, recall of mental "maps" of familiar places, systematic familiarization to new places, and effectively soliciting aid to obtain orientation information. Using one or more of these strategies, visually impaired travelers usually are able to travel efficiently in their homes and communities. The problems of spatial orientation and the strategies to solve them provide the framework for this chapter.

SPATIAL ORIENTATION: AN INTRODUCTION

The term *spatial orientation* has its origins in research literature in the field of cognitive psychology. A substantial body of psychological research has developed during the past 50 years about various aspects of spatial orientation, both in humans and animals (Rieser & Garing, 1994; Schone, 1984). Psychologists who study perception and cognition use the term spatial orientation in a relatively narrow sense to refer to knowledge of the spatial relationship (e.g., the alignment or position) of one's entire body, or part of the body, to objects or locations. Environmental psychologists and others use the term *wayfinding* to refer more broadly to the process of navigating through an environment and traveling to places by relatively direct paths. Spatial orientation is considered one component of successful wayfinding. The student of orientation and mobility (O&M) instruction may refer to the environmental psychological literature on way-

The authors gratefully acknowledge the assistance of Professor John Rieser of Peabody College, Nashville, in preparing this chapter.

finding and the psychological literature on spatial orientation for more information on these topics.

Spatial orientation is an important topic to people who are blind or visually impaired, to orientation and mobility (O&M) specialists who provide services to them, and to researchers who seek to understand the problems and strategies for orientation used by blind and low vision individuals. Spatial orientation is broadly defined in the field of O&M as "the process of using the senses to establish one's position and relationship to all other significant objects in one's environment" (Hill & Ponder, 1976, p. 3), "the ability to use one's remaining senses to understand one's location in the environment at any given time" (Jacobson, 1993, p. 3), and "the ability to establish and maintain an awareness of one's position in space" (LaGrow and Weessies, 1994, p. 9). The focus of these definitions is on an individual's current location or position in space relative to other locations or places. The Jacobson and LaGrow and Weessies definitions also acknowledge the importance of updating, or keeping track of spatial relationships as one moves.

Two terms are important for understanding spatial orientation of visually impaired travelers because they form the basis for communication about the process. These terms are *self-to-object* and *object-to-object spatial relationships.* Self-to-object spatial relationships refer to an individual's alignment or position relative to objects or locations in an environment. These objects or places might be on a tabletop, across a room, on another floor of a building, or several blocks away. Object-to-object spatial relationships refers to knowledge of the spatial relationship of two or more objects or places, independent of the individual's position in space. Although object-to-object spatial relationships are not included explicitly in the definitions of orientation, their importance in efficient travel is clear to O&M instructors and their learners. The ability to acquire accurate object-to-object relationships, for example, aids the traveler in acquiring mental representations of larger-space environment.

The terminology used to describe self-to-object and object-to-object relationships is important in O&M instruction because it provides a basis of communication and understanding among O&M specialists, O&M specialists and students, and between students. According to Blasch, Welsh, and Davidson (1973), self-to-object relationships can be described using egocentric, topocentric, cartographic, and polarcentric terms. One commonly used egocentric reference system is lateral position, indicated by the terms left and right ("The desk is to my right; I am to the left of the bakery"). Self-to-object relationships also can be described with topocentric terminology, using prepositions such as over, behind, or between (e.g., "I am between the bakery and the cleaners; I am beside the bakery"). In addition, they can be described using cartographic or polarcentric terminology. Cartographic terms refer to systematic spatial arrangements of places in an environment. This may include patterns of street names (e.g., alphabetized or numbered) and the organization of building and street numbering systems. As discussed later in this chapter, using orientation strategies based on cartographic spatial knowledge can aid travelers in precisely locating specific travel objectives ("I am located at 648 Dogwood Road, in apartment 104"). Polarcentric terminology uses compass directions ("I am south of the bakery").

The above terminology, with the exception of egocentric terminology, can also be used to describe object-to-object relationships. For example, object-to-object spatial relationships can be expressed in prepositional or topocentric terms ("The bakery is beside the drugstore"). They can also be expressed in cartographic terms ("The department store is at the corner of Smith and Main Streets"). Polarcentric terminology is especially useful in describing object-to-object relationships ("The department store is west of the subway entrance").

Many of the terms used to describe self-to-object and object-to-object spatial relationships can be somewhat ambiguous and imprecise. The terms right and left, for example, can be undependable if one's facing direction changes. An object on the right is on the left after turning around. Cardinal directions (or polarcentric terminology) are unique as a spatial reference system because they have a fixed, constant reference point (i.e., magnetic north). As a result, cardinal directions are unambiguous. They are the same regardless of one's point of view (e.g., the bakery is always north of the drugstore, regardless of a traveler's perspective). As anyone who uses cardinal directions as a strategy for efficient wayfinding would attest, their unambiguous nature makes them extremely valuable in describing spatial relationships.

Just like the terms for self-to-object relationships, terms used to describe object-to-object distances can also be ambiguous and imprecise. The degree of precision or ambiguity depends in part on whether relative or absolute terms are used. For example, it often is useful to describe self-to-object and object-to-object distances in precise terms ("The bakery is three blocks from here") rather than by relative terms such as "far away" or "close" (e.g., "The bakery is far from here"). The more precise and unambiguous the distance and direction terms used in communicating spatial information to travelers with impaired vision, the more valuable they will be.

In the definitions of spatial orientation used in O&M cited earlier, spatial updating was noted to be an important characteristic of self-to-object spatial relations. In contrast, object-to-object spatial relationships are unaffected by an observer's movement in an environment, while self-to-object relationships change as one moves through space. Consider the problem of maintaining self-to-object spatial relationships: Maintaining self-to-object spatial relationships requires that individuals know how their movement through the environment affects the distances and directions to places beyond their reach. To illustrate how self-to-object spatial relationships change depending on an observer's point-of-view, imagine a large room with an object in the middle of the room. An individual explores the object, then moves so that she is standing with her back to one wall and facing the object. The object is in front of her. If she then moves to the opposite wall of the room and maintains her original facing direction, the object now is behind her. If she then points to the rear when asked to locate the object, her response indicates that she knows how her self-movement (i.e., walking across the room) has changed the self-to-object spatial relationship (from in front to behind). However, if she points straight ahead after movement across the room, she may not understand how her movement affects her position relative to the object in the center of the room. People usually keep track of changing distances and directions to places out of view as they walk, because doing so aids in moving about efficiently, or by relatively direct routes. They usually expend relatively little conscious mental effort to keep track of these relationships while traveling familiar routes.

Now consider the nature of object-to-object spatial relationships. To continue the example above, imagine an individual in a large room containing two objects. One object is near the door and the other is in the center of the room. Regardless of where a person is located in the room, the spatial relationship of the two objects to each other is the same. The relationship can be described in cardinal directions independent of the person's perspective (e.g., the object near the door is always north of the object in the center of the room). A person's knowledge of object-to-object spatial relationships can aid in planning efficient routes from place to place. Knowledge of these spatial relationships is sometimes characterized as a *cognitive or mental map.* This metaphor is used in part because maps preserve the relationships between objects and places, and also because maps are familiar ways to depict object-to-object spatial relationships.

ORIENTATION IN O&M: LANDMARKS AND INFORMATION POINTS

Visually impaired persons use their senses to learn about their surroundings and then use their cognitive abilities, especially reasoning and memory, to determine what the sensory information "means" for spatial orientation. In short, they listen, touch, smell, and feel as they move about, and they associate certain sensory and perceptual experiences with locations along a route. *Landmark* is the term used to describe perceptible features of environments that permit travelers to know their precise location in a known environment. Hill and Ponder (1976) define landmarks as any familiar object, sound, odor, temperature, tactile, or visual clue that is easily recognized, is constant, and has a discrete, permanent location in the environment that is known to the traveler. *Information points* are two or more sensory stimuli that, when linked, allow a traveler to determine his or her exact location. Information points have been labeled by various authors as cues, clues, and dominant clues.

The quality or usefulness of sensory information for orientation depends in part on (1) the likelihood that the traveler will perceive the sensory information and (2) the specificity of the information provided by the input. Landmarks and information points differ on these two factors. As noted above, landmarks are spatial "anchors" because they provide precise information about one's location. A box for depositing books after-hours at a library in a particular neighborhood, for example, might serve as a landmark. It is easily distinguished from a mailbox. It is not easily moveable. Perhaps most important, it is unique; there is not another box of similar size and shape nearby. Each of these characteristics aids the traveler who contacts the box in determining or confirming that he is at the library.

Landmarks are always recognizable or identifiable when encountered, and they always provide relatively precise information for orientation. Some landmarks are always present while others, like the sound of a fan in a water fountain, are intermittent. Even if landmarks are always present, they may not always be encountered by travelers every time they travel the same route. For example, if a traveler walks on the left side of a wide sidewalk and misses a distinctive break in the sidewalk on the right, she has not encountered a landmark that is always present. Prior literature has not sufficiently differentiated these two types of landmarks. To improve the terminology of O&M, landmarks that are always present and always encountered by travelers will be called *primary landmarks.* An example of a primary landmark may be a series of missing slabs of concrete along a path. Landmarks that are not always present or for some reason are not always encountered will be termed *secondary landmarks.* Although they can provide the traveler with precise information about her unique location, they can not always be counted upon. Examples include information that is intermittent or easily missed by a traveler. Both primary and secondary landmarks are critical to visually impaired travelers because they are one of the most important ways to confirm one's location in an environment.

Travelers vary on the number of landmarks they know in a particular travel environment, and they vary on the amount and type of information they have about landmarks. They may, for example, simply be able to recognize an environmental feature and recall its location along a route without knowing what the feature is. Conversely, they may know both the name and function of a landmark and may be able to describe it in detail. A person who uses a statue as a landmark may know the name of the person on the statue, and may know that the person is mounted on a horse. This knowledge may help him solicit aid from a passerby to locate this particular statue if he becomes disoriented while in the park. A store might be known by its location (e.g., address, proximity to another store) and its name; its distinguishing visual, auditory, or tactile features (e.g., pink shutters, distinctive music, carpeted entryway); and its contents (e.g., the smell of coffee beans roasting). As noted earlier, secondary landmarks, while distinctive, may not always be present or may not always be encountered by travelers. In the example above the smell of coffee beans roasting may only be present at certain times of the day.

Information points differ from landmarks. Like landmarks, information points are sounds, odors, temperatures, or visual or tactual stimuli. A single information point does not provide sufficient information to identify the exact position of the traveler by itself. However, when the spatial information of two or more information points is linked, a traveler can determine her precise location. For instance, there are many features found in a variety of locations in large indoor and outdoor environments. Because the features are common, they do not provide precise location information, although they can aid in determining one's general location along a route. When linked spatially with other information points, they may indeed permit a person to determine his exact location. For example, a traveler moving along the sidewalk may encounter a series of bushes followed by a curb cut. Taken by themselves the bushes may suggest several possible locations along a route. When found in proximity to the curb cut, the unique combination alerts the traveler to the precise location of Main and Maple Streets. Because both bushes and curb cuts are common in the environment, neither of them alone is adequate for determining one's precise location. However, when spatially linking the bushes to the curb cut, he has successfully combined the pair of information points to determine precise location.

COMPONENTS OF SPATIAL ORIENTATION IN O&M

As noted earlier, the ability to establish and maintain self-to-object and object-to object spatial relationships and to use landmarks and information points to travel efficiently from place to place is based on the complex interaction of a traveler's perceptual and cognitive abilities. The ability to extract spatial "meaning" from sensory information and to move purposefully and efficiently toward a travel objective is the essence of spatial orientation. This section provides a brief overview of the perceptual and cognitive components of orientation.

Perceptual-Motor Components

Several chapters in this volume provide detailed descriptions of perception as it affects orientation of visually impaired persons. As Warren (1994) has summarized, vision has significant advantages over other senses for perceiving environmental information and forming object-to-object spatial relationships. Vision permits simultaneous perceptions of the locations of several objects or landmarks. Sighted pedestrians often simply see a destination in the distance and maintain visual contact with it and with intermediate landmarks as they travel toward it. Vision is an efficient sense for identifying landmarks and information points. It also permits perception of objects at substantial distances from the viewer. Another advantage of vision for spatial orientation is that visual stimuli are abundant in most travel environments. Many visual stimuli are available to the individual with very low vision. Critical visual features in the environment often can be identified and used as landmarks along a route.

When vision is absent or impaired, other senses are used to acquire information about one's surroundings. These include the senses of touch, smell, proprioception, and hearing. One fundamental aspect of these nonvisual sensations is they typically do not have the range, richness, or flexibility of vision for acquiring spatial information. Consider, for example, a tactual information point such as a metal plate on a sidewalk. When combined with another information point such as a slope, a blind traveler may use these information points to determine or confirm where he or she is along a route. There is a possibility, however, given the relatively incomplete surface preview provided by the sense of touch via the long cane a traveler might walk beside the plate in the sidewalk without detecting it. Auditory information also provides cues to orientation. Pedestrians sometimes listen for the sound of moving traffic beside them, and align themselves parallel to the sound of that traffic by mentally tracing its movement. Guth, Hill, and Rieser

(1989) and Wiener & Lawson (Chapter 4) provide more information about using auditory information for alignment at street crossings. Also, secondary landmarks, such as certain sounds or textures, may be present in a given place along a walk on one occasion, but not present on a subsequent walk. Auditory and tactile information can be difficult to interpret when the environment is rich in sounds and tactile cues, or when such information is scarce.

Perceptual-motor information is useful to visually impaired travelers in a variety of ways. Proprioception and kinesthesis, the sensation of body position or movement that results from neural stimulation in muscles and joints, can be linked to other sensory information to aid orientation. For example, as a individual in a quiet residential area approaches an intersection and plans to cross the perpendicular street (i.e., the street in front of her), she "monitors," either consciously or subconsciously, the rotation of her body as she stops and waits for a safe time to cross. She knows that the line of direction she was walking is the correct line for crossing the street to the opposite corner, and she does not want to turn even slightly to the right or left. If she does, she may walk into the perpendicular street but away from the corner, or into the parallel street (i..e., the street to her side). She maintains her line of direction by using kinesthetic feedback to determine that her body alignment has not changed. Kinesthetic information may also be useful in a situation where a traveler must turn corners. O&M specialists, particularly those working with congenitally blind individuals often have clients practice turning precise quarter turns. Practice allows them to "remember" the "feel" of this particular amount of rotation around a vertical axis. Ninety- and 180-degree turns are especially important in independent travel because many of the rotations used when traveling in built environments are made up of these turns (e.g., turning from one street onto a perpendicular street). Despite the relative disadvantage incurred by reliance on nonvisual cues for spatial orientation, individuals who are blind or severely visually impaired use these cues successfully to move about independently and remain oriented in both familiar and unfamiliar places.

Cognitive Components

Body Concepts

Concepts are fundamental components of spatial orientation. Hill and Blasch (1980) define concepts broadly as mental representations, images, or ideas, and they classify concepts in three categories: (1) body concepts, (2) object and environmental concepts, and (3) spatial concepts. Frostig and Horne (1964) differentiate between body image, body concept, and body schemata. *Body image* includes the subjective feelings associated with a person's body while *body concept* refers to understanding the potential positions of the body. Body concept has been evaluated in children who are blind or visually impaired in various ways, including asking them to touch or name body parts and planes on themselves and others, identify the function of body parts, and to draw or model one's body. Warren (1994) in reviewing research literature about body concepts, including the landmark study in this area by Cratty and Sams (1968), describes the age-related progression of development of body concepts. He notes that children with partial vision and higher intelligence tend to have better body concepts than blind children or children with lower intelligence of similar age. Knowledge of body planes is also an important aspect of body concept. Children who can touch the front, sides, back, top, and bottom of their various body parts on request demonstrate an understanding of the planes of their body. Knowledge of body parts and planes is important for spatial orientation. For example, travelers often must align planes of their bodies with landmarks (e.g., "the mailbox is on my side and the street is in front of me"). O&M specialists and teachers of visually impaired children often work with young blind and low vision children to help them form the body concepts that are critical to establishing and maintaining orientation.

Object and Environmental Concepts

Object concepts refer to basic knowledge that objects have mass and occupy space, and to knowledge about various physical and functional properties of objects. For example, children learn that some objects can move, some always remain stationary, and some either can move or be stationary. Objects can be classified by their physical characteristics (e.g., shape, texture, color), their functional uses, and the actions they make or that can be made with them. The ability, for example, to identify a residential mailbox by its characteristic shape, despite variations in mailboxes, would be useful in using mailboxes as landmarks for orientation.

Environmental concepts refer to knowledge of environmental features (e.g., size, shape, color, and texture of telephone poles, parking meters, sidewalks) and to knowledge of spatial regularities of these features in built environments. Examples of environmental regularities include the location of parking meters, which are usually between the sidewalk and the street and in a line parallel to the street and the sidewalk. Curbs are in predictable locations in most outdoor environments (e.g., parallel to streets and lie between the sidewalk and the street). Environmental regularity and predictability often is useful in orientation for individuals who are blind or visually impaired. It allows them to determine accurately what is ahead on or beside the travel path and which way they are facing. Knowledge of environmental features such as terrain, slope, and physical characteristics of various walking surfaces can be useful. For example, curbs often have downward sloping ramps to accommodate travelers using wheelchairs. Visually impaired travelers often anticipate arrival at a curb by the downward slope of the sidewalk.

Spatial Concepts

Spatial concepts include knowledge of shape, size, and location. These concepts are based largely on early sensorimotor experiences involving cycles of perception and action (Chapter 1). Shape concepts are important components for orientation during mobility. For example, the knowledge that city blocks are usually rectangular (and knowledge of the characteristic features of rectangles) can aid in remaining oriented while traveling around a block. As Guth and Rieser (Chapter 1) note, this type of spatial knowledge usually is referred to as conceptual or semantic knowledge. Good concepts of size, like those of shape and mass, likely influence spatial orientation during mobility. For example, knowledge that buses are almost always larger than cars, or that two-lane streets are narrower than four-lane streets, can be useful in travel.

Concepts of position or location, including laterality and directionality, are also important cognitive components for orientation during mobility. Positional or topocentric concepts often are described with prepositions such as "toward," "away from," "up," "down," "behind," "in front of," and "near." Warren (1994) reviews research on laterality and directionality in visually impaired children. He notes they have difficulty in moving from understanding location from an egocentric reference system (i.e., laterality or self-to-object) to understanding spatial relationships of external objects independent of the child's own body. For example, children may readily learn that an object is to their right or left, but may have difficulty understanding that one object is next to another object. Fluency in laterality and directionality is a key building block for orientation, as it aids travelers in following directions and reading maps as they move about.

Generalizing Conceptual Knowledge

To effectively use concepts for orientation, blind travelers must be able to generalize their conceptual knowledge to new places and situations. Children, for example, learn to generalize their knowledge of the concept of shape to many objects and many situations, selecting salient perceptual features to make judgments about whether this particular concept describes a spatial arrangement. The streets in a neighborhood might form a rectangle, and a table in the cafeteria at school might also be a rectangle. From experience with a variety of objects and movements, children develop generalized notions of various concepts. Concepts often are defined with some degree of imprecision. For example, while shape concepts may be relatively precisely defined, object classes and spatial concepts may be more difficult to define precisely. There are "gray areas" in assigning objects to conceptual categories, especially when objects function in a particular way but do not have features characteristic of other objects that function similarly. Objects can be classified with varying degrees of precision in terms of attributes, function, or meaning (Lydon & McGraw, 1973). Is a beanbag a chair, albeit a relatively poor example? Spatial concepts can also be ambiguous. Is six blocks considered "far away?" Is 12 blocks? An understanding of the characteristics of concepts is a fundamental cognitive building block for spatial orientation.

Application of Conceptual Knowledge During Travel

Memory

Memory is an important cognitive component for spatial orientation. It is an important element in the development of a cognitive map or mental image of the layout of a place. The map consists of spatial arrangement remembered in an organized fashion. Short-term memory is necessary to recall the order or sequence of perceptual events occurring during travel (e.g., "I crossed Inkster, Creston, Edgemore, but have not yet crossed Montrose"). Long-term memory is necessary to recall the specific landmarks or features, referred to by Guth and Rieser (Chapter 1) as "episodic knowledge." It is also important when remembering how to perform motor movements necessary in travel (called *procedural memory*). Finally, it is necessary to retain a conceptual knowledge of the environment. A traveler may, for example, recall that sidewalks are typically parallel to the street, or that numbering systems proceed in a predictable fashion as one moves from north to south or east to west in a town. For more information on memory see Jacobson and Bradley (Chapter 11).

Cognitive Maps

Guth and Rieser (Chapter 1) provide an overview of two other components for orientation: cognitive mapping and spatial updating. The term *cognitive map* was coined by psychologists as a metaphor for the way object-to-object spatial relationships might be learned and represented mentally. A cognitive map is a mental image of the relationship and distances between objects in a place. There has been considerable research about the ability of blind and low vision individuals to update and to form cognitive maps of new places, and to use mental maps to remain oriented during mobility.

To illustrate how a traveler might use cognitive mapping, imagine a blind individual standing on a sidewalk in a typical urban environment. She is near an intersection of two streets. She has been at this location many times before. There is a bakery to her right and a drugstore across the street and to her left. She knows where she is in relation to the bakery because of the smell of bread baking. She also knows she is facing north because she recalls that the bakery is on the east side of the street, and the bakery is to her right. She hears the sound of cars on the street ahead of her and the street beside her. Although she cannot directly perceive the drugstore across the street, she recalls it is there because of her cognitive map. She knows her location, facing direction, and the location of places around her. She can demonstrate her spatial knowledge of the self-to-object spatial relationships by pointing directly to the bakery and the drugstore. She can travel to either of these places using her knowledge of facing directions and her ability to make precise turns and estimate distances walked to update her position. She can describe her location using egocentric, topocentric, cartographic, or polarcentric terms. She even can imagine herself standing at the drugstore facing north, and can indicate which direction the bakery is from her imagined position. These abilities to recall and describe spatial relationships and to move efficiently are indicators of her cognitive mapping abilities. She even may be able to draw or make a model of the place that depicts accurately these self-to-object and object-to-object spatial relationships.

Spatial Updating

Spatial updating refers to the ability to keep track of the spatial arrangements of places in an environment, including those along one's current path. It focuses on maintaining self-to-object spatial relationships as one moves. Rieser (1991) provides an overview of many of the important issues concerning spatial updating of blind and low vision individuals. For example, he discusses environmental flow, or the lawful changes in the distances and directions to features in one's surroundings that occur while moving. He analyzes how perceiving environmental flow might be affected by total or partial impairment of sight. Rieser, Guth, and Hill (1982; 1986) conducted several studies to explore basic developmental issues and acquire practical information leading to more effective interventions for orientation-related problems among visually impaired individuals. Specifically, they were interested in whether or not a period of visual experience early in life conferred advantages in acquiring and using spatial knowledge. The results of their study, and the work of many other researchers, indicate that a period of early visual experience confers an advantage on spatial tasks such as walking or pointing to objects out of reach. However, these and other authors have noted wide individual differences among both early-blind and late-blind individuals, and have concluded that early visual experience alone does not always explain the variation in performance usually found by researchers (Warren, 1994; Klatzky et al., 1990).

STRATEGIES FOR ESTABLISHING AND MAINTAINING ORIENTATION

Problem Solving, Reasoning, and Decision Making

At the beginning of this chapter some of the spatial "questions" travelers must answer were noted. Some of the perceptual and cognitive components that make up the foundation for successful orientation were then briefly discussed. In the remainder of the chapter we discuss how perceptual and cognitive information is used by individuals who are blind or visually impaired for maintaining orientation during mobility. Orientation for visually impaired individuals involves a cycle of perception, reasoning, problem solving, and goal-directed action. It should be noted that in this process, action usually leads to new perceptions and problem-solving activity. Good orientation is fundamentally akin to hypothesis testing—the ability to perceive information; make informed choices about one's location and desired direction of travel based on perceived information; move efficiently based on one's decision; and analyze the effectiveness of one's action. All travelers must make orientation-related decisions. They must, for example, determine the initial direction they need to walk in order to move toward a distant travel goal that cannot be seen, heard, felt, or smelled. They often must use sensory information such as sights, sounds, textures, and smells, to identify landmarks and information points as they walk. They must note the self-to-object position of landmarks as they encounter them, and perform spatial updating as they move toward a destination. Finally, they must solve the problem of disorientation that all travelers experience from time to time, such as being unable to locate a landmark, destination or the travel path itself.

Reestablishing orientation can be characterized as a problem-solving or decision-making activity. It can be described in four stages: (1) identifying the nature of an orientation problem;

(2) identifying alternative strategies for solving problems; (3) selecting a strategy from the available alternatives and implementing it; and (4) evaluating the effectiveness of the selected strategy. These four stages are applicable to activities as diverse as learning to play chess, assembling a swing set, or writing a short story. Psychologists have used this four-stage schema to study problem solving for a variety of everyday tasks, and it is applicable to orientation problem solving as well (Bransford & Stein, 1984; Hayes, 1988).

The first stage of problem solving requires identifying that a problem exists and analyzing the nature or characteristics of the problem. How do visually impaired individuals recognize they have an orientation-related problem? What problems must visually impaired individuals sometimes solve when traveling? First, they must determine their location in a place, usually by locating a familiar landmark (e.g., "I am at the fountain located in the center of the mall"). After establishing orientation, they must decide on a general direction of travel that will lead toward a destination. As they move, travelers must periodically locate and identify landmarks and information points that allow them to confirm that they are moving toward the destination. Travelers also must recognize when they have arrived at points along a walk where turns or changes in direction are possible, and they must turn in the correct direction when required. In the absence of expected landmarks and information points, they may conclude that they are not on their desired path or not traveling in the desired direction. They must recognize that they have arrived at their destination. If they become disoriented at some point along a walk, they must relocate the travel path if they have veered from it, reestablish their location and facing direction relative to a landmark, and begin again to travel toward a destination.

Often these orientation-related activities are performed effortlessly, with little mental effort required to move efficiently from place to place. Landmarks and information points are plentiful and easily recognized, walls or edges are available for trailing, and the space is familiar and regular. Under these circumstances a traveler simply follows the sequence of walks and turns he has followed many times before to reach a destination. Sometimes, however, if places are unfamiliar or confusing, or if secondary landmarks are missed, travelers become disoriented. For visually impaired travelers and sighted travelers alike, the realization that they are disoriented occurs when their perceptions of the surroundings, and the self-to-object spatial relationships they perceive, do not fit with their expectations based on prior experience or knowledge. As noted earlier, much of the mental activity for visually impaired travelers involves hypothesis testing. Travelers periodically test whether their perceptions of landmarks and information points (e.g., what they see, feel underfoot, hear, or smell) fit with their recollection of the percepts they should be experiencing if they are on the correct path and moving toward their desired destination. Hearing an escalator on the right when, from past experience in the store, a person knows it should be on the left is an example of problem identification based on sensory information. Contacting an object unexpectedly is another indication that a traveler may be disoriented, and that memory and problem-solving skills must be brought to bear in order to become reoriented.

When percepts do not fit expectations, what strategies do individuals consider in an effort to solve orientation-related problems? How do they reestablish orientation when they become disoriented? Visually impaired individuals have a number of strategies at their disposal. First, they may simply stop and take "inventory" of the perceptual information available, and form a hypothesis about where they likely are, where the travel path probably is if they have deviated from it, what might have caused them to deviate, and then determine the direction they need to move in order to resume walking toward their destination. Travelers may attend consciously to the available perceptual information (e.g., slope of ground, sound of traffic) to determine the location of the travel path or desired destination. They also may move about in order to locate a familiar landmark or information point that provides information about their location in a place. To do this they may follow a naturally occurring line or border, such as a wall or a grassline, in a direction most likely to lead to a familiar landmark. Often they are able to reestablish orientation once a landmark is located ("I am at the corner of Third Street and Sunrise Drive") and recall the location of the destination relative to the landmark ("My destination is north of here, along this sidewalk and on my left"). Once a landmark is located, travelers may recall from memory the direction of travel and the sequence of turns and walks that leads to a destination. Asking others for help or consulting a map are other strategies that may be employed. Individuals may even use a strategy of making an educated guess about where a destination is located based on general knowledge of the environmental regularity of places. For example, elevators are often in the center of office buildings, particularly if the hallways are laid out in an "H" configuration. If no other strategy for establishing orientation is useful, an individual simply may travel toward the center of the building in an effort to locate the elevator.

In the final stage of problem solving, individuals evaluate the effectiveness of their chosen strategies in solving the orientation-related problems they face. Sometimes strategies fail. For example, sometimes travelers are unable to locate a landmark or information point. When strategies fail, individuals must recognize the failure and identify, implement, and evaluate alternative strategies to solve their orientation problems. Sometimes individuals elect to use several strategies simultaneously. For example, an individual may travel toward a distant object she can hear and also may use the regularities in an address numbering system to help her remain oriented. As she moves, she must evaluate each of the strategies to determine how to proceed.

Now consider a brief example of an orientation-related problem and the application of the four-stage problem-solving schema. A visually impaired pedestrian realizes he is disoriented; he no longer knows where he is relative to any landmark in the environment. In addition, he realizes that the perceptual information he is "receiving" does not "fit" with what he expected to find on this particular five-block route. He must reestablish his orientation and determine which direction to walk to continue traveling toward his destination. He thinks the problem has occurred because he has veered off the sidewalk. After exploring for a few moments, he unexpectedly contacts a parking meter with his long cane. He perceives from the sound of traffic that the parking meter is not between him and the street; instead, he is between the parking meter and the street. He relocates the sidewalk by walking away from the street. Once reoriented to the sidewalk, he recalls from memory that he was on the east side of the street when he became disoriented, and he also recalls that parking meters are only on the east side of this particular street for one block. With the parking meter on his left, he knows he is facing north. He knows where he is within one block ("I am on the east side of Hillsboro Street between Linden and Maple, facing north") and knows his destination is straight ahead. He has solved his disorientation problem by first identifying that he is disoriented, determining what strategies he has at his disposal, and selecting a strategy, implementing it successfully, presumably evaluating it. Effective problem solving is always hypothesis testing.

Using Rote Travel

Some people are limited in their ability to take alternate routes when they travel. O&M specialists often use the term *rote traveler* when they refer to an individual who does not have the spatial knowledge and spatial problem-solving ability to deviate from the known route. They are considered "locked in" to particular routes. Rote travelers recognize when they have reached choice points where alternative paths of travel are possible. They recognize these choice points either because there is sensory information that "alerts" them or because, in the absence of such information, they recognize that they have walked approximately the correct distance. At choice points they recall the direction they must travel to reach their destination, and they change their direction of travel if necessary. They also recognize when the desired destination has been reached. The ability to travel a known route efficiently requires only the ability to perceive when points are reached along the walk where choices must be made about the direction of travel, the ability to recall and execute the correct choices at these points, and the ability to recognize when a destination has been reached. Travelers on familiar routes perceive both external objects or landmarks, and they also are sensitive to kinesthetic feedback from their own body. These perceptions permit them to update their position along the route. Individuals who know only certain routes from various places in an environment and who have little understanding of object-to-object spatial relationships may be limited in their ability to imagine detours to known routes or to "mentally map" new routes between familiar places that they have never traveled before.

There are at least several potential causes of disorientation for visually impaired individuals who are travelers. Travelers may become disoriented if they fail to recognize an intersection or choice point. If a traveler is blind, for example, he may miss an important tactile landmark underfoot that indicates he has reached his destination. This could occur as a result of veer on the travel path that results in a line of travel to one side or the other of a secondary landmark. Another possibility is that the traveler may feel the landmark underfoot, but may not remember that it means he has reached his destination. In either case, rote travelers may become disoriented and may be unable to locate their destination. They may also have difficulty relocating the travel path if they veer from it.

Soliciting Aid to Create a Cognitive Map

Planning a route involves finding out the location of a destination and determining the route from the starting point to the desired destination. This process is enhanced by developing a cognitive map of the area to be traveled. Such maps are usually developed by walking through an area and gaining information about the environment through firsthand experiences with landmarks, information points, objectives, and object-to-object relationships. Another way of adding to a cognitive map is by soliciting information before traveling. This information can then be organized into a cognitive map that can be used to plan a route of travel. The traveler constructs this map by calling businesses or other destinations and asking for the address, the nearest cross street, whether or not the business is on the corner or mid-block, and which side of the street the business is on. They may also call providers of public transportation to obtain information about the location of transit stops and information about transit routes. From a practical point of view, a traveler may use each of these strategies for soliciting aid in order to develop an accurate cognitive map.

Soliciting Aid for Spatial Updating

Travelers can also update their spatial information by interacting with the public while traveling. When soliciting assistance, individuals who are blind or visually impaired often must ask very specific questions about location landmarks, or information points that will enable them to locate a choice point or destination. For example, blind individuals may ask how many doorways from the corner to aid in locating the entrance to a business or residence. Sighted individuals or those with low vision may be able to rely on visual landmarks, such as the color of a building. Because blind individuals cannot see signs or street numbers, it is often beneficial for them to know the cardinal direction from an intersection or bus stop to a particular destination. Knowing, for example, that the bus stops on the northwest corner of the street and that the desired destination is on the northeast corner may be very useful information to a blind person.

Individuals in outdoor situations most often find it easiest to solicit assistance at intersections or large commercial establishments where people are likely to congregate. Footsteps or conversation generally are clues that someone is nearby who may be able to provide orientation information. Blind individuals are taught during O&M training to ask for confirmatory information as they get directions from others, as pedestrians often are not skilled at direction giving or they may make mistakes. If a person giving directions says "Go to the right," it often is useful for the blind person to point in that direction and say "This way?" in order to confirm that he or she understands the directions.

Maintaining Orientation by Judging Distance Walked

Making accurate judgment of distances traveled also can serve as an orientation strategy. Imagine an individual traveling in a large open area in a rapid rail station. She must walk halfway through the open area and then turn to travel towards her destination. In order to accomplish this route without becoming disoriented, she must be able to accurately estimate the distance she has walked. The ability to make accurate distance estimations facilitates establishment and maintenance of orientation, especially in places where few landmarks exist. This ability is based largely on kinesthetic memory (see Chapter 5). Blind travelers rely heavily on the ability to judge distance walked in situations where sensory information is not adequate to aid in orientation. For example, when walking through a large open area and then turning towards a turnstile, an individual who is blind or visually impaired often can walk an appropriate distance and make the necessary turn. He is able to accomplish this because of precise kinesthetic memory for the distance walked without counting steps. Although the public generally believes that blind people stay oriented by counting steps, this is usually not the case. Only on rare occasions, when other sensory stimulation is not available, is counting steps necessary.

Environmental Regularities

Using Environmental Regularity to Solve Orientation Problems

In the earlier discussion of environmental concepts, it was noted that regularity and predictability of environments provided information for orientation. Streets often run at 90-degree or right angles to one another. Street surfaces typically have a crown, meaning they are slightly elevated in the middle and slope toward each side in order to facilitate water runoff. Parking meters often are in a line running parallel to the direction of traffic movement on a street and are located between the sidewalk and the street. Sidewalks sometimes are alternatively level and sloping. Visually impaired individuals often can rely on their knowledge of environmental regularities like these to formulate hypotheses about their location in a place and their direction of travel. They know at corners they must usually turn 90 degrees in order to change their direction of travel and move perpendicular to their former line. They know that, while crossing a street, they usually should feel the rising slope of the crown, followed by a gentle descent to the opposite corner. If they feel the rising slope but no descent, this may alert them that they are walking down the middle of the street rather than crossing it to the other side. Contacting two parking meters in quick succession is an information point alerting a person that he is walking parallel to a street. Streets, curbs, and sidewalks have predictable relationships to one another. Visually impaired individuals who are knowledgeable about the usual "arrangement" of the built environment can use this knowledge for establishing and maintaining spatial orientation. Environmental regularities also may be useful indoors. Men's and women's rest rooms in an office building, for example, often share a common interior wall, and typically there is a water fountain near the rest rooms. Rest rooms in a multistoried building tend to be directly underneath one another. A visually impaired individual who has been told that a particular office is three floors up and next to the rest room may be able to travel directly to this office even though he has never traveled on this particular floor. To do this, he makes an educated guess that the spatial relationship of the elevator to the bathroom is the same on the floor he knows and the floor he has not traveled before. Experience tells him this guess will be correct most of the time. If it is not, he must fall back on another strategy to solve the resulting problem of disorientation. Environmental regularities, in combination with landmark knowledge, are probably the most commonly used orientation strategy by travelers with visual impairment.

Using Numbering Systems to Solve Orientation Problems

As noted earlier, environmental regularity or predictability often is an important source of information for orientation. One example of environmental regularity is the numbering system usually used in buildings and street addresses. Rooms on a given floor of an office building usually have a common number in the leftmost digit that corresponds to the number of the floor. The numbers on a floor generally change in a predictable fashion as one moves from one end of the building to another. Some buildings use a focal point system, in which numbers increase as one moves away in any direction from the lowest numbered room (or focal point). Other buildings use a reference line system, where two hallways serve as reference lines from which all numbers increase. In a reference line system, the easternmost and southernmost hallways may serve as the origin of the numbering system, and all numbers would begin at these hallways. This system allows interior hallways to be numbered in a logical fashion relative to exterior hallways. In both systems, odd-numbered offices are usually on one side of the hall and even numbers on the other.

When using street addresses as a strategy for orientation, individuals know that addresses typically get smaller as one moves toward the central business district of a city. If a person is at 1302 Adeline Street and wants to go to 1200 Adeline Street, he knows that he usually needs to travel toward the central business district rather than away from it. Also, he may know that even-numbered addresses are on one side of the street and odd-numbered addresses on the other. His knowledge of the systematic arrangement of numbering systems provides information for orientation while traveling. Numbering systems, for example, may permit a disoriented individual to make an educated guess about which direction to move to reach his destination ("I know that my destination is somewhere east of here, and I know that I am east of the central business district. I know that I need to travel away from the central business district and not toward it in order to move toward my destination"). In many areas residential or business blocks are organized by number. For example, a traveler may be able to predict that a store will be in the third block from Central Square if the address is in the 300 range.

Familiarization: The Effect of Systematic Exploration Strategies on Orientation

Learning the self-to-object and object-to-object spatial relationships in an unfamiliar place is a problem experienced from time to time by all travelers. Strategies for solving this problem include consulting a map; exploring the place systematically, either alone or with a guide; or following verbal or written directions. Each of these strategies might be used by a traveler who is visually impaired. O&M specialists sometimes help visually impaired individuals learn new routes, either by guiding them and pointing out landmarks and information points in the environment or by providing tactile, auditory, or large-print maps. Sometimes friends and family members help by guiding visually impaired individuals or by pointing out features along the route. Many visually impaired individuals quickly learn simple routes after being shown them, either by maps or computer simulations, or by actually being guided through the space.

Visually impaired individuals often use procedures to independently learn about their environment. Self-exploration is often accomplished by using maps or physical exploration with and without a cane and sometimes with the use of an electronic travel aid. Several studies have been conducted about the effectiveness of strategies for learning new places. Zimmerman (1990) compared two strategies for learning self-to-object spatial relationships in an unfamiliar place. One strategy involved use of a microcomputer-based simulation and the other involved use of a tactile map. No clear evidence was obtained for the superiority of either mode of learning spatial information, although there were indications that the tactile graphic may have yielded better knowledge of the space. In his discussion Zimmerman speculates on the reasons for this finding and points out that the tactile graphic, because of its compact size, permitted participants to locate landmarks from the first trial of the study. They perhaps could get a better overview of the space from the tactile graphic, which translated into modestly improved performance.

Two other studies have been conducted recently about strategies for learning the spatial layout of new places. Three primary exploration strategies are used by travelers who are blind or visually impaired for self-familiarization: perimeter, gridline, and reference point (Hill & Ponder, 1976). In a *perimeter strategy* the traveler walks the outside border of a space. In a *gridline strategy* a traveler crosses back and forth in the interior of a space in order to locate landmarks in the space systematically. In a *reference point strategy* a traveler explores a place by walking from a known location (i.e., home base) to various landmarks, returning to home base before walking to another landmark. Tellevik (1992) hypothesized that the way an individual approaches a wayfinding task may influence what he or she learns and remembers about a space. He further hypothesized that movement with the goal of learning as much as possible about the self-to-object relationships in a place is more likely to result in the ability to recall spatial relationships than movement without the expressed purpose of learning a place. Also, he believed that systematic patterns of locomotion would be more useful in acquiring spatial information than locomotion without a systematic pattern. He conducted a study to investigate whether different exploration strategies may yield different kinds of knowledge and, consequently, whether specific strategies should be encouraged when one wants to learn as much as possible about the layout of a place. In his study, Tellevik evaluated perimeter strategies, gridline strategies, and reference point strategies. He asked the ten participants, who were sighted, blindfolded O&M specialists, to find four objects in a room under each of two conditions. Videotapes were analyzed to learn about self-exploration strategies and their relationship to spatial layout knowledge. The author found that exploration with perimeter and gridline strategies may be more effective for learning object-to-object relationships than a reference point strategy.

Hill et al. (1993) extended Tellevik's work on self-familiarization strategies. They investigated the relationship of exploration patterns in new places to spatial knowledge of the places. They videotaped 65 early- and late-blind adults as they explored a 15-foot by 15-foot space for 7 minutes. The participants' task was to learn the location of five objects by exploring the area later to estimate directions from one object to another. Perimeter, gridline, and reference point all were used, although not all participants used all of the strategies. The top 25% of performers and bottom 25% of performers on spatial layout knowledge (as measured by the distance estimation task) were evaluated for frequency of strategy use (both reported and observed). The authors hypothesized that participants with higher scores on the distance estimation task would use strategies more often and more efficiently. They found that the strategies participants reported using, and the strategies they were observed to use, affected their ability to estimate distances to objects in the space. The subjects with highest performance on a distance estimation task used more types of strategies than lower performing participants. They also used strategies that linked objects to reference points. In general, higher performing participants located the five objects more quickly and tended to use linking strategies rather than perimeter search strategies. Interestingly, they reported that 6 of the high performing group had early onset of vision loss, and 14 of 15 in the worst group were early onset. This finding is evidence of the fact that individuals who are blind from birth often, but not always, perform more poorly on spatial task performance than individuals with late onset of vision loss.

The work of Zimmerman (1990), Tellevik (1992), and Hill et al. (1993) in the area of self-familiarization illustrates several important points in research about spatial orientation. First, each of these studies addressed an important practical problem in spatial orientation. A traveler's familiarity with a place and the movement experiences used when becoming familiar with it are likely to play a key role in development of self-to-object and object-to-object relationships and in learning routes from place to place. Second, the importance of individual differences was recognized, particularly in Zimmerman's single-subject research. Further research is needed to learn more about sources of individual differences in other subpopulations of individuals who are blind or visually impaired (e.g., children). Studies also should consider exploration of large outdoor places. There also is a need to determine the degree to which visually impaired individuals find themselves in travel situations that demand self-familiarization skills, and investigate the skills they bring to bear in these situations. Such studies should be useful to O&M specialists and visually impaired travelers.

Problem Solving: The Drop-Off Lesson as an Integrated Example of Strategies Used in Orientation

One avenue for discussing strategies for orientation of visually impaired individuals as a problem-solving activity is to consider the problems posed by *drop-off lessons.* Drop-off lessons often are included in instruction of visually impaired individuals. There are various versions of drop-off lessons; often they are graduated in difficulty beginning with an indoor lesson and leading to more complex drop-offs outdoors. In the less complex lessons, partial information may be provided or the traveler may be encouraged to solicit assistance to gain information.

Identifying Orientation Problems on a Drop-Off Lesson

At the highest level of difficulty the lesson is conducted in neighborhoods that are relatively familiar. Learners are blindfolded and driven on a circuitous route until they become disoriented, and then "dropped off" at some point in the familiar neighborhood. They are not told where in the neighborhood they are dropped off. The goal of a drop-off lesson is simply to travel from the point where one is dropped off to a known destination. One of the greatest sources of difficulty in these lessons is that students do not know, other than in very general terms, where they are as they begin the lesson. In addition to not knowing where they are in the neighborhood, they may not know what direction they are facing. Students on drop-off lessons presumably have learned, during previous routes through the area, the location of several landmarks and information points in the environment relative to one another. Often they can travel directly to various places once they have determined their initial location and their facing direction. Determining initial location and facing direction thus is the primary challenge of a drop-off lesson.

Sometimes students can "solve" the problems posed during drop-off lessons easily. On the other hand, drop-off lessons sometimes can be very difficult, particularly if the students cannot locate a landmark from which to establish initial orientation. Drop-off lessons are sometimes used as a "final exam" in orientation instruction because students who can solve drop-off problems presumably can identify and solve other less demanding travel problems, such as maintaining orientation while traveling to a destination in a familiar place from a known starting point (e.g., from home to work). Drop-offs also can be very useful in teaching new learners to gather sensory information and test hypotheses about where they are and how to get to a destination efficiently. When designed properly, drop-off lessons can be great confidence-builders for students learning orientation strategies.

As noted earlier, the spatial problems to be solved and the strategies to solve them depend on the demands of the situation. To identify relevant problems for a particular travel situation, individuals presumably draw on their own experiences and from their knowledge of the experiences of others. In other words, they apply their experience and knowledge in selecting, implementing, and evaluating various problem-solving strategies. In essence the drop-off is an exercise in hypothesis testing. The individual collects information to verify her hypothesis about her location. If the data "fits," she will locate her objective. If the data does not confirm her location, she must try another hypothesis.

Identifying Strategies for Problem Solving on a Drop-Off Lesson

The main task of the drop-off lesson is to identify alternative strategies for locating one's position in the environment. The most likely strategy used to solve a drop-off problem is to locate and identify a landmark at or near the beginning point of the drop-off lesson. At the beginning of a drop-off lesson, the student likely will stand on the sidewalk, listen, feel what is underfoot, and determine whether or not this information provides assistance in locating her present position. One of the most helpful pieces of information, depending on the time of day, is the position of the sun. The sun can be used to establish direction and is most useful in the early morning and the late afternoon, and least helpful around the noon hour. Once the direction of the sun is identified, the traveler can then determine her current facing direction. Another important strategy is the use of traffic sound. If the traveler is standing at an intersection, she may listen for the sound of traffic to determine which way cars are moving on the street beside her (the parallel street) and in front of her (the perpendicular street). She may be able to use the direction of movement of traffic to provide orientation. Suppose, for example, that there is only one street in the area that has one-way traffic. If she determines that traffic is moving in only one direction on the street beside her, she should know what street she on. At the start of a drop-off lesson the student may find that traffic is not present. In this case another useful approach may be to move toward the sound of distant traffic to try and identify the street where the traffic is moving. Finally, if an orientation information point is not readily available when the student begins the drop-off lesson, she may use the strategy of moving systematically, using a search pattern, to establish initial orientation by looking for landmarks and information points.

Strategies similar to those used for establishing initial location may be applied to the problem of determining the direction of movement that will lead to the destination. To travel efficiently to a specific destination, the individual must know both where she is and where the destination is relative to her current location. How does the student accomplish this? Often, she simply remembers the direction that she must face (and move) to go toward the destination from the landmark she has located, and then faces and moves in that direction. Establishing facing direction often requires that the student locates a landmark or a series of information points and recalls the direction from the landmark to the destination. Consider, for example, a student standing at the newspaper box at the intersection of Fifth and Broad. In order to ultimately move toward her destination, she must first determine whether she is facing Fifth Street (east), or facing Broad Street (north). Relating another landmark to the newspaper box is one way to determine this. She may recall that the front of the paper box is closer to Broad Street than Fifth Street, and that Broad Street runs north–south. Using the combination of sensory information and her memory of the place, she determines that she is on the southwest corner of Fifth and Broad, facing east. She then recalls that her destination is directly in front of her (east), three blocks away on the south side of Fifth Street and at the corner of Fifth Street and Sunrise Drive. The problem, "Which way do I move?" in this case is solved simply by walking in the facing direction.

As she moves, the student also must keep track of her location relative to the destination so she can travel to it efficiently. To accomplish this, she may remember the number of blocks she has walked in one direction, and recall that she must turn in a certain direction at a certain point along the walk in order to continue walking toward the destination. She likely uses landmarks or information points as she moves along to check her progress. A landmark or information points may alert her that a change in direction is required (e.g., "I feel the gravel under my feet and know my turn is coming soon"), or she may simply recall the approximate length of time she needs to walk prior to turning (e.g., "I've walked about as far as I usually walk to reach the next turn"). The absence of an expected landmark or information point can prompt hypothesis testing about whether she is moving toward the goal or in some other direction. Mentally keeping track of the approximate distance and direction one has walked toward a destination and one's position relative to intermediate landmarks are important strategies used in maintaining self-to-object orientation and successfully completing a drop-off lesson. The strategy of using environmental regularity is useful as well. A line of parking meters or a grass shoreline, for example, can often provide a rich source of information for maintaining spatial orientation. Jansson (1991) refers to movement along a path toward a destination that cannot be directly perceived as "walking along," meaning that a student is guided by "some elongated feature in the environment" (p. 335). In walking along, a traveler must simply maintain contact, either tactually or auditorially, with a feature such as a wall, a grass shoreline, or the sound of moving cars, and follow along the path delineated by the feature.

Selecting and Evaluating Strategies While on a Drop-Off Lesson

Strategies for solving orientation-related problems are more effective in some situations than others. Visually impaired individuals must decide which of the possible strategies will likely be most effective for solving the particular orientation problems they face. Deciding which strategy is best sometimes is easy. If there are other pedestrians around, then soliciting aid likely is a useful strategy (although O&M specialists sometimes ask learners not to use this strategy on a drop-off because they want them to rely on what they perceive and what they know). There usually is a strategy that is best for a given individual in a particular situation, although most experienced travelers have several strategies at their disposal. They likely select strategies based on judgments of their relative effectiveness and the amount of effort required to implement a strategy. Experience in "managing" problems that arise during independent travel provides a rich source of data about the relative effectiveness of various strategies. For example, the likelihood that an individual would choose to move about in an attempt to locate a familiar landmark probably would depend in part on his assessment of the likelihood of success in doing so. If he knows the general area he is in, and knows he recognizes few landmarks in the area, he may decide that a search would be unproductive and if permitted may choose to solicit aid. Propensity for risk taking and his inclination to approach strangers and solicit help also influence choice of strategy for information about wayfinding. Individuals also need to recognize when strategies have failed and need to try new ones. Some must resist the tendency to perseverate in using a strategy that is not working.

SPATIAL ORIENTATION AND PROBLEM SOLVING

This chapter has briefly discussed some of the principal cognitive and perceptual components that result in efficient travel from place to place. This chapter adopts the approach that spatial orientation is fundamentally a practical problem-solving activity and has illustrated some of the problems and solutions encountered in moving from place to place efficiently and the strategies useful in solving these problems. By the use of examples, the chapter has shown how orientation is achieved through hypothesis testing. Strategies are employed and evaluated according to how well they help an individual gain an understanding of his relationship to significant objects in the environment. This problem-solving approach is a useful way to understand how travelers establish and maintain orientation.

Well-elaborated theories about spatial orientation in general and for individuals who are blind or visually impaired in particular do not exist. As they emerge in the future, however, they will benefit practitioners in three ways. First, they will aid in identifying those factors which lead to skilled performance in a traveler. Second, spatial orientation theories can lead to a more precise method for developing instructional goals. Finally, theories about spatial orientation can lead to improved methods of instruction of strategies for orientation. Comprehensive theory is usually built upon individual studies that each examine a part of the larger picture. To date, various components have been examined but a comprehensive theory has not yet emerged. Although much is known about spatial orientation, further study will lead to better theory and ultimately to better practice.

Suggestions/Implications for O&M Specialists

1. Establishing orientation and maintaining orientation as one moves toward a desired goal are critical components of successful travel.
2. Low vision and blindness result in limitations in acquiring information useful for orientation.
3. Individuals who are blind must use auditory, tactile, kinesthetic, proprioceptive, vestibular, and olfactory information to maintain orientation. Persons with low vision usually can use visual information as well.
4. Travelers who are well oriented know the distances and directions to places they cannot directly perceive and how self-movement changes the relative locations of places.
5. Individuals who have accurate cognitive maps of places know the distances and directions from place to place, and can mentally construct routes between places they have never traveled.
6. Primary landmarks are objects or environmental features that are detectable by visually impaired travelers, always present, and always encountered. They convey spatial information to travelers, in that they provide information about one's present location in a place. When travelers mentally link their present location to another location in order to travel efficiently, they

(continued on next page)

Suggestions/Implications for O&M Specialists (continued)

are using their knowledge of self-to-object as an aid to orientation.

7. Secondary landmarks are objects or environmental features that may not always be present or are not always encountered by a traveler.
8. Information points are two or more sensory stimuli that, when linked, allow travelers to determine their exact location.
9. Sensory information and cognitive abilities such as body, object, and environmental concepts, along with one's ability to recall spatial information and solve spatial problems, are the basis for efficient orientation.
10. Many of the more complex orientation-related activities, such as recovering from disorientation after veering from the travel path after veering or planning a new route, are problem-solving activities. They require that travelers identify the nature of the spatial problems to be solved and the strategies that may be useful in solving them. After they implement strategies, travelers must evaluate them to determine their effectiveness. Understanding spatial orientation of blind and low vision travelers is aided by understanding the problems they encounter and the strategies they use to solve them.
11. Strategies for reorientation include searching systematically for a landmark, consulting a map, and soliciting aid from others.
12. Some visually impaired travelers are rote travelers who travel efficiently from place to place in familiar environments, but who have poor cognitive mapping abilities and do not understand the spatial relationships of the routes or places in the environment. These travelers have difficulty with problem solving and usually are relatively inflexible in their travel patterns.
13. To solicit aid that is useful for wayfinding, travelers must know the kinds of information they need and be able to request it. Wayfinding needs of visually impaired travelers often differs from those of sighted individuals.
14. The ability to judge distances walked and the degree to which one has turned is very useful in maintaining spatial orientation, particularly in situations where landmarks are not available to establish orientation.
15. Numbering systems for buildings and offices, because they usually are regular and predictable, offer information useful for wayfinding if the visually impaired traveler has access to the numbers and knows the conventions related to their use.
16. Different strategies for self-familiarization to a new environment have been shown to be associated with differences in one's knowledge of object-to-object spatial relationships in the environment. Tactile maps, auditory maps, and guided exploration have also been shown to be effective means of learning the spatial layout of new places.
17. A drop-off lesson, in which a traveler is required to determine his or her location in a familiar area and locate a destination, often is an excellent tool for assessing problem-solving abilities related to spatial orientation.

ACTIVITIES FOR REVIEW

1. Differentiate between primary and secondary landmarks.
2. Explain the importance of information points.
3. Describe the components of the problem-solving cycle and how they can be applied to spatial orientation of visually impaired persons.
4. Explain spatial updating.
5. Cite four examples of sensory information that may be useful for orientation.
6. Cite three strategies that may be useful in recovering from disorientation.
7. Name two problems that visually impaired travelers may encounter on a drop-off lesson and describe the strategies they may use to solve the problems.
8. Name three cognitive components of good spatial orientation.
9. Describe the characteristics of a route traveler.
10. Explain how the ability to judge distances walked and degrees turned relate to spatial orientation.
11. List three important considerations when soliciting assistance for orientation.
12. Define a search strategy. Consult the research literature to determine the relationship of search strategies to spatial knowledge.
13. Explain how numbering systems can be useful in orientation.
14. Describe a cognitive map.

CHAPTER 3

Low Vision and Mobility

Duane Geruschat and Audrey J. Smith

Vision is not a requirement for independent mobility. Safe and independent travel is possible with or without sight. However, significant differences exist in the way information is obtained for those who are sighted or blind, and these are reflected as different styles of travel.

How does vision contribute to mobility? What are the differences between mobility for those who are fully sighted, partially sighted, and totally blind? The human species has evolved to rely principally on sight for movement and orientation. Estimates suggest that as much as 80 to 90 percent of information is obtained through vision. There is no other sense that can gather and process the same volume and richness of information as quickly as sight. In addition to the *speed* and *volume* of information obtained through sight is the *distance* from which the information can be obtained. In a mobility context, distance means anticipation, the ability to preview the travel path, which provides the individual with the ability to be proactive through the avoidance of obstacles and the identification of a curb or stairs before arriving at them. Distance, as offered through vision, also permits quick and easy orientation. For example, walking into an unfamiliar room, the sighted student quickly scans the room to find a chair, phone, or desk. Outdoors, looking at a flock of flying birds, the color of flowers in a window box, cars coming over a hill, and the identification of a curb—all occur instantaneously. Thus the sighted traveler utilizes an anticipatory, proactive style of mobility that is characterized by quickly obtaining and processing critical information.

By way of comparison, the student who is totally blind obtains the information required for independent travel through a combination of the remaining sensory information, principally auditory and tactile. For the purpose of being mobile, auditory, tactile, and other sensory information provides all the critical information required for independent travel. The primary differences between sighted and blind travel are the speed, volume, and distance from which auditory and tactile information is obtained and processed. These differences combine to make blind mobility fundamentally different from sighted mobility. The traveler who is totally blind utilizes the sounds of cars, other pedestrians, the bark of a dog, and the touch of the cane and the feet to identify such surfaces as gravel from grass, the incline and decline of the travel path, or the apex of the street during a crossing—to obtain and process the critical information that is required for safe and independent travel without sight. Although the traveler who is blind may have at times less volume of information available with regard to speed and distance, nevertheless, in general, the available auditory and tactual information is sufficient for safe and independent travel. It is important to recognize that travel with or without sight works, and that one style is not necessarily better than the other—they are just different.

Low vision mobility offers both challenges and opportunities. All students with low vision will experience fluctuations in the quality and clarity of what they see, caused by internal and external factors. Examples of internal fluctuations include changes in vision caused by diseases such as diabetes or retinitis pigmentosa, and visual fatigue caused by continuous visual demands. External factors resulting in vision changes may be attributed to such variables as side effects from ocular or systemic medications. The external fluctuations can also be environmentally influenced by rapid or extreme changes in lighting or contrast or even subtle changes in lighting occasioned by walking through the shadow of a tree can influence what the individual sees. Fluctuations can also be a combination of both internal and environmental sources. Regardless of the reason, coping with fluctuations in visual information and sifting through all the additional sensory information to make safe decisions are the defining characteristics of independent travel for the student with low vision.

For the student who accepts the challenges imposed by fluctuations of visual information come many benefits and opportunities. As an example, one student looks for Tulpehocken Street but cannot read the entire street sign. She does see a letter "T" with lots of smaller letters to follow and can reasonably assume this is the correct street. Another example would be the student who can see the golden arches of McDonald's and knows the identity of the store without ever reading the name. Visually trailing a shoreline to stay on a path, knowing the color of a building as a landmark, and following the lights in a hallway to assist in a straight line of travel are some anticipatory visual cues and behaviors a traveler can use. The challenges facing the student with low vision: deciding when visual information is reliable and when a combination of visual, auditory, and tactile information is the best way to make a safe decision. Ultimately the challenge for low vision students is the same as that of the person who is fully sighted or totally blind—the sorting of sensory information into a picture of the environment accurate enough for the purposes of safe travel.

HISTORY OF LOW VISION AND MOBILITY

The term *low vision* has many definitions, all of which depend on the purpose for which the definition is developed: legal, clinical, educational, or international. Over the years many have attempted to develop one widely accepted definition, a noble goal as yet not achieved (Apple, Apple, & Blasch, 1980; Colenbrander, 1977; Corn, 1983, 1986; Corn & Koenig, 1996; Faye, 1984; Genensky, 1983; Jose, 1983; Kirchner & Lowman, 1988; Mehr & Freid, 1975; Smith, 1990).

For the purposes of this chapter, the term low vision encompasses persons with usable vision, not fully correctable by standard eyeglasses, who experience difficulty performing visual tasks. Persons with low vision exist somewhere along the continuum between total blindness and fully sighted. Orientation and mobility (O&M) specialists frequently work with the low vision population who are considered legally blind, with these individuals as the majority of their students.

Though the formal instruction of O&M with long canes began in the 1940s, it has only been within the past few decades that O&M specialists have turned their attention to the majority of the blind population—those with low vision. Before this, evaluation and training techniques based on the mobility needs of the totally blind population were used for those with low vision. Although many of the techniques were useful for both populations, the unique visual needs and varying visual performance levels of persons with low vision remained unaddressed.

The pioneering work of Barraga (1964) challenged the previous concepts of sight saving and conserving vision. She demonstrated that, with a training program of sequential vision stimulation, children manifested increased levels of visual functioning. In the 1960s and 1970s others in the field began to call for more attention to the unique mobility needs of the low vision population. They cited the inappropriateness of some of the accepted mobility techniques and the need for better methods of visual training designed specifically for those with low vision (Blasch & Apple, 1976; Hughes, 1967; Richterman, 1966). Apple and Blasch (1976) were among the early pioneers who called to O&M specialists to join with other disciplines to develop a more systematic body of knowledge that would serve the special needs of this population.

The first national low vision mobility conference was held in 1971 in San Francisco, bringing together professionals from many disciplines to address the mobility needs of the low vision population and stimulate an interest in low vision mobility research. In 1972 the first course on low vision was required by Western Michigan University's orientation and mobility professional preparation program. Five years later, a second national multidisciplinary conference on low vision mobility was held to pull together state-of-the-art information and chart a course for future efforts in this area (Apple & Blasch, 1976). The 1970s also witnessed the publication of *Distance Vision and Perceptual Training* (Apple & May, 1970) and, under Apple's impetus, the launching of *Low Vision Abstracts* in 1971, which emphasized literature related to low vision mobility and served as a stimulus for low vision mobility research. Some of the early mobility studies and reports on the low vision population included children's concept development (Hill, 1971); distance visual training (Davidson, 1973; Dyer & Smith, 1972; Mattingly, 1976; Shibata, 1976); and the combined use of low vision and the long cane (Blasch, 1975). In 1977 Allen emphasized the need for further research and stressed the benefits of O&M programs specifically designed to meet the needs of persons with low vision.

The mid-1970s to mid-1980s witnessed the most productive period to date, with professionals from eyecare, psychology, education, and rehabilitation merging interests, articles, and research that targeted various aspects of the multidimensional needs of the low vision population (Ault, 1976; Beliveau-Tobey & Smith, 1980; Berg, Jose, & Carter, 1983; De l'Aune, 1980; Faye, 1984; Genensky, Barry, Bikson, & Bikson, 1979; Geruschat, 1985; Jose & Springer, 1975; Marron & Bailey, 1982; Reiser et al., 1985; Smith, 1976), to name but a handful of the many contributions during this period.

In 1983 the Pennsylvania College of Optometry, in cooperation with Peabody College of Vanderbilt University, received the first Research and Demonstration Project on orientation and mobility for low vision individuals from the National Institute for Handicapped Research. The goal of this project was to develop a theory of low vision mobility. Various research topics, including spatial orientation, locomotion, mobility hazards, lighting, optical devices, etc., were studied. Factors hampering one unified theory included the lack of standardized assessment instruments for this population, the variable nature of low vision, and visual fluctuations in the environment. Smith (1987) further discussed the difficulty in establishing one unified theory of low vision mobility due to the multiple factors impinging upon the person's mobility. The 1980s and early 1990s also witnessed research interest in the relationship of clinical vision measurements and mobility performance (Brabyn & Brown, 1990; Long, 1985; Long, Reiser, & Hill, 1990; Marron & Bailey, 1982; Pelli, 1986). Specifically, visual acuities, visual fields, and contrast sensitivity were evaluated for their relationship to mobility performance. Two complications are especially pertinent to these studies. One is the difficulty of objectively measuring mobility performance, and the second is controlling all the individual variables that persons with low vision and the environment bring to the mobility setting. Together they underscore the problems faced by O&M specialists attempting to generalize results to their individual students (Geruschat & De l'Aune, 1989; Smith, 1987). Nevertheless, the field has progressed—with information, guidelines, and training curricula materials—from a quarter of a century ago, when Blasch (1971) noted the field had barely scratched the surface, and Apple (1971) stated, "Low vision is the single greatest unmet need in the field of Orientation and Mobility today" (p. 128).

National and international mobility survey studies of the late 1980s and early 1990s

(Beliveau-Tobey & De l'Aune, 1991; Cory et al., 1992; Geruschat, Neustadt-Noy, & Cory, 1994; Uslan, Hill, & Peck, 1989) continue to highlight the area of low vision as a major interest for continuing education by O&M specialists. Many members of the Association for Education and Rehabilitation of the Blind and Visually Impaired's Mobility Division #9 also are members of its multidisciplinary Low Vision Division #7, which underscores the convergence of disciplines that are contributing their findings to address the needs of the low vision population. Although low vision mobility has covered considerable ground since the initial call for information, it remains at the early stages of knowledge, which need to be studied, synthesized, and disseminated to O&M specialists who still struggle for the best ways to assist their students with low vision.

FUNCTIONAL LOW VISION MOBILITY PROBLEMS

There is a great deal of commonality in the mobility problems experienced by students, whether they are totally blind or have low vision. The major problems include detecting changes in terrain and depth, avoiding unwanted contact (bumping), negotiating street crossings, and having insufficient auditory and tactile information for decision making. One unique problem area for those with low vision is dealing with the effects of changing lighting conditions and glare.

Lighting Conditions and Glare

The most frequently reported mobility problem area for persons with low vision is lighting, inclusive of glare; light adaptation from outdoors to indoors and vice versa; dim and night lighting; and frequent changes in lighting while moving through the same or within different environments. Understanding and dealing with the varying effects of lighting on functional vision performance is the primary difference between travel for students with low vision and those who are totally blind.

Several authors have documented the role that lighting plays on the visual performance levels of persons with low vision (Genensky et al., 1979; Geruschat, 1985; LaGrow, 1986; Long, Reiser, & Hill 1990; Smith, 1990; Smith, De l'Aune, & Geruschat, 1992; Waiss & Cohen, 1992). In Genensky et al.'s 1979 landmark study on the visual environmental adaptation problems of the partially sighted, the majority of subjects reported problems with illumination, especially adjusting to rapid or sharp lighting changes, such as those encountered when moving from daylight to a room with darker lighting. Smith (1990) conducted a national study on the mobility problems of persons with low vision as reported by clients and mobility practitioners. Results of this study indicate lighting conditions and adaptation to lighting changes to be the highest rated area of difficulty in mobility, with glare as the most frequently reported mobility problem in both bright and dimly lit conditions. Daylight examples of glare include light reflection from a shiny floor or walking while facing toward the direction of the late afternoon sun. Nighttime examples include glare from oncoming headlights or streetlight reflecting off storefront windows. Related to mobility performance, conditions of dim lighting were viewed as significantly worse than those of bright lighting, echoing Long et al.'s 1990 study, which cited the negative effect of reduced lighting on mobility.

Changes in Terrain and Depth

Another mobility problem frequently cited involves the detection and negotiation of depth, including stairs, curbs, and uneven terrain (Genensky et al., 1979; Long, 1985; Smith, 1990; Smith et al., 1992). Students report that steps and curbs sometimes appear as blended ramps and other times as flat surfaces. With regard to stairs, the location of the first and last steps seem to present the most difficulty. Students with low vision also report difficulty identifying raised slabs of sidewalk, as well as distinguishing and interpreting puddles, shadows, and terrain changes. Couple these with the problems of visually detecting low-lying objects, and the lower area of visual field constitutes an area that is particularly hazardous and frequently misjudged.

Problems with detecting changes in terrain, such as broken sidewalks, curbs, and stairs, are also difficult for persons who are totally blind. The difference for travelers with low vision, especially if they are not using assistive devices such as long canes or dog guides, is that they sometimes have problems because they have visually misinterpreted the ground surface and either totally miss depth or misjudge visual cues.

Unwanted Contacts (Bumping)

Bumping into objects or obstacles is a frequently reported mobility problem. This is true whether the person is totally blind or has low vision. This problem is especially true when walking in cluttered or crowded areas. Studies of low vision mobility indicate both head-height and low-lying objects cause the greatest difficulty, with head-height objects cited as a more difficult problem than low-lying objects (Genensky et al., 1979; Long et al., 1990; Smith et al., 1992).

Street Crossings

Another problem of note for both types of students is the difficulty of negotiating street crossings. Specific problems include general anxiety; judgments of speed, distance, and best time to cross; and concern and confusion caused by cars turning on a red signal. Unique to the student with low vision is the visual identification of traffic light color, and the opportunity to identify crosswalk lines, see the opposite corner, and visually identify traffic. Problematic to students with low vision is the inconsistency in their ability to discern the color of traffic lights. Sometimes they can rely on vision to see traffic lights (e.g., on a cloudy day), while at other times they are not able to distinguish the color at all (e.g., when they are facing toward the sun).

The combined problems of lighting, depth perception, and terrain changes; bumping into objects or obstacles; and street crossings head the list of the most critical mobility problems that students with low vision face.

Differences between Reduced Acuity and Restricted Fields

Some problems are more often reported by individuals with restricted visual fields versus those with reduced acuity. In particular, gatherings such as parties, concerts, and crowded stores present greater problems for persons with restricted fields who miss details in their periphery, whereas those with reduced acuity are more apt to report difficulty with discerning fine details, such as reading signs or recognizing faces. In addition, those with reduced visual fields generally report greater difficulty with light adaptation problems, especially adjusting from outdoor to indoor lighting. Because of their loss of peripheral retinal cells, which function in dim lighting and for night vision, these individuals experience decreased visual functioning to total blindness, depending on the level of lighting and extent of their pathology.

A final consideration is the amount of information in the environment and the speed with which it changes. Visual clutter, fine details, and movement are confusing for the person with low vision who tries to identify, interpret, and plan movement. This is especially problematic for the individual with severely constricted fields who has a significantly smaller "visual window" for making fast and efficient mobility decisions.

In conclusion, students with low vision face a greater variety of environmental factors that affect travel than students who are totally blind. In addition they are continually dealing with fluctuations in visual performance. This combination of factors demands additional flexibility and creativity when developing strategies for mobility instruction.

ANATOMY, PHYSIOLOGY, AND FUNCTIONAL IMPLICATIONS

Part of the body of knowledge required to be an O&M specialist includes basic anatomy and pathology of the human eye, with emphasis on the progression of pathology and anticipated functional problems commonly associated with each pathology. For an introduction to anatomy or for a review of this material, texts by the following authors are suggested: Chalkley (1982); Corn and Koenig (1996); Jose (1983); Vaughn, Asbury, and Riordan-Eva (1995).

Knowledge of anatomy and pathology increases the O&M specialist's ability to understand or anticipate the types of functional problems that students with low vision may exhibit. This understanding could result in more efficient functional evaluations and in the identification and presentation of functional solutions for mobility purposes. For example, if a client has aniridia, knowledge of the purpose of the iris (to control the amount of light entering the eye) enables the O&M specialist to design an assessment that specifically evaluates the effects of various types and amounts of lighting on functional vision. This illustrates how information on visual pathology can be integrated within a mobility evaluation to save time and improve the quality of the evaluation and the obtained information.

For the purposes of mobility instruction there are two primary categories of visual pathology: reduced visual acuity and restricted visual fields. Reduced visual acuity is more common and the category most people think of when asked to describe a student with low vision. Table 3.1 is a quick summary of the most common patholo-

Table 3.1. Common Pathologies and Their Functional Problems

Pathology	Glare	Visual Field Loss	Scotoma	Night Blindness	Light Adaptation	Refractive Error	Nystagmus	Fluctuating Vision	Depth Perception
Achromatopsia	X			X	X		X		
Albinism	X				X	X	X		
Aniridia	X				X				
Aphakia	X					X			X
Cataracts	X				X			X	
Coloboma	X	X							
Diabetes	X	X	X		X			X	X
Glaucoma	X	X		X	X			X	X
Hemianopsia			X						
High myopia	X	X						X	X
Keratoconus	X					X		X	X
Macular deg.	X		X						X
Optic atrophy	X	X	X				X	X	X
Retinal detachment	X	X						X	
ROP	X	X	X				X	X	X
Retinitis pigmentosa	X	X		X	X			X	X

gies and their functional problems. Although each student's functional mobility performance will be affected by multiple visual and nonvisual factors, the general categories of visual problems in this table are usually present to some degree.

This table clearly indicates that lighting and depth perception are the most common functional problems experienced in mobility. Although light is a basic requirement for sight, too much light, or frequently or quickly changing light can be disabling. Therefore the primary functional problem O&M specialists must address when teaching a student with low vision is lighting. Strategies for both increasing and decreasing light and decreasing glare are a basic requirement for maximizing remaining vision for most, if not all, students of mobility with low vision.

CLINICAL LOW VISION ASSESSMENT

The clinical low vision examination is completed by a qualified ophthalmologist or optometrist. Although certification as a low vision specialist is not a requirement, the professional organizations representing these professions do have diplomate programs that offer this specialty. The role of the eye care specialist is to complete the clinical assessment, including the prescription of low vision devices when appropriate. This professional can also be quite helpful in counseling the student with regard to medical treatments that may be available as well as situations where further treatment cannot restore lost sight.

The clinical low vision examination has five primary components:

1. Visual acuity
2. Visual field
3. Refractive error
4. Ocular health
5. Response to optical devices

The clinical exam attempts to describe, under ideal conditions, what the student can see. The examiner attempts to control all factors that may cause the student to see less than his or her best. This includes control of overall illumination such as extraneous sources of glare, and the use of high quality single-letter or number charts.

Visual Acuity

Measurement of visual acuity defines the smallest size print or picture the student can see at a distance (see Figure 3.1). The resulting fraction for visual acuity notation, provides a general sense of the amount of remaining clarity the student possesses when looking at objects. In the visual acuity fraction the numerator represents the distance at which the student views the target, and the denominator represents the smallest size the person can identify. Functionally this means that a person with 20/200 visual acuity must stand approximately 20 feet from an object that a person with no visual impairment can see from 200 feet. However, many factors affect the functional ability of a mobility student when actually looking at a target such as a street sign (figure/ground, contrast, angle of viewing). The measure of visual acuity nevertheless increases the O&M specialist's ability to anticipate the student's chances of seeing the fine detail of distant objects (e.g., street signs, bus numbers) and performing tasks (e.g., reading bus schedules and maps).

Visual Field

Mapping the visual field is especially useful for mobility instruction. While visual mobility does require a minimum level of visual acuity, the visual field plays a significant role in movement. The student with macular degeneration, 20/200 acuity, and no peripheral field loss will, in general, travel with greater ease than the student with 20/20 acuity and 5–10 degrees of remaining central visual field.

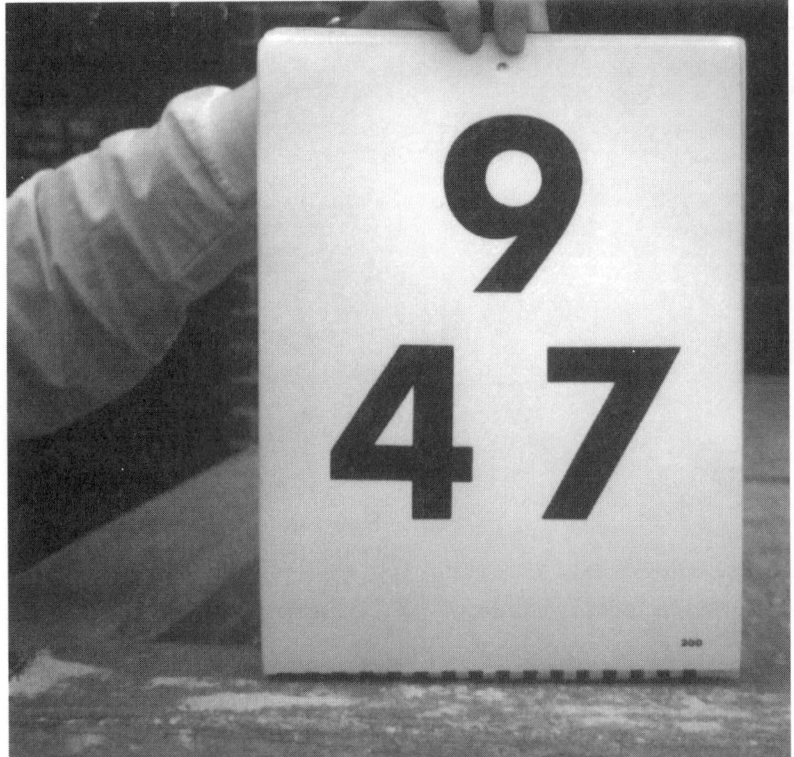

A

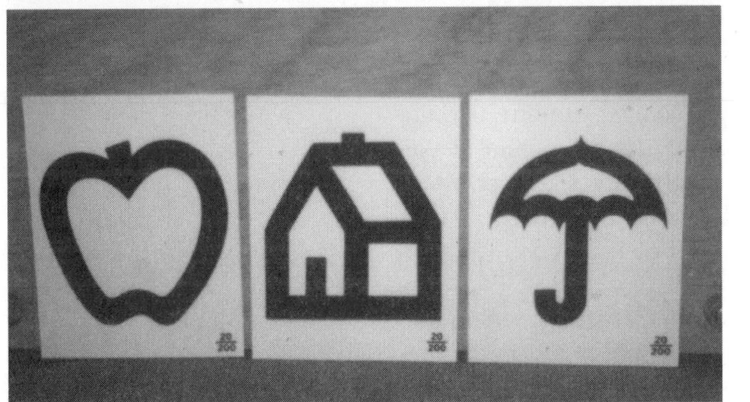

B

Figure 3.1. Visual acuity can be tested by (A) a high-quality letter chart or (B) a picture chart for near and distance viewing.

Four different clinical visual field tests can be administered: (1) confrontation; (2) Amsler grid (Figure 3.2); (3) tangent screen; and (4) perimetry. The *confrontation* visual field is a screening procedure involving lights or objects that are presented from the periphery and gradually moved in toward the central field. This test yields practical information rather than clinical measurement. This provides a gross estimate of the size and location of peripheral field losses. For the practicing O&M specialist this screening is especially valuable since it is easily administered, requires little equipment, and evaluates the peripheral visual field, which is of particular importance to mobility. This approach is also useful with young children and individuals with severe

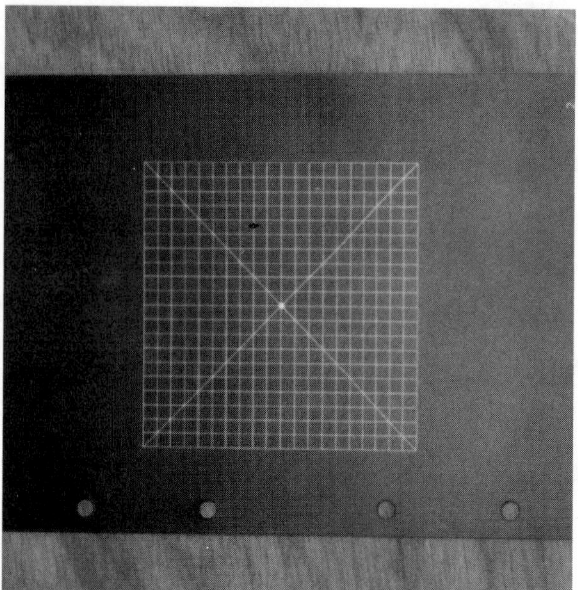

Figure 3.2. The Amsler grid is a tool used to test the area of central vision.

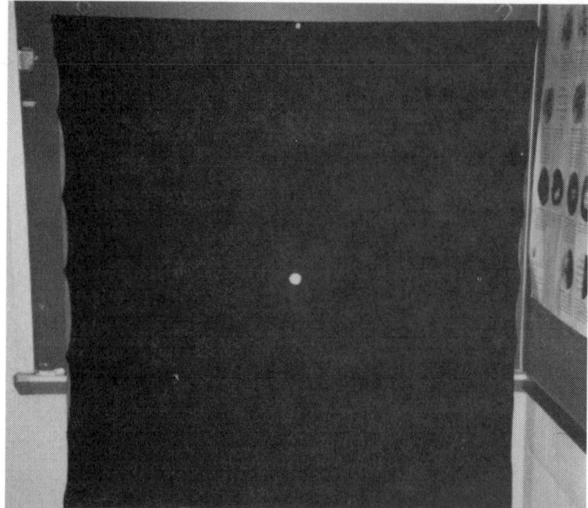

Figure 3.3. The tangent screen is used to test the visual field within 25–30 degrees of fixation.

multiple impairments, and as a quick screening for use at school, home, or the workplace.

This screening procedure requires the student to fix their vision on an object in the distance. The O&M specialist, standing behind the student, presents a light or small, brightly colored target in various areas of the peripheral visual field. As the students see the target, they point to or touch the target. This screening procedure can be used effectively for identifying large defects of the peripheral visual field.

The Amsler grid is a clinical assessment of the central 10 degrees of the visual field (see Figure 3.2). It is especially useful for identifying the size and location of a central scotoma caused by pathologies such as age-related maculopathy (ARM). The Amsler grid answers questions related to fine detail activities such as reading a bus schedule or using a telescope to read a street sign.

The Amsler grid requires students to fix their vision on the center black dot of the grid. Without moving their eyes, the students must indicate where parts of the grid are missing or where the horizontal and vertical lines are not straight. This test requires a high degree of cooperation and the ability to respond to the tester's questions.

The *tangent screen* is the most common type of clinical field assessment for low vision, testing the central 25–30 degrees of the visual field (see Figure 3.3). Because it describes both the central and midperipheral visual fields, the tangent screen results can address both near point and distance activities.

With the student seated 1 meter from the test screen, the student is required to fix her vision on the white button that is in the center of the screen. Standing to one side, the examiner holds a black rod with a small white target attached to the end. The examiner slowly moves the small white target toward the center of the screen. When the student sees the white target, she signals by raising a hand or looking at the target. The examiner records the responses along all meridians to plot the visual field.

The *arc perimeter* evaluates the entire 180 degrees of the visual field (see Figure 3.4). This test is particularly useful for mobility instruction as its results often identify areas of significant field loss, such as hemianopsia and restricted fields due to advanced glaucoma or retinitis pigmentosa.

The requirements for administering this test are similar to the tangent screen. The student must look directly at the center of the screen. The

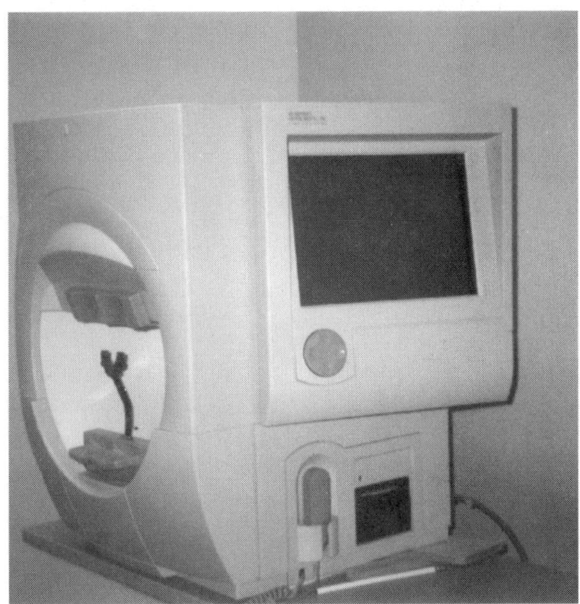

Figure 3.4. The arc perimeter is used to evaluate the entire visual field and identify significant vision losses.

examiner presents targets in all areas of the visual field. The student signals when the target is seen, with the response being plotted by the examiner.

The identification of field loss helps to explain the travel difficulties of many students, which is especially important information for the O&M specialist. One challenge for O&M specialists is knowing which field test to request. The different visual field assessments can be remembered through a common example of route planning. The use of road maps to help plan before and navigate during a trip is analogous to the use of field tests to help plan for understanding potential mobility performance. For example, when planning to travel from Chicago to Washington, D.C., you would begin by looking at a map of the United States (arc perimeter). This map would allow you to determine the interstate roads between Illinois and Washington. To identify the specific road for entering Washington, D.C., you would need a map of Virginia, Maryland, and the District of Columbia (tangent screen). The exact roads for entering Washington, D.C., and the location of the Capitol would require a detailed map of the District of Columbia (Amsler grid). Which map you choose involves identifying the question you want to answer. Similarly, which field test you choose involves determining what area of the visual field is required to complete the functional task. For example, reading a street map or train schedule involves the central visual field, which is best described by the Amsler grid or tangent screen, while walking on the sidewalk is a general task involving the entire visual field, which is best evaluated by the arc perimeter and tangent screen. Just as a map of the District of Columbia will not answer the question of how to travel from Chicago to Washington, D.C., the Amsler grid will not answer the question of why someone is consistently bumping objects on the left side.

Refractive Error

Testing for refractive error is performed to determine if the eye has either too much or not enough bending power, and what prescription eyeglasses will correct this condition. There are three primary types of refractive error: hyperopia, myopia, and astigmatism (see Figure 3.5). Briefly, *hyperopia,* or farsightedness, is when a distant image focuses at a point behind the retina, requiring a plus- (convex) shaped lens to shift the image forward so that it is focused onto the retina. Functionally, the person with hyperopia will experience difficulty clearly seeing objects up close, such as reading a bus schedule. *Myopia,* or nearsightededness, is when a distant image focuses at a point in front of the retina, requiring a minus- (convex) shaped lens to focus the image farther back onto the retina. Functionally the person with myopia will experience difficulty seeing objects or reading signs in the distance, such as reading a street sign. Both hyperopia and myopia are corrected with a spherical lens, offering the necessary plus or minus correction in all planes of the lens. *Astigmatism* is an irregular or uneven shape of the cornea, lens, or both. This irregularity is similar to looking through a window pane of very old glass. As you scan through the glass a thin line of irregularity may appear. This irregularity in the window is similar to the problem of astigmatism. It is corrected with a cylindrical lens

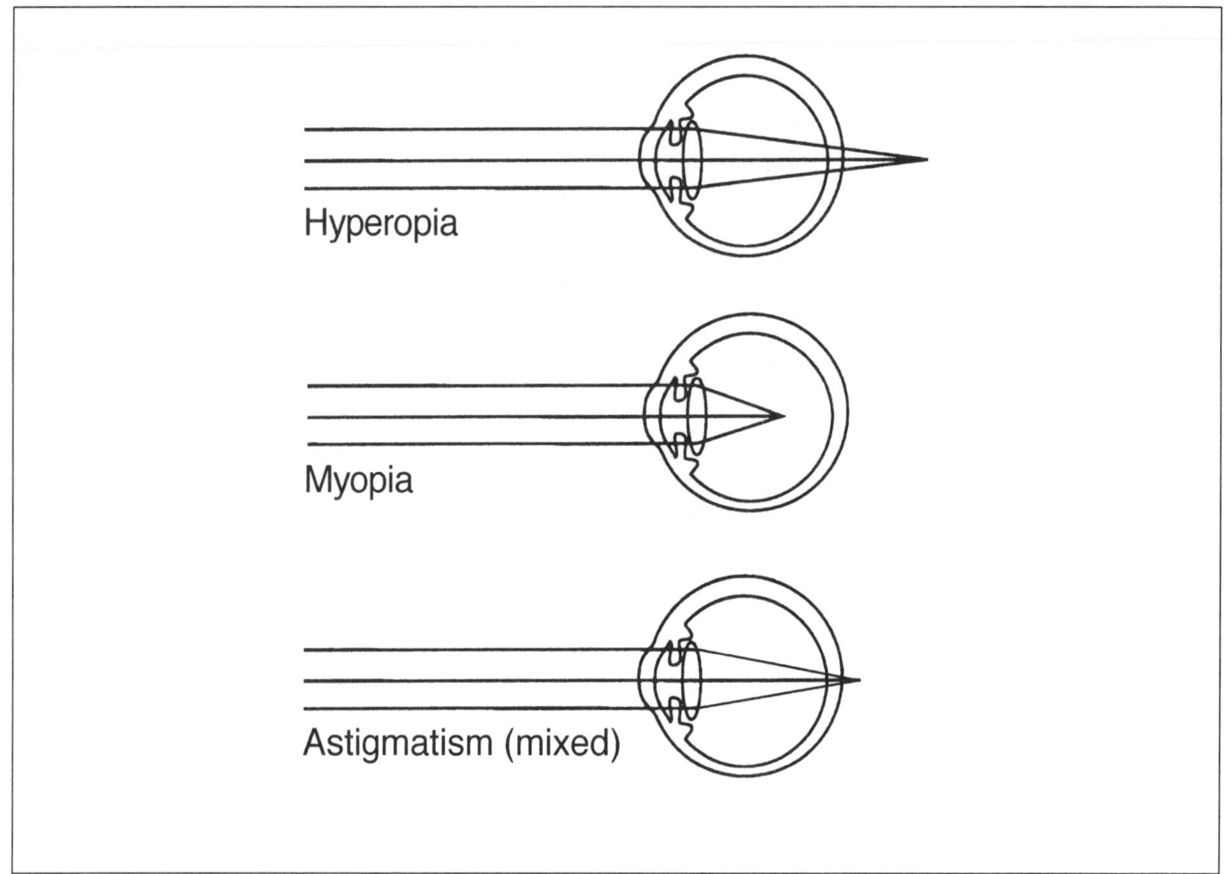

Figure 3.5. The three most common types of refractive error: hyperopia, myopia, and astigmatism.

that offers correction in only one plane of the lens, corresponding to the identified plane of irregularity. A comprehensive explanation of refractive errors is available in Jose (1983).

For the O&M specialist it is important to understand the difference between eyeglasses that correct for refractive error and eyeglasses that are prescribed for magnification. Eyeglasses which correct for refractive error can be worn for most mobility activities, while eyeglasses for magnification (microscopic spectacles) are only worn to see things at a close distance when the student is stationary, usually sitting.

Specialized Testing

Binocularity

Binocularity is the ability of the two eyes to work together. Functionally, this allows the brain to fuse the information from the two eyes into one image, providing depth perception. Binocularity primarily involves central vision, which is usually reduced in the students seen by a mobility specialist. In addition, the majority of students whom we see for mobility have unequal acuities between the two eyes, or have a significant eye turn (esotropia, exotropia) that precludes any possibility for the eyes to work together in a binocular fashion.

Many students have remaining vision in both eyes, but with unequal acuities such that the brain cannot merge the two images into one. These students are described as biocular. In these students both eyes work; however, they do not work together to form one image. In a mobility situation the peripheral vision of both eyes will provide critical information regardless of whether the student is biocular or binocular.

One of the most common tests for binocularity which is administered to a person with low vision is known as the Worth 4 dot. In this test the student wears a pair of eyeglasses in which one eye looks through a red lens while the second eye looks through a green lens. The eye care specialist directs a flashlight that emits four dots of light at the student. The four dots of light include one red, one green, and two white lights. Depending on the light combinations seen by the student, a determination of whether the student is using both eyes or one eye can be made.

Color Testing

Color vision screening is accomplished with isochromatic plates. In this screening the student is required to look at a card containing small circles of various colors. In the center of the card is either a number or a letter that can be seen if the student sees the specific color. The complete screening involves a series of plates with varying colors. If the student cannot distinguish the letters or numbers, then a comprehensive vision test may 1be ordered. The comprehensive color vision test is called the Farnsworth D-15 test of color vision. This test requires the student to sequence various shadings of one area of the color spectrum. The sequence is recorded on a score sheet, which provides an analysis of any color deficit. The time required to complete this test limits its use with persons who have low vision. In a mobility context color identification and color cues are useful to identify landmarks as well as the function of a landmark. For example, an object near the street corner that is slightly higher than head height and is seen as "red," even if the shape and letters cannot be identified, is usually a stop sign.

Contrast Sensitivity Function

Contrast sensitivity function (CSF) measures the ability to discriminate various shades of grey. This test involves identifying letters that begin as high contrast black letters on a white background and gradually reduce in contrast. The requirement for the student is to read the lightest shade of letters possible. This is an estimate of the student's contrast function or peak contrast. Contrast is quite useful in mobility; the environment consists of shades of grey such as curbs or outdoor stairs. This type of testing has been shown to be highly predictive of mobility performance (see Figure 3.6).

Ocular Health

The examination procedures for ocular health are the same for students with low vision as for the general public. More extensive examinations may occur if there is concern for a specific pathology. This component of the eye exam begins with analysis of the external eye. Examination of eyelids, eye alignment, and response of the pupils to light are the most common elements. Next is the examination of the internal structures of the eye. The cornea, aqueous, and front portion of the lens are evaluated with a biomicroscope (see Figure 3.7). Examination of the retina is the final step. In the general examination the direct ophthalmoscope is often the instrument of choice. If the pupil is dilated, both the direct and the indirect ophthalmoscopes can be used to perform a comprehensive examination of the periphery of the retina.

The clinical low vision assessment provides the O&M specialist with a baseline of the student's visual status. By obtaining clinical information under ideal viewing conditions in which all visual factors that often degrade functional vision are controlled, the eye care specialist serves a valuable role in describing the visual status of the student. Measures of visual acuity, visual field, refractive error, the health status of the eye, and the student's response to optical devices are useful precursors to effective rehabilitation.

FUNCTIONAL LOW VISION MOBILITY ASSESSMENT

There are three components to a low vision mobility assessment. These include (1) a review of information from the clinical examination, (2) an

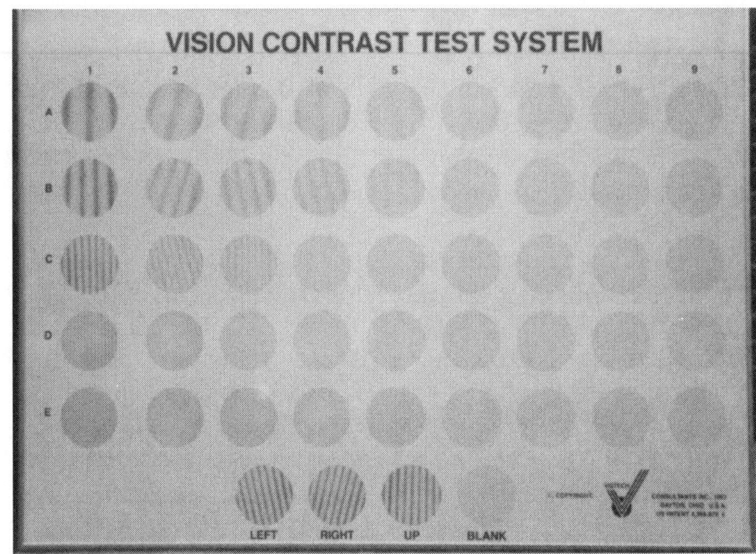

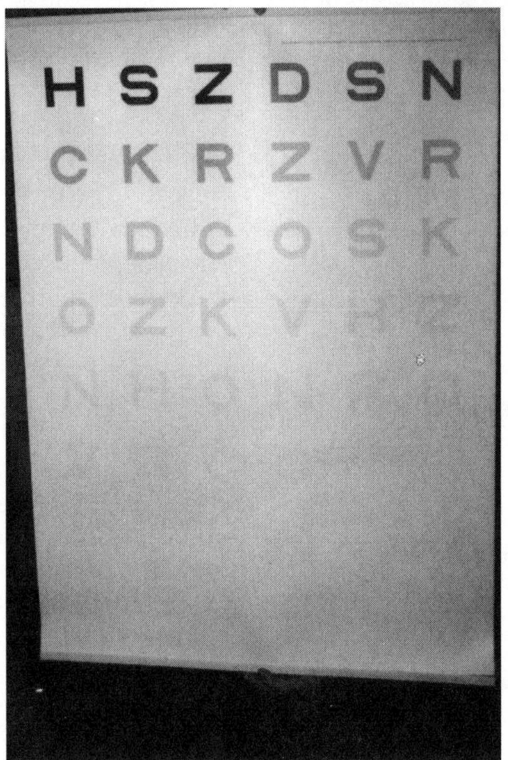

Figure 3.6. Two examples of charts used to test contrast sensitivity.

assessment of the student's functional vision, (3) an assessment of the student's mobility in different travel environments, and (4) an assessment of the travel environment itself. Each component of the assessment contributes pieces to a puzzle that ultimately forms a comprehensive understanding of the student's use of vision during mobility.

Although clinical information is a valuable resource, the student's performance in real-world

A

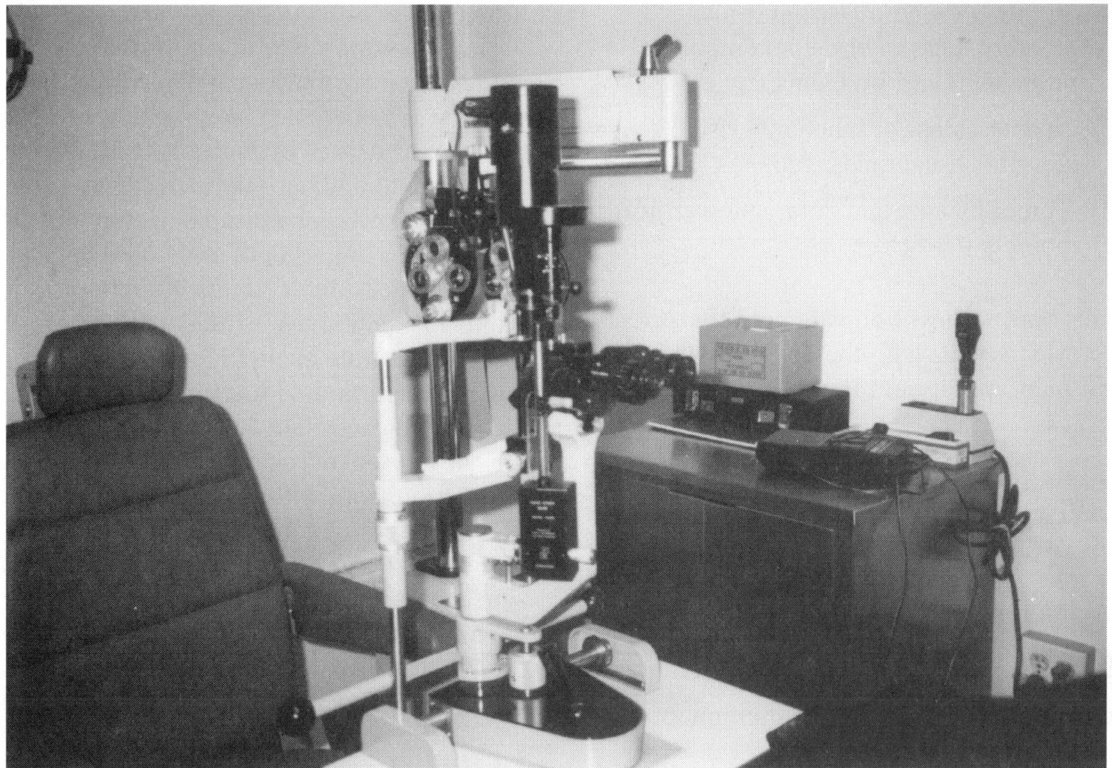

B

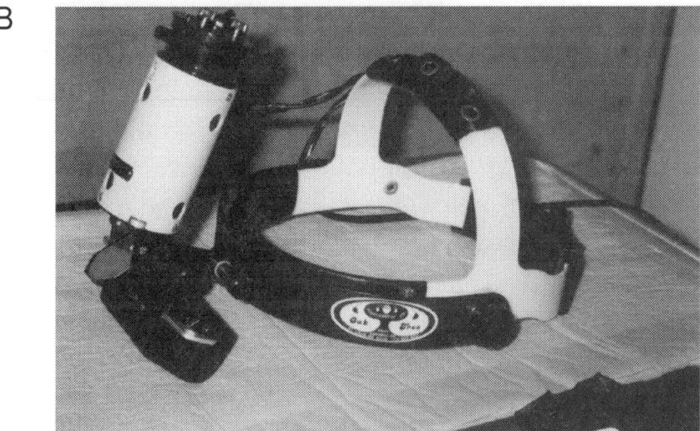

C

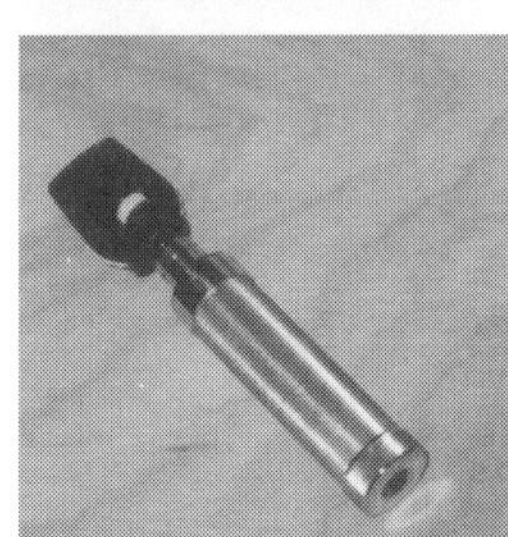

Figure 3.7. The three most commonly used instruments in a general eye examination are the (A) biomicroscope, (B) indirect ophthalmoscope, and (C) direct ophthalmoscope.

mobility situations is central to what the O&M specialist needs to assess. Clinical reports assist the O&M specialist in quantifying the level of visual functioning under static conditions using standardized charts and stimuli. What remains to be determined is the functional level of vision under everyday dynamic situations with real-world objects of various sizes and contrast, and in varying lighting conditions.

The beginning steps in bridging clinical reports to functional performance for mobility purposes are:

1. An interview emphasizing student-reported areas of visual and mobility proficiency and problems;
2. An assessment of functional visual acuities and visual fields; and
3. A mobility assessment targeting critical mobility problem areas.

This approach will provide both the student and O&M specialist with the necessary information to plan appropriate intervention strategies.

Low Vision Mobility Assessment Interview

Depending on the style and personality of the O&M specialist and student, the interview can be based on a variety of forms. The following areas are suggested for obtaining a minimum amount of information:

- Student needs/concerns/goals
- Demographic information and emergency contacts
- Diagnostic information, including visual and medical diagnoses, as well as medications and their systemic and visual side effects
- Previous mobility instruction
- Self-reported areas of proficiency and problems regarding vision and mobility performance
- Use of assistive devices—cane; dog guide; optical, nonoptical, and electronic travel aids
- Questions/comments

Functional Visual Acuities

Clinical measures of visual acuity are obtained in a static, controlled environment. By comparison, functional acuity encompasses a variable range of visual environments and performance for each student. During the course of a typical walk, students will experience varying levels of visual functioning caused by movement (self-, obstacle, and people), and variations in target size, lighting, and so on. For example, it may not be uncommon for one student to demonstrate a range from no measurable acuity (functioning totally blind) to the abilities to see small cracks in the sidewalk and the changing of a traffic light from red to green, and to identify people moving at distances greater than 100 feet. Three differences are all caused by changes in contrast and illumination, and by the effects of glare.

Because functional visual performance fluctuates, it is important to determine functional vision acuities in a variety of environments and under a variety of lighting conditions. Assessment of functional visual acuities involves the following:

Awareness acuity—The farthest possible distance at which the presence of any form is first detected.

Ask the student to look as far away as possible and indicate when the presence of any form is first detected. Examples may include building shapes contrasted against the sky, blobs or blurs of colors, indistinguishable specific objects, etc.

Identification acuity—The farthest possible distance at which a detected form is first correctly identified.

Ask the student to slowly move forward and identify the same detected form from the farthest possible distance. As an example, the student may say, "That red blob is beginning to look like a car."

Preferred viewing distance—The most comfortable distance for identifying a detected form.

Ask the student to continue to move forward until he is at a distance comfortable enough to provide sure identification (e.g., "I'm definitely sure now that that's a car").

Many students with reduced visual acuities can detect and identify the presence of objects at greater distances, yet feel more comfortable working at shorter, preferred distances. The exceptions are students with severely constricted visual fields who need to work at greater distances to fit more detail into their narrow fields of view.

Since interaction with the environment occurs at different distances and with objects of various sizes, choose tasks and objects that will reflect these situations. For example, activities that are typically completed at near and intermediate ranges, such as reading a bus schedule, building directories, or menus in fast-food restaurants, can be introduced along with those involving the detection and identification of traffic lights, people, and curbs at farther distances.

Conduct this assessment in both familiar and unfamiliar environments, and under different real-world lighting conditions. The nature of a functional acuity assessment necessitates repeated measures at different times on different days, in both indoor and outdoor environments. In essence, the O&M specialist takes advantage of different settings, cloudy and sunny conditions, bright and dim lighting—the stuff of real life. The pieces of the puzzle are gradually assembled to understand the range of visual acuity, and which factors facilitate or hinder visual functioning.

An excerpt from a sample report may read:

> Optimum visual acuity occurs on cloudy days when student is first able to detect the presence of cars, trees, and larger objects at distances of 80–100 feet. Student first correctly identifies these objects at 50–60 feet, but feels most comfortable identifying them at approximately 20 feet.
>
> On sunny days, student's functional acuity is reduced to 40 feet for awareness of large objects and to 15 feet before they are first correctly identified. The presence of glare, directly from the sun or indirectly from reflective surfaces, further reduces the functional acuity to a range of 1–5 feet, depending on the size and contrast of the object being viewed.
>
> Indoors, under overhead fluorescent lighting, awareness acuity for presence of a person is 35 feet, with identification of the person by facial detail correctly occurring at 6–8 feet. A posted bus schedule in the main terminal was identified from 6 feet and read with a 4× short-focus telescope from 30 inches.
>
> The student also demonstrates significant reduction in acuity when adapting to lighting changes: outdoors to indoors (30 seconds to 1 minute), indoors to outdoors (1 to 2 minutes) before acuity stabilizes.

Functional Visual Fields

As with visual acuities, assessment of functional visual fields occurs in a variety of environments and lighting conditions. A reduction in lighting will usually result in a reduction of the functional field, especially for individuals with severely constricted visual fields. Similar to clinical testing of acuity, clinical assessment of the visual field occurs in a setting that controls for illumination, the size of the target, and the distance at which the test is completed. Functional field assessment, by comparison, uses real-world settings with everyday objects such as people, cars, signs, and objects that vary in size.

To measure a functional visual field, assess the following:

Static visual field—A measure of the outermost boundaries of the visual field performed in everyday environments, with the person in a static position, keeping her head and eyes still.

Tell the student to stand still. Keeping head and eyes still, the student fixates straight ahead on a distant target. The student points to or describes objects seen at the highest, lowest, and farthest boundaries to the left and right.

An excerpt from a sample report may read:

> Student appears to have relatively full visual fields. She noted the ceiling and floor, as well as objects on both sides against the wall from 1 to 20 feet.

Dynamic visual field—A measure of the outermost boundaries of the visual field performed in everyday environments, with the person moving forward while keeping her head and eyes still.

Tell the student to commence moving forward. Keeping her head and eyes still while continuing to fixate ahead on distant targets, the student points to or describes objects at the highest, lowest, and farthest boundaries to the left and right. Remind the student to keep changing targets as she moves to ensure that the targets are at least 20 feet away.

An excerpt from a sample report may read:

> While moving, the same student appears to be using less functional field area, noting objects to the side at only 3–20 feet away. Objects, previously noted during static field assessment, within 1–3 feet on either side were frequently ignored while she was moving.

Preferred visual field—A dynamic measure of a person's regular pattern of viewing in everyday environments, with no limitations on head or eye movement, and emphasis on where visual information is most often obtained.

Ask the student to walk forward and tell you everything that he or she sees. Tell the student to look around as they normally would. Do not pose limitations on head or eye movements. Observe the student's regular pattern of viewing (e.g., frequent scanning, consistent gazes downward, etc.), and where visual information about the environment is obtained (e.g., only notices objects on right side). Using the chart in Figure 3.8A, mark an X corresponding to where each object or person is noted by your student. By the end of your session a pattern will emerge, indicating preferred visual field use.

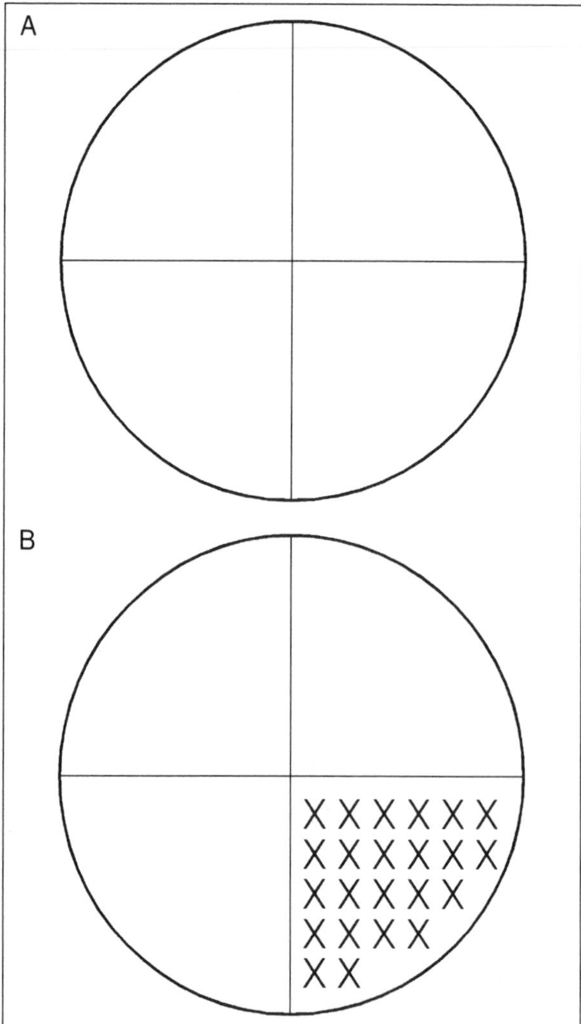

Figure 3.8. Examples of a (A) blank and a (B) completed chart on which a student's preferred vision field is plotted.

An excerpt from a sample report may read:

> Student consistently gazes downward and ahead. He noted most objects in the lower field of view and within 3–6 feet ahead. Some objects were noted infrequently on the lower right side, but no objects were noted on student's left side (see Figure 3.8B).

The first two measurements, static and dynamic, tell you about the potential area of visual field available to the student. The preferred field assessment tells you what the student is actually using, given a dynamic situation with no restrictions on how or where looking occurs. This estimates the student's use of potential functional field. Conducting a preferred visual field assessment yields the most significant information for the O&M specialist, as it more accurately reflects how the student uses their vision for mobility purposes, regardless of what the clinical field may imply.

A final functional field assessment is recommended for students with known or suspected constricted fields. It is particularly helpful for determining how much of a functionally blind area is affecting early detection of objects or people on either side of the student.

Peripheral constriction or *early warning field*—A measure of peripheral or side vision performed in everyday environments, with the person in a static position, keeping his head and eyes still.

Ask the student to stand still, fixate straight ahead on a distant object, and tell you when he or she first notes you passing on either side. You begin at your student's side, and continue walking a straight line (parallel to student's line of sight) until the student is able to detect your presence. Repeat this same procedure on the other side. This assessment provides information on the amount of field restriction to each side and estimates the extent of the functional blind area.

An excerpt from a sample report may read:

> He was unaware of me passing by his right side until I was approximately 3 feet away. After 3 feet, he was consistently able to detect the presence of myself and other objects on his right. On the left side, he demonstrated less field awareness, as was only able to detect me passing by after I was 6–8 feet away. This may help explain his frequent bumping into objects, especially on his left side.

Upon examination of clinical findings and completion of functional acuity and field assessments, the O&M specialist understands the capability and functional use of the student's vision. This information, obtained in various settings and under different lighting conditions, enables the O&M specialist and student to predict visual functioning. In addition, the O&M specialist is now better able to assist the student in understanding what frequently has seemed a puzzling, inconsistent visual picture, thus knowing when vision may or may not be relied on for various mobility purposes.

The O&M specialist can then assist the student in becoming more proactive about visual awareness and identification for increased safety and mobility efficiency. Before leaving this topic, it is important for the O&M specialist to recommend a comprehensive low vision clinical evaluation, including evaluation for optical devices. If the student is currently using optical devices, they should be included in the functional evaluation. If the student does not use optical devices, he or she should be informed of the options and potential benefits of a complete evaluation and the possible use of both optical and nonoptical devices to enhance visual functioning.

Other mobility devices such as a cane, electronic travel aids, and so on, should also be included in the dynamic assessments. When possible, compare visual efficiency, with and without optical and other assistive mobility devices. Many students do not realize the extent of increase in visual functioning, for instance, when a cane is used to detect depth, thus freeing vision for object identification, orientation purposes, and for viewing at greater distances.

Critical Incidents Mobility Assessment

A comprehensive mobility assessment is accomplished over a number of hours on different days. It involves assessment in both familiar and unfamiliar areas, indoor and outdoor settings, under varying lighting conditions, and at different times of the day.

Whether the O&M specialist has the time to complete a comprehensive or only a brief assessment, the use of the critical incidents approach is germane to both. As opposed to working with prearranged forms that direct the O&M specialist's attention toward collating information for prescribed assessment items, the Critical Incidents approach individualizes the assessment through observation of the student, with no predetermined areas to "fit" the student into.

When conducting a Critical Incidents Assessment, the O&M specialist observes the student's mobility performance, noting mobility problems (critical incidents) in the order they naturally occur. The O&M specialist starts a tally each time a critical incident (e.g., bumping into an object, missing a step or curb, shuffling the feet, underreaching, considerably slowing the pace, misjudging a street crossing, becoming disoriented, etc.) occurs. Where appropriate, the incident is followed by more detailed information, such as: "bumped into shoulder-high object on right side, tripped down a 6-inch curb, did not see turning car from left before stepping into the street (no side-to-side scanning)," etc. In addition, environmental conditions relative to lighting, contrast, glare, etc., are noted. It is conceivable that a student may exhibit different abilities to negotiate the same mobility routes at different times of the day or under different conditions of direct and reflecting glare.

What emerges are clusters of the most frequently occurring critical incidents or mobility problems unique to each student, as well as student behaviors and environmental variables that contribute to them. An individualized plan can then be developed, plotting the direction of intervention to address specific mobility problem areas.

COMBINING CLINICAL RESULTS WITH THE FUNCTIONAL ASSESSMENT

Results from the clinical examination may offer explanations and insights about the functional vision characteristics observed during the functional mobility assessment. For example, the clinical examination from a student may read: "Albinism, visual acuity of 10/400 without eyeglasses and 10/120 OU with corrective eyeglasses, and a refractive error of +4.50 − 2.75 × 120 OU." The mobility assessment indicated that this student's functional visual acuity was better with eyeglasses, that functional visual fields were full, and that the biggest problem was traveling in brightly lit areas, specifically outdoors on a sunny day. A review of Table 3.1 reveals the information that students with albinism have problems with glare and a significant refractive error. These characteristics have been confirmed in the functional assessment, and indicate the importance of working with the student to cope with the issue of lighting, and the importance of wearing corrective lenses to achieve best visual acuity.

A second example is the student with a diagnosed retinal detachment. The clinical exam reports:

> Visual acuity of 10/100 OU, an inferior temporal field loss OD with no significant refractive error. During the mobility assessment, the functional visual field confirms the absence of vision in the lower right field of the right eye. In the critical incidents assessment, the student consistently misses objects in the lower right field. For example, garbage cans, bicycles, and low-lying shrubs on the right side incur the highest number of critical incidents.

Both of these examples illustrate how the clinical and functional assessments can be analyzed to confirm the functional characteristics of the clinical findings. In addition, the clinical findings offer the O&M specialist insights into the types of problems the student may experience, allowing for the individualization of the functional assessment to specifically evaluate the anticipated areas of concern.

ASSESSING THE ENVIRONMENT

Independent function depends on two main factors: the ability of the student and the demands of the environment. As long as the student's ability is equal to or exceeds the demand, independence can be maintained. Problems occur when the demands of the environment exceed the abilities of the student. This relationship is dynamic and will change as the environment or the student's skills change.

Determining the impact of the environment on mobility involves analysis of several environmental characteristics such as space layout, movement patterns, and objects in the environment. Mobility lessons are contingent on the specific environment in which the student is traveling. For example, lessons are sequenced from indoors to outdoors, residential to small business, and quiet areas to crowded city centers. These sequences recognize the effects of changes in pedestrian and vehicular traffic, weather, and so on. Lessons are specifically sequenced to gradually increase the amount and complexity of environmental characteristics. The O&M specialist is constantly analyzing the environment to determine the cause of, and solutions to, problems. For example, after crossing a series of streets with accuracy, the student may become confused because of an offset intersection. In this example the O&M specialist attributes the problem to the uniqueness of the intersection, not a specific deficit in travel skills of the student. This type of environmental analysis is an important component of all mobility instruction, whether the student has low vision or is totally blind or fully sighted.

When considering the environment to be used by a student with low vision, special emphasis is placed on significant visual environmental characteristics, such as illumination, color, and contrast. The following factors are of specific importance:

1. *Amount of light.* This includes analysis of the following:
   - The overall lighting in the area (bus terminal)
   - Lighting on the specific task area (e.g., schedule information board)
2. *Type of light.* This includes identification of:
   - Different light sources such as natural, incandescent, or fluorescent
   - Type of light source student prefers and types that hinder performance
3. *Light angle and location.* This includes descriptions of:
   - Relationship of natural and artificial light sources to student
   - Effect of different light positions on mobility performance
4. *Light adaptation.* This includes evaluating:
   - Changes in functional vision from indoors to outdoors and vice versa
   - Changes in functional vision from one level of lighting to another (e.g., shade to sun, hallway to classroom, and so on)
   - Amount of time student needs to adapt to lighting change
5. *Glare.* This includes determination of:
   - Sources of glare (e.g., reflections off windows, shiny walls, floors, or puddles of water)
   - Effect of sunwear and other eyeshades, such as hats and visors, on functional vision performance
6. *Color or contrast.* This includes identification of:
   - Color and contrast cues available to assist orientation (e.g., crosswalk lines, church steeples, and so on)
   - Changes in terrain color and contrast (e.g., broken sidewalks, puddles, curbs, stairs, potholes, and so on)

An excerpt from a sample report may read:

Student moves with ease in the brightly lit bus terminal; however, experiences problems reading the information board due to insufficient amount of light on the board. Natural sunlight is preferred while fluorescent lights cause visual discomfort. Moving into the bus terminal, the student experienced approximately 30 seconds of decreased vision. In response to this the student stood to the side until her eyes adapted to the new light level. In the terminal's fast-food restaurant, the student experienced difficulty reading the overhead food menu due to glare reflecting from fluorescent lights. The student was able to locate the first and last steps to the train platform due to high-contrast colored strips on the steps (normally the student experiences difficulty identifying the first step, consequently shuffling her feet to detect the edge of the step).

Assessment of the student (clinical assessment of vision, functional assessment of vision, critical incidents) combined with assessment of the visual demands of the environment and the student's functioning in the environment provides the O&M specialist with the amount and quality of information from which an instructional program can be developed. This comprehensive point of view is fundamental to the provision of quality services in low vision mobility.

In the field of low vision, optical solutions are too often viewed as the primary or only solution to the problems resulting from impaired vision. As O&M specialists, our experience clearly indicates there is more to independence than 20/20 visual acuity. Systematic analysis of environmental factors is a reflection of the importance attributed to the effects of the environment on functional vision. Analyzing and teaching students about environmental effects can improve their understanding of how environmental changes affect vision. They, in turn, can use this information to become better consumers and increase their independence.

IMPROVING FUNCTIONAL USE OF VISION

Congenital versus Adventitious Vision Loss

Whether the student is born with low vision or acquires low vision later in life is significant with regard to the type and extent of visual stimulation and efficiency instruction. Unlike those who acquire vision loss after experiencing unimpaired visual concepts and memory, children born with low vision have different levels of visual memory, from little to a significantly useful amount. However, they cannot be described as having vision losses, since they cannot "lose" vision they never had. It is critical to take these differences into account when tailoring programs for improving functional vision.

Although many functional vision enhancement techniques are similar for both populations, the student with congenital low vision requires considerably more time and effort in the formation of a visual language and memory (usually taken for granted in the situation of student with adventitious vision loss). A common mistake is the assumption that children with severely reduced visual acuity, because they cannot see clearly, lack the potential to more effectively and efficiently interpret visual cues for mobility or other purposes. Equally common is the assumption that students with higher levels of visual acuity do not necessarily need mobility instruction because they appear to be moving about with relatively few problems in familiar areas.

Both of these cases are examples of students who may "fall between the cracks" due to assumptions on the part of the O&M specialist. In addition, many students with adventitious vision loss at low and high extremes frequently fall between the same cracks in rehabilitation service delivery systems. An advisable rule of thumb is to assess all students for visual and mobility proficiency and problems, and to plan a range of low vision mobility instruction from basic to advanced, depending on the student's assessed needs.

In the case of the student with congenital low vision, a program of vision stimulation, started as early as possible, is recommended to assure instruction at vision developmental levels the student is capable of achieving. Without this instruction many students may not acquire the basic skills to interpret visual stimuli and make judgments concerning important pieces of visual information available to them. A vision stimulation program helps the student learn about and develop labels for critical visual features such as lines, angles, curves, and colors; how to identify them separately and as parts of common shapes and objects; and how to piece together missing details from what is seen to better interpret an incomplete visual picture of the environment.

Barraga and Morris (1980), Levack (1991), Smith and Cote (1982), and Smith and O'Donnell (1991) are but a few of the references available to assist in sequential vision stimulation programming for students with visual and multiple impairments. This instruction enhances eventual mobility performance, and, when combined with a systematic exposure to environmental and other sensory concepts, ensures a comprehensive approach to mobility instruction.

Visual Efficiency without Optical Devices

Having attained basic visual concepts commensurate with the student's cognitive and visual potential, the O&M specialist further assists the student in visual interpretation and movement through the environment. This is accomplished through lessons geared toward maximizing visual efficiency, in conjunction with instruction in other sensory training and mobility tools such as long canes and electronic aids, and travel techniques that maximize safety and efficiency of movement.

A starting point for maximizing visual efficiency is a discussion with the student about his or her visual condition(s) and functional implications. This necessitates familiarization with the student's record, including the results of the clinical examination. Do not be surprised if the student is either unaware of, or confused about, his or her visual condition and functional performance. Remember that both internal and external variables affect visual performance from day to day and, in some cases, from one minute to the next. Your role is to assist the student in understanding this information and to teach the student when and when not to rely on visual information for decision making while mobile.

In assisting the student to understand the functional implications of visual impairment, one should neither bombard nor overwhelm them with information. Many children with congenital low vision lack an understanding of their vision because no one has taken the time to provide them with a meaningful description of and discussion about their vision. Explaining how the eye works, which part of their eye is affected, and how this effects their functional vision (e.g., a sensitivity to light, the need to wear eyeglasses, bumping into objects on the side, and so on) helps children to better understand what they are experiencing. Erin and Corn (1994) reported on children's first understanding of being visually impaired. Their findings indicate that for children, low vision is a more complex concept than blindness. Detailed explanations, at a pace and level each child can appreciate, are recommended to enable the child to understand the functional implications of their eye condition and how this affects mobility performance. It is also recommended that children keep a mobility diary or journal which includes, but is not limited to, the following:

1. a functional description of their eye condition(s) and its effects
2. best and worst times of day and weather conditions affecting their visual performance
3. best and worst lighting conditions (indoor and outside)
4. medications taken and any visual side effects
5. most common mobility problems which can or cannot be visually remediated
6. optical and nonoptical devices used and how they assist in mobility.

Whether for a child or adult, young or old, this diary or journal enables students to get a better handle on their vision, and the internal and external variations that affect day-to-day mobility. In addition, it can serve as a monitor of progress, concepts learned, descriptions of techniques mastered (both visual and nonvisual), orientation tips, etc.

For those with adventitious low vision (usually adults and the elderly), the O&M specialist helps them understand the visual *changes* they experience, as compared to their prior experiences with full sight. The O&M specialist still needs to review the same steps outlined for the younger student. These include a review of the eye's condition and its effect on vision, internal and external variables affecting visual performance, and when or when not to rely on visual information for mobility decisions. In addition, instructions for new ways of using vision, such as eccentric viewing for those with age-related maculopathy, or new scanning techniques for those with advanced glaucoma or retinitis pigmentosa, need to be emphasized. The mobility diary or journal is also recommended for adult students, especially as it relates to new vision information (both clinical and functional), changes in visual behavior, and new visual skills.

Timing your presentation of this material is important. This may not be the most critical information to address if, for instance, the person is experiencing a difficult adjustment to vision loss or is resistant to the idea of mobility instruction. A holistic look at the person, his or her individual situation and unique personality factors, and consultation with other appropriate professionals enables the O&M specialist to successfully time and sequence this information.

Long Cane Use and Visual Instruction

The long cane, besides assisting in general mobility travel, can be one of the most important tools for enhancing visual efficiency. If the student relies on the cane for overall detection of depth and terrain changes, vision is then free for orientation and more detailed viewing of the general environment, in addition to visual aesthetics. Many students who do not use long canes spend a considerable amount of time looking down to detect changes in depth and uneven surfaces. Vision is used exclusively for safety issues rather than detection of the whole range of visual cues that are available in the environment to enhance the travel experience.

There are many instances in which a student with low vision does not require the use of a long cane. Conversely there are many environmental conditions such as lighting, time of day, or crowds that warrant the use of the long cane for effective travel. One of the most important features of instruction in low vision mobility is teaching each student the critical variables he or she must assess to make this determination. Just as learning to use your vision more efficiently is important to mobility, learning when vision is not effective for travel decisions is equally as important. At these times the use of the long cane augments travel safety and efficiency.

Basic Visual Motor Skills

After assisting in understanding functional implications of the student's vision, instruction or review in basic visual motor skills is advised. Basic visual motor skills such as scanning, tracing, and tracking are the foundation upon which instruction in the use of vision for mobility is built. The following section provides selected examples of visual motor skills use for orientation and mobility purposes, with references that address these skills in greater detail.

Tracing, or visually following a stationary line, is particularly useful for orientation purposes. In effect it is the visual counterpart of trailing with one's hand or cane. Compared to tactile methods, however, it affords a greater reach, because of the visual ability to project farther in space. Practice in tracing various environmental lines such as grasslines and other shorelines, the tops of hedgelines, baseboards, and so on, enhances orientation. Perhaps a student can only discern contrast. She can trace along a baseboard (contrasted to the floor coloring), and know that an office is located at the fourth break in the baseboard. Another student with similarly decreased vision can trace along and count six breaks in the hedgeline, signaling the path to the house he wishes to locate. A student may only have light projection, yet could use this vision to trace a line of fluorescent lights along the ceiling to maintain a straight line of direction. In addition, when the line of lights ceases, this may be used as an additional clue to indicate the intersecting hallway.

For some younger students, placing objects at the end of short, then gradually lengthening, lines of brightly colored yarn or rope is effective for teaching the skill of tracing. This establishes head and eye movement patterns. Gradually increasing the length of yarn and complexity of the surrounding environment teaches the student to search ahead for environmental lines of borders, lights, colors, and so on, which assist in orientation and maintaining a desired line of travel.

Tracking, or visually following a moving target, can be a particularly helpful skill for both maintaining orientation and locating targets. Teach your students to follow the shoulderline of a person walking in front of them, and watch for a raising or lowering of this person's shoulderline. This might indicate up or down steps, or any raised or dropped level of terrain, be it a raised sidewalk or hole in the ground. When going out to a dimly lit restaurant, the student may ask his or her companion to wear a light or bright shirt, blouse, or jacket. By walking slightly ahead of the student, the companion's clothing serves as an orientation cue the student can use to track a path through the dimly lit area.

Perhaps one of the more common uses of tracking is at street crossings or corners while waiting for the bus. Have the student practice tracking cars through busy intersections. Determine if the student can follow movement and discern turning cars from those continuing through the intersection. Good tracking skills can significantly augment safety and decision-making skills when crossing streets.

For anyone experiencing difficulty with tracking, the sequence should begin with head and eye tracking and progress to refining eye movement tracking as the student's skills improve. Keep the student seated at first while following moving targets such as people. Then have the student begin to walk and look for moving targets. Gradually increase the complexity of the task until the student is able to follow other pedestrians in crowded situations such as moving through crowded stores.

This combination of systematic tracing and tracking skills contributes to the proactive use of vision, as opposed to simply moving without using vision to its fullest extent. They serve as advanced problem solving and safety cues for more effective decision making, especially for orientation purposes.

Scanning is the systematic use of head and eye movement to search for targets. This skill can be used for a variety of purposes including locating targets, establishing and reestablishing lines of direction, and finding landmarks. The O&M specialist's role is to convert random patterns into systematic and goal-specific visual scanning behavior. Most students display random and unsystematic patterns of scanning. Random scanning patterns can be observed regardless of age, amount of vision loss, or cognitive abilities. The example that follows briefly describes questions followed by a teaching example.

Initially, ask the student to visually locate a number of different targets or landmarks in indoor and outdoor environments. Observe for a specific search pattern. Are some areas missed completely while others are repeatedly checked? Is scanning overly time-consuming or time-efficient? If the answer to either question is yes, then the student would benefit from basic instruction in patterns of scanning. Begin by asking the student to search a wall or any large surface for a specific sign, clock, etc. If necessary, direct the student's head and eyes to the top left corner of the wall. Then have the student begin to trace from the left to the right corner, then lower the head slightly and trace back to the left side, again lower the head and trace to the right side, and continued this pattern until the target is located. This will ensure that no area is either missed or repeated, because of the systematic nature of the scanning pattern (see Figure 3.9A). As an example, this pattern can be used in stores when scanning for overhead signs or attempting to locate specific food items.

If objects or targets are typically located around borders or walls of a room, then a perimeter scanning pattern along the outer walls is more appropriate (see Figure 3.9B). Higher objects, such as hanging plants, require upper field scanning, whereas a floor pillow against the wall will be more quickly located by a lower field perimeter scanning pattern. Many congenitally vi-

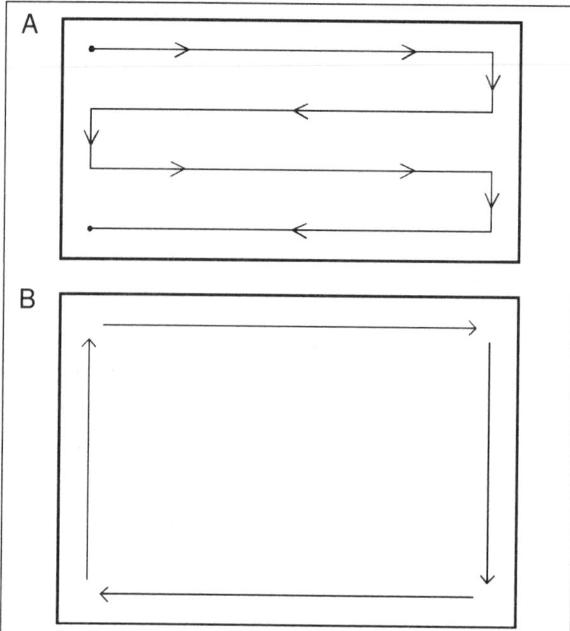

Figure 3.9. (A) Gridline scanning pattern; (B) perimeter scanning pattern.

sually impaired students benefit from systematic instruction in the positional locations of common environmental objects. It should not be assumed that students will automatically know where and how to look for targets; this is why an initial evaluation is helpful in planning instruction.

One general rule to emphasize for scanning is that when students are looking for vertical targets, they should scan horizontally, and when looking for horizontal targets, they need to scan vertically. As an example, when looking ahead for a street sign, scan horizontally along the curb or sidewalk border to locate the bottom of the intersecting vertical pole. Then scan vertically up the pole to locate the intersecting horizontal street sign. This increases the chance of locating the target quickly and efficiently.

Students should also learn that a combination of scanning techniques are sometimes needed. A good example of this is a house address. Some are on the mailbox or beside the front door or on the step, while other addresses are painted on the front curbs. Systematic use of visual scanning saves time and contributes to more proactive and efficient mobility.

Other mobility areas lending themselves to the need for scanning instruction are general orientation, street crossings, and maintaining and reestablishing a line of direction. As an example for *general orientation* purposes, instruct the student to scan for a series of visual landmarks along a new route. The student then writes, brailles, or records these landmarks and their positional location (e.g., "fire hydrant, lower left side"), and uses this list to assist in scanning until they are committed to memory. The student will learn that, while the upper and lower locations will not change, opposite sides will need to be scanned when reversing the route (e.g., "fire hydrant, lower right side"). At *street crossings,* students should be instructed in scanning for traffic lights and walk–don't walk signs (horizontally along ground, vertically up light pole), as well as for traffic and pedestrian movement. As the street crossing begins, the student should scan for turning cars on the parallel street. This will involve scanning behind the shoulder nearest the parallel street, since the car in that position poses the most immediate danger. Approaching the middle of the street, the student scans to the parallel street slightly ahead, since the turning car from the other side of the intersection now poses more danger. Systematic scanning will significantly enhance safety at busy intersections. Unfortunately many students do not use scanning at intersections beyond looking for traffic lights. Some may scan for cars only before crossing, and discontinue once they step off the curb. For younger students, lessons in the concept of traffic and intersections may be necessary first, whereas for older students, reminders of the safety hazards and the need for more effective and systematic scanning may need to be emphasized.

A scanning example for *establishing and reestablishing a line of direction* is the student traveling in a new location. She could begin by scanning down the street as far as possible to look for a distinctive landmark (e.g., the blue mailbox or the colorful bed of flowers up ahead on the right). If she becomes disoriented after veering up a driveway, she would stop, turn her head, and scan for the street. In addition to the sound and movement of cars, the bushes or tree at the edge of the sidewalk may provide the necessary cues to change direction and return toward the sidewalk. Once back on the sidewalk, she could gradually scan the area in either direction to search for the initial landmark and realign her direction of travel. As she continues walking, she can search for other landmarks to maintain her line of travel.

Although some of us automatically employ scanning for landmarks (e.g., the *red* floor in a parking garage, or the third car after the *green 2A sign* in the mall parking lot), many students with congenital low vision may require instruction in systematic scanning to establish and reestablish orientation cues.

Eye-hand and eye-foot coordination are frequently lacking in students with low vision. It is not unusual for students to misjudge distances of objects by over- or underreaching and groping with the hands to locate objects, or to misjudge steps and shuffle the feet to locate the first step. This is because the eyes, hands, or feet are functioning independently of each other. For instance, the object or target may first be located visually, then identified tactually, independent of vision. Through instruction and practice of reaching for objects while keeping the hand in view, this problem can be minimized. As an example, ask the student to visually locate a series of doorknobs. Then ask the student to place his hand between his eyes and the doorknob, and watch his hand as it approaches the doorknob. This should reduce groping and enable the student to achieve greater accuracy when reaching for targets. Students should also be instructed to watch their feet as they approach stairs to enable them to more accurately judge the location of the first step.

Eccentric viewing is the use of the off-center or paramacular ("para" meaning near or beside) area of vision for a clearer view. Children with a loss of central vision, due to Best's or Stargardt's disease or any condition that results in a central scotoma or blind spot, typically develop eccentric viewing postures automatically. This involves a tilt of the head or eye or a combination of both to view around the scotoma. Adults who lose their central vision to age-related maculopathy, for example, may need instruction in locating and maintaining the best eccentric area for fixating and viewing.

The clinical report may provide information as to how the student eccentrically views. If this information is not available, one method for establishing the best viewing position is to ask the student to cover one eye, look directly at your face and describe what she sees. Have the student shift the eye up, down, to the right, and to the left as she describes your face. When the best angle of viewing is reached, double check by moving the eye slightly around this position to assure clearest possible vision. A clock on the wall could also be used for demonstration of eccentric viewing position. If the student looks straight ahead at the clock, its middle section will appear to be missing. The student can then experiment with different head and eye positions as above, until the face of the clock is more clearly seen. Once this position is learned the student can use it for short-term tasks such as reading signs with or without telescopes, or long-term viewing such as watching television.

Depth Perception Cues

Difficulty judging depth is a universal problem for persons with low vision. This is especially true when some visual cues, such as the appearance of a gradual slope or apparently flat area, are actually masking steps or curbs. Nevertheless, there are a host of visual cues that can be used to enhance depth perception. Examples of cues that assist in locating stairs include:

- the *slope of a railing* indicates whether the stairs are going up or down
- the *height change of persons* in front of you indicates up or down stairs, depending on whether they are slowly rising or descending in your field of view
- the *feet or lower body of persons are blocked* when approaching downward steps; one may only notice, for example,

the upper body of a person coming up those same stairs

- *jagged or broken edged shadows* cast from objects indicate the presence of steps
- *right angles or triangular shapes* along the side border where the riser and adjoining step meet indicate steps, with a long succession of these angles indicating a long flight of steps
- *contrasting color strips at the edge of steps* assist in detecting their presence

In addition, sounds emanating from above or below, such as voices or footsteps, indicate oncoming up or down steps. Practice in looking and listening purposefully for these cues helps the student to become more visually proactive about potentially dangerous areas of depth.

Examples of cues that assist in locating curbs include:

- *crosswalk lines*
- *vehicles* (parked or moving) *on a nearby perpendicular street*
- *visual contrast of street to street pavement and/or curb*
- *end of building, grassline, or other continuous shoreline,* indicating the presence of an intersecting sidewalk and potential intersecting street
- *curbs painted in contrasting colors* (e.g., yellow and blue)
- *broken shadows at curb* from light poles or other objects near the corner

In addition, pedestrians suddenly stopping or congregating at a corner, as well as the presence of various objects such as newspaper stands, traffic light control boxes, and so on, at corners indicate oncoming intersections. The sounds of cars traveling perpendicular to the student's line of travel, even before they can be seen, provide another sensory cue for detecting an oncoming curb area.

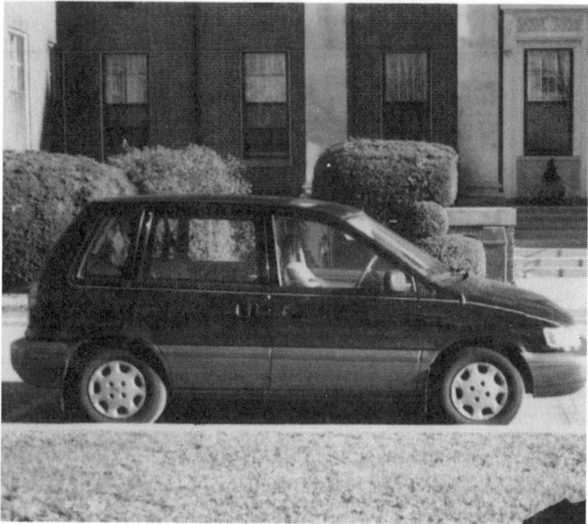

Figure 3.10. The depth of a curb can be determined by observing the extent to which the curb obscures the bottom of a car's tires.

The long cane represents one of the best tools for detecting depth. Its use in conjunction with active visual scanning for depth cues assures the best level of safety and efficiency in traveling. Although visual cues alone may enable the student to detect the presence of stairs and curbs, the exact amount of depth is frequently difficult to judge without the use of a cane. One visual cue that does assist in judging the depth of curbs involves scanning for tires of parked cars. By seeing how much of the bottom of the tire is blocked or obscured by the curb, the student can establish a relatively accurate estimation of the depth of the curb (see Figure 3.10).

Terrain Changes

Abrupt terrain changes are one of the most difficult areas for the student with low vision. For those with sufficient vision, the following cues may prove helpful:

- For detecting *missing slabs of sidewalk,* a change in color from light to darker or vice versa, as well as the presence of dirt that gives a granular or bumpy appearance may be useful cues;

- For detecting *puddles,* reflections on the ground or a broken or ripple effect from raindrops may be helpful;
- *Wet cement* may be detected by noticing a darker shade underfoot or the presence of construction by contrasting strips or ropes sectioning off newly finished areas;
- *Raised slabs of cement* are detected by darkly lined, uneven, or thick sections of sidewalk, which indicate the raised section or slab;
- *Broken sidewalks* are indicated by color or shading changes in the broken areas, as well as additional lines bordering the broken areas.

Visual Landmarks

Orientation can be greatly facilitated by the use of visual landmarks. The following represent a few of the many landmarks and techniques that can assist the person with low vision to use his or her vision more effectively while traveling.

- *Distinctive shapes*—such as McDonald's arches, a steeply sloped roof along a street with flat roofed buildings, or an oddly shaped lawn sculpture—if scanned for, can reduce the amount of time it takes to locate objectives or areas near them;
- *Distinctive colors,* such as a bright red door, the color yellow along a row of condiments to signal mustard, the color purple to signal cabbage in the vegetable section of a store, or the blue arrow line along the floor to signal the route through a cafeteria;
- *Scanning the upper field of view* for landmarks, such as different heights of buildings or church steeples, or the top of a silo, to establish or reestablish one's direction;
- Remembering *forward and reverse sequences of visual landmarks,* along with anticipating which visual cue is next, to facilitate learning routes and maintaining orientation.

The key is to choose distinctive visual landmarks that enhance the proactive use of vision as opposed to simply reacting to whatever visual stimuli is stumbled upon. Active looking and the use of visual landmarks enhances mobility skills, especially as they relate to orientation and efficient use of time while traveling.

Glare and Light Adaptation

As previously discussed, lighting (i.e., glare, light adaptation, and dim lighting), represents the single most critical problem area for persons with low vision. The following strategies will assist the student who experiences problems with lighting:

- wear appropriate *absorptive sun filters* to shield from glare-producing light. Sun lens evaluation should include exposure to different color tints and light transmission levels, to determine which provide the most comfort from glare and improve visual detail. Lenses with top and side filters are especially effective for protection from glare.
- With or without sun lenses, wear *visors, wide brimmed hats,* or *billed hats* such as baseball caps to eliminate glare from above and improve visual detail.
- If the student is unable to distinguish a sign because of glare or bright light, a *change of the angle of viewing* avoids the effect of harsh light and improves the ability to read print.
- If the student is unable to distinguish the color of a traffic light due to glare, he should *turn to view the opposite traffic.*
- *Conduct mobility lessons in dim and nighttime conditions* when many students' mobility is more severely affected. Additional cane training may be necessary, especially as many students experience anything from significantly decreased to a total loss of visual cues.

- *Evaluate light adaptation times* from indoors to outdoors and vice versa. Note how long and to what degree visual functioning is affected. Some students may only experience a few seconds of adjustment, others a few minutes, and others longer still. Some students may experience periods of nonvisual functioning and may need to step aside and wait, use a sighted guide, or use a folding cane to maneuver safely. The O&M specialist shouldhelpstudentsunderstandthe conditions under which these changes occur, their effect on functional vision, and the different strategies to cope effectively.
- Use sun lenses of different transmissions to *simulate dim or nighttime conditions,* if an immediate evaluation is called for and is not possible in these conditions at the time of your evaluation.

O&M specialists can also assess the effectiveness of different light sources (e.g., fluorescent, incandescent, overhead, and natural light) for near tasks, such as reading maps, bus schedules, or menus. The student can be advised to carry a small, portable flashlight in addition to portable magnifying devices such as microscopic reading glasses or hand or stand magnifiers.

It is important to keep in mind that students are constantly dealing with the changing effects of a variety of everyday lighting situations, and require different strategies for varying conditions, including the use of nonvisual cues when vision is not effective enough for making sound mobility decisions.

A number of references provide more extensive coverage of low vision mobility. *The Interdisciplinary Approach to Low Vision Rehabilitation* (Beliveau-Tobey & Smith, 1980) offers techniques for enhancement of unaided vision, instruction with telescopes, and environmental modifications to increase visual efficiency. *A Curriculum for Teaching Clients to Use Landmarks while Traveling* (MacWilliam, 1980) provides instruction in the use of visual landmarks. *Beyond Arm's Reach* (Smith & O'Donnell, 1991) is a sequential curriculum for enhancing distance visual efficiency. *Suggested Curriculum for Distance Vision Training with Optical Aids* (Wiener & Vopata, 1980) presents a curriculum for introducing handheld telescopes for mobility.

Whether the students are children or adults, the O&M specialist helps provide the tools for them to enhance mobility performance by concentrating on their visual capabilities, and incorporating these within the broader array of nonvisual techniques, including the use of other senses and assistive devices such as the long cane and electronic travel devices. This combination of visual and nonvisual information affords the person a more complete understanding of the environment from which more comfortable, efficient, pleasurable, and safe mobility skills can emerge.

OPTICAL DEVICES FOR MOBILITY

In the broadest of contexts, mobility involves near, intermediate, and distance activities. Optical devices support the student in completing a variety of mobility activities, from near to far. They are categorized as near, intermediate, and distance devices. As the distance requirements of a task change, the optical device is usually changed. Although this statement is not true for more advanced optical systems, it is true for most devices that mobility students obtain through a local low vision clinic.

Types of Magnification

The purose for using magnification is to make the perceived image large enough on the retina so that the image can be resolved by the brain. While the functional experience of magnification is always the same (i.e., the size of the image is increased), there are four different types of magnification: (1) relative size magnification, (2) relative distance magnification, (3) angular magnification, and (4) electro-optical magnification.

Relative size magnification does not require lenses; this involves simply changing the actual size of the image so as to make it more visible. The most common example of relative size magnification is large print.

Relative distance magnification involves bringing the object closer to the eye. As the distance from the eye to the object decreases, the size of the image on the retina increases. For example, when trying to read a street sign, if the sign cannot be seen from the opposite side of the street, the student can cross the street, getting closer to the street sign. In a reading example, when a student uses a pair of high plus reading eyeglasses, the distance to the reading material is closer, and the primary effect of the eyeglasses is to focus the image from the reading material onto the retina.

Angular magnification involves combining lenses, and at times prisms and lenses, to optically increase the apparent size of an image. This is the type of magnification that occurs within a telescope.

Electro-optical magnification involves the basic principle of magnification (increasing size) in combination with the advantages of cameras and television. The most common example of electro-optical magnification is the closed-circuit television (CCTV).

Magnifiers and Telemicroscopes

The common optical devices for near activities are handheld magnifiers, stand magnifiers, and reading microscopes (see Figure 3.11). These devices have a critical fixed distance at which they will focus (usually between $\frac{1}{4}$ and 3 inches). If the device is not held at the exact distance, images will not be in focus. Auxiliary lighting is typically required when working with these devices in the form of a flex-arm lamp or by having a source of illumination incorporated into the design.

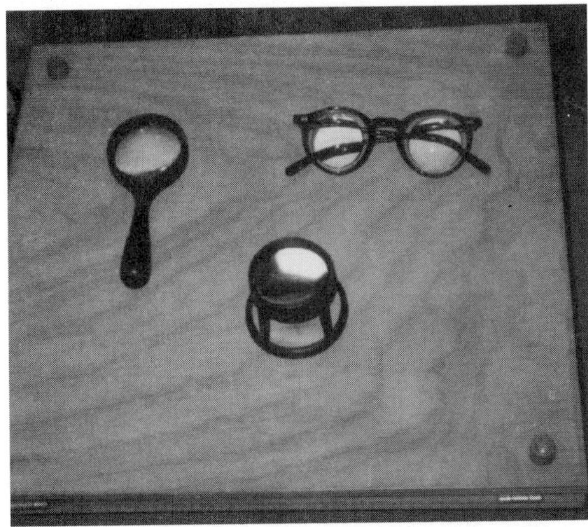

Figure 3.11. Examples of optical devices that magnify images.

Intermediate devices are known as *telemicroscopes,* as they have the characteristic of telescopes for distance viewing and the characteristic of microscopes for viewing small details (see Figure 3.12). The intermediate working distance offered by this device is of particular importance for tasks that involve safety such as looking at the side of a bus which has stopped to discharge passengers. The primary disadvantages of telemicroscopes include a critical depth of focus for near tasks (if it is less than $\frac{1}{4}$ inch too close or too far, the image is blurred) and a small field of view.

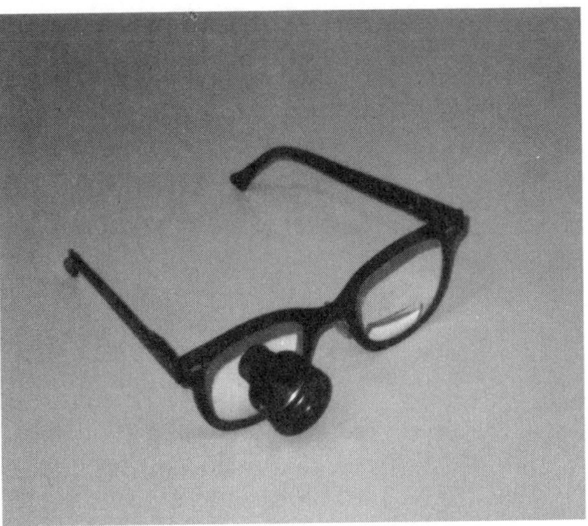

Figure 3.12. Telemicroscopes enhance distance viewing and the perception of detail.

Telescopes

Because the majority of students with low vision have reduced visual acuity, the most common optical device the O&M specialist will work with is the telescope. Telescopes can be handheld or mounted in a spectacle (see Figure 3.13).

There are advantages and disadvantages to both handheld and spectacle-mounted telescopes, although which one is selected will depend primarily on the student's goals and motivation.

The primary advantages of the handheld telescope is the ease with which it can be purchased from a low vision specialist or catalog. Telescopes are now very small, making them lightweight and cosmetically appealing. If the student is not well motivated or is unsure of when to use the telescope, the handheld telescope may be the preferred device. By comparison, the spectacle-mounted telescope is usually placed very close to the eye, offering an increased field of view; is quick and easy to use; and, for the student who is seeking a driver's license, is the only optical device approved for drivers with low vision. In addition, the student's prescriptive lenses can be incorporated into the telescope. The primary disadvantages are its cosmetic effect, as the device is quite noticeable; its relatively high cost as compared to the handheld telescope; and the difficulty of finding an eye care specialist who is skilled in prescribing the system.

With both the handheld and spectacle-mounted telescopes the student must stand still when using the telescope, as the image may be blurred if the user is moving; the visual field is severely restricted and safe travel can be compromised. The exception to this is driving, where it is possible to use a spectacle-mounted telescope safely while operating a motor vehicle. As pedestrians, students are commonly instructed to stop to use the telescope to reduce blur and attain maximum acuity.

Telescopes for students with low vision have the same functional optical characteristics as the binoculars used by baseball fans or birdwatchers. They improve visual acuity while re-

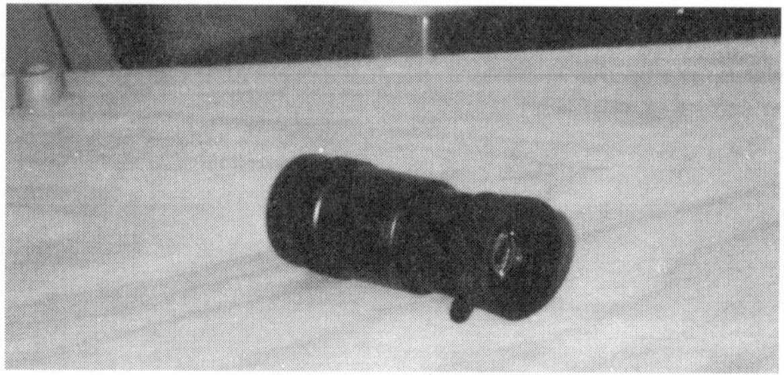

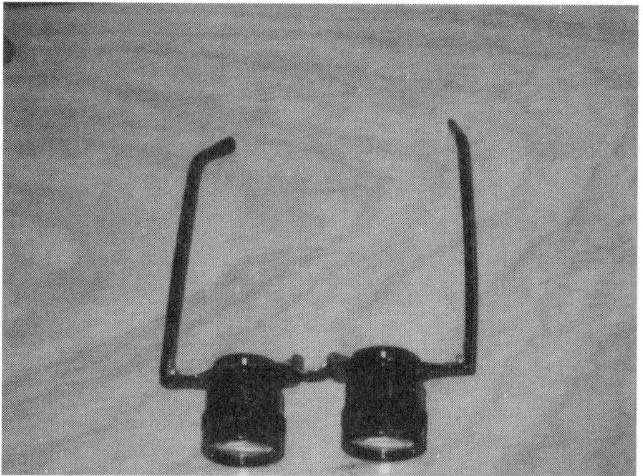

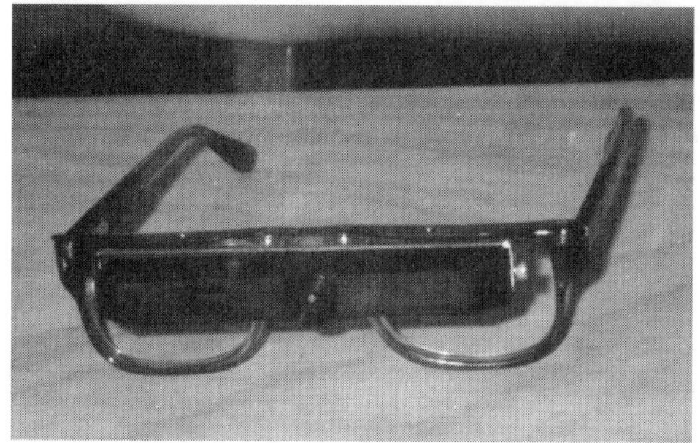

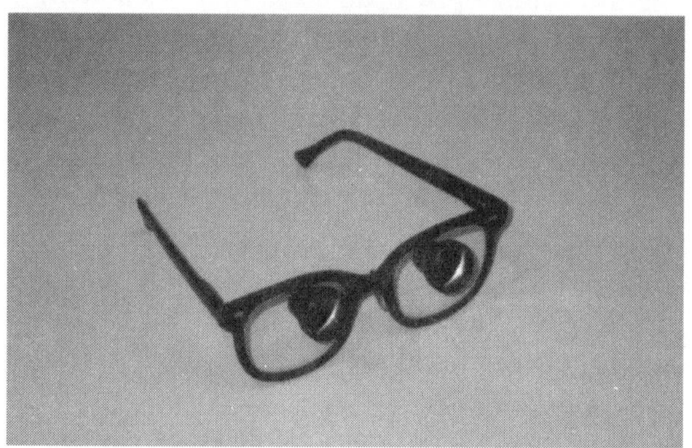

Figure 3.13. Four examples of telescopes, both handheld and mounted.

ducing the visual field. In general, the higher the magnification, the smaller the visual field. Telescopes also typically reduce the amount of light entering the eye. To best address the needs of students with low vision, manufacturers produce monoculars because few students with low vision have equal acuities in both eyes; they instead use one eye at a time or see with a dominant eye. The advantages of monoculars are reduced weight, smaller size, and lower cost. Monoculars are designed to fit discretely in the hand, improving its cosmetic appearance. Most monoculars sold today have one primary optical difference from binoculars, the ability to focus at close range. These are known as short-focus telescopes. Although both binoculars and monoculars can focus at far distances, standard binoculars cannot focus closer than approximately 5 to 10 feet. Monoculars with the short-focus feature, however, can focus as close as 10 inches. This feature is particularly useful for mobility purposes as it allows the student to accomplish short-term reading without an additional optical reading device. For example, the same telescope that enables the student to read the bus number or street sign can also be used to read menus or small print on bus schedules.

The optical characteristics of telescopes fall into two primary categories: Galilean, also known as terrestrial telescopes, and Keplerian, or astronomical telescopes. The Galilean telescope, named for its inventor, Galileo, contains a plus and minus lens with an airspace between them. The advantages of the Galilean telescope are a large field of view, the ease with which it focuses (known as depth of focus), and the low purchase price. The disadvantage is that they are not commonly prescribed in high powers, generally not over 3×.

The Keplerian telescope, also named for its inventor, Kepler, consists of a series of lenses and prisms which have high amounts of magnification (up to 10×), a rapidly changing and critical depth of focus, and a higher cost. The other main feature of the newer astronomical telescopes is known as extra-short focus. The standard telescope cannot focus closer than 6 to 10 feet; any object that is closer than these distances will be blurry. The extra-short focus enables the user to focus to distances as close as 10 inches. Thus the extra-short focus telescope can be used for short-term or spot reading for menus, addresses, phone numbers, and so on.

Two relationships will affect the student's ability to use the telescope: the relationship between the power of the telescope and the field of view, and the relationship between the distance of the target and the field of view. The general approach for addressing reduced visual acuity is to make the image bigger. The larger the image, the easier it is to see it. Following this logic, the bigger the better. However, while seeing objects is easily accomplished with telescopes, finding objects is the challenge. The problems associated with finding objects are related to the field of view. It is important to remember that the higher the power of the telescope, the smaller the field of view, and the closer the target, the smaller the field of view. These relationships are critical to the successful use of the telescope, since the telescope's ease of use is a function of the field of view. For example, a student who needs a 4× telescope should not be using a 6× telescope since it has a smaller field of view, therefore creating more difficulties with localization.

Visual Field Enhancement Devices

The mobility student with good visual acuity and severely restricted visual fields has a different problem that is addressed by different types of optical devices. Two of the more common optical approaches for students with severely restricted visual fields are reverse telescopes and fresnel prisms. The *reverse telescope* is based on the same concept as the fish-eye lens in the door of a hotel room: minifying the image enables the student with a restricted visual field to "see" farther toward the side where peripheral vision is no longer functioning.

A *Fresnel prism* is a series of prisms compressed into a transparent, thin, plastic membrane. It is placed on the lens of a pair of eye-

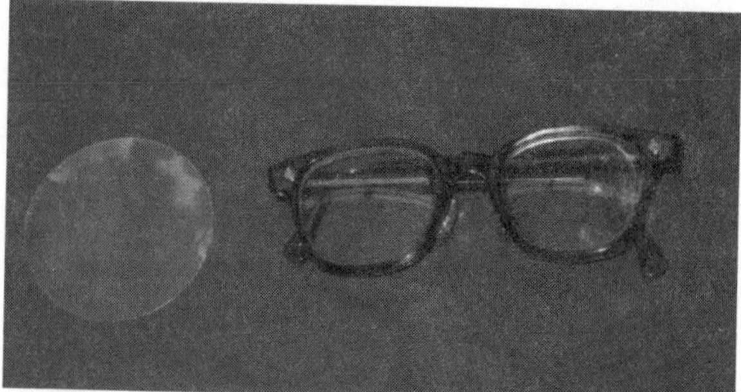

Figure 3.14. A Fresnel prism is a series of plastic prisms applied to regular eyeglasses to help correct the wearer's peripheral vision loss.

glasses, in the area corresponding to the nonfunctional field of view. The basic philosophy of this approach is the recognition that a student with severely restricted visual fields, despite the amount of head or eye movement, cannot take in information fast enough to absorb what is necessary for safe and efficient travel. With a Fresnel prism placed on the periphery of a lens, the student with peripheral field loss glances behind the prism and can see objects 80–90 degrees over to the side. This is because light rays are displaced by the prism, causing objects at the side to be displaced in toward the viewer (see Figure 3.14).

Nonoptical Devices

Nonoptical devices can also have a significant effect on the use of remaining vision. A review of the functional problems associated with the common visual pathologies reveals that lighting is the major issue with which students have to manage. The O&M specialist can provide important information and materials on nonoptical solutions to this primary functional problem. Sun lenses are the most common approach to light adjustment. Today a number of companies produce sun lenses that are especially designed to meet the needs of the student with low vision. Their design affords the student maximum protection from ultraviolet and infrared light entering from the most disabling angles, the top and side. For example, light from above or light from the side is usually more disabling than light that enters the

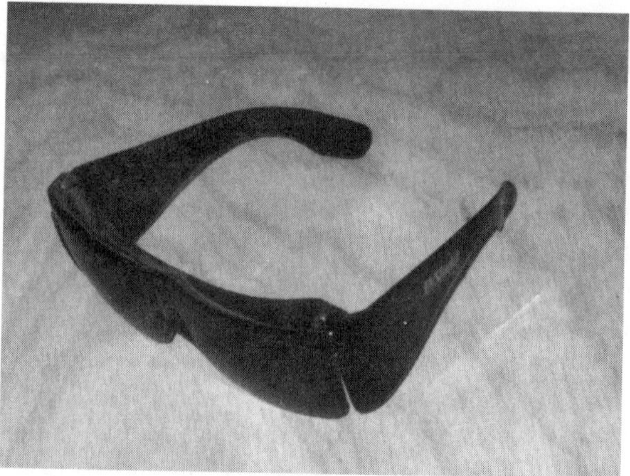

Figure 3.15. Lighting can present many problems for some individuals with low vision. Special sun lenses can be used to shield the wearer from light, particularly from above or from the sides.

eye straight on. Thus the design characteristic of top and side shields is an important benefit for the student with low vision. They are available in a variety of colors ranging from yellow and amber to green and gray. The grade of tint can also vary widely from allowing as much as 40% to as little as 1% of total light to pass through the lens (see Figure 3.15). The primary disadvantage of these lenses is their appearance. They are large and not particularly stylish. This leads some people to resist the design advantages and to maintain their current pair of sunglasses. In this case the use of a baseball cap, sunhat, or visor will complement the sunglasses, or, if worn alone, will assist in limiting the effects of glare, especially from above.

At the other extreme is the situation of insufficient light. Auxiliary light sources range from lights on a keychain for spotting purposes to standard flashlights. One product specifically marketed for students who experience night blindness is the Wide Angle Mobility Light (WAML). The WAML is actually a diver's light that provides a very wide and bright beam, which are its advantages. The disadvantage is its size and weight. The unit is approximately the size of a Volkswagen headlight and requires a shoulder harness to reduce the weight in the user's hand.

The long cane is also considered a useful nonoptical device for the student with low vision. The biggest concerns for most travelers with low vision is falling or tripping. As an O&M specialist, you may observe students looking down most of the time. The visual posture of looking down affects orientation skills and can affect the safety of the student who is not attending to visual information from the side. One primary feature of the long cane is surface preview (i.e., the identification of drop-offs). When used for touch technique, the long cane locates drop-offs, and students can use their vision to scan the entire environment. This affords greater safety and enhanced orientation. The development of an effective touch technique allows the student the opportunity to visually scan the entire environment, with the long cane dedicated to locating surface changes such as drop-offs, textures, slopes, and so on.

INSTRUCTIONAL CONSIDERATIONS FOR LOW VISION MOBILITY

Basic Introduction to Teaching the Use of Telescopes

In comparison to optical devices for reading, the telescope, whether handheld or spectacle-mounted, is relatively simple to teach. This is because of the optical characteristics of telescopes, particularly the ease of maintaining and changing focus, and because many students have prior experiences with binoculars. Additionally, as young children many of us took the paper towel tube and "played pirate," experiencing one of the primary functional characteristics of telescopes, a reduced visual field.

Instruction with telescopes involves six basic steps: (1) familiarization, (2) localization, (3) focusing, (4) scanning, (5) tracing, (6) tracking.

The purpose of instruction with a telescope is to familiarize the student with its structure and focusing mechanism, offer tips on the five skills (localization, focusing, scanning, tracing, and tracking), and suggest a few strategies for increasing the ease of use and problem solving when problems arise. Many adults may already be familiar with telescopes and require little to no instruction. The following section is designed for those unfamiliar with telescopes, particularly children.

Familiarization

The development of a common nomenclature is critical. The student should be able to identify the various parts of the telescope so that a common language can be used. Begin with the student visually and tactilely identifying the *ocular* (closest to the eye) and *objective* (closest to the target) lenses. Without looking through the telescope, the student should demonstrate the full range of the focusing mechanism. Two key points are being made. First, recognize whether the student is either looking through the telescope or listening to your instructions. From the point of view of the student, the magnified image is usually more interesting than your instructions. Initially, talking should occur only when the telescope is away from the eye. Second, when the student is holding the telescope to his or her eye, a common difficulty is turning the focusing mechanism through its full range. Introducing the motor skills of focusing when the student is not looking though the telescope can facilitate the transition to focusing while viewing through the telescope. This approach allows the student to experience the full range of turning the focusing mechanism from far left to far right both with and without viewing through the telescope.

Localization and Stabilization

This involves alignment of the eye, telescope, and object. Experience suggests that the majority of students will be able to find and localize a target through the telescope. The concept of looking for the object without the telescope, then identifying the object through the telescope is important for the acquisition of this skill. Many students begin to localize an object by immediately looking through the telescope. Because of the magnified image and restricted visual field of the telescope, this can make finding the object more difficult. Teach the student to look for the object without the telescope. Once the object, or an area where it is most likely situated, has been grossly identified, the telescope can be placed in front of the eye for positive identification. If localization is a problem, it is typically caused by one of three reasons:

1. The student cannot find or maintain a straight line of the eye-telescope-target;
2. The student has motor difficulties that impair her ability to control the telescope; or
3. The student has a large scotoma and is not eccentrically viewing.

Stabilization is the ability to maintain the image in the telescope once the target is localized. Stabilization requires the student to maintain a steady balance and consistent grip, which may sometimes require the student to rest his or her elbows on a hard surface or hold the telescope with both hands. While stable, the student has the best visual acuity and the greatest opportunity to see the target.

Focusing

Begin with a brief review of the motor skill required to focus the telescope. Once an object is successfully localized, the student turns the focusing mechanism slightly to the right. Determine if the image has increased or decreased in clarity. If the image has increased in clarity, continue with another turn to the right. Continue this pattern until the image is worse. Instruct the student to next turn the focusing mechanism slightly to the left which is, in fact, returning to the previous focus. The general concept taught here is that the identification of best focus is achieved by turning the focusing mechanism in the direction that improves the image. Once the image starts to blur, the focusing mechanism is rotated to return to the prior focus, which provides the sharpest image. A good analogy is the tuning of an analog radio: most people tune a station by passing the best reception, then returning to the strongest signal.

The second concept relates the distance of the target to the length of the telescope. The short-focus telescope can vary its length by a factor of approximately 2×. For example, a 4× short-focus telescope, when used for distance purposes, is approximately 3 inches in length. This same telescope can extend to 6 inches when used for reading something at a short distance. The rule of thumb to teach the student is: the closer the target, the longer the telescope. Conversely, the farther the target, the shorter the telescope. This rule is especially important for targets that are 5 feet or closer. In general, the student will localize distance targets with the telescope extended slightly (less than $\frac{1}{4}$ inch). Once the target is localized, the focus can be refined. As the target gets closer and closer, the student engages the short-focus mechanism by extending the length of the telescope until the desired focus is achieved.

Scanning

The key concept for successful scanning is the importance of being *systematic*. Strategies for teaching or improving scanning skills are the development of different scanning patterns, depending on the location and orientation of the target. This orientation can benefit students who know the primary orientation of the target they are attempting to find. For example, the pole that holds a street sign has a primarily vertical orientation. Thus scanning in the opposite, or horizontal, direction will provide the quickest approach to locating the pole. The opposite is also true: if the student is looking for the name of a business along a building line, scanning vertically will allow the quickest approach to *locating* signs, while scanning horizontally facilitates *reading* each sign.

Tracing

Visual tracing involves following one or more stationary lines in the environment. It is a precursor for tracking moving people or vehicles. Students are asked to view through the telescope while moving their heads to trace along lines such as baseboards, grasslines, and so on. Students can also trace along the outlines of houses, furniture, and storefronts.

Tracking

This skill involves maintaining a consistent alignment of the eye, telescope, and the object being viewed while the object is moving. Tracking is easiest when looking at objects at a far distance. The closer an object to the student, the more challenging the tracking task. This is because of the relationship between functional visual field and distance. When viewed through a telescope, objects are magnified but only with a limited field of view. The greater the distance between the telescope and the object, the greater the amount of the object that will be seen through the telescope. As an object gets closer, the acuity will increase while the amount of the object seen will decrease.

Environmental Sequencing and Instructional Considerations

The teaching approach with telescopes involves five basic skills and the appropriate sequencing of the environmental and visual environmental factors to enhance the successful development of those skills. When teaching the use of the long cane, the basic skill of touch technique is often isolated and practiced until a basic level of competence is achieved. The skill of touch technique is then applied to indoor and outdoor, residential and small and large business environments. This same approach works well when introducing telescopes. Specifically begin the observation and teaching of concepts indoors. As success is demonstrated, move to an outdoor residential and then a business environment. An exception to this rule is when students require the increased lighting experienced outdoors before they are able to use the telescope effectively.

Target selection is critical to the successful development of these skills. Three variables should be considered when selecting targets: (1) size, (2) distance, and (3) contrast.

The importance of *size* is self-evident. In general, the larger the target, the easier it is to see or read. There is a constant inverse relationship between size and *distance.* As distance decreases, relative size increases. As distance increases, relative size decreases. Therefore size and viewing distance are both considered when selecting targets. The third variable, *contrast,* is essential for viewing a target and can be more important than size. For example, with camouflage (which is a form of low contrast) it is possible to hide large objects, while a single candle on an overcast night (high contrast) can be seen from great distances. For mobility purposes the higher the contrast, the more quickly the target will be located and identified. Pay particular attention to figure–ground relationship of targets and their location.

The eye care specialist will typically prescribe a telescope that achieves 20/20 to 20/40 visual acuity. This is the amount of clarity required to view most street signs and bus numbers from a distance. At times the visual field of the higher power telescopes will be too restrictive for the beginning student to even localize a target. This may result in the student's ability to read the sign clearly, but the student may have difficulty in finding the sign. The eye care specialist's role is to provide the necessary magnification for the student to see signs. It is our job, as O&M specialists, to teach the skills necessary for the student to find the sign. Some students will simply not be able to localize a sign with a 6× or more powerful telescope. In this situation, reduce the power of the telescope for the purpose of instruction. For example, working with a 2.8× or 4× telescope will give the student a larger field of view, making localization, tracing, tracking, and scanning easier to accomplish. This is analogous to lifting weights: if a student cannot lift 100 pounds, the teacher will begin with 25 pounds and work toward a goal of 100 pounds. The same is true with telescopes. Selecting a low power telescope and working to the high power telescope develops skills and gives the student the basis for a successful experience. Recognize that a low power telescope reduces visual acuity. Therefore either larger targets need to be selected or the student must be closer to the target to resolve its image.

Many people wear prescriptive lenses, including students with low vision. When a student tries to look through a telescope while wearing prescriptive lenses, two problems often occur. First is the absence of eye/telescope information that is received when the telescope is placed directly against the cheek and skin surrounding the eye. Second is the reduced field of view caused by the increased distance from the eye to the telescope. Often students will independently solve this problem by simply removing their eyeglasses, increasing eye/telescope information and increasing the visual field.

Basic Introduction to Fresnel Prisms

The student with good visual acuity but severely constricted visual fields (less than 10 degrees) may experience serious problems with mobility. Frequently this student cannot turn her eyes or head fast enough to obtain the information needed for safe travel. For example, when the student with severely restricted visual fields is looking left, she does not obtain information from straight ahead or to the right, the functional result of her visual field loss. When looking straight ahead, she does not see things to the left or right. Thus this student is missing significant portions of critical information needed for safe mobility.

Fresnel prisms specifically address the problem of eye scanning by assisting the student in obtaining information from a much larger area of the visual field with only a slight increase in eye movement. As explained before with eye scanning, the Fresnel prism provides a functional view of objects off to the side in the 80–90 degree area for a total field of approximately 160 degrees, if the prisms are worn bilaterally. Fresnel prisms therefore enable the student to obtain significantly more peripheral information quickly and efficiently.

The keys to success with Fresnel prisms include:

1. A highly motivated student who bumps into objects because of visual field constriction.
2. Good visual acuity (20/100 or better) and severely constricted visual field (less than 10 degrees).
3. Accurate placement of the prism that reflects the natural eye scanning patterns of the student.
4. Sequential instruction for adapting to the displacement of objects that occurs when viewing through the prism.
5. Sequential exposure to increasingly complex and crowded travel environments.

The instructional program involves establishing a baseline of natural eye and head scanning so the prism can be placed on the lens temporally enough to be outside of the student's natural eye scanning. This approach enhances the student's natural scanning ability by encouraging increased scanning. It also allows the student to control viewing through the prism. The only time the student will see objects through the prism is when a definite increase in scanning to the side occurs. This reduces visual confusion and problems with double vision.

As with all mobility instruction, sequencing of the environment is critical to a positive experience and ultimately a successful outcome. The sequence begins with indoor seated activities that introduce the student to the effects of the displacement of objects while looking through the prism. As the student becomes more accurate touching objects while viewing through the prism, movement can be introduced. Beginning in quiet hallways and gradually working toward shopping malls or cafeterias increases complexity, while building on positive experiences. These indoor experiences will involve frequent viewing through the prism and touching objects to connect the apparent visual location of objects with their actual location. As the student demonstrates successful adaptation to object displacement, outdoor travel in increasingly complex areas can be introduced. Through frequent comparisons of both straight ahead and prism vision, and, when possible, touching to confirm the location of objects, the student can gradually adapt to the effects of displacement. Ultimately, improved mobility will be demonstrated as the student is capable of efficiently scanning for information in the far periphery with a simple eye scan. Evaluation and training lesson plans for Fresnel prism use are detailed in Smith and Geruschat (1983).

Driving with Low Vision

Obtaining a driver's license is a rite of passage for most young adults. Similarly, losing a license because of visual loss often has an equal, yet negative impact on one's life and lifestyle. For the fastest growing segment of the low vision population, the elderly, driving is viewed as critical for autonomy and for avoiding social isolation (Corn & Sacks, 1994). Control of transportation has a major impact on many aspects of life.

In the United States, driving is controlled by each state. States permit driving with low vision either through legislation that specifically outlines the low vision requirements or by default where the law does not describe nor disallow driving with low vision. The standard in most states is to require a minimum of 20/40 visual acuity for obtaining a driver's permit and a license, with many states offering a restricted daytime-driving-only license for those with 20/70 visual acuity. Currently there are 26 states that allow driving with bioptic telescopes. This includes states in which driving with low vision is possible, either because of a specific law or by default.

The most commonly asked question regarding driving with low vision relates to the issue of driving safely with less than 20/20 or 20/40 visual acuity. Examination of the visual requirements of driving suggests that peripheral vision dominates the driving task, with good acuity a requirement for relatively specific activities. For example, staying in the correct lane, and seeing traffic flow of oncoming vehicles and vehicles on cross streets involves more peripheral rather than central vision. Good central visual acuity is important for specific activities such as identifying traffic controls at intersections, reading information signs on expressway exits, and determining whether the small brown item on the road ahead is a paper bag or a small dog. In recognition of the fact that the majority of driving occurs in familiar areas, most drivers use more visible landmarks, rather than informational signs and the location and type of traffic controls are known, leaving the unexpected event as the primary area of need for good visual acuity. Thus, it could be argued that approximately 90 percent of all driving involves peripheral vision, with good acuity required for the remaining 10 percent (Huss, 1988).

Further documentation that 20/40 visual acuity is not required for safe driving occurs on a daily basis. Driving in early evening as the sun sets, at night, and on rainy days are a few examples of the frequency with which driving occurs with reduced visual acuity. Physiological factors also contribute to functionally reduced vision. For example, the older driver is more sensitive to glare, does not recover as quickly from rapid changes in light, and does not see as well at night compared to the younger driver. Thus, although driving does require vision, an analysis of the task from a visual point of view indicates that peripheral vision is more involved than central vision, and that an acuity requirement of 20/40 is not required for safe driving, as documented by the safe driving of many older drivers and by all drivers ability to drive in less-than-ideal environmental conditions.

The use of a bioptic telescope enables many students with low vision to drive. The telescope is used for specific situations that require good visual acuity. Think of the telescope as being similar to a rearview mirror: the driver periodically looks in the rearview mirror and specifically looks at critical times—when changing lanes, braking, and turning. The bioptic telescope is used in a very similar fashion, although identifyication of traffic controls, unknown objects, traffic sign information, and landmarks constitute the majority of its use. At all other times drivers with low vision use their regular vision to drive. Although their vision is less than 20/40 during the day, this in many cases may be analogous to the driving experience of those with good visual acuity who drive at night.

The role of the O&M specialist in driving with bioptics has been evolving. The traditional role was to provide instruction on the use of the bioptic telescope, including training in bioptic use with the student as a passenger in a car. As skills with the telescope developed, referral to a driver's education program was often recommended. This role has now expanded in some facilities so that agencies for those who are blind and visually impaired now offer comprehensive instructional programs in the area of driving with bioptics (Huss, 1984, 1988).

THE O&M SPECIALIST'S ROLE WITH OPTICAL DEVICES

The array of optical devices to enhance mobility is as broad as the wide range of visual tasks that make up the mobility experience. Traditionally O&M specialists are associated with distance vision activities and distance optical devices such as telescopes; however, many near tasks such as reading maps, bus and subway schedules, and phone numbers are germane to the mobility experience.

It is the O&M specialist's role to familiarize the student with the prescribed optical devices and to offer instruction with near, distance, and field enhancement devices. The role of the O&M specialist entails assuring that devices which have been prescribed in the ideal clinical setting can be used effectively in the real world, where less-than-ideal conditions are experienced.

Understanding Low Vision (Jose, 1983) offers more in-depth treatment of this topic. It discusses low vision optics and instructional strategies with near, intermediate, and distance optical devices. *The Interdisciplinary Approach to Low Vision Rehabilitation* (Beliveau-Tobey & Smith, 1980) presents assessment and instructional strategies in low vision.

LOW VISION MOBILITY ISSUES

Although a number of questions in low vision mobility have emerged over this field's short history, two of the more common involve the use of the long cane by persons with low vision and instruction while blindfolded for students with low vision.

Canes and Vision

"Should my student use a cane or use vision?" "Why not use both?" may be the most appropriate answer, as opposed to choosing one at the exclusion of the other. When the O&M specialist is teaching a student with low vision, instruction in the use of a long cane as well as the use of existing vision is often recommended.

A long cane actually facilitates visual efficiency, freeing the student to use vision for decision making, orientation, and aesthetic purposes. Without the cane, vision is frequently used to gaze downward for depth perception concerns such as steps, curbs, and terrain changes. This affects the overall safety of the person, who is not attending to visual information from the side. Additionally, just as the use of other senses should be stressed, the use of a long cane becomes one more compensatory mechanism to augment independent mobility.

Some people with greater amounts of vision may only require the cane for night travel, or in unfamiliar areas, or for travel in conditions of dim lighting or heavy glare. Others may benefit from its more consistent use during travel. Emphasis is placed on teaching the student when to use the cane, or when visual and other sensory cues are sufficient for safe mobility.

If the individual is receptive, the authors suggest that the use of a long cane, in conjunction with vision, offers a greater assurance of travel ease and safety. As previously stated, it also enables the student to be more proactive in decision making and, ultimately, more confident and independent in mobility.

Blindfolding

To blindfold or not to blindfold? This question represents a long-standing controversy in the field of O&M. Surveys of O&M specialists (Smith, 1976, 1990) have demonstrated a 50/50 to 30/70 split of opinion as to whether or not blindfolds should be used on a regular or periodic basis, or not at all.

Proponents of blindfolding on a regular basis believe that it builds confidence, develops important nonvisual skills, and helps people realize that they can travel independently regardless of the extent of remaining vision. Some feel blindfolding is an important tool to prepare students for eventual blindness, and for building their skills as soon as possible. Other O&M specialists use blindfolds to simulate nighttime travel or help sharpen other sensory skills. Some use blindfolds at street crossings to refine traffic and crossing judgments and build confidence in students' abilities to handle potentially dangerous mobility situations.

Those who do not use blindfolds believe that this process, in fact, ignores the student's vision, and that visual override will occur when the blindfold is removed. They think it is important to teach students under the low vision circumstances they will be experiencing in their everyday lives. Some use dark filters or partial occlusion to simulate evening conditions if night lessons are not possible. Others do not use blindfolds because of some students' fear of total blindness, and the difficult psychosocial overlay that complicates blindfold use, rather than facilitating the O&M instructional process.

It is important not to view blindfolding as an "either we do or do not use them" process. In some cases, if the student is willing, blindfolding can enhance other sensory training, particularly judging traffic sounds and alignment skills. In some instances, it can be effective in helping the student concentrate on specific cane skills. In still other circumstances, it can provide students who are curious about whether they could maneuver independently without vision, an opportunity to experiment and gain confidence in this area.

The judicious use of blindfolds should be considered for these purposes, as long as the student does not object or fear their use. In addition, after training in areas such as sensory development or street crossing skills, it is important to follow or interweave training in the combined use of vision and other sensory skills. This is critical, as vision usually dominates, and students will need skills in acting on their visual interpretations. The majority, if not all, of the training should emphasize the evaluation and use of existing vision and skills for determining when vision is or is not reliable for mobility judgments. Generally, the student who is trained in a combined use of sensory input is the student who will be better equipped to deal with all functioning senses.

FUTURE IMPLICATIONS

By definition, discussions of the future are rather speculative, at times a risk to the author. Nevertheless an attempt to look into the future, perhaps to the early part of the next century, may offer some guidance and support to those who are interested in advancing the field of low vision mobility.

Providers of mobility services need to objectively identify the problems of students with low vision, which then enables the O&M specialist to objectively measure improvements in travel through instruction. Unfortunately the literature is very limited, which leaves many questions unanswered. How do we measure the performance of mobility? Can the principles of testing and measurement, such as reliability and validity testing, be applied to measures of performance? Assuming there is a reduction of performance as eyesight decreases, how does this reduction of eyesight affect mobility performance? What is the exact nature of this problem? Literature reviewed earlier suggested that illumination and changes of depth were the variables that affected mobility, that is, they are the causes of bumping or stumbling. Are these the only variables that are affected? Can this reduction in performance be objectively measured? As the age of limited funding and questions regarding the effectiveness of O&M services continues, O&M specialists may feel increasing pressure to develop and apply standardized measures of pre- and post-instruction performance.

In the area of low vision technology, head-mounted displays have been recently introduced that may offer the potential for improving the mobility of students with low vision. Two systems will be briefly described: the Low Vision Enhancement System (LVES) manufactured by Visionics and a prototype device by Innoventions (Littleton, CO) (see Figure 3.16). LVES is a head-mounted display with three cameras, specifically two locating cameras that provide regular visual acuity and a single magnifying camera with variable magnification. The system is analogous to a head-mounted closed-circuit television. For mobility it offers two opportunities, control of illumination and variable magnification for distance viewing. To address the major problem with changing illumination for mobility with low vision, the LVES electronically maintains a consistent level of illumination regardless of the brightness or dimness of the actual environment. LVES also provides from 2× to 10× magnification. This variation is significant as the field of view with a low-power telescope is significantly larger and therefore easier to use than the field from a 10× telescope. Thus the student can vary magnification depending on the viewing distance and size of the target while maintaining maximum field of view by using the least amount of magnification required to view the target. The primary disadvantages of the LVES are cosmetics and restrictions of the visual field. According to the manufacturer, LVES has a fixed 50-degree visual field when no magnification is used. This may have significant implications on safe mobility be-

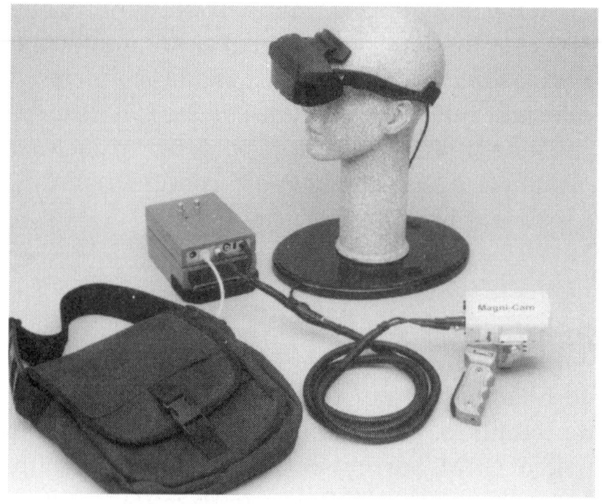

A

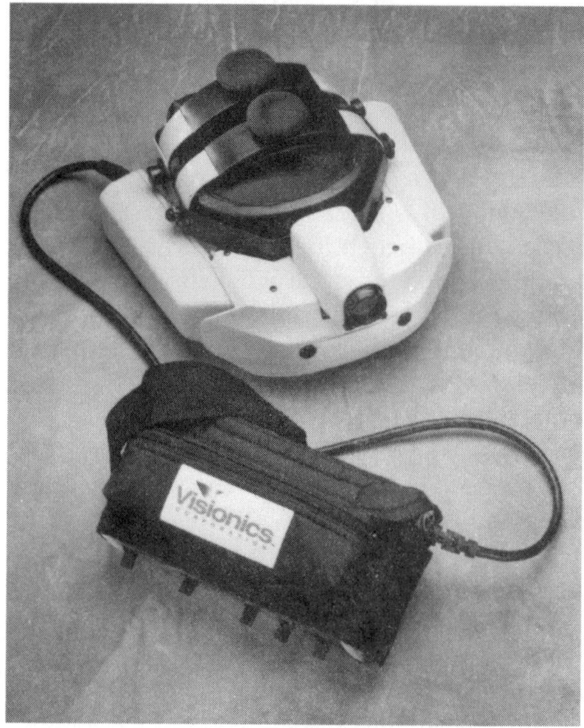

B

Figure 3.16. Two examples of head-mounted displays for persons with low vision: (A) the Low Vision Enhancement System; (B) the prototype device by Innoventions.

Source: Reproduced, with permission, from Visionics.

cause the student is always looking through LVES when wearing it, as the system surrounds the eyes. Studies are currently being conducted that will identify the positive and negative effects of both illumination and visual field on the potential mobility applications of LVES.

The prototype device from Innoventions is a head-mounted display connected to a small handheld camera. The system is lightweight, comfortable to wear, and provides unimpeded vision for the lower visual field, an important consideration for mobility. The user walks along using his regular vision by holding his head up, similiar to using a bioptic telescope. When an object needs to be magnified, the handheld camera is pointed toward the object, and the user looks into the glasses and sees the magnified image. This system has a 25-degree visual field when no magnification is used. This device can offer up to 12.5× magnification. Both the prototype device from Innoventions and LVES can enhance images electronically. For example, enhanced contrast, edge enhancement, and reverse polarity are all possible. At present, the LVES display is black and white, while the Innoventions device can be black and white or color, changed with a simple flip of a switch. Head-mounted displays offer an exciting new application with multiple opportunities for improved mobility. Other technologies offer potential for low vision mobility. Global Positioning Satellites (GPS) is a system that permits highly accurate definition to the user's position on Earth (see Chapter 9). At present, prototypes and models have been developed for experimental purposes for use with those who are totally blind. Although this technology may indeed offer opportunities for those who are totally blind, a more immediate benefit may be available to those with low vision. For example, a student may have excellent travel skills but may not be particularly skilled with a handheld or spectacle-mounted telescope. A voice output GPS that states "you are at 14th and Connecticut Avenues" would be of tremendous benefit.

Eye-tracking technology has been successfully applied to the mapping of scotomas in age-related maculopathy and recording the eye movements of persons with low vision while they read. As this technology becomes more portable, the application to mobility could help identify the critical environmental features to which a low vision traveler attends. Similarly, this technology might be applied to the development of standards related to the Americans with Disabilities Act and the types of environmental modifications that would be most helpful to the low vision traveler.

Although the population of persons with low vision has existed for a long time, the field of low vision mobility is less than three decades old. As the population ages, O&M specialists will be faced with burgeoning numbers of persons with low vision. Although we have gone beyond merely scratching the surface, the O&M profession has also have quite a way to go to achieve the legitimacy, stature, and research level to affirm that the mobility needs of the population of students with low vision are adequately identifed and significantly addressed.

Suggestions/Implications for O&M Specialists

1. Remaining vision offers both opportunities and challenges for the student with low vision. The O&M specialist needs to evaluate how the student functions with their remaining vision in a variety of settings.
2. The term *low vision* has many definitions—legal, clinical, educational, or international. The use of functional vision is actually along a continuum such that the student may experience difficulty with one visual requirement of mobility—reading a street sign, for example—yet is able to use remaining vision to see a curb.
3. Research and practice have identified the following common functional mobility problems for students with low vision: lighting and glare, changes in terrain and depth, unwanted contacts, and street crossings. The comprehensive mobility evaluation will evaluate all of these components.
4. There may be a significant difference between the mobility problems associated with reduced visual acuity and reduced visual fields. The O&M specialist will evaluate how these different conditions affect visual performance.
5. The clinical low vision assessment can offer important information when working with a student who has low vision. Visual acuity, visual fields, pathology, and refractive error are all important pieces of information for understanding the visual performance of the mobility student.
6. Eyeglasses can serve two very different purposes: to correct for refractive error or to magnify an image. It is important for the O&M specialist to know why eyeglasses have been prescribed and for what purpose, as magnifying eyeglasses can only be worn when seated and are for looking at very close distances.
7. The functional low vision mobility assessment begins with an interview. This interview establishes the student's needs and goals, identifies areas of self-reported problems and proficiency, and describes any previous O&M instruction.
8. Functional visual acuities and visual fields offer the O&M specialist insights into how the student is using remaining vision.
9. The environment plays a significant role in the student's ability to use remaining vision. Assessing the environment is therefore critical if the O&M specialist is to understand and anticipate the performance of their student.
10. The student with congenital vision loss does not have a visual memory and many visual concepts that the student with adventitious vision loss maintains. The O&M specialist may need to teach basic visual skills to the student with a congenital loss of vision, who has had no previous instruction.
11. Visual strategies such as eccentric viewing and monocular depth perception cues are useful skills for the student with low vision. The O&M specialist can teach these skills in a systematic method to improve the student's mobility performance.
12. Telescopes can assist the student with orientation by improving distance visual acuity for spotting purposes. The O&M specialist can provide a sequence of instruction to the student.

(*continued on next page*)

Suggestions/Implications for O&M Specialists (continued)

13. Nonoptical devices to control illumination can be provided by the O&M specialist.
14. For students with severely restricted visual fields and good visual acuity, reverse telescopes and Fresnel prisms may assist the student to increase visual scanning and widen the viewing area.
15. Driving with low vision is possible in many states. The O&M specialist can support this by teaching the use of bioptic telescopes, which then can be used with a driving instructor.
16. Electronic Travel Aids for low vision are still being developed. Head-mounted displays may provide an important contribution to improving the mobility of students with low vision.

ACTIVITIES FOR REVIEW

1. Describe the most frequently reported mobility problem areas for persons with low vision.
2. Describe the functional differences between travel with reduced visual acuity and travel with reduced visual fields.
3. List the five major components to a clinical low vision examination and explain the purpose of each?
4. Describe the various clinical visual fields and how they can be applied to assist the O&M specialist.
5. List the components of a functional low vision mobility assessment.
6. Define the three types of functional visual acuities, and describe how you would administer this section of a functional assessment.
7. Review the procedure for evaluation of the early warning visual field?
8. Describe the visual skills that form the basis for enhanced visual performance.
9. List and describe the principal skills to be developed when working with a handheld telescope.
10. Describe the four types of magnification, with one functional example for each type of magnification.

CHAPTER 4

Audition for the Traveler Who Is Visually Impaired

William R. Wiener and Gary D. Lawson

Chapter 3 of this volume explored the ways in which vision plays a central role in helping a person with low vision learn about the environment. In a similar way hearing, or audition, helps people without vision or with greatly reduced vision gain information about the environment. Audition is particularly important to persons with visual impairments not only because it facilitates spoken communication, but because it assists with orientation and mobility (O&M) as well. Hearing, like sight, is a distance sense that can provide information about objects with which one does not have direct contact. It helps one to appreciate depth by identifying the existence of space and the distance through space to a reflecting surface or a sound-emitting object. Hearing also enables comprehension of some of the characteristics of the environment. Auditory cues make it possible not only to determine and maintain one's position or orientation in the environment, but also to move independently, even in complex environments.

To determine and maintain one's position or orientation in the environment, an individual must be aware of self-to-object and object-to-object relationships. Hearing facilitates this awareness by providing information to help identify known landmarks and information points. In a public building, for example, a person may identify a sound from a ventilator fan that could signify one's position within a particular hallway. One's position relative to an elevator door can be determined by localizing the sound of the opening door. A person entering a room can learn to use reflected sound to determine whether the room is large or small and what type of furnishings are present. Once inside the room, reflected sound helps a person to avoid contact with obstacles or walls. Reflected sound may also provide the clue that the traveler is approaching the end of a corridor or a large object within the corridor. Similarly, walls and objects beside an individual can reflect sound that will make their presence known. Using this information, a visually impaired person can determine when a particular intersecting hallway is reached by noting the absence of reflected sound at the junction.

Hearing may be used also to determine the type of environment through which one is navigating outdoors. The sound of heavy traffic, for example, may identify a business area. The sound of moving and stationary vehicles make it possible to localize and identify one's position relative to a busy downtown intersection. Accelerating traffic parallel to one's direction of travel indicates that the light has changed, and it is safe to cross the street. At a residential intersection the absence of sound provides the necessary cue that it is safe to cross. One can determine position at a street corner by localizing the sounds of the cars stopped behind the crosswalk. One may be able to verify a position in the environment by identifying other sounds as well; for example, the sounds of children playing on a playground. The ability to make fine discriminations to differentiate between similar sounds also may enable the traveler to determine personal location more accurately. It may be useful, for example, to recognize that the sound heard is coming from the fan at the drugstore and not from the air conditioner at the restaurant next door.

In order to understand the auditory functioning of the person who is visually impaired, the O&M specialist must comprehend audition itself and the special uses of audition in independent travel. This chapter is therefore divided into four parts. The first part examines the physical and biological basis for hearing; the second focuses upon identifying, quantifying, and classifying hearing loss; the third covers the use of auditory skills by people who are visually impaired; and the fourth discusses how to facilitate the use of audition in the rehabilitation of people who are visually impaired.

FUNDAMENTALS OF SOUND AND AUDITION

Auditory perception unfolds as a child begins to associate meaning with various auditory stimuli and starts to seek out and classify sound. As the child matures, various perceptual skills emerge that make interpretation of acoustic information possible (Sanders, 1971; Gibson, 1966). Auditory perception includes such processes as awareness, recognition, discrimination, figure–ground perception, sound localization, closure, and perceptual constancy. The interpretation of sound is based not only on mechanical generation and biological reaction, but also upon active cognitive processes dependent upon the individual's past and present experiences. In order to more fully understand these issues of hearing development, one must first understand the basics of sound. This section provides an introductory definition and description of sound, an explanation of how hearing sensitivity is quantified by decibels and frequency, and a description of the structure and function of the auditory system. Later in the section "Development and Use of Special Auditory Skills" the development of hearing in a child is explored.

Characteristics of Sound

Sound Propagation

Sound may be defined as a disturbance in the density of the particles or masses in an elastic medium (e.g., air) through which the disturbance travels. In order for sound to occur, a sufficient force (push or pull) must be applied to a vibrator, which must transfer energy to particles in an elastic medium such as air.

When a force is applied to a tuning fork (i.e., a vibrating source), its tines (prongs) vibrate back and forth around their undisturbed positions, that is, their points of rest or equilibrium. This vibration disturbs the surrounding air, transferring energy from the vibrator to the air (see Figure 4.1). As the tines move away from each other toward nearby air particles, the particles are forced to move away from the tines toward more distant particles. As the displaced particles move away from their undisturbed positions, they create an area of reduced density and pressure in the medium (i.e., a *rarefaction*); as they approach nearby but more distant particles, the particles come closer together, creating an increase in the density and pressure of the medium (i.e., a *compression*).

Elasticity can be thought of as the medium's tendency to resist deformation or return to its original state after removal or reduction of a force. Imagine the elasticity of the medium as a series of springs connecting the particles together. As a vibrator pushes a particle away from the vibrator, the spring between the vibrator and the particle is stretched, creating a pull, and the spring between that particle and the next is compressed, creating a push. It is this elasticity or stretching and compressing of springs that causes the particles to move back and forth about their points of rest. Sound energy is transferred from one particle to the next as the particles vi-

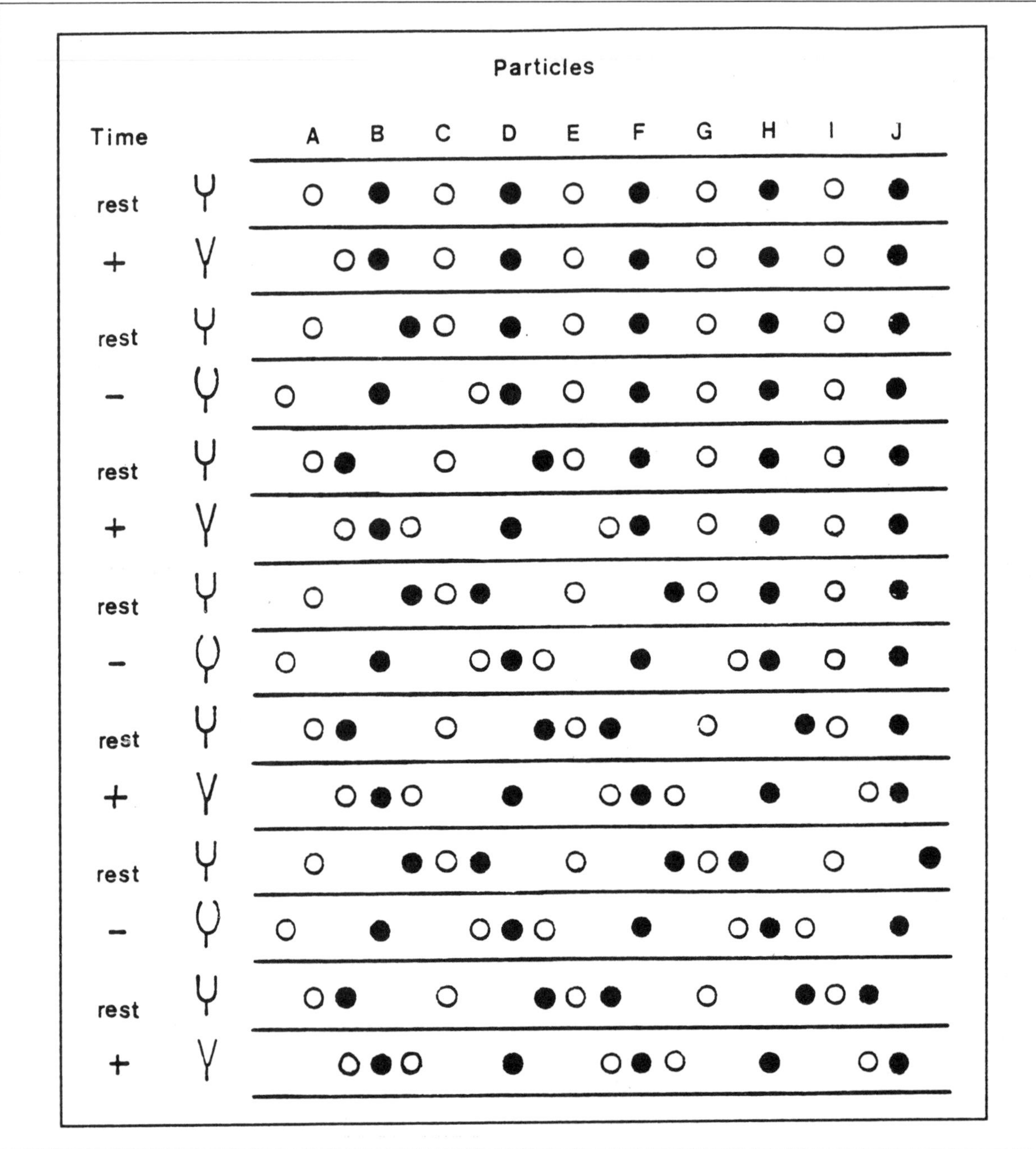

Figure 4.1. Displacement of individual air particles due to the vibratory motion of a tuning fork.
Source: Reprinted with permission from C. E. Speaks, *Introduction to Sound: Acoustics for the Hearing and Speech Sciences* (San Diego, CA: Singular Publishing Group, 1992), Fig. 1-3, p. 11.

brate around their points of rest. This is how sound moves from the source to a receiver.

Collectively, the particle vibrations create alternating concentric spheres of rarefactions and compressions (Figure 4.2). If undisturbed by objects or other sounds, energy that is transferred to the medium from the vibrator travels equally well in all directions; the strength of particle vibration,

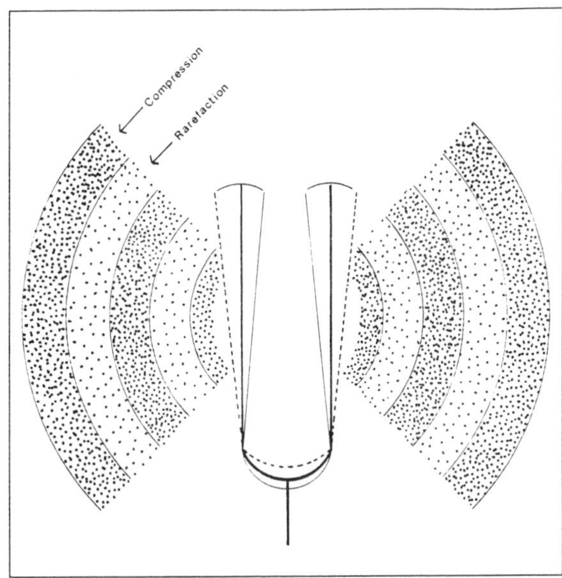

Figure 4.2. Alternate regions of compression (condensation) and rarefaction moving outward through an air mass, caused by the vibratory motion of a tuning fork.

Source: Reprinted with permission from C. E. Speaks, *Introduction to Sound: Acoustics for the Hearing and Speech Sciences* (San Diego, CA: Singular Publishing Group, 1992), Fig. 1-4, p. 13.

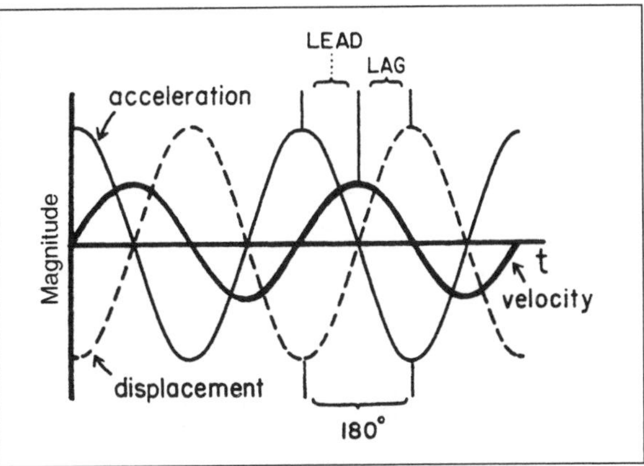

Figure 4.3. Decay of sound pressure with increasing distance from the source.

Source: Adapted from J. D. Durrant, "Simulation of Sound Waves on the Oscilloscope," *Journal of the Acoustic Society of America, 57* (1975), 1558–1559.

and therefore sound intensity, becomes weaker as distance from the vibrator increases.

The characteristics of the medium affect the speed of sound. The influence of density and elasticity is such that the speed of sound is typically faster in solids than in liquids and faster in liquids than in gases. The speed of sound is much slower (about 1/1,000,000th) than is the speed of light. Thus at great distances a sound source can be seen before it is heard. This is why we see lightning before we hear the accompanying thunder. With reduced vision, however, recognition of a sound may occur before it is visually perceived.

Intensity, Frequency, and Phase

Three important characteristics of sound are intensity, frequency, and phase (Martin, 1994). The *intensity* of a sound, perceived as loudness, is related to the amplitude of particle vibration—the distance a particle in the medium travels from its resting position during sound propagation. When the particle's amplitude of vibratory displacement is great, the intensity will also be great. Increased amplitude of displacement, and therefore increased intensity and increased loudness, is achieved when the energy moving the particles is increased. In a free field, sound intensity becomes predictably weaker as the distance from the sound source increases (Figure 4.3).

Frequency, perceived as pitch, is the rate of particle vibration or the number of compressions and rarefactions that take place within 1 second. It is related to *wavelength,* that is, the distance covered by one complete cycle of a sound wave. More short wavelengths than long wavelengths can occur in a unit of time. Thus, high frequencies are associated with short wavelengths and low frequencies with long wavelengths. In the past, frequency was described in cycles per second (cps). Currently frequency is measured in Hertz (Hz), after the German physicist Heinrich Hertz. If a tone is identified as having a frequency of 1,000 Hz, it is completing 1,000 compressions and rarefactions in 1 second. The time required to complete one cycle is called the *period.* Any tone that is composed of one and only one frequency is called a *pure tone.* Pure tones rarely exist in nature. It is more common to encounter complex sounds, which consist of many pure tones.

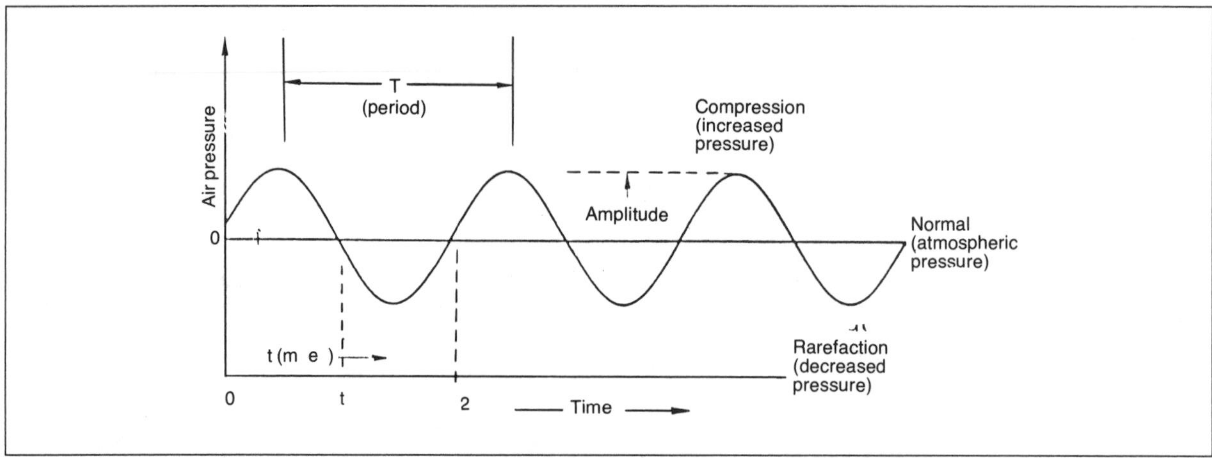

Figure 4.4. A sine function showing compressions and rarefactions in sound waves.
Source: From W. R. Wiener, "Audition." In R. L. Welsh & B. B. Blasch (Eds.), *Foundations of Orientation and Mobility* (New York: American Foundation for the Blind, 1980), Fig. 1-6, p. 119.

The *phase* of a sound refers to the position of a particle within its vibratory cycle or the position of pressure change that occurs within a complete cycle of a sound wave. Phase can be explained through a graphic representation of intensity and frequency over time. The points used to determine the curve shown in Figure 4.4 (a sine function) represent a mathematical description of the movement of particles in the medium as they vibrate around their positions of rest. This curve also can be used to represent compressions (pressure increases) and rarefactions (pressure decreases) in a sound wave over time. Compressions are represented by the upward or positive portions of the curves, while rarefactions are represented by the downward or negative portions of the curves. The height of the curve from the baseline represents a particle's amplitude of vibration or the sound's intensity. When the curve's peaks and valleys are closer together, more compressions and rarefactions occur within a given amount of time. Since a compression and rarefaction represent one complete cycle, it is easy to see that a larger number of cycles means a higher frequency while a lower number means a lower frequency (Figures 4.5 and 4.6).

Although phase can be measured in units of time or angles, it is easiest to understand when quantified in degrees of a circle. Although an inexact analogy, the sine wave may be thought of as representing a circle whose lower half is disconnected and rotated. Degrees can be assigned to the wave as depicted in Figure 4.7. The start of the curve at the baseline is 0 degrees (the particle's

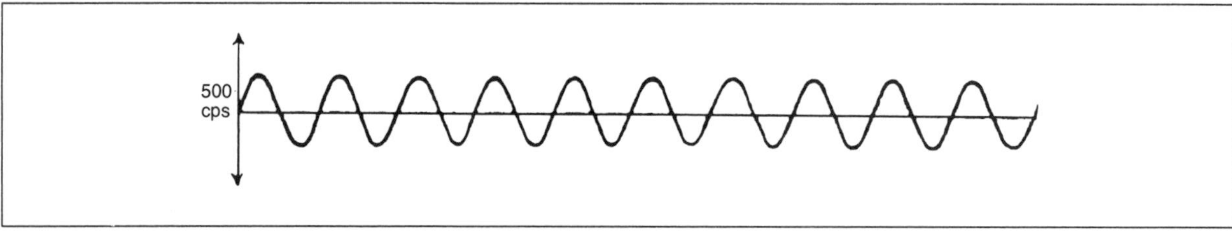

Figure 4.5. A sine function showing a high frequency (500 cycles per second).
Source: From W. R. Wiener, "Audition." In R. L. Welsh and B. B. Blasch (Eds.), *Foundations of Orientation and Mobility* (New York: American Foundation for the Blind, 1980), Fig. 2-6, p. 120.

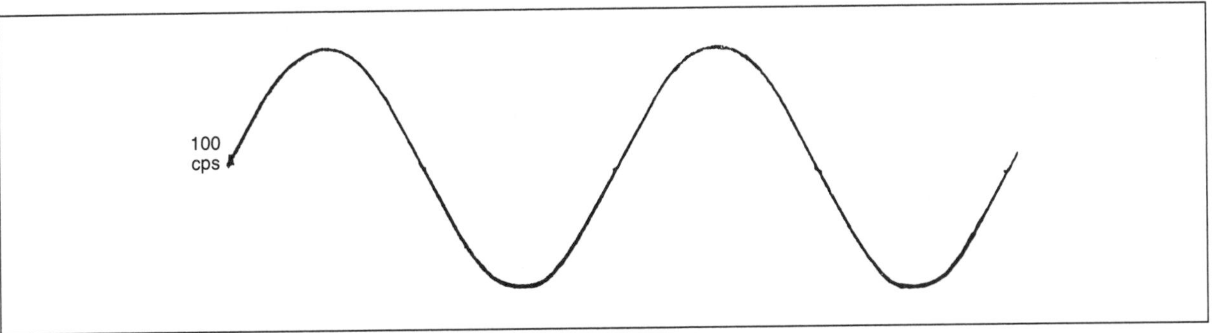

Figure 4.6. A sine function showing a low frequency (100 cycles per second).
Source: From W. R. Wiener, "Audition." In R. L. Welsh and B. B. Blasch (Eds.), *Foundations of Orientation and Mobility* (New York: American Foundation for the Blind, 1980), Fig. 3-6, p. 120.

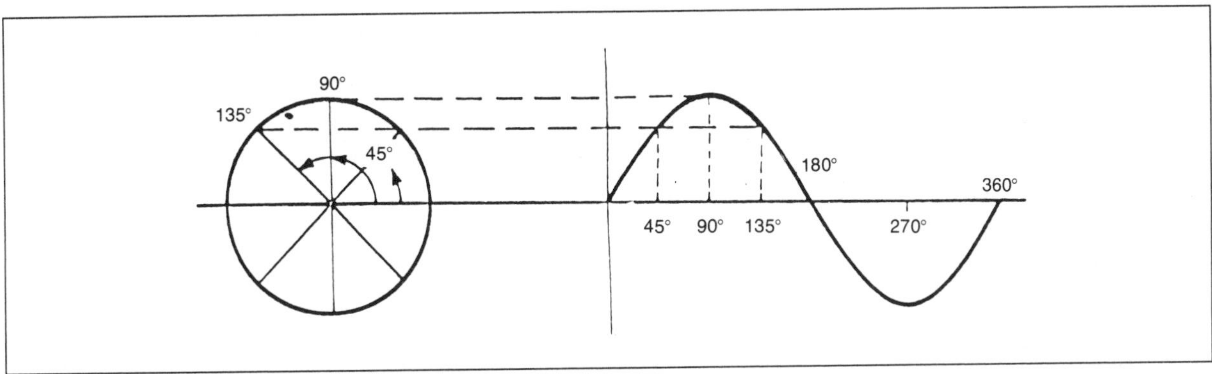

Figure 4.7. A sine function labeled in degrees.
Source: From W. R. Wiener, "Audition." In R. L. Welsh and B. B. Blasch (Eds.), *Foundations of Orientation and Mobility* (New York: American Foundation for the Blind, 1980), Fig. 4-6, p. 120.

position at rest). The point where the upward slope or compression peaks is 90 degrees. The point where the curve returns to the baseline (the particle's point of rest or equilibrium) is 180 degrees. The point of greatest depression in the rarefaction curve is 270 degrees. Finally, the return from rarefaction to the resting position is 360 degrees. The total circle represents one complete cycle of particle vibration. Phase is the relative position of a vibrating particle or the accompanying pressure change in the sound wave at a given time in the cycle. It is often used as a comparative measure to describe the position of a vibrating particle or pressure change in one sound wave relative to the position of a vibrating particle or pressure change in another.

Sound Wave Phenomena in a Sound Field

A *sound field* is a space where sound waves are present. It is not uncommon that sound waves in a sound field interfere with each other. When two sounds of the same frequency and phase occur in the same space, the compressions and rarefactions of the two waves occur at the same time. Figure 4.8A shows the wave forms for two tones of the same frequency, amplitude, and phase; their positive and negative pressures add to form a new wave with twice the amplitude. When the compression of one tone occurs with the rarefaction of another, the two tones are said to be *out of phase.* When two tones are 180 degrees out of phase and are of the same frequency and ampli-

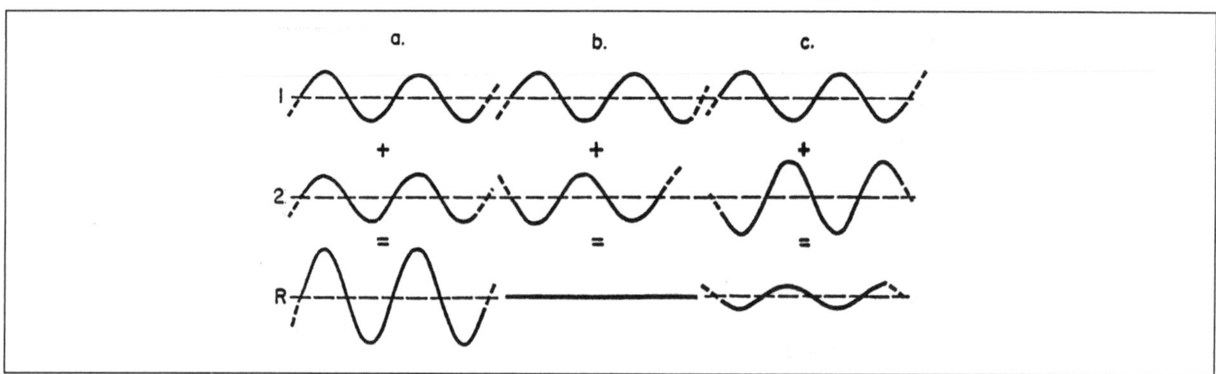

Figure 4.8. The result of adding two sine waves that have the same frequency but different phase relationships (wave 1 + wave 2 = wave R). (A) in-phase relation, identical amplitudes = doubling of resultant amplitude; (B) phase opposition, identical amplitudes = cancellation of resultant amplitude; (C) phase opposition, unequal amplitudes = partial cancellation of resultant amplitude.

Source: Adapted with permission from J. Tonndorf, "Introduction to Acoustics." In A. Glorig (Ed.), *Audiometry: Principles and Practices* (Baltimore: Williams & Wilkins, 1965), Fig. 2.4, p. 19.

tude (Figure 4.8B), the compressions of one wave add to the rarefactions of the other, and they cancel each other, leaving an absence of sound. Figure 4.8C shows an example where two tones of the same frequency are 180 degrees out of phase and different in amplitude. In this case the pressures of the two tones summate to produce a wave whose frequency is the same, but whose amplitude is altered. The cancellation principle is used by engineers to reduce sound levels in luxury automobiles. Figures 4.9A and 4.9B show two cases where the wave forms for two pure tones differ in their frequencies, amplitudes, and phase relationships. In both cases the summation of the pressures produces a complex wave form, one with more than one frequency component; the resultant wave forms differ from each other. Most sounds are not simple, but complex in nature, consisting of a combination of pure tone components of different frequencies, amplitudes, and phase relationships.

When a sound in the environment strikes a *baffle* (e.g., an object or a wall), a variety of events can occur. Sound energy can be transmitted through the baffle, absorbed by the baffle, reflected by the baffle, diffracted by the baffle, refracted by the baffle, or it can undergo a combination of these processes. What actually happens when a sound meets a baffle depends partly upon the wavelengths present in the sound and the nature of the baffle. Relatively high frequencies whose wave lengths are short relative to the size of the baffle tend to be absorbed or reflected; relatively low frequencies (long wavelengths) tend to be transmitted or diffracted. The

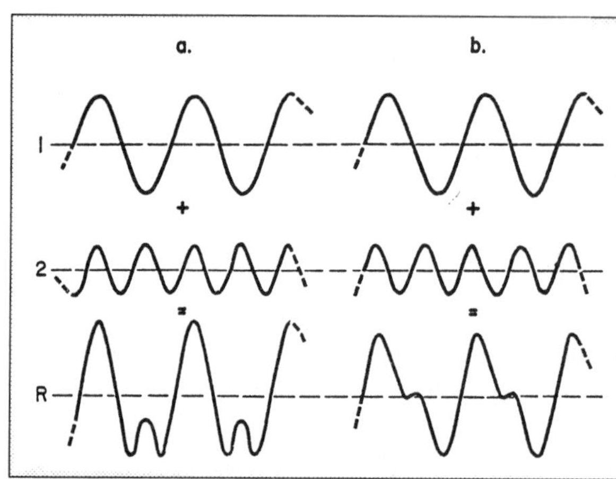

Figure 4.9. The result of adding two sine waves, one with twice the frequency of the other (wave 1 + wave 2 = wave R). Differences in the resultant complex waveforms (waves RA and RB) are due to the different phase relationships between wave 1 and wave 2.

Source: Adapted with permission from J. Tonndorf, "Introduction to Acoustics." In A. Glorig (Ed.), *Audiometry: Principles and Practices* (Baltimore: Williams & Wilkins, 1965), Fig. 2.5, p. 21.

material constituting the baffle will also affect its ability to reflect, diffract, refract, or absorb sound energy. *Reflection* occurs when sound energy bounces off a baffle, changing its direction and perhaps its phase. Reflected sound can interfere with the incident sound. *Absorption,* the acoustic analog of friction, occurs when sound energy is dissipated in the form of heat. If a great deal of sound energy is reflected and/or absorbed, the result will be a *sound shadow,* an area of reduced sound energy, on the side of the baffle opposite the sound source. In mobility a sound shadow is often created when the sound from passing cars is reflected and/or absorbed by poles, phone booths, or bus shelters. *Diffraction* (the scattering of energy in the wave front) occurs when sound scatters around a baffle that is smaller than the wavelength of the sound, or scatters through a hole in the baffle that is smaller than the wavelength of the sound. Refraction occurs when a sound is forced to change its direction of propagation because of a change in speed while passing through the baffle.

Refraction can also occur without sound striking an object or a wall. As sound is transmitted from one medium through another, its speed may change, producing a change in the direction of sound wave propagation. Outdoors the direction and distance of sound travel will vary, depending upon the the presence or absence of windy conditions (Figure 4.10). In the absence of wind the direction of travel should be unaltered (Figure 4.10A). When conditions are windy, however, wind speed increases with height above the ground (Figure 4.10B). Thus, as a sound wave travels against the wind, the speed of the upper portions of the wave front will be slowed more than the speed of the lower portions, and the sound will be turned upward (Figure 4.10C). On the other hand, if a sound travels with the wind, the wind will increase the speed of the upper portions of the sound's wave front more than the lower portions, and the sound will be turned downward, reflecting off the ground (Figure 4.10D); it is partly because the sound wave is repeatedly bent downward by the wind after being

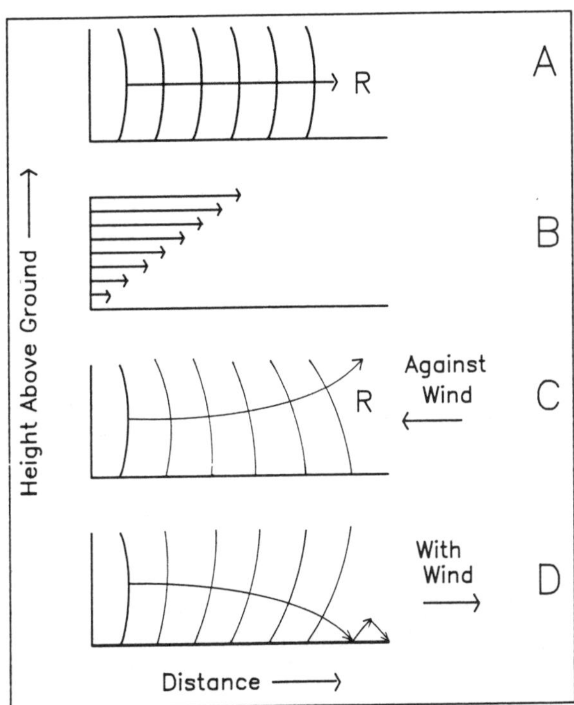

Figure 4.10. Differences in refraction and travel distance for a sound wave propagated under different wind conditions.

Source: reprinted with permission from C. E. Speaks, *Introduction to Sound: Acoustics for the Hearing and Speech Sciences* (San Diego, CA: Singular Publishing Group, 1992), Fig. 8-12, p. 282.

reflected upward by the ground that sound travels farther with, rather than against, the wind (Speaks, 1992).

Differences in air temperature can also affect how far sound carries (Speaks, 1992). Since air temperature typically differs with the time of day, the transmission of sound may also vary with the time of day. In the morning, air temperature is cooler and the speed of sound is slower near the ground; because the speed of sound is faster in the warmer air above, sound waves are refracted downward until striking the ground, where they are reflected upward (Figure 4.11A). Sound is repeatedly refracted and reflected, causing the sound to travel a greater distance than if the air temperature were constant. This is why sound travels so well in winter when the earth's surface is typically cooler than the air, and also over wa-

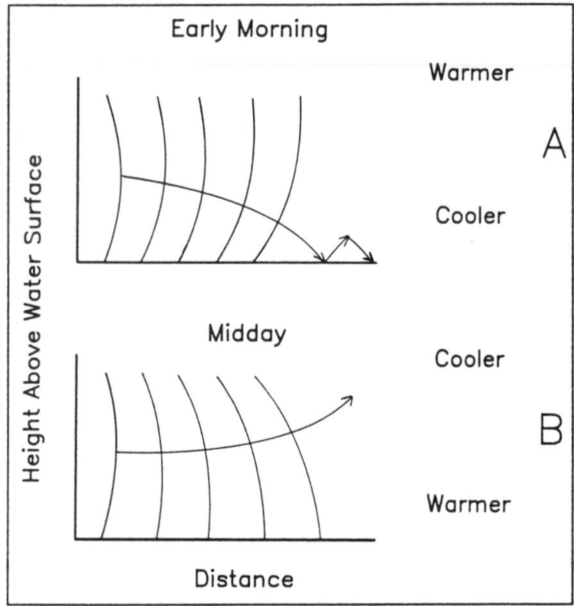

Figure 4.11. Differences in refraction and travel distance for sound propagated in the early morning and at midday.

Source: Reprinted with permission from C. E. Speaks, *Introduction to Sound: Acoustics for the Hearing and Speech Sciences* (San Diego, CA: Singular Publishing Group, 1992), Fig. 8-13, p. 284.

ter, which is typically cooler than the air. At midday, when the temperature is warmer near the Earth's surface and cooler above, the speed of sound is faster in the warmer air near the ground than in the cooler air above, and sound is refracted upward where it is not reflected (Figure 4.11B). Thus sound tends to carry farther in the morning than at midday.

As already described, when sound strikes a baffle or is affected by wind or differences in air temperature, it will most likely change in some way. Outdoors, wind conditions may affect the speed of sound; one may learn to judge distance differently, depending upon the speed and direction of the wind and upon differences in air temperature. Traffic sounds, for example, may be more quickly detected in some conditions than in others. Changes may also occur in the frequency, intensity, and/or phase of the sounds in the environment based upon weather conditions. In general, changes in sound provide useful information for someone who learns to notice the differences.

Changes in sound can also help one to determine the characteristics of the indoor environment. For example, the material in a room may alter sound by transmitting, reflecting, diffracting, absorbing, or refracting it to varying degrees. If a room has a great deal of carpeting, drapery, or upholstery, some of the sound, particularly high frequencies, will be absorbed, resulting in what is commonly called a *dead room*. A room without such soft, absorbing material will reflect more of the sound, creating acoustic reverberation—the prolongation of the sound after the source has stopped vibrating; the result will be an acoustically *live room*. The sound quality resulting from either of these situations may help the person with visual impairment to determine the nature of the room's walls and floors, its furnishings, and its approximate size. A small room has fewer reflections than does a larger room. Often distortion in the returning sound occurs because the materials in a room are frequency specific, reflecting and absorbing some frequencies more than others.

Hearing Sensitivity with Decibels and Frequency

It is common practice to describe an individual's sensitivity to intensity by the sound level used to measure the sensitivity for a particular signal. The intensive unit for quantifying sound level is the decibel (dB), which is one-tenth of a Bel, a unit named after Alexander Graham Bell. The decibel is a unit on a logarithmic scale, which involves taking the log of a ratio between the intensity or pressure of the sound being heard and a corresponding reference intensity or pressure.

An audiologist uses an audiometer (Figure 4.12) to estimate a person's *threshold of sensitivity* to sound by measuring, typically in 5-dB steps, the lowest intensity or dB level at which the subject hears a test signal 50 percent of the time. Threshold can be measured for words or for spe-

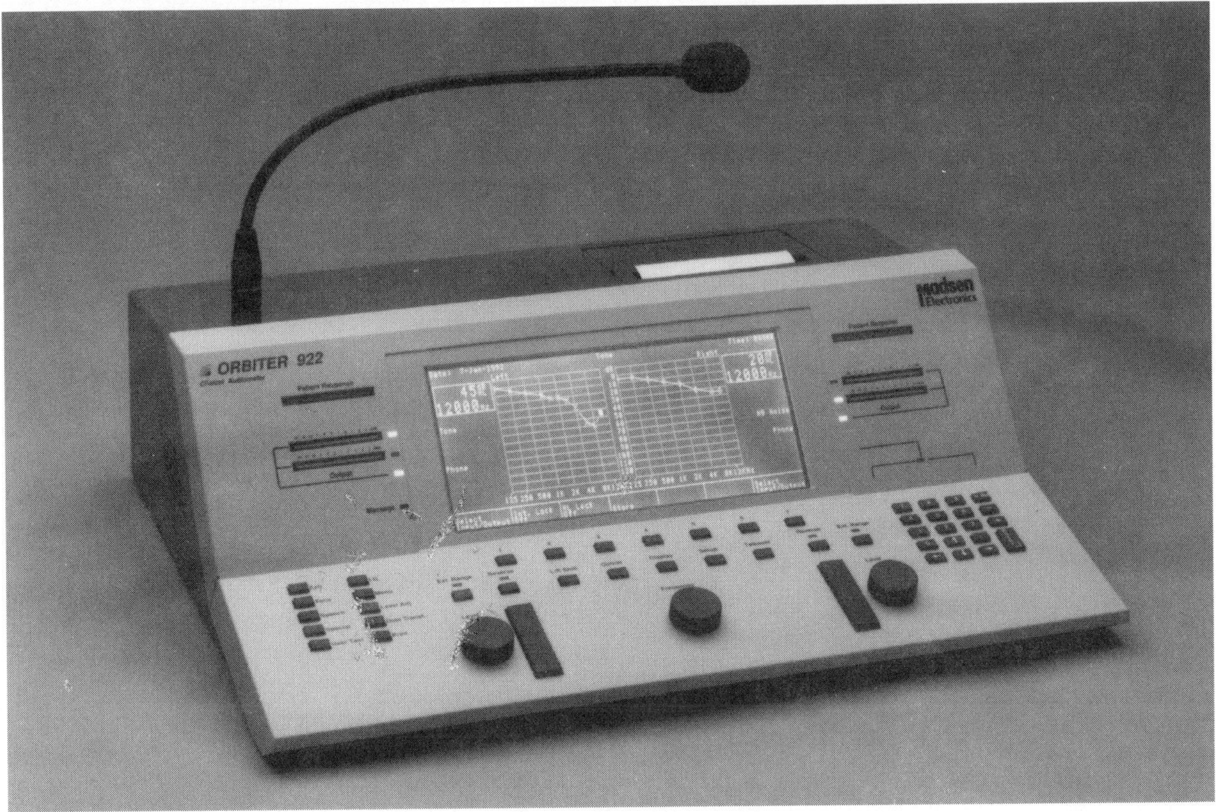

Figure 4.12. A diagnostic audiometer.
Source: Reprinted with permission of Madsen Electronics, Minnetonka, MN.

cific frequencies. For the threshold measurements to have meaning, however, they must be interpreted in comparison to normative data. Currently audiometers in this country are calibrated to the 1969 American National Standards Institute (ANSI) standard. Audiometers are calibrated so that the actual sound pressure level (SPL) needed for the average person with normal hearing to detect a test signal 50 percent of the time is labeled 0 dB hearing level (HL). At 0 dB HL on the audiometer dial, the SPL generated for speech is about 20 dB, and the SPL generated for pure tones is different for each frequency tested. Table 4.1 (American National Standards Institute, 1989a) shows the amount of intensity (SPL) required to make each frequency audible for the average normal hearing person.

Thus, under the ANSI standard the average person with normal hearing will require 11.5 dB of actual intensity or SPL to make a 500-Hz tone barely audible and 7 dB SPL to make a 1000-Hz tone barely audible. In both instances, however, the threshold of audibility would be 0 dB HL. In other words, the hearing level in dB HL indicates an adjusted level and not the actual SPL being generated by the audiometer. In testing hearing, an audiologist may indicate an individual's threshold for a frequency of 1000 Hz to be, let us say, 10 dB HL. In reality, however, the audiometer is putting out 17 dB SPL (7 + 10 dB) to produce 10 dB HL at 1000 Hz. The typical clinical audiometer is calibrated to produce intensities beginning below 0 dB HL and extending to 110 dB HL.

To interpret audiologic data, it is necessary to have some perspective about environmental sound levels and the sensitivity limits of the hu-

Table 4.1. Reference Sound Pressure Levels for 0 dB Hearing Level as a Function of Frequency

	Frequency (Hz)									
	125	250	500	1000	1500	2000	3000	4000	6000	8000
dB SPL	45	25.5	11.5	7	6.5	9	10	9.5	15.5	13

man hearing mechanism. At a distance of 1 meter faint speech would measure approximately 25 dB HL, average conversation would be about 45 dB HL, and loud speech would be about 65 dB HL. Although some individuals have sensitivity thresholds as low as −5 dB HL, −10 dB HL, or perhaps even lower, the average *threshold of audibility* for persons with normal hearing should be about 0 dB HL for pure tones or speech. At the upper end of the dynamic range the normal *threshold of discomfort* begins at about 100 dB HL. For the average person with normal hearing the practical limits of the dynamic range for speech (threshold of discomfort minus threshold of audibility) would most likely be over 100 dB HL (Martin, 1994).

In terms of frequency sensitivity, the human ear can perceive pitch for frequencies of 20 Hz to 20,000 Hz. Sounds below 20 Hz, termed *infrasonic,* are inaudible to most individuals. Sounds above 20,000 Hz are also usually inaudible, and are termed *ultrasonic.* The frequencies most likely to be tested by the audiologist are 125, 250, 500, 1000, 2000, 4000, and 8000 Hz. Each doubling of frequency is called an *octave.* On occasion the audiologist may test sensitivity at 3000 and 6000 Hz when there is particular concern about detailed hearing for the upper frequencies. Traditionally, special importance has been given to thresholds for 500, 1000, and 2000 Hz, because of their importance for understanding speech. Although these frequencies are widely used to determine the severity of loss, higher frequencies are also important for understanding speech. O&M specialists must be concerned with all frequencies tested, not just the speech frequencies. Losses for lower or higher frequencies will certainly have an impact upon O&M.

Structure and Function of the Auditory System

A general understanding of the peripheral and central auditory systems will help the O&M specialist understand the functioning of the hearing mechanism and the nature of hearing losses. The peripheral auditory system consists of the outer ear, middle ear, inner ear, and the auditory or cochlear portion of the cranial nerve (CN VIII); the central auditory system consists of the auditory neural pathways, nuclei, and centers in the brain beyond the synapse of the eighth nerve fibers in the cochlear nuclei of the brainstem. The types of hearing losses correspond to disease processes found in the various portions of the auditory system. Audiometric tests, in effect, assess the amount of hearing loss that may result from problems in the various parts of the auditory system.

The Outer Ear

The outer ear consists of the *pinna* and the external auditory meatus or *ear canal.* The pinna (Figure 4.13) is a cartilaginous structure composed of grooves and depressions. The deep depression leading to the meatus is called the *concha.* The outer ear collects and conducts airborne sound waves to the *eardrum,* a part of the middle ear. In animals the pinna is movable and quite helpful in localizing sounds; in man, the pinna is generally immovable, but still offers some assistance in localization (Zemlin, 1988).

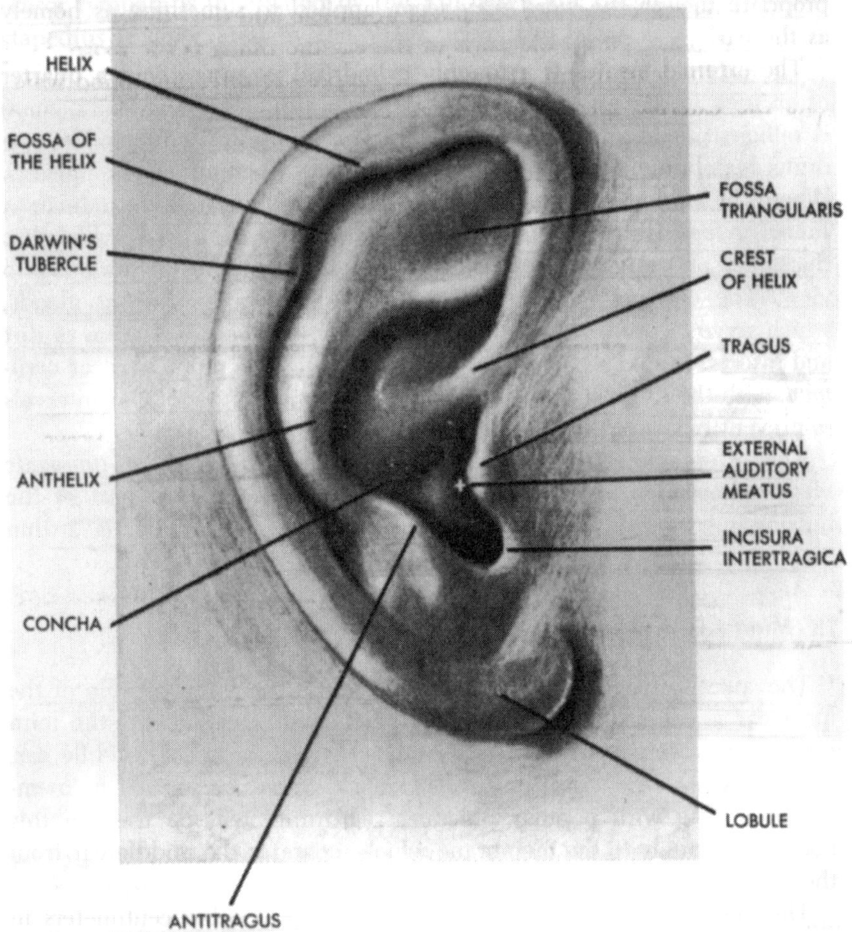

Figure 4.13. The pinna.
Source: Reprinted with permission from F. L. Lederer and A. R. Hollender, *Textbook of the Ear, Nose, and Throat* (Philadelphia: F. A. Davis, 1947).

The Middle Ear

The middle ear (Figures 4.14 and 4.15) consists of the eardrum or the tympanic membrane; the three ossicles, or the middle ear bones, and their attachments; and the eustachian tube (Gelfand, 1990). The *tympanic membrane* is roughly circular, layered tissue attached to the wall of the osseous portion of the ear canal. The space between the tympanic membrane and the inner ear is called the middle ear cavity, tympanic cavity, or tympanum. The tympanic membrane on the lateral wall of the cavity is connected to the medial or labyrinthine wall of the cavity by a chain of three bones or ossicles. The first bone, the *malleus* or hammer, attaches to the upper portion of the drum, pulling it medialward (toward the body midline) and giving it somewhat of a conical shape. The malleus articulates with the next ossicle called the *incus* or anvil which, in turn, articulates with the *stapes* or stirrup. The footplate of the stapes attaches to the *oval window,* an opening into the inner ear. Also located within the middle ear cavity is the opening of the *eustachian tube,* a structure that connects the middle ear cavity to the nasopharynx. The eustachian tube permits changes in outside air pressure to influence or equalize air pressure within the middle ear cavity. In addition, it allows drainage to the

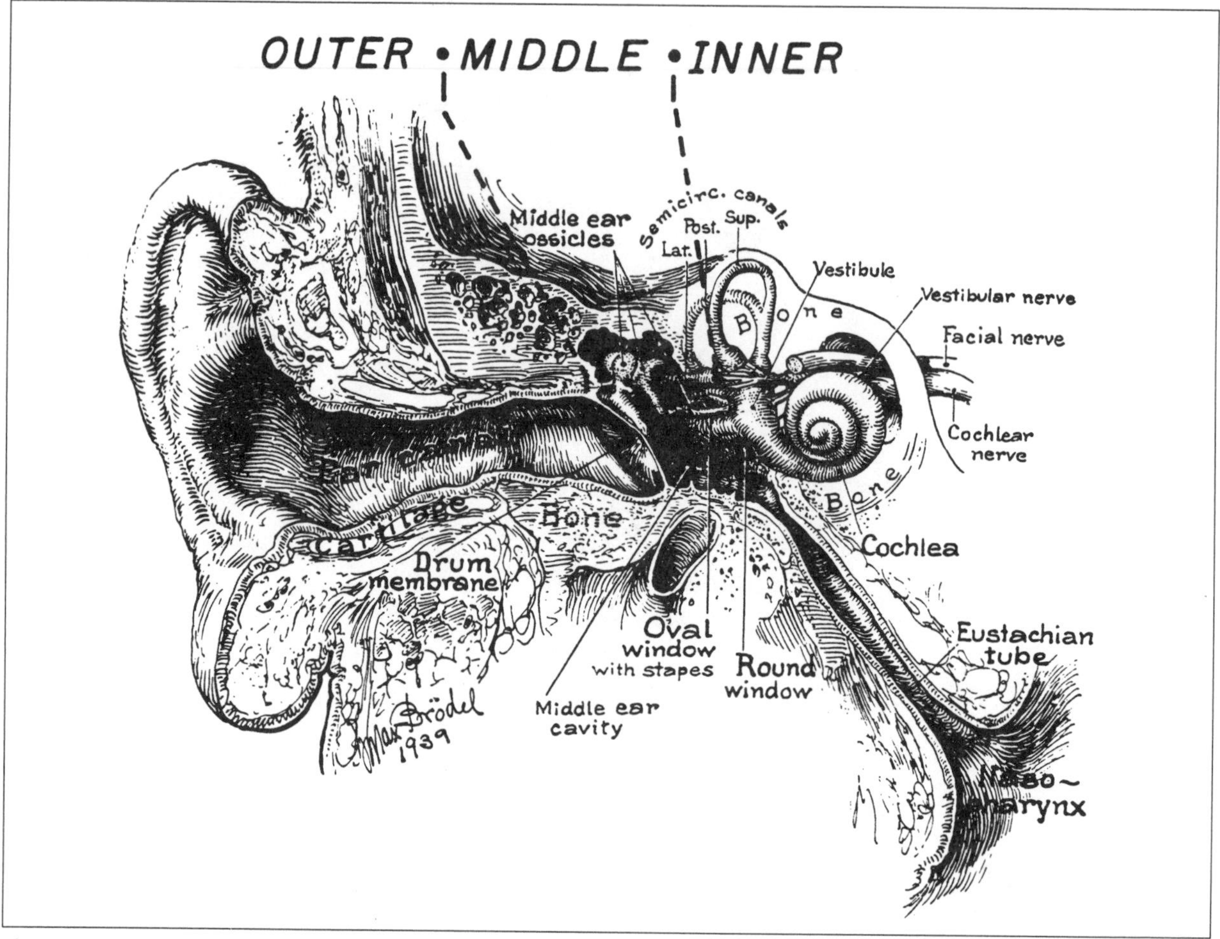

Figure 4.14. Drawing of the outer, middle, and inner ear based upon a frontal section of the head.
Source: Adapted from M. Brodel, *Three Unpublished Drawings of the Anatomy of the Human Ear* (Philadelphia: W. B. Saunders, 1946).

throat of secretions that sometimes occur within the middle ear.

The middle ear contains two muscles (Figure 4.16) which are believed to protect the inner ear, to a limited extent, from excessively loud noise. The *stapedius muscle* responds at lower intensities than does the *tensor tympani* and is thus the primary contributor to the acoustic reflex. The stapedius muscle pulls the stapes posteriorly (toward back) away from the oval window, while the tensor tympani pulls the malleus anteriorly toward the inner ear. The action of these two muscles changes the tension and the balance of the ossicles, reducing the transmission of intense sound (Zemlin, 1988).

The middle ear changes the airborne sound transmitted from the outer ear into a mechanical vibration that is passed to the inner ear through the motion of the ossicles. In doing so, it acts as a transformer—it increases the energy reaching the inner ear over what it would be if there were no middle ear and airborne sound were to directly strike the inner ear fluid.

The Inner Ear

The inner ear consists of two systems—one concerned with hearing and the other with balance. This chapter covers only the structures responsible for hearing; refer to Chapter 5 in this volume

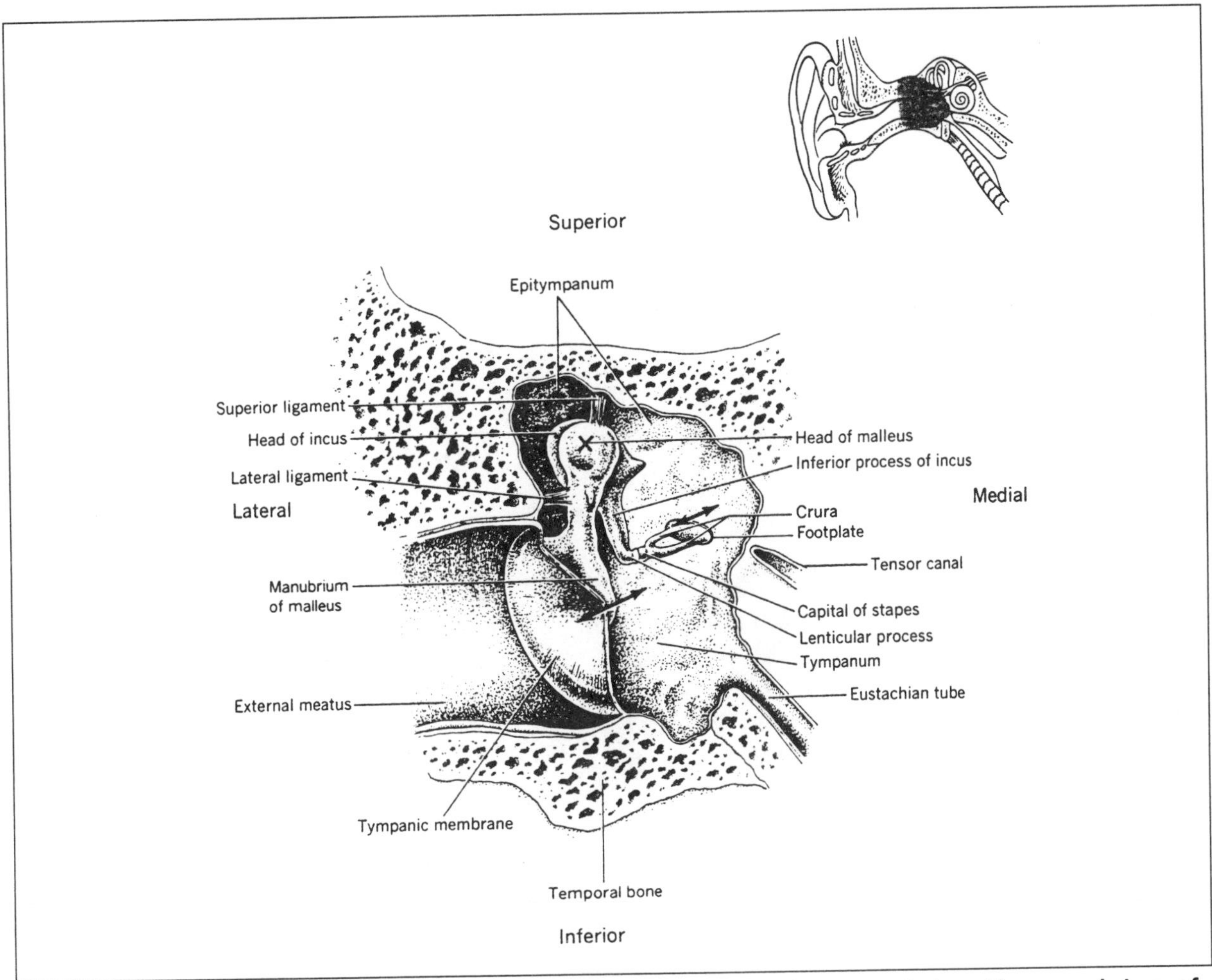

Figure 4.15. The general structures of the right middle ear seen in the coronal view. The manubrium of the malleus, the inferior process of the incus, and the stapes all move to and fro along a medial-lateral line, as shown by the double-headed arrows. The ossicular chain as a whole oscillates about an anterior-posterior axis that runs through the heads of the malleus and incus, as shown by the X.

Source: Reprinted with permission from W. L. Gullick, G. A. Gescheider, and R. D. Frisina, *Hearing: Physiological Acoustics, Neural Coding, and Psychoacoustics* (New York: Oxford University Press, 1989), Fig. 4.3, p. 79.

for information about balance-related functions of the ear. The auditory portion of the inner ear, located in the petrous portion of the temporal bone, is called the *cochlea* because of its winding construction (Figure 4.17). It is a snail-like chamber composed of $2\frac{3}{4}$ turns that spiral around the modiolus, a bony core which houses the cell bodies of the auditory portion of CN VIII. The cochlea consists of a bony labyrinth within the temporal bone and a membraneous labyrinth within the bony labyrinth. The membranous labyrinth is bounded on three sides by Reissner's membrane above, by the *basilar membrane* below, and by the tissues on the outer bony wall, which form a roughly triangular shape in a cross-sectional view (Figure 4.18). The boundaries of the membraneous labyrinth form the cochlear duct, or *scala media,* within the bony labyrinth. The scala media contains a fluid called endolymph and partitions the bony labyrinth into up-

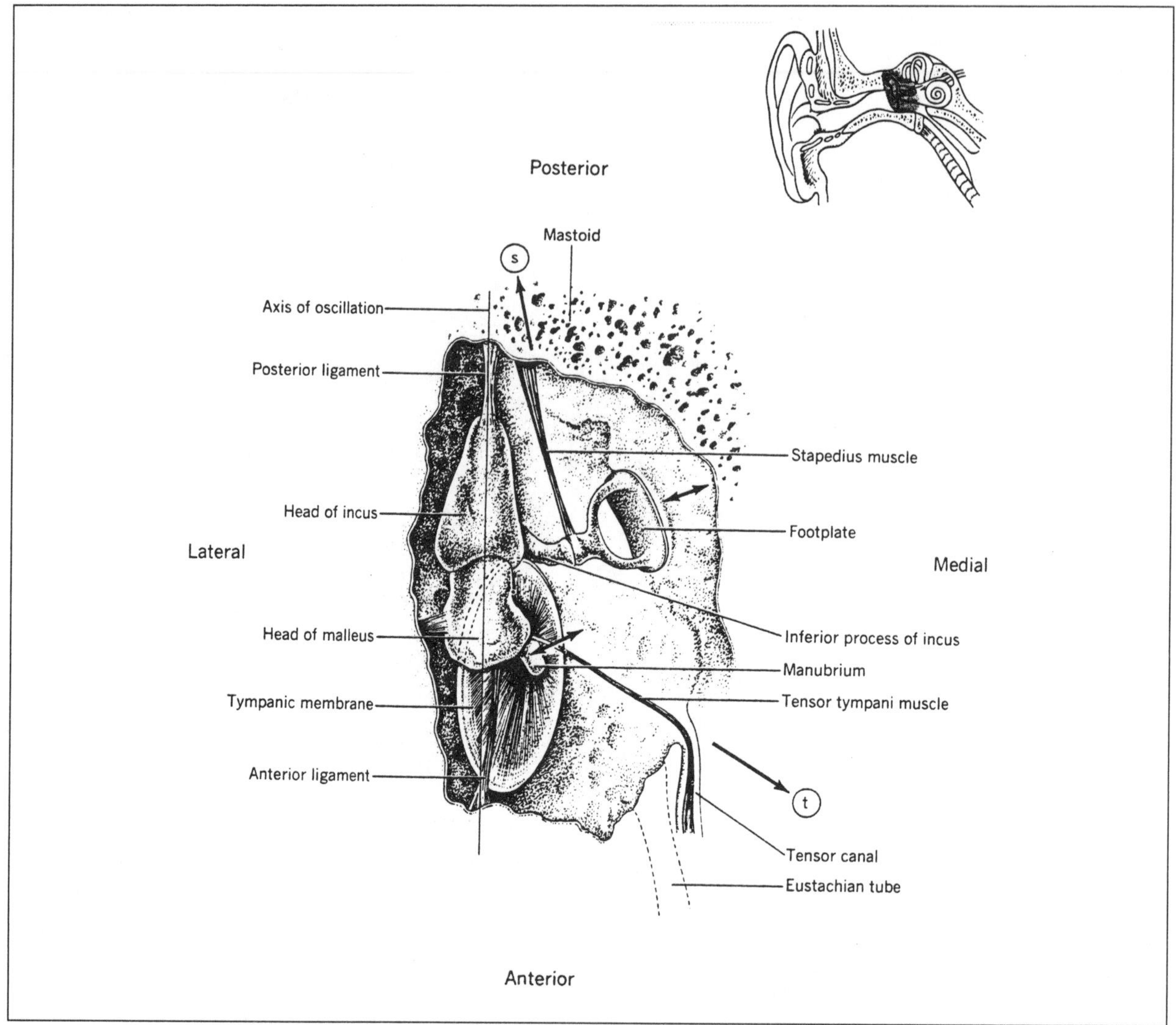

Figure 4.16. The general structures of the right middle ear seen in the superior view. The manubrium of the malleus, the inferior process of the incus, and the tympanic membrane are all partly obscured in this view by the heads of the ossicles. Arrows *s* and *t* indicate the direction of tension imposed by the stapedius and tensor tympani muscles relative to the axis of oscillation.

Source: Reprinted with permission from W. L. Gullick, G. A. Gescheider, and R. D. Frisina, *Hearing: Physiological Acoustics, Neural Coding, and Psychoacoustics* (New York: Oxford University Press, 1989), Fig. 4.6, p. 84.

per and lower chambers, which are filled with a spinal-like fluid called *perilymph* (Figure 4.19). The upper chamber is called the *scala vestibuli* because it opens into a portion of the bony labyrinth called the vestibule, a space separated from the middle ear (tympanum) by the oval window. The lower chamber is called the scala tympani because it ends at the *round window membrane,* a structure that separates the middle ear from the inner ear. The two chambers or scalae connect at the apex of the labyrinth in a junction called the helicotrema. At this junction the perilymph from both chambers is continuous.

Lying on the basilar membrane within the scala media is the *organ of Corti. Hair cells* in the organ of Corti are so named because cilia extend

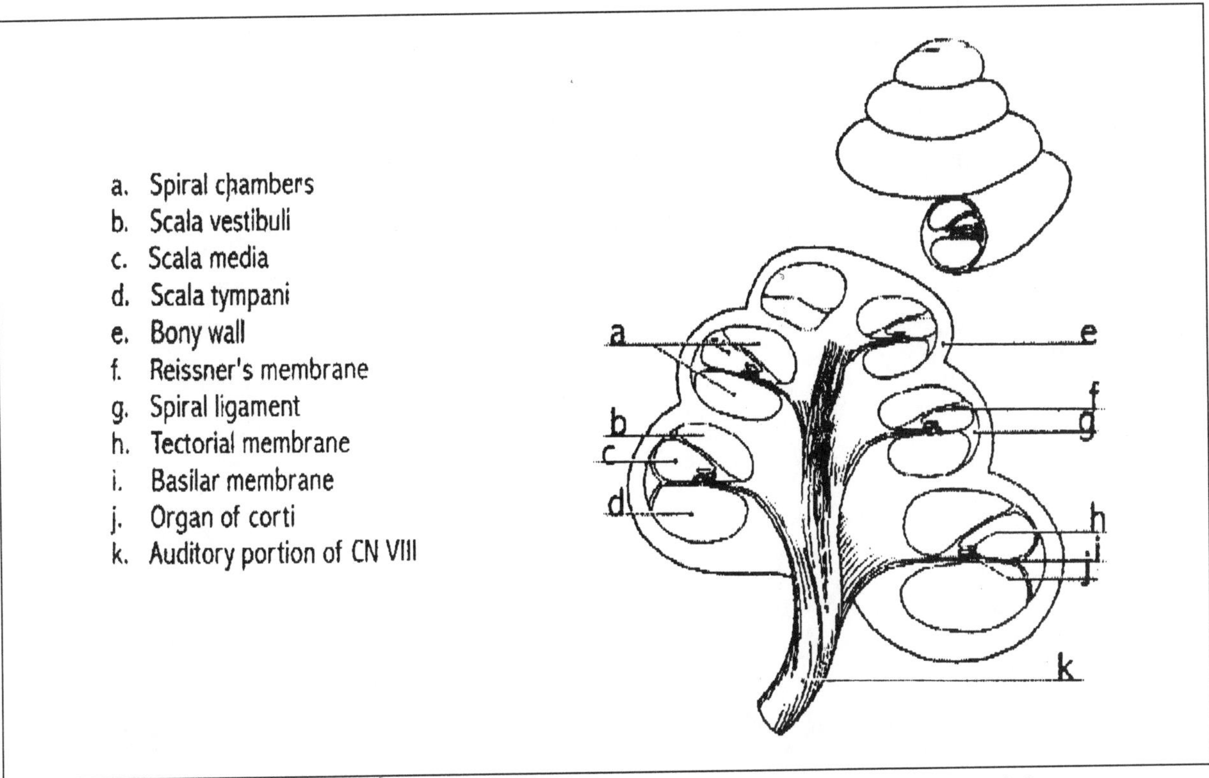

Figure 4.17. Cross-section of the cochlea, illustrating the scalae through each of the turns.

from their tops somewhat like hair extending from the head. The rows of hair cells are separated by the rods or Corti's cells. Two columns of Corti's cells are in contact with each other at their tops and separated at their bases on the basilar membrane; a cross-sectional view shows a triangular space that is called Corti's Tunnel and is filled with a fluid called perilymph. On the inner side of the inner Corti's cells is a single row of inner hair cells, and on the outer side of the outer Corti's cells are three rows of outer hair cells. The top of each hair cell accommodates a number of cilia that are connected together. Only the longest cilia of the outer hair cells are in contact with the overlying tectorial membrane. At the bases of the hair cells is a complex arrangement of nerve fibers, which form the ascending and descending auditory portions of CN VIII. After leaving the inner ear, these auditory nerve fibers terminate in the cochlear nuclei of the brainstem (Figure 4.20).

The primary functions of the inner ear are to transform mechanical energy into electrochemical energy and to perform a frequency analysis of the incoming signal. As the stapes footplate moves in the oval window, it creates a disturbance of the perilymph in the scala vestibuli. Given that the inner ear fluids are relatively noncompressible, an inward movement of the footplate leads to a downward movement of the cochlear duct and an increase in pressure in the scala tympani (Figure 4.19). The increased pressure in the scala tympani is released by an outward bulging of the round window membrane. These events lead to an up-and-down wavelike motion that travels from the base to the apex of the cochlear duct. Up-and-down movements of the cochlear partition result in a bending of the cilia on the tops of the outer hair cells. Cilia on the tops of the inner hair cells may be stimulated by fluid movements beneath the tectorial membrane. The modern view is that the outer hair cells shorten and elongate themselves in response to stimulation, alter-

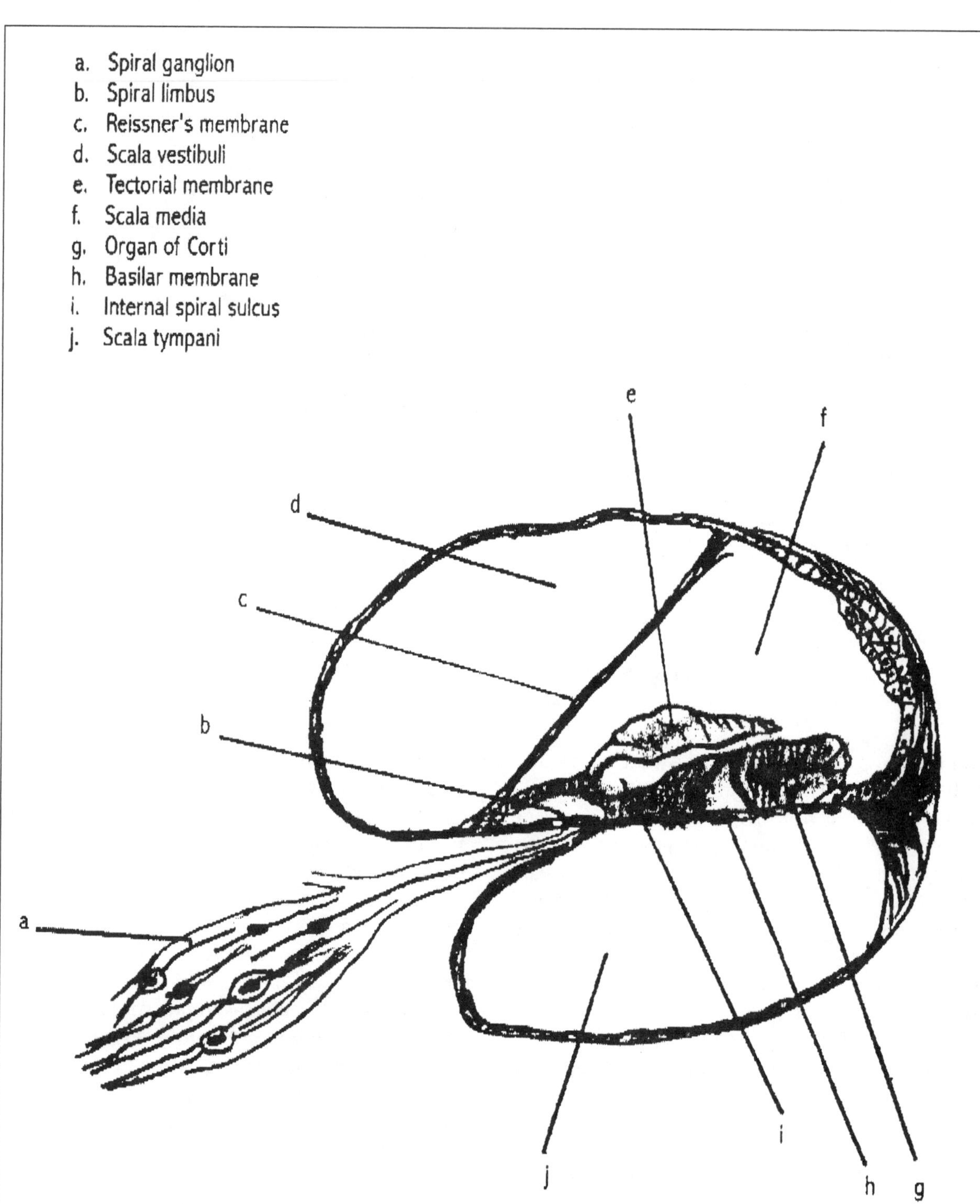

Figure 4.18. Cross-section of the cochlea showing the boundaries of the cochlear duct.

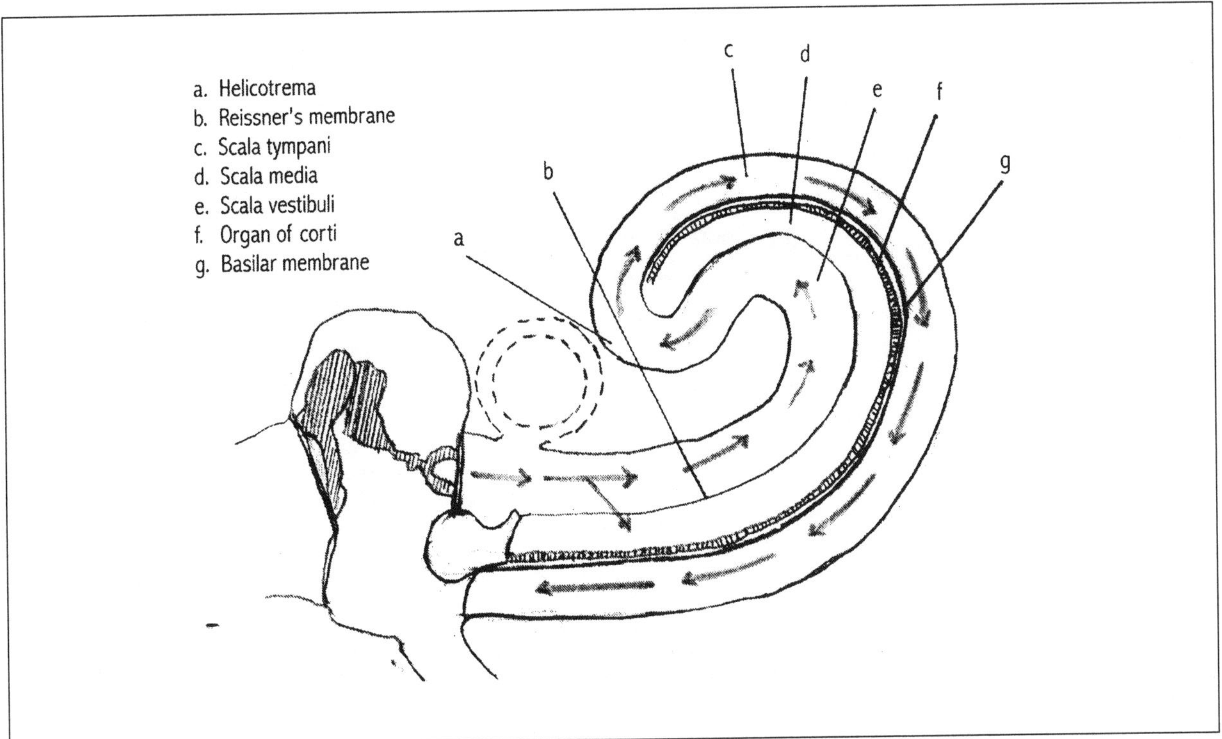

Figure 4.19. Schematic of the middle and inner ear showing the cochlea uncoiled.

ing the movement of the basilar membrane and subsequently altering the stimulation of the inner hair cells (Burch-Sims & Ochs, 1992). Thus movement of the outer hair cells may facilitate the stimulation of the inner hair cells. Stimulation of the hair cells results in the release of a chemical across the synaptic space at the base of the hair cells to initiate impulses in the auditory nerve fibers leading to the brain.

Central Auditory Pathways

The central auditory pathways (Figure 4.20) begin at the synapse of the eighth nerve fibers in cochlear nuclei. The pathways ascend ipsilaterally (same side) and contralaterally (opposite side) through the brainstem to the auditory cortex. Impulses from one ear stimulate both sides of the brain, including the auditory cortex. Descending pathways from both sides of the brain provide a means of altering function in both cochleas. No doubt the nuclei and centers connected by the neural tracts recode and process signals all through the system. The system is even more complex than indicated by most schematics, and its detailed description is beyond the scope of this chapter.

Frequency Encoding

Several theories attempt to explain frequency perception primarily on the basis of what happens in the inner ear. Support for a *traveling wave form of place theory* (Bekesy, 1928) is based largely on three observations: (1) the basilar membrane is differentially responsive to frequency such that the wave traveling from base to apex reaches its maximum amplitude near the base for high-frequency sounds and progressively nearer the apex for lower-frequency sounds; (2) the neurons at the bases of the hair cells along the basilar membrane respond differentially to frequency such that those near the base respond best to high frequencies and those progressively

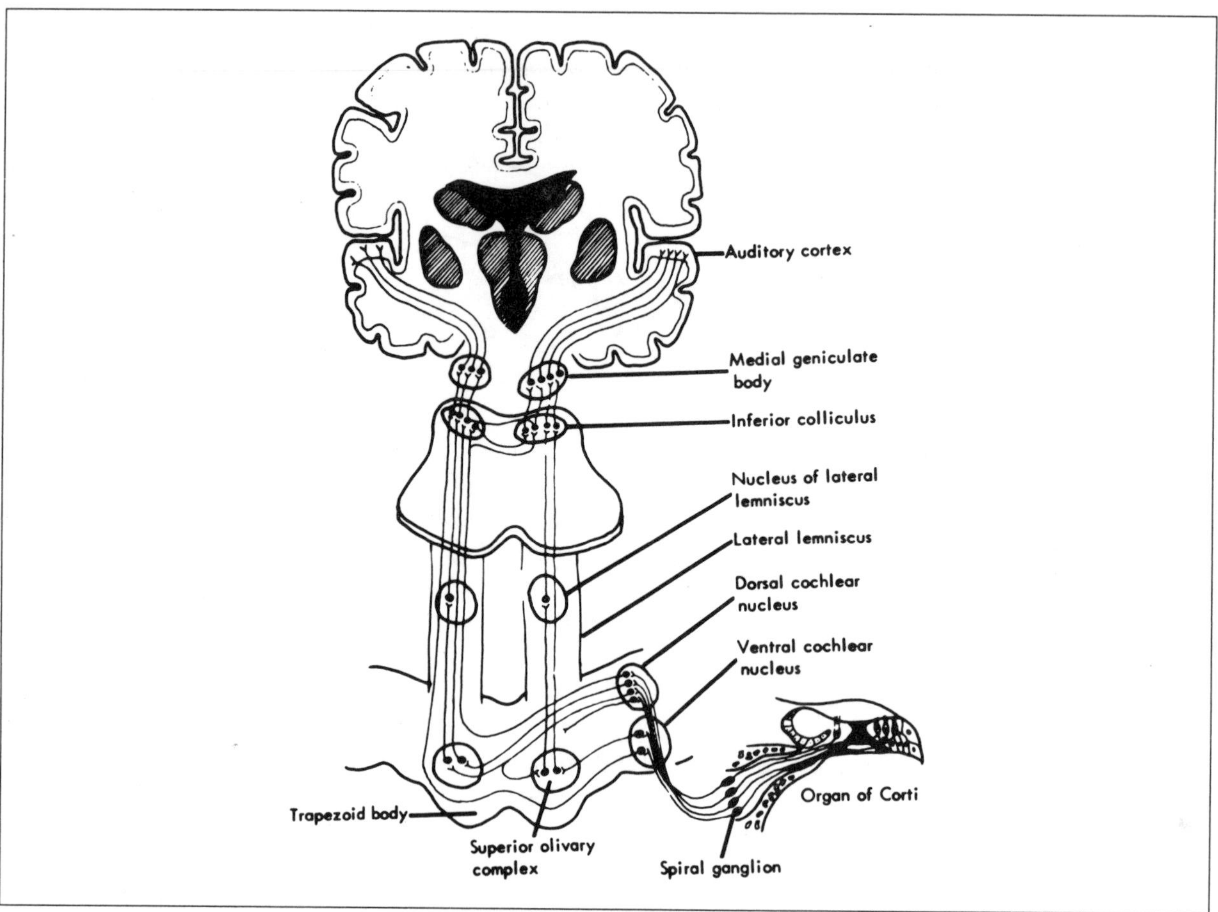

Figure 4.20. Ascending auditory neural pathways.
Source: From W. R. Zemlin, *Speech and Hearing Science: Anatomy and Physiology* (Englewood Cliffs, NJ: Prentice-Hall, 1968), p. 414.

near the apex respond best to low frequencies; and (3) differential sensitivity to frequency occurs at various levels in the central auditory nervous system. A traveling wave theory, however, can only account for encoding of high frequencies because the envelope of the traveling wave is too broad to allow for refined encoding at low frequencies. A *frequency theory of frequency encoding* (Rutherford, 1886) is based on the notion that vibration of the basilar membrane leads to neural discharges at rates corresponding to the frequency of the stimulus. This principle is plausible only for low frequencies because of the inability of individual neurons to discharge at high rates. According to Wever's *Volley Theory* (1949), a number of neurons may fire together so that a continuous series of discharges is maintained even during periods when individual neurons must rest before firing again. For example, ten neurons firing 500 times per second will add up to 5000 Hz. A combination of these principles may provide the best account for frequency perception.

Intensity Encoding

The basis of intensity encoding for a given input frequency appears to be the number of neural discharges reaching the brainstem per unit of time (Durrant & Lovrinic, 1995). A single neuron is most sensitive to, or fires at the lowest stimulus intensity for, a particular stimulus frequency (i.e., the characteristic frequency of the neuron). However, individual neurons cannot discharge rapidly enough to account for the wide dynamic range of intensity to which humans are sensitive. To account for this wide dynamic range, the central nervous system (CNS) must use discharges from nerve fibers whose characteristic frequencies (CFs) differ from the frequency of the stimulus. At stimulus intensities sufficient only to reach threshold for nerve fibers whose CFs match the stimulus frequency, relatively few fibers will fire. As the intensity increases, it eventually reaches a level sufficient to discharge nearby fibers which have CFs that differ from the frequency of the stimulus. The firing of these additional fibers leads to an increase in the number of neural discharges per unit of time and to a perception of increased loudness.

IDENTIFICATION OF HEARING LOSS

In some instances hearing tests are used for screening, for identifying—among persons who apparently have normal hearing—those who have a reasonably high probability for having a hearing disorder, impairment, or disability, so that they may be referred for further evaluation by appropriate professionals. In audiologic screening protocols, screening for hearing disorders is usually limited to looking for obvious structural defects and otitis media (inflammation of the middle ear); screening for impairment usually means presenting pure tones at a single intensity at a limited number of frequencies in each ear; and screening for a hearing disability usually means administering a questionnaire to detect restricted ability to perform activities of work or daily living (see Table 4.6). In order to classify and quantify hearing loss, a more complete evaluation is required.

Because persons who are visually impaired are very dependent upon audition for O&M as well as for communication, they should have regular hearing evaluations and take special care to conserve their hearing. All newborn children should be screened for hearing loss. Children known to be at risk for hearing loss should be rescreened for hearing loss annually. Children found to have normal hearing should be rescreened before starting school, whenever they are at risk for hearing loss, and at intervals established by the school system. Adults thought to have normal hearing should be rescreened for hearing loss at least once every 10 years until age 50 and at least once every 3 years after age 50 (American Speech-Langauge-Hearing Association, 1997). All persons known to have hearing loss or special risk factors should have their hearing evaluated according to the schedule recommended by their physician or audiologist.

Classification of hearing loss can be based upon the site of disease or breakdown in particular anatomic sites in the hearing mechanism. If the site of lesion or disease is located in the outer ear or in the middle ear, the loss is classified as *conductive.* If the dysfunction lies somewhere within the inner ear or beyond, any resulting loss is classified as *sensorineural.* Although a cochlear abnormality is typically the cause of a sensorineural hearing loss, a retrocochlear abnormality (beyond the cochlea) could also be the cause. If on the basis of test results it is possible to identify the cochlea as the specific site of lesion, the loss could be classified as sensory (or cochlear), and if it is possible to identify the site of lesion as the eighth nerve, the loss could be identified as neural. Lesions of the auditory neural pathways in the brainstem may or may not cause a loss of hearing sensitivity for pure tones; lesions of the auditory cortex typically do not cause a loss of sensitivity for pure tones. Generally speaking, the symptoms associated with central auditory nervous system involvement are more subtle than those associated with involvement of the peripheral auditory system. Central auditory involvement is likely to affect speech-language processing in some way.

The O&M specialist, however, needs only to be concerned primarily with differentiating between the conductive loss, the sensorineural loss, or a combination of the two, which is called a *mixed loss.* An understanding of the differences between these categories will help the specialist to interpret basic audiometric test results and to understand the student's auditory functioning.

The Basic Audiologic Test Battery

The basic audiologic test battery typically consists of pure tone air and bone conduction threshold tests, speech recognition threshold tests, suprathreshold speech recognition tests, and immittance tests. This is a relatively efficient battery for identifying hearing loss; distinguishing between conductive, sensorineural, and mixed hearing loss; and estimating the degree of loss.

Pure Tone Thresholds and the Audiogram

A *pure tone threshold* is obtained by determining the lowest level of a tone one can detect 50 percent of the time. *Air conduction thresholds* are determined by presenting the tones through earphones. *Bone conduction thresholds* are determined by presenting the tones through a bone conduction vibrator placed on the forehead or, more typically, on the mastoid of the skull (a portion of the skull behind the ear). As each pure tone threshold is obtained, it is usually recorded on an *audiogram.* Figure 4.21 shows an audiogram form like those typically used for graphically recording hearing thresholds and other hearing test results. Test frequencies are shown on the horizontal axis, and hearing level is shown on the vertical axis. The 0 dB hearing level line (based upon different SPL values at each frequency) represents the hearing sensitivity of the average young adult with normal hearing. In Figure 4.21 each pure tone air conduction threshold is recorded with a circle for the right ear and with an X for the left ear. A threshold symbol is placed on the audiogram at the hearing level indicating threshold for each test frequency. Each pure tone bone conduction threshold is recorded with a carat open to the right for the right ear and open to the left for the left ear. Pure tone thresholds provide a basis for identifying the degree and type of any hearing loss present.

The various symbols used to plot test results on an audiogram are explained by the symbol key to the right of the audiogram in Figure 4.21. It should be noted that some symbols indicate *masked thresholds.* Use of these symbols indicates that it was necessary to do the threshold testing with a masking noise in the nontest ear to insure that signals presented to the test ear were not heard in the nontest ear. As noted on the key, the masking symbol for pure tone thresholds is a triangle for the right ear and a box for the left ear. When masking is used in the left (nontest) ear to obtain bone condition thresholds for the right ear, each threshold is indicated by a bracket that is open to the right. When masking is used in the right (nontest) ear to obtain bone condition thresholds for the left ear, each threshold is indicated by a bracket that is open to the left. Note that some symbols are drawn with a downward arrow. These symbols are placed at the intensity limits of the audiometer for the test signal when there is "no response" to the signal, indicating that threshold cannot be obtained due the severity of the loss and limitations of the equipment. Although the key shows other symbols, those explained here are the most widely used.

Typically the pure tone thresholds at 500, 1000, and 2000 Hz are averaged for use in estimating degree of hearing loss for each ear. In Figure 4.21 the pure tone threshold average is 5 dB HL for each ear, suggesting bilateral normal hearing sensitivity. Figure 4.21 shows the severiy of hearing loss categories to the right of the audiogram. These categories were modified by Clark (1981) from Goodman (1965). Goodman's normal hearing category ranged from −10 to 25 dB HL; Clark divided Goodman's normal hearing category into a normal hearing category that ranged from −10 to 15 dB HL, and a slight hearing loss (near normal or normal for many situations) category that ranged from 16 to 25 dB HL. Some audiologists find Clark's categories to be particularly useful when dealing with children. Using these categories, a pure tone air conduction threshold average of 35 dB HL would indicate a mild degree of hearing loss. Typically, categories of hearing loss roughly estimate disability based on lost ability to understand speech. There has been no research that relates categories of hearing loss with the ability to interpret environmental sounds for O&M.

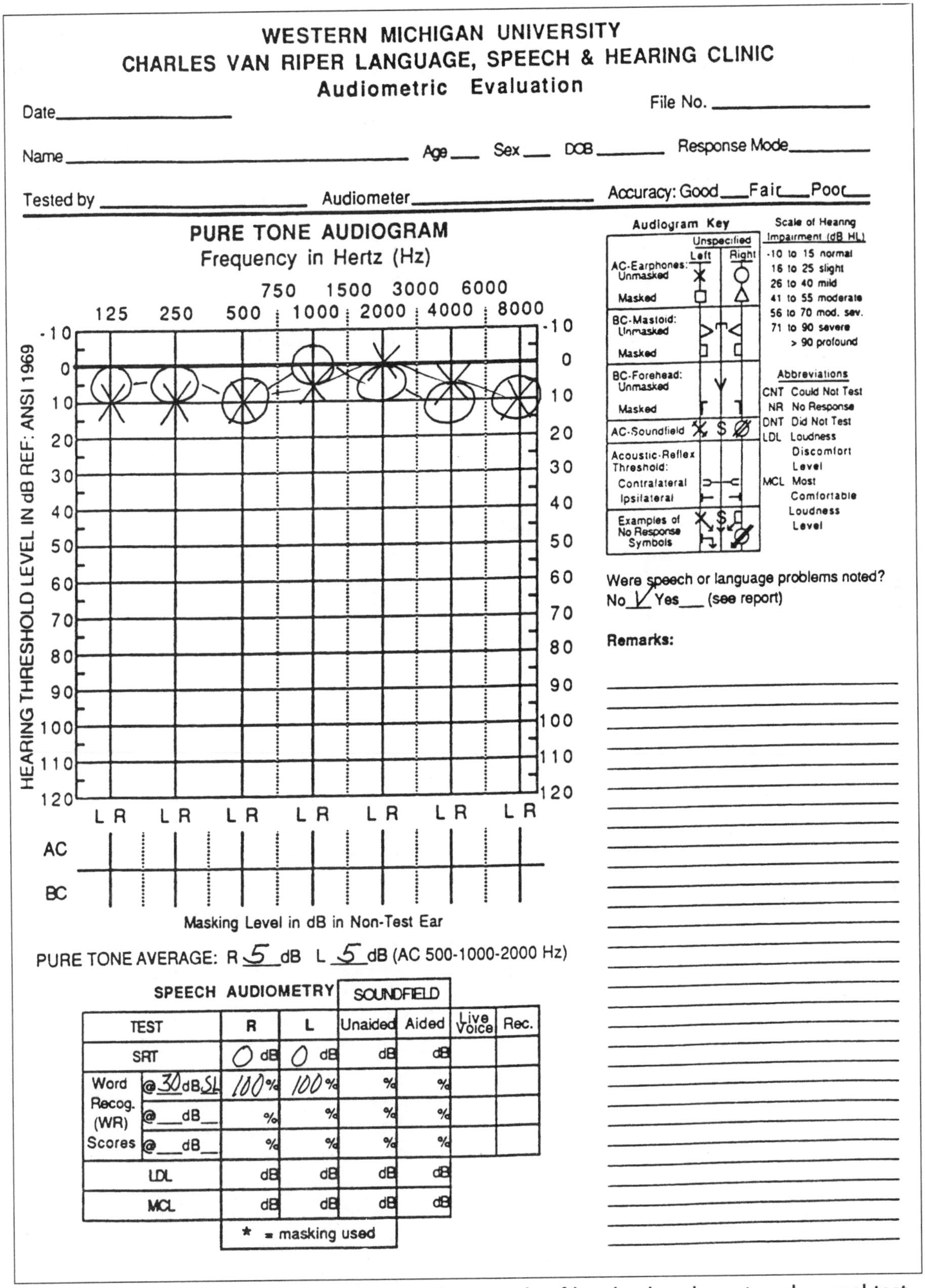

WESTERN MICHIGAN UNIVERSITY
CHARLES VAN RIPER LANGUAGE, SPEECH & HEARING CLINIC
Audiometric Evaluation

Date________________ File No. ____________

Name______________________ Age___ Sex___ DOB______ Response Mode________

Tested by ______________ Audiometer______________ Accuracy: Good___Fair___Poor___

PURE TONE AUDIOGRAM

Frequency in Hertz (Hz)

750 1500 3000 6000

125 250 500 1000 2000 4000 8000

HEARING THRESHOLD LEVEL IN dB REF: ANSI 1969

-10 0 10 20 30 40 50 60 70 80 90 100 110 120

L R L R L R L R L R L R L R

AC

BC

Masking Level in dB in Non-Test Ear

Audiogram Key	Unspecified	Left	Right
AC-Earphones: Unmasked		X	O
Masked		□	△
BC-Mastoid: Unmasked		>	<
Masked		]	[
BC-Forehead: Unmasked	↓		
Masked		┌	┐
AC-Soundfield	X	$	Ø
Acoustic-Reflex Threshold: Contralateral		⊃—	—⊂
Ipsilateral		⊢	⊣
Examples of No Response Symbols			

Scale of Hearing Impairment (dB HL)
- -10 to 15 normal
- 16 to 25 slight
- 26 to 40 mild
- 41 to 55 moderate
- 56 to 70 mod. sev.
- 71 to 90 severe
- > 90 profound

Abbreviations
- CNT Could Not Test
- NR No Response
- DNT Did Not Test
- LDL Loudness Discomfort Level
- MCL Most Comfortable Loudness Level

Were speech or language problems noted?
No ✓ Yes___ (see report)

Remarks:

PURE TONE AVERAGE: R 5 dB L 5 dB (AC 500-1000-2000 Hz)

SPEECH AUDIOMETRY

TEST		R	L	SOUNDFIELD Unaided	SOUNDFIELD Aided	Live Voice	Rec.
SRT		0 dB	0 dB	dB	dB		
Word Recog. (WR) Scores	@ 30 dB SL	100 %	100 %	%	%		
	@___dB___	%	%	%	%		
	@___dB___	%	%	%	%		
LDL		dB	dB	dB	dB		
MCL		dB	dB	dB	dB		

* = masking used

Figure 4.21. An audiogram showing a symbol key, a scale of hearing impairment, and normal test results.

Goodman (1965) warned that it is not helpful to interpret the categories too strictly because different types of hearing loss may impose different degrees of disability and the dB loss by itself can be only one source of information used to determine disability. With this qualification it is possible to use the classifications for cautious estimation of the probable disability and the needs of the individual. Someone with a *mild hearing loss* may have some difficulty hearing faint or distant speech. A person with a *moderate hearing loss* may be able to understand conversational speech only in close proximity of approximately 3 to 5 feet (90 to 150 cm) and have great difficulty in a group discussion. An individual with a *moderately severe hearing loss* may find that conversation must be very loud for comprehension and that he or she generally cannot participate in group communication. Someone with a *severe hearing loss* may be able to hear a loud voice approximately 1 foot (30 cm) from the ear, and may be able to identify environmental sounds. A person with a *profound hearing loss* may hear various loud sounds, but cannot rely upon them consistently as a primary channel for communication.

A traditional definition of *deafness* is defined according to the Conference of Executives of American Schools for the Deaf, as hearing that is nonfunctional for ordinary purposes of life. A newer definition by the same organization states that a deaf person is one whose hearing disability precludes successful processing of linguistic information through audition, with or without a hearing aid (Newby and Popelka, 1985).

The rationale for categorizing hearing loss by type is based on the anatomic structures tested by air and bone conduction tests. The air conduction threshold test examines the combined sensitivity of all the peripheral structures at once. Bone conducted signals, for the most part, bypass the outer and middle ear conductive mechanism and directly stimulate the cochlea. If air and bone conduction sensitivity are the same (within 10 dB), any hearing loss present is considered to be of the sensorineural type. If air- and bone-conducted signals reach the cochlea equally well, the loss is assumed to be due to a problem in the sensorineural mechanism. On the other hand, if the air conduction sensitivity shows a significant hearing loss and the bone conduction sensitivity is normal and at least 15 dB better than the air conduction sensitivity, a conductive hearing loss is present. The reason for the poorer air conduction sensitivity is assumed to be a problem in the outer or middle ear that reduces the level of the signal reaching the cochlea. If the air and bone conduction sensitivity show a significant hearing loss and the bone conduction sensitivity is at least 15 dB better than the air conduction sensitivity, a mixed hearing loss is present. This would be due to involvement in both the conductive and sensorineural portions of the hearing mechanism.

Figures 4.22, 4.23, 4.24, and 4.25 illustrate the major types of hearing loss as they appear on audiograms. Figure 4.22 illustrates *bilateral sensorineural hearing loss.* Note the agreement (within 10 dB) between the air conduction thresholds (circles and Xs) and the bone conduction thresholds (carats) and the loss of sensitivity for both air and bone conduction test signals. Figure 4.23 illustrates *bilateral conductive hearing loss.* In this case the bone conduction thresholds (brackets) indicate normal sensitivity, while the air conduction thresholds (circles and Xs) indicate that the sensitivity is 15 dB poorer. Note that it is possible for a conductive problem to exist even when air conduction thresholds are within the range of normal sensitivity (e.g., at 1000–4000 Hz). Figure 4.24 illustrates a *mixed hearing loss.* Both the air (circles and Xs) and bone conduction thresholds (brackets) show a loss of sensitivity, with the air conduction thresholds at least 15 dB greater than the loss for bone conduction signals at specific frequencies.

The pure tone thresholds recorded on the audiogram in Figure 4.25 illustrate all three types of hearing loss described above. At the right ear, thresholds obtained for low frequencies show a loss of sensitivity by air conduction (circles or triangles) and normal sensitivity by bone conduction (carets or brackets), indicating a conductive hearing loss; thresholds obtained for high fre-

WESTERN MICHIGAN UNIVERSITY
CHARLES VAN RIPER LANGUAGE, SPEECH & HEARING CLINIC
Audiometric Evaluation

Date________ File No. ________

Name________ Age___ Sex___ DOB______ Response Mode______

Tested by ________ Audiometer________ Accuracy: Good ✓ Fair___ Poor___

PURE TONE AUDIOGRAM

Frequency in Hertz (Hz)

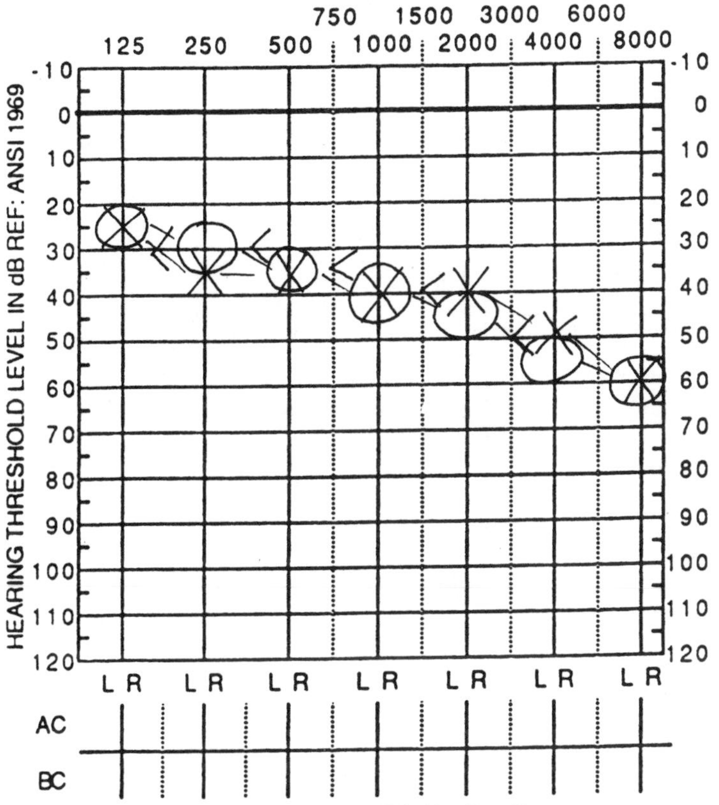

125 250 500 750 1000 1500 2000 3000 4000 6000 8000

HEARING THRESHOLD LEVEL IN dB REF: ANSI 1969

-10 0 10 20 30 40 50 60 70 80 90 100 110 120

L R L R L R L R L R L R L R

AC

BC

Masking Level in dB in Non-Test Ear

PURE TONE AVERAGE: R 40 dB L 37 dB (AC 500-1000-2000 Hz)

Audiogram Key

	Unspecified	Left	Right
AC-Earphones: Unmasked		X	O
Masked		□	△
BC-Mastoid: Unmasked		>	<
Masked		]	[
BC-Forehead: Unmasked	V		
Masked		⌈	⌉
AC-Soundfield		$	Ø
Acoustic-Reflex Threshold: Contralateral			
Ipsilateral			
Examples of No Response Symbols			

Scale of Hearing Impairment (dB HL)

- -10 to 15 normal
- 16 to 25 slight
- 26 to 40 mild
- 41 to 55 moderate
- 56 to 70 mod. sev.
- 71 to 90 severe
- > 90 profound

Abbreviations

- CNT Could Not Test
- NR No Response
- DNT Did Not Test
- LDL Loudness Discomfort Level
- MCL Most Comfortable Loudness Level

Were speech or language problems noted? No ✓ Yes___ (see report)

Remarks:

SPEECH AUDIOMETRY

TEST		R	L	SOUNDFIELD Unaided	SOUNDFIELD Aided	Live Voice	Rec.
SRT		40 dB	40 dB	dB	dB		
Word Recog. (WR) Scores	@ 30 dB SL	90 %	92 %	%	%		
	@___dB___	%	%	%	%		
	@___dB___	%	%	%	%		
LDL		dB	dB	dB	dB		
MCL		dB	dB	dB	dB		

* = masking used

Figure 4.22. Audiogram illustrating sensorineural hearing loss.

WESTERN MICHIGAN UNIVERSITY
CHARLES VAN RIPER LANGUAGE, SPEECH & HEARING CLINIC
Audiometric Evaluation

Date________ File No. ________

Name________ Age___ Sex___ DOB____ Response Mode____

Tested by ________ Audiometer________ Accuracy: Good___Fair___Poor___

PURE TONE AUDIOGRAM
Frequency in Hertz (Hz)

750 1500 3000 6000
125 250 500 1000 2000 4000 8000

HEARING THRESHOLD LEVEL IN dB REF: ANSI 1969

-10 0 10 20 30 40 50 60 70 80 90 100 110 120

L R L R L R L R L R L R L R

AC

BC

Masking Level in dB in Non-Test Ear

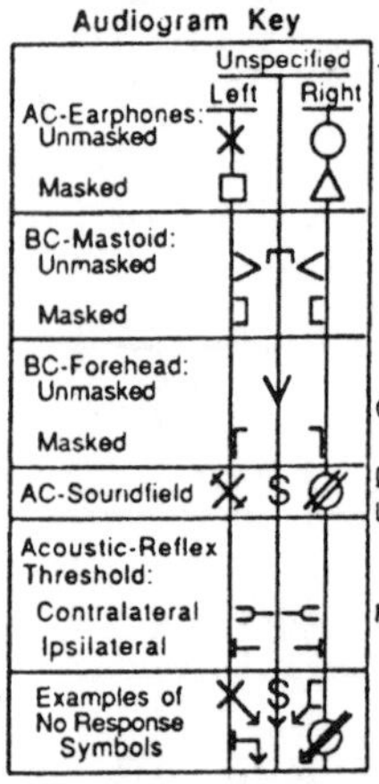

PURE TONE AVERAGE: R 22 dB L 18 dB (AC 500-1000-2000 Hz)

Audiogram Key

	Unspecified Left	Unspecified Right
AC-Earphones: Unmasked	X	O
Masked	□	△
BC-Mastoid: Unmasked	>	<
Masked	]	[
BC-Forehead: Unmasked	↓	
Masked	⌐	¬
AC-Soundfield	X	$ Ø
Acoustic-Reflex Threshold: Contralateral	⊐—	—⊏
Ipsilateral	⊢	⊣
Examples of No Response Symbols		

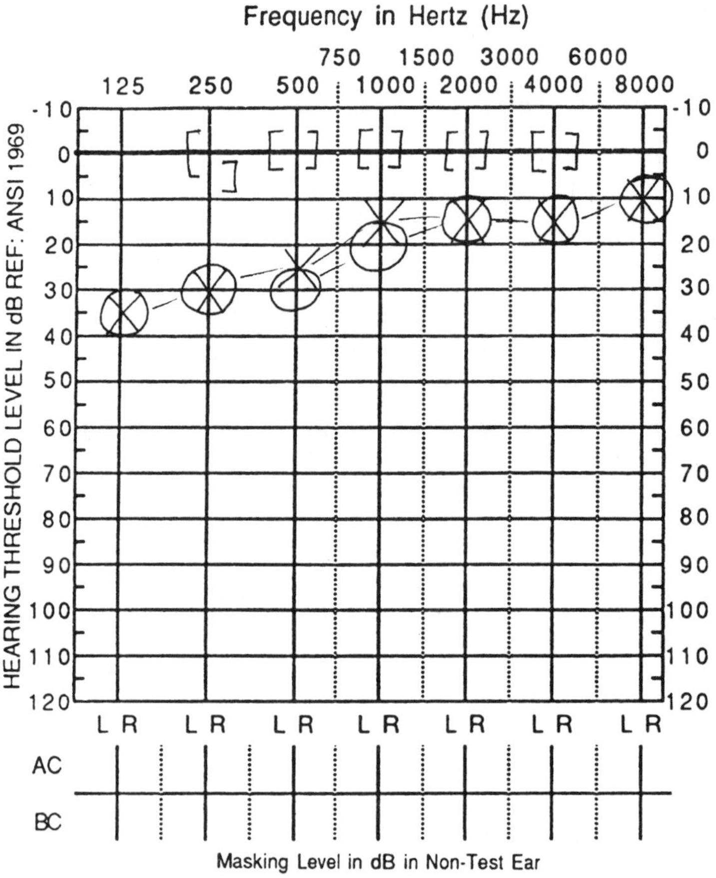

Scale of Hearing Impairment (dB HL)
-10 to 15 normal
16 to 25 slight
26 to 40 mild
41 to 55 moderate
56 to 70 mod. sev.
71 to 90 severe
> 90 profound

Abbreviations
CNT Could Not Test
NR No Response
DNT Did Not Test
LDL Loudness Discomfort Level
MCL Most Comfortable Loudness Level

Were speech or language problems noted?
No ✓ Yes___ (see report)

Remarks:

SPEECH AUDIOMETRY

TEST		R	L	SOUNDFIELD Unaided	SOUNDFIELD Aided	Live Voice	Rec.
SRT		20 dB	15 dB	dB	dB		
Word Recog. (WR) Scores	@ 30 dB SL	100 %	100 %	%	%		
	@___dB__	%	%	%	%		
	@___dB__	%	%	%	%		
LDL		dB	dB	dB	dB		
MCL		dB	dB	dB	dB		

* = masking used

Figure 4.23. Audiogram illustrating conductive hearing loss.

WESTERN MICHIGAN UNIVERSITY
CHARLES VAN RIPER LANGUAGE, SPEECH & HEARING CLINIC
Audiometric Evaluation

Date________ File No. ________

Name________ Age___ Sex___ DOB_______ Response Mode________

Tested by ________ Audiometer________ Accuracy: Good___Fair___Poor___

PURE TONE AUDIOGRAM
Frequency in Hertz (Hz)

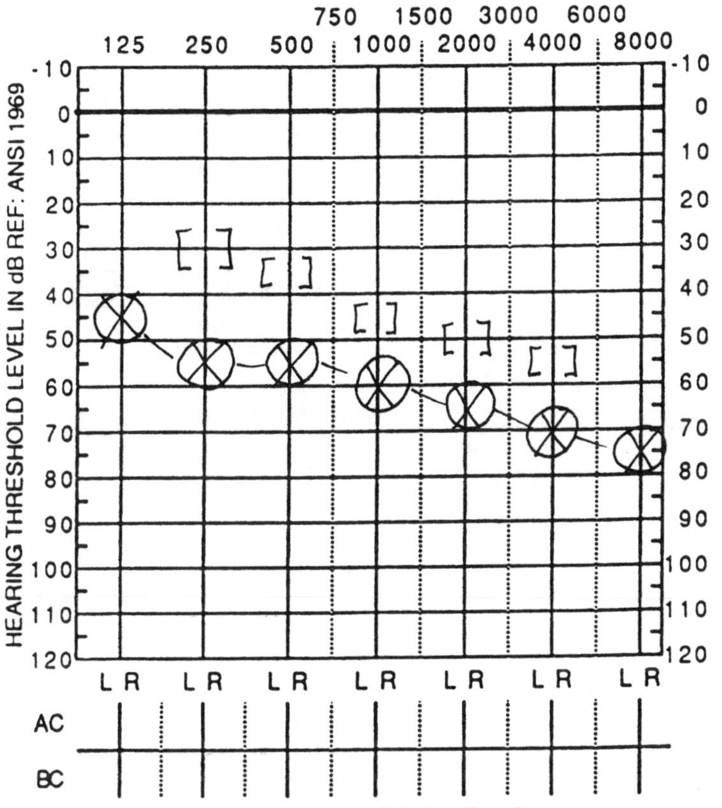

125 250 500 750 1000 1500 2000 3000 4000 6000 8000

HEARING THRESHOLD LEVEL IN dB REF: ANSI 1969

-10 0 10 20 30 40 50 60 70 80 90 100 110 120

L R L R L R L R L R L R L R

AC

BC

Masking Level in dB in Non-Test Ear

Audiogram Key

	Unspecified	Left	Right
AC-Earphones: Unmasked		X	O
Masked		□	△
BC-Mastoid: Unmasked		>	<
Masked		]	[
BC-Forehead: Unmasked	V		
Masked		⌐	¬
AC-Soundfield		X	Ø
Acoustic-Reflex Threshold: Contralateral			
Ipsilateral			
Examples of No Response Symbols			

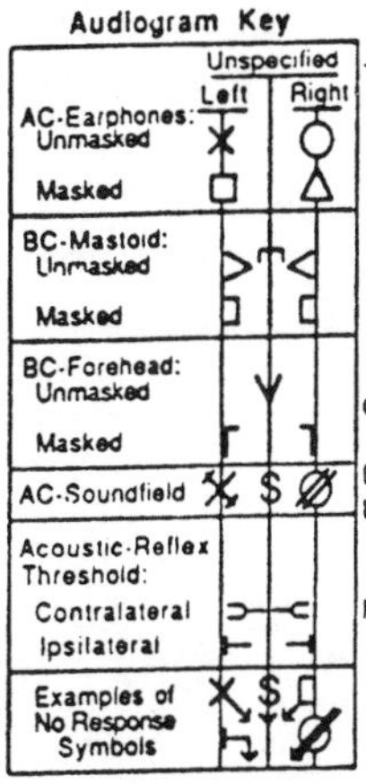

Scale of Hearing Impairment (dB HL)

-10 to 15 normal
16 to 25 slight
26 to 40 mild
41 to 55 moderate
56 to 70 mod. sev.
71 to 90 severe
> 90 profound

Abbreviations

CNT Could Not Test
NR No Response
DNT Did Not Test
LDL Loudness Discomfort Level
MCL Most Comfortable Loudness Level

Were speech or language problems noted?
No ✓ Yes___ (see report)

Remarks:

PURE TONE AVERAGE: R 60 dB L 60 dB (AC 500-1000-2000 Hz)

SPEECH AUDIOMETRY			SOUNDFIELD			
TEST	R	L	Unaided	Aided	Live Voice	Rec.
SRT	60 dB	60 dB	dB	dB		
Word Recog. (WR) Scores @ 25 dB SL	84 %	86 %	%	%		
@___dB___	%	%	%	%		
@___dB___	%	%	%	%		
LDL	dB	dB	dB	dB		
MCL	dB	dB	dB	dB		

* = masking used

Figure 4.24. Audiogram illustrating mixed hearing loss.

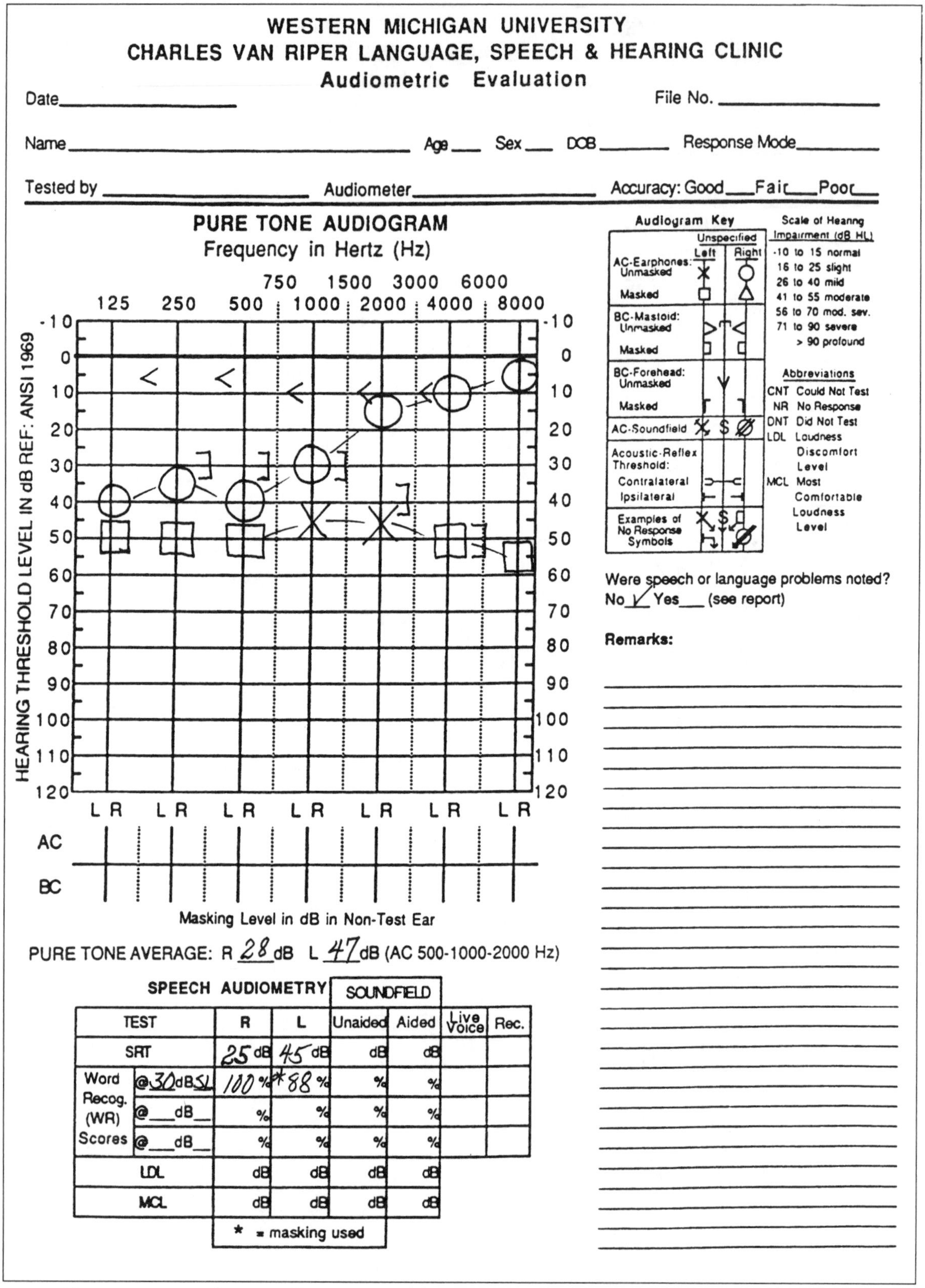

WESTERN MICHIGAN UNIVERSITY
CHARLES VAN RIPER LANGUAGE, SPEECH & HEARING CLINIC
Audiometric Evaluation

Date________ File No. ________

Name________ Age___ Sex___ DOB_______ Response Mode________

Tested by ________ Audiometer________ Accuracy: Good___ Fair___ Poor___

PURE TONE AUDIOGRAM
Frequency in Hertz (Hz)

Audiogram Key

	Unspecified Left	Unspecified Right
AC-Earphones: Unmasked	X	O
Masked	□	△
BC-Mastoid: Unmasked	>	<
Masked	]	[
BC-Forehead: Unmasked	↓	
Masked		
AC-Soundfield		$
Acoustic-Reflex Threshold: Contralateral		
Ipsilateral		
Examples of No Response Symbols		

Scale of Hearing Impairment (dB HL)
- -10 to 15 normal
- 16 to 25 slight
- 26 to 40 mild
- 41 to 55 moderate
- 56 to 70 mod. sev.
- 71 to 90 severe
- > 90 profound

Abbreviations
- CNT Could Not Test
- NR No Response
- DNT Did Not Test
- LDL Loudness Discomfort Level
- MCL Most Comfortable Loudness Level

Were speech or language problems noted?
No ✓ Yes___ (see report)

Remarks:

PURE TONE AVERAGE: R 28 dB L 47 dB (AC 500-1000-2000 Hz)

SPEECH AUDIOMETRY

TEST		R	L	SOUNDFIELD Unaided	SOUNDFIELD Aided	Live Voice	Rec.
SRT		25 dB	45 dB	dB	dB		
Word Recog. (WR) Scores	@ 30 dB SL	100 %	*88 %	%	%		
	@___dB___	%	%	%	%		
	@___dB___	%	%	%	%		
LDL		dB	dB	dB	dB		
MCL		dB	dB	dB	dB		

* = masking used

Figure 4.25. Audiogram illustrating sensorineural, conductive, and mixed hearing loss.

quencies are the same for air and bone conduction and show normal sensitivity, indicating no hearing loss. At the left ear, thresholds show a loss of sensitivity by air conduction (Xs or boxes) and bone conduction (carats or brackets) at all test frequencies; the bone conduction thresholds are better than the air conduction thresholds by 15 dB or more at low frequencies, indicating a mixed loss; the air and bone conduction thresholds are the same (within 10 dB) for high frequencies, indicating a sensorineural loss.

Speech Recognition Tests

The most widely used speech audiometric tests are (a) the *speech recognition threshold test*, formerly called the speech reception threshold test, and (b) the *suprathreshold speech recognition test*, formerly called the speech discrimination test. Speech recognition tests provide information about a person's functional ability to hear and understand speech. While the pure tone audiogram provides information about threshold responses to pure tone signals, speech recognition procedures test the individual's ability to receive complex signals.

A speech recognition threshold (SRT), the lowest level at which 50 percent of two-syllable words can be recognized, is usually determined for each ear using earphones. The SRT is an estimate of the lowest level at which the listener can just start to follow the meaning of running speech. The SRT is expected to agree within about 10 dB with the pure tone threshold average (PTA) that is typically reported on the audiogram for each ear. Large discrepancies between the SRT and the PTA for a given ear may indicate unreliable test results. Given reliable results, the SRT can be used in the same way the pure tone threshold average is used to categorize the degree of hearing loss. Besides offering a way of estimating sensitivity for speech, checking the reliability of test results, and categorizing the degree of hearing loss, SRT can also be used to choose a level at which to administer the suprathreshold speech recognition test (percent correct word recognition tests).

Suprathreshold speech recognition tests may be administered using a variety of stimuli at a variety of test levels, depending upon the goal of the audiologist. Most frequently, however, the best percent correct score possible is estimated by presenting specially constructed monosyllabic word lists through earphones at a single level 20–40 dB above the SRT, that is, at a 20–40 dB sensation level (SL) relative to the SRT. The percentage of words repeated correctly by the subject (the speech recognition score), provides functional information regarding one's ability to receive communication auditorily. Goetzinger (1978) offered the following general guidelines for evaluation of word recognition scores: A score between 90 and 100 percent indicates an understanding ability within normal limits. A score between 75 and 90 percent indicates a slight difficulty comparable to listening over a telephone. A score between 60 and 75 percent indicates moderate difficulty. A score between 50 and 60 percent may indicate poor speech recognition with marked difficulty in following a conversation. Finally, a score less than 50 percent indicates very poor speech recognition with probable inability to follow the meaning of running speech.

Immittance Tests

Immittance tests (tympanometry and acoustic reflex tests) are electroacoustic tests that require no behavioral response from the subject. *Tympanometry* evaluates middle ear function by measuring the mobility of the tympanic membrane and ossicular chain in response to sound presented in the external ear canal under varying air pressures in the canal. Some pathologies (e.g., a disruption of the ossicular chair), show abnormally increased mobility whereas others (e.g., stiffening of the joints between the ossicles), show abnormally reduced mobility. *Acoustic reflex testing* also aids the assessment of middle ear function and, in some instances, provides information about cochlear, eighth nerve, facial nerve, and lower brainstem function. In our earlier discussion of the middle ear it was noted that the stapedius muscle is a primary contributor to the acoustic reflex, which reduces the transmission of sound through the middle ear. The presence or absence of this reflex, the intensity required to illicit the reflex, and the ability to sustain the reflex over time are diagnostic cues for the audiologist.

Tests Beyond the Routine Battery

Brainstem Auditory Evoked Response Tests

In brainstem auditory-evoked response (BAER) testing, also called auditory brainstem response (ABR) testing, or brainstem-evoked response (BSER) testing, acoustic stimuli are presented through earphones to evoke electrical activity in the auditory portion of the eighth nerve and brainstem. This electrical activity is picked up by electrodes placed on the head and the earlobes so that it can be processed by a computer and compared to norms. Although the BAER test is not a hearing test per se, the test does assess the function of the structures required for normal auditory function and can be used to estimate hearing sensitivity. It is particularly useful because it assesses the function of the eighth nerve and the auditory brainstem pathways without requiring behavioral responses from the person being tested.

Otoacoustic Emissions Tests

Otoacoustic emissions (OAEs) are sounds generated by movement of the outer hair cells in the cochlea and are transmitted through the normal middle ear to the external ear canal, where they can be measured by special equipment. OAEs are evoked by introducing test signals into the external ear canal for transmission through the middle ear to the inner ear. Assuming that middle ear function is normal, measurement of evoked OAEs provides a way of evaluating cochlear function. Evoked OAEs are used in screening protocols to identify hearing loss and in evaluation protocols to help distinguish between cochlear and retrocochlear involvement in cases of sensorineural hearing loss.

Other Tests

A variety of other tests are used by audiologists as needed. For example, some tests are designed to provide information about central auditory processing, and some are designed to assess psuedohypacusis (false hearing loss). Discussion of these tests is beyond the scope of this chapter.

Characteristics of Conductive and Sensorineural Hearing Loss

Conductive and sensorineural hearing losses present hearing characteristics that are generally different from each other. People with conductive hearing losses generally have somewhat poorer hearing in the low frequencies or hearing loss that is relatively equal across frequencies. Conductive losses result primarily in a reduction in the intensity that reaches the cochlea, and so people with conductive hearing losses generally benefit from increased volume. Although hearing aid amplification can be helpful in some instances, surgery and medication are the usually preferred remedies. People with conductive losses tend to talk either softer than usual or with normal intensity because they hear their own voices through bone conduction, but they do not hear competing noise. They may hear better in loud, noisy environments than they do in quieter environments, because the level of the noise reaching the cochlea is reduced by the conductive problem, and other people in the environment speak louder to be heard over the noise.

The audiograms of people with sensorineural losses generally have sloping curves. The amount of hearing loss typically, but not always, is more severe at the upper frequencies. Sound will arrive at the cochlea at a normal level, but will appear to be softer and distorted to some degree because of damage to cochlear or retrocohlear structures. In most instances surgery cannot remediate this type of loss, and increased volume alone cannot entirely make up the deficit. Hearing aids that amplify sounds and augment upper frequencies are helpful but do not restore perfect hearing. Before obtaining hearing aids, people with sensorineural losses often talk louder than normal since they may not be able to hear their own voices as loudly through bone conduction as they talk. To compensate, they speak up. People with this type of loss tend to hear more poorly in noisy environments than in quiet environments. Communicating with such an individual is facilitated by speaking distinctly, because much of normal speech is received as though it had been mumbled or muffled. In general, it is helpful for a hearing impaired person to be positioned to best take advantage of auditory cues and make the best use of residual vision to see the speaker's face and lips.

The pure tone thresholds and the results of speech recognition tests are used to determine what difficulty, if any, the individual will have in following conversation. In some cases test results are used to recommend hearing devices that will help to make up for the deficits in hearing and improve the reception of aural communication. The O&M specialist must be able to interpret the audiometric data in order to understand the student's ability to follow speech. This understanding is important so that the O&M specialist will not be surprised by communication problems and will be better able to communicate with the student. Some situations may require the use of manual communication skills or an interpreter. Equally important is the O&M specialist's sensitivity to communication problems that the student may have with the sighted public. As will be seen later in this chapter, audiometric data can also be used to help the O&M specialist to evaluate the use of sound for independent travel.

USE OF SPECIAL AUDITORY SKILLS BY PERSONS WITH VISUAL IMPAIRMENTS

This section begins with the development of hearing in children. The functions of hearing that are used specifically by visually impaired persons for independent travel are then examined.

Development of Hearing in Children

When do we first hear and how does hearing develop? The hearing mechanism appears to be ready at 6 to 7 months of gestation. Even some premature newborns respond to sound by 25 weeks.

During pregnancy, sound intensity inside the womb averages 85 dB SPL (Walker, Grimwade, & Wood, 1971). Although the intensity of external sounds, especially those above 800 Hz, are reduced by the intrauterine surroundings, voices that are close by or other loud sounds may be heard by the fetus (Armitage, Baldwin, & Vince, 1980). These first sounds are most likely low frequency components of the mother's voice and physiologic noise. These sounds may help to fine tune the development of the auditory mechanism and pathways (Fifer & Moon, 1988). Because of the internal environment, the fetus' first sound experience may be closer to that of bone conduction hearing than air conduction hearing (Rubel, 1985).

After a child is born, his or her hearing switches from fluid and tissue conducted sound to air conducted sound (Peck, 1994). Auditory brainstem response audiometry (discussed in the section "Tests Beyond the Routine Battery," above) has shown that a newborn's thresholds for clicking sounds are approximately 17 dB poorer than adult thresholds (Hecox, 1975; Schulman-Galambos & Galambos, 1979). It is also clear through observation of the child's startle response and other reflexive responses that newborns respond to intense sounds. Using a behavioral approach to assessing auditory ability, it has also been observed that infants between 2 and 5 weeks of age have thresholds to sound of 55 and 60 dB SPL at 500 and 4000 Hz (Werner & Gillenwater, 1990). The gap between the hearing sensitivity of the adult and the child continues to close with the growth of the child (Trehub, Schneider, Morrongiello, & Thorpe, 1988, 1989). Children reach adult sensitivity by the age of 4 or 5 years for frequencies around 10,000 Hz; by age 8 for the 2000 to 4000 Hz range; and by the age of 10 for the 400 to 1000 Hz range. By 7 years of age, children actually are more sensitive than adults for 20,000 Hz and gradually lose sensitivity in that range as they mature to adulthood.

Sound localization in infants develops first in the horizontal plane and later in the vertical plane. As an orienting reaction to sound, infants turn their heads to the right or the left of their midline (Clifton et al., 1981). As the infant matures, the speed of localization improves and reflexive localization becomes voluntary behavior (Morrongiello & Clifton, 1984; Morrongiello & Gotowiec, 1990). In the horizontal plane, the smallest detectable angle of localization change moves from 27 degrees at 8 weeks to 14 degrees by 6 months, 8 degrees by 12 months, and 4 degrees by 18 months (Morrongiello, 1988a). Localization in the vertical plane is less accurate than in the horizontal plane by 1 or 2 degrees (Morrongiello & Rocca, 1987b). Vertical localization seems to depend on high frequency sounds, which are affected by the shape of the pinna. It may be that as the child matures and the pinnae develop, high frequency cues can be better utilized. According to Morrongiello and Gotowiec (1990), early localization is accompanied by visual searching activities. Beyond the second month, babies combine the use of the auditory and visual senses to locate objects. It has been observed that an infant who is blind is less likely to localize than a sighted child during the first 6 months (Muir, 1985).

Recognition of specific sounds has been observed in neonates as young as 3 days old (DeCasper & Fifer, 1980). It has been shown that babies of that age are able to identify their own mother's voices. Infants are also able to recognize specific kinds of vocalizations. For example, they tend to prefer vocal patterns that adults typically use when speaking to babies. Such language, often referred to as "motherese," is characterized as language consisting of slow tempo, high frequency, and well-differentiated intonations (Aslin, Pisoni, & Jusezyk, 1983; Fernald, 1992). These vocalizations transmit the feelings and mood of the parent. Later other vocalizations begin to carry more sophisticated meanings that are associated with the circumstances of the environment and situation.

Discrimination of sounds is also possible for neonates (Papousek, 1961; Siqueland & Lipsitt, 1966). Infants can discriminate between differences in time and frequencies of various sounds. This ability allows the infant during the first year of life to achieve discriminations that make the acquisition of language possible (Kuhl, 1987). It has been hypothesized that listening to prenatal low-frequency sound prepares the infant for this later discrimination (Peck, 1995).

The development of perceptual hearing skills is a complex phenomenon that may occur through the interaction of biology and experience. It appears that infants may be biologically designed to process speech, but that experience is needed by 6 months of age for that capability to unfold (Kuhl, 1987). For example, a child with profound congenital deafness usually will be unable to learn aural–oral communication without an intervention program. There are a number of theories that try to define how genetics and experience interact to establish perceptual development (Werker & Tees, 1992). At one end of the continuum is the theory that maturation alone may account for the emergence of perceptual skills without any experience. Other theories suggest that experience is necessary to maintain perceptual skills, facilitate those skills, or attune the perceptual mechanism. At the other end of the continuum is the theory which states that the skills are latent and the development of the skills is totally dependent upon environmental experience.

In all likelihood, an interaction between genetics and environmental experiences are responsible for the development of perceptual hearing capabilities. This has implications for the development of perceptual hearing skills for children who are blind. It is clear that development of localization in a sighted child occurs through a bimodal model that depends upon the integration of vision and hearing. It is clear that without vision, localization skills may be delayed. It may be that vision also plays a supporting role in the development of other hearing skills. If this is the case, it becomes necessary to help children with visual impairment to combine all of their senses with hearing so that they can develop their perceptual hearing capabilities as quickly as fully sighted children. For example, toys that emit sounds should be visually stimulating and/or tactilely interesting so that infants will have as much information as possible to combine with hearing. It is important to provide practice with sound localization to help the child establish ear–hand coordination. It should also be noted that the mother's or father's touch, when paired with their vocalizations, serves to stimulate the development of sound recognition and discrimination. The visually impaired toddler may benefit by being introduced to environmental sounds by the parent or through games and recordings.

Binaural Sound Localization by the Visually Impaired Traveler

The visually impaired traveler benefits greatly from the reception of acoustic cues through both ears. Differences in the signal characteristics reaching each ear make it possible to localize the sound source. Thus it is important to understand the basic principles of sound localization. To a visually impaired traveler, sound localization emerges as a perceptual skill of paramount importance that goes beyond the usual listening skills of a sighted person. It allows the visually impaired traveler to locate objects within the environment and travel safely through that environment.

Signal Differences at the Two Ears: An Overview

According to Carhart (1958), the listener uses both ears to obtain an auditory triangulation (left ear, right ear, sound source) that enables localization of the sound source on the basis of signal differences at the two ears. Carhart (1958), Bergman (1957), and Sayers and Cherry (1957) all report four characteristic differences between signals reaching the ears. The first difference between incoming signals is the time of arrival at the two ears. The second difference in signal reception between the two ears is signal intensity. The ear closest to the sound source will receive a more intense signal because of the separation of the ears and the defraction effect of the head, which tends to reduce the intensity to the far ear. The third difference is found in the phase relationship of the signals reaching the ears. Again, because of the distance between the ears, the phase position of the sound wave reaching the farther ear will be different from the phase of the signal reaching the closer ear. The fourth and final difference between signals is the spectral composition. According to Wiener (1947), and Perrott and Elfner (1968), the head acts as a filter, reducing high frequency sound as the signal moves around the head. Low frequency sounds with wavelengths longer than the diameter of the head tend to bend around the head, while high frequency sounds with wavelengths shorter than the diameter of the head tend to be reflected rather than scattered around the head. As a result, the ear away from the sound source will receive fewer high frequency components. Furthermore, Sayers and Cherry (1957) state that additional spectral differences may be perceived due to the reflective properties of the environment and different angles-of-incidence of sound waves as they strike the various parts of the pinna.

Head and Pinna Shadow

When a signal comes from the side, one of the ears receives the signal earlier and with more intensity than the other ear. Phase and spectral differences are also present. All these differences permit the individual to localize the position of the sound source accurately. If the sound comes from directly in front of or behind the individual, the signals to the two ears will be very similar and will complicate the distinction between front and rear sound sources (especially for one who is visually impaired). In this situation, a person may turn the head slightly to create a difference between the signals that enables localization. According to Noble (1975), spectral components may also help one to localize sound where the source is directly ahead of or behind the person. According to the "pinna-shadow hypothesis," the pinna acts to shadow the ear canal when the signal approaches from the rear, allowing passage of low frequencies more easily than high frequencies. Therefore, a complex sound will provide different spectral components to the inner ear, depending upon whether it is emanating from in front of or behind the individual. Furthermore, Hirsh (1950a) explains that the pinna may also serve to reduce the overall intensity of a sound approaching the ear from the rear relative to the intensity of sounds approaching from the front. A similar intensity reduction theory was postulated earlier by Stevens and Newman (1936). Intensity reduction theories state that the pinna, by altering spectrum and intensity, helps a person to determine whether a sound is coming from the front or the rear.

Role of Frequency, Phase, Time, and Intensity in Localization

Certain signal differences become more important for sound localization at specific frequency ranges. According to Stevens and Newman (1936) and Harris et al. (1974), the time of arrival and phase differences at the two ears are most important for localizing frequencies below 1500 Hz. Harris notes that the value of phase differences diminishes to 0 as the frequency increases to about 1500 Hz. At frequencies above 1500 Hz intensity cues become more important. Mills (1960) reported the minimum perceptible difference in interaural intensity to be as small as 0.5 dB at 1500 Hz and above. Although both time and intensity differences may be available for localization over a wide range of frequencies, time and phase differences are most useful at low frequencies, and intensity differences are most useful at high frequencies. Data from Stevens and Newman (1936) indicate that localization errors are more frequent for frequencies in the 2000 to 4000 Hz range and less frequent for frequencies above and below this range. Thus localization is somewhat dependent on a sound's spectral content.

Reverberant spaces, those in which reflective surfaces produce multiple reflections or echos of sound, in essence produce multiple "sources" of the original incident sound. Because the first sound wave reaching the ears is usually the incident sound, it dominates or takes precedence over echoes in localizing the sound source. Localization is toward the first side or ear to receive the first wave front. This phenomenon, sometimes called the *principle* or *law of the first wave front* or the *precedence effect,* helps one to localize sound under reverberant conditions (Durrant & Lovrinic, 1995; Gelfand, 1990).

Localization of Direction and Estimation of Distance

Localization of a sound source goes hand in hand with determining its distance. Very little research has dealt with the ability to judge the distance of a sound. According to Whetnall (1964) estimation of distance to a sound source is determined by the ratio of reflected sound to direct sound reaching the ears. When the sound source is nearby, a greater proportion of the sound comes directly from the source. When the sound source is farther away, more of the sound comes from reflection. An automobile may be heard directly when it is close, but a car farther off in the distance is identified by its direct sound as well as the sound reflected from buildings. Furthermore, a given source sounds louder if it is nearby compared to when it is far away.

Accuracy of Localization

Mills (1958) reported on the minimum audible angle, the smallest difference in azimuth to the sound source (a clockwise angle in a horizontal plane) that a listener can discriminate with the head restrained facing straight ahead. Mills reported minimum audible angles to be smallest when sound was directly in front of the head (1–2 degrees) and largest when sound was at the side of the head. In actual field testing it is not uncommon, however, to find 15-degree errors in localization.

The ability to localize sound in a vertical direction can be studied by varying the elevation of a sound source in a median plane midway between the ears. Such study shows that vertical localization requires that the listener have an intact pinna and that the sound source contain energy at frequencies greater than 4000 Hz. Because of its small size, the pinna effectively contributes to localization only at high frequencies, those frequencies that have short wavelengths. Vertical localization is typically poorer than localization in a horizontal plane.

When the head is stationary, different sound locations can produce the same interaural time and intensity differences. For example, Feddersen, Sandel, Teas, and Jeffress (1957) found that at 0 and 180-degree azimuths, interaural time and intensity differences are negligible. Thus it is often difficult to determine whether a sound is coming from the front or the rear. In the real world, a sound source can be in any direction at any angle, and the head is typically free to move.

Role of Head Movement in Localization

Movement of the head plays an important role in localization of sound. Hirsh (1950b) indicates that localization effects are the greatest when the individual moves his head to use both ears. According to Briskey (1972), sounds of long duration may require head movements to maximize localization by utilizing the head-shadow effect to identify sound intensity differences. According to Koenig (1950) our directional perception is in part related to our ability to analyze the way binaural sounds are affected by head movements. He noted that in an experiment using a binaural telephone system, localization to the right and left were possible, but the listener seemed to identify all sounds as emanating from a semicircle behind his head. Similar experiments using binaural tapes with subjects who were blind by Norton (1960) resulted in the same confusion when head movements did not make changes in the signals reaching the two ears. Sayers and Cherry (1957) explained that physical acoustic clues may be correlated with kinesthetic neck muscle clues to further process direction. The brain may analyze the sound and correlate it with kinesthetic clues as it attempts to fuse the signals from the two ears.

Hearing Loss and Localization

Often when there is unilateral hearing loss or when the ears have different thresholds, there are implications for sound localization. Bergman (1957) indicates that when individuals have markedly different thresholds between the two ears, localization ability depends primarily upon the level of intensity of the sound. He performed a study in which he tested localization of hearing impaired individuals by continually raising the sound stimulation in steps of 5 dB, beginning 10 dB above the speech detection threshold for spondee words in a free-field presentation. His results showed that the ability to localize in a person with a significantly better ear occurred when the level of sound was sufficient to stimulate the poorer ear as well. It was found that at low sensation levels the subjects tended to judge the sounds to be emanating from the side near the better ear or from in front of them. The subject was able to localize more accurately only when the sounds reached the level above auditory threshold of the poorer ear.

Sound Localization with Monaural Hearing

Wright and Carhart (1960) found that some individuals were able to localize monaurally. Perrott and Elfner (1968) noted that although sound localization is primarily a binaural process, monaural localization is possible, particularly when the sound source is persistent and the head can be moved. Monaural localization is facilitated, for example, if a person who is unilaterally deaf moves his or her head to seek out the area of maximum intensity for a stable sound source. Perrott and Elfner further reported that some subjects were able to demonstrate monaural localization without head movements. Generally the performance of these subjects was poorer than normal, but still significantly better than predicted by chance, and performance for some subjects was nearly as good as that of individuals who used binaural hearing.

Use of Traffic Sounds for Orientation and Mobility in Independent Travel

One of the main concerns of the O&M specialist is how well the person who is visually impaired will be able to interpret traffic sounds. Audiometric data must be used not just to understand the student's communication ability, but to assess the student's potential for independent travel. The ability to use auditory cues will help determine how successful a traveler can become. It is therefore important to understand the hearing sensitivity of the traveler and the nature and audibility of traffic sounds.

Spectral Characteristics of Traffic Sounds

A *sound level meter* is an instrument used to measure sound levels. It can measure the overall sound pressure level, an A-weighted level that reduces the low frequences, and with a filter attached to it can be used to measure the sound level in individual bands of frequencies. The overall sound pressure level is a linear measurement that gives equal importance to all frequencies. The A-weighted sound level (dBA) is a measurement obtained by filtering out low frequencies that generally correspond with the frequency responsiveness of the human ear. Spectral analysis is accomplished by measuring the sound energy in selected bands of frequencies while filtering out energy outside the bands. Usually, energy is measured within individual *octave* bands named for their center frequencies (e.g., 16, 32, 64, 125, 250, 500, 1000, 2000, 4000, and 8000 Hz.).

Frequency and Intensity of Traffic Sounds

The frequency and intensity of traffic sounds are affected by various conditions (Bugliarello, Alexandre, Barnes, and Wakstein, 1976). When a car is operating in low gear, the overall noise output is mainly produced by the engine and connecting parts (Nelson, 1987) . However, when a car is in the highest gear, the overall noise output is mainly generated by the tires. With each doubling of speed the tire noise increases by about 9 dB. Tire noise covers the entire audible frequency range from 20 to 20,000 Hz. Acceleration of vehicles can increase intensity 10 to 20 dB beyond that of normal driving at a constant speed. Pavement surfaces can cause variations of 5 to 7 dB (Hamilton, 1980). Rough pavement can increase the sound intensity by about 12 dBA in the frequency range from 100 to 1000 Hz.

Weather and traffic conditions also affect the sound. A car riding in the rain can produce a sound 10 dBA greater than would be produced on dry pavement. Snow tends to reduce intensity. The average sound intensity of traffic becomes greater when the number of vehicles increases. The sound level is 10 dB greater for the average heavy truck than for the average car.

In an unpublished study, Wiener and Goldstein (1977) measured approximate traffic intensities in different settings to examine the relationship between auditory thresholds at various frequencies and the ability to use traffic sounds for independent travel. Measurements of sounds were made as cars passed by in a quiet residential area with intermittent traffic, a residential area with continuous traffic, a small business area, and in a downtown metropolitan area. The overall measurements were 72 dBA, 71 dBA, 76 dBA, and 84 dBA respectively. Octave band analysis of these traffic sounds showed that levels were generally greater for low frequency than for high frequency components.

Wiener et al. (1997) measured the range of intensity of traffic sounds in situations where vehicles were accelerating at residential and small business intersections. In the residential area 40 recordings were made as various single vehicles accelerated from a stop sign. In the small business area 40 recordings were made as groups of vehicles in multiple lanes accelerated from a traffic light. In the small business area twenty measurements were made on a two way street with a total of four lanes of traffic and another twenty measurements were made on a street with four lanes of traffic all moving in one direction. Recordings were analyzed to determine intensity in each octave band (16 Hz to 8000 Hz). Octave band levels were determined for sound generated during the first 5 seconds of vehicle acceleration. Five seconds was an estimation of the time necessary for a person to determine if a vehicle was going straight through an intersection or turning.

Data from Wiener et al. (1997) is shown in Tables 4.2–4.5. Octave band noise levels (traffic sounds), minimum audible field values for pure tones, and estimated hearing levels (HL) for noise necessary to detect traffic at each octave band center frequency are shown. Minimum audible field values (db SPL) in Tables 4.2–4.5 represent pure tone levels that are just audible to the average normal hearing listener in a standard test environment. These minimum audible field values represent correction factors which can be subtracted from the octave band measures to estimate the audiometric hearing level (HL) needed to hear the traffic noise present in each octave band. In Tables 4.2–4.5 minimum audible field values are subtracted from the minimum octave band noise levels to estimate noise hearing levels (HL) that can be compared with hearing thresholds on the audiogram. The threshold of audibility should be better for noise than for pure tones. However, Tables 4.2–4.5 compare octave band noise levels of traffic to thresholds of audibility for tones in a standard (quiet) test environment rather than a traffic environment. Therefore, the audibility of the noise may vary depending upon the environment.

Detection of Accelerating Vehicles

According to Wiener et al. (1997), although accelerating vehicles produce the greatest amount of energy in the lower frequencies, the human hearing mechanism is best designed to respond to intensity in the upper frequencies. In a residential setting the intensity of vehicles accelerating from a stop ranged from 77.8 dB SPL to 90.4 dB SPL with a mean of 86 dB SPL. In the small business setting the intensity of two-way traffic accelerating from a traffic light ranged from 88.8 dB SPL to 102.4 dB SPL with a mean of 94 dB SPL. In the small business setting with four lanes of one-way traffic, intensity ranged from 80.6 dB SPL to 103.5 dB SPL with a mean of 88 dB SPL. The greater intensity on the two-way street in the small business area can be explained by the double acceleration of traffic from the same light during the 5-second period. As can be seen by the octave band levels (Tables 4.2–4.4), most of the energy in the traffic sounds was concentrated in the low frequencies. However, as can be seen by the minimum audible field values, the auditory system is less sensitive to frequencies below 500 Hz, and most sensitive in the 500 Hz to 4000 Hz range. This means that audiometric thresholds in the 500 Hz to 4000 Hz range may be particularly important in assessing one's ability to detect traffic. Generally speaking, hearing impaired individuals who have threshold averages of 55 dB HL or better in the 500 Hz to 4000 Hz range may be able to detect the acceleration of vehicles from a stop in a residential area. Threshold averages of 65 dB HL or better in the 500 Hz range may be needed to detect acceleration of vehicles in a business area, where the noise is more intense. Some individuals who are seen by the O&M specialist will be wearing hearing aids that augment frequencies in the 500 Hz to

Table 4.2. Octave Band (OB) Sound Levels for Traffic Acceleration from a Stop Sign in a Residential Area

OB Center Frequencies	32 Hz	63 Hz	125 Hz	250 Hz	500 Hz	1000 Hz	2000 Hz	4000 Hz	8000 Hz	Overall SPL	Overall dBA
OB levels (dB SPL)											
Mean	74.8	81.1	77.5	73.2	71.2	71.3	69.8	68.6	63.7	86.0	77.4
Minimum value	68.7	71.0	67.5	63.2	61.2	60.5	57.3	59.4	56.6	77.8	66.9
Maximum value	81.4	92.3	85.1	82.3	79.8	79.2	84.3	77.2	73.7	90.4	84.6
SD	3.5	4.9	4.6	4.7	4.6	4.6	4.8	4.6	4.9	3.4	4.2
Minimum audible field (dB SPL)[a]	**78.2[b]**	**43.7[c]**	**22.2**	**11.1**	**4.0**	**1.9**	**−1.6**	**−6.4**	**11.5**		
Estimated hearing levels (dB HL)											
Mean	−3.4	37.3	55.3	62.1	67.2	69.4	71.4	75.0	52.2		
Minimum value	**−9.5**	**27.3**	**45.3**	**52.1**	**57.2**	**58.6**	**58.9**	**65.8**	**45.1**		
Maximum value	3.2	48.6	62.9	71.2	75.8	77.3	85.9	83.6	62.2		

[a]ISO/R225-1985: ISO Normal Equal-Loudness Contours for Pure Tones under Free-field Listening Conditions-with low-frequency corrections as suggested by Killion (1978). Adapted from Yost (1994, p. 139).

[b]The minimal audible field measurement of 78.2 is for a frequency of 20 Hz.

[c]The minimal audible field measurement of 43.7 is for a frequency of 50 Hz.

Table 4.3. Octave Band (OB) Sound Levels for Traffic Accelerating from a Stop Light in a Small Business Area on a Two-Way (four lane) Street

OB Center Frequencies	32 Hz	63 Hz	125 Hz	250 Hz	500 Hz	1000 Hz	2000 Hz	4000 Hz	8000 Hz	Overall SPL	Overall dBA
OB levels (dB SPL)											
Mean	85.6	88.3	85.2	78.2	75.8	75.3	73.3	71.8	66.8	94.0	81.4
Minimum	80.4	80.8	77.7	73.2	73.2	68.0	65.0	64.4	61.2	88.8	74.6
Maximum	92.3	97.5	98.1	84.9	83.3	82.9	83.0	81.3	76.1	102.4	88.4
SD	4.3	4.5	4.9	3.5	3.4	3.4	4.1	4.8	4.0	3.4	3.5
Minimum audible field (dB SPL)[a]	**78.2[b]**	**43.7[c]**	**22.2**	**11.1**	**4.0**	**1.9**	**−1.6**	**−6.4**	**11.5**		
Estimated hearing levels (dB HL)											
Mean	7.4	44.6	63.0	67.1	71.8	73.4	74.9	78.2	55.3		
Minimum value	**2.2**	**37.1**	**55.5**	**62.1**	**69.2**	**66.6**	**66.6**	**70.8**	**49.7**		
Maximum value	14.1	53.8	75.9	73.8	79.3	84.6	84.6	87.7	64.6		

[a]ISO/R255-1985: ISO Normal Equal-Loudness Contours for Pure Tones under Free-field Listening Conditions-with low-frequency corrections as suggested by Killion (1978). Adapted from Yost (1994, p. 139).

[b]The minimal audible field measurement of 78.2 is for a frequency of 20 Hz.

[c]The minimal audible field measurement of 43.7 is for a frequency of 50 Hz.

Table 4.4. Octave Band (OB) Sound Levels for Traffic Accelerating from a Stop Light in a Small Business Area on a One-Way (four lane) Street

OB Center Frequencies	32 Hz	63 Hz	125 Hz	250 Hz	500 Hz	1000 Hz	2000 Hz	4000 Hz	8000 Hz	Overall SPL	Overall dBA
OB levels (dB SPL)											
Mean	80.5	83.2	80.2	74.0	71.2	70.5	68.2	65.3	60.6	88.0	76.2
Min	71.5	74.3	72.3	66.6	67.2	68.0	66.5	62.8	53.8	80.6	69.7
Max	97.8	100.5	94.4	89.9	82.1	84.2	84.1	80.5	74.7	103.5	90.3
SD	7.1	6.5	6.8	6.3	4.9	5.7	5.7	6.4	6.1	6.1	5.5
Minimum audible field (dB SPL)[a]	**78.2**[b]	**43.7**[c]	**22.2**	**11.1**	**4.0**	**1.9**	**−1.6**	**−6.4**	**11.5**		
Estimated hearing levels (dB HL)											
Mean	2.3	39.5	58.0	62.9	67.2	68.6	69.8	71.7	49.1		
Minimum value	**−6.7**	**30.6**	**50.1**	**55.5**	**63.2**	**66.1**	**68.1**	**69.2**	**42.3**		
Maximum value	19.6	56.8	72.2	78.8	78.1	82.3	85.7	86.9	63.2		

[a]ISO/R225-1985: ISO Normal Equal-Loudness Countours for Pure Tones under Free-field Listening Conditions-with low-frequency corrections as suggested by Killion (1978). Adapted from Yost (1994, p. 139).
[b]The minimal audible field measurement of 78.2 is for a frequency of 20 Hz.
[c]The minimal audible field measurement of 43.7 is for a frequency of 50 Hz.

4000 Hz range. Energy for frequencies at 125 and 250 Hz is also typically audible. Individuals who have relatively good hearing at these low frequencies and significantly impaired hearing for high frequencies may still be able to use traffic sounds for orientation and mobility. While these generalizations may apply to many individuals, comparing the traveler's frequency specific thresholds with the noise hearing levels needed to detect traffic (Tables 4.2–4.5), will provide a better indication of one's ability to travel in traffic. This process must be accompanied by clinical trials in a variety of travel environments.

Detection of Approaching Traffic

Wiener et al. (1997) gathered further information to determine the intensity that may be needed to detect an oncoming car in a residential neighborhood. Measurements of intensity were recorded at 110 feet as 24 individual cars approached a sound level meter and Digital Audio Tape recorder positioned at a street corner controlled by a stop sign (Table 4.5). This distance was chosen because the American Automobile Association (1957) indicates that a car traveling 30 mph requires 78 feet to stop (33 feet of reaction distance and 45 feet of braking distance) under clear conditions. To provide a safety margin and to allow for a car going faster than 30 mph, the distance of 110 feet was chosen to assure that a pedestrian could hear the car from a far enough distance to avoid injury. Wiener et al. found that traffic intensity levels for individual cars at a distance of 110 feet (Table 4.5) ranged from 70 dB SPL to 83.1 dB SPL with a mean of 74.4 dB SPL. Again, as seen in the minimum audible field values, the auditory system is most sensitive in the 500 Hz to 4000 Hz range. By subtracting the minimum audible field values from the minimum traffic noise levels at each octave band, it is possible to estimate the auditory thresholds (in dB HL levels) needed to detect approaching vehicles. Generally speaking, detection of a vehicle approaching from 110 feet

Table 4.5. Octave Band (OB) Sound Levels for Traffic Approaching from 110 feet in a Residential Area

OB Center Frequencies	32 Hz	63 Hz	125 Hz	250 Hz	500 Hz	1000 Hz	2000 Hz	4000 Hz	8000 Hz	Overall SPL	Overall dBA
OB levels (dB SPL)											
Mean	68.9	69.8	64.7	58.0	57.9	61.6	61.9	55.1	48.4	74.4	66.8
Minimum	63.6	63.7	58.1	51.4	50.5	54.4	55.3	48.3	42.0	70.0	60.7
Maximum	75.5	81.1	74.0	72.2	72.8	69.8	73.7	61.6	62.2	83.1	77.3
SD	3.3	3.7	4.4	5.0	4.7	3.9	4.5	3.3	4.8	3.0	3.9
Minimum audible field (dB SPL)[a]	**78.2**[b]	**43.7**[c]	**22.2**	**11.1**	**4.0**	**1.9**	**−1.6**	**−6.4**	**11.5**		
Estimated hearing levels (dB HL)											
Mean	−9.3	26.1	42.5	46.9	53.9	59.7	63.5	61.5	36.9		
Minimum value	**−14.6**	**20.0**	**35.9**	**40.3**	**46.5**	**52.5**	**56.9**	**54.7**	**30.5**		
Maximum value	−2.7	37.4	51.8	61.1	68.8	67.9	75.3	68.0	50.7		

[a]ISO/R225-1985: ISO Normal Equal-Loudness Contours for Pure Tones under Free-field Listening Conditions-with low-frequency corrections as suggested by Killion (1978). Adapted from Yost (1994, p. 139).
[b]The minimal audible field measurement of 78.2 is for a frequency of 20 Hz.
[c]The minimal audible field measurement of 43.7 is for a frequency of 50 Hz.

away in a residential area would require thresholds of 45 dB HL or better in the 500 Hz to 4000 Hz range. However, it may also be possible for an individual who has significant hearing loss in the upper frequencies and fairly good hearing thresholds in the lower frequencies to detect traffic. Again, it is best to consult the traveler's audiogram relative to the noise hearing levels and to conduct clinical trials in the travel environment rather than relying solely on the above generalizations.

Comparison of a Traveler's Audiogram to Traffic Noise Hearing Levels

A traveler's hearing thresholds can be compared to traffic noise hearing levels to estimate how audible the noise would be. Figures 4.26 and 4.27 show sound field hearing threholds (S) for the same individual with and without hearing aids. Sound field thresholds are obtained by presenting warble tones (tones which vary around a center frequency) through a sound field speaker (ears uncovered). Sound field thresholds that are not ear specific are indicated by S's. Warble tone thresholds in a sound field generally produce similar thresholds to pure tones presented through head phones. Individuals who wear hearing aids are sometimes tested in a sound field with and without hearing aids. According to Figure 4.26, the individual's unaided thresholds are 55 dB HL at 500 Hz, 60 dB HL at 1000 Hz, 65 dB HL at 2000 Hz, and 70 dB HL at 4000 Hz. Without hearing aids, the individual probably can not detect vehicles approaching from 110 feet away in a residential area (Table 4.5). According to Table 4.5, hearing threshold levels must be 46.5 dB or better for 500 Hz, 52.5 dB or better for 1000 Hz, 56.9 dB or better for 2000 Hz, and 54.7 db or better for 4000 Hz for approaching traffic to be heard in the residential neighborhood at 110 feet. In the case of accelerating vehicles, however, the individual's thresholds may be low enough to recognize accelerating vehicles (Tables 4.2–4.4).

Figure 4.27 shows thresholds (S) for the same

WESTERN MICHIGAN UNIVERSITY
CHARLES VAN RIPER LANGUAGE, SPEECH & HEARING CLINIC
Audiometric Evaluation

Date________ File No. ________

Name________ Age___ Sex___ DOB______ Response Mode______

Tested by ________ Audiometer________ Accuracy: Good___Fair___Poor___

PURE TONE AUDIOGRAM

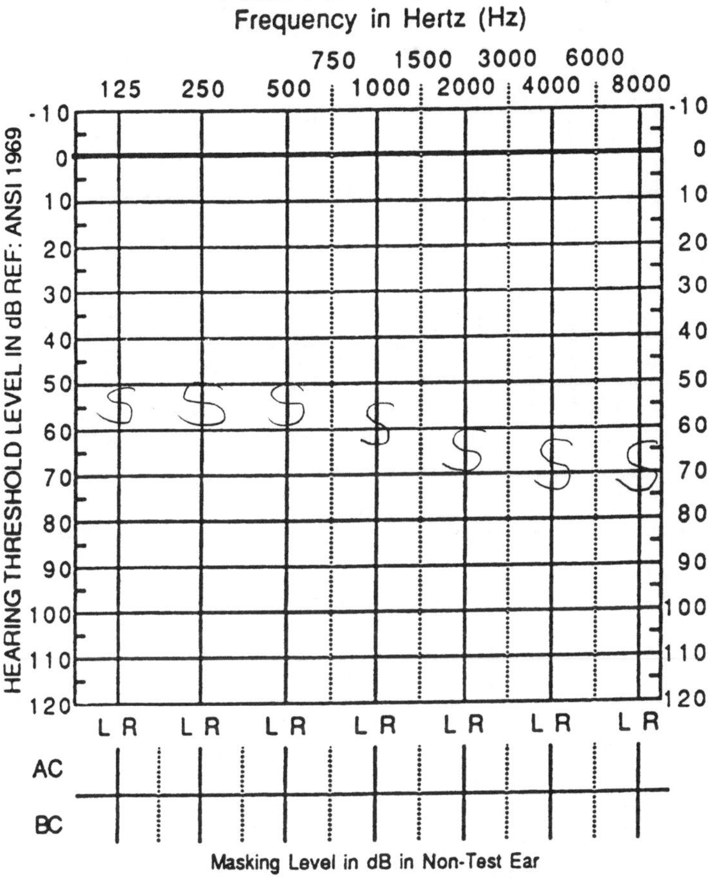

Frequency in Hertz (Hz)

Masking Level in dB in Non-Test Ear

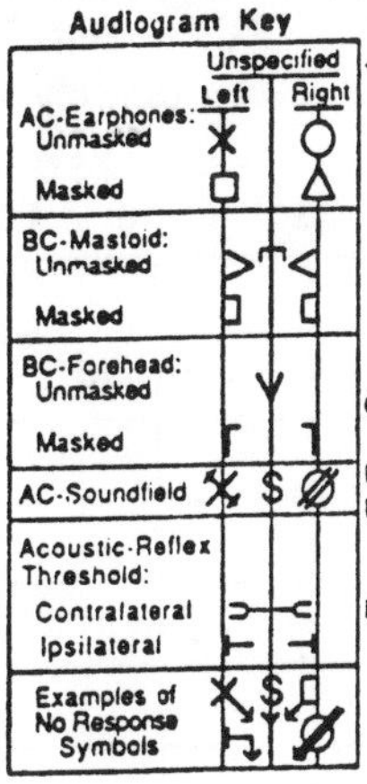

PURE TONE AVERAGE: R ____dB L ____dB (AC 500-1000-2000 Hz)

Audiogram Key

	Unspecified Left	Right
AC-Earphones: Unmasked	X	O
Masked	□	△
BC-Mastoid: Unmasked	>	<
Masked	[	]
BC-Forehead: Unmasked	V	
Masked	[	]
AC-Soundfield	X	S Ø
Acoustic-Reflex Threshold: Contralateral	⊃—	—⊂
Ipsilateral	⊢	⊣
Examples of No Response Symbols		

Scale of Hearing Impairment (dB HL)

-10 to 15 normal
16 to 25 slight
26 to 40 mild
41 to 55 moderate
56 to 70 mod. sev.
71 to 90 severe
> 90 profound

Abbreviations

CNT Could Not Test
NR No Response
DNT Did Not Test
LDL Loudness Discomfort Level
MCL Most Comfortable Loudness Level

Were speech or language problems noted?
No___ Yes___ (see report)

Remarks:

SPEECH AUDIOMETRY

TEST		R	L	SOUNDFIELD Unaided	SOUNDFIELD Aided	Live Voice	Rec.
SRT		dB	dB	dB	dB		
Word Recog. (WR) Scores	@___dB___	%	%	%	%		
	@___dB___	%	%	%	%		
	@___dB___	%	%	%	%		
LDL		dB	dB	dB	dB		
MCL		dB	dB	dB	dB		

* = masking used

Figure 4.26. Audiogram illustrating sound field hearing thresholds without hearing aid.

WESTERN MICHIGAN UNIVERSITY
CHARLES VAN RIPER LANGUAGE, SPEECH & HEARING CLINIC
Audiometric Evaluation

Date________ File No. ________

Name________ Age___ Sex___ DOB______ Response Mode______

Tested by ________ Audiometer________ Accuracy: Good___Fair___Poor___

PURE TONE AUDIOGRAM
Frequency in Hertz (Hz)

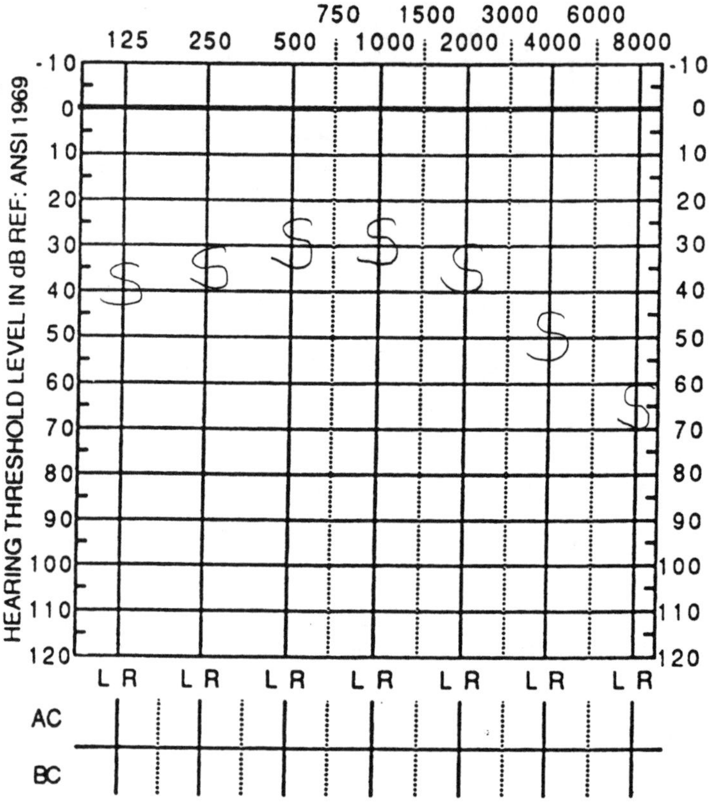

125 250 500 750 1000 1500 2000 3000 4000 6000 8000

HEARING THRESHOLD LEVEL IN dB REF: ANSI 1969

-10 0 10 20 30 40 50 60 70 80 90 100 110 120

S S S S S S S

L R L R L R L R L R L R L R

AC

BC

Masking Level in dB in Non-Test Ear

PURE TONE AVERAGE: R ____dB L ____dB (AC 500-1000-2000 Hz)

Audiogram Key

	Unspecified Left	Unspecified Right
AC-Earphones: Unmasked	X	O
Masked	□	△
BC-Mastoid: Unmasked	>	<
Masked	⊐	⊏
BC-Forehead: Unmasked	∨	
Masked	⌐	¬
AC-Soundfield	X S Ø	
Acoustic-Reflex Threshold: Contralateral		
Ipsilateral		
Examples of No Response Symbols		

Scale of Hearing Impairment (dB HL)
-10 to 15 normal
16 to 25 slight
26 to 40 mild
41 to 55 moderate
56 to 70 mod. sev.
71 to 90 severe
> 90 profound

Abbreviations
CNT Could Not Test
NR No Response
DNT Did Not Test
LDL Loudness Discomfort Level
MCL Most Comfortable Loudness Level

Were speech or language problems noted?
No_✓_Yes___ (see report)

Remarks:

SPEECH AUDIOMETRY

TEST		R	L	SOUNDFIELD Unaided	SOUNDFIELD Aided	Live Voice	Rec.
SRT		dB	dB	dB	dB		
Word Recog. (WR) Scores	@___dB___	%	%	%	%		
	@___dB___	%	%	%	%		
	@___dB___	%	%	%	%		
LDL		dB	dB	dB	dB		
MCL		dB	dB	dB	dB		

* = masking used

Figure 4.27. Audiogram illustrating sound field hearing thresholds with hearing aid.

individual evaluated with hearing aids. Hearing appears to be adequate for detecting both accelerating (Tables 4.2–4.4) and approaching vehicles (Table 4.5). Improved sensitivity for the upper frequencies improves thresholds to levels that permit the individual to perceive traffic sounds in all four conditions (Tables 4.2–4.5). A note of caution is necessary here. The use of hearing aids complicates one's ability to localize the direction and distance of traffic sounds. Some complicating factors may be the hearing aid's automatic gain control, potential lack of balanced binaural reception, and possible distortion in phase, amplitude, and frequency. Hearing aids may have a type of compression which systematically adds less gain as input levels increase in order to protect the individual from excessively intense sounds. Compression amplifiers add gain so that the output is amplified, but the range of output intensities is reduced relative to the range of input intensities. The result may be reduced accuracy in judging distances. Furthermore, even aided hearing may not be the same in both ears.

Possible Changes of Intensity in Traffic Sounds

The amount of audible vehicle information available to the visually impaired pedestrian may be reduced in the future. Over the years the level of noise produced by cars has been gradually reduced. Prior to 1972 the federal government did not have regulations regarding traffic noise levels. In 1972 the Federal Noise Control Act required cars to make changes to quiet their total noise output. Prior to 1972 moving vehicle output was commonly 90dB (Nelson, 1987). Presently the maximum noise output for a passenger car must not exceed 78dB and cars account for 80 percent of all traffic noise. Worldwide, there are 10 vehicles for every 100 individuals, and in America there are 70 vehicles for every 100 people (Sperling, 1995). This proliferation of the internal combustion engine causes air pollution, damages the ozone layer, and contributes to the greenhouse effect. It is predicted that attempts to solve these problems may lead to a technological revolution which will direct us to electric vehicles. In addition to having reduced emissions, these vehicles will have greatly reduced noise output. The quietest electric vehicles produce an output level of 58 dBSPL while traveling at 30 mph and an acceleration output level of 61 dBSPL (Hamilton, 1980; Society of Automotive Engineers of Japan, 1977). Because of the reduction in noise output, "electric vehicles are a greater danger to pedestrians than are conventional automobiles" (Whitener, 1981). They certainly will reduce audible information that is used by travelers who are visually impaired. A dangerous complication may be the masking of electric vehicles by louder combustion engine vehicles when they are traveling together on our roads in this country.

Use of Reflected Sound

While the visual system is tailored for the appreciation of patterns that vary in space and time, the auditory system may provide similar information through various patterns in frequency, intensity, and time (Barth & Foulke, 1979). The visually impaired traveler who is able to make good use of reflected sound learns to travel in a more sophisticated, more graceful manner than those who cannot. The use of reflected sound, known as *echolocation,* enables a person to gain an understanding of nonvisual spatial perception. It enables a traveler to avoid large obstacles before making contact; use sound to trail a wall or other surface; locate alleyways and recesses for purposes of orientation; detect corners by the absence of reflected sound from buildings; and make turns within a complicated building without physically contacting the walls. Originally the ability to use reflected sound was not understood by the public, and misconceptions persist to this day. A survey of the research on the use of reflected sound will help us to understand the current status of our knowledge on O&M.

Early Bat Studies

The first investigation into the use of reflected sound centered on the ability of bats to avoid bumping into obstacles (Griffin, 1958). In 1793 the natural scientist Lazzaro Spallanzani learned that bats that were blinded were able to remain oriented and avoid obstacles. In 1794 Charles Jurine demonstrated that when a bat's ears were tightly plugged with wax or other material, it crashed helplessly.

Roughly 100 years later, others concluded (Hahn, 1908; Maxim, 1912; Hartridge, 1920) that bats emit sounds that are used for navigation. Griffin (1958), using a "sonic detector," found that bats produce ultrasonic frequencies as they approach objects, and that when reflected off the objects, these frequencies—particularly those around 50,000 Hz—can be detected and used for navigation. Whales, porpoises, sea lions, and some nocturnal birds also use ultrasonic echoes in similar ways.

Early Studies on Facial Vision

Investigators studying the use of reflected sound for persons who were blind were not familiar with Spallanzani's or Jurine's experiments with bats and had to build a base of knowledge without the benefit of the bat experiments. As early as 1749, Diderot (trans. Jourdian, 1916) reported that a blind friend had the ability to perceive the presence of objects and determine their distance accurately. His explanation of this phenomenon was that the objects were perceived because they compressed a column of air against the individual's face as he walked toward the object. He felt that persons who were blind might have increased sensitivity of facial nerves and end organs, and his explanation was accepted by contemporaries. According to a summary by Burklen (1924), Zeune in 1808 and Knie in 1821 said that blind people used their cheeks and foreheads as feelers, with air pressure being the stimulus. Levy (1872) named this ability "perceptio facialis" or facial perception or vision, and described the performance of remarkable feats.

Investigators began experimenting to find a more accurate explanation for the ability to perceive obstacles. Heller (1904) stated that obstacle detection was a twofold process. He believed that the traveler used changes in the sound of his own footsteps in order to alert himself to sensations of pressure against his forehead. He believed the sound of the footsteps served to inhibit other processes that could interfere with full attention. At the same time, James (1890) suggested that the awareness of obstacles might result from pressure sensations against the tympanic membrane that far exceeded the amount actually present from the air-wave pressure caused by the approach toward an object. Dressler (1893) did further research by covering the face of his subjects as they approached obstacles. He concluded that perception of obstacles was due to differences in sound. Javal (1905) introduced the phrase "the sixth sense of the blind." He believed that this sense was similar to touch but was aroused by ether waves. Truschel (1906) believed that detection resulted from a rising pitch in the sound of footsteps as a person approached an obstacle. He also concluded that localization of stationary objects outside of the path of the individual was due to reflected sounds. In 1918, Villey (1930) concluded that the ears were responsible for the avoidance of obstacles by those who were blind. He stated that sounds are present around us all the time and that when there is some change in these sounds, they are interpreted as an object present between the traveler and the sound source. He explained the feelings of pressure upon the face as an auditory illusion.

In a dramatic step backward, Romains (1924) said that people who were blind detected obstacles through what he called "vestigial ranvier corpuscles," or little eyes located in the forehead of an individual that were brought into function by those who were blind. (He did not present his method of experiment.) Dolanski (1931) experimented by covering subjects' faces and later their ears in an attempt to discover the source of obstacle perception. He concluded with a physiologic theory that any clues from any sense cause contraction of small muscles in the skin. Mouchet (1938) determined that an auditory process involving subliminal auditory stimuli was involved in obstacle perception.

The Cornell Experiments

Facial Vision. In the 1940s a series of modern scientific experiments called the Cornell Experiments investigated the obstacle perception phenomenon. In "'Facial vision:' The perception of obstacles by the blind," Supa, Cotzin, and Dallenbach (1944) reported an experiment designed to determine whether sound was the explanation for the phenomenon. They used a long hallway over 60 feet (18 m) in length and conducted experiments asking subjects who were blind or blindfolded to detect a masonite board $\frac{1}{4}$ inch (6 mm) thick, 4 feet (120 cm) wide and 4 feet 10 inches (145 cm) high. They had each subject walk on a hard floor with hard-soled shoes, stopping when an object was perceived. The subjects were then to walk as close as possible to the object without touching it. Sighted subjects wearing a blindfold could not detect the board well at first, but began having some success after the ninth trial. The blind subjects picked up the presence of the board much sooner, but did not get closer without touching. When the same experiment was tried on soft carpet with bare feet the performances of all subjects were poorer, but they could still locate the board. Next, the facial areas were covered and the subjects could still detect the board, suggesting that air waves or pressure against the skin were not necessary for this detection. Next, the ears of the subjects were plugged and it was found that none could detect the board. In fact, they began veering into the walls.

The experiment was repeated using a 1000-Hz masking sound to eliminate the use of auditory cues. Again the subjects were unable to detect the board. Next, any possible air or pressure waves against the skin were eliminated by isolating the subjects in sound attenuation rooms while having them wear headphones and listening to the sounds made by another individual as he walked down the hallway toward the board carrying a microphone. They reported that the microphone had a dynamic range of between 70 and 9000 Hz. The subjects in the sound attenuation room could detect the board by listening to the changes in sound as perceived over the headphones. This experiment more credibly ruled out air pressure as the source of obstacle detection. Later, the subject walked down the hall in a monaural experiment to determine if a blocked ear would interfere with detection of the object; it was found that it did not interfere. A final experiment used pseudophones to switch the sound from one side of the head to the other by rerouting the stimulus before it could affect the ears; these did not affect obstacle detection.

Kohler (1964) carried on further experiments to determine whether the facial area had any role in obstacle perception. He used novocaine to anesthetize the facial area, and found that in spite of the anesthetic his subjects still reported skin perception when approaching an object. He later used pseudophones and found that the subjects experienced skin sensations on the sides opposite from what would normally be expected based on the acoustic cues. Therefore the sound was responsible for detection, but was perceived as facial pressure.

In another experiment, Worchel and Dallenbach (1947) found that subjects who were deaf and blind were unable to detect obstacles and therefore concluded that neither pressure on the surfaces of the ear canal nor the tympanic membrane was responsible for obstacle detection.

Pitch and Loudness. Cotzin and Dallenbach (1950) investigated the role of pitch and loudness in perception of obstacles by those who were blind. The purpose of the study was to determine which frequencies were involved in obstacle perception. The subjects were placed in sound attenuation rooms and fitted with earphones that were connected to a microphone with an upper frequency limit of 12,000 Hz. A sound stimulus was moved toward the test object on a trolley suspended from the ceiling and could be accelerated, decelerated, or stopped by the subject. A

10,000- to 12,000-Hz hissing sound was generated as the trolley and microphone approached the test object. All subjects did well in locating the board. Each noted a rise in pitch as the noise approached the object. The noise worked better than the footsteps had. Next, 125-, 250-, 500-, 1000-, 2000-, 4000-, 8000-, and 10,000-Hz pure tones were used separately for each trial. Collisions were numerous during the trials when stimulus tones of 8000 Hz and less were presented. Between 65 and 75 percent of the trials resulted in collisions and no improvement was evident. At 10,000 Hz the results changed and the subjects did much better. The loudness of the sounds did not affect the perception of obstacles, but frequencies of 10,000 Hz and higher were needed for effective obstacle perception. The authors concluded that the high frequencies allowed for a rise in pitch as the object was approached, a phenomenon known as the *Doppler effect.* That this phenomenon is actually due to the Doppler effect has not been verified. In the Doppler effect, a sound appears to have a slightly higher frequency if heard by a listener who is moving toward its source. Conversely, a listener who is receding will hear the sound at a distinctly lower pitch. For example, a train presents a higher frequency when approaching and a lower frequency after it has passed. The magnitude of the Doppler effect depends upon the ratio between the velocity of the individual and that of the sound wave. If the Doppler effect were responsible for obstacle perception, higher frequencies would be necessary because the sound at such frequencies travels fast enough to reflect off the object and return to the listener soon enough for the Doppler effect to be perceived while a person walks at normal speeds.

Effects of Practice on Obstacle Perception. Worchel and Mauney (1950) conducted a study to determine the effect of practice on the perception of obstacles. They selected 7 of 34 students who had failed to develop obstacle perception in a study conducted at the Texas State School for the Blind, to determine whether those who had failed could develop this ability with proper training. Training and testing of the seven subjects took place outdoors on a concrete walk 65 feet (19.5 m) long and 8 feet (2.4 m) wide. The subjects improved considerably, and all showed striking improvements within the first 30 to 60 training trials. They concluded that systematic training made the difference. The trial-and-error procedures naturally resorted to by people who are blind are not always efficient.

The results of the Texas State experiment were similar to the data on the amount of practice necessary to acquire object perception in two other studies. Supa, Cotzin, and Dallenbach (1944), while working with two sighted persons, found that they were able to achieve 25 successes in 44 trials. In another study with ten sighted subjects, Worchel and Ammons (1953) found that 30 to 90 trials were needed to obtain success in 25 out of 30 cases. Implications for training based on these studies indicates that O&M specialists should not give up prematurely in training efforts and should make more systematic efforts at teaching echolocation.

Juurmaa (1965), in a study at the Institute of Occupational Health in Helsinki, revealed that object perception was demonstrably present in about 85 percent of people who are blind. Obstacle perception correlated with the early onset and long duration of blindness, and was independent of intelligence. Juurmaa also gave an explanation for the subjective facial pressure that has been associated with obstacle perception. He felt that because the head is likely to be injured first, the person unconsciously detecting a wall due to reflected sound will also experience a tenseness in his or her face due to an associated rise in the tension of the facial muscles.

Differences in Proficiency between Blind and Blindfolded Persons

As a byproduct of various studies it has been learned that persons who are congenitally blind make more effective use of echolocation (object perception) than do blindfolded subjects (Supa, Cotzin, & Dallenbach, 1944; Strelow & Brabyn,

1982). It has even been reported that blind people exhibit superior performance in central auditory functioning as detected through Brainstem-evoked responses (Arias, Curet, Moyano, Joekes, & Blanch, 1993). Boehm (1986) directly studied the superiority of echolocation of blind subjects by comparing the accuracy of spatial data between blind subjects and blindfolded subjects. Using a handheld clicker to scan the environment while walking with a sighted guide through a hall, the blind subjects identified nearly three times as many reference points as the blindfolded subjects. It is clear, however, that while blind subjects function at a higher level, the skill of echolocation can be learned by sighted persons and individuals who recently became blind (Worchel & Ammons, 1953; Supa, Cotzin, & Dallenbach, 1944).

Target Discrimination and Echolocation

Kellog (1962) investigated the size, distance, and material of objects that could be perceived auditorally. He stationed his subjects in a sound attenuation room with small plywood disks capable of holding targets. The disks would move noiselessly toward or away from the subjects. The subjects were allowed to make any noise they wanted to help them to detect the object. Seven distances were measured between 12 inches (30 cm) and 48 inches (120 cm). In comparing the size of the test objects, the subjects who were blind revealed discrimination ability at 12 inches, (30 cm) but this became worse with increasing distance. Objects between 6 inches (15 cm) and 12 inches (30 cm) in diameter were used for this phase of the experiment. Later, in material discrimination, disks that measured 12 inches (30 cm) in diameter and were made of six different materials were compared. The subjects were able to distinguish metals from all materials except glass. Glass was confused with both metal and wood; plain wood and painted wood were indistinguishable; and velvet and denim were distinguishable from the four previously mentioned materials. Discriminations between hard and soft materials were made with 99 percent accuracy. When evaluating the above results, one must remember that the subjects were allowed to generate artificial sounds to help them with the differentiations. Ambient sound may not allow for such fine discrimination.

Rice (1967/1965) investigated the influence of target shape on target detectability. Rice found that there were fewer detections of the rectangular objects as the ratio of the object's width-to-length dimensions increased. For example, a 2- by 8-inch (5- by 20-cm) target was detected less often than a 4- by 4-inch (10- by 10-cm) target, and a 1- by 16-inch (2.5- by 40.6-cm) target was detected less often than a 2- by 8-inch (5- by 20-cm) target. No increase in detections was noted when the longer dimensions were changed to either a horizontal or vertical plane. These findings should heighten the O&M specialist's awareness that very thin objects, such as the edge of a door left ajar, a pole, or a thin shelf may go undetected. When the shape of the targets was changed, it was found that concave targets reflected more sound and could be detected more easily, while convex objects reflected less sound and were the most difficult to detect. Round objects, therefore, may also be difficult to detect.

Strelow and Brabyn (1982) investigated the parameters of echolocation of subjects who were blind or sighted and blindfolded as they walked along a solid wall, and also as they moved in the presence of small objects. In one condition the subjects were asked to walk along an indoor path with fiberboards that made up a solid continuous shoreline. In two other conditions rows of 15- and 5-centimeter poles replaced the wall. It was found that the blind subjects had poorer performances when walking along the poles in comparison to the walls. The blind subjects, however, experienced greater success than the blindfolded subjects. They concluded that locomotor accuracy can be affected by the size and spacing of targets. Since the larger poles were similar in size to a telephone pole, they further concluded that such poles would pose a danger to the unaided traveler.

In England Myers and Jones (1958) presented different sized objects at different distances to gather data about echolocation. When the subject was silent, he or she did poorly in detecting the object, but did much better when generating artificial noise—clicking proved an excellent sound source. They concluded that most people who are blind could detect while stationary an object 2 feet (60 cm) wide at 6 feet (180 cm). Some could even detect an object 2 inches (5 cm) wide at 6 feet (1.8 m). Young blind children can develop this ability by 4 years of age. According to the results from various studies, it seems that artificially generated noise increases the chances of perception. This may be the reason that young blind children click or snap their fingers when they are not sure of their orientation.

Schenkman and Jansson (1986) studied the use of sounds produced by the cane as a source for echolocation. Specifically they investigated whether objects can be detected and localized solely with the aid of long-cane tapping sounds, and the effect of the size of the objects to be detected and localized. Three subjects, each using ten different types of canes, attempted to detect the presence of objects suspended from the ceiling. No significant differences in target identification between the canes were found. Although detection and localization of objects using solely cane tapping sounds were possible, it was a difficult task. They did report that the subjects had greater success with the larger targets.

Ashmead, Hill, and Talor, (1989) conducted a study which concluded that children who are blind naturally acquire echolocation skills during their early developmental years through the spontaneous use of audition. Children 4 to 12 years of age who had minimal or no training in O&M were observed while they walked an outdoor path that contained boxes 2 and 4 feet tall. A similar group was also asked to identify the presence of circular disks alongside them that ranged from 2 to 20 inches in size. The children in the first experiment were typically able to identify the box from 5 feet away. In the second experiment, disks as small as 12 inches could be readily identified by the majority of children. Based on the observations of Ashmead et al., it seems that congenitally blind children learn to attach "visual" spatial meaning to the sound patterns to which they are exposed, and that this can occur without specific training.

Alternative Theories for Echolocation

Echolocation as a Result of Differences in Frequency and Intensity

Kohler (1964) conducted a study to determine the correlation between auditory thresholds of frequencies up to 8000 Hz and the ability to detect obstacles. He found a low correlation between the thresholds and performance in obstacle detection, which ranged from 0.20 for the low to middle frequencies to 0.40 at 8000 Hz. He also investigated the age of subjects and obstacle detection performance to see if good performance would correlate strongly with youth, since younger people usually have better thresholds in the upper frequencies. He found poor correlation between the age of the subjects and obstacle detection performance, which resulted in a −0.30 value. Furthermore, Kohler found that those with equally good hearing who participated in training courses for obstacle detection developed very different levels of performance in the skill. Kohler concluded, therefore, that while hearing capacity is crucial to the ability to detect obstacles, hearing capacity may involve two different, separate faculties.

Kohler (1964) hypothesized that obstacle detection may be more directly related to the ability to detect small differences in sound than to the actual hearing threshold of the individual. In order to prove his hypotheses, Kohler constructed a sound modifier that emitted a constant hissing noise at an intensity of about 30 dB. The device produced fluctuation of sound intensity that increased or decreased in response to a button pressed by subjects. The subjects were asked each time the fluctuations became less obvious to press the button to increase the differentiation.

When they felt they could detect the fluctuations again, they pressed the button again, decreasing the differentiation. A recording device automatically recorded the subjects' sensitivity to small differences in sound. Results obtained from 48 subjects led to a correlation of +0.74 between sensitivity to fluctuations and obstacle detection performance. Kohler concluded that an individual's ability to detect variations in sound is more important than their absolute threshold.

Bassett and Eastmond (1964), like Kohler, explained the basis of echolocation in terms of the ability to detect a change in the pitch (frequency) of available sound cues. When a complex sound (i.e., one containing multiple frequencies) is reflected from an obstacle with a flat surface, a subject in the field of both the incident and reflected sounds is made aware of the presence and distance of the obstacle by detecting a broad tone with a pitch that varies inversely with the distance from the surface of the obstacle. The particular pitch heard at a given point is the result of interference between incident and reflected waves, which causes a cancellation of certain frequencies and an augmentation of others. In effect, this explanation rules out the possibility that the Doppler effect is responsible for echolocation. Finally it was concluded that echolocation is most easily noticed with a frequency band of 200 to 2000 Hz and does not depend upon frequencies above 10,000 Hz.

Arias et al. (1993), in studying echolocation in relation to central auditory processing, stated that low and middle frequencies seem to be mainly responsible for the ability to detect obstacles. They based their conclusion on theoretical studies on the perception of pitch. They also identified two basic modalities of echolocation. With long-distance echolocation between distances of 2 and 5 meters, the authors concluded that the traveler hears two separate signals: the directly emitted signal and the reflected signal. They hypothesized that the change in loudness of the returning signal may be responsible for the detection of an obstacle. At short distances of less than 2 meters, they hypothesized that the individual does not perceive two separate signals but instead receives a single fused stimulus that provides information about periodicity.

Recent Data and Implications for Echolocation

Carlson-Smith and Wiener (1996) studied the relationship between selected audiometrical measures and echolocation performance. The subjects were nine graduate students who had normal middle ear status, essentially normal hearing for octave frequencies 250–8000 Hz, and vision that was normal when bilaterally corrected by lenses. Audiometric measures included scores on a Detection of Change in Intensity (DCI) test, scores on a Detection of Frequency Modulation (DFM) test, and pure tone thresholds for 8, 10, and 12 kHz. The DCI test assessed the ability to detect small increments in intensity for 45 dB HL tones at 500 and 2000 Hz, and the DFM test assessed the ability to detect small modulations in frequency for 30 dB HL tones at 500 and 2000 Hz. Echolocation performance was measured on an obstacle detection test and a doorway-detection test; the subjects wore blindfolds. At 500 Hz both DCI and DFM scores were significantly correlated with scores on the doorway-detection test, and on the obstacle detection test in the range of + 72 to + 79. No correlations were significant at 2000 Hz. Thresholds for high frequencies were not significantly correlated with scores on the doorway-detection test or the obstacle detection test.

Carlson-Smith and Wiener reported that the two subjects with the worst high-frequency hearing loss at 10–12 kHz demonstrated performance that was superior to the performance of more than half of the other subjects who had better high-frequency hearing sensitivity. Similarly, some of the subjects who had the worst performances on the echolocation tests had very good pure tone thresholds at 10,000 and 12,000 Hz.

It is clear that in echolocation tasks like those used by Wiener and Carlson-Smith, lower-frequency hearing and lower-frequency sound cues are important and that high frequency hearing and sound cues in the range of 10,000–12,000 Hz are not required. This is not to say that these higher frequencies are not useful when they are available and audible, but simply that information in these frequency regions is not *necessary* for echolocation to occur.

Since auditory cues from random ambient noise, footsteps, and cane tapping are all complex sounds (i.e., comprising many different frequencies), it is quite likely that at least some useful auditory cues will be available even to those with hearing loss. The number of individuals who are blind who also are truly deaf (i.e., who have profound bilateral hearing loss) is quite small. For many blind individuals with less severe hearing loss, it is likely that their sensitivity will be adequate at low frequencies for the detection of small frequency and intensity changes related to the detection of obstacles and openings; if this is the case, the potential for developing echolocation skills would be sufficient justification for echolocation training.

OPTIMIZATION OF AUDITION

Development of Auditory Skills for O&M

Effective use of sound is essential for the person with visual impairment in order to become a well-oriented and successful traveler. O&M specialists concerned with helping their students to develop auditory skills have provided auditory training for them. An audiologist defines auditory training as a systematic attempt to improve communication techniques such as lipreading, auditory training, speech and language therapy, counseling, and hearing aid fitting and orientation. The O&M specialist, however, provides a different type of auditory training that focuses on the auditory skills necessary for independent movement.

The first and most widely used approach to auditory training is done in natural settings. It is generally recognized that actual experience coupled with immediate feedback is the most effective method for improving auditory functioning. O&M specialists, therefore, have developed training procedures that use real environments and actual sounds. Two approaches to this type of training have evolved. The O&M specialist may provide auditory training using (1) one-to-one student–teacher interactions to provide auditory training as part of active travel lessons or (2) auditory training that is separate from the active travel lessons. The first approach is conducted with a one-to-one student–teacher ratio to insure safety, while the second approach can be conducted with an individual or with a group of people. Both approaches have advantages and disadvantages. In the first approach, exercises are given to teach the student to use specific auditory skills that relate directly to travel situations. Usually the use of an auditory skill and the actual travel procedure are taught together, which has the advantage of illustrating to the student in the most direct way the actual use to which auditory skills can be put. This procedure may increase motivation by showing the relevance of the auditory skill. In addition, working one-to-one, the O&M specialist is able to individualize training, taking into consideration the abilities and needs of each student.

Separating auditory training from the actual travel lesson also has advantages. In such an approach the student is free to concentrate fully upon the sounds without worrying about related wayfinding skills or being inhibited by a fear of dangerous situations. Another advantage is that auditory training can precede formal travel lessons and prepare the individual for travel before actually taking part in such a program. This allows the building of essential skills in young children before teaching wayfinding. It also permits group lessons, which can have the effect of building self-efficacy through observation and interaction with other successful learners.

It is part of the role of the certified O&M assistant to provide practice in using auditory information (Wiener et al., 1990; see Chapter 20 on the growth of this profession). In this model the assistant uses sighted guide technique to guide the individual through the environment while monitoring the student's ability to interpret pertinent auditory information.

Training in Natural Settings

Whether auditory training is taught as part of the travel lesson or is separated from it, there are many important skills that must be learned. Wiener et al. (1991), in the Association for Education and Rehabilitation of the Blind and Visually Impaired trainer-supervisor manual for O&M assistants, presented a series of auditory training exercises for sharpening skills and enhancing confidence. Some of the exercises include the following:

Sound Localization.

- Practice sound localization in a large room. Have the student stand in the center of the room while the instructor moves around the student, claps at different positions, and asks the student to point to the instructor.
- Practice sound localization with coin localization or with games involving an audible ball.

Indoor Sound Identification and Discrimination.

- Practice sound identification indoors by walking a student through a building and having him identify varying sounds such as phones ringing, doors opening, people walking, people keyboarding, and elevator doors opening.
- Practice determining room characteristics by having the student listen to the ambient sound in rooms as the student and instructor walk through acoustically live rooms (no sound-absorbing materials) and through acoustically dampened rooms (drapes, soft chairs, or thick carpets present).
- Practice interpretation of the indoor environment by creating common sounds that represent everyday activities such as dialing a number on the phone, opening and closing drawers, opening books, moving materials, and turning on lights, and having the student identify these.
- Practice sound identification with the cane by striking many common objects with the cane and asking the student to identify the objects.

Indoor Echolocation.

- Practice echolocation by asking the student to identify the presence of boards that are brought in close to the individual's face while he or she is seated.
- Practice using echolocation while the student walks to locate boards and other surfaces that are in his or her travel path.
- Practice using echolocation during indoor travel—identifying open doorways, intersecting corridors, and walls at the end of a hallway.

Outdoor Sensorium.

- Practice sound identification and localization outdoors by walking a student through a residential neighborhood and having her determine the location of pedestrians, positions of cars, locations of streets, and identification of other sound-producing objects.
- In a small business area, take the student for a walk to identify and localize sounds of buses, trucks, cars, motorcycles, people entering cars, cars pulling away from traffic lights, cars slowing down, and other typical sounds.
- Practice using sound shadows to locate objects between a sound source and the student, such as poles, bus shelters, and parked cars along a street or at a corner.
- Practice sound tracking by having the student trace the movement of the instructor by pointing as he or she walks various paths.
- Practice sound tracking by mentally tracing the paths of moving vehicles, having

the student point to them as they go through intersections.

- Practice lining up with traffic by having the student mentally trace the path of vehicles and changing his or her position so that their facing position is parallel to the moving traffic.
- Practice using echolocation outdoors by guiding the student along a street and having him or her identify buildings that are close to the sidewalk and alleys or recesses in the building line.

Auditory training skills can be practiced with students who are totally blind or when appropriate with low vision students. The question always arises as to whether or not it would be beneficial to blindfold those with low vision to assist them in learning to use their hearing more effectively. Experience shows that it is better not to blindfold, but instead to teach the student how to use hearing to interact with residual vision. Only when vision interferes or when there is the prognosis of continued reduction in vision is it helpful to blindfold.

Training with Recorded Sounds

The second and less widely used approach to auditory training involves the use of recorded sounds for improving auditory skills. Training may be done with binaural tapes using headphones and/or monaural tapes played through speakers in a controlled sound field. The procedure used for binaural training is to record environmental sounds on a multitrack tape recorder, with each track recording the sound received at ear level for the respective ear. The recording microphones are placed in positions that correspond to each ear. They may either be implanted in an artificial head at ear position or worn at ear level by a person. The separation of the microphones coupled with the head-shadow effect combine to create authentic recordings for practice in localization of sounds. With high quality equipment having a wide frequency response, fidelity approaches realistic levels. Reproduction is accomplished by amplifying the sounds and playing them back over headphones.

There are many advantages to such a system. Tapes provide sounds of the environment without the fear usually associated with traffic and other hazardous situations. Tapes also allow better control of environmental sounds for training situations. Instead of random experiences that are often encountered in on-the-spot training procedures, tapes permit planned sequencing of principles in an order that will facilitate learning. Also, tapes can be replayed for repeated study and can be used as a supplement to the actual travel training on the street.

There are also disadvantages to the use of training tapes. When used as a substitute for practice with actual environmental sounds, tapes deprive the student of necessary experience with using sound cues during actual travel. Another drawback concerns problems with front–rear localization, which seems to be inherent in such prerecorded tapes. Many students undergoing such training have reported that although they could easily distinguish between sounds coming from the left versus the right, they had difficulty determining whether some sounds originated from the front or the rear. This difficulty occurs often enough to be considered a serious problem. Because localization is due to differences in the time of arrival, phase, intensity, and spectral components between the two ears, sounds coming directly from either the front or rear are easily confused in a live listening situation until the head is moved slightly. Head movement changes these interaural differences enough to permit accurate localization. In a taped situation using headphones, turning the head does not change the signals of the two ears and does not resolve localization problems. Instead, the auditory environment turns with the head via the headphones. Some individuals rely more heavily upon head movements to localize sound than others. Those who are more dependent on such movement find difficulty in localization with tapes. They report hearing all sounds as coming either from the front or the rear.

Hearing Aids

Most of the many devices that can be used to enhance communication by those with hearing loss fall into three categories: conventional and special feature hearing aids, alternative hearing aids, and assistive devices and systems. Alternative hearing aids, such as cochlear implants and tactile devices other than bone conduction hearing aids, pick up speech signals and amplify or process them for transmission to the patient in some nonacoustic manner. Assistive devices or systems, for example, an alarm clock signaler or a hearing dog, may pick up information other than oral speech and send it to one or more of the sensory systems. The reader is referred to Newby and Popelka (1992) and to Hnath-Chisolm (1994) for information on cochlear implants and tactile devices, and to Tyler and Schum (1995) for information on assistive devices and systems. The emphasis here will be on conventional hearing aids.

For those who do not have normal hearing, a conventional hearing aid is the most widely used tool for improving their ability to process auditory information. Appropriate instruction by an audiologist in the use of hearing aids and improvement of auditory communication skills is a prerequisite for training in the use of auditory cues for independent travel. Nevertheless, an O&M specialist should have basic knowledge about hearing aid amplification and its use by the blind and hearing impaired traveler.

Basic Components of Hearing Aids

All hearing aids generally have at least four components in common: an input device, an amplifier, a power source, and an output transducer; most aids have at least one control, a volume control (Figure 4.28). The input device is either a microphone that converts airborne sound into electrical energy or a telecoil in which a voltage is induced by electromagnetic energy from a telephone or other induction loop. The amplifier receives weak energy from the input device and amplifies it by adding energy from the power source, a power cell popularly referred to as a battery. A volume control adjusts how much energy is added to the weak input signal. Energy from the amplifier is sent to an output transducer. The output transducer is typically an air conduction receiver that converts the amplified electrical energy to amplified acoustic energy, but in some cases the output transducer may be a bone conduction receiver that converts the amplified electrical energy to mechanical vibrations which are transmitted through the bones of the head to the inner ear.

Microphones may be of the directional or omnidirectional type. When tested in a standard

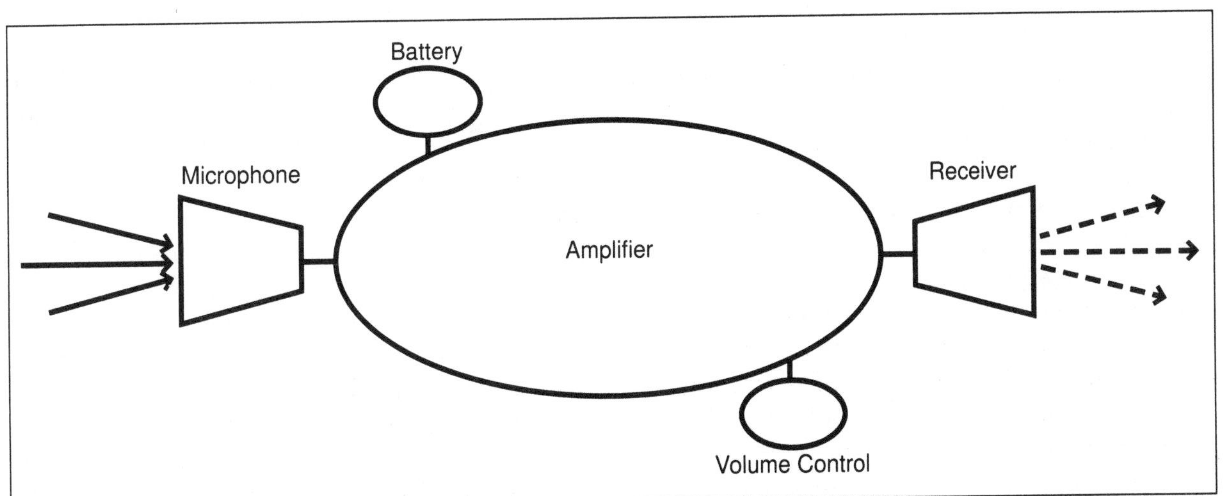

Figure 4.28. Block diagram of a simple hearing aid.

test space, the omnidirectional microphone picks up sound from all directions equally well, and the directional microphone picks up better those sounds emanating from the front and positions 45 degrees to the right and left of straight ahead. When worn, however, all hearing aids become somewhat directional, those having directional microphones being more directional than those with omnidirectional microphones. Binaural hearing aids with either type of microphone have directional advantages. Not all hearing aid users prefer directional hearing aids (Mueller, Grimes, & Erdman, 1983), but those who use directional aids successfully do so as a result of improved pickup of sound from the front and reduced pickup of background noise (Staab, 1978).

Electroacoustic Characteristics of Hearing Aids

Four electroacoustic characteristics are essential in considerations of hearing aid amplification: maximum power output (MPO) or saturation sound pressure level (SSPL), gain, frequency response, and distortion (Pollack, 1975). The *saturation sound pressure level* (American National Stan dards Institute, 1989b) is an estimate of the MPO—the highest output level the hearing aid can produce, regardless of how high the input level to the aid may be. The MPO or SSPL is typically set at the upper limit of the individual's comfort range for loud sounds. The goal is to provide the maximum range of amplification possible while protecting the user from discomfort and perhaps damage to their hearing from overly intense amplification. *Gain* is the amount of amplification. It is the difference between the input and output levels of the hearing aid at individual frequencies or averaged across particular frequencies. Varying degrees of gain are prescribed for varying degrees of hearing loss. *Frequency response* is a curve representing relative gain as a function of frequency. Hearing aid fittings attempt to enhance those frequencies at which hearing loss exists. It has been estimated that low frequencies between 62 and 500 Hz supply 60 percent of the intensity for speech, but only 5 percent of the information for intelligibility; conversely, the frequencies between 500 and 8000 Hz supply only 40 percent of the intensity for speech, but they supply only 95 percent of the information for intelligibility (Gerber, 1974). The upper frequencies provide more information for communication, while the lower frequencies provide more environmental noise. Therefore most hearing aids are designed for some degree of high frequency emphasis. *Distortion* is an unplanned difference between the original input signal and the amplified output. It may occur as a degradation of frequency, intensity, or phase, and is generally thought to negatively affect the listener's subjective impressions and communicative performance.

Traditional Linear Hearing Aids Versus Signal Processing Aids

Hearing aids have sometimes been classified as linear or nonlinear, depending upon the manner in which the hearing aid output is limited. *Linear hearing* aids limit their output by *peak clipping*, which means that the output increases linearly with increased input up to a point where the peak amplitudes are clipped, causing distortion. The level at which peak clipping occurs is ideally a level that allows as much usable amplified sound as possible without exceeding the listener's loudness discomfort level. So-called *nonlinear hearing* aids are those that limit their output by compression. *Compression* results when the amount of gain added to a wide range of possible input levels is reduced in a way that results in an amplified but narrower range of output levels. Again, the output levels for intense sounds should not exceed the listener's loudness discomfort level. In reality, the output of the compression system over a given range of inputs may be just as linear as that of a peak clipping aid without introducing the distortion associated with peak clipping. Therefore some form of compression is probably the preferred method of limiting output.

The term *signal processing* is an interesting one when applied to hearing aids. Fundamentally, a hearing aid whose output differs from its input—essentially any hearing aid, could be thought of as a signal processor. A useful scheme by Killion, Staab, and Preves (1990) classifies automatic signal processing aids as either fixed-frequency response aids (FFR) or level-dependent frequency response aids (LDFR). The FFR processors use compression to limit hearing aid output without affecting the frequency response of the aid. The LDFR processors automatically change the frequency response as well as introduce compression, depending on the input levels to the aid. There are three types of LDFR instruments. For Type 1, bass increases at low levels (BILL). So, in relatively noise-free environments, low frequency response would be increased, while in places where low frequency noise predominates, the low frequency response would be reduced. For Type 2, treble increases at low levels (TILL). Listeners with high-frequency hearing loss typically need more gain for high frequencies when inputs are low and less when inputs are high. These listeners may find help in the automatic reduction of high frequency response when input levels are high. Type 3 allows programmable increases at low levels (PILL), which means that it can exhibit either BILL or TILL type processing. The challenge is to determine what type of signal processing will best serve the traveler who is blind in O&M. Most visually impaired persons probably should be fit with easy-to-use programmable hearing aids that allow flexibility for choosing amplification characteristics to meet changing needs. Frequency response characteristics of an aid can be changed by a switch on the aid itself, or in some instances by remote control.

Hearing Aid Candidates

Being a hearing aid candidate means that one should be evaluated to assess the need for and potential benefits from amplification. Hearing aid candidacy is typically based on audiometric and motivational factors.

Audiometric factors include the type and degree of loss shown on pure tone tests, speech recognition thresholds, the percent-correct speech recognition scores, and the dynamic range or range of useable hearing. Most hearing aid users have sensorineural hearing loss, and relatively few have conductive loss since most conductive losses can be remediated medically. High speech recognition scores and wide dynamic ranges suggest more benefits from amplification; low speech recognition scores and narrow dynamic ranges suggest less benefits. A variety of rules have been proposed for deciding what degree of hearing loss indicates a need for amplification. For example, it has sometimes been said that anyone whose average hearing loss or speech recognition threshold is worse than 25 dB HL in the better ear is a candidate for a hearing aid. Simply put, however, anyone who has difficulty with speech communication due to a hearing problem should be considered a candidate for hearing aid use. Even those with unilateral losses or very severe bilateral losses should be considered as candidates. Hearing aids may make listening and localization easier even for persons with mild impairments; they may improve sound detection and speech-reading (lipreading) even for those whose hearing loss is so severe (greater than 85 dB HL) that their speech recognition scores are not improved with amplification. Perhaps in situations with persons who are blind, anyone whose hearing problem causes difficulty with the use of auditory cues in O&M should also be considered a candidate for hearing aid use.

Motivational factors are represented by one's desire to alleviate a hearing disability, that is, the impact of one's impairment or deviation from normal hearing on the ability to communicate and participate in other desired activities (e.g., independent travel). Although audiometric factors may suggest possible benefit from hearing aid use, one must be or become somewhat motivated in order to use amplification successfully.

Alternative Approaches

A cochlear implant is a device that is surgically implanted so that wire electrodes inserted directly into a nonfunctional cochlea can electrically stimulate a healthy auditory nerve when the implant is activated by sound. Candidates for cochlear implants typically have pure tone thresholds in the 90–109 dB HL range, no open-set word recognition with appropriately fitted hearing aids, and no apparent physical or mental contraindications for having the surgery and benefiting from the results (Hnath-Chisolm, 1994). Exceptionally successful implant users are able to use timing and voice cues to aid speech-reading and may even have some limited success in telephone listening. At the very least, implant users usually benefit from an awareness of sound. According to Hnath-Chisolm (1994), improvements in speech production are greater for children who have implantation during early childhood.

Those with profound hearing loss who do not receive adequate assistance from the use of conventional amplification may be candidates for using vibrotactile aids. These devices provide limited information about speech and have been used primarily as aids to speech-reading (Hnath-Chisolm, 1994).

Types of Hearing Aids

A variety of hearing aid types are shown in Figure 4.29. According to Kirkwood (1990) the three most common types of hearing aids based on percentage of sales, are the in-the-ear aids (47.2

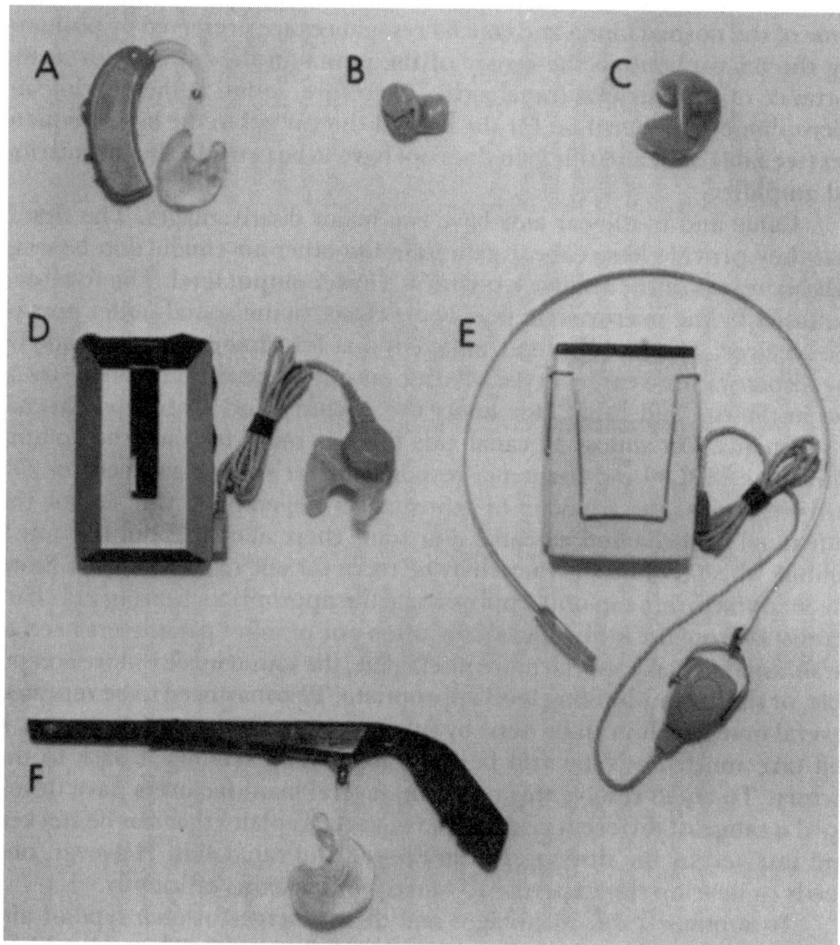

Figure 4.29. Types of hearing aids. (A) Behind-the-ear aid; (B) in-the-canal aid; (C) in-the-ear aid; (D) body aid with external receiver; (E) body aid with bone conduction vibrator; (F) eyeglass aid.

Source: Reprinted with permission from M. W. Skinner, *Hearing Aid Evaluation* (Englewood Cliffs, NJ: Prentice Hall, 1988), Fig. 8.1, p. 211.

percent), in-the-canal aids (31.2 percent), and behind-the-ear devices (21.1 percent), while both body-worn and eyeglass aids combined represent less than 1 percent of sales.

In-the-Ear and In-the-Canal Devices. Most in-the-ear (ITE) aids and in-the-canal (ITC) aids (Figures 4.29, B and C) are of the custom variety in which electronic components are built into an acrylic shell made by the manufacturer from the audiologist's impression of the user's ear. The ITE shell fits into the ear canal and the concha. ITE aids are called full concha, low profile, or half concha instruments, depending upon the degree to which they fill and protrude from the concha. ITC aids are located mostly or entirely within the external ear canal; completely-in-the-canal (CIC) aids have recently achieved considerable popularity. While most of CIC aids require screwdriver adjustment of the gain control, persons who are visually impaired may find remote control to be more satisfactory. The probability for successful use of ITE aids is reduced for average hearing losses (500, 1000, or 2000 Hz) of less than 35 dB HL (Staab & Lybarger, 1994) or greater than 70 dB HL (Wernick, 1985). Similar results are likely for ITC aids. Nevertheless, there are successful ITE and ITC hearing aid users whose hearing loss falls outside the 35–70 dB HL range.

Behind-the-Ear Aid. The postaural or behind-the-ear (BTE) aid is contoured to fit behind the ear (Figure 4.29A). All components are typically contained within the unit behind the pinna and amplification is sent from an air conduction receiver through tubing to an earmold. When two aids are used together to fit symmetrical losses, true binaural amplification can be attained, permitting accurate localization in many instances. Ample space is available on BTE aids for a variety of controls; a variety of appropriate frequency response, gain, and output characteristics are available in BTE aids for fitting a variety of hearing losses that range from mild to profound.

Eyeglass Aids. The eyeglass (EG) aid (Figure 4.29F; Figure 4.30) is similar in design to the BTE. The components of the EG are enclosed within

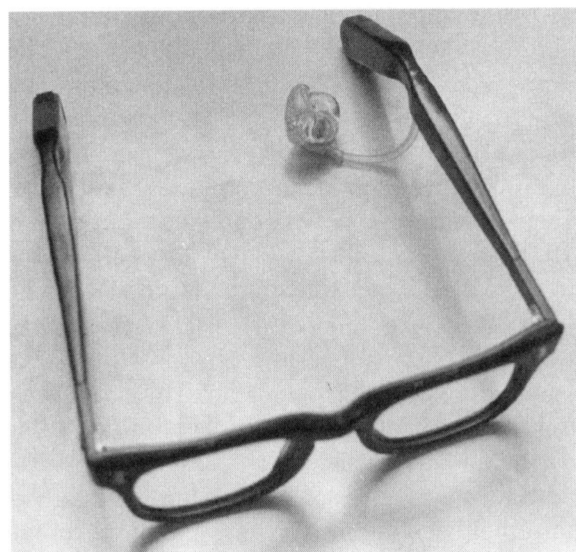

Figure 4.30. Eyeglass hearing aid.

Source: From W. R. Wiener. (1980). "Audition." In R. L. Welsh and B. B. Blasch (Eds.), *Foundations of Orientation and Mobility* (New York: American Foundation for the Blind, 1980), Fig. 26-6, p. 176.

the temple of the eyeglasses, and can be installed in any pair of eyeglasses with a 5- or 7-barrel bridge. Assuming similar microphone locations, the advantages of the BTE aid are also applicable for the EG aid. EG aids may be more comfortable than BTE aids for the visually impaired individual who must wear eyeglasses and a hearing aid. This issue can typically be avoided, however, by careful selection of a BTE with a small case and templates (which do require a large space); if appropriate, this issue could also be avoided by using an ITE or ITC aid. EG aids have a disadvantage: the user may need an extra pair of eyeglasses for times when the hearing aid is being repaired.

Contralateral-Routing-of-Sound Aids. Contralateral-routing-of-sound (CROS) aids often represent variations of BTE and EG aids. The classic CROS aid (Harford & Barry, 1965) and its power CROS variation consist of the electronics for one complete BTE hearing aid housed in two cases; one contains the amplifier and receiver, the other contains the microphone. These CROS aids, as well others that route signals from one side of the head to the other, can transmit the signal by wire, but radio frequency transmission appears be the more common mode.

Although a variety of CROS-type hearing aids are possible, Figure 4.31 illustrates the major types. The *classic CROS aid* picks up sound at a nonhearing ear and routes it to an amplifier and receiver at a near-normal ear. The near-normal ear is fit with a tube or a nonoccluding earmold to keep the ear open to environmental sound. This arrangement eliminates head shadow on the hearing side when the sound source is on the nonhearing side. The *power CROS,* used in cases of severe bilateral hearing loss, also routes the sound from one side to the other. The side receiving the amplified sound is fit with an occluding earmold. This arrangement uses head shadow advantageously: sound leaking from the aid on the amplifier side reaches the microphone on the opposite side at a reduced level, diminishing the probability of feedback. The advantage of this arrangement is that a high-gain hearing aid can be used in cases where feedback is a potential problem. The *bilateral–contralateral-routing-of-sound (BICROS)* aid also consists of two hearing aid cases, one containing a complete hearing aid coupled to an occluding earmold and the other containing only a microphone with an on–off switch. The BICROS aid can be fitted for a bilateral hearing loss in which one ear is functional and the other is not. The complete hearing aid is fit to the hearing side and the microphone to the nonhearing side to eliminate head shadow. The *ipsilateral-routing-of-sound (IROS) aid* is not a true CROS aid. It is a monaural hearing aid that is coupled to a nonoccluding earmold to avoid too much low frequency amplification in cases of near-normal low-frequency hearing and mild-to-moderate high-frequency hearing loss. The *multiCROS aid* is another system that consists of two cases, one containing a complete hearing aid with an on–off switch on the microphone, and the other containing a microphone with an on–off switch. The multiCROS device can be manipulated by switches to achieve CROS, BICROS, or monaural amplification. The *transcranial CROS aid* (Sullivan, 1988) is a BTE hearing aid with an air conduction receiver that puts out enough intensity to vibrate the bones of the skull, producing a bone conduction signal. It should be noted that bone conduction signals reach both cochleas equally or almost equally well. The transcranial CROS aid can be fitted for a nonhearing ear in order to overcome head shadow by providing bone conduction amplification to the ear with normal or near-normal hearing on the opposite side of the head. The fitting of CROS aids should be considered for persons who are blind since they can have an enhancing effect on sound localization.

Body Aids. The microphone and amplifier of the body aid are contained in a case that is placed in a pocket, clipped to the user's clothing, or worn in a harness on the torso; the external receiver is connected to the amplifier in the case by a wire and snapped to the earmold (Figure 4.29D). The location of the microphone in a body-worn case makes it susceptible to clothing noise and body baffle and shadow effects that are more undesirable than those associated with ear level aids. Furthermore, even when two aids are used and placed far apart on the body, true binaural amplification is not obtained because the microphones are not at ear level. The relatively large external receivers used with body aids typically have a poorer high frequency response range than do smaller receivers in ear level aids. Today such aids are rarely used. Their advantages over aids worn at the ear may include increased gain with less chance of acoustic feedback, larger controls and batteries, room for more controls, and better ruggedness and durability. They are occasionally recommended for geriatric clients with poor manual dexterity or very young, active children who have a hearing loss of 85 to 100 dB HL.

Hearing Aids That Utilize Bone Conduction Receivers

Although the vast majority of hearing aids (described above) amplify by an air conduction receiver, a small number do so by a bone conduction receiver (e.g., Figure 4.29E). Bone conduction receivers are typically used in rare situations where an ITE or an earmold cannot be put into the ear canal for medical reasons or where a large

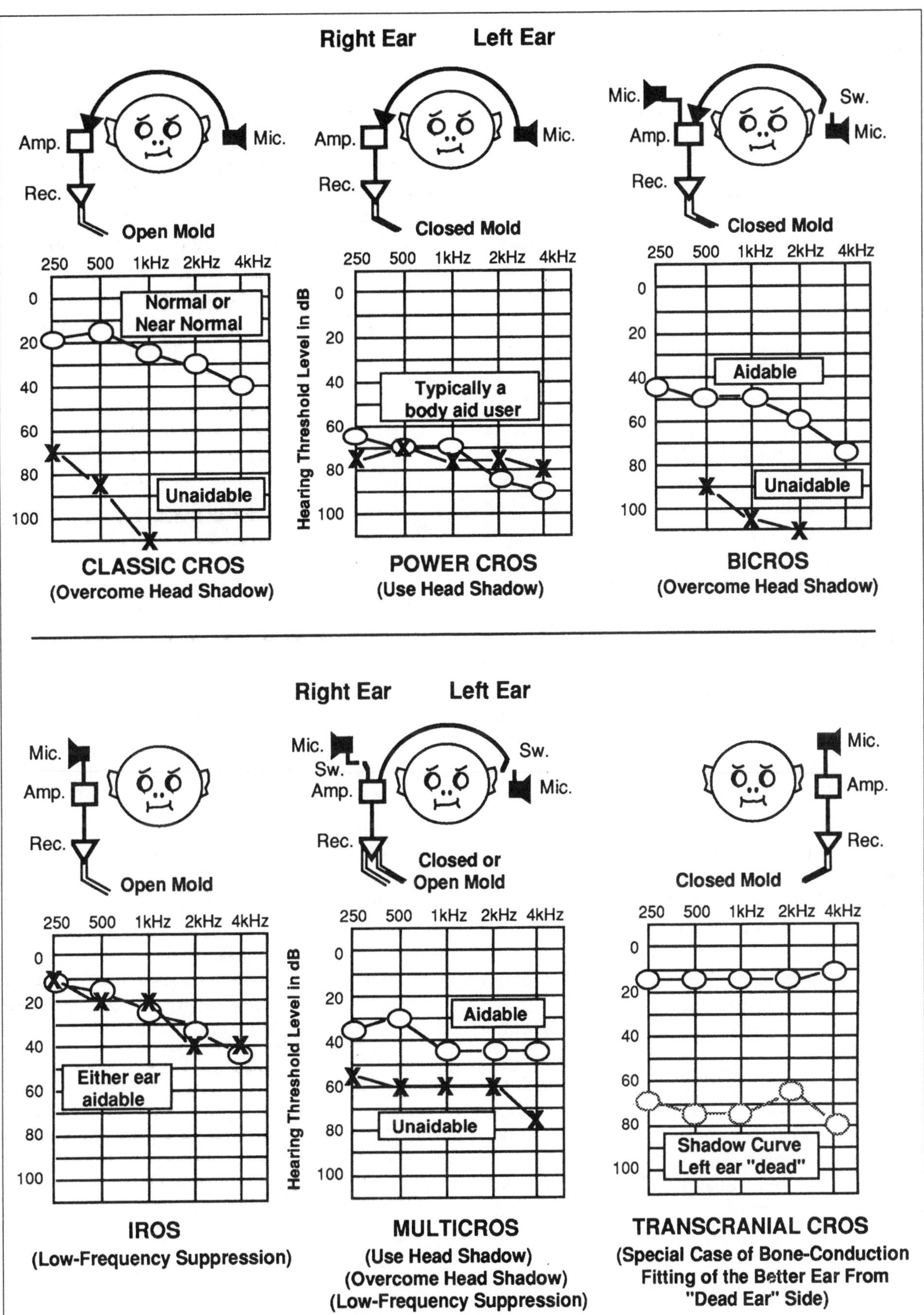

Figure 4.31. Major types of CROS hearing aids.

Source: From W. J. Staab and S. F. Lybarger, "Characteristics and Use of Hearing Aids." In J. Katz (Ed.), *Handbook of Clinical Audiology* (Baltimore: Williams & Wilkins, 1994), Fig. 43.4, p. 662.

conductive component to a hearing loss exists. For BTE and body aids the bone conduction receiver is attached to a headband placed on the mastoid on the opposite side of the head from the other components; the receiver is connected to the hearing aid case by a wire. For an eyeglass aid the bone conduction vibrator is part of the eyeglass template that fits behind the pinna, and the remaining components are located in the template on the opposite of the head; the wire connecting the receiver to the amplifier can be very conveniently routed through the frame of the eyeglasses. Generally speaking, a significant amount of force must be amplified to the vibrator; because this force is more easily applied by a headband rather than by spring-loaded eyeglass templates, eyeglass aids tend to have lower vibrator outputs than do BTE aids (Staab & Lybarger, 1994).

Recommendation of Hearing Aid Types

The fitting of special types of hearing aids may be particularly challenging for some dispensers because of infrequent experience with such aids. In general, the smaller aids (in-the-canal and in-the-ear) have less electronic flexibility, require smaller controls, can accommodate fewer controls, allow fewer modifications, and require a smaller battery than do larger aids. Nevertheless, they are often adequately adjustable; they require less power than larger aids for achieving a given result because the internal receiver is located relatively close to the tympanic membrane; their use provides possible benefits from the natural resonances of the external ear; they facilitate localization; they are typically easier to insert and remove; and, cosmetically speaking, they are typically more appealing than larger aids. Although cosmetic judgments are an individual matter, it is not surprising that collectively ITE and ITC aids represent over 75 percent of hearing aid sales. Although small hearing aids are often the instruments of choice, when selecting the type of device, hearing aid users and fitters should carefully consider the individual's needs.

Hearing Aids as a Rehabilitation Tool

The hearing aid industry is largely market driven. Manufacturers would like to sell products that are in demand, and most hearing aid dispensers would like to fit reasonably priced products that are beneficial and in demand. Nevertheless the selection and fitting of hearing aids is not an exact science, and manufacturers must deal with the challenge of providing the best technology at a marketable price. The nature of the tools available for aural rehabilitation is determined to some extent by market forces.

Traditionally, most hearing aids have been fixed-frequency response devices that limit their maximum output by distortion-causing peak clipping. Typically they have been built to function within a limited frequency range of about 400 to 4000 Hz, and fitting trends have emphasized amplification for frequencies of about 1000 to 4000 Hz, a range that is particularly important to the intelligibility of speech. Frequencies beyond this range could, in theory, contribute additional cues for speech intelligibility and for O&M. However, lower frequencies are generally not amplified as much as the higher frequencies because they are the major carriers of noise, and enhancing them generally makes communication more difficult. More gain may be needed for greater hearing loss, and hearing loss tends to be greater at higher frequencies. The increase of gain at high frequencies (even at 4000 Hz) is sometimes limited by problems with *feedback,* a squealing sound produced by the reamplification of sound leaking from the system. In other words, there is a limit to the amount of gain possible before feedback. The amount of gain possible at a given frequency is also limited by the difference between the level of the input signal to the hearing aid and the user's loudness discomfort level, both of which can vary with frequency. Recall that gain equals input plus output and that output should not equal or exceed the loudness discomfort level. Less gain can be added to high input levels than to low input levels before reaching a given loudness discomfort level. Because of physical and physiological limitations it may be impossible, particularly with traditional technology, to provide all of the perceptual cues above the threshold level that ordinarily is necessary for understanding speech or for O&M.

In spite of their limitations, hearing aids have great potential as a rehabilitation tool for the traveler who is blind and hearing impaired. Rehabilitation should include improvement of O&M skills as well as communication skills. Traditional hearing aid technology provides significant benefits for many hearing impaired users. However, newer technologies should be considered as options. Newer aids can provide programmed options between a variety of linear responses with activation of compression at high levels or automatic increases in amplification for low level inputs of high and/or low frequencies. If appropriate for a given individual, such aids could provide some degree of flexibility for experiencing different amplification options for changing needs.

Amplification of Traffic Sounds. A spectral analysis of traffic sounds (Wiener & Goldstein, 1977; Wiener et al., 1996) found the greatest absolute intensity to be in the lower frequencies. When the sensitivity of the human ear to different frequencies is considered, it becomes evident that the greatest traffic-sound intensity available to the individual is between 500 and 4000 Hz. Although these mid- to upper frequencies play the greatest role in the audibility of traffic sounds, frequencies between 125 and 500 Hz also contain energy that is sufficiently audible for use in O&M. Most indivduals who are hearing impaired have better hearing for low frequencies than for high frequencies. Therefore a hearing aid that emphasizes only frequencies above 1000 Hz may fail to provide some useful information for interpretation of traffic sounds. Assume for a moment that a traveler in an outdoor area near traffic would like to optimize reception of low frequency cues. A programmable hearing aid could allow the traveler to select a predominantly low frequency response, or a broad frequency response. The result should be better reception of low frequency traffic cues. Now assume that the traveler reaches his or her desk in a quiet office environment and wishes to eliminate low frequency noise and maximize reception of speech cues. He or she could now select a predominantly high frequency response. The flexibility offered by programmable hearing aids may be important to visually and hearing impaired travelers.

Sound localization has been shown to be more accurate in both the lower and higher frequencies than in the middle frequencies. Given that the ability to localize sound is critical for acquisition of good mobility skills, it is important that hearing aids have the capability of amplifying both lower and higher frequencies.

According to De l'Aune et al. (1976), the ability to judge the distance of a sound-emitting object may be impaired by some hearing aids. They explain that environmental sounds that are closer to the individual have higher frequency components than sounds which are farther away. The more distant sounds lose high frequencies as they travel through the air. Hearing aids that do not have a sufficient high frequency response may not allow the individual to receive the high frequencies necessary for distance judgment. De l'Aune et al. also state that hearing aids which are designed to limit gain in response to loud sounds may also make distance judgment difficult. Although this usually is not the case, an automatic volume control (AVC) in a hearing aid may reduce the intensity differences between the near and far sounds while preventing user discomfort from overamplification. For those who need large amounts of amplification and have a narrow range of usable hearing, hearing aids may be specifically designed to greatly limit gain at high input levels. Therefore intense sounds from objects nearby may be transmitted at a softer level and judged by the individual as being farther away than they really are. In the case of a fast moving automobile, this could be a dangerous situation. AVC or compression hearing aids have traditionally limited hearing aid output across the frequency range by adding progressively less gain to the input as input levels increase. Today, some multichannel hearing aids are capable of using this technique to differentially limit output in particular frequency bands. Such aids might retain some of the frequency cues that would assist in distance judgment. De l'Aune et al. recommend that hearing aids have an AVC switch that would permit turning off output limitation circuitry during travel times. Although such hearing aids are currently possible, user-operated output controls are not common.

Unilateral vs. Bilateral Loss. Hearing aids should help persons who are hearing impaired improve their sound localization skills. Unilateral hearing loss disrupts the natural balance of acoustic cues arriving at the two ears. As reported by Bergman (1957), when sound levels reach the threshold of the ear with a greater hearing loss, the ability to determine the direction of the sound is greatly improved. The closer the sensitivity of the two ears, the better the localization will be. Therefore a hearing aid that provides more intensity to the ear with a greater hearing loss should help to improve localization.

Whenever bilateral hearing loss is a factor, binaural hearing aids should be used when possible to balance the hearing sensitivity of the two ears. Although binaural amplification helps to determine whether a sound is coming from the right or left, it may also lead to front–rear reversals. As noted by Yost (1994), there are a number of directional sound locations that would produce the same interaural time and intensity differences. One example would be sound locations directly in front of and behind the listener; this is why a sound from the front is sometimes thought to be coming from the rear. Without head movement, only pinna effects differentiate sound from the front and rear. Reversals are not a severe problem for sighted people because vision is used to verify sound origin. The traveler who is blind who experiences these reversals, however, cannot use sight to help localize the sound.

Keane (1965) suggested that these reversals might be due to the location of the microphone port in most BTE hearing devices. The microphone port is behind or above the pinna of the ear and is not shadowed from the rear by the pinna. ITE or ITC hearing aids may provide a solution to this problem.

Because of sound localizing difficulties with hearing aids, De l'Aune et al. (1976) suggested that visually impaired individuals with mild hearing losses who experience this might do better to remove their hearing aids for travel purposes. They caution, however, that such a decision be made only in collaboration with an audiologist. Those with more severe losses will have to depend upon hearing aids.

When hearing aids are worn for localization, every attempt should be made to provide localization training coupled with immediate feedback to improve accuracy. Often, when inaccuracies are found in distinguishing sounds coming from the right or left, the difficulty can be overcome by adjusting the gain control of the hearing aid. A simple "fusion test" can help a person to adjust the gain control or other controls to equalize the sensitivity of the two ears more closely and thus improve localization (Keane, 1965). The O&M specialist should stand directly in front of the student and instruct him or her to adjust the gain control on the aid or aids until the specialist's voice sounds as though it is coming from directly ahead. Noting the control position at this point will facilitate returning to it when necessary.

A person with one near-normal ear and one totally deaf ear may have trouble localizing sound accurately. If so, localization can often be greatly improved with a CROS hearing aid. Successful use of this aid for independent travel has been documented (Rintelmann, Harford, & Burchfield, 1970). The reality is that some audiologists see very few people who are blind and may not be immediately aware of a given blind person's auditory needs. If the audiologist is concerned only with helping someone to understand speech, he or she may not consider all the options for amplification. The use of the CROS aid, for example, might not be considered worth the effort. Interpreting information with CROS aids takes practice. The necessity for a blind person to be able to localize traffic and other environmental sounds, however, may make the extra time needed to learn to use a CROS aid well worthwhile. a

Table 4.6. Hearing Handicap Inventory for the Elderly—Screening Version

	Yes	Sometimes	No
1. Do you experience communication difficulties when speaking with one other person? (for example, at home, at work, in a social situation, with a waitress, a store clerk, with a spouse, boss, etc.)	( )	( )	( )
2. Do you experience communication difficulties in situations when conversing with a small group of several persons? (for example, with friends or family, coworkers, in meetings or casual conversations, over dinner or while playing cards, etc.)	( )	( )	( )
3. Do you experience communication difficulties while listening to someone speak to a large group? (for example, at church or in a civic meeting, in a fraternal or women's club, at an educational lecture, etc.)	( )	( )	( )
4. Do you experience communication difficulties while participating in various types of entertainment? (for example, movies, TV, radio, plays, nightclubs, musical entertainment, etc.)	( )	( )	( )
5. Do you experience communication difficulties when using or listening to various communication devices (for example, telephone, telephone ring, doorbell, public address system, warning signals, alarms, etc.)	( )	( )	( )
6. Do you experience communication difficulties when you are in an unfavorable listening environment? (for example, at a noisy party, where there is background music, when riding in an auto or bus, when someone whispers or talks from across the room, etc.)	( )	( )	( )
7. Do you feel that any difficulty with your hearing limits or hampers your personal or social life?	( )	( )	( )
8. Does any problem or difficulty with your hearing upset you?	( )	( )	( )
9. Do others suggest that you have a hearing problem?	( )	( )	( )
10. Do others leave you out of conversations or become annoyed because of your hearing?	( )	( )	( )

From I. M. Ventry and B. E. Weinstein, "The Hearing Handicap Inventory for the Elderly: A New Tool," *Ear and Hearing, 3* (1982), 128–134.

BICROS aid, on the other hand, is not recommended for people who are blind. It reduces directional information and makes localization more difficult.

The O&M Specialist's Role

In order to prepare students for independent travel, the O&M specialist must have a realistic understanding of the auditory functioning of each individual. The specialist should ensure that in addition to a battery of social, medical, and ophthalmologic information, each student's file includes valid audiometric information. The specialist should be sufficiently skilled in the interpretation of audiograms to evaluate general auditory function as a starting point in communication with the student. Audiometric data are useful, but must be combined with observation of auditory functioning in natural environments because people with very similar audiograms can function very differently. It is a known fact that some learn to use hearing more effectively than others; therefore, actual observation is necessary. Speech recognition scores can be a useful supplementary tool for assessing speech comprehension. Pathology and type of hearing loss may give the O&M Specialist some rough idea about functional expectations. For example, conductive losses are relatively free from distortion. Sensorineural losses, on the other hand, are prone to distortion even with hearing aids.

The O&M Specialist should be constantly alert to the possibility of hearing problems. Observation of the student's use of hearing during travel is a good method for determining if difficulties exist. An auditory questionnaire can also be useful as an aid in determining when to refer for an audiometric examination (see Table 4.6). Each item is scored 0 for a "no" response, 2 for a "sometimes" response, and 4 for a "yes" response. Total scores range from 0 to 40. Table 4.7 provides information on how to score the results. If a hearing loss is suspected, the student should be referred to an audiologist or otolaryngologist. When such referral leads to the discovery of a hearing loss, the O&M Specialist is in a position to work with the audiologist to describe functional difficulties and acquaint the audiologist with the special auditory needs of people who are blind. The audiologist and the O&M Specialist can then work together to follow the hearing aid fitting with an appraisal of the individual's functioning with the aid, both in communication and orientation. Together the O&M Specialist and the audiologist can help the visually and hearing impaired person to achieve a higher level of rehabilitation.

Table 4.7. Probability of Hearing Impairment Based Upon the Hearing Handicap Inventory for the Elderly (HHIE-S)

HHIE-S Score	Probability of Hearing Impairment (%)
0–8	13
10–24	50
26–40	84

Source: Adapted from M. J. Lichtenstein, F. H. Bess, and S. A. Logan, "Validation of Screening Tools for Identifying Hearing-Impaired Elderly in Primary Care." *Journal of the American Medical Association, 259* (1988), 2875–2878.

The O&M specialist is responsible for developing a training program to teach the necessary auditory skills for independent travel. As indicated earlier, the auditory skills program may be implemented before formal training in travel techniques, concurrently with but separate from such training, or as an integral part of it. The training may be provided in natural settings or in a combination of natural settings and recorded sound settings. The O&M Specialist is often in a position to consult with family and teachers on auditory training activities. Explaining to family members the necessity for stimulating the child with auditory toys and games to initiate ear–hand coordination, exploration of the environment, and auditory development is most helpful. Providing auditory training suggestions to the classroom teacher is also beneficial. All in all, the O&M specialist should function as a member of the auditory rehabilitation team, working alongside the otolaryngologist, audiologist, and the family.

Suggestions/Implications for O&M Specialists

1. Sound is characterized by intensity measured in decibels (dB) and perceived as loudness; frequency measured in cycles per second (Hz) and perceived as pitch; and phase or position of the vibrating molecules measured in degrees. These characteristics contribute to sound identification, discrimination, and localization.
2. Hearing sensitivity is represented by a dynamic range of about 100 dB (threshold of discomfort minus the threshold for sound audibility) and a frequency range of 20 to 20,000 Hz. Within the typical hearing test range (500–8000 Hz), normal hearing thresholds are usually 15 dB HL or lower.
3. Dysfunction in the outer and/or middle ear results in conductive hearing loss while dysfunction in the remainder of the system results in sensorineural hearing loss.
4. Classifying and quantifying hearing loss is accomplished through a test battery consisting of pure tone air and bone conduction tests, speech recognition threshold tests, suprathreshold speech recognition tests, and immittance tests. Together these tests distinguish between conductive loss, sensorineural loss, or a combination of the two, called a mixed loss.
5. During pure tone testing of individuals with hearing loss, differences between air conduction and bone conduction thresholds of 15 dB or more are typically associated with a conductive or mixed hearing loss, while differences of 10 dB or less are typically associated with sensorineural loss. If bone conduction thresholds are in the normal range and 15 dB better than the air conduction thresholds, the loss is conductive; if bone conduction thresholds show a loss and are 15 dB better than the air conduction thresholds, the loss is mixed.
6. The speech recognition threshold test is designed to determine the lowest level at which individuals can just start to understand speech, while the suprathesold speech recognition test provides a functional evaluation of the individual's ability to understand speech at intensity levels above threshold.
7. Individuals with conductive hearing loss usually have losses in the lower frequencies or have a more or less equal loss across the frequencies, while individuals with sensorineural loss usually have loss in the upper frequencies. People with conductive loss often can be helped through medical management, while people with sensorineural loss must rely on hearing aids.
8. Children achieve adult sensitivity to sounds between the ages of 4 and 10 years.
9. Binaural sound localization depends upon differences in the time of arrival, intensity, phase, and spectral characteristics of the sound reaching the two ears. Localization is enhanced when the individual moves his head to use both ears.
10. The intensity of traffic sounds is greater for low to middle frequencies than for high frequencies. Due to one's differential sensitivity to frequency, sound energy present in the 500 to 4000 Hz range is important in assessing the ability to use

(*continued on next page*)

Suggestions/Implications for O&M Specialists (continued)

traffic sounds for orientation and mobility. Typically, however, energy present at 125 and 250 Hz is also audible and should be considered for individuals with losses above this range.

11. Hearing impaired individuals who have threshold averages of 55 dB HL or better in the 500 Hz to 4000 Hz range may be able to detect the acceleration of vehicles from a stop in a residential area, while averages of 65 or better would be needed to detect acceleration of a vehicles in a business area. Detection of a vehicle approaching from the distance of 110 feet in a residential area would require thresholds 45 dB HL or better. Such determinations must be verified through functional experience.
12. Echolocation can help a visually impaired person avoid large obstacles and locate openings along walls or other surfaces before making contact with them.
13. The Cornell Experiments demonstrated that reflected sound was the underlying mechanism responsible for echolocation. These experiments led practitioners to believe that frequencies of 10,000 Hz and higher were necessary for echolocation.
14. Current research indicates that echolocation may be dependent upon small interaural differences in the intensity and frequency of reflected sound. Lower frequency sound cues are particularly important in echolocation, while high-frequency sound cues in the range of 10,000–12,000 Hz are useful but not required.
15. Adults are more typically taught auditory skills during active travel instruction in O&M. Sensory training classes are a less frequently used approach with adults. Children often first learn these skills through play, incidental learning, and structured learning experiences.
16. Hearing aids are designed to amplify frequencies at which the individual experiences hearing loss. Typically 95% of the energy needed for speech intelligibility is available for frequencies in the 500–8000 Hz range. These frequencies are amplified to the extent practical for a particular hearing loss and electroacoustic limitations.
17. In order to prevent reaching the level of discomfort, linear hearing aids use a peak clipping approach to limit the output of the aid, while signal processing aids limit output by compression.
18. Conventional hearing aids include in-the-ear (ITE), in-the-canal (ITC), behind-the-ear (BTE), eyeglass (EG), contralateral routing of signals (CROS), and body aids.
19. Signal-processing hearing aids with level-dependent frequency response (LDFR) can be classified as either those in which base increases at low levels (BILL), those in which treble increases as low levels (TILL), and those which have programmable increases at low levels (PILL). The PILL category allows users who are blind to select characteristics that are likely to meet both communication and travel needs.

ACTIVITIES FOR REVIEW

1. Explain how the characteristics of sound affect its use for O&M.
2. How do temperature and wind affect the transmission of sound?
3. Create audiograms to illustrate a conductive hearing loss, a sensorineural hearing loss, and a mixed loss.
4. Discuss how the various categories of hearing loss affect communication skills.
5. Identify how a problem in each portion of the ear would affect hearing.
6. What functional hearing characteristics would you expect to find with a conductive loss, a sensorineural loss, and a mixed loss?
7. Describe how sound localization works and how it unfolds in the child.
8. Describe how an O&M specialist would evaluate an audiogram of an individual with a hearing loss to predict possible ability for making street crossings.
9. Discuss the underlying mechanisms that allow individuals who are blind to use echolocation.
10. What information should be provided to the audiologist who will prescribe hearing aids for an individual who is blind?

CHAPTER 5

Kinesiology and Sensorimotor Function

Sandra Rosen

Movement is life. It is in all we do on a daily basis, from brushing our teeth to crossing the street. For children, movement is also the natural learning medium. It is the means by which they explore the environment, learn how it functions, and interact with it.

This chapter explores sensorimotor development and functioning in children and adults who are visually impaired. This consideration includes the role of sensorimotor skills in independent mobility and the impact of visual impairment on their development. Kinesiology, the study of movement, provides the structure for categorizing, analyzing, understanding, and communicating about sensorimotor skills.

KINESIOLOGY

Highly defined kinesiological terms describe movement so precisely, even complex motor acts can be broken down into small, easily handled components. Through an understanding of these basic terms, orientation and mobility (O&M) specialists can analyze the performance of mobility and other motor skills. They can precisely identify which components are being correctly or incorrectly performed, and focus their intervention directly on the source of the problem. By using kinesiological terms to describe movement, O&M specialists can also exchange information most efficiently among themselves and with health care professionals such as occupational and physical therapists. Table 5.1 lists common kinesiological terms.

On a physical level, movement is the interdependent action by the body's skeletal, muscular, and neurological systems. The *skeletal system* consists of 206 bones. In much the same way that the wooden frame of a house provides the structure upon which the walls hang and the roof rests, the skeletal system provides the supporting framework for the operation of many of the body's operating systems.

The *muscular system* consists of elastic cells bound into specific groups called muscles. There are three basic muscle types: cardiac, visceral (digestive), and skeletal. Skeletal muscles are responsible for voluntary movement. They consist of elastic centers that taper at the ends to thin, fibrous bands called *tendons* which, in turn, attach to the bones on each side of a joint. Muscles operate in opposing pairs and can span one or more joints. As one muscle contracts, the points where tendons attach to bone pull closer together, resulting in motion at the joint(s) (see Figure 5.1). Simultaneously, the opposing muscle relaxes, stretching to allow smooth motion at the joint(s).

The *nervous system* consists of two primary subsystems: the central and peripheral nervous systems. The central nervous system (CNS) con-

Table 5.1. Definitions of Kinesiologic Terms

Term	Definition
Flexion	Bending of a joint; forward motion at the shoulder/hip
Extension	Straightening of a joint; backward motion at the shoulder/hip
Dorsiflexion	Bending at ankle to point foot upward
Plantar flexion	Bending at ankle to point foot downward
Lateral flexion	Bending head/trunk to the side
Abduction	Sideward motion of upper arm/thigh away from midline
Adduction	Sideward motion of upper arm/thigh toward midline or across body
Internal Rotation	Rotation of arm about its axis to point inner aspect of upper arm backward Rotation of leg about its axis to point toes toward midline
External rotation	Rotation of arm about its axis to point inner aspect of upper arm forward Rotation of leg about its axis to point toes away from midline
Pronation	Rotation of forearm, turning palm downward or backward
Supination	Rotation of forearm, turning palm upward or forward
Ulnar deviation	Bending of wrist toward the little finger side
Radial deviation	Bending of wrist toward the thumb side
Inversion	Motion of foot facing sole toward midline
Eversion	Motion of foot facing sole away from midline
Horizontal abduction	Abduction from a previously flexed position
Horizontal adduction	Adduction from a previously flexed position
Circumduction	Circular motion of arm/leg/head; combination of all of the above motions

sists of the brain and spinal cord; the peripheral nervous system (PNS) consists of the nerves that leave the spinal cord and travel to the distant body parts. Sensory receptors in the body carry impulses from the peripheral nerves through the spinal cord, and then to the brain for interpretation. Similarly, motor commands originate in the brain and travel down the spinal cord through the peripheral nerves to the appropriate body part(s).

At its most basic level, movement is the result of two intertwined physical functions—sensory input and motor output. Sensory input includes visual, auditory, tactile, vestibular, and proprioceptive functions. Motor output consists of muscle tone and a complex array of motor reflexes (primitive, involuntary responses) and reactions (mature motor responses) to environmental stimuli. Operating as a feedback loop, this interaction is seen when people perform any motor skill, even one as simple as picking up a pen from the table. To pick up the pen, they use visual feedback to identify its location, motor coordination to bring their hand to it, and proprioception (awareness of body position) to verify that their hand is moving through space as desired. The diagram in Figure 5.2 illustrates this feedback loop.

The integration of these functions (known

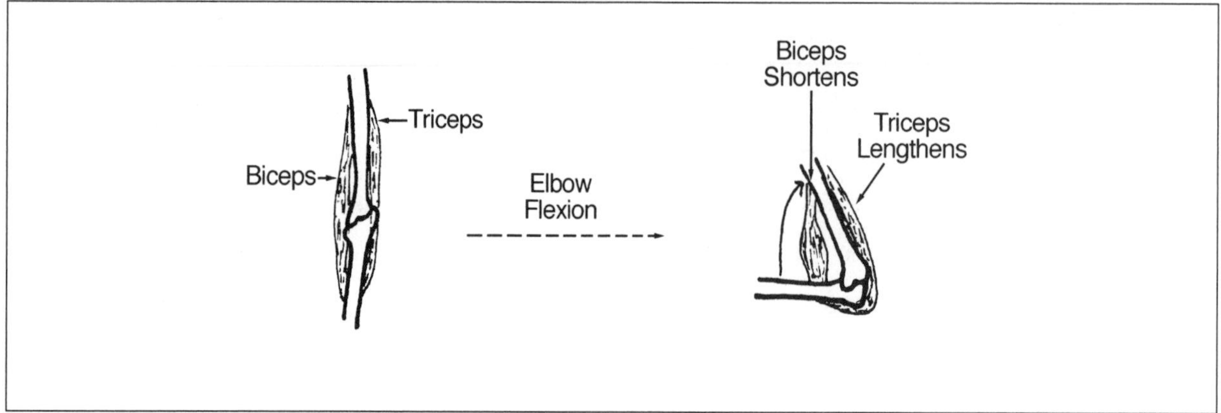

Figure 5.1. Muscle contraction surrounding the elbow joint.

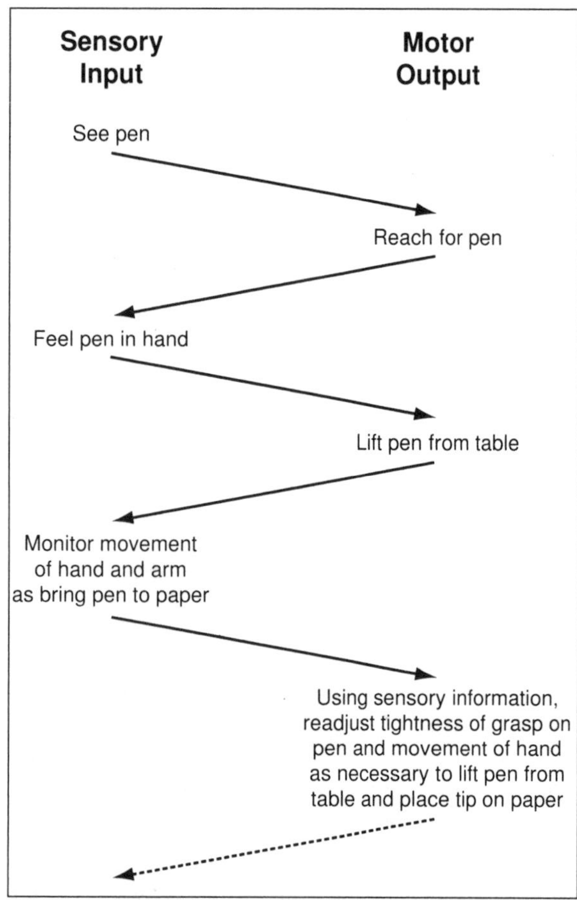

Figure 5.2. Sensory feedback loop.

collectively as sensorimotor functions) determines the physical efficiency and effectiveness with which we perform everything we do. It begins at birth and occurs every time infants or toddlers move in response to sensory stimulation. It continues as children grow and interact with the environment. Due to the degree of interaction between visual, vestibular, and reflex sensory inputs in the CNS, when one of these systems is slow to develop, usually one or both of the others also demonstrate delay (Pyfer, 1988). Additionally, children who lag in development in any of the sensory or motor systems seem to progress less rapidly in perceptual cognitive areas (Barraga, 1986; Scholl, 1986).

To best understand sensorimotor integration and functioning, and its role in mobility, it helps to break it down into its building blocks: muscle tone, sensory awareness, and coordination. These elements form the foundation for all gross and fine motor skills used in travel as well as in daily life. As shown in Figure 5.3, each level of motor functioning depends upon optimum development of precursor skills and, in turn, of the basic building blocks.

Sensory Awareness

The quality of both controlled and spontaneous movement depends on the ability to interpret sensory information accurately. There are seven major types of sensory input to the brain: visual, tactile, vestibular, proprioceptive, auditory, olfactory, and gustatory. The first five play a special role in sensorimotor development and functioning. Vision enables children to learn motor skills through visual imitation. The proprioceptive, tac-

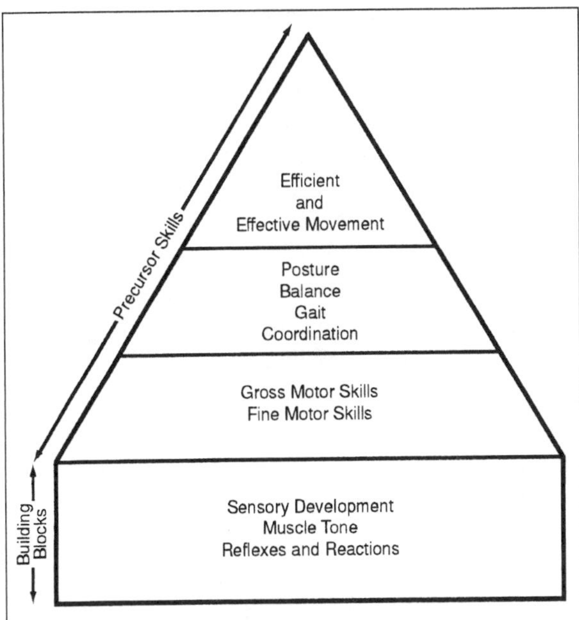

Figure 5.3. Hierarchy of motor abilities.

tual, and auditory systems help children to form concepts about themselves and their environment. Vision, together with the vestibular and proprioceptive systems, provide the feedback mechanism by which children develop, self-monitor, refine, and integrate sensorimotor skills into daily functioning. A detailed look at each of the first five sensory systems and their role in sensorimotor functioning will demonstrate this.

Visual System

When observing an infant who is sighted or who has low vision, one can immediately see the role vision plays in facilitating sensorimotor development. Vision stimulates, guides, and verifies infants' interaction with the environment. It stimulates motor activities and the development of cognitive relationships. Children with low vision or those who become visually impaired later in life are able to develop a basic sensorimotor foundation upon which to build later skills. Without this stimulation, children who are functionally blind often experience a delay in the development of fine and gross motor skills.

Tactile System

Nerve endings located in the skin transmit tactile sensory information through the peripheral nerves to the spinal cord, and then to the brain for interpretation. The sense of touch can detect six types of sensory information: deep touch (awareness of touch), light touch (textures), vibration, pain, temperature, and two-point touch (i.e., identification of the number of points of contact an object has with the skin at any given time). Braille readers use two-point touch to identify the shape of braille characters by distinguishing the number of dots contacting the skin at one time. Touch serves as an interface between one and the environment. It provides information about items that one touches and one's location in space relative to those items.

Vestibular System

The vestibular system, located in the inner ear, consists of two parts. One part, called the *static utricle*, signals the position of the head in space. It responds to sudden tilting movements of the head as well as to linear acceleration and deceleration. It also largely influences muscle tone throughout the body and plays a role in neurological reactions (discussed in the section "Coordination," below) that are fundamental to mature motor functioning. The second part of the vestibular system, the *kinetic labyrinth* (see Figure 5.4), consists of three semicircular ducts and registers other head movements. The three semicircular ducts are attached to the utricle and each lie in a different plane: perpendicular posterior and anterior vertical planes, and a more horizontal plane. Rather than lying perfectly vertical and horizontal, however, the lateral semicircular duct slopes downward and backward at a 30-degree angle. The ducts of each ear also form spatial pairs: the horizontal ducts lie in the same plane; the anterior duct of the left ear lies in a corresponding plane to the posterior duct of the right ear, and vice versa. This arrangement provides optimal awareness of head position in space and movement. Each duct expands slightly at one end to form an *ampulla* that contains sensory *hair*

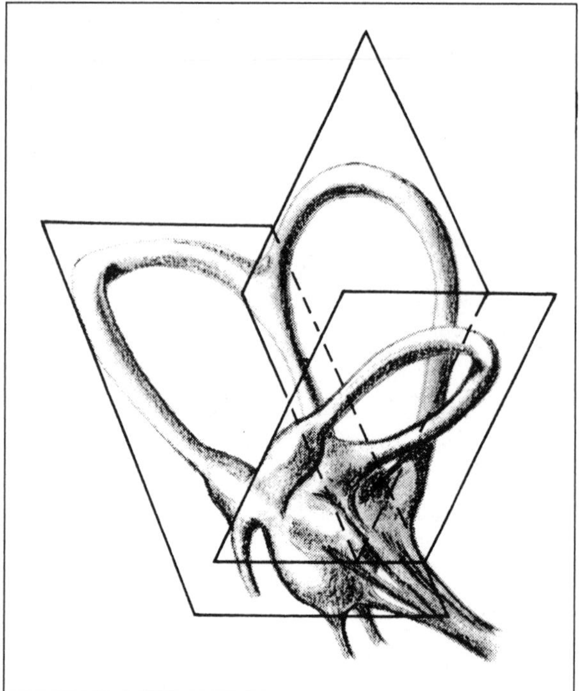

Figure 5.4. Kinetic labyrinth.

Source: Reprinted with permission from R. L. Welsh and B. B. Blasch (Eds.), *Foundations of Orientation and Mobility* (New York: American Foundation for the Blind, 1980), p. 76.

cells, the other ends of which lie in a gelatinous material called *endolymph.* When the head moves, relative movement of the endolymph stimulates the hair cells to provide information about the direction of movement. This labyrinthine system has a special relationship to ocular movements, allowing one to maintain visual fixation despite head movement. It is this function that allows one to fixate on a landmark while walking either toward it or perpendicular to it.

Children learn to use vestibular sensory information efficiently through motor activities that provide the opportunity to match vestibular inputs to visual, proprioceptive, and tactile sensory inputs. Without these opportunities, children with visual impairments may not be able to fully develop their ability to use vestibular information. This has implications for their lives both as children and adults. Studies have shown that children who have not learned to use vestibular input are delayed in gross motor activities requiring coordination of both sides of the body, the ability to balance on one foot or on a balance beam, eye–hand coordination, and fine motor control (Pyfer, 1988). These children may also show poor muscle tone, delayed postural reactions, and delayed mobility (Jan, Freeman, & Scott, 1977; Jan, Robinson, Scott, & Kinnis, 1975). Studies of adults who are blind have shown that unless the vestibular system is functioning within normal limits, the development of mobility, vocational, and self-help skills can be delayed (Pyfer, 1988).

Activities that provide age-appropriate vestibular experience such as rocking, swinging, roughhousing, and riding merry-go-rounds facilitate its development. Studies of children with Down's syndrome and other developmental delays have shown that brief periods of vestibular stimulation also positively affect muscle tone, gross motor skills, fine motor skills, and reflexive behavior (Humphries, Snider, & McDougall, 1993; Kantner, Clark, Allen, & Chase, 1976; MacLean & Baumeister, 1982).

Proprioceptive System

The proprioceptive sensory system provides information about body position in space. Proprioceptive sensory receptors are located in the muscles, tendons, and joints of the body; they provide an awareness of static body position at any given moment. Successive proprioceptive inputs provide awareness of movement. Kinesthesia, a term commonly used to describe awareness of movement, is actually the interaction of tactile, proprioceptive, and vestibular inputs and provides further awareness of body movement in space. As such, proprioception and kinesthesia play a vital role in the movement of people who are visually impaired. Since all movement operates on a feedback system, either visual or proprioceptive, the latter sense provides the only means by which people who are blind can identify and precisely coordinate movement.

In nondisabled children, proprioceptive development begins in infancy and occurs through a combination of movement experiences and visual feedback. Family members and other caregivers repeatedly move infants' bodies throughout the day. Stimulating the proprioceptive system with such passive movement is similar to stimulating the visual system with illumination (Barraga, 1986). When infants voluntarily move their extremities and trunk, this further stimulates the receptor systems in the muscles, tendons, and joints, providing an additional interface between touch and movement (Schiff & Foulke, 1982). In addition, infants watch each body movement with interest, fine-tuning proprioceptive awareness through visual feedback. Observation of infants playing with their feet, watching every movement intently, bears witness to this.

Children who are blind, however, lack this opportunity for visual feedback. As a result, they are often unable to fine-tune their use of this system and consequently develop inefficient movement skills that impact directly upon mobility. For example, blind children may have difficulty maintaining the elbow bent to 120 degrees when performing the upperhand and forearm technique; they may have difficulty maintaining a consistent and centered arc when performing the touch technique. Without the ability to discriminate between a wrist that is bent slightly backward or forward, or is in neutral, it is especially difficult for children with visual impairments to self-monitor their cane techniques. Furthermore, they often lack opportunities for much physical activity, which further limits the avenue for proprioceptive development. In fact, studies comparing the proprioceptive abilities of people who are sighted with those who are visually impaired have found that those with visual impairment are more variable in reproducing movements (suggesting less proprioceptive precision) (Toole, McColskey, & Rider, 1984).

Proprioceptive sensory ability additionally plays a major role in several other areas of motor functioning. It provides a foundation upon which body awareness can develop and secondarily contributes to laterality, directionality, and spatial awareness. It is also a vital element in what is termed haptic perception. *Haptic perception* is the ability to identify objects by size, shape, and feel. It results from the integration of tactile and proprioceptive inputs and is the means by which people who are blind identify and manipulate objects in their environment. Proprioception also plays a vital role in muscle tone and balance as well as the development and maintenance of good posture. Research with congenitally blind children has subsequently documented difficulties in areas such as body awareness, muscle tone, coordination, posture, gait, and balance that depend upon proprioceptive awareness for their own optimum development (Jan et al., 1975; Rosen, 1986; Rosen, 1989).

Muscle Tone

Closely related to the development of proprioception, muscle tone can be viewed as a motoric "readiness for movement." The nervous system continually sends a low level flow of neural impulses into the muscles, maintaining them at a baseline level of tension. For movement to occur, the brain only needs to send a few additional impulses to the muscles to have them contract (many impulses will cause a stronger contraction). This process is depicted in Figure 5.5A.

Muscle tone development is a recognized problem for children with congenital visual impairment (Jan et al., 1977). Many children who are congenitally blind have *hypotonia,* or abnormally low muscle tone. In hypotonia, the flow of neural impulses from the brain to the muscles is insufficient to maintain them in a state of readiness. When the muscles need to move, the brain must send a higher level of neural impulses to bring the muscles to a state of readiness, and then send additional impulses to stimulate movement (see Figure 5.5B).

A study of children who are blind in Canada (Jan et al., 1975) examined 101 children with visual impairment, each with intelligence quotients (IQ's) above 80 and without clinical diagnosis of neurological system damage that would cause hypotonia. The study found that 30 of 91

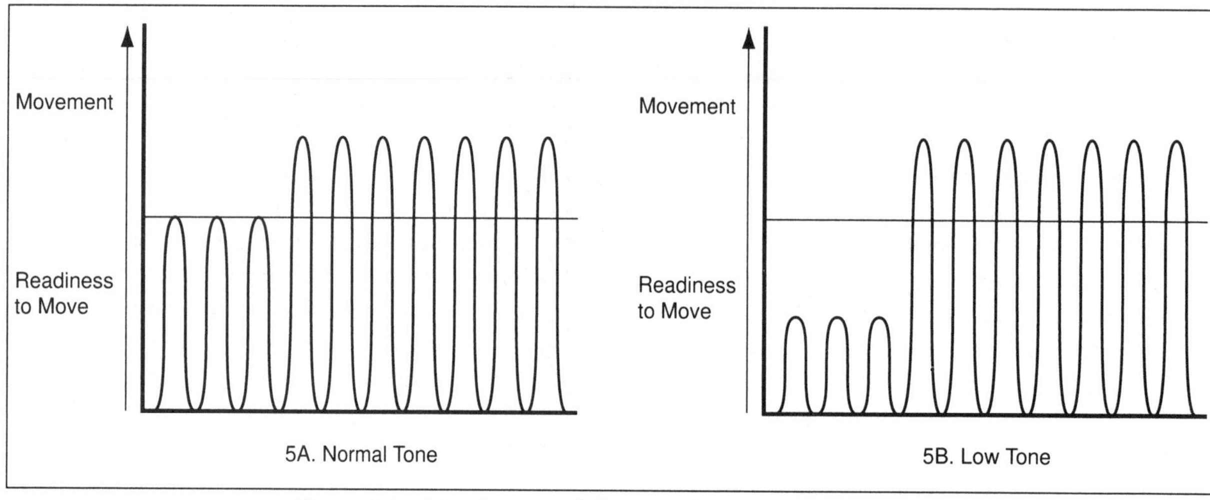

Figure 5.5. Muscle tone. (A) Normal tone; (B) low tone.

congenitally visually impaired children demonstrated hypotonia; none of the 10 adventitiously visually impaired children did. Less hypotonia was also present in blind children who were more mobile. Finally, hypotonia was related to age and the degree of visual impairment. There was a greater tendency in younger children (50 vs. 21 percent) and in those with severe visual impairment (61 vs. 21 percent) to have hypotonia.

Without sufficient muscle tone to support efficient movement, children who are visually impaired demonstrate motor skill delays. In their study comparing children with and without hypotonia, Jan et al. (1975) found that about 80 percent of nonhypotonic children achieve unassisted sitting, crawling, and walking within normal age limits as noted in parent reports, whereas only 30–40 percent of those with hypotonia achieve these milestones within normal age ranges. Furthermore, when motor skills do develop, children with visual impairments also often demonstrate many tone-related postural and movement problems. These include decreased endurance in activity, a tendency not to hold the head erect, poor shoulder girdle and abdominal strength, and varying degrees of out-toeing.

To compensate for these problems, children with visual impairments may use abnormal postural adjustments to maintain a position or to support movement. Examples of these adjustments include elevating the shoulders to provide neck stability and rotating the pelvis anteriorly to lock the hips in place and maintain an erect posture. These positions, in turn, interfere with such motor activities as moving the head when scanning visually and auditorily and when using the arms to reach. They also interfere with normal posture and gait development, balance, and straight-line travel. Clinical examination of coordination and gait patterns has, in fact, shown abnormalities for 40 to 75 percent of those in the hypotonic group, but only for 5 percent of those in the nonhypotonic group (Jan et al., 1975).

One possible explanation why many children who are blind are hypotonic is based on the role visual impairment plays in infant development and the correlation between proprioception and muscle tone development. Visual impairment limits opportunities during infancy for visual feedback of motor skills, making it difficult for children to practice proprioceptive awareness and develop related muscle tone. A second explanation centers on the passivity of many children with visual impairments. Comparisons of young children in the United States with those in other countries highlight the role of this passivity. In many cultures, mothers or caregivers carry infants on their bodies while going about their daily activities. Mexican families carry a baby in a *rebozo;* Japanese and Tibetan caregivers shop with infants strapped on their backs. In China, parents will often make a cradle of hands behind their backs and carry a youngster piggyback style. A study of children raised in one such culture found that babies who were hypotonic at birth made significant motor advances in the first two weeks of life (Brazelton, 1977). It is this movement experience that serves to develop muscle tone. In the United States, however, visually impaired children often lack incentives and opportunity to explore their environment and experience movement. An aggressive program of sensorimotor development and physical activity, started long before children enter school, could therefore benefit visually impaired children.

Coordination

Coordination is essentially the neurological system's co-ordering of activity to organize movement. Higgins (1985) described coordination as the capacity to integrate internal states and processes with external demands. Essentially, the sensorimotor system processes information about environmental conditions and task requirements and then provides neuromotor control to execute the task at hand.

At a neurological level, the development of coordinated movement begins with primitive reflexes that exert much control over infants' movements during the early months. These movements, in turn, provide tactile, proprioceptive, and kinesthetic stimulation as the children interact with their environment.

As infants gain movement experience these primitive reflexes soon integrate into a higher level of CNS control and give way to mature, voluntary reactions beginning at about 3 months of age. Major reflexes and reactions that impact upon motor development are shown in Table 5.2.

While reflexes can be somewhat rigid and strongly influence movement, reactions are never rigid. To illustrate this difference, consider the comparative movements of children at 1 month, 4–6 months, and 1 year of age. At 1 month of age, the asymmetrical tonic neck reflex (ATNR) (see Figure 5.6) exerts a strong influence over infants' movements. Moving the head from side to side is often accompanied by an associated movement of the arms and legs. At 4–6 months of age, however, the ATNR has integrated and the body-on-body and neck-righting reactions needed for rolling are firmly in place. Infants learn to roll by turning the head to the side, allowing the neck-righting reaction to pull the shoulders over to begin the roll. At the same time, the body-on-body righting reaction aligns the pelvis with the shoulders, completing the roll. The end result appears much like a log roll in which the children appear to roll over rigidly, almost as if flopping over unintentionally. In this process the children continue to develop muscle tone and the proprioceptive awareness of rolling. By approximately 1 year, they are able to use the righting reactions or inhibit them, allowing them voluntarily to assist in rolling as necessary, but maintaining the ability to isolate the movement of one section of the body from the other, rolling segmentally. As motor patterns gradually come under voluntary control, infants and young children begin to feel the relative positions of their body parts and their movements. In so doing, they learn about their bodies in relation to space. Table 5.3 shows the ages at which reflexes and reactions appear and disappear in children who are not disabled.

Each reflex and reaction plays a unique and important role in the development of motor abilities. The symmetrical tonic neck reflex (STNR), for example, facilitates the initial development of head and trunk extension. The Landau reaction stimulates the development of muscle tone and strength in the neck, back, and hip muscles. Equilibrium reactions aid in maintaining the upright posture and are constantly active as we move through space.

If, in the course of development, the primitive reflexes fail to integrate and mature reactions fail to develop, coordination difficulties result. For example, if the STNR is retained and the righting and equilibrium reactions do not develop, children will have difficulty raising their heads, rolling, and balancing on all fours. Without well-developed equilibrium reactions, children

Table 5.2. Major Neurological Reflexes and Reactions

Term	Definition
Reflexes	
Asymmetrical tonic neck (ATNR)	Flexion of arm and leg on side toward which head turns; extension of arm and leg on side away from which head turns
Symmetrical tonic neck (STNR)	Flexion of arms and head with extension of legs; extension of arms and head with flexion of legs
Tonic labyrinthine	Increased flexor tone in the prone (lying on stomach) position; increased extensor tone in the supine (lying on back) position
Primary standing	Increased extensor tone in legs upon weight-bearing
Automatic walking	Forward "walking" movement of legs when infant is held in standing position with trunk leaning forward
Grasp reflex (hand)	Closing of hand around an object touching palm; grasp remains as long as object touches palm
Reactions	
Neck righting	Trunk rotation in response to head rotation (or vice versa) to maintain forward alignment of head and trunk
Body-on-body righting	Pelvic rotation in response to trunk rotation (or vice versa) to maintain forward alignment of pelvis and trunk
Labyrinthine righting	Movement of head to regain upright position; occurs in response to vestibular sensory information
Optical righting	Movement of head to regain upright position; occurs in response to visual sensory information
Landau	Increased extensor tone in the body when infant is held prone in the air with support under the trunk
Protective extension	Extension and abduction of the arms/legs in response to a sudden loss of balance (e.g., when falling)
Equilibrium	Muscle tone changes to maintain balance in response to slow changes in support (e.g., when walking, riding on a boat)

demonstrate an immature gait pattern and have difficulty maintaining balance when required to shift direction quickly. If the protective extension reactions do not develop well, the children may fail to extend their arms to break a fall, increasing the possibility of injury.

Anecdotal evidence suggests that some of the coordination difficulties experienced by children who are born with visual impairments may be related to poor sensorimotor integration of primitive reflexes and development of mature neurological reactions. A common example of this is the influence of the ATNR in performing the touch technique. The ATNR normally integrates at 4–6 months of age. When it fails to integrate fully, however, it can increase the difficulty some children have in centering the cane hand. The touch technique requires children to reach the

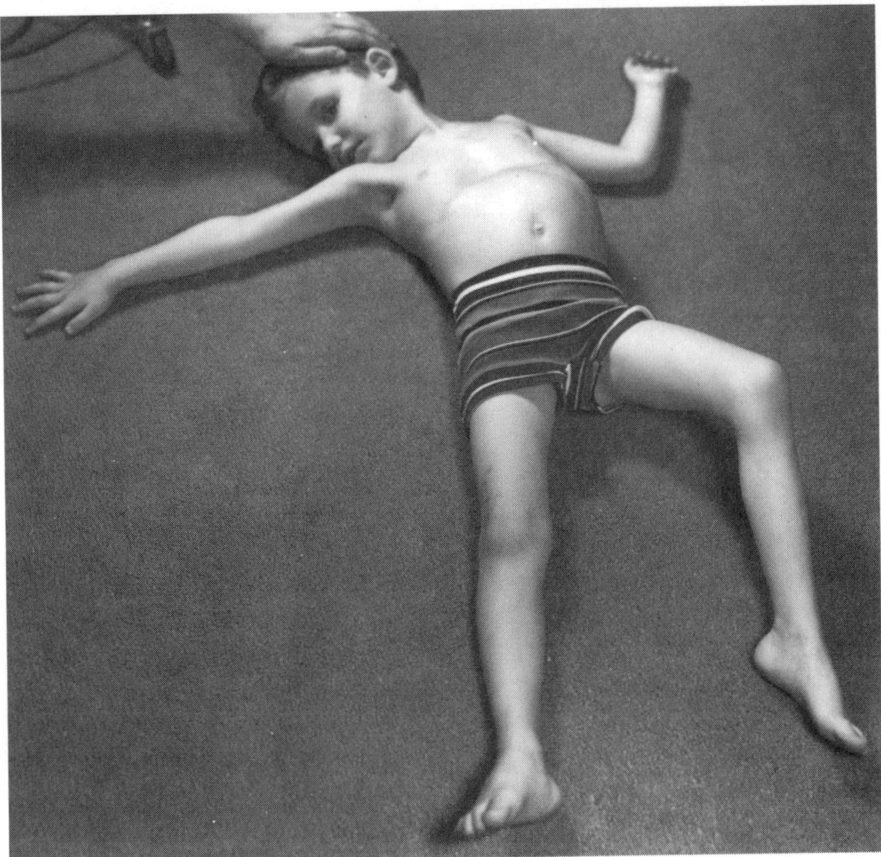

Figure 5.6. Asymmetrical tonic neck reflex.
Source: Reprinted with permission from R. L. Welsh and B. B. Blasch (Eds.), *Foundations of Orientation and Mobility* (New York: American Foundation for the Blind, 1980), p. 59.

cane arm forward while facing the head in the same direction (Figure 5.6). This position stimulates the primitive ATNR reflex, complete with its helpful component of extending the arm and facing the head forward. However, it also stimulates the interfering component of pulling the opposite shoulder backward. This interfering component not only increases the tendency to veer, but also increases the energy expenditure required to perform the cane technique.

Another aspect of coordination related to the integration of reflexes and reactions is the ability to perform isolated motions. These are motions in which one joint or body part is able to move without concomitant movement of another; for example, flexing and extending the wrist when performing the touch technique without simultaneously supinating or pronating the forearm. Due to residual primitive reflex activity and inadequate proprioceptive development, students who are congenitally blind often have difficulty learning body awareness and developing isolated motions; they develop movement "patterns" instead. Examples of functional problems caused by lack of isolated motion include poor supination or pronation for stirring, turning doorknobs, and so on. Similarly, pelvic, trunk, and limb rotation, which are prerequisite to good locomotor ability (Ferrell, 1985), are also frequently undeveloped or missing altogether in young children who have several visual impairments. Opportunities to develop and practice skills requiring isolated motions are critically important for young blind children.

Table 5.3. Ages at Which Reflexes and Reactions Appear and Disappear in Nondisabled Children

Responses	1–4 Weeks	2 Months	4–6 Months	7–12 Months	12–14 Months	18 Months to 5 Years	After 5 Years
Reflexes							
Asymmetrical tonic neck (ATNR)	±	+	±				
Symmetrical tonic neck (STNR)		±	±	±			
Primary standing	+	+					
Automatic walking	+	±					
Grasp reflex (hand)	+	+	±				
Reactions							
Neck righting	±	+	±	±	±	±	
Body-on-body righting			±	+	±	±	
Labyrinthine righting (plus optical righting)	±	+	+	+	+	+	+
Landau			+	+	+		
Protective extension			±	+	+	+	+
Equilibrium							
Prone			±	+	+	+	+
Supine				+	+	+	+
Sitting				+	+	+	+
Standing						+	+

± Transitional—reflex/reaction developing or disappearing.
+ Reflex/reaction present.

Furthermore, while mature reactions provide the foundation for coordinated movement, primitive reflexes can be called into play unconsciously when people are under physical or emotional stress (Pyfer, 1988). This can be seen when people try to push a heavy piece of furniture across a room. They typically bend the knees slightly and extend the head backward while pushing forward with fully extended arms (the STNR position). Stress may facilitate the influence of the ATNR on children's ability to center the hand in the touch technique. For many children with visual impairments independent travel imposes an underlying level of stress, including increased physical demands exacerbated by the presence of hypotonia, a poorly tuned proprioceptive system, and the increased level of concentration required by the travel. Hence the potential for unwanted reflex activity is enhanced. This problem further points out the importance of teaching activities that facilitate integration of neurological reflexes and reactions (see the section "The Role of the O&M Specialist" for sample activities).

IMPACT OF VISUAL IMPAIRMENT ON SENSORIMOTOR DEVELOPMENT

In nondisabled infants and children, vision plays a primary role in the development of sensorimotor skills. Nondisabled infants hold their heads up to enjoy the visual world around them. Infants with visual impairments, however, do not get the visual reward that comes from lifting their heads and thus often lack the motivation to do so (Hill, Rosen, Correa, & Langley, 1984; Schneekloth, 1989; Scholl, 1986). Consequently they often fail to develop normal strength and muscular control of the head, neck, and trunk. Similarly, visual input stimulates infants to reach in order to obtain objects across a room. Without this stimulation, children with visual impairments may not readily initiate creeping or crawling and may be slow to explore their surroundings. It is a documented fact that self-initiated exploration and movement in the environment are notably decreased in children with visual impairments (Hill, Dodson-Burk, & Smith, 1989; Jan, Sykanda, & Groenveld, 1990). This lack of physical activity, in turn, delays the later acquisition of such motor skills as walking and fine motor coordination. Furthermore, such delays are critical because reaching, crawling, and walking are young children's means of interacting with the environment, and it is motor activity that largely forms the foundation for cognitive (Thompson, 1993) and perceptual (Bushnell & Boudreau, 1993) development. In fact, the absence of active interaction has been found to be more detrimental than visual deprivation itself in enabling children to construct sensorimotor schema (Millar, 1981).

The level of delay, however, is not a simple linear relationship. In fact, both children who are blind and those who are sighted follow the same sequence in motor development during the first few months of life, and there are no significant differences in their development. Major delays in gross motor milestones occur, however, after the first 4–6 months, especially in children without functional vision (Adelson & Fraiberg, 1974; Palazesi, 1986; Schneekloth, 1989). These delays, which can range from 3–6 months, are most evident in skills such as reaching, crawling, and walking, which involve locomotion and interaction with the environment (see Table 5.4). Delays are also visible on a microlevel in the integration of the ATNR; head-lifting and weight-bearing on the hands when prone; and the development of postural responses, head- and trunk-righting responses, Landau reaction, protective extension reactions, and equilibrium reactions (Sonksen, Levitt, & Kitzinger, 1981).

In a study of infants who were blind, Fraiberg (cited in Warren, 1984) noted a marked delay in the coordination of the two hands. She reported the inability of blind infants to bring the two hands together at midline, and consequently retardation in their ability to use their hands together when exploring and manipulating objects tactilely. In another study, Adelson and Fraiberg (1974) compared the early development of ten blind babies (aged birth to 2 years) to normative data on nondisabled infants. They found that the children who were blind sat, stood, and walked (with hands held) close to the expected age of achievement for nondisabled children. Motor skills requiring independent movement in the environment, with the exception of rolling over, however, were significantly delayed. Fraiberg (1977) later characterized the development of blind children in terms of "developmental arrests" in which the infants would develop well during the early months and then encounter "roadblocks" that temporarily delayed further development.

Fraiberg proposed that children may not move through space readily because they don't understand that objects exist to which they could have access. In children who are sighted, the emergence of locomotor skills appears to precede object permanence (Bigelow, 1992; Zelazo, 1984). Studies of sighted infants (Campos, Hiatt, Ramsay, Henderson, & Svejda, 1978; Kermoian & Campos, 1988) demonstrated this most clearly when they showed that prelocomotor infants of-

Table 5.4. Motor Development Milestones: Comparison of Children Who Are Sighted and Visually Impaired

Motor Skill	Sighted Children	Children with Visual Impairment†
Exercises head control		
Vertical	1 month	1 month
In prone	2 months	2 months
Pulled from supine	4 months	4 months
In supine	5 months	5 months
Rolls (supine to prone)	3–4 months	7 months
Sits unsupported	6–7 months	9–10 months
Pushes to sit	8 months	10 months
Creeps*	8 months	13 months (or later)
Pulls to stand	9 months	11 months
Walks with hands held	9–10 months	10–11 months
Stands unsupported	10–11 months	11–12 months
Walks unsupported*	11–12 months	18 months (or later)

*Motor skills involving independent movement into environment.
†From S. Fraiberg, *Insights from the Blind* (New York: Basic Books, 1977).

ten had difficulty searching for partially hidden objects, whereas locomotor infants of the same age did not. But in her study of children who were blind, Fraiberg found that the children only became mobile after demonstrating the ability to reach to a sound. Thus Fraiberg proposed that for blind children, object permanence precedes locomotion. In reality, there is likely a cyclical relationship between self-initiated movement and increased knowledge about the environment. As children who are blind learn more about their environment, they are more motivated to move within it; this increased ease of movement in space further increases motivation to explore and learn about the environment. Bigelow (1992) showed just this in her study of three boys who were congenitally blind without multiple impairments. She found that there was indeed a sustained relationship between advancement in locomotive skills and object knowledge.

Similarly, so much of what young children learn is through imitation, primarily visual imitation (Miller, 1983). For children with visual impairments, however, opportunities for imitative learning are limited or absent (Scholl, 1986). The children may not be able to visually observe erect posture, crawling and creeping, normal gait patterns, and so on. This lack of access to visual imitation therefore makes it more difficult to develop optimum physical skills. As a result, not only are some aspects of motor development often delayed in children with visual impairments, but they may actually arrest at immature levels of skill achievement. It is therefore important for O&M specialists to help children with visual impairments develop many of the sensorimotor skills that their peers who are sighted learn through visual imitation. Specialists can do this by encouraging meaningful movement, demonstrating skills using kinesthetic and visual modeling, and assisting children to perform motor skills while emphasizing the host of auditory, olfactory, tactile, vestibular, and other sensory inputs that are part of such experiences.

Finally, children with visual impairments also often engage in what are termed stereotypical movement patterns, sometimes called *blindisms* or *stereotypies.* Commonly seen in children with developmental disabilities, and to a lesser degree in all children, these are repetitive movement patterns that, on the surface, appear to serve no useful function. Patterns typically demonstrated by some children who are born with impaired vision include rocking their trunk back and forth or rubbing their eyes. Professionals have speculated on the causes of stereotypies for years. Some see stereotypies as a means of supplying movement experience when external opportunities for physical and motor activity are limited (Burlingham, 1965; Hoshmand, 1975; Tait, 1972). Others see them as learned motor behaviors (Blasch, 1978), the result of social deprivation (Berkson, 1973, as cited in Scholl, 1986), inadequate primary caregiver–child relationships (Hoshmand, 1975; Tait, 1972), or lack of ability to visually imitate appropriate social behavior (Smith, Chetnik, & Adelson, 1969). Some postulate that stereotypies may be an attempt to provide sensory input that will increase muscle tone (Lewis, 1978; Montgomery, 1981). Still others consider stereotypies to be the means by which children provide sensory stimulation when external stimulation is insufficient (Knight, 1972; Scott, 1962; Warren, 1984). This latter explanation is of particular interest when considering the impact of limited sensory awareness on sensorimotor development in children with visual impairments. It is interesting that the most common stereotypies seen in children who are born with a significant visual impairment are trunk rocking, head rolling, eye rubbing, and hand flapping. These behaviors specifically stimulate the vestibular, proprioceptive, and perhaps the visual system (or at least the tactile components within it). Perhaps stereotypies do serve an important function in sensorimotor development, whether it be to provide some stimulation, or perhaps only to alert family members and professionals of the children's need for specific additional sensory stimulation. Whatever the true cause of stereotypical movement patterns, research and a greater understanding of their nature and function is needed.

Taking sensorimotor development to the next level, we also see a strong impact of visual impairment on development of specific motor areas that play primary roles in mobility. These areas include posture, balance, and gait (walking) patterns.

Posture

Several fundamental concepts underlie the development of good posture. The first concept is that of *body planes.* As seen in Figure 5.7, the frontal plane bisects the body into front and rear sections. The transverse plane (passing horizontally through the body at any level) divides the body into top and bottom parts. The sagittal plane divides the body into left and right sides.

Body segments (e.g., head, shoulders, pelvis) are aligned with respect to each other in the three planes. In proper posture, key body segments align themselves, one directly above the other, in the sagittal and frontal planes, and directly across from each other in the transverse plane. Figure 5.8 shows the ideal alignment of body parts in the frontal plane.

The second concept is *center of gravity.* Specifically, each body segment has a point within it, which if supported, would then support the rest of the segment without toppling. As an analogy, if one balanced a plate on the end of a pencil, the plate would balance without toppling if the pencil was directly in the center of the plate. Similarly, every body segment has a center of gravity.

In optimal posture, body segments are aligned one on top of the other, so that the center of gravity of each segment is directly above the center of gravity of the one below. Taken as a whole, the body's center of gravity is at the intersection of the three body planes at the upper sacral region of the pelvis, just in front of the second

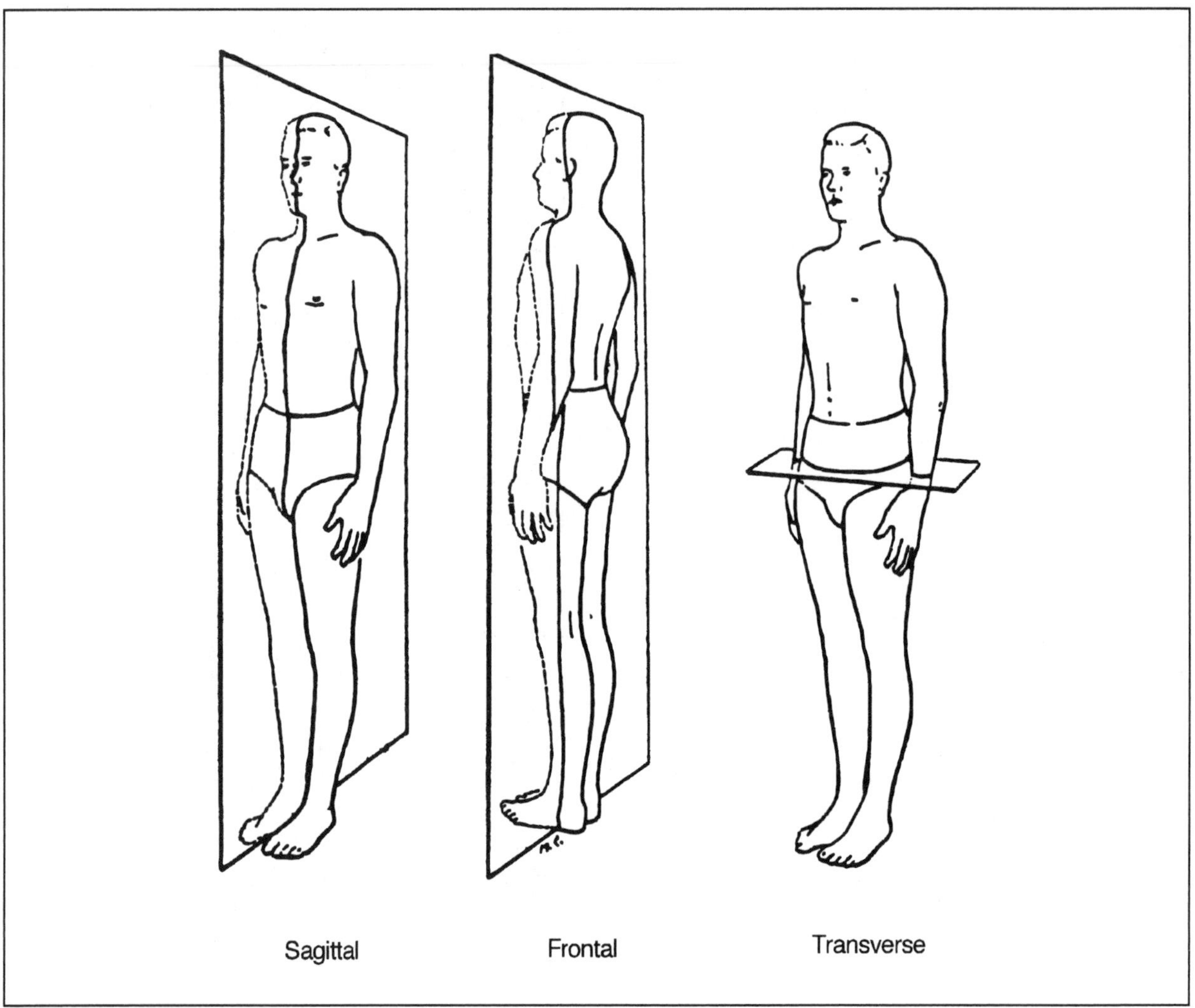

Figure 5.7. Body planes.

Source: Reprinted, with permission of the authors and the publisher, from K. F. Wells and K. Luttgens, *Kinesiology,* 6th ed. Copyright © 1976 by W. B. Saunders Company.

sacral vertebra. In adult men, this is approximately 56–57 percent of their standing height from the floor; in adult women, about 55 percent (Rasch & Burke, 1965). In fact, this posture is so optimum that studies of electromyography (EMG) have shown the muscles of the body to be at rest when standing with this alignment.

In real life, however, body segments are rarely completely balanced. The phenomenon of *postural sway* demonstrates this. Observe people standing perfectly erect and still. One will see that they are not truly still, but that their bodies tend to move in a slightly pendular, "figure 8" motion. To avoid tipping over with the slightest misalignment of centers of gravity, the muscles react to bring the body back into alignment, continually compensating for any changes in alignment of body segments. Even in movement, the body tries to maintain a posture as close to this optimal balance as possible. This serves to reduce wear on joints and optimizes the functioning of internal organs, while providing a foundation for efficient movement that requires a minimum of effort.

What is "proper" alignment? If one suspends a vertical line (often referred to as a plumb line)

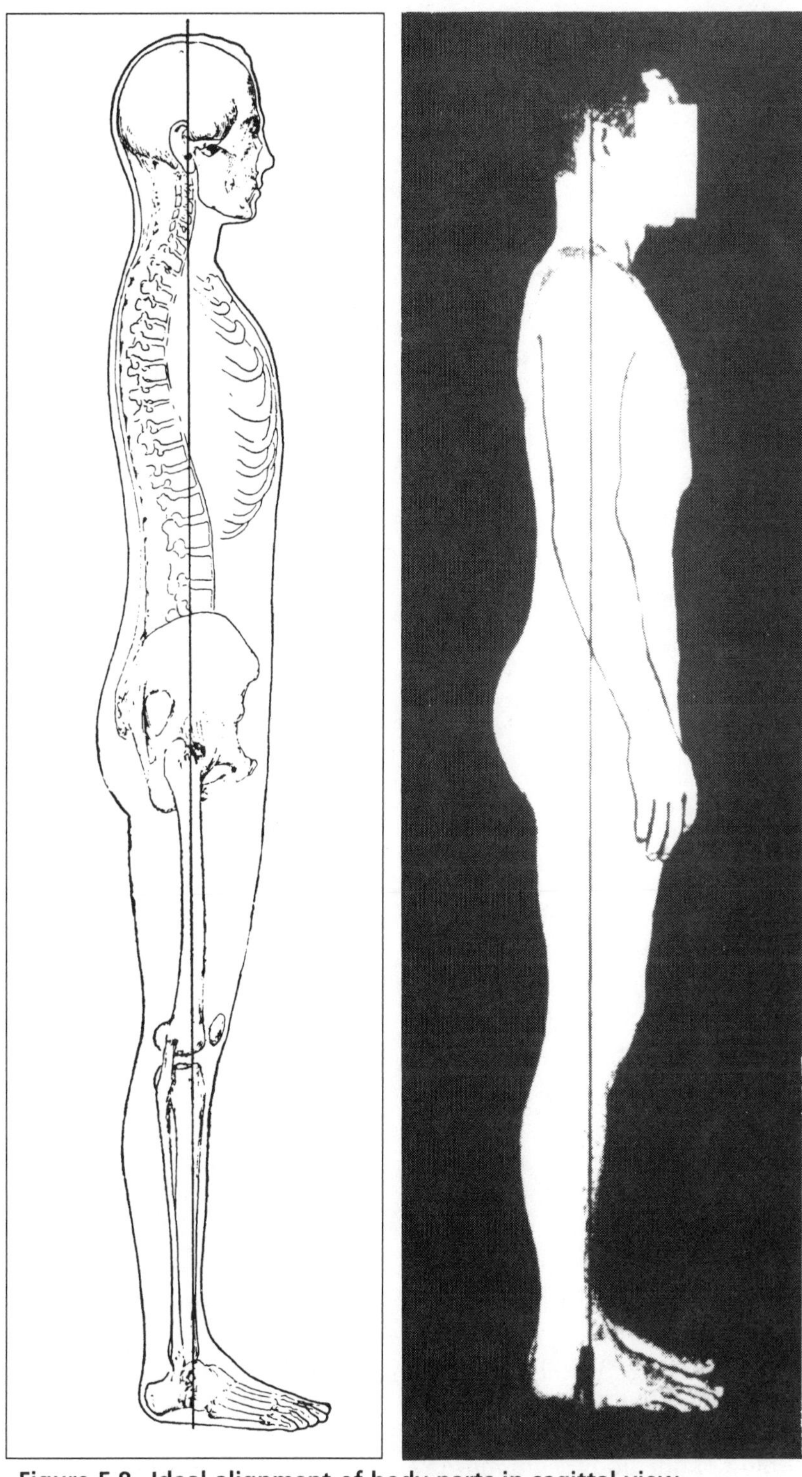

Figure 5.8. Ideal alignment of body parts in sagittal view.

Source: Reprinted with permission from R. L. Welsh and B. B. Blasch (Eds.), *Foundations of Orientation and Mobility* (New York: American Foundation for the Blind, 1980), p. 55.

from the ceiling directly in front of the ankle bone, the plumb line will pass through the following body landmarks:

Frontal View (Sagittal Plane)

The line directly bisects the body from head to toe (see Figure 5.7).

Sagittal (Side) View (Frontal Plane)

1. Through the ear lobe or through the mastoid bone (just behind the earlobe) (see Figure 5.8);
2. Through the tip of the shoulder;
3. Just behind the greater trochanter of the hip (the greater trochanter is the large protrusion at the top of the thigh bone and lies approximately at the middle thigh, measured from front to back);
4. Just behind the knee cap.

It is important to remember, however, that what is considered good posture may vary at different ages. It is natural for toddlers to incline the body slightly forward and have a protruding abdomen, knock-knees, and flat feet. Similarly a mild dorsal kyphosis (excessive forward rounding of the spine in the upper back), forward head tilt, and mild hip and knee flexion may be seen in some elderly people for reasons related to thinning bones and decreased physical activity.

To a degree, children learn correct posture through visual modeling of people around them. To a much larger degree, however, posture depends on the interplay of sensory information, coordination, and muscle tone. With regard to sensory information, posture requires the integration of visual and proprioceptive information. Vision yields information about posture every time one looks in a mirror; proprioception tells one the relative position of one body segment to the next, helping one make ongoing adjustments through a feedback loop. Coordination operates through the optical righting reflex to maintain the head in an erect position. Normal muscle tone supports erect posture, enabling one to remain erect even when the centers of gravity are slightly misaligned.

Many people in the world have less than ideal posture and suffer its consequences. Chronically poor posture has been implicated in low-back pain, arthritis, limited endurance, and a host of other ailments. Research has shown that children and adults who are congenitally blind demonstrate very specific postural deviations (Aust, 1980). As shown in Figure 5.9A–J, common postural deviations among congenitally blind people include:

1. Lumbar lordosis (swayback)
2. Excess flexion (bending) of the hips
3. Dorsal kyphosis (excessive forward bending of the upper spine)
4. Scoliosis (sideways curvature of the spine)
5. Excess neck flexion or anterior head tilt (head hanging down)
6. Rounded shoulders
7. Backward lean of the trunk
8. Pes planus (flat feet)
9. Excess knee flexion, or sometimes hyperextension (back-kneeing)
10. Foot eversion (outward rotation of the ankles, placing the body's weight on the instep)

Interestingly, these postural deviations rarely occur in isolation; in some cases, they even contribute to the development of one another. For example, lumbar lordosis is generally associated with weak abdominal muscles, which some relate to a lack of physical activity. Dorsal kyphosis, in turn, often develops in response to lordosis. In addition, rounded shoulders often accompany dorsal kyphosis because the shoulder girdle and the dorsal spine are mechanically related.

Many views and theories, both social and medical, have been put forth to explain why people with congenital visual impairments often show these characteristic postural deviations. One commonly held belief among professionals

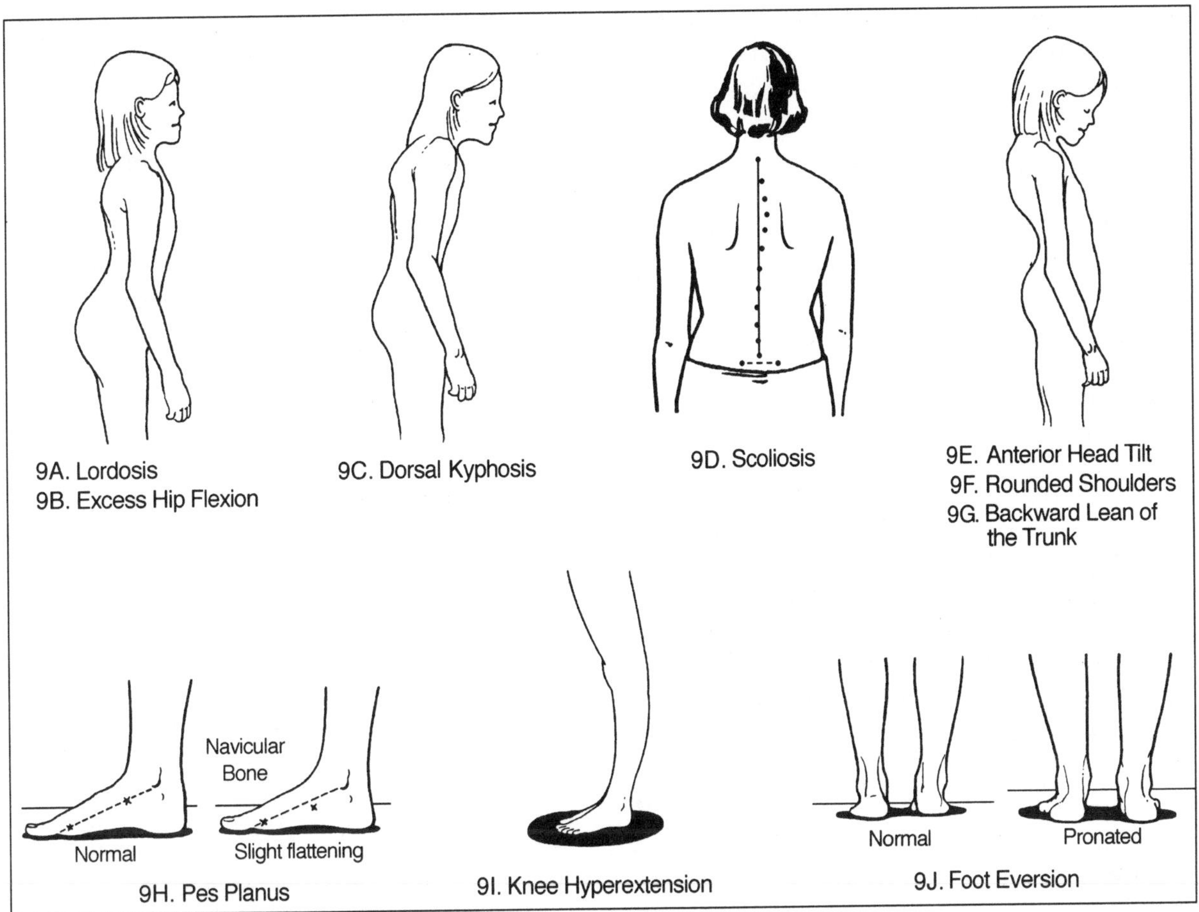

Figure 5.9. Common postural deviations.

Source: Parts A, B, C, E, F, and G are reprinted with permission from R. L. Welsh and B. B. Blasch (Eds.), *Foundations of Orientation and Mobility.* (New York: American Foundation for the Blind, 1980), p. 67.

is that without visual feedback, children who are congenitally blind are unable to learn proper posture through visual imitation as effectively as their sighted peers do. Other theories suggest a lack of physical activity and the need to assume a "protective" posture against unexpected encounters in the environment. For example, some view an anterior head tilt as a protective mechanism from "face-on" collisions with objects. Other theories (Miller, 1967) suggest that it compensates for the backward lean of the trunk during gait. Similarly, many congenitally blind people tend to stand with their hips and knees slightly bent. They may even keep them slightly bent as they walk, rather than bending and straightening them with each step as sighted people normally do. This tendency to keep the hips and knees bent has been associated with both long periods of sitting and a defensive posture in case one encounters unexpected drop-offs (Aust, 1980).

There are other possible explanations yet to be explored that, when taken in conjunction with the above, may provide yet a clearer understanding of postural deviations in people who are congenitally blind. One such explanation seeks to relate the postural deviations to the motor components of muscle tone and balance, since many postural deviations are rooted in these components. When viewed in this way, each specific deviation can be seen as serving one of two functions: to either lower the center of gravity (minimizing demands on the proprioceptive system to maintain equilibrium) or minimize demands on muscle activity to maintain the alignment of body parts. For example, excessive hip and knee flexion lower the center of gravity, thereby compensating for limited dynamic balance. Lordosis is the body's natural reaction as it tries to keep the trunk erect in the presence of excessive hip flexion. As stated above, kyphosis and rounded shoulders naturally occur in the presence of lordosis. Hyperextension of the knees and backward lean of the trunk may be an effort to maintain an upright posture with a minimum of muscular exertion. By leaning the trunk backward, for example, the body shifts its center of gravity backward. Strong ligaments that connect the pelvis to the thigh bone, however, keep the trunk from extending too far back. This posture greatly reduces the demand on hypotonic hip extensors. This posture is commonly seen in children with muscular dystrophy, whose hip extensors have weakened beyond the point where they can help the child maintain an upright position; the child compensates by leaning the trunk backward and "hanging on the hip ligaments."

Several researchers have noted pes planus (flat feet) and foot eversion (outward rotation of the ankles, which places the body's weight on the instep) in children and adults who are congenitally blind (Jan et al., 1975; Rosen, 1989; Rosen & Pogrund, 1994; Siegel, 1970). These deviations might be related to hypotonia (insufficient muscle tone to support the ankles and the arches of the feet) and to out-toeing (which shifts the weight to the inside edge of the foot and over time stretches the long and transverse arches of the foot).

Similarly, scoliosis may be related to hypotonia. Muscles run alongside the vertebral column and normally maintain an erect posture. When these muscles are low in tone they do not maintain an erect, symmetrical posture easily. The vertebrae shift position, "hanging on the ligaments" that connect each to the one below it. Support for this explanation can be seen in the comparatively good posture seen in people who are congenitally blind who were physically active (and consequently developed their equilibrium reactions and muscle tone more fully) during their growing years.

Throughout the years many researchers and authors have emphasized the role of good posture in endurance, comfort, and efficiency in mobility. Siegel and Murphy (1970) studied 45 students with visual impairments, ranging in age from 17–58 years, all of whom showed postural deviations and mobility deficiencies. Following a 12-week intervention, two-thirds of the students showed an improvement in mobility. Gender, age, and IQ were eliminated as relevant variables. Although the data were correlational in nature, a strong argument was made that correcting postural difficulties leads to more efficient mobility. Additional research in this area is needed to identify any true causal relationships and evaluate the effectiveness of postural remediation on mobility.

Balance

There are two types of balance—static and dynamic. Static balance is used to maintain a static posture such as sitting or standing. Dynamic balance is used during movement, such as when walking or running. Dynamic balance results from the integration of several sensory and motor functions, including vestibular, proprioceptive, and visual inputs (Woollacott, Debu, & Mowatt, 1987); muscle tone; and neurological equilibrium reactions. Vestibular information tells one when the head is no longer upright and is linked to the protective extension responses that play a role in recovery from a sudden loss of balance. The proprioceptive sense reacts to slow changes in balance and is vital in maintaining balance during movement. Muscle tone provides the foundation for a rapid response to the above sensory information, and the equilibrium reactions provide the neurological foundation for maintaining dynamic balance. Vision plays a major role in both the maintenance of balance and its recovery.

Dynamic balance, as will be discussed later, is often not fully developed in those who are congenitally blind. It can also be impaired in the presence of certain physical disabilities, and even some hearing impairments. Research has also shown that dynamic balance is impaired in elderly people, whether or not they are visually impaired or have additional disabilities. Stelmach, Teasdale, DiFabio, and Phillips (cited in Manchester, Woollacott, Zederbauer-Hylton, & Marin, 1989) showed that older adults have difficulty with high-level sensory integration of vestibular, visual, and proprioceptive information used for balance. Horak, Shupert, and Mirka (1989) reported that elderly people have slow muscle response when their balance is challenged, decreased muscle strength, limited range of motion, and changes in sensory integration (including a decreased sensitivity to proprioceptive information). Furthermore, medications such as some antihypertensive drugs (Gerson, Jarjoura, & McCord, 1989), altered mental ability, and decreased vision are major contributors to impaired balance (Manchester et al., 1989; Pyykko, Jantti, & Aalto, 1990). In the elderly, vision normally plays a major role (Pyykko et al., 1990). When their vision is impaired, the elderly are even more prone to having difficulty maintaining their balance and can be more likely to fall than their sighted counterparts. Moreover, falls among the elderly more often result in broken bones and serious injury than do falls in the young.

In a study of 95 residents of a hostel for the aging, Lord, Clark, and Webster (1991) showed that poor dynamic balance was associated with poor visual acuity and contrast sensitivity. They found that residents who fell one or more times a year had significantly poorer contrast sensitivity than those who did not fall. Contrast sensitivity was tested using the Melbourne Edge Test which consists of 20 circular test patches (25 mm in diameter) that contain a series of edges of gradually reduced contrast. In this study, those who had greater difficulty on the Melbourne Edge Test experienced significantly more falls. Correlational data from these and similar studies have led many researchers to conclude that impaired vision is a predisposing factor to falls in the elderly. Although reduced ability to discriminate fine detail may not put the elderly at risk for falls, impaired detection of objects and hazards, such as steps and cracked pavement that contrast poorly with their surrounding environment, may contribute to falls (Felson et al., 1989; Owen, 1985; Owsley, Sekuler, & Siemsen, 1983). To minimize the potential for falls among the elderly, good mobility skills, high visual contrast in the home and other controlled surroundings, elimination of household hazards such as loose rugs, and good illumination are important.

Studies throughout the years have shown that dynamic balance is also impaired in children who have congenital visual impairment (Gipsman, 1981; Leonard, 1969; Periera, 1990; Rosen, 1989). Leonard and Gipsman assessed dynamic balance in children who varied widely in age and residual vision. They found poor dynamic balance in students of varying ages who were blind and in many who had low vision. Rosen found that not only was dynamic balance impaired in children and adolescents aged 6–18 years, but that limited balance correlated significantly with the presence of selected immature gait characteristics such as out-toeing and short stride lengths. Periera evaluated the dynamic balance of blind and sighted children, and those with low vision. She found balance difficulties in blind and visually impaired children to be related to low visual acuity, and altered and reduced visual fields.

Gait

Gait is the normal manner of walking. One's *gait pattern* is one's collection of specific gait characteristics. When standing, the body strives to maintain the center of gravity within the base of support. In walking, however, the center of gravity is repeatedly moved outside the base of support, and the body moves in that direction to realign the center of gravity within the base of support. In this sense, walking is the ongoing process of repeatedly losing and regaining balance.

Gait consists of two phases: stance and swing. Each phase is distinct, yet the two phases function in concert. The stance phase begins with

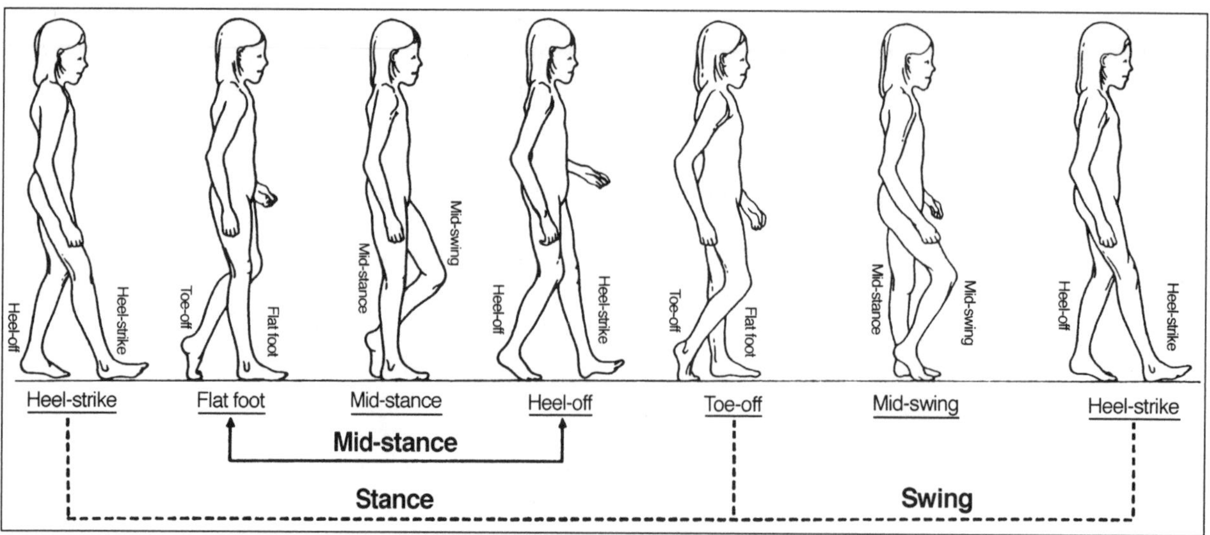

Figure 5.10. Phases of the gait cycle.

heel-strike and progresses through flat-foot, mid-stance, heel-off, and finally toe-off. During mid-stance the body's weight is immediately over the flat foot. The swing phase begins with toe-off, proceeds through mid-swing, and ends at the moment of heel-strike. During mid-swing, the knee and ankle bend and the leg passes underneath the pelvis and the hip. Figure 5.10 shows the components of each phase. Eighty percent of the stride phase is single-support stance. During the 10 percent double-support stance periods, both feet are not flat on the ground.

Gait patterns can also be broken down into specific spatial components within the two phases that indicate the quality and efficiency of gait. The development of these components have their roots in childhood and include stride width (the distance between the feet in a plane perpendicular to the line of travel), stride length, degree of out-toeing (see Figure 5.11), arm swing, trunk rotation, and knee flexion. As infants learn to walk, their gait patterns go through specific stages of development until stabilizing in their adult form, usually by the age of 7 years. The gait pattern of toddlers is generally characterized by short stride lengths, a wide stride width, an initial lack of significant out-toeing, and a lack of reciprocal arm swing. Initially the arms are held in the "high guard" position, then gradually move through "medium guard" to a "low guard" position (see Figure 5.12) before a reciprocal arm swing develops. As the gait patterns mature, the stride length increases, stride width decreases, reciprocal arm swing develops, the knees extend fully during mid-stance, and the feet develop a mild out-toeing position that averages 7.5 degrees (range: 0–15 degrees) (Rasch & Burke, 1965; Rosen, 1986).

People who are congenitally blind often show characteristic differences from people who are sighted in many specific gait pattern components. This is particularly true of those without functional vision. Typically, for people without functional vision during their early years of life, the spatial gait pattern does not fully develop, but rather plateaus at an immature level that is characteristic of the sighted toddler. It consists of short stride lengths, a wide stride width, flexed knees even during stance, a slower speed, decreased heel-strike that results in a "shuffling" step, and no reciprocal arm swing (Rosen, 1986). In addition, congenitally blind people show a larger than normal degree of out-toeing.

Several explanations have been presented over the years to account for immature gait pattern development in people who are congenitally

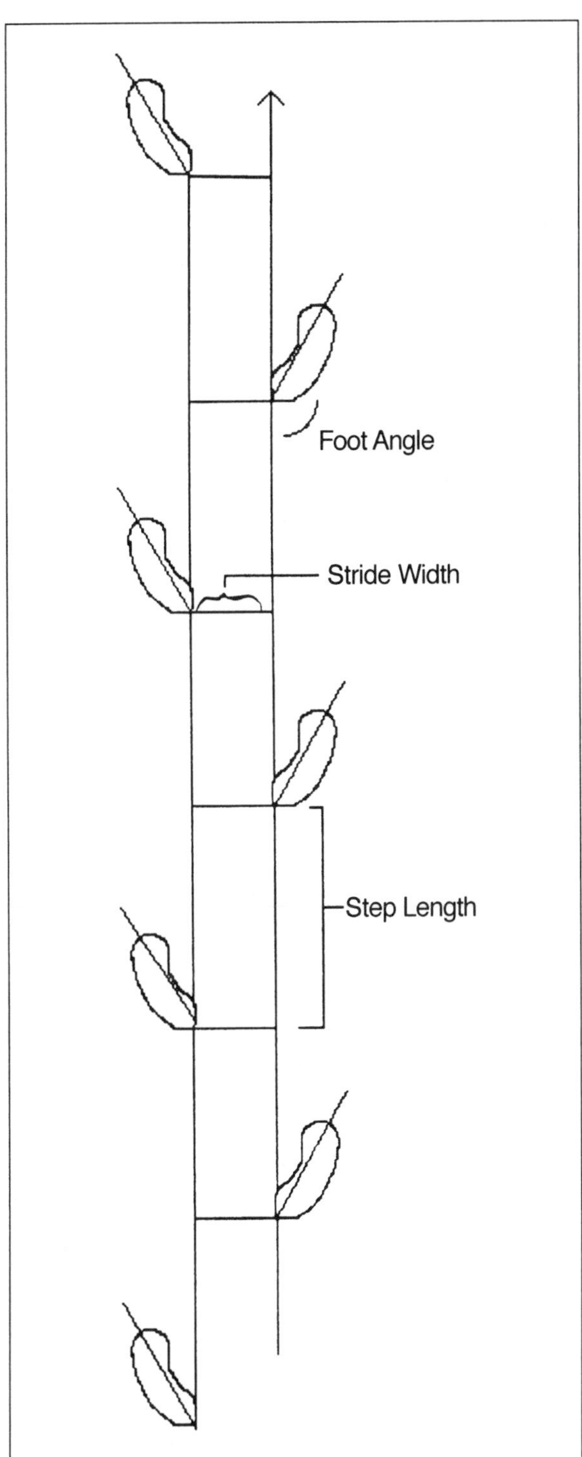

Figure 5.11. Components of the gait cycle.

blind. Miller (1967) wrote that visual impairment affects gait in three ways: a loss of sensory data needed to time steps, impoverished balance, and a deficiency of protective reactions. Others have blamed poor maturation of gait patterns on a lack of visual modeling. In addition, tension, fear, and anxiety are also factors often credited (or blamed) for the differences between the gait patterns of congenitally blind people and sighted people (Aust, 1980). When a person is tense, fearful, or anxious, gait patterns may become more rigid and less fluid, and muscle fatigue occurs more quickly. The shortened stride length, in particular, has been attributed to a fear of walking into objects (Aust, 1980).

On a motoric level, hypotonia, limited proprioceptive awareness, and poor integration of primitive reflexes and mature reactions may also account for some of the gait patterns characteristic of people who are congenitally blind. An example of how poor integration of neurological reflexes and reactions can affect gait patterns can be seen in trunk rotation. Efficient gait patterns require good trunk rotation to keep the trunk facing forward while rotating the pelvis and bringing a leg forward. Such rotation is frequently underdeveloped or absent in young children with visual impairments (Ferrell, 1985). This lack of rotation may stem from the fact that infants and young children with visual impairments, unlike their sighted counterparts, do not turn their heads repeatedly to follow visual targets and therefore do not gain head and neck balance in rotation. Similarly, when sitting on the floor, blind children are not necessarily enticed to reach for objects near them by extending one arm for support and bringing the other arm around to reach, thus rotating their trunks. Lastly, because many visually impaired children often do not creep on all fours before learning to walk, they lack yet another opportunity to develop trunk rotation and reciprocal arm movements. As a result, the ATNR may not always fully integrate and the children's bodies may retain a resistance to rotation. Also, due to the poor development of proprioceptive awareness, low muscle tone, and resultant poor development of balance, many children do not incorporate rotation into their gait patterns (perhaps because rotation places additional demands on balance for which they would have

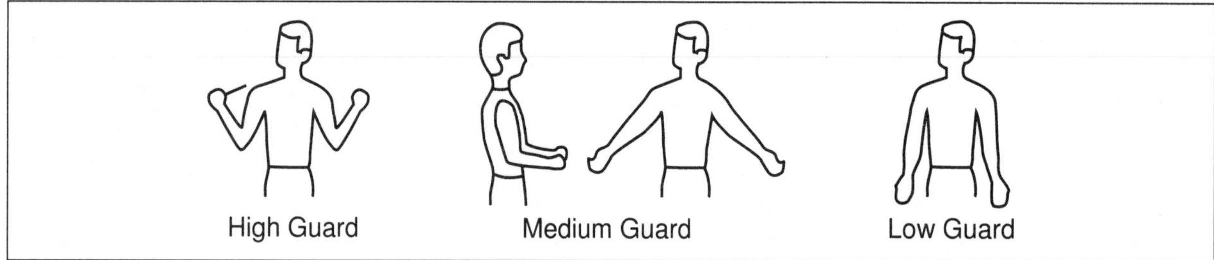

Figure 5.12. Guard positions.

to compensate). As a result, congenitally blind children often do not develop the same fluid and efficient gait patterns as do their sighted peers.

Many of the immature gait patterns characteristic of people who are congenitally blind can also be seen as having their roots in the lack of well-developed dynamic balance (Gipsman, 1981; Rosen, 1989). Short stride lengths limit the amount of time one needs to support oneself on one foot before bringing the other foot down to regain double support. A decreased heel-strike with more of a flat-footed step, a wide stride width, and out-toeing increase the base of support (see Figure 5.13). Knee flexion lowers the center of gravity of the entire body, and a lack of reciprocal arm swing limits challenges to balance caused by varying relative locations of the centers of gravity of each arm.

It is not only children who are congenitally blind, however, who may demonstrate characteristics similar to the immature gait pattern of sighted toddlers. Often the gait patterns of the elderly (aged 65 years and over) demonstrate many of the same characteristics: shorter stride lengths, a wider base of support, slower speed, a flatter step with decreased heel-strike, as well as increased knee and hip flexion (Azar & Lawton, 1964; Finley, Cody, & Finizie, 1969; Manchester et al., 1989; Murray, Kory, & Clarkson, 1969; Winter, Patia, Frank, & Walt, 1990). Studies of gait patterns in the elderly have made inferences about the reasons for observed changes in gait patterns from typical mature patterns to the less mature patterns described above. The suggested reasons for the change in gait patterns generally imply a degeneration of balance, combined with a general loss of muscle strength. In a study comparing the gait patterns of 15 healthy elderly adults (aged 62 to 78 years) to those historically documented in healthy younger adults, Winter et al. (1990) found shorter stride lengths, an increase in

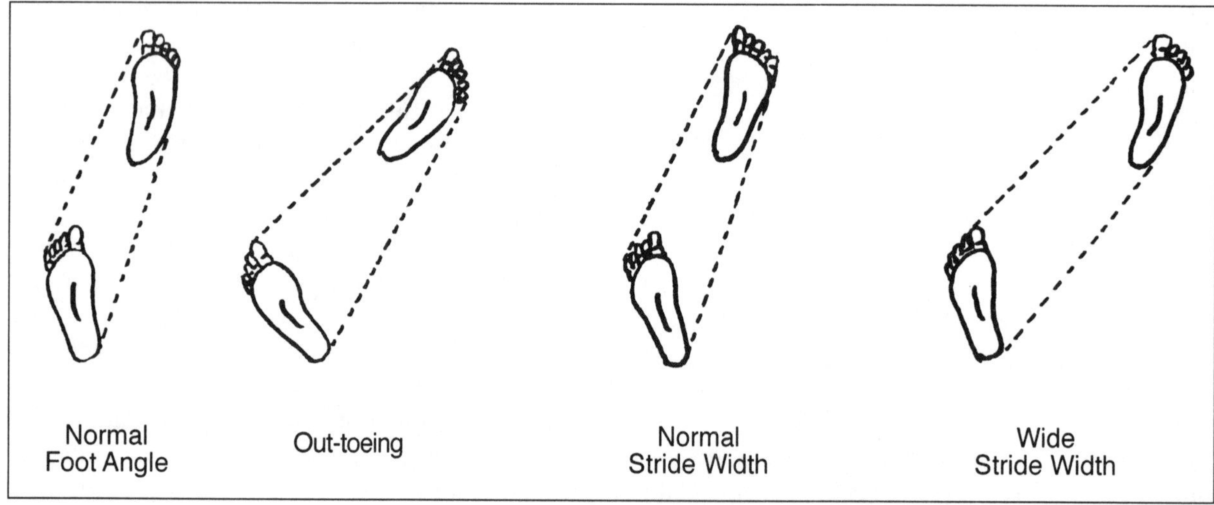

Figure 5.13. Base of support.

double-support stance time, and a more flat-footed walk among the elderly. They attributed these differences to an adaptation to a safer (less destabilizing) gait. Yet, just as a lack of exercise causes muscles to lose strength, it is a well-known fact that regular physical activity helps muscles maintain their strength. O&M instruction becomes especially important to the elderly in this regard. Not only does it provide elderly people who have visual impairments the means to travel safely in their environments, but it gives them the ability to get out of their homes, be involved in their communities, and be physically active. Taking daily walks is a common way in which elderly people try to keep fit. O&M instruction can make this possible for elderly people with visual impairments.

The development and retention of mature gait patterns is important in several ways. Immature gait patterns have been shown to negatively impact mobility. Evidence indicates that as speed is decreased and out-toeing occurs, there is an increase in the tendency to veer from a straight line of travel (Rosen, 1989). Also, anecdotal evidence suggests that immature gait patterns are associated with decreased endurance in travel (logically due to the higher energy demands of less efficient motor performance).

However, regardless of why the gait patterns of people who are congenitally blind and elderly people who are blind differ from the standard, some important questions for the mobility specialist are: (a) do the gait patterns interfere with safe, efficient, and independent mobility for a given person, and (b) can the gait patterns be changed? Unfortunately, because the gait pattern changes of both congenitally blind children and the elderly have their roots not merely in outward behavior, but also in accommodation to motor limitations, they are very resistant to change. Furthermore, since developing gait patterns stabilize around 7 years of age (Sutherland, Olshen, Cooper, & Woo, 1980), they become increasingly difficult to change in school-aged children with each successive year. That is why it is important to address motor and gait pattern development during the preschool years. Fortunately there is some anecdotal evidence suggesting that providing motor development activities which emphasize balance and neurological integration during the preschool years can positively impact the maturation of gait patterns (along with the development of posture and coordination). Physical therapists can also provide valuable input on strategies to facilitate the development of mature gait patterns in specific children.

THE ROLE OF THE O&M SPECIALIST IN SENSORIMOTOR FACILITATION

O&M specialists play a vital role in facilitating sensorimotor functioning of people with visual impairments. This is true whether it involves teaching new motor skills (such as those that use a long cane) to adults or giving elderly people the skills to travel independently and thereby remain active and more physically fit. It is most notably true in the sensorimotor development of children. In fact, the role of the O&M specialist begins in infancy when early intervention can do much to minimize sensorimotor delays and alleviate their impact on other areas of development.

We have seen that motor development is sequential (children must sit before they can walk) and that visual impairment affects the development of most motor skills, including those that we most readily associate with successful travel—posture, gait, and balance. We have also seen that the optimal performance of sensorimotor skills relies not only on the previous development of lower level skills, but also on the adequate development of fundamental sensorimotor elements—sensory awareness, muscle tone, and coordination. Therefore, when choosing and designing sensorimotor activities for children who are visually impaired, it is important for the O&M specialist to consider what functional skills the children need and what prerequisite abilities they must have, and to choose activities that facilitate:

1. Normal muscle tone in children who are hypotonic (e.g., weight-bearing on the

arms and legs; activities in which the muscles move against resistance such as tug-of-war, using a scooterboard, etc.).

2. Sensory development, including proprioception (e.g., swinging and playing on a merry-go-round for vestibular stimulation; weight-bearing and resistive activities such as wheelbarrow games, swimming, push–pull games, climbing on playground equipment, jumping, and marching, for proprioceptive stimulation; identification and localization activities for auditory and visual skill development).
3. The integration of primitive reflexes; activities that require one to perform a skill contrary to the action of the reflex will help to integrate it. For example, the ATNR reflex places the extremities on one side in extension and those on the other side in flexion. Activities requiring children to use both hands together (e.g., puzzles, some musical instruments, some ball activities) and/or to keep their hand(s) in midline will help to integrate the ATNR. The STNR links neck flexion with arm flexion and leg extension. Activities such as crawling, climbing, and propelling forward and backward on a scooterboard while keeping one's head up call for arm and head movements contrary to those seen in the STNR and will help integrate it.
4. The fine-tuning of balance and other mature neurological reactions (e.g., segmental rolling and climbing to facilitate the development of trunk rotation and isolated motions; balancing on a rocker board to strengthen balance reactions; jumping, hopping, and gymnastics to facilitate balance and protective extension reactions).

Adapted physical education specialists can recommend a variety of general motor development activities for children. Also, physical and occupational therapists can suggest activities and provide advice in planning and implementing motor programs for specific children.

Finally, when planning activities to facilitate sensorimotor development in children, it is crucial to remember the following key words: active movement, quality of movement, timing of movement, integration of movement, and families.

Active Movement

Self-initiated movement, not passive movement, is essential for developing motor skills. Only through active movement can children develop muscle tone, proprioceptive awareness, and coordination. Only through active interaction with the environment can children learn how to function within it. Although some children may fear moving in the environment due to the potential for injury (Burlingham, 1965; Griffin, 1981; Hill et al., 1984; Schneekloth, 1989), it is through movement experience that they are able to decrease this anxiety. Increasingly, O&M specialists advocate teaching young children to use a cane or an alternative mobility device during the preschool years in order to reduce any movement apprehension and enable the children to feel protected while moving.

Quality of Movement

For people with visual impairments, quality is as important as function. True, there may be times when the need for function outweighs the need for quality in performing a task. For example, a student may need to learn a route or how to perform a self-help task immediately, whether or not it is done with the highest level of grace or coordination. However, in the area of sensorimotor development and functioning, quality cannot always be ignored in a rush for function. Because the acquisition of higher level motor skills relies so heavily on the development of lower level skills and abilities, it is important to weigh immediate need against the long-term benefit of emphasizing quality in movement. For example, a child may be delayed in walking. Rather than just practicing how to walk, however, it may be important to encourage the child to creep first. It has been suggested that a lack of creeping experience may be related to hypotonia and a decreased ability to stabilize neck and shoulder girdle muscles (Lampert, 1991). Without creeping experience a child will also likely have difficulty developing trunk rotation, which is an essential component of mature, efficient gait patterns. This in turn can then potentially limit the efficiency of the child's mobility later in life. Similarly, for children who are already walking, but have not yet reached the age when gait patterns have stabilized, practicing age-appropriate motor skills that incorporate trunk rotation such as climbing or dancing may enable the children to refine their gait patterns and increase their body awareness and coordination.

It is also important to consider the impact of any additional disabilities. Cognitive impairments, for example, may limit the children's potential to learn some skills precisely. In this case it may be more important to achieve any level of skill performance quickly, regardless of quality, in order to allow the children to go on to learn other things. Working closely with professionals who serve these children, such as teachers of children who have severe disabilities, is important in determining goals for students with significant cognitive impairments. Similarly, some physical disabilities may limit the ability of children to develop the same level of quality in movement as their peers. When working with children who have physical impairments it is important to consult a physical and/or occupational therapist before engaging in motor development activities. The therapist can determine the best motor activities for the children as well as provide information on which activities to avoid in the presence of specific physical disabilities.

Timing of Movement

Specific skills are learned best during their "critical periods" when the appropriate sensory and motor inputs are coming together (Langley, 1980). Greenough, Black, and Wallace (1987) proposed a neurophysiological mechanism to explain the role of what they termed "sensitive periods" for the development of certain types of abilities. They organized their model around the concept of experience–expectancy. They proposed that during such periods an excess number of synaptic connections among brain neurons generates. As children develop, those synapses that are activated by sensory or motor experiences survive; the rest are lost through disuse. If it takes longer to acquire a certain skill, or if the acquisition of a skill begins after the "critical period," higher level skills based on that first skill will be delayed even further. Furthermore, if these critical periods are missed, some skills might never be learned, or if they are learned out of sequence, higher level skills may rest on a faulty foundation (Langley, 1980; Moore, 1984; Scott, 1962). The consequences of missing such periods can be seen in children with visual impairments who skip the creeping stage, for example, and therefore do not have the opportunity to practice weight shifting, reciprocal balance, and hip and trunk rotation. As a result, their gait often lacks fluidity and they may walk stiff-legged, shifting weight from one leg to the other with feet spread wide apart (Ferrell, 1985).

In planning motor and mobility goals for young children with visual impairments, it is therefore vital to encourage the sequential development of sensorimotor skills at normal developmental ages. By continually emphasizing age-appropriate sensorimotor functioning throughout O&M instruction with infants, toddlers, and preschool and young school-age children, one can build foundations to support the development of effective functional motor and mobility skills later on.

Integration of Movement

In addition to sensorimotor activities done in the context of an O&M lesson, it is important to integrate new sensorimotor activities into children's everyday lives. Working with parents, family members, and other members of the children's educational team, motor activities can be taught, practiced, and easily incorporated into all aspects of children's lives. For example, activities and games that incorporate coordination, proprioception, and muscle tone development, such as swinging, climbing, riding a tricycle, using playground equipment, running relay races, going through obstacle courses, and orienteering, can be part of activities done on family outings. These activities also provide a common ground for playing and interacting with other children and for developing social skills.

Parents and Families

Parents and families are generally eager to do everything that will benefit their child. Some parents, however, may not know the importance of motor behavior and learning (Periera, 1990) or understand that young children with visual impairments need many structured opportunities to learn to use their bodies effectively in exploring their world (Hill et al., 1984; Schneekloth, 1989; Warren, 1984). Other parents, fearing for the children's safety, may unintentionally overprotect their children and thereby fail to provide opportunities for them to learn and practice motor skills. Parents often need encouragement and support in learning the motor needs and abilities of their visually impaired children. Inviting parents and families to observe mobility lessons and videotaping children engaging in play and exploratory experiences can show parents and families what is possible despite visual impairment, even for very young children. Inviting parents and families to also observe other, perhaps more experienced children (who are confident and effective in their play and exploratory skills) can also be a means of showing parents and families what is possible. Setting up support groups, in which parents and family members can share mutual concerns, learn from each other's experiences, and encourage one another, can also be immensely effective.

SUMMARY

Sensorimotor skills are fundamental for functioning in life and are especially important in O&M. Because of the major role that vision plays in sensorimotor development, however, people who are born with a visual impairment often have difficulty in this area of development. Through attention to sensorimotor needs and by providing structured sensorimotor development activities, the O&M specialist can do much to help those they serve overcome sensorimotor difficulties and delays, and in turn, develop effective, efficient, and independent mobility skills.

Suggestions/Implications for O&M Specialists

1. Sensorimotor skills are fundamental for functioning in life and are especially important in O&M.
2. Sensory input includes visual, auditory, tactile, vestibular, and proprioceptive functions. Motor output consists of muscle tone and a complex array of motor reflexes (primitive, involuntary responses) and reactions (mature motor responses) to environmental stimuli.
3. The integration of sensory inputs and motor outputs determines the physical efficiency and effectiveness with which one performs a given task.
4. Sensorimotor integration begins at birth and continues as children grow and interact with the environment. Due to the degree of interaction between visual, vestibular, and reflex sensory inputs in the CNS, when one of these systems is slow to develop, usually one or both of the others also demonstrate delay.
5. The building blocks of sensorimotor functioning are: sensory awareness, muscle tone, and coordination.
6. There are seven major types of sensory input to the brain: visual, tactile, vestibular, proprioceptive, auditory, olfactory, and gustatory. The first five play a special role in sensorimotor development and functioning.
7. Muscle tone can be viewed as a motoric "readiness for movement." Many children who are congenitally blind have hypotonia, or abnormally low muscle tone. As a result, many demonstrate motor skill delays and tone-related postural and movement problems.
8. Possible contributors to the hypotonia of children who are congenitally blind include: (a) missed opportunities during infancy for visual feedback of motor skills, which make it difficult for children to practice proprioceptive awareness and develop related muscle tone, and (b) lack of incentives and opportunity to explore their environment and experience movement
9. The development of coordinated movement begins with primitive reflexes that in turn soon give way to mature, voluntary reactions that support coordinated movement.
10. Anecdotal evidence suggests that some of the coordination difficulties experienced by children who are born with visual impairments may be related to poor sensorimotor integration of primitive reflexes and development of mature neurologic reactions.
11. In nondisabled infants and children, vision plays a primary role in the development of sensorimotor skills. Much of what young children learn is through visual imitation. Children with visual impairments, however, miss opportunities for imitative learning.
12. Self-initiated exploration and movement in the environment are notably decreased in children with visual impairments. This lack of physical activity, in turn, delays the later acquisition of motor skills and can in turn impact cognitive and perceptual development.
13. Children with visual impairments sometimes engage in stereotypies. Speculated causes of stereotypies include: (a) a means of supplying movement experience when external opportunities for physical and motor activity are limited, (b) learned motor behaviors, (c) the result of

(*continued on next page*)

Suggestions/Implications for O&M Specialists (continued)

social deprivation, (d) inadequate primary caregiver–child relationships, (e) lack of ability to visually imitate appropriate social behavior, (f) an attempt to provide sensory input that will increase muscle tone and stimulate sensory integration.

14. Research has shown that children and adults who are congenitally blind often demonstrate specific postural deviations including: (a) lordosis (swayback), (b) excess flexion (bending) of the hips, (c) dorsal kyphosis (excessive forward bending of the upper spine), (d) scoliosis (sideways curvature of the spine), (e) excess neck flexion/anterior head tilt (head hanging down), (f) rounded shoulders, (g) backward lean of the trunk, (h) pes planus (flat feet), (i) excess knee flexion, or sometimes hyperextension (back-kneeing), (j) foot eversion (outward rolling of the ankles, placing body weight on the instep).

15. Dynamic balance results from the integration of several sensory and motor functions, including vestibular, proprioceptive, and visual inputs; muscle tone; and neurologic equilibrium reactions. Studies have shown dynamic balance to be impaired in children with congenital visual impairment.

16. Research has shown that dynamic balance is impaired in elderly people, whether or not they are visually impaired. Moreover, research has shown that poor dynamic balance in the elderly is associated with poor visual acuity and contrast sensitivity. For minimizing the potential for falls among the elderly, good mobility skills, elimination of household hazards, and good illumination are important.

17. Typically, for persons without functional vision during their early years of life, the spatial gait pattern does not fully develop, but rather plateaus at an immature level that is characteristic of the sighted toddler.

18. Immature gait patterns have been shown to negatively impact mobility. Evidence indicates that as speed is decreased and out-toeing occurs, there is an increased tendency to veer from a straight line of travel. Also, anecdotal evidence suggests that immature gait patterns are associated with decreased endurance in travel.

19. When choosing and designing sensorimotor activities for children who are visually impaired, it is important to consider activities that facilitate: (a) normal muscle tone in children who are hypotonic, (b) sensory development, including proprioception, (c) the integration of primitive reflexes, and (d) the fine-tuning of balance and other mature neurologic reactions.

20. In planning effective activities to facilitate sensorimotor development in children, it is crucial to remember the following keys:

    a. Active movement.

    b. Quality of movement.

    c. Timing of skill development.

    d. Integration of skills into daily life.

    e. Involvement of parents and families.

ACTIVITIES FOR REVIEW

1. Define the term "feedback loop?" Give an example of a feedback loop in mobility.
2. What is meant by "sensorimotor" integration?
3. What can happen when motor skills develop out of sequence or lower level skills fail to develop fully.
4. Describe the role each of the following sensory systems plays in sensorimotor functioning.
   a. visual
   b. tactile
   c. proprioceptive
   d. auditory
   e. vestibular
5. Explain why many children who are congenitally blind have difficulty developing finely tuned proprioceptive awareness. How does this decreased proprioceptive awareness affect mobility. Cite an example.
6. Define "muscle tone" and explain how visual impairment affects its development. How does low muscle tone impact motor functioning.
7. Describe how reduced dynamic balance impacts spatial gait patterns.
8. Explain the importance of addressing problems with gait maturation before a child reaches 7 years of age.
9. How can immature gait patterns impact independent travel by people who have visual impairments.
10. What role can O&M services play in the motor functioning of elderly people who have visual impairments?

CHAPTER 6

The Psychosocial Dimensions of Orientation and Mobility

Richard L. Welsh

A person's ability to move through the environment without vision or with seriously reduced vision is affected by numerous psychological and social factors. These factors can have a positive or negative impact. They may act alone or in combination with one another. They can be influenced by the environment in which the person is traveling. These psychological and social factors include elements such as: motivation, self-confidence, anxiety, attitudes, family dynamics, and stigmatization to name a few. Despite general agreement about their significance, there is little empirical research clarifying their impact on orientation and mobility (O&M).

Even without the guidance of definitive research, the methods of teaching O&M developed by professionals in this field collaborating with people who are blind have taken many of these factors into consideration. These approaches reflect a strong orientation of "putting the person first," which characterized mobility instruction's origins at Valley Forge Hospital and Hines Veterans Administration Hospital (Bledsoe, 1980). In doing so, these methods effectively address many of the psychological and social barriers that inhibit independent mobility for some blind people. They also harness positive factors that facilitate travel.

Explanations for the success of these teaching methods can be inferred from a review of theories and research in the area of personality psychology. The study of O&M in light of these theories can suggest hypotheses and research methodologies that can help to further develop the knowledge base for understanding and managing the psychosocial dimensions of O&M.

THEORIES OF PERSONALITY DEVELOPMENT

Most approaches to the study of personality come from one of four traditions: psychoanalytic, dispositional, cognitive or behavioral. (Some reviews consider existential theories as a separate tradition. However, in this chapter, existential theories are grouped within the cognitive tradition.) Each of these traditions has contributed concepts that are helpful to the study of how individuals respond to the loss of vision and the challenge of independent travel. None has produced a unified theory that satisfactorily explains and predicts the reactions of every person who experiences vision loss; nor is such a theory likely.

The psychoanalytic approach emphasizes the role of early developmental experiences and unconscious forces on personality development and behavior. The dispositional approach focuses on the role of fairly stable and impelling traits within the individual to explain and predict behavior. On the other hand, the cognitive and existential approaches introduced the role of the conscious "self" for interpreting and planning behavior. The behavioral strategy stresses the effectiveness of outside reinforcers as an explanation for how and why people act the way they do. Each of these approaches will be discussed in this chapter, but no one theory explains all behavior; nor does any one theory suggest approaches that the practitioner can use to help every client change ineffective behaviors related to orientation and mobility.

Some of the most promising trends in personality psychology are integrating concepts from various schools of thought in an effort to develop more comprehensive and therefore more useful theories of behavior (Krahe, 1992). According to Ekehammer (1975), neither the "psychic structures" of the person nor the situational and environmental factors can adequately explain behavior by themselves. However, the interaction of these factors is more likely to explain individual behaviors.

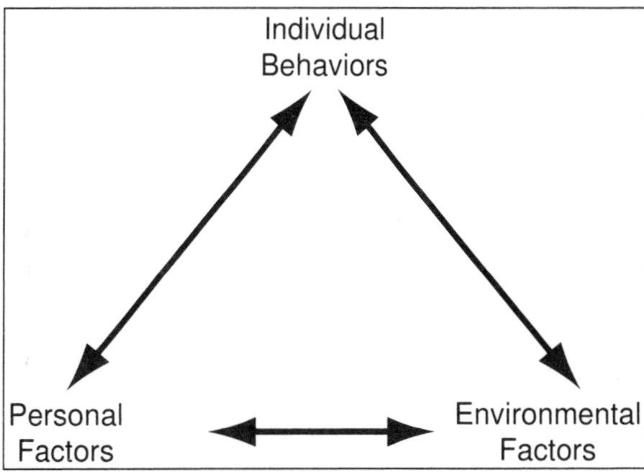

Figure 6.1. Bandura's (1986) three-sided model of reciprocal determinism.

Social Cognitive Theory

The work of one theorist, Albert Bandura (1986), integrates cognitive and other personal factors with the role of social and environmental influences in his efforts to explain, predict, and change behavior. He also provides research models that can be useful in further developing information about how these approaches work and how they can be improved. Central to Bandura's *social cognitive theory* is the concept that personality develops through a process of "reciprocal determinism," which refers to the continuous interaction of personal and environmental factors and the person's own behavior.

In Bandura's three-sided model, the action between each of the three elements is continuous and reciprocal. In other words, an individual's behavior is influenced by personal factors such as anxiety or self-confidence, just as these personal factors are influenced by his behavior. Similarly, the environment influences behavior and the environment changes as a result of the person's behavior. To complete the third dimension of the model, the environment can impact an individual's personal factors and can be influenced by the personal factors of individuals as well (see Figure 6.1).

The interactions between successful orientation and mobility and the self-concept, motivation for rehabilitation, the attitude of the family, and the ability to cope effectively with people on the street are continuous and reciprocal. A positive self-concept can be both a cause and an effect of success in mobility. On the other hand, a negative self-image can result from a lack of independent mobility or can make progress toward independent functioning more difficult.

Bandura (1986) was quick to point out that the tools for researching how the three-way interactions among the elements of social cognitive theory operate are not yet available. "This is a formidable task not only because the triadic systems are interactive, but because each subsystem itself contains multiple reciprocal processes" (Bandura, 1986, p. 28). Many factors working together in different blends influence particular behaviors in each situation.

And yet this is precisely the challenge facing the orientation and mobility specialist. How can she most effectively help a specific person who is visually impaired cope with a particular situation in which multiple psychosocial and environmental factors are operating?

Current knowledge is inadequate to predict

the impact of all variables for specific individuals in specific situations. However, there is a considerable body of information about how individual factors operate or the interaction of individual factors with one another or in specific environmental situations.

The following discussion of these concepts is organized in a manner consistent with Bandura's three-sided model of reciprocal determinism. First, information will be presented about the range of *personal factors* that influence O&M. This will be followed by a review of some of the *environmental factors* that impact on the travel of a person who is blind. Finally, there will be a discussion of the behaviors of the blind person who is traveling and the effect of those *behaviors* on his personal factors and the environment. The discussion of these elements will necessarily overlap, reflecting the complexities of the psychosocial aspects of human behavior.

A Note About Motivation

In the everyday language of O&M specialists, motivation is the psychosocial factor referred to most frequently. When a student appears to be having difficulty beginning or progressing in mobility training and there are no other obvious explanations, there is a tendency to regard him as being not "motivated." Similarly, if a student is progressing very well, he is considered to be highly motivated.

This reflects an early stage in our understanding of human behavior, which is parallel to the history of psychology itself. Some of the earliest theorists, such as James, Freud, and Hull, focused their efforts on discovering or articulating a grand theory of human behavior, and especially what "motivated" behavior. However, the grand theories of motivation were eventually recognized as too simplistic (Reeve, 1992). One term, motivation, was recognized as inadequate to explain the complex and varied ways in which behavior is energized and directed.

In spite of the popularity of the term in the language of mobility instructors, this chapter will not address the issue of motivation separately. Rather, the entire chapter is focused on efforts to understand, explain, and predict the causes and direction of O&M behavior. What we routinely think of as "motivation" is manifested in one way or another in practically every concept that will be discussed, and especially in their interactions.

PERSONAL FACTORS

Many personal factors have been proposed and researched by personality psychologists from different theoretical perspectives as explanations for behavior. Taken by themselves, they have usually proven inadequate in predicting behavior in complex real-life situations. However, to understand how these factors interact with environmental situations and human behavior, it is necessary to review what is known through empirical research and common-sense practice about some of these factors themselves.

Psychoanalytic Theory

As developed by Freud (1961), psychoanalytic theory represented the first formal approach to the study of personality. It has had a broad impact on basic concepts about human behavior. It holds that behavior is determined largely by unconscious forces that trace their source to early developmental experiences. All behavior has some meaning for the person, but frequently the person is unaware of the significance of, or the reasons for, the behavior because the forces are subconscious.

Occasionally it happens that a person's hesitancy or resistance to begin O&M training or proceed with a particularly threatening part of the training will have unconscious roots that are associated with early life experiences that have been repressed. This may be hypothesized by the O&M specialist when the student does not respond to the usual cognitive and behavioral strategies used to encourage hesitant students to attempt the training. When this seems to be the case, the O&M specialist will have to refer the student to an appropriately trained counselor who can help the student understand and find a way to cope with these dynamics. However, this is a rare event in current mobility practice.

Another application of psychoanalytic concepts to the issue of adjustment to blindness has been offered by Blank (1957), Cholden (1958), and Schulz (1977). They suggest that the reluctance of some individuals to participate in rehabilitation training following the news that their blindness is permanent and irreversible can be explained by the existence of a "shock stage" followed by depression and the need for a period of mourning. The purpose of this stage is to enable the ego to deal with this radical change in identity and to integrate this information at a pace that it can handle. The implications are that the person will not be ready to participate in rehabilitation activities until the impact of the loss of vision is absorbed.

These concepts are also related to the "loss model" articulated by Carroll (1961). In this model, the focus of the person who is blind is on a number of negative changes, or losses, that have occurred as a result of his blindness. This leads to a period of grieving and the need for emotional recoupment before rehabilitation can proceed.

Dodds (1989) suggests that the loss model and the need for grief counseling has had a dominant influence on the thinking of those who deliver rehabilitation services for people with visual disabilities. However, Bledsoe (1980) described how the development of rehabilitation training programs for military personnel following World War II marked a drastic change in this approach to rehabilitation training. There was neither the time nor the counseling resources to encourage a focus on grieving and loss. Instead, recently blinded veterans were quickly introduced to the techniques of learning how to function without vision, sometimes within days of having lost their vision on the battlefield. This change with its emphasis on learning alternative skills instead of spending time grieving—when considered in the light of Bandura's self-efficacy theory (1977), which will be discussed later in this chapter—may explain the successes achieved by O&M instruction as developed in the army and Veterans Administration programs.

Disposition Theories

Dispositional psychologists (Cattell, 1965; Allport, 1961) have focused their research on identifying personal factors that are relatively stable in people and can explain an individual's consistency in actions and behavior. These factors have been called dispositions or traits. To the extent that some of the traits of an individual can be known, a teacher working with that individual can understand or predict subsequent behavior.

Dispositional-oriented research (De l'Aune, Lewis, Needham, & Nelson, 1977) has attempted to identify the traits of individuals who are especially successful in coping with blindness. The hope behind such research is not to select only the most promising clients to receive the services, but to try to understand how to approach people with different patterns of traits differently in order to achieve positive rehabilitation outcomes.

Throughout the history of dispositional research there have been efforts to identify recurring patterns or clusters among groups of traits that can account for almost all of the adjectives used to described stable personality factors. Using factor analysis, numerous research studies have consistently identified similar clusters of traits. The consistency of these recurring factors has helped to focus dispositional research and improve efforts to understand the existence and impact of different personality types. McCrae and Costa (1987) have shown that five factors appear consistently. The factors have been labeled as: (1) neuroticism/stability, (2) extroversion/introversion, (3) openness, (4) agreeableness/antagonism, and (5) conscientiousness/undirectedness. As methods of assessing these factors continue to progress, research relating them to other personal and environmental factors and behavior will be better understood.

Wright and Mischel (1987) demonstrated the validity of the "conditional dispositional construct." This concept suggests that the most promising way to understand the role of dispositions or traits is to understand the "if–then" link between certain clusters of situations and clusters of behaviors. In this view a particular trait—for example, aggressiveness—in a mobility student would not suggest the likelihood that this person would behave aggressively across all mobility situations. Instead, it should be understood as a person's tendency to respond to certain situations, such as being confused or frustrated, with certain behaviors, such as lashing out verbally. In the absence of the relevant situations, the person high in the trait of aggressiveness would be no more likely to behave aggressively than the person who is not high in the trait.

Anxiety

Spielberger (1972) has contributed to the more sophisticated understanding of one specific trait, anxiety, which is frequently a concern of O&M specialists. Anxiety has been defined as a diffuse reaction to a vague or not clearly perceived threat. Unlike fear, which is a reaction to a specific threat or danger and usually generates some type of avoidance behavior such as flight, anxiety is a reaction to a less intense threat in which the reason for the discomfort is not well understood. It does not usually result in flight, but usually occurs in situations where the person cannot escape.

Spielberger proposed a two-factor theory of anxiety, differentiating between state anxiety and trait anxiety. *State anxiety* was conceptualized as a transitory experience of unpleasant, consciously perceived feelings of tension and apprehension. This is an experience that affects most people at certain times to a greater or lesser degree and varies from moment to moment and day to day. *Trait anxiety* was described as a more stable disposition of certain individuals who are prone to experience anxiety more frequently and more intensely in response to a wider range of situations.

Spielberger's model fueled the criticism of the "trait approach" to the study of personality in its conceptualization of anxiety as a unidimensional construct. In effect, Spielberger said that a person's likelihood of experiencing state anxiety in a wider variety of situations was related to the strength of the underlying trait of anxiety. However, Endler (1980) cited a number of studies which showed that individual differences in trait anxiety predicted corresponding differences in state anxiety for only certain types of situations. There was a high correspondence between trait anxiety and subjects experiencing the state of anxiety in situations containing threats to self-esteem or interpersonal threats. However, for other situations, especially those containing physical danger, the level of trait anxiety failed to predict the intensity of state anxiety.

Endler (1983) went on to develop an interactionist model of anxiety that identified five dimensions of trait anxiety relating to different types of anxiety-provoking situations. The five dimensions are:

1. Interpersonal anxiety: activated by situations involving interactions with other people
2. Physical danger anxiety: activated by situations in which the person faces the probability of physical injury
3. Ambiguous anxiety: activated by threatening situations in which the person does not know what is going to happen
4. Social evaluation anxiety: activated by situations that involve threats to a person's self-esteem as a result of being evaluated by other people
5. Daily routines anxiety: activated by circumstances encountered in routine, everyday situations

These differentiations can be of particular value to O&M specialists who frequently encounter anxiety in their students. Sometimes this anxiety prevents a person from beginning mobility instruction, and sometimes it appears at various points along the way. In the first case, the anxiety might be a manifestation of "ambiguous anxiety" in which the person reacts to a situation in which he does not know what is going to happen. In this case the O&M specialist may want to provide more information about each new step in the training process so that the student has the maximum amount of information available as he thinks about what comes next. Other students may begin to show anxiety as stair travel or street crossings are approached, which represent physical dangers. Still others may show the greatest amount of anxiety as the lessons bring them into interaction with people on the street. This may suggest a high level of "interpersonal anxiety." These observations can better focus the O&M specialist's responses to the student.

Anxiety in O&M

Helping students use and cope with anxiety and with the stress caused by anxiety has been of great concern to O&M specialists. Mandler and Sarason (1952) have shown how limited amounts of anxiety can be helpful in assisting learning and in completing challenging tasks. Generally speaking, however, research suggests that anxiety interferes with learning and task accomplishment, especially for complex tasks. Easterbrook (1959) demonstrated that increased anxiety affects learning and performance by decreasing the number of cues that a person attends to and uses. Fluharty, McHugh, McHugh, Willits, and Wood (1976) cited research which showed that for highly anxious subjects learning was slower and the retention of what was learned was less; judgments of time and distance were distorted; and efficiency in the performance of complex motor tasks was diminished. Mandler and Sarason (1952) described how anxiety lessens learning by producing responses not directly related to the task at hand, such as feelings of inadequacy, hopelessness, helplessness, anticipated negative outcomes, and attempts to leave the scene.

Fluharty et al. (1976) presented a number of practical suggestions for ways in which orientation and mobility specialists can help students cope with anxiety. These included:

- exposing the student to a variety of situations to lessen the impact of totally new situations after training;
- distracting the student from the most anxiety-producing aspects of the training while providing instruction and practice with skills;
- supplying modes of dependence during the training and gradually removing them as the student becomes accustomed to the threatening situation; and
- reassuring the student of the instructor's presence during especially threatening situations.

O'Donnell (1988) reviewed the literature related to anxiety and stress in mobility training and travel situations and advocated the use of modern stress reduction techniques such as muscle relaxation, meditation, and biofeedback by students receiving mobility training.

Cognitive and Existential Theories

Another set of personal factors that influence behavior have been studied by theorists identified with cognitive psychology and existential theory. According to these theories, human behavior is motivated by feelings and mental processes, chief among which are self-related thoughts such as the self-concept and self-esteem. Cognitive and existential psychologists focus on how sensory information is processed by the central nervous system, which includes organizing it, categorizing it, and comparing it to information that is contained in memory. This information then leads to certain expectations in the person that contribute to the process of making choices, developing plans, setting goals, and, in general, consciously directing behavior.

Tolman (1932) is credited with launching the cognitive approach to understanding behavior with his observation that behavior "reeks of purpose," that it is goal-directed and gives evidence of being based on cognition or knowledge. Through experience people learn what behaviors lead to the satisfaction of needs. When presented with the same or a similar need in the same or a similar environment, the person draws upon his knowledge to direct his purposeful behavior to satisfy the need.

Lewin (1936) added to the development of a cognitive view of motivation by defining the concept of "valence," as the amount of positive or negative value possessed by an object related to its ability to satisfy a particular need. Lewin introduced the notion that behavior was not influenced exclusively by the person's past history of learning and reinforcement, but was also affected by the current judgment about the ability of environmental objects to satisfy present needs. He viewed the person as an independent actor who could make new decisions that would lead to the satisfaction of needs in new ways.

Plans and Goals

Miller, Galanter, and Pribram (1960) illustrated the operation of cognitive mechanisms in directing behavior through their analysis of planning. When a person compares a current situation with her ideal or preferred notion of what that situation ought to be, she may find a mismatch between the two. This incongruity can motivate a plan of action to bring the current situation into conformity with the ideal. The action plan is implemented to correct the incongruity, and then the situation is retested until congruity is achieved.

Goal setting is a similar process of comparing a present state of affairs with an ideal state. Many studies have demonstrated the motivational value of explicit goal setting (Weinberg, Bruya, Longino, & Jackson, 1988). To enhance performance, goals need to be specific, difficult, and challenging (Locke, Shaw, Saari, & Latham, 1981). Goals that are vague and easy are not effective. Locke and Latham (1985) identified four reasons why goal setting improves performance.

1. Goals direct a performer's attention to the task at hand.
2. Goals mobilize effort. The harder the goal, the greater the effort expended.
3. Goals increase persistence since the performer is less likely to give up until the goal is reached.
4. Goals promote the development of new strategies for improving performance until the goal is reached.

Goals also add the helpful mechanism of feedback. Goal setting only works if there is timely feedback documenting progress in relation to the goal (Locke et al., 1981).

Vallerand, Deci, and Ryan (1985) clarified the impact of short-term versus long-term goal setting on the development of intrinsic motivation. They demonstrated that a performer's initial level of motivation toward a task is the key variable. When performers begin an activity with a relatively low intrinsic motivation, short-term goals enhance motivation by enhancing the performer's sense of competence that results from achieving the short-term goals. However, when performers begin an activity with relatively high intrinsic motivation for the task, short-term goals are considered intrusive, apparently because feedback about competence is not as important. If the person is highly motivated, long-term goals provide more of a challenge and are not regarded as controlling.

The O&M specialist should note the strong support for the impact of explicit planning and goal setting on the motivation of the student for the task at hand. This reinforces the value of having the student involved in the planning of the mobility program and the need for individualizing the development of each person's plan.

The Self-Concept

Central to most cognitive theories is the construct of the self-concept. The self-concept is defined as a collection of thoughts and feelings one has about oneself (Ross, 1992). While most theorists consider it to include both thoughts and feelings about the self, some (Tuttle, 1984) use the term "self-esteem" to refer specifically to the affective dimensions of the self-concept.

People acquire a concept of themselves through their interactions with their physical and social environments. One's self-concept influences how one acts and how one acts influences how one perceives oneself (Ross, 1992). Knowing something about a person's self-concept is helpful in understanding that person's behavior. The self is a cognitive structure that reflects a present state of being but is capable of imagining possible future states. In this regard, a discrepancy between a "present self" and an ideal "possible self" can operate much like a plan or a goal by initiating behavior designed to reduce the discrepancy between the present self and the ideal possible self (Markus & Nurius, 1986). A second way in which the self-concept can motivate behavior is in a person's effort to seek feedback that is consistent with his self-concept and avoid information that is contradictory (Markus, 1977).

Both of the ways in which self-concept discrepant information can motivate behavior can be of potential value to the O&M specialist. The person who is blind or visually impaired who is immobile and thinks of himself as necessarily dependent may have to be helped to envision a possible self that is more independent. But since a person's self-concept is resistant to change, this goal may not be as easily reached as the O&M specialist might expect. Embracing the goal of a more independent self may be a risky option for the visually impaired person, no matter how inconvenient his present dependency.

On the other hand, a person who is blind who thinks of himself as sufficiently independent may not be easily convinced that his level of independence is less than what he might accomplish with additional instruction. If his self-concept as a capable person is strongly reinforced by those around him who don't mind providing the assistance he might need, he may not be open to hearing the O&M specialist's observation that he really could be accomplishing much more for himself.

The Self-Concept and Blindness

Efforts to establish empirical evidence of a consistent impact of blindness on the self-concept of people who lose their vision or who grow up without vision when compared with sighted controls has produced contradictory results (Meighan, 1971; Cowen, Underberg, Verillo, & Benham, 1961; Jervis, 1959; Head, 1979; Coker, 1979). Such research inevitably encounters confounding variables related to the measuring instruments, the length of time that the blind subjects have experienced vision loss, the diverse coping mechanisms they have used, the ability of people to adjust their concepts of themselves to the conditions in which they find themselves, and the fact that there is no consistent psychology of blindness.

Tuttle (1984) has produced an extensive catalog of the many possible discrepancies that persons with visual disabilities might encounter between and among the ways they see themselves, and how they are seen by significant others. These discrepancies give rise to an equally wide range of possible resolutions that have been used by different individuals or by the same person in different situations. Tuttle (1987) summarized four problems facing the person who is blind that relate to the challenge of developing self-esteem: (1) in order to feel competent, the blind person must develop good coping skills and adaptive behaviors; (2) the blind person has to maintain a sense of high self-esteem in the face of predominantly negative reflections from the general public; (3) the blind person is especially challenged to maintain control over situations, perceive alternative courses of action, and make decisions or choices regarding events in his life; and (4) the blind person must maintain positive self-esteem even while still having to depend on others for the accomplishment of some daily tasks. From this analysis, it is possible to conclude that self-concept–related discrepancies are highly likely to occur and that the blind person's efforts to resolve such discrepancies are likely to have a major impact on his adjustment.

Self-Efficacy

The concept of self-efficacy, introduced by Bandura (1977) as one particular type of self-referencing activity, has generated a significant amount of empirical support for its effect on behavior and motivation (Bandura, 1986). The concept of self-efficacy is one of two elements in the emerging study of "expectancy motivation," which focuses on the effect that our expectations have on our motives and behavior. As Reeve (1992) described it, "If we expect our coping efforts to be futile, we tend to give up and behave listlessly. If we expect our coping efforts to provide us the means to control our environment, we tend to persist in coping and actively work to adjust to our surroundings." (p. 205)

Dodds (1989) first proposed the usefulness of the concept of self-efficacy for rehabilitation personnel struggling with unmotivated or under-motivated clients. Dodds noted the criticism of Smedslund (1978), that Bandura's theory of self-efficacy consists of self-evident truths which could be discovered by logic and common sense just as easily as by empirical research. Part of the appeal of the theory, however, is that while possessing a practical face validity, it lends itself to empirical validation in both a laboratory setting and the world of rehabilitation programs. It also provides support for the motivational success of the teaching methodology, with its emphasis on practical problem solving in real situations that has been used in O&M programs.

Efficacy in dealing with one's environment not only requires a knowledge of what to do and the skill to carry out the necessary deeds, but also a belief that one is up to the task. From watching professional athletes perform, the general public realizes that different people with very similar skills or the same person on different occasions may perform poorly, adequately, or extremely well. O&M specialists have also experienced this phenomenon in observing the performance of their students. Bandura (1977) has demonstrated that a person's perceived self-efficacy in relation to the task at hand plays a major role in these performance differences. Perceived self-efficacy is defined as "people's judgments of their capabilities to organize and execute courses of action required to attain designated types of performances" (Bandura, 1986, p. 391). Translating this into ordinary language, Smedslund (1978) described perceived self-efficacy as a person's belief in what he can do and how strongly he believes it. A person's beliefs in what he can do determine whether he will try to do it, how hard he will try, and how long he will keep trying even though obstacles and unpleasant experiences are encountered.

According to Bandura (1986), perceived self-efficacy develops from one or more of four principal sources: (1) performance accomplishments, (2) vicarious experiences, (3) verbal persuasion, and (4) monitoring of one's own physiological states.

Performance Accomplishments. The most significant of the four sources of self-efficacy is the direct personal experience of successfully performing the task at hand. Nothing is more effective in convincing a person that he is up to handling a challenge than past success at doing so, nor is there anything more motivating for the future. Successes raise efficacy judgments and repeated failures lower them, especially if the failures occur early in the course of events and do not reflect lack of effort or adverse external circumstances.

The extent to which people change their perceived self-efficacy through performance experiences will depend upon the difficulty of the task, the amount of effort they expend, the amount of external aid they receive, the circumstances under which they perform, and the temporal pattern of their successes and failures (Bandura, 1986). This supports the importance attached by O&M specialists to the sequence of lessons and challenges provided to their students if success at those lessons is to have a positive impact on a student's perceived self-efficacy to handle future mobility tasks. If the task is too easy or too difficult, or if the student receives too much help or too little, success at handling the task will not have the same effect on his perceived self-efficacy and therefore on his motivation and self-confidence.

Vicarious Experience. A second source of perceived self-efficacy is the observation of others performing the same behavior, or what Bandura calls vicarious experiences. Seeing other people adequately perform a behavior encourages the observer to feel that he can too. Vicarious experience also works the other way: seeing someone being unable to perform can decrease an observer's belief in his own ability. Bandura's studies (1986) indicate that the impact of the vicarious experience is stronger if the observer considers the actor to be similar to himself. Also, the less experienced the observer is in relation to the task, the more powerful the impact of the vicarious experience. In other words, vicarious experience can have a powerful impact on efficacy expectations for inexperienced observers watching others whom they perceive to be similar to themselves. Vicarious experience, on the other hand, is less powerful for experienced observers who are watching others dissimilar to themselves.

The mobility specialist can see in these findings confirmation for the value of having beginning mobility students associate with other students who are also beginning or slightly ahead of them in their training. Frequently, the small accomplishments of similar beginning students can have a more motivating impact on other students than the smooth and easy skill of the experienced staff member who is blind, who may appear dissimilar to the students.

Verbal Persuasion. A third source for increasing a person's perceived self-efficacy is verbal encouragement from others. This is a widely used technique by coaches, teachers, parents, employers, and friends. By itself or when it is unrealistic, this approach is of limited value in producing lasting changes in a person's perceived self-efficacy. When the encouragement is realistically based, however, it can have the effect of encouraging the person to mobilize greater sustained effort to succeed. On the other hand, the raising of unrealistic beliefs of personal competence invites failure that will discredit the persuaders and undermine the recipient's perceived self-efficacy.

In the mobility training model, the instructor frequently encourages the student and helps him pull together the courage to try his skill in new situations or with less supervision. The quality of the relationship between the instructor and the student will have an impact on the instructor's effectiveness in persuading the student to take the next steps. A relationship that is characterized by genuine caring and accurate, concrete feedback is more likely to be effective in its impact.

Monitoring Physiological Feedback. Most people are aware of and influenced by their state of arousal as they approach new or threatening tasks. They are sensitive to the arousal signals from the autonomic nervous system, which include a more rapid heart rate, changes in breathing, sweating, muscle tension, and any number of idiosyncratic mannerisms. When a person approaches a task for which he does not have a sense of efficacy, he is not surprised to experience many of these symptoms. One's awareness of these symptoms as he approaches a task may alert him to his lessened sense of efficacy for that task. On the other hand, Bandura and Adams (1977) demonstrated that treatments which eliminate emotional arousal in response to subjective threats can heighten a person's sense of self-efficacy in approaching the threatening task and lead to corresponding improved performance.

The O&M specialist frequently uses this same insight by attending to behavioral manifestations of nervousness or fear in students who are approaching a new or difficult part of the training. The signal may be a slower walking pace, a tightened grip on the instructor's arm, a clenched fist, or the appearance of a rocking mannerism or noticeable tremors. When these signals appear, the O&M specialist may choose to restructure a lesson, alter the level of difficulty, or make some other adjustment that keeps the level of challenge appropriate without overwhelming the individual. According to Bandura's theory, the more these arousal symptoms are managed and kept in check, the more likely it is that the student will perceive a sense of self-efficacy for the task at hand.

Self-Efficacy and Adjustment to Blindness

Dodds et al., (1994) provided support for the importance of the concept of perceived self-efficacy along with the concept of internal self-worth in understanding adjustment to the loss of sight. They analyzed responses to the Nottingham Adjustment Scale from clients of the Royal National Institute for the Blind. Using structural modeling techniques, the researchers studied the relationships between the cognitive and emotional factors represented by the scale items and developed a model of the relationship between the cognitive and emotional factors. This model identifies two factors, which are not assessed directly by the scale, but appear as latent factors resulting from the study of intercorrelations. These factors, "self as agent" and "internal self worth," seem to explain the high interrelationships among factors assessed by the scale (see Figure 6.2).

Based upon this research, Dodds et al. offered suggestions for how the relationships between these factors might influence rehabilitation practice. For example, they found that acceptance of vision loss is strongly related to the factor "self as agent" but only weakly to "internal self worth." From this they concluded that counseling may not directly lead to measurable improvements in self-worth, but it may lead to improved motivation for the individual to act in ways that will bring about successful outcomes. It is the experience of the successful outcomes that leads to a sense of improved self-worth. This theory is similar to Bandura's (1977) notion that verbal persuasion may only serve to encourage attempts at the desired behavior, but it is the experience of the successful behavior itself that has the greatest impact on motivation and future behavior.

Dodds et al. (1994) also suggest that when counseling is a part of rehabilitation services, there should not be a presumption that it must focus on grief work or acceptance of blindness. Although there may be some students who need this kind of support, many are ready to go directly into skill training. The data support the notion that when counseling is provided, it might be more effective to draw upon some of the cognitive approaches that focus on helping the student see that success in rehabilitation is due to his own efforts and thereby reinforce the student's perception of his own self-efficacy in relation to the tasks of rehabilitation. Bandura, Reese, and Adams (1982) pointed out that similar performance successes had variable effects on the perceived self-efficacy that performers took away from their experiences. As a result, they concluded that how people understand their performance successes rather than just the successes themselves was an important determiner of cognitive and behavioral changes. This supports the recommendation that counseling be used to reinforce the student's perception that it was his own effort and skill that resulted in the successes.

Outcome Expectations

The second major element of "expectancy motivation" is outcome expectations. While efficacy expectations involve a person's judgment of how well she can perform a particular behavior, outcome expectations refer to the person's assessment of how likely a particular behavior is to produce a particular outcome. Both elements are important to understanding motivation. People are more likely to pursue goals which, in their view, they can accomplish and, once accomplished, have a high probability of leading to a desired outcome.

Reeve (1992) identified four determinants of the strength of outcome expectancies: (1) outcome feedback; (2) task difficulty; (3) social comparison information; and (4) personality differences.

Outcome Feedback. Past experience of success or failure following the performance of a particular behavior has the most direct impact on the acquisition or change of an outcome expectancy.

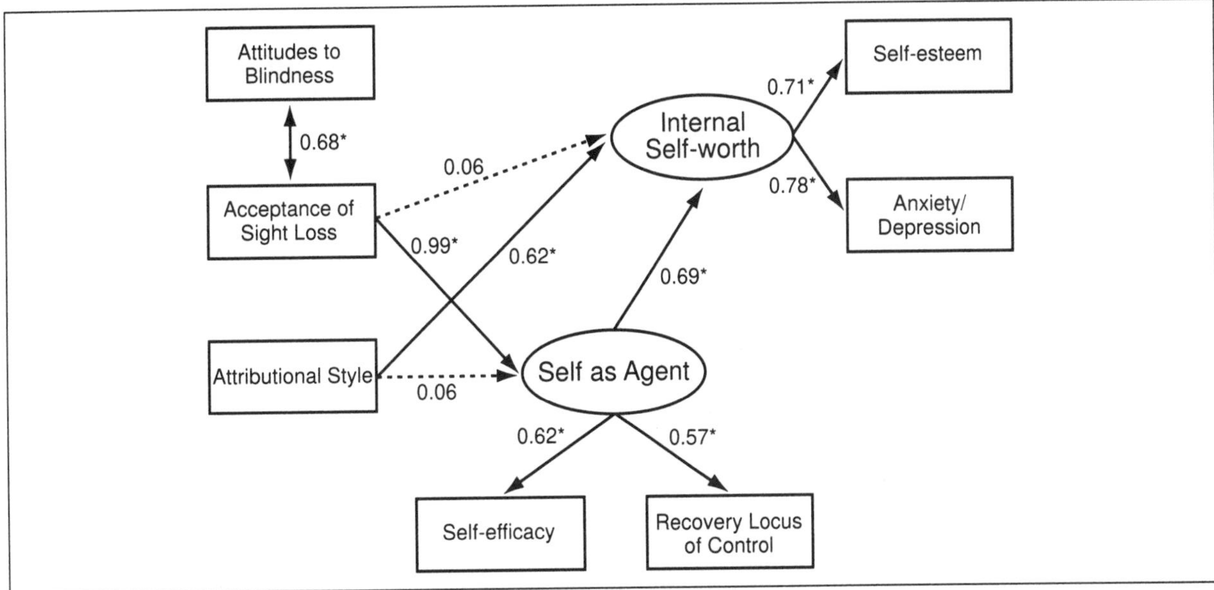

Figure 6.2. LISREL (Linear Structural Relations) structural model with path coefficients (* = $p < 0.05$).

Feather (1966) illustrated this effect by having subjects work on a series of 15 anagrams. For one group, the first five were very difficult, leading to initial failure, and for the other group they were easy, leading to initial success. For the remainder of the study, all of the subjects worked on the same ten puzzles, recording their expectations of success or failure. Data demonstrated that the subjects' expectations were significantly affected by the experience of initial success or failure. Those who were initially successful expected to do well and those who initially failed expected to do poorly even though their objective performance on the remaining anagrams was about equal. This concept suggests that it is important for mobility students to experience successful outcomes in their early learning and travel opportunities, which sets a tone for what follows.

Task Difficulty. Outcome expectations are also determined by perceptions of task difficulty. Each task has specific salient characteristics that influence the judgment of difficulty. Difficult tasks give rise to low expectancies of success and easy tasks generate high expectancies. It helps to have complex tasks understood in terms of manageable subcomponents that appear doable to the mobility student.

Social Comparison Information. Outcome expectancies are also affected by the observation of which outcomes others have attained on the task under consideration. This can be a limiting factor for individuals considering mobility training because of the likelihood that they have no comparison group from which to draw expectancies. In this case, the opportunity to interact with others who have had successful experiences with rehabilitation and specifically mobility training may be an essential part of developing appropriate outcome expectancies.

Personality Differences. Certain personal traits or dispositions can have a significant influence on an individual's outcome expectancies. Wiener (1974) has shown that persons high in need achievement tend to overestimate their chances for success and make overly optimistic outcome expectancies. On the other hand, low need-achievers tend to be pessimistic in their outcome expectations. McFarlin and Blascovich (1981) related outcome expectancies to level of self-esteem. Individuals with high self-esteem overestimated their outcome expectations while those with low self-esteem underestimated.

Another characteristic identified as having an impact on outcome expectancies is learned helplessness. It is defined as a psychological state which results when an individual perceives that events in his environment are uncontrollable (Seligman, 1975). The effects of learned helplessness were described by Alloy and Seligman (1979) as leading to three kinds of functional deficits. Motivational deficits result in the person showing an unwillingness to try new behaviors to solve problems or achieve certain outcomes. Cognitive deficits result in a person's having a difficult time learning that a response can have an impact on outcomes in the future. Affective deficits lead to depressive reactions when it becomes clear that there is nothing that the person can do to control or predict his situation.

Still another personality characteristic that affects outcome expectancies has to do with attributional style. Rotter (1966) identified the existence of fairly stable characteristic ways in which people view the source of the outcomes they experience. He called this characteristic the "locus of control" and developed a method of measuring it. According to Rotter, a person with a predominantly internal locus of control views reinforcements or punishments as results from her own efforts. On the other hand, a person with a predominantly external locus of control considers that her reinforcements and punishments are due to outside forces such as luck, chance, or fate, over which she has no control. Regardless of an objective analysis of the actual source of an outcome, it is the person's subjective locus of control that affects how she behaves.

People with an internal locus of control, when compared to externals, tend to be higher in information seeking and achievement, are more cooperative, participate in more health-promoting behaviors, and experience better psychological adjustment (Phares, 1976). In spite of these advantages for internals, there are some situations in which an external orientation can be more adaptive. Felton and Kahana (1974) demonstrated that among elderly persons in an institution, persons characterized by an external locus of control seemed to experience better adjustment and more feelings of satisfaction than did those who had an internal locus of control. Wolk and Kurtz (1975) found that the reverse was true among a group of noninstitutionalized elderly people. In that group, internal locus of control was more likely to be associated with better adjustment and satisfaction.

Research on the effects of locus of control on the behavior of people entering rehabilitation settings (MacDonald & Hall, 1971) suggests that an internally controlled person may be better motivated through an appeal to his desire for competence, while an external may be motivated more by praise from people in authority or peer support. Diamond, Weiss, and Grynbaum (1968) showed that resigned attitudes concerning a disability and excessive guilt feelings were associated with individuals who could not be influenced to participate in a rehabilitation program. Hyman (1972) found that attributing illness to supernatural causes was one of several factors that impaired the motivation of persons entering a stroke rehabilitation program.

Summary of Cognitive Theories

While the O&M specialist cannot discount the influences of the unconscious determinants of behavior identified by psychoanalytic theorists nor the impact of drives and needs identified by dispositional psychologists, the concepts and theories of cognitive psychologists have the greatest relevance for day-to-day practice. Cognitive theories developed for understanding and changing behavior in counseling settings also lend themselves to an understanding of the motivations and behaviors that are characteristic of O&M instruction.

ENVIRONMENTAL FACTORS

A thorough understanding, explanation, and prediction of human behavior require a review of the effect of environmental factors on the behavior of people with visual disabilities. Because we are concerned in this chapter with psychological and social factors that affect O&M, the focus will be on the social environment through which the traveler passes and the effects of that environment on mobility behavior.

Behavior Theory

Some of the social learning theories discussed earlier, including Bandura's social cognitive theory, reflect a basic behavioral strategy. They were included in the discussion of personal factors because they integrate cognitive and other personal constructs with behaviorism within their theories of personality. However, behavior theory, as reflected in the work of Skinner (1974), holds that behavior is primarily determined by external environmental influences, particularly by the consequences of one's actions as one operates on the environment. He challenged the notion that behavior is influenced by internal factors such as unconscious impulses, traits, and concepts of the self. Skinner (1953) did not go so far as to claim that inner states do not exist—he felt that they are not relevant to the study of behavior. The psychosocial variables that are the focus of this chapter (i.e., self-concept, anxiety, motivation, etc.) are outside of the domain of the operant approach. Many of the concepts and procedures developed by Skinner and other behaviorists have been integrated into a wide variety of educational programming, including the teaching of O&M. These concepts are fully explained in this volume (Chapter 11) and will not be repeated here.

An O&M specialist using a behavioral approach to address a student's lack of willingness to engage in mobility training would do a thorough analysis of the environmental factors which are affecting the student in that situation in an attempt to determine which reinforcers are supporting the student's avoidance of the training situation. Similarly, she would assess which reinforcers are available in that environment that could be manipulated to bring about a behavioral change. Secondary reinforcers might have to be used at first, later replaced by naturally occurring reinforcers in order to sustain the travel behavior without the intervention of the instructor.

The eclectic nature of most O&M specialists very rarely results in the use of a pure behavioral approach. The most likely occasion for such an approach may be in the teaching of individuals with severe and profound developmental disabilities. It is more common that formal behavioral techniques are used to supplement a more cognitively oriented approach. For example, the systematic use of reinforcers and rewards in a token economy is sometimes used to supplement other kinds of motivational approaches for a variety of clients, especially children. The concepts of shaping and fading might be used in the development of cane techniques or the elimination of mannerisms that interfere with the acceptance of the student in public situations.

An example of the use of a behavioral approach in relation to orientation and mobility is the use of systematic desensitization techniques (Wolpe & Lazarus, 1966) to help individuals with extreme anxiety or fear reactions related to mobility situations. This is done not by the mobility instructor, but by appropriately trained psychologists. Thyer and Stocks (1986) present a case study in which a therapist used "real-life exposure therapy" to help a woman who was blind overcome her phobia of elevators.

The Social Environment and Attitudes toward Blindness

The most salient features of the environments in which people with visual disabilities must learn to function are the attitudes of people toward blindness and people who are blind. These attitudes are responsible for the feedback that the blind person receives and uses in the development and refinement of his self-concept and perceptions of self-efficacy. They influence his judgments of the attainability of desired outcomes, and affect the quality and the amount of help offered as he travels. Their effect is pervasive in the blind person's life, and the power of their influence should not be underestimated.

Monbeck (1973) summarized the long history of attitudes toward blindness and toward people who are blind as reflected in the literature of centuries. Most of the reactions and attitudes have been negative or demeaning. Blindness elicits pity, sympathy, fear, and avoidance responses from people. Some project misery and unhappiness on blind people while others feel that blind people are helpless. There are a few examples in the literature of positive attitudes toward blindness. These include the association of special abilities with visual impairment, and the desire to help blind people and to be associated with them. Tuttle (1984) generated a similar list of attitudes containing mostly negative reactions but with some positive biases as well.

Empirical efforts to discover how people regard blindness have been confounded by a variety of measuring instruments, different eliciting stimuli, and confusion regarding whether the research was measuring attitudes toward blindness or toward people who are blind (Lukoff, 1972). Many of the confusing and discrepant findings might also be explained by the fact that attitudes toward blindness are not unidimensional, as some measuring instruments suggest, but multidimensional.

Whiteman and Lukoff (1965) identified five factors or dimensions of attitudes toward blindness:

1. Personal attributes, which reflect a negative view of the emotional life and general competence of people who are blind
2. Social attributes, which reflect a readiness for interactions with people who are blind and a positive view of the social competence of blind people
3. Evaluation of blindness—the degree to which blindness is perceived as threatening and uniquely frustrating to one's self and others
4. Nonprotectiveness, reflecting a lack of protectiveness and sympathy
5. Interpersonal acceptance, reflecting an emotional acceptance of people who are blind in interpersonal situations

Assuming the accuracy of Whiteman and Lukoff's five identified characteristics of people that influence their interactions with people who are blind, four of which appear to be negative, it is easy to see how such attitudes can create a barrier to normal interactions and have a negative impact on the blind person's confidence in himself. The strained interactions are also disrupted by the blind person's lack of eye contact, atypical gestures and facial expressions, and inability to pick up on visual conversational cues used by the sighted person (Monbeck, 1973). The blind traveler, as perceived by the general public, may be regarded as incompetent and unable to function on his own, or he may be regarded as exceptionally talented even though, in his own mind, he is performing routinely. He may be ignored or helped in an oversolicitous manner. One thing is certain, the blind traveler is a strong stimulus to other people in the situation and he, in turn, has to be ready and able to respond to a wide variety of reactions.

Family Interactions

Many of the attitudes toward blindness and people who are blind identified in the previous section as being characteristic of the general public are also found among the families of people with visual disabilities. When the family's attitudes are negative and rejecting, the impact on the blind person can be especially devastating. Conversely, when they are positive and accepting, the blind person can be helped tremendously. Large (1982) documented the powerful influence of family members on blind individuals. Tuttle (1986) reviewed the reactions of families to the visual disability of their members as found in biographies and autobiographies of people with visual disabilities.

Even more important than the impact of family attitudes is the effect of the behaviors of family members on the education and rehabilitation process. Neff (1979) and McPhee and Magleby (1960) demonstrated a positive correlation between success in rehabilitation and stable family relationships. On the other hand, Olshansky and Beach (1975) and Wardlow (1974) indicated an association between lack of success in rehabilitation and poor or disrupted family relationships.

The family of the person with a visual disability is a salient feature of the environment in which mobility training and independent travel occur, as is the culture that family developed within (see Chapter 12 and Chapter 13). If the family understands the practical aspects of travel without vision and if they are confident in the student's ability to handle it, they can be a strong positive force in support of the process. Moore (1984) concluded that the family serves as a major source of interpersonal influences that affect what blindness means to the person who is blind and what he does with it. For this reason, time spent informing the family and encouraging their observation of mobility lessons is a good investment. On the other hand, a family that manifests a lot of anxiety and skepticism about the student's skill can become a formidable barrier.

Klausner (1969) and Fordyce (1971) highlighted the powerful dynamics which occur in some families that seem to be held together by the need for family members to care for one "sick" or "dependent" member. When it begins to appear that the dependent member may no longer need the other members of the family to fill their care-giving roles, the family feels threatened and behaviors may occur that are designed to consciously or unconsciously sabotage the rehabilitation or education process. In such a situation, it may be the introduction of mobility training with its strong emphasis on independence that activates a family crisis. In cases where these dynamics are especially strong or not conscious, formal counseling, provided by a professionally trained counselor, may be needed to address them. In less intense situations, empathetic listening and feedback from the O&M specialist and time to get used to the changing dynamics may be all that is necessary to help the family past this change.

Many of the psychosocial dynamics that affect the student learning mobility without vision may also affect the family. One of these is the impact of the social environment. When the student is learning to travel while attending a rehabilitation center or a residential school at some distance from her home, the family may be quite supportive of the process. However, when the student is ready to use these skills in her home community, either independently or as the training is brought to her home neighborhood, the family's support may be replaced by active resistance. When this occurs, it is sometimes occasioned by the embarrassment that family members anticipate as the member who is blind is seen traveling with a cane in the neighborhood (Seybold, 1993). In another case, the family was not open in talking to neighbors about the seriousness of the blind member's disability and they minimized the problem in an effort to protect their own self-esteem. The possibility of the family member advertising her disability by traveling through the neighborhood with a long cane set off a credibility crisis.

Some family members may also experience fear or anxiety as they think about the person who is blind traveling with a cane through the community. When such a reaction is noted in a student, a great deal of care is taken to provide an appropriate sequence of lessons in a supportive atmosphere in order to help the student learn to overcome the fear or cope with the anxiety. A similar carefully planned sequence of exposures may be needed for family members. They may need opportunities to see the blind student travel safely first in less threatening areas before they are ready to think of her traveling independently in their own neighborhood with its particular level of difficulty.

Observing mobility lessons provides family members with good opportunities to ask the O&M specialist about concerns that they have. Sometimes these concerns are a generalized anxiety that is not well formulated in their minds, but the opportunity to observe lessons in real travel environments makes the threats, as well as the solutions, more concrete.

Dependence vs. Independence

In the previous discussion of the environment created by the families of visually impaired travelers, a central concept was the issue of dependency. While the degree of dependence or independence felt by the student is not an environmental factor, to a large extent it results from and is reinforced by the environment created by the family or those close to the student. It also serves to structure that social environment.

Bandura and Walters (1963) defined dependency as a class of behaviors that are capable of eliciting positive attending and ministering responses from others. A person's characteristic level of independence or dependence is not innate, but is a learned response that develops from an individual's past experiences, especially with significant others in his environment.

Vision loss, as well as other disabilities, are likely to cause at least temporary disturbances in the individual's balance between independence and dependence. In some, the problems that arise are quite natural and temporary. In others, they may be pathological and enduring. Until the person learns techniques for functioning without vision, he will have to depend to a greater degree on others to assist him in performing many tasks of daily living and especially for help in travel. This can lead to a serious problem if an individual has had dependency conflicts throughout his life. The loss of vision can be the excuse a person uses to move into a socially acceptable dependent role that he previously was unable to assume. Other individuals may be threatened by even the necessary and natural short-term dependency that accompanies vision loss. These persons' responses may be to strongly resist any assistance and insist that they need neither help nor any rehabilitation service.

While the problem of finding an acceptable balance is an issue faced by everyone, it is more serious for the person with a disability. He finds himself in a society that generally encourages independence, but discourages it in subtle ways for people with disabilities. He may find himself caught between his family, which encourages and rewards dependence, and his own need for more freedom. Or his family and friends may be feeling burdened by his dependence, while the individual himself is reluctant to learn to function on his own.

For the person who initially responds to his dependency with comfortable acceptance, the movement toward greater independence may begin with the experience of "dependency dissatisfaction" (Havens, 1967). This occurs as the person discovers that depending on others leads to outcomes that are dissatisfying. In the area of mobility, the dependent person may find that he has to adjust his schedule for coming and going to meet the schedule of the person or persons on whom he depends for a ride. Or the person who is supposed to provide a ride forgets and leaves the person who is blind stranded or late for a critical appointment. A sufficient number of such experiences may eventually convince the person that he should learn to function on his own. Corn and Sacks (1994) documented the lifestyle changes that result when people with visual disabilities must depend on other people for transportation and recommended a number of strategies that can be used to lessen some of the frustrations that result from not driving.

A standard of absolute independence for a visually impaired traveler is neither feasible nor desirable. Inevitably, he will encounter situations in which he will have to obtain assistance. When this happens, the student may have to learn that the judicious use of help is not a threat to his independence.

O&M BEHAVIORS

Using Bandura's (1986) three-sided interactive model of reciprocal determinism, this chapter has reviewed information about personal factors and environmental factors that might influence the psychological and social aspects of the O&M behavior of people who are blind. Now it is time to look at the impact that mobility behavior, as well as the learning and teaching of mobility, have on personal and environmental factors.

As a person with a visual disability moves through the environment, there are multiple effects on the person as well as on the environment, especially the social environment. These effects can be positive or negative and can have an impact on the person's willingness or ability to travel in that environment. According to Stotland and Canon (1972), a person's sense of competence or self-esteem can be affected by (1) his perception of the effectiveness of his own actions, (2) his perceived freedom to select from a number of possible actions, (3) his sense of similarity with others, and (4) the communications he receives about his competence. When the person with a visual disability has the option of traveling independently to accomplish his goals, this can contribute to his sense of competence and self-esteem.

Baker (1973) extended this effect to the attitudes and behaviors of other people. Using the image of a circular process (Figure 6.3), Baker proposed that the behavior of the person who is blind, who in this case is moving independently and successfully through the environment, has an impact on the attitudes of others who observe his behavior. This impact is usually a positive one of increased respect for the blind person and a greater likelihood of the observer seeing the blind person as being more like himself. This leads to a change in attitude that usually also leads to a change in behavior toward the blind person. When the sighted observer reacts to the blind person with more respect and treats him more like a peer, this has a positive impact on the self-esteem and sense of self-efficacy of the blind person.

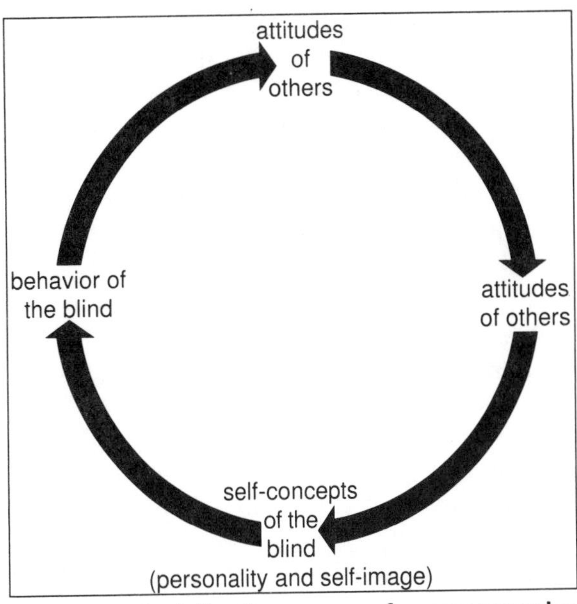

Figure 6.3. Socialization process for persons who are blind.

Interactions with the Public

Many visually impaired people are stigmatized when they travel in public. In this context, "stigma" does not refer to its primary meaning as a "mark of infamy," but rather to a more general sense of a label or behavior that indicates some deviation from a norm or standard. Some persons are stigmatized by their appearance, perhaps resulting from the eye condition that led to the vision loss. Others may be stigmatized by the equipment they use or the behaviors they adopt to cope with the vision loss. Some persons with low vision only become stigmatized when they are forced to solicit assistance in a situation where a person with normal vision would be able to function independently (Wainapel, 1989; Emerson, 1981).

Goffman (1963) and Friedson (1965) theorized about the effects of stigma on human interactions. In their theories, it is clear that the problem does not reside in the person who possesses the stigma nor in the persons who react to the stigma, but in the interaction between these two sets of actors.

People who are stigmatized elicit atypical, although often predictable, reactions and behaviors from the general public. These reactions can impact the self-concept of the person with the disability as well as his behavior. Wright (1960) pointed out that the reactions that an impaired person has to an exchange with members of the public can go a long way toward making the exchange worse, controlling it, or even turning it into a positive experience and changing the attitude and future behavior of both parties.

The treatment of persons with disabilities has been documented in a number of studies. Farina, Holland, and Ring (1966) demonstrated how the perception of a person as mentally ill can influence the behavior and attitudes of others. When a coworker was viewed as mentally ill, subjects preferred to work alone rather then with him and blame him for experimentally manipulated inadequacies in the joint performance. Kleck, Ono, and Hastorf (1966) discovered that subjects interacting with a stimulus person who had a physical disability (1) tended to demonstrate less variability in their behavior than did subjects interacting with a physically normal person; (2) tended to terminate the interaction sooner; (3) expressed opinions that were less representative of their actual beliefs than those expressed by subjects in the nondisabled group.

Three concepts are useful in understanding these interactions: A *new psychological situation* (Lewin, 1936; Barker, Wright, Meyerson, & Gonick, 1953) is one in which the location of positive goals and the path by which they can be reached are not clearly perceived by the person. Entering a new psychological situation both attracts and repels a person, because of the uncertain location of the positive goals. A person will engage in trial and error behavior and will experience frustration as a result of the searching. The person will feel conflict as he simultaneously tries to reach the goal of the new situation and then withdraw to the safety of the old.

Visually impaired persons and people with other visible disabilities more frequently experience new psychological situations than do persons without disabilities (Barker et al., 1953). This is often due to the person lacking a necessary tool for dealing with the situation, usually a tool that is closely related to the disability. Without vision as a tool, which people use to learn about and adjust to changes in the environment, the person enters more situations in which he may not have information about changes that have taken place.

Other situations are "new" for the person with a disability as a result of the stimulus value that the disability represents for others in the situation. According to Meyerson, "Disability has many meanings to others. The disabled person often does not know when he enters a social situation whether he will be an object of curiosity or be pitied, sympathized with, helped, patronized, exhibited, praised for his spunk, avoided, or actively rejected" (Meyerson, 1963, p. 41). What is reasonably certain is that the disabled person will elicit a strong reaction of some sort. What is uncertain is the direction and type of reaction to expect.

The concept of *overlapping roles* arises from the realization that each person simultaneously belongs to many different groups and must play multiple roles (Meyerson, 1963). There are four types of overlaping roles. First, many overlapping roles are compatible and can be handled simultaneously. Second, others may be interfering and can be resolved simply by choosing one or the other. Third, some overlapping roles are antagonistic, and responding to one automatically rules out the other. Frequently persons who are visually impaired have to choose between the antagonistic roles of either a dependent person who relies on help or an independent person who functions without help. Sometimes it is difficult to get just a little help without being compelled to take more than is actually needed.

A fourth type of overlapping role is that of excluding roles. The disabled person finds himself torn between the roles of the disabled person and a physically normal person. Stonequist (1937) was one of the first to identify this situation, which he described as the condition of the "marginal man." This referred to an individual whose salient identity has elements that burden him or put him at a disadvantage. Consequently, this marginal individual may have ambivalent feelings about his identity, and he may wish to reject it. If a person acts appropriately for a disabled person in a situation—for example, using a cane for mobility—he will automatically surrender the possibility of being considered a nondisabled person. This conflict frequently surfaces in social situations where the rewards for being a "normal" person are greatest and the negative effects for deviating from the norm are most potent.

The struggle to manage this conflict can put the person with a disability under considerable strain and lead to strong resistance to being identified as a disabled person in public, particularly through the advertisement of a long cane (Wainapel, 1989). The pressures associated with trying to resolve the conflict of excluding roles may lead to the phenomenon of "passing."

Passing has been defined by Goffman (1963) as behavior by a person designed to conceal a salient aspect of her identity. This may be particularly appealing for persons with low vision who are able to frequently conceal the fact of their vision loss. According to Goffman, passing may begin when a person discovers that she has passed accidentally, realizing that others have treated her as not having a disability that she actually possesses. She may progress through the stages of passing for the "fun of it," passing on vacations, passing in situations involving people with whom she frequently interacts, and finally passing completely and being able to entirely conceal the disability portion of her identity. Goffman also discusses some of the strains associated with passing. He notes the anxiety associated with always having to be alert to all of the details of a situation that might be responsible for unveiling the hidden aspect of the disabled person's identity. There is also the strain associated with explaining the ruse when the hidden aspect of her identity comes to be revealed one way or another.

For many persons with low vision, their disability may not be obvious. It becomes apparent in some situations and not in others. This variability leaves them with decisions to make concerning how they present themselves. Freeman, Goetz, Richards, and Groenveld (1991) documented the fact that many of the people with low vision interviewed in their long-term follow-up study rarely or never used a cane because of their wish to avoid the stigma of being identified as blind. This same study also documented that 40 percent of the responders reported having been hit by a vehicle on at least one occasion.

If persons with low vision choose to conceal the disability components of their identities, they are spared some of the difficulties in those situations in which their vision loss does not matter. However, when they encounter situations where they cannot function visually, their inability to function or their need for assistance may then stigmatize them and cause interaction problems.

For persons who choose the first alternative—identifying themselves as being visually impaired in mobility situations—it is frequently recommended that this can be most effectively accomplished through the use of, or merely carrying, a long cane, usually of the collapsible variety. This results in these persons being identified as visually impaired more than is necessary, but when they do need assistance, their reasons for asking are obvious to others and the situation is made more comfortable for themselves. For those who choose to remain unidentified, they frequently can be assisted in developing ways to approach others in situations where help is needed. These strategies, such as preceding a request for information with acknowledgment of the vision loss, usually require some revelation that a disability is present, but this can be done in a more focused and less public way than by carrying a cane. Persons choosing either alternative might benefit from the opportunity to role-play and rehearse responses for those situations when the alternative aspect of their identity is discovered in a social situation.

It is not the role of the O&M specialist to decide for the person who has low vision how she wants to present herself. This can only be decided by the person herself. The O&M specialist has the responsibility to help the person consider all of the factors associated with one approach or the other in travel situations; these include both psychosocial and safety factors. Once the person has made a decision or is in the process of making a decision, the O&M specialist should expose the person to the full range of possible situations she will encounter. He should structure practice opportunities during which the student can try out a variety of solutions to the safety, psychosocial, and orientation problems that might arise.

For many people with visual disabilities, mobility training situations might be the first that bring to light the problems associated with interacting with other people. A child who is congenitally blind may have been protected from these encounters by parents and family members. The child's social experiences may have been entirely with close friends and neighbors who are "in the know" about the disability. The adventitiously blind person may also have had family members "running interference" in social situations since the disability occurred, preventing others from approaching and offering assistance or expressing curiosity. However, mobility training will require that the visually impaired person move through environments on his own and be exposed to the unpredictability of these interactions with the public. The O&M specialist has to be sensitive to how the student is handling the anxieties and frustrations that often accompany these encounters. If necessary, the sequence of lessons may have to be modified to provide a gradient of more demanding involvement with other people for students who need time to develop these skills.

Offers of Help

One particular type of interaction with the public are offers of help. There are three types of offers: those that are unsolicited and unnecessary, those that are unsolicited and necessary, and those that are solicited. Each of these types may have a different effect on the student, depending on how he is coping with his identity as a person with a disability.

The person who is feeling the conflict of excluding overlapping roles is likely to be further frustrated by offers of help, whether needed or not, and whether accepted or not. Such a person is also less likely to solicit assistance when it is needed, which may further aggravate a frustrating situation. The person who reacts to new psychological situations with a great amount of anxiety or emotion may be more upset by offers of help and less likely to solicit assistance when necessary because of the uncertainty of how people are going to respond.

Both of these types of persons may be helped through role-playing a variety of situations that occur during travel and rehearsing different responses to each. Being prepared and having confidence in the effectiveness of certain responses will help to reduce the newness of new psychological situations and the anxiety associated with them. For the person struggling with excluding overlapping roles, having effective responses to use in interactions with the public may help the person maintain her self-esteem as a disabled person, and reduce the conflicts associated with the struggle to function as a nondisabled person in situations where the disability excludes normal functioning.

Certain responses to unnecessary and unwanted offers of help are more effective than others in getting rid of it. An effective response for one student may be ineffective for another. The role of the O&M specialist is to discuss the variety of responses that are possible and help the person who is visually impaired select those that she would prefer to use in future situations.

Extracting necessary assistance from sighted pedestrians once a contact has been made is a skill. Since this is usually a new situation for the sighted person, he may not know what information is useful, or because of his own anxiety, he may make rather basic errors. The person who is visually impaired must learn how to take charge of the interaction to assure that she gets the information she needs. She must learn how to ask specific, open-ended questions that will elicit responses from the helper, other than "yes" or "no." She must be able to break down requests for information into manageable units that the helper can provide in a way which will result in the visually impaired person getting thorough and accurate information. This structuring of the interaction by the visually impaired person will take some of the newness and uncertainty out of it for both persons, which will result in less anxiety and frustration for both.

Other types of interactions may also cause problems. People may approach the person who is visually impaired with expressions of sympathy or inappropriate curiosity. This can produce anxiety and frustration if the visually impaired person is unprepared. The O&M specialist should help the student cope with the emotions that such remarks may generate and assist the student through discussion and perhaps role-play. If a student can understand these remarks in the context of how disabilities are perceived and misunderstood by the general public, she can better prevent the negative impact of these experiences on her self-esteem and on her attitude and willingness to travel through the community.

While interactions with the public can be negative and can present challenges to the visually impaired traveler, the student can do a lot to structure and better manage them. In addition, the successful handling of these interactions can go a long way toward reinforcing the sense of self-efficacy that comes with success in mobility and in maintaining high motivation for further independent travel.

Psychosocial Elements of the Training Situation

Two elements of the traditional approach to the teaching of O&M have a significant impact on the psychological and social factors that affect independent mobility with a visual disability. These elements are (1) the use of a logical and client-sensitive learning sequence that features a pattern of success experiences and increased problem-solving by the student and (2) the development of an effective helping relationship between the student and the instructor.

These elements trace their origins to the earliest days of mobility training at Valley Forge and Hines (Apple, 1962; Williams, 1965). They have been incorporated in university training programs that require O&M specialists to learn how to travel while blindfolded. Some of these elements, which are also included in Mettler's (1995) "new paradigm," have been used by O&M specialists since the early days of the Hines program (Malamazian, 1970; Welsh, 1972) to develop what they called "self-confidence," before Bandura (1977) empirically verified the importance of the closely related concept of self-efficacy.

The Learning Sequence

Most O&M training services are built around an ideal structure of lessons, which serves as a basic curriculum for the instruction. This concept is traceable to the Valley Forge program directed by Richard Hoover (Ball, 1964); it was further refined at Hines (Malamazian, 1970) and continues to this day (Hill & Ponder, 1976; Jacobsen, 1993; LaGrow & Weessies, 1994). However, LaGrow and Weessies (1994) point out that the ideal sequence envisioned by the written curriculum is usually modified by the demands of each situation. For example, in an itinerant program the ideal learning environments may not be available, or the special needs of an individual may be to learn his way around the residential center where the program is being offered or around his apartment building. Other necessary modifications result from characteristics of the learner, including other disabilities, such as developmental delays or severe neuropathy of the feet, or limited interests that result in very narrow learning goals, such as the need to only get to a neighbor's house or a neighborhood store.

Each student's learning sequence typically reflects a certain logical order, even though that order and the considerations that shape it may vary from student to student. To some extent the sequence is determined by a natural hierarchy of skills in which later skills presuppose the presence of more basic skills. For example, the ability to cross a street effectively requires prior skill in straight-line walking and detecting veering.

Each individual's sequence also usually reflects a logical progression in relation to psychosocial factors. For a student who lacks sufficient motivation for mobility training, the sequence may include a progression of increasing success in performing travel skills. This direct experience of success is the primary way in which an individual's perception of self-efficacy can be developed, leading to increased motivation to continue the training (Bandura, 1977).

For some students there may be a need for a sequence of lessened dependency on the instructor. Frequently the student depends quite a lot on the instructor, even to the point of using her as a sighted guide in the beginning lessons. However, it is important for the typical student who eventually will be capable of independent travel that the transition to depending on oneself starts during the very first lesson. For this reason the instructor talks to the student in terms of learning to *use a guide* instead of *being guided,* and the student is expected to start using his own hearing and other senses to stay oriented, even while using a guide during the early lessons.

Another progression that may be necessary for some students is to increasing their interactions with other people. Students who have a particularly strong anxiety response to new situations involving interacting with other people will need to be sensitively exposed to situations of increasing interaction, but with preparation to structure and manage the interactions.

Still another sequence may reflect increasing requirements in the area of problem solving. The instructor builds in graduated levels of expectations in this area, beginning with the student planning alternate and return routes to and from the travel objectives. This progresses to the expectation that the student will learn how to recognize when orientation mistakes have been made and then decide how to get back on track. This approach was used in the early mobility training at Hines (Malamazian, 1970). Mettler (1995) relates it to current theories in the area of cognitive psychology referred to as "discovery learning."

In the traditional use of a problem-solving sequence, the student is exposed to problems of orientation from the earliest lessons in the sequence and is asked to solve these problems. Initially, these are simple and basic problems related to remaining oriented while traveling with a sighted guide, but as the training progresses, they become more complex. As the student begins to travel by himself, he is required to make more decisions on his own and cope with the consequences of these decisions, including the new problems that incorrect decisions bring.

The O&M specialist typically tries to control the complexity of the problems that the student must confront through the structuring of lessons and through her own decisions about when to step into a situation and provide additional assistance. In this way the instructor has some discretion relative to how complex the problems become. She decides when to terminate a lesson or when to let it continue. Through an effective relationship with the student, the instructor learns to evaluate how much frustration a student can tolerate and how to keep the focus on successful experiences. It is unlikely that a student will develop more confidence in his ability to solve problems if the problems presented do not represent a reasonable challenge, but the problem also has to be solvable by the student at the student's current level of skill. Ultimately, the problem-solving sequence may lead to the use of drop-off lessons as described in Chapter 2.

Mettler (1995) emphasizes the importance of the instructor's discussion with the student following the lesson. It is helpful to lead the student through a review of his problem-solving and decision-making processes to make conscious and reinforce the successful methods used by the student. This is consistent with the findings of Bandura et al. (1982) and the suggestions of Dodds et al. (1994), that it is not merely the experience of success which has an impact on a person's perception of his own self-efficacy, but it is also important that he consciously understands and emotionally appreciates that his success was due to his own efforts.

The Helping Relationship

Because O&M is taught using a one-on-one teaching approach and the process frequently involves the confronting of significant personal challenges by the student, the relationship that develops between the student and instructor is especially important. This factor was recognized by the pioneers of mobility training. Bledsoe (1980) quotes from an unpublished paper by Richard Hoover in which Hoover's concept of the appropriate relationship between the student and the instructor reflects the need for collaboration between the two, each learning from the other. He also stressed the need to accept the student and his feelings, to communicate genuine caring for him, and to speak the truth, especially with regard to the student's actual ability and potential for independent travel.

In reflecting on the principles needed to run a center for the rehabilitation of people who are blind, Williams (1965) summarized them this way:

> (The principles) are: the real meaning of a success pattern in activities that are tried; the kind of observations which tell when success is really being achieved; the subordination of certain basic needs on the part of the staff in favor of the satisfaction of needs on the part of a client who after all, is the one struggling for growth; the real principles behind sensitive observation or evaluation of a person; the gradation of activity so that there is enough to be challenging and satisfying when achieved but not so much as to bring about the negative effects resulting from failure. (p. 33)

These expectations of the kind of relationship that should exist between the O&M specialist and the student were inculcated in the early instructors at Hines by Bledsoe, Hoover, and Williams. They represent the basis for the teaching methodology that emanated from Hines and has become the psychosocial basis of professional O&M instruction.

The type of instructor–student relationship described by Hoover is very similar to the client-centered approach to counseling developed by Rogers (1951), refined for the use of teachers, rehabilitation specialists, and other helpers by Carkhuff (1972), and specifically suggested for teachers of the visually impaired by Welsh (1972) and Tuttle (1987). According to Carkhuff's theory, the O&M specialist must be honest and genuine with the student. At some point it may be necessary for the student to place his trust in the specialist at a time of high anxiety. When that happens, the student should have no reason to doubt that the O&M specialist is trustworthy. The specialist should share openly with the student where she will be during the lesson and whether or not she will be in a position to intervene to prevent injury or embarrassment. The student should know when he is being observed and when he is functioning on his own. The O&M specialist must communicate a positive acceptance of the student, regardless of his success or failure, and a respect for the student's right to be involved in planning and decision making about his own program of instruction.

Risk Evaluation

One aspect of the relationship between the mobility instructor and her student is highlighted by the emerging interest in the determination and disclosure of risks for a person that might result from services rendered by a professional. Debate about the intersection of patient autonomy and professional responsibility has increased during the past 10 years in the field of health care. Some of these concepts have been related to the field of O&M by Banja (1994) following the development by Blasch and De l'Aune (1992) of a computerized model for evaluating the effectiveness of cane technique coverage.

The Blasch and De l'Aune Mobility Coverage Profile and Safety Index modeling process, referred to as RoboCane®, challenged some of the generally held understandings of the effectiveness of some aspects of the standard long-cane techniques. The possibility that the standard touch technique may result in less effective coverage than previously assumed by O&M specialists has focused attention on the instructor's responsibility for adequately informing the student of the risks associated with mobility training and independent travel.

The information obtained through the use of the RoboCane® with an individual student relates to one specific component of the process of independent travel. As Blasch and De l'Aune (1992) point out, the process of predicting risk for any aspect of independent travel, even a component as specific as the adequacy of cane coverage, is very complex. The RoboCane® does not take into consideration the impact of factors such as residual vision, auditory perception, reaction time, orientation, level of attention, and motivation in determining the actual risk associated with a specific level of cane coverage given the complexity and hazards of a particular environment. However, RoboCane® does represent a first step toward developing a more objective process of describing behaviors more precisely and making an objective presentation to a student about the level of risks that he might encounter in traveling independently.

The instructor has to decide how to approach the discussion of the potential risks of mobility training with her students. The need for an honest and trusting relationship would seem to require that the instructor fully discuss her understanding of the risks associated with independent travel. The possibility that such a discussion may dissuade a student from participating in training is not a sufficient reason to avoid it. On the other hand, it is probably most helpful for the process of encouraging clients whose motivation is marginal at the beginning to pace the discussion of the level of risk according to the individual student's skill and the environment that he will encounter in each successive phase of training, rather than laying out all of the possible risks that lie ahead. Naturally, the potential for risk typically increases as the student moves into more complex and challenging areas of travel. However, if an appropriate learning sequence has been followed, the student should not move into more complex areas until he has demonstrated the skills to handle the next level of difficulty.

SUMMARY

The psychological and social factors that influence the mobility behavior of a person with a visual disability are very significant to the outcome of the process and difficult to understand and control. The difficulty is explained by the complexity that results from the three-way interaction of personal factors, environmental factors, and behavior. Although research methodologies that can empirically describe the reciprocal effect of these factors are not easy to conceptualize and implement, the common-sense approaches which have been characteristic of formal mobility training since World War II are effective in helping students cope with these complex psychosocial variables and experience success in learning to travel. Recent trends in the study of personality, such as the growing focus on interactionism and the emergence of social cognitive theory, combine the strengths of behaviorism and cognitive psychology, and hold promise for empirically validating the common-sense practice methodologies of mobility instruction in the future.

Suggestions/Implications for O&M Specialists

1. Theories and research in the field of personality psychology can suggest to O&M specialists hypotheses and research methodologies for better understanding the psychosocial dimensions of independent travel with reduced vision.
2. Some of the most promising emerging theories of human behavior emphasize the complex interaction of personal factors, environmental factors, and individual behaviors. O&M specialists should be cautious about accepting simplistic explanations of mobility problems that focus on just one factor or element.
3. Even when a mobility client appears to have a strong trait or disposition that may affect mobility performance, the O&M specialist needs to understand the environmental situations that are the most likely to interact in positive or negative ways with this trait.
4. Student or client involvement in selecting and approving individualized education or rehabilitation plans not only meets legal and bureaucratic requirements, but can also have an impact on a person's motivation for the mobility instruction that follows.
5. As described by Tuttle (1987), persons who are blind face naturally occurring situations that challenge their ability to develop and maintain self-esteem. All of these situations can be positively impacted by successful O&M.
6. Bandura's (1986) research on self-efficacy provides empirical explanations for the positive impact on motivation of the teaching methodology that has been used in O&M programs since their development by the Veterans Administration following World War II. This methodology emphasizes practical problem solving in real situations that require a managed sequence of lessons of graduated difficulty and challenge.
7. A student's or client's outcome expectations are likely to affect his or her motivation for mobility instruction. These outcome expectations can be influenced by the teaching methods used by the O&M specialist.
8. Because the attitudes of the general public about blindness can represent a major barrier with which the traveler who is blind has to contend, the O&M specialist needs to understand how these attitudes manifest themselves and how to help a client cope with them.
9. The attitudes and behaviors of family members can have significant positive or negative effects on the mobility training of a person who is blind. The O&M specialist needs to assess the role of family members and design interventions to change negative factors when they are present.
10. The person who is visually impaired or blind who travels through the environment with a cane is a significant social stimulus that can create positive, negative, or ambiguous situations. The mobility specialist has to be aware of how the blind traveler handles these different circumstances and structure learning experiences to improve these skills if necessary.
11. The person with low vision frequently has the option of making his or her visual disability more or less apparent when traveling. The O&M specialist tries to

(*continued on next page*)

Suggestions/Implications for O&M Specialists (continued)

structure a thorough range of travel experiences that enable the person with low vision to evaluate the effectiveness of the travel method he chooses.

12. Handling offers of help requires special skills of the person who is blind. The O&M specialist has to understand the full range of help interactions that might occur and the impact of each type on students with different personality characteristics.
13. The sequence of learning experiences traditionally used by O&M specialists is instrumental in addressing many psychosocial factors. It can contribute to improved motivation, a greater sense of self-efficacy, lessened dependence, and more effective problem-solving.
14. The professional helping relationship that typically develops between the O&M specialist and her students can itself be a tool that the instructor uses to address some of the psychosocial issues a mobility student faces. The O&M specialist has to understand how to develop and maintain an appropriate and effective helping relationship and how to use the power of this relationship to help clients accomplish their goals.

ACTIVITIES FOR REVIEW

1. Review an autobiography of a person who is blind to identify how some of the psychosocial dimensions identified in this chapter affected that person's efforts to function independently.
2. Review a sample of initial assessments or final reports written by O&M specialists and identify issues described as "motivation" by the writer, but which might better be described as one of the more specific elements discussed in this chapter.
3. Develop a comprehensive list of mobility situations that might be likely to activate each dimension of trait anxiety identified by Endler (1983). For each mobility situation, suggest steps that can be taken by the O&M specialist to counter the anxiety.
4. Describe how O&M instruction and success in independent travel can have a positive impact on the challenges to developing self-esteem as described by Tuttle (1987).
5. Analyze three mobility vignettes for evidence of any of the four principal sources of perceived self-efficacy as described by Bandura (1986).
6. Compare Bandura's (1986) four principal sources of perceived self-efficacy to Reeve's (1992) four determinants of the strength of outcome expectancies.
7. What differences in methodology might be required when teaching persons with a primarily external locus of control compared to persons with an internal locus of control?
8. Interview three people who have no direct involvement with people who are blind and identify which of the Whiteman and Lukoff (1965) dimensions of attitudes toward blindness best characterizes each person.
9. Review the biography or autobiography of a person who is blind and identify the posi-

tive contributions made by family members to the blind person's independence.

10. Relate Baker's (1973) image of the circular effect of independent travel on a person's self-concept to Bandura's concept of self-efficacy.

11. Interview travelers who have low vision and identify some of the situations in which they have the most difficulty from a psychosocial perspective.

12. Role-play the range of "help" interactions that a traveler who is blind or has low vision is likely to encounter and develop possible strategies for handling each.

13. Discuss with travelers who are blind the impact of their mobility instruction on the development of their self-confidence as travelers.

14. Videotape role-playing with other students of typical interactions between O&M specialists and clients and analyze behaviors that reflect genuine caring and honest feedback of information.

PART TWO
Mobility Systems

CHAPTER 7

Adaptive Technology

Leicester W. Farmer and Daniel L. Smith

People who are visually impaired have used many methods and devices to aid in mobility. Over time, animals, sighted people, and devices (such as sticks or canes) have been used to achieve varying levels of safety in independent travel. Today there are basically four types of mobility systems or tools for getting about. The first is the human guide. The other three most accepted and proven types of mobility systems or tools include canes, dog guides, and electronic travel aids (ETAs).

The function of these mobility systems or tools is to provide information about the travel path in advance of entrance into a space. When using the long cane and ETA, the individual must be concerned about the type and amount of coverage the specific device provides. Mobility coverage is a broad concept relating to a three-dimensional area in which detection of objects and drop-offs is important and recognition of various types of environmental information should be obtained. Therefore, mobility coverage, as defined by Blasch, LaGrow, and De l'Aune (1996), is:

> The scope or range of environmental preview of clear path information provided to the traveler. The area of coverage provided, however, is dependent upon the unique functions of each of the devices or techniques used. The amount of protection or safety is dependent on variables specific to the traveler (e.g., ability to respond to the detection of information, reaction time, degree of vision).

The function of a mobility device, such as a cane, is to preview the immediate environment for (1) objects in the path of travel (i.e., object preview), (2) changes in the surface of travel (i.e., surface preview), and (3) the integrity of the surface upon which the foot is to be placed when brought forward (i.e., foot placement preview). As adaptive technology is discussed, it is important to consider this technology in relation to the mobility coverage and preview they provide.

Mobility training, as discussed in other chapters of this volume, encompasses many components; however, in the area of adaptive technology there is a focus on three general areas: devices, skills, and strategies. This chapter will present mobility devices such as ETAs, long canes, and adaptive mobility systems (dog guides as a mobility system are presented in Chapter 8 of this volume). When one is considering devices, as an example, the cane by itself is just a piece of pipe or fiberglass and will not make a person independently mobile. It is the strategies of using the cane in a systematic fashion that gives the significance to the long cane. Once the strategies have been taught through a systematic curriculum of instruction (see Hill & Ponder, 1976; Jacobsen, 1993; Weessies & LaGrow, 1994), the individual then develops skill and proficiency in the application of these strategies for using the long cane as a device (Blasch, 1994). The following sections present information about canes and classifies ETAs according to their functional importance to orientation and mobility (O&M).

CANES

Several types of canes and walking aids are manufactured to meet the varied needs and demands of persons with visual impairments. The rigid long canes, folding or collapsible canes, white wooden canes (not generally recommended by O&M specialists), and orthopedic support canes, used in conjunction with travel canes, are the most commonly used (see Figure 7.1). Canes are fabricated from such products as wood, aluminum alloy, fiberglass, carbon fibers, composites of various materials, plastic, and stainless steel.

The cane serves to provide detection or preview by extending the tactile sense of the user. This is accomplished by transmitting information about the environment and, in some cases, providing physical support.

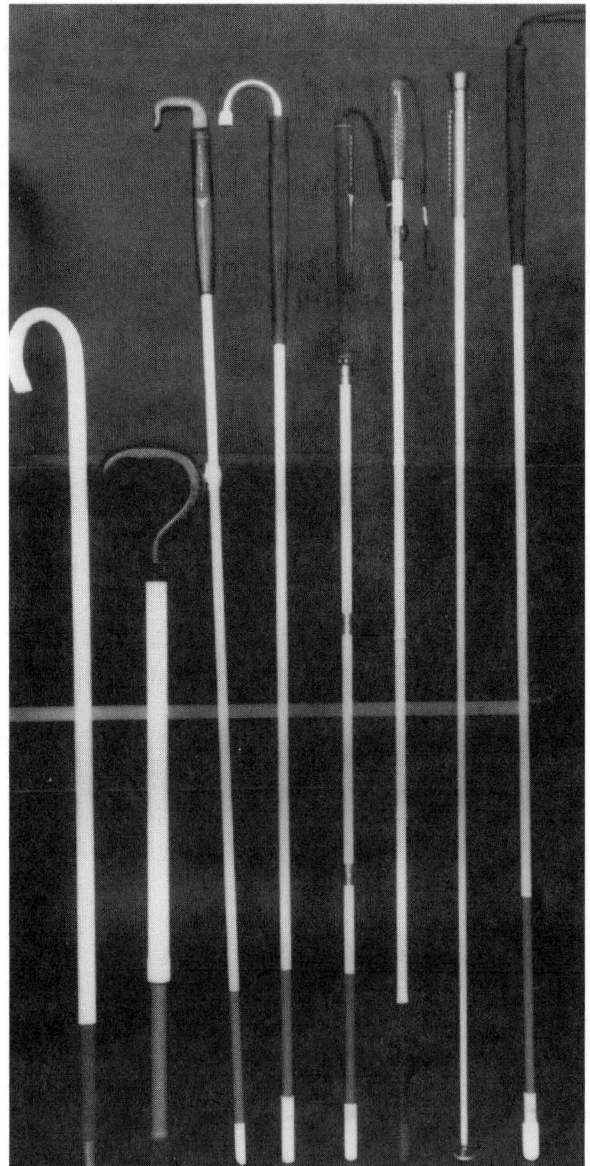

Figure 7.1. A wide range of canes is available to the traveler with a visual impairment.
Source: VA Medical Department.

The Long Cane

Following Hoover's pioneering efforts, consumers, engineers, manufacturers, and mobility specialists have since worked in concert toward the continued development of the long cane and refinement of the techniques and strategies employed in its use.

The most desirable characteristics of a cane include:

1 Conductivity of vibrations and tactile information, but not of thermal or electrical energy.
2. Good weight distribution (balance).
3. Lightweight, but not like a feather in the breeze.
4. Strong, durable, rigid, and resilient.
5. High visibility to drivers and pedestrians both in daylight and darkness, when illuminated by vehicle headlights.

Most requirements and specifications for a folding or collapsible long cane mirror those of the rigid cane. Conferences in the early to mid-1960s (MIT, 1963) resulted in essential and unique specifications for folding or collapsible canes as follows:

1. Cane must be collapsible to pocket size.
2. Design must include provisions for supplying cane assembly in 2-inch (5 cm) increments of length over a range of 36 to 70 inches (91 cm to 178 cm).
3. Cane should be easy to open and close, lock, and store with one hand, and should survive 5,000 fold–extend cycles based on 1 year of use by an active traveler.
4. Cane must have a simple overall design with assembly of component parts that do not require specialized techniques.
5. Tip should be sensitive and durable, and constructed so as not to stick or catch in cracks or on rough surfaces.
6. Joints should be self-cleaning.
7. Cane should not require retraining to use.

Cane Tips

The first long cane tips were manufactured from readily available wooden dowels. Users found the wooden tips inconvenient because of their tendency to stick on rough surfaces and tendency to fall out of the cane if they dried out.

Years of experience since the first attempt at standardization by the Veterans Administration have yielded many types and styles of cane tips. The original VA specifications described a $3\frac{1}{4}$-inch (8.25-cm) long, $\frac{1}{2}$-inch (1.27-cm) diameter nylon rod, with $1\frac{1}{4}$ inches (3.18 cm) of screw threads for insertion into the cane, leaving 2 inches (5.08 cm) exposed. The above specifications describe today's cane tip, with the exception of the threaded end. Many currently available canes are provided with a nylon tip with a split in one end, which is fitted with a rubber wedge that spreads the split to provide a snug frictioned fit for insertion into the cane tubing.

Another common cane tip is a larger $\frac{5}{8}$-inch (1.6-cm) diameter, drilled nylon tip that slips over the shaft of the cane. There are many other types of cane tips on the market, as described below:

1. A larger diameter nylon tip with a shape similar to a marshmallow or mushroom.
2. A curved version of the $\frac{1}{2}$-inch (1.27-cm) diameter nylon tip in which the tip is heated and bent at a 100-degree angle so that the curved elbow, rather than the tip, rides on the ground (LaGrow, Kjeldstad, & Lewandowski, 1988).
3. A metal glide tip, which resembles a chair glide, that attaches to the cane via a rubber connector. This tip is often supplied with the fiberglass canes and can be fit with an adapter onto other long canes.
4. A marshmallow-shaped tip mounted on a roller bearing so that the tip rolls instead of slides as it swings back and forth in front of the user.
5. A marshmallow-shaped tip mounted with a recoil spring that collapses toward the cane if the tip sticks in a crack.
6. A larger 2-inch (5.08-cm) outside diameter (OD) ball tip, which slides over the standard nylon tip.

Travelers with visual impairments often express a strong preference for one of the above-mentioned cane tips, but there is little empirical evidence to support the choice of the best cane tip. Fisk (1986) collected information concerning visually impaired travelers' opinions about the "marshmallow" tip's function. All of his subjects expressed positive opinions about the tip's usefulness in travel situations that used the constant contact technique. Although all of the subjects stated that they would purchase and continue to use the marshmallow tip, the study only sought consumer opinion. No data was collected as to the actual effectiveness of the tip or cane technique.

LaGrow et al. (1988) conducted a study with 15 blindfolded subjects who were sighted and found a lack of statistical significance between the performance of the curved, rounded (marshmallow), and cylindrical (*chalk-shaped*) tips. The three variables tested were sticking, curb detection, and continuous travel. The lack of statistical significance could well be the result of an underpowered study with only 15 subjects. There was statistical significance supporting the opinion of the subjects who favored the curved cane tip over the cylindrical tip, and then next the marshmallow tip.

Cane Grips

Manufacturers have utilized various types of cane grips for long cane production, including rubber golf grips, flexible plastic, leather and leatherlike wraps, and various types of tape. User preference varies for cane selection and may be based partially upon the grip style. Instructors have a responsibility for acquainting students with the various available cane styles.

High Visibility Canes

Ideally, all canes should be designed to be visible during the day, at night, and under hazardous weather conditions such as rain, fog, and snow. Although "white cane laws" mandate that canes be white with a red tip, a cane's visibility at night is dependent upon reflectivity or possibly internal illumination.

Franck (1990) studied the visibility of canes at night with drivers in a rural setting. He found that canes coated with Reflexite AP 1000M microprism reflecting tape were visible at virtually twice the distance (up to $\frac{1}{5}$ mile) of canes coated with Scotchlite glass-beaded reflecting tape.

One cane incorporated a bright strobe light, with claims to increase visibility up to 2 miles. Other inventors have attempted to utilize illuminated fiber optics to enhance visibility. Whether or not these methods of illumination are utilized, the traveler should not relinquish the responsibility for safety and environmental awareness to the observer. Many people have designed innovative devices to meet the needs of people with visual impairments. The majority of these devices have not gone beyond the prototype stage because of a lack of knowledge concerning mobility, ill-conceived ideas, or a lack of research and field testing.

Advantages and Disadvantages

The long cane, including the rigid style and collapsible long cane, is the most commonly used mobility device and facilitates safe, independent travel by the majority of people with visual impairments. When used with the proper training, it is an effective and efficient mobility device. It is a highly maneuverable aid that allows investigation of the environment without actual hand contact.

The long cane is reliable, long-lasting, and largely unaffected by unfavorable weather and temperature conditions. Most require no accessories, and virtually no maintenance except the occasional replacement of a worn tip and cords for the collapsible style long cane. The cane can be accommodated to most users' physical specifications and, in some instances, their special needs.

There are, however, some disadvantages peculiar to the long cane and its use. It does not provide adequate protection against collision to the upper part of the body (Suterko, 1967). In a recent study, LaGrow, Blasch, and De l'Aune (1997) studied the efficacy of the touch technique for surface and foot placement preview. They defined foot placement preview as a dichotomous variable in which "foot placement preview is said to have occurred if the foot was placed on the surface previewed by the cane tip." Preview is afforded by direct contact with the surface by the cane tip and evaluated for each step and foot placement. The study, using biomechanical analysis, found that foot placement preview was not accomplished at any time for any of the participants in the study. The subjects were certified O&M specialists using the touch technique as described by Hill and Ponder (1976). Even if constant contact were used, the exact correspondence of foot and cane tip placement would have been achieved only rarely. Even though there was obstacle and surface preview, there was seldom foot placement preview. This deficiency appears to be attributable to shortcomings in the consideration of the cane length and stride length rather than an inadequacy of the traveler's use of the technique or the cane. Continued objective analysis with the software modeling program, RoboCane®, indicates that the cane and the techniques are very complex. As stated by Blasch and De l'Aune (1992), with objective evaluation it is apparent that there is not a single technique that is best. Instead, the cane technique is a dynamic interaction of variables. Stated differently, with each modification there are tradeoffs in object, surface, and foot placement previews; discrimination; and drop-off detectability and reaction time. According to Blasch & De l'Aune (1992), a cane user cannot obtain complete mobility coverage with only a cane, no matter how the cane is used (Figure 7.2).

Another disadvantage is that the rigid-style long cane is noncollapsible, and storing it at social gatherings, on public or private transportation, or when using a sighted guide may present a problem. Furthermore, there is also the danger of tripping pedestrians in congested areas.

Cane tips that break or wear out must be replaced. High winds can interfere with maneuverability of the cane, and the long cane is not designed as a weight-bearing or support cane. Improperly fitted canes (too long or too short) may give inadequate preview and detection information. In addition, learning to use the long cane effectively requires extensive training.

ADAPTIVE MOBILITY DEVICES

O&M specialists first used adaptive mobility devices (AMDs) before they introduced the long cane. These "precanes" were used for two main purposes: as a protective device for children whose use was easy to learn (Bosbach, 1988; Foy, Kirchner, & Waple, 1991; Kronick, 1987; Clarke, Sainato, & Ward, 1994) and as a way to begin skill development that would later transfer to use of the long cane (Kronick, 1987; Foy et al., 1991) (see Chapter 13). Later, AMDs were used as permanent mobility devices for individuals who were unable to use a long cane, such as individuals with multiple impairments or elderly visually impaired individuals. Populations specifically considered for adaptive devices include those with limited strength, diminished coordination, limited cognitive abilities, and impaired proprioceptive and kinesthetic abilities (see Chapters 14 and 16).

Basically, the AMD is designed to provide full coverage across the width of the body and constant contact with the ground, providing optimum tactile and audio feedback. Most designs have a bumper bar across the bottom to clear a wide path and absorb impact. The user pushes the AMD in the direction of travel and does not need the strength and coordination required by the long cane. Figure 7.3 illustrates some of the designs reported at conferences, in literature, and in research proposals. AMDs include those that are made by O&M specialists and, to a lesser degree, commercially manufactured devices such as the WalkAlone™ and the Adaptive Cane produced by Autofold.

Some specialists provide students with push-broom–shaped "T-Cane" devices which include optional "T"-shaped handle and wheels, while other specialists provide miniature shopping carts or other pushcarts. The AMD by Autofold is produced in two "knock-down," adjustable sizes (for adults and children). They are constructed of aircraft-grade aluminum, with the wheels spaced 12 inches apart. Interchangeable equipment includes 2-inch ball-bearing wheels, eurowheels or larger diameter wheels for cobblestone environments, and curved nylon tips.

In some cases, individuals with poor gait have experienced significant improvement in gait

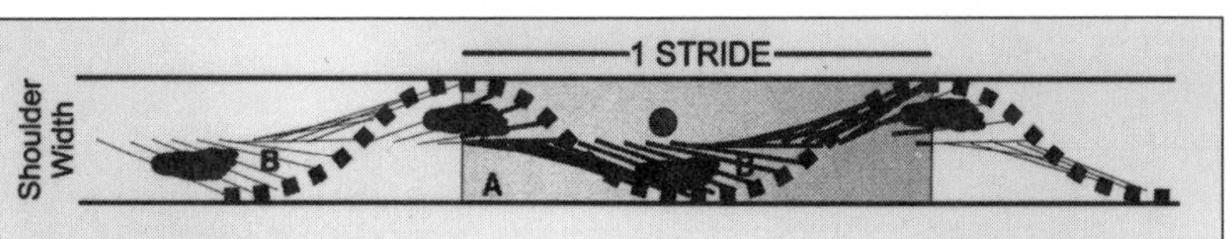

Figure 7.2. The shaded area (A) indicates the three-dimensional area requiring coverage by the cane less the three-dimensional area that is covered by the cane (B). The percentage of coverage is calculated as follows: 100% × B / (A+B).

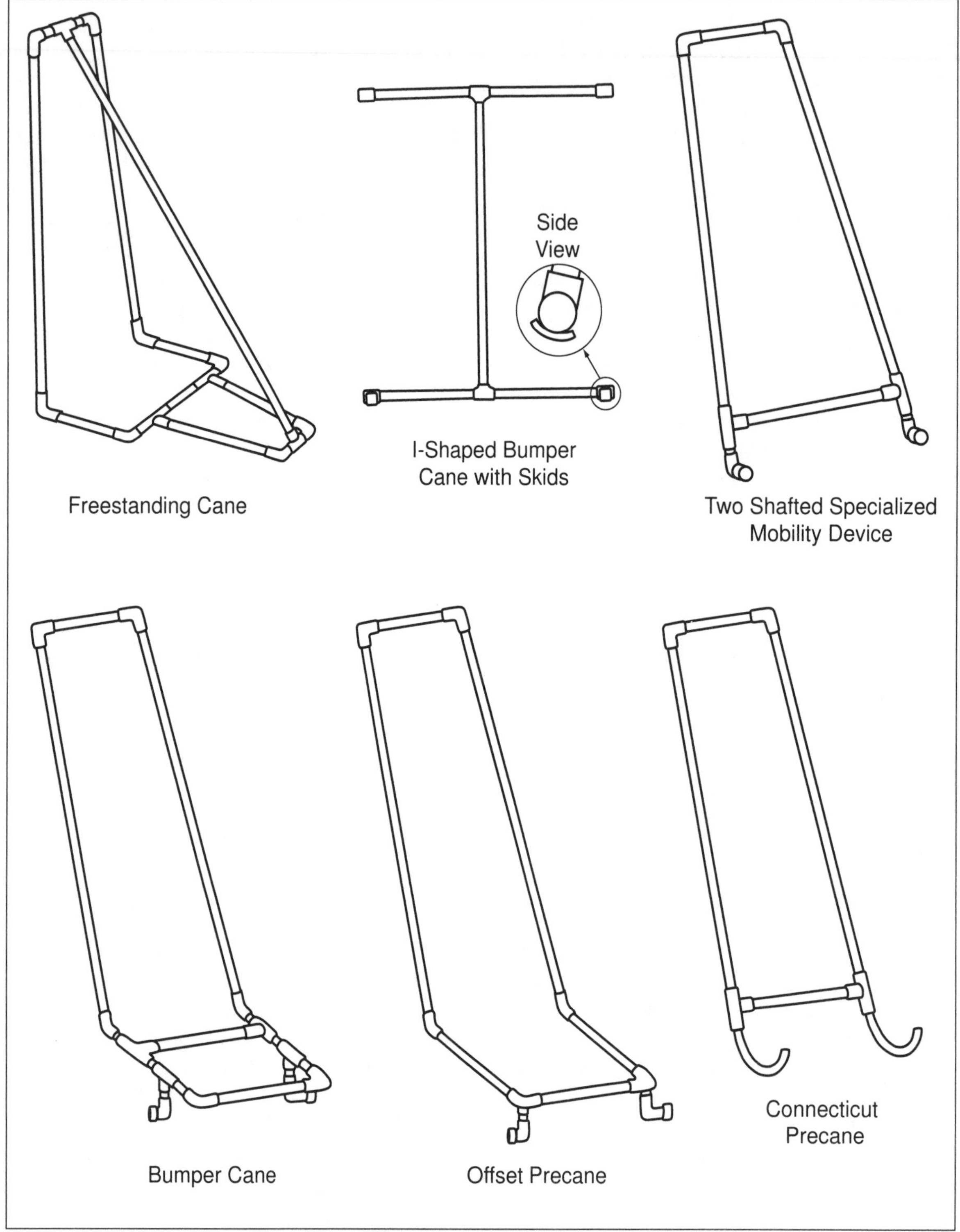

(*continued on next page*)

Figure 7.3. Examples of adaptive mobility devices.

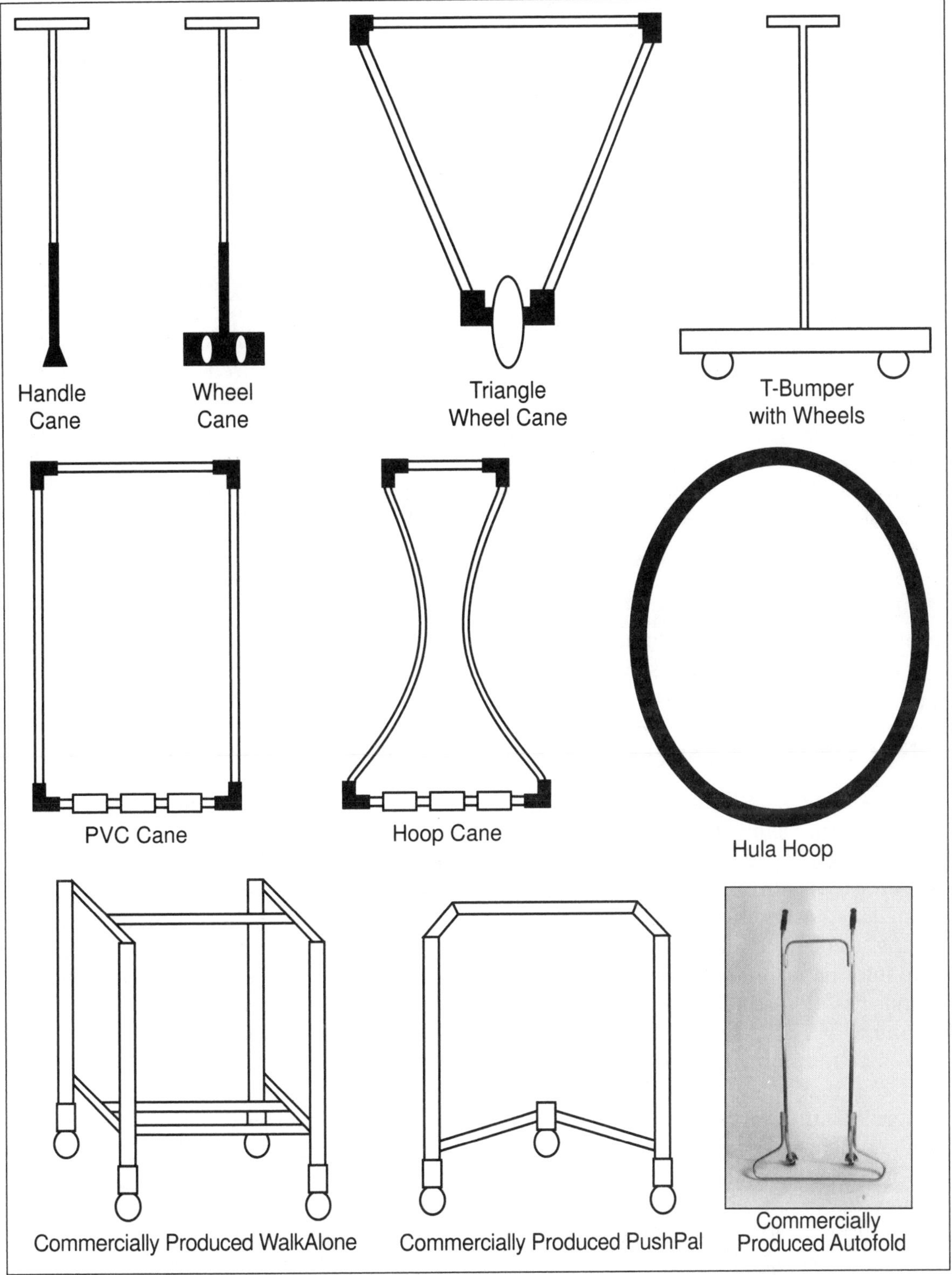

Figure 7.3. Examples of adaptive mobility devices. (*continued*)

when using an AMD (Kronick, 1987). O&M specialists have also reported increased travel abilities among preschoolers (Foy et al., 1991; Kronick, 1987; Clarke et al., 1994).

Advantages and Disadvantages

Adaptive mobility devices have many of the same advantages and disadvantages as the long cane. The major disadvantage is the cumbersomeness of the device. This relates to the maneuverability and storage of the device. The AMD produced by Autofold has interchangeable nylon runners or wheels that allow for greater longevity of the tip, depending on the environment where it is used.

The long cane and adaptive mobility devices share two common disadvantages: the inability to scan the entirety of space through which the body travels (the area above the hands) and transmission of information at the moment of contact with objects—not before! If greater mobility coverage is desired, electronic travel aids and sensory systems offer some solutions.

ELECTRONIC TRAVEL AIDS

An ETA is a device that emits energy waves to detect the environment within a certain range or distance, processes reflected information, and furnishes the user with certain information about the immediate environment. The device should probe the immediate area and present the detected information to the traveler in an intelligible and useful manner. Blasch, Long, and Griffin-Shirley (1989) state further that ETAs are "devices that transform information about the environment that would normally be relayed through vision into a form that can be conveyed through another sensory modality."

Experience, evaluation, and consumer interviews show that improvement in mobility performance by using an ETA can be very difficult to demonstrate. The evaluation of an ETA should consider at least three separate but related areas: the functions that the aid was engineered to perform for the consumer, the benefits that consumers feel they receive from using the device, and the coverage limitations of the long cane. ETAs are generally categorized into four types, which are reviewed later in this discussion.

Acquisition and Display of Environmental Information

Although some ETAs have been designed to respond to ambient light or sound reflected from detected objects, most of the attention is presently focused on active energy radiating systems. The energy used by these aids is either acoustic or electromagnetic.

Researchers have also investigated using more easily implemented sources of infrared light, light-emitting diodes (LEDs). Mims (1972) implemented infrared LEDs in an eyeglass-mounted aid which did not reach production. This attempt at utilization of LED technology could have been a stepping stone toward inexpensive ETAs in the future. There may still be room for research with this technology.

Two opposing viewpoints relative to device display and output have been expressed by Russell (1966), developer of the Lindsay Russell Pathsounder, and Kay (1974), developer of the Binaural Sensory Aid (BSA), the Sonicguide Mark 11, the Trisensor, and Kaspa. Both Kay and Russell's devices use ultrasonic acoustic energy for object detection and environmental sensing. Russell stated that an aid should not burden the user with complex sounds; it should simply display information indicating to the traveler whether the travel path is or is not clear; a "go-no-go system." The Pathsounder, therefore, strips away all complexity from the signal by processing or codifying the echoes it receives. Russell refers to the display concept as a "language system," because the presentation consists of a language of discrete sounds. He suggests that it is a question of giving either the headlines or the text. He has chosen to give the headlines.

Kay's approach, in contrast, has been to design an aid that displays the maximum amount of environmental information that the auditory channel can effectively transmit, and to do this in such a way as to enable the user to readily disregard both redundant and unwanted information merely by focusing attention on pertinent information (analog system).

Benjamin and his staff developed the Laser Cane, which employs electromagnetic (light) energy. While the Russell and Kay devices emit a wide ultrasonic cone in the forward and peripheral fields to get environmental information, the earlier Laser Canes emitted three pencil-thin beams of invisible infrared (IR) light for target detection.

Function

An ETA can provide a degree of sensory information about the environment which, even under the most ideal circumstances, would not be possible to obtain when using only a long cane or dog guide. A sensory aid may detect and locate objects, and provide information that allows the user to determine (within acceptable tolerances) range, direction, and dimension and height of objects. It makes noncontact trailing and tracking possible, enabling the traveler to receive directional indications from physical structures that have strategic locations in the environment. With the Sonicguide it is even possible to achieve a degree of primitive object identification because the timbre of the auditory signal may give clues about the nature of the surface being detected.

Guidelines

Before 1970, various investigators, developers, and engineers designed devices according to their own perceptions of the needs of persons with visual impairments. Also, there was little communication and cooperation among developers, consumers, and mobility specialists regarding ideas, input, and preferences. Furthermore, many sensory devices failed to meet even the most fundamental travel needs of consumers with visual impairments because of a lack of uniform guidelines for baseline functions.

While sensory devices differ in principle, design, display, and output, there are many similar functions that they must perform as secondary travel aids. At the present, no one device meets all of the baseline requirements for a travel aid, but guidelines for an ETA can be set forth for the typical user. Special considerations must always be given for the exceptional user.

The National Research Council (1986) published a comprehensive review of strengths and weaknesses of technology for information acquisition and display and made recommendations for further development, utilizing current and future technology. The most essential information needs of the pedestrian include

1. Detection of obstacles in the travel path from ground level to head height for the full body width.
2. Travel surface information including textures and discontinuities.
3. Detection of objects bordering the travel path for shorelining and projection.
4. Distant object and cardinal direction information for projection of a straight line.
5. Landmark location and identification information.
6. Information enabling self-familiarization and mental mapping of an environment.

Ergonomics must be a prime consideration in the development of travel devices. Benjamin (1968) stated that a device "should be small, light in weight, easily stored when not in use, and easily picked up and put down."

An ETA should operate with minimum interference to the natural sensory channels and interface with the environment. It should be self-contained as a single unit, with user choice of auditory or tactile modalities. It must be reliable, durable, and reflect good quality control. Repairs, if needed, should be infrequent and with a minimum turnaround time. The device should not be damaged by moisture and should operate in adverse environmental conditions. Utilization of standard, user-replaceable, rechargeable batteries with a minimum of 5 hours continuous use

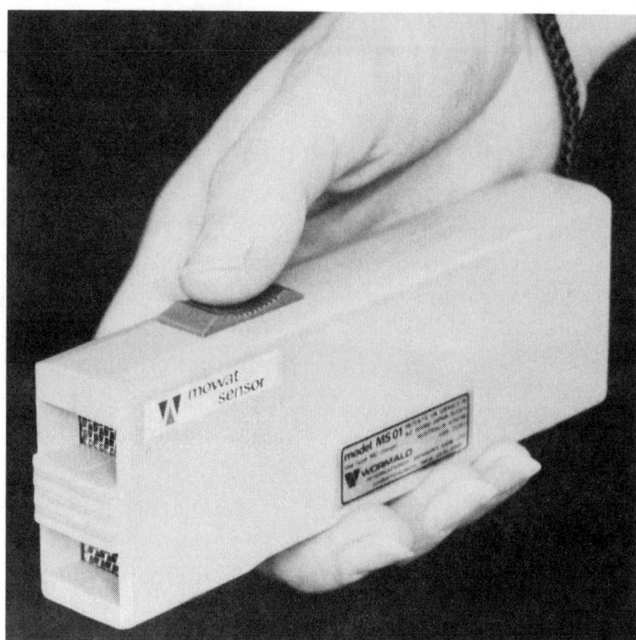

Figure 7.4. The Mowat Sensor.

is a major consideration. Finally, but by no means less important, ETAs must be cosmetically acceptable. In an effort to categorize the devices, they have been grouped into four types. There are several Type I ETAs that are commercially available.

Type I Devices

Type I devices (single output for object preview) provide clear-path information. These devices provide obstacle preview. They are considered a go-no-go system and provide limited information about the attributes of the object or surface in one's path. Type I ETA devices include the Pathsounder, Mowat Sensor, Polaron, and Sensory 6.

Lindsay Russell E Model Pathsounder

The Pathsounder was invented by Lindsay Russell. The Pathsounder is mentioned because it was one of the first commercially available ETAs and paved the way for future developments. It is currently out of commercial production but will be supplied in cases of special need. Those in use are maintained by the inventor. (For a complete description of this device, refer to Farmer [1980].)

Mowat Sensor

Geoff C. Mowat of New Zealand began experiments with electronic travel aids in 1970, and by 1972 he had settled on the fundamentals of the current handheld Mowat in the form of a black metal case (Figure 7.4). The Mowat Sensor is currently manufactured by Pulse Data International Ltd. of New Zealand and Australia. The sensor measures 6 × 2 × 1 inches (15 × 5 × 2.5 cm), weighs 6.5 ounces (184.2 g), is handheld, has a vibratory output, and can be easily carried in a pocket or purse. If an audible output is desired, an earphone is available.

The device emits an elliptical ultrasonic cone 15 degrees wide and 30 degrees high, approximating the form of a human body. There is a single control (three-position slide switch) on top of the unit to enable the user to operate the Mowat Sensor at two ranges. A range of 13.2 feet (4 m) may be selected by pushing the slide switch forward from the center position (Off). A shorter range of 3.3 feet (1 m) is attained by moving the control backward from the center position.

The Mowat Sensor is silent in free space and detects only the nearest object within beam range. When an object is detected, the Mowat

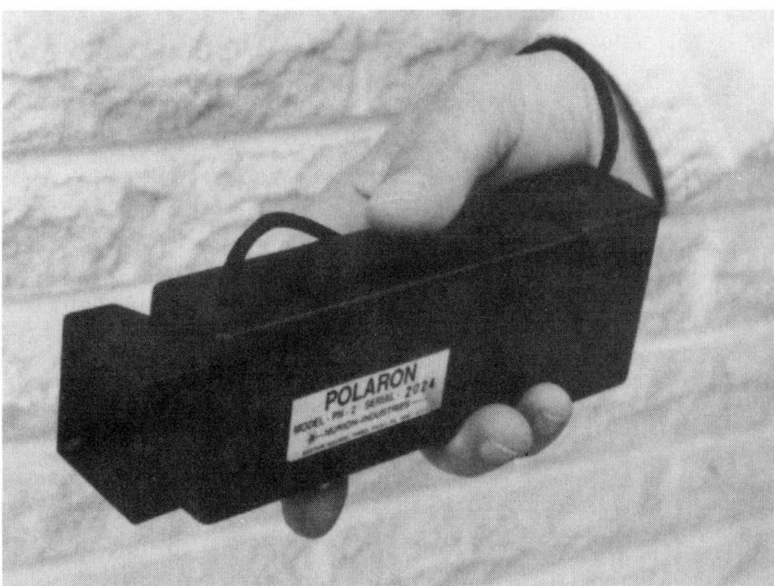

Figure 7.5. The Polaron.

Sensor vibrates at a rate inversely related to the distance from the object; at 13.2 feet (4 m) from a target, the aid vibrates at a rate of 10 pulses per second and increases to a vibratory rate of 40 pulses per second when the traveler advances to within 3.3 feet (1 m) of the target. The device is powered by a supplied rechargeable 9-volt battery, or 9-volt nonrechargeable batteries can also be used. A fully charged battery will provide 8 hours of use, after which it must be recharged for 14 hours.

Benefits. The Mowat Sensor is easily pointed to locate landmarks and objects not directly in the travel path. As a result of its small size (it fits in a pocket or purse) and the relative ease of learning how to use it, it may be appropriate for situational use by those who have some remaining vision. The larger beam size at long range affords the user with simultaneous protection from overhead and knee-high objects, even at rapid walking speeds.

Limitations. The Mowat Sensor requires dedicated use of the free hand. Thus, it is not useful to the support cane user or those with amputations or unilateral impairment (due to stroke or other etiology), although some specialists have experimented with mounting the Mowat Sensor on wheelchairs and walkers. The user may encounter difficulty when carrying packages, or maintaining balance on slippery surfaces. It may pose some difficulty during the winter months because the user's wearing of heavy gloves may make the vibrations less detectable, and cold temperatures will reduce the output of the battery to as little as half the rated capacity. As with the other ETAs, significant amounts of snow or rain may result in continuous (false) warning signals (Farmer, 1975).

Polaron

With the advent of the Polaroid Automatic Focusing System and the company's willingness to share the ranging system with developers of new technology, the Polaron became a reality in the early 1980s. Nurion Industries was able to control development costs by incorporating the Polaroid ranging module into a handheld/chest-mounted ETA (Figure 7.5).

The Polaron utilizes the ultrasonic sound navigation and ranging (sonar) system to detect objects at ranges of up to 16 feet (4.9 m). By means of three slide switches the user chooses ranges of 4, 8, or 16 feet (1.2, 2.4, or 4.9 m); turns the power on and off; and selects between vibrotactile or audible warning signals (at one of two volume levels).

Although the warning signal is constant for objects between 16 and 8 feet (4.9 and 2.4 m), changes in perceived pitch of the tone or the frequency of the vibration, a function of the distance, occur when objects are closer than 8 feet (2.4 m).

There are two modes for operation: handheld like a flashlight, or suspended from the neck at chest level. During handheld use, the case vibrates, and when chest-mounted, a miniaturized vibrator on the neck loop vibrates. The user can also select 4- and 8-foot (1.2- and 2.4-m) ranges, and receive vibratory or tonal information at varying rates or pitch to represent the range.

Power is supplied by a 9-volt Ni-Cad, alkaline, or lithium battery. With an overnight recharge the nicad battery will provide up to 3 hours of continuous use (Nurion Industries, 1992).

Benefits. The Polaron's benefits include dual handheld and chest-mounted modes of operation; three range selections; and the option of vibratory or sound output. When used in the handheld mode, the Polaron can be used to locate landmarks at up to 16 feet (4.9 m).

Limitations. There are several limitations of the Polaron that should be considered. First, there is some inconsistency in signal reception, particularly at close range with specular (mirrorlike) objects. Second, the volume control is limited to two intensity levels, which may not be appropriate for the situation. Finally, the 3-hour battery life between charges may be insufficient to last for a normal day's use, thus requiring the user to carry a replacement battery.

Sensory 6

The Sensory 6 is a spectacle-mounted ETA that utilizes the Polaroid Ultrasonic Ranging System. (Brytech, a division of E.L. Bryenton and Associates Inc. in Ottawa, Ontario, Canada, manufactures the Sensory 6.) The device is composed of three detachable cable-connected parts: eyeglass frames, stereo headphones, and a base unit. The eyeglass frames resemble dark sunglasses with two black fabric-covered transducers instead of lenses. Lightweight stereo headphones provide sound information to the user, and the control box houses the major electronics, range and volume controls, and the battery pack (see Figure 7.6).

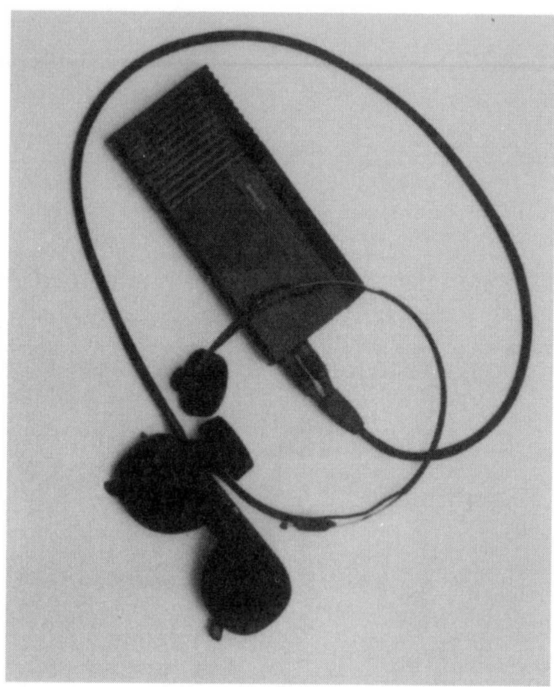

Figure 7.6. The Sensory 6.

Source: Reprinted with permission of Brytech Inc., Ottawa, Canada.

The Sensory 6 detects objects at ranges of up to 6.56 feet (2 m) at short range and up to 11.48 feet (3.5 m) at long range. Tones emitted from the headphones alert the user to the range of the nearest object detected; the nearer the object, the higher the pitch. Objects directly in the travel path will be heard in both ears, while objects to the side are heard only in the ear adjacent to the object.

Power is supplied by a rechargeable battery pack, which provides up to 8 hours of continuous operation on a 14-hour charge. The user can carry a spare battery pack, available from the manufacturer only, for convenience.

Benefits. Since the Sensory 6 is worn on the head, it does not require the use of the free hand. With a relatively simple output it can be used with limited training.

Limitations. Detection of overhead or waist-high objects is dependent on head position, forcing the user to situationally chose the protection zone by modifying head position. This could result in head contact with objects. Since the Walkman-like headphones will attenuate the hearing, perception of environmental auditory information may be compromised. Since the transducers are mounted in front of the eyes, some potential users may complain of the cosmetic effect, and any remaining vision will be occluded.

WalkMate

The WalkMate (produced by Safe Tech International, Inc. [1993]) is a Type I device developed after the others described. The WalkMate ultrasonic sonar modules are packaged in a 10-ounce plastic box, 3 × 5 × 2 inches (7.62 × 12.7 × 5.08 cm), and can be worn at waist level suspended from the neck loop, or it may be handheld like a flashlight. A 9-volt rechargeable battery powers the WalkMate and a 1.5-volt AA battery powers the cable-connected vibrator.

Upon choosing vibration or sound for a warning signal, the user hears beeps or feels vibrations that represent objects in the travel path. The WalkMate has two range zones, 7 and 4 feet (2.13 and 1.22 m). Objects within the 7-foot (2.13-m) range zone will trigger a slowly pulsed (about 4 pulses per second) beep and vibration. Objects within the 4-foot (1.22-m) range zone will trigger a more rapid beep and vibration.

The manufacturer suggests that the transmission pattern of the ultrasonic beam is "U"-shaped rather than the conventional cone-shaped beam used by the other ultrasonic ETAs. Nominal beam dimensions are 6 feet (1.83 m) tall by 2.31 feet (0.704 m) wide at 4 feet (1.22 m) of range and 6 feet 3 inches (1.90 m) tall by 2.31 feet (0.704 m) wide at 6 feet (1.83 m) of range. Due to the wide beam coverage, the manufacturer recommends the device for outdoor use only.

Benefits. The WalkMate's low cost and pleasant cosmetic features are attractive. The broad beam coverage may be of benefit for detection of objects in outdoor travel situations.

Limitations. Initial engineering bench testing of this device found a great variability in beam configuration and reliability (Blasch, Kynast, & Manuel, 1995). There is no research to support the claims made by the manufacturer and the device has yet to be objectively validated by research, the O&M profession, and consumers. The availability of this device is in question.

Benefits of Type I ETAs

ETA users will particularly appreciate the early warning nature of the ETA. Simon (1984) noted correction of veer and increased pace as benefits mentioned by respondents to her survey. Protection against overhangs and advance warning of objects are benefits noted by Blasch et al. (1989). In the Blasch et al. (1989) study of all identifiable ETA users, respondents stated that primary benefits of using ETAs were "increased knowledge, awareness of the environment, safety, and greater travel confidence." Some users indicated that for the first time in their experience as travelers, they had the option to either avoid or make contact with objects, or simply use them for orientation and reference points. There are many times when contact is desirable, and it is gratifying to know when one is within range of the target and can follow the electronic signal to within cane-reaching or hand-touching distance.

Type II Devices

Type II devices (multiple outputs for object preview) provide multiple or complex outputs that indicate clear-path information. The distinction between Type I and Type II devices involves the use of lasers for object preview. In addition, these devices may be used in conjunction with or as a part of a wheelchair or long cane. They are considered a go-no-go system and provide limited information about the attributes of the object or surface in one's path. Type II ETAs include Wheelchair Pathfinder and the Laser Cane.

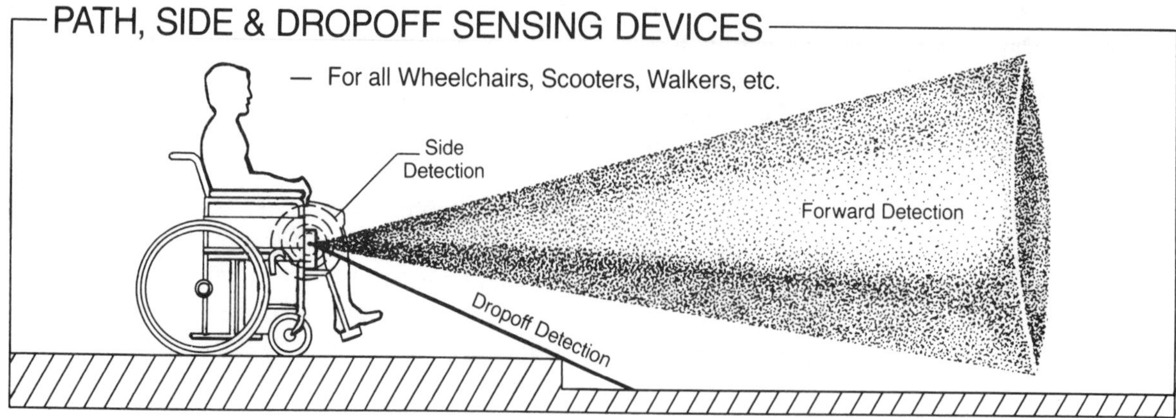

Figure 7.7. The Wheelchair Pathfinder.

Wheelchair Pathfinder

The Wheelchair Pathfinder was designed as a result of consumer demand by individuals with visual impairments and ambulatory limitations that required the use of a wheelchair. The Wheelchair Pathfinder (see Figure 7.7) can be configured to meet the needs of the user, offering forward protection and optional side, drop-off, and backup protection.

The Wheelchair Pathfinder is an ETA that utilizes both ultrasonic (forward, side, and backup detection) and laser (drop-off detection) signals to provide wheelchair travelers with increased safety and information. Detection ranges of 4 or 8 feet (1.2 or 2.4 m) may be selected for the forward beam. Maximum side detection range is up to 12 inches (30.4 cm) and drop-off protection ranges up to 4 feet (1.2 m). Differently pitched tones and optional multibeaded vibrating neckbands or straps offer warnings to the user, generating different signals for each of the protection beams. The Wheelchair Pathfinder is powered by rechargeable batteries and, depending upon the battery option, offers at least 1 day of operation prior to an overnight recharge.

Benefits. The Wheelchair Pathfinder's benefits include the relative ease of learning how to use it and simultaneous forward, side, and drop-off protection. Since this wheelchair device does not require hand manipulation of the ETA, it is useful to those who have motor limitations.

Limitations. The potential sphere of independent travel varies among individuals, but it infrequently happens that an individual will be an independent traveler in an unfamiliar outdoor setting. In some cases the long cane is utilized alone or in conjunction with the wheelchair ETA (see Rosen, Chapter 15).

Laser Canes

The Laser (light amplification by stimulated emission of radiation) Cane (originally developed and manufactured by J. Malvern Benjamin and his colleagues at Bionic Instruments, Inc.) is a product of the combined efforts of private enterprise and government. It evolved from a series of efforts using optical principles implemented with progressively better components. The use of the Laser Cane by following detection information of the laser beams is based on the cane being used in the traditional touch-technique fashion.

Beginning with Lawrence Cranberg's handheld sensory aid for the U.S. Signal Corps in 1943, a progression of devices, which included the G-5 Obstacle detector and early Laser Cane prototypes, led to the introduction of the newest N8 Laser Cane in 1992. The foundation for the Laser Cane operating system is the Cranberg principle

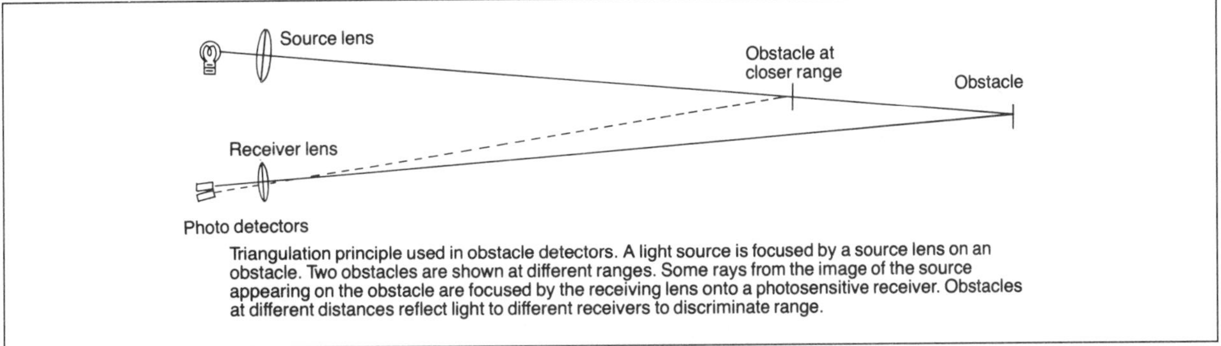

Triangulation principle used in obstacle detectors. A light source is focused by a source lens on an obstacle. Two obstacles are shown at different ranges. Some rays from the image of the source appearing on the obstacle are focused by the receiving lens onto a photosensitive receiver. Obstacles at different distances reflect light to different receivers to discriminate range.

Figure 7.8. Optical triangulation.

of optical triangulation, wherein the device emits pulses of infrared light, and reflections from an object in the path of the light are detected by photodetectors behind the receiving lens. The angle made by the diffusely reflected ray as it passes through a receiving lens is an indication of the distance to the object detected (Figure 7.8).

The current model, the N8 (Figure 7.9), reflects miniaturization and refinement based upon results of a survey of consumers by Blasch et al. (1989). One result was the elimination of the drop-off detection system of the previous models. Consumers reported that the use of this and the upper beam were less important than the forward beam. However, elimination of the lower beam would also reduce the cost by almost one-third. The old crook and body of the C-5 through ND-7 canes, which were formed from a single section of 1-inch (2.54-cm) diameter aluminum tubing, have been replaced by a plastic crook attached to an 0.875-inch (2.22-cm) aluminum body.

The N8 crook now houses a standard size rechargeable C cell instead of the curved custom battery utilized by former models. The lower fiberglass section (staff) of the N8 cane is attached by an elastic cord, which differs from the completely removable metal staff utilized by prior models.

The N8 Laser Cane utilizes two gallium-arsenide (GaAs) room-temperature injection lasers to project beams upward and forward for detection of objects in the path of the user. The

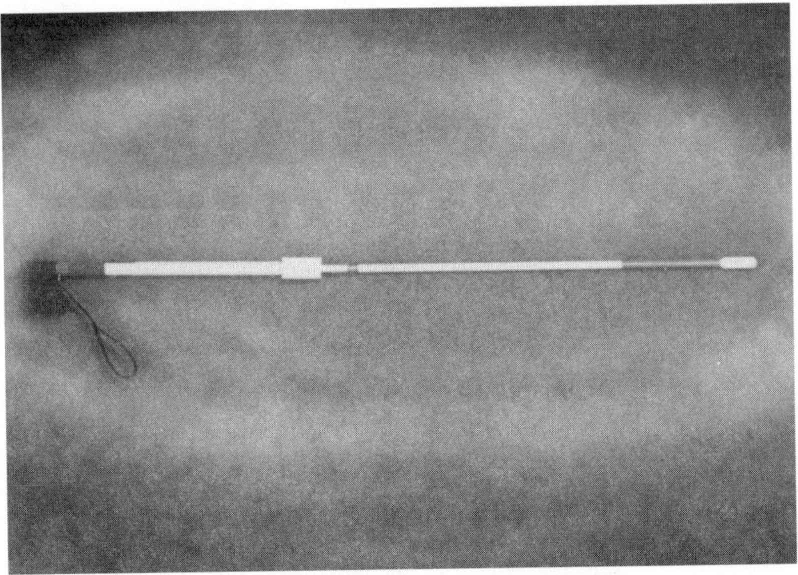

Figure 7.9. The Laser Cane, model N8.

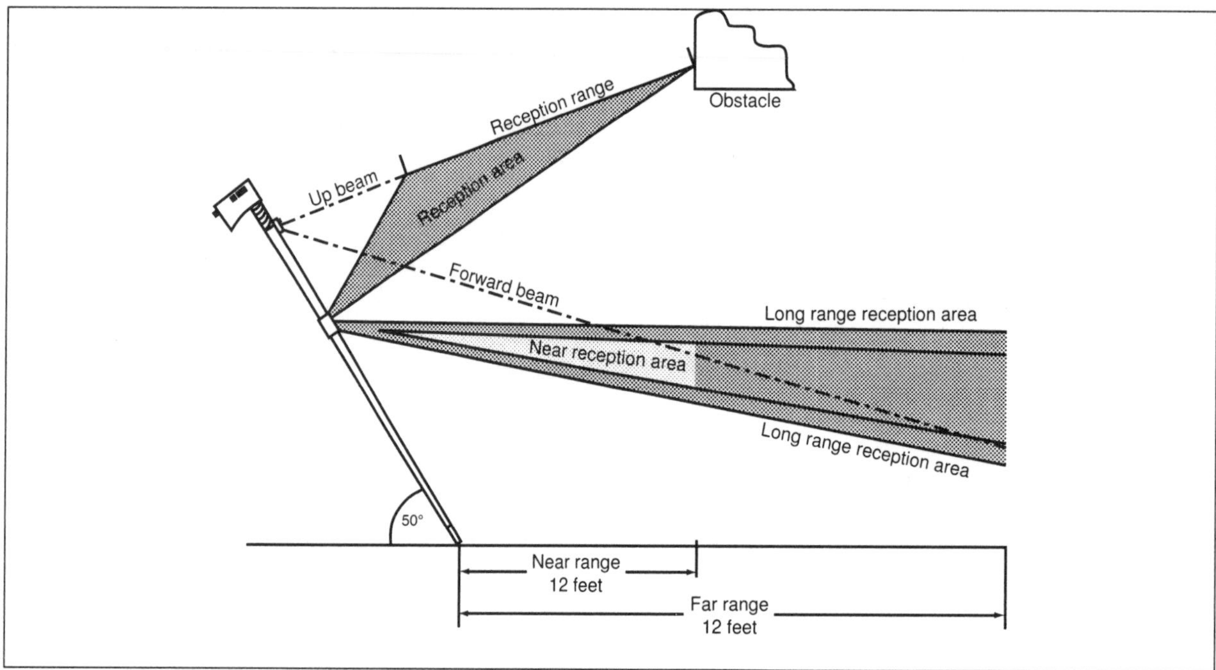

Figure 7.10. The Laser Cane beam path.

lasers emit 180-nanosecond pulses 80 times per second, with a wavelength of 905 nanometers. These tiny beams of invisible light have maximum dimensions of .25 inch (0.64 cm) high by 5 inches (12.7 cm) wide by 12 feet (3.66 m) long. The forward-projecting beam gives information about objects in the travel path and the immediate periphery, and the upward-projecting beam gives the user information about objects in the vicinity of the head (Figure 7.10).

The forward beam detects objects extending upward about 2 feet (0.60 m) from the walking surface. The forward channel has a range control that can be set to detect objects from a distance of 5 feet (1.50 m) to a maximum of 12 feet (3.60 m) from the cane tip. The range potential of the Laser Cane may be limited by the size, shape, or color (especially dark colors) of the object, or angle of approach to the object. When a maximum range is designated, it means that it was on the best possible target, a large and light-colored one. The forward-channel signal couples a medium pitch, 1800 Hz tone with a vibration of the lower tactile stimulator against the index finger.

The up-channel signal is a high-pitched tone of 2600 Hz coupled with a vibration of the upper tactile stimulator. The warning is activated by objects up to 30 inches (76 cm) in front of the cane tip and as high as 73 inches (1.85 m) above it. In addition to detecting overhangs, the up channel will respond to objects that extend from the walking surface up to head level. When the Laser Cane approaches a vertical surface, the forward-channel signal activates first at 12 or 5 feet (3.66 or 1.52 m), depending on the range selected. The up-channel signal activates 30 inches (76 cm) in front of the cane tip. Although the user can turn the auditory signal volume down or off, the tactile signal remains ready to respond.

When in use, the Laser Cane is pivoted laterally like the conventional long cane, with certain modifications of the long cane technique. This enables the user to receive peripheral information beyond the cane tip or to monitor pedestrians, guidelines, or automobiles. If the electronic elements fail to function, the traveler is still able to use the Laser Cane as a conventional, although somewhat heavier, long cane. The N8 weighs approximately 16 ounces (0.45 kg) compared to the long cane, which is approximately 8 ounces (0.225 kg).

The N8 Laser Cane disconnects and folds at approximately the middle for easy carrying or storage. The lower section contains no electronics and is made from a light fiberglass material. The cane is available in lengths from 42 to 54 inches (106 to 137 cm) in 1-inch (2.54 cm) increments. The lasers and transmitting optics, miniature electromagnetic speaker, tactile stimulators, laser-pulse drive circuits, sound-output volume control, receiving optics, printed circuit boards, and other electronics are housed in the upper section.

A 1.2-volt, 200-amp-hour, Ni-Cad rechargeable battery powers the N8 system and is located in the crook. The battery is user-replaceable, takes up to 15 hours to recharge, and provides for approximately 7 hours of continuous use between charges. A small battery charger is included with the cane. The N8 cane has a battery test switch that activates a high-pitched tone when the battery reserve is diminished to less than 1 hour of remaining operation.

Laser Hazard. When Laser Canes were introduced, the hazard of radiation exposure to the user was questioned. However, studies indicated that gallium-arsenide (GaAs) lasers used in the Laser Canes are of such low power that the radiation danger is negligible (Epstein & Meyer, 1970; Sliney & Freasier, 1969).

Benefits. The Laser Cane is more effective than the ultrasonic devices at locating objects at obtuse angles, due to the shorter energy wavelength. As a combined manual cane and ETA, the Laser Cane is the only device that can be used without an additional mobility device. With a narrow energy beam, the Laser Cane offers high precision for object location.

Limitations. Because the infrared beam is very narrow, one must be certain to keep the Laser Cane pointed in the direction of travel and have a consistent movement involving flexion-hyperextension of the wrist. Some potential users may not possess adequate motor and cane skills to utilize the Laser Cane, and its cost may prevent even the best candidate from acquiring the device.

Limitations of Type II Devices

Type II devices will not receive reflections from clear plate glass in windows and doors unless there is dirt on the glass or some object is within range behind the glass. However, it will detect door handles, frames, and kick plates. The beam will not pick up objects less than 9 to 18 inches (22.9 to 45.8 cm) high. Glossy and highly polished surfaces, particularly black, risk oblique reflection of the beam with consequent failure of forward-channel detection at maximum range. Heavy precipitation (particularly snow) causes the up- and forward-channel signals to go off constantly. Because the infrared beam is very narrow, it must be pointed in the direction of travel.

Type III Devices

Type III Devices (object preview and environmental information) provide environmental information in addition to object preview. A device in this category provides information about the characteristics of the objects detected.

Sonicguide

The Sonicguide, a derivation of the Binaural Sensory Aid (BSA), was developed by Dr. Leslie Kay at the University of Canterbury, Christchurch, New Zealand. Dr. Derek Rowell's collaborative and other research (1970) resulted in improvements in the auditory display of spatial information.

The Sonicguide exemplifies the analog system (that is, it emits a continuously variable signal), collecting and displaying an abundance of environmental information to the user with the option of using all or whatever part of the messages one wishes to use, or is capable of using. As

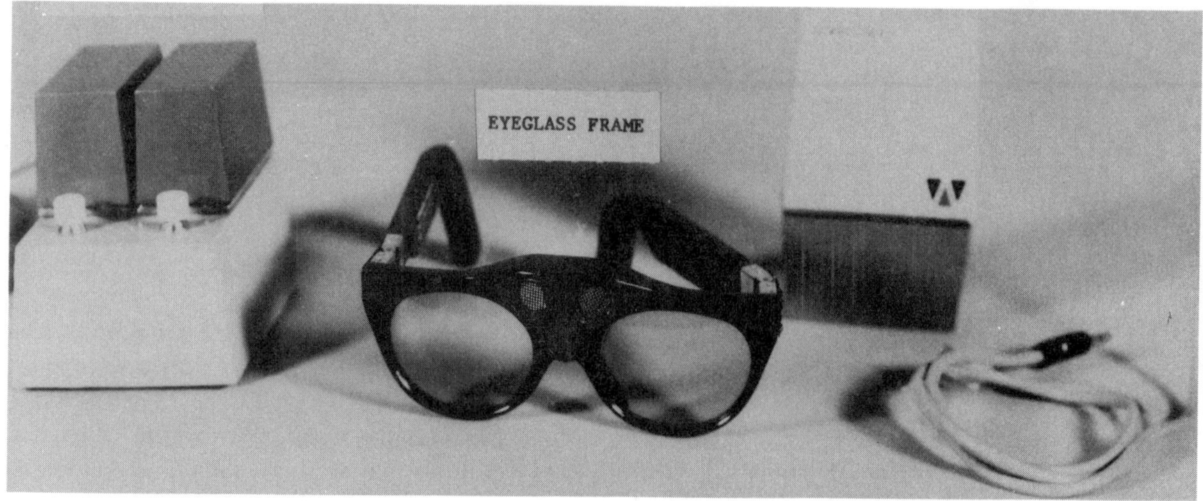

Figure 7.11. The Sonicguide.

Russell (1966) suggests, the Sonicguide gives the text rather than the headlines delivered by such go-no-go ETAs. The aid was designed to give the user who is visually impaired greater perception of the environment through the auditory sense (Kay, et al., 1971). It supplies the user with three kinds of information: distance estimation, directional appreciation, and interpretation of tonal characteristics that make primitive object identification possible; the latter, however, is possible only with much practice and experience.

The Sonicguide detects objects from above the head to about knee height. The sides of the body are more than adequately protected by the very wide sonic cone, which exceeds 45 degrees to the right and left of the body's medial plane.

The Sonicguide is a secondary ETA to be used in conjunction with either a dog guide or long cane (Figure 7.11). The electronics, which consist of three miniature, wide-band transducers (a central tiny ultrasonic transmitter located just above the bridge of the nose), and two small microphones (receivers) above and on each side of the loudspeaker (transmitter), are housed in a pair of spectacles and a control box. The auditory output is directed into the ears by means of custom-fitted ear molds that result in minimal obstruction (5 to 10 decibels) of ambient sound. Echos coming from the right side are heard by the right ear and echos coming from the left side are heard by the left ear. Sounds coming from straight ahead are heard in both ears simultaneously (Figure 7.12).

The Sonicguide signals enable the user to estimate distance by relating it to pitch. The transmitting transducer generates electrical signals that are converted into ultrasonic waves and pulsed out into the environment. At the nominal 13.1-foot (4-m) range, users with good hearing can detect specular targets (large, smooth surfaces such as walls or plate glass) at a maximum range of 20 feet (6 m). The effective range with diffuse objects (smaller or rough surfaces such as trees or foliage) is 12 to 15 feet (3.6 to 4.5 m).

Object Identification by Signal Timbre. The Sonicguide enables perception of tonal characteristics that give information about the nature of the presenting surface, whether it is specular or diffuse, as well as its range, direction, and dimensions. If a user "looks" at a smooth, round aluminum post, the reflected echoes will have a single-frequency, pure-tone quality. However, a tree presents many branches and leaves with multiple-frequency components. The echoes reflected from these surfaces will be scattered, presenting an electronic image of the complexity of a tree through signals with a scratchy, harsh quality.

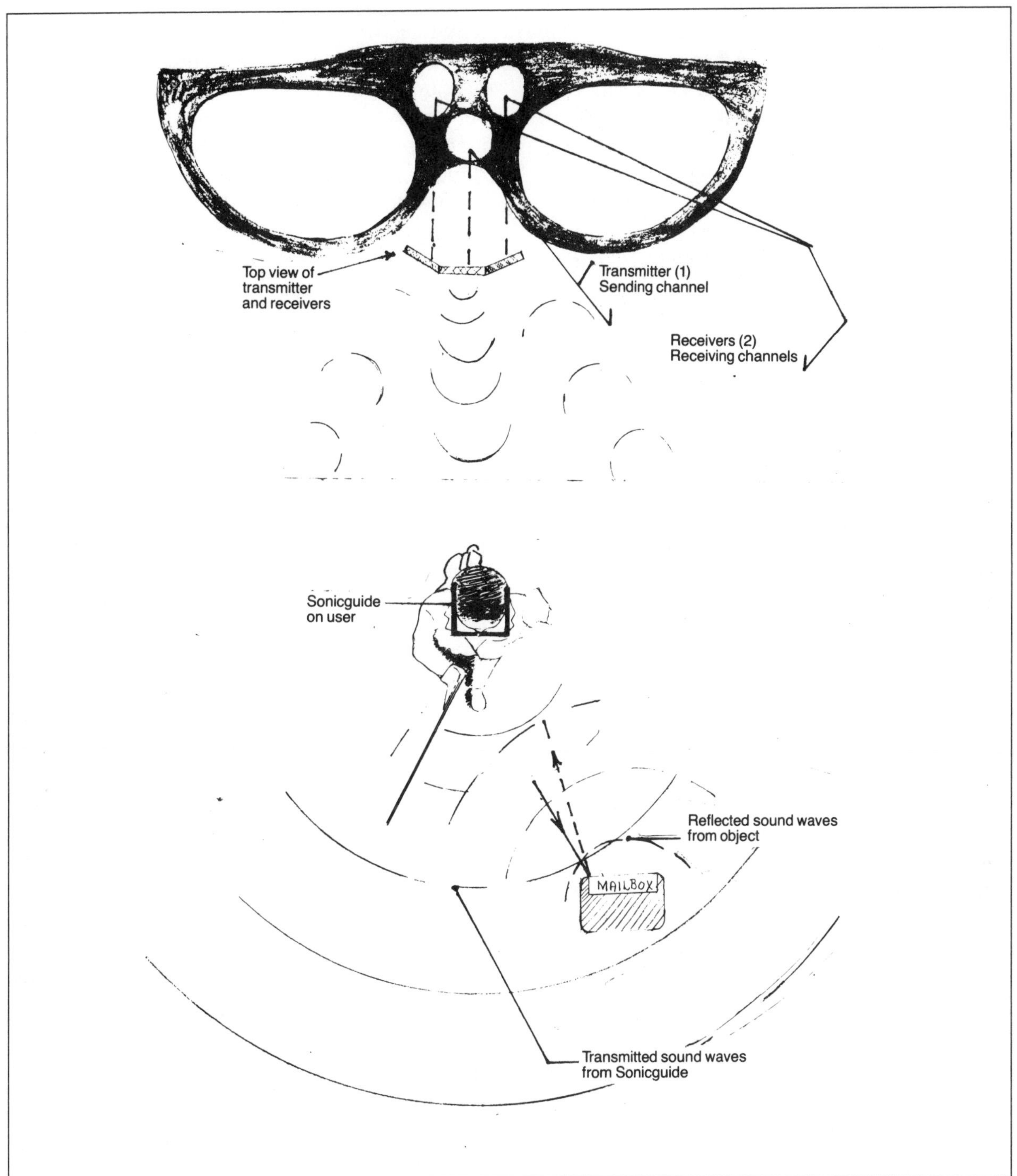

Figure 7.12. Diagram of Sonicguide signals.

Power. The power supply is housed in a small control box, not much larger than a deck of cards, with an On–Off/volume control knob. The control box is connected to the left temple of the spectacle frame by a flexible cable. A battery charger supplied with the Sonicguide accommodates two rechargeable Ni-Cad batteries. A fully charged battery lasts 5 hours, and a 14-hour recharge will restore a totally discharged battery.

The Sonicguide Training Aid for Children incorporates smaller eyeglass frames with adjustable temples. The aid was designed for use in concept development, and as an environmental training aid to enhance spatial awareness and sound localization skills in children who are visually impaired. Strelow (1983) observed that children with visual impairments were able to improve their distance awareness and object categorization skills with the use of the Sonicguide for Children. A more recent study (Hill, Dodson-Burk, Hill, & Fox, 1995) has shown the Sonicguide's effectiveness at helping teach children with visual impairments and developmental delays to reach out and locate objects.

Benefits. The Sonicguide is the only device that offers the user information about the character of the environment, from texture to shape and relative size. The ability to simultaneously detect objects at multiple ranges with the same energy beacon is unique to the Sonicguide and the Kaspa (see below).

Limitations. In addition to the fact that the Sonicguide does not offer detection of drop-offs and is expensive, there are other limitations. High winds can affect reception, and it may lose sensitivity in heavy rains or become inoperable in snowstorms because of constant echoes from snowflakes. Users will encounter ambient disturbances from neon signs, although they could be used as landmarks in areas frequented by a traveler. Electronic security systems utilized by many retail establishments, particularly in shopping malls, might present so many unexplained signals that it could render the device ineffective. The Sonicguide output is auditory, and the signals quite possibly could be masked in certain very noisy situations. In addition, hearing losses associated with aging may make this device difficult for some elderly people to use. Another serious limitation is that the Sonicguide may interfere with ambient environmental sounds. Finally, at this time the Sonicguide may not be available for purchase.

The Next Generation. The Sonicguide has been taken out of production at the time of this writing. Dr. Kay has continued development with a new generation of devices. His research with a post-Sonicguide prototype device called the Trisensor has continued with the advent of Kaspa. The Kaspa incorporates the wide-angle (up to 80 degrees wide), binaural channels of the Sonicguide with a narrow-angle (6 degrees wide), central channel. Dr. Kay correlates this three-channel system to the central and peripheral fields of the visual pathway. The user can focus the central beam on an object, such as a light pole, for exact location, while still monitoring the peripheral information from the wide binaural channels. The Kaspa, according to Dr. Kay, has increased directional coding and has lower background noise than the Sonicguide.

Type IV Devices

Type IV mobility devices (obstacle preview and artificial intelligence) differ from Types I, II, and III in that artificial intelligence is a component. This addition has been accomplished by having the device controlled by a computer. The only device in this category is the Sonic Pathfinder.

Sonic Pathfinder

During the mid-1970s Dr. Tony Heyes and other researchers at Nottingham University developed an ETA called the Nottingham Obstacle Detector (NOD). Although the NOD was never produced in large quantities, its design provided the founda-

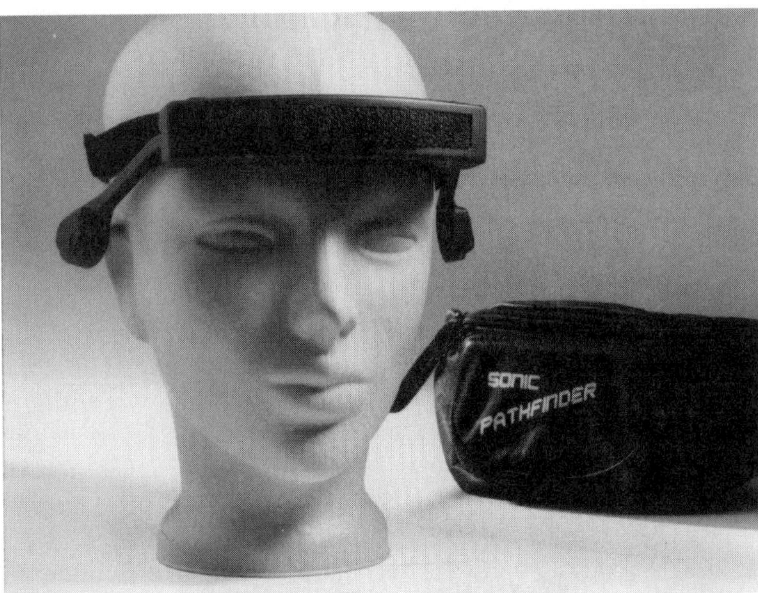

Figure 7.13. The Sonic Pathfinder.

tion for the Sonic Pathfinder, which defines a new class of computer-controlled ETAs that utilize what Dr. Heyes refers to as "artificial intelligence" (1993).

The Sonic Pathfinder (Figure 7.13) is an ultrasonic sonar device with two transmitting and three receiving transducers mounted within a molded plastic headband. The two transmitters flood the user's path with a wide beam of ultrasonic energy. Three ultrasonic receivers detect ultrasound echoed from objects in the pathway. A ribbon cable connects the headband to a control box that houses the microcomputer control circuitry and the Ni-Cad rechargeable battery. An overnight charge enables the battery to provide 30 hours of continuous use. A 9-volt alkaline battery can be plugged into the recharging socket for backup power. The control box is housed in a waist-belted, compartmentalized carrying case (hip pack). Since ranging is automatic, the only external control is a power/volume knob.

Once processed by a microcomputer, the echoes are encoded to notes on a major musical scale. The musical notes vary as a function of distance: high-pitched notes for distant objects and low-pitched notes for near objects. The musical notes sound from miniature speakers mounted in arms (earpieces) that are hinged to the headband at an adjustable angle to hang in front of the ears. The Sonic Pathfinder alerts the user to objects directly in front with a tone to both ears, and objects to the side with a tone to only the corresponding ear.

In the absence of an object in the direct travel path, the device displays objects to the side with a tone to only the corresponding ear. The artificial intelligence within the device continuously adjusts the range of the device to suit the walking speed of the user. Information overload is eliminated by restricting the display to only those objects that will be encountered during the next 2 seconds of travel.

Benefits. The Sonic Pathfinder provides the user with clear pathway information. Its "artificial intelligence" shields the user from confusing information about objects out of the pathway or beyond 2 seconds of travel time. This simplification of information presentation may enhance the user's rate of travel and make the Sonic Pathfinder useful with less training.

Limitations. Some users may be confused by the "artificially intelligent" ranging adjustments. Familiar objects and landmarks may become momentarily undetectable if the range has been automatically shortened either in crowded areas or when the user looks at a close object for an extended period of time.

The chart (see Figure 7.14) represents a summary of the four types of ETAs and some of the characteristics that are relevant for students.

ELECTRONIC ORIENTATION AIDS

Electronic orientation aids (EOAs) are used for orientation and navigation enhancement. This is a new category of devices used for the purpose of providing orientation to the environment prior to or during travel. Some of these devices may be external to the user and mounted on poles or walls while other devices are carried with the traveler.

Talking Signs®

Smith Kettlewell Institute of Visual Sciences developed a navigation aid (Talking Signs®) that utilizes infrared light transmitters and handheld receivers. Brief spoken auditory messages are encoded in the invisible infrared broadcast signal. When the user aims the 2.4 × 3.8 inch (6.1 × 9.7 cm) receivers at a Talking Sign® transmitter within 10 to 60 feet (3 to 18.3 m) of its range, the speech message can be heard. In a study comparing the Talking Sign® system with the Verbal Landmarks system, Bentzen and Mitchell (1993) found that the Talking Sign® system decreased the need for assistance and time to locate a destination in unfamiliar settings.

Marco

Marco is another infrared light transmitter and receiver system that has more recently become available. Marco is comparable with Talking Signs® systems and provides similar benefits for navigation. Receivers with a range of up to 50 feet (15.2 m) measure 5 × 3 inches (12.7 × 7.62 cm) and weighs 7 ounces (198 g).

Verbal Landmarks

Verbal Landmarks is a wayfinding tool that utilizes inductive loop radio signals. The user hears a spoken message when the portable receiver is within 5 feet (1.5 m) of the transmitter. While the infrared system relies upon line-of-sight transmission, the inductive loop system can transmit through obstacles such as people. Verbal Landmarks systems will often broadcast extensive messages that offer a more comprehensive introduction to the environment.

POSITION LOCATOR DEVICES

Directional Sensors

Compasses, either manual or electronic, have a place in the travel schemes of some persons with visual impairments. Compasses are used for establishing a line of travel and verifying the integrity of one's directional orientation while the user is stationary.

Electronic compasses provide the user with eight possible spoken announcements, including the cardinal directions and intermediate compass points. Experimentation is continuing with gyroscopic compasses, which are currently priced beyond the means of the average traveler. Although the electronic compass may be less accurate, requires battery power, and is more likely to be effected by temperature changes and environmental magnetic fields, it has some advantages. The electronic compass may be less susceptible to user errors through improper positioning or manipulation, and may be more useful to those users with impaired tactile sensitivity, due to its audible output.

Type	Device	Cost	Display Output	Energy System	Beam Coverage	Range Selections	Short Range Coverage Height/Width (ft.)	Long Range Coverage Height/Width (ft.)	Mounting	Battery Type	Hours of Use per Charge	Recharge Time	Learning Difficulty	Student Characteristics: Unilateral Impairment	Non-Ambulatory	Support Cane	Sensory Integration Impairment	Residual Vision	Hearing Impairment	Rapid Walking	Motor Impairment
TYPE I	Pathsounder	$1300	DV DS	US	U	2.7/6	NA	2/2	Neck Worn	Perm NC	2–5	14	↑	↑	↑	↑	↑	→	↑	→	↑
TYPE I	Mowat Sensor	$850	CV	US	K H	3/13	1.75/.86	7/3.5	Hand Held	NC/Alk 9V	8	12	↑	↓	↓	↓	↑	↑	↑	↑	→
TYPE I	Polaron	$870	CV CS	US	K H	4/8/16	1.5/1.5	5/5	Hand Held/ Neck Worn	NC/Alk 9V	3	14	↑	↑	↑	↑	→	↑	↑	↑	→
TYPE I	Sensory 6	$895	DS	US	U	6/11	.75/1.5	1.5/3	Head Worn	NC 5V	8	14	→	↑	↑	↑	→	↓	↓	↑	↓
TYPE I	Walkmate	$185	DV DS	US	K H	7.3	NA	7/2	Body Worn	NC 9V & Alk 1.5V	10	14	↑	↑	↓	→	↑	→	↑	→	↑
TYPE II	Wheelchair Pathfinder	$3500	FS *FV	US &L	F	***1/ 4/4/8	F2.2/2.5	F4.5/2.8	W/C Mount	NC 9V	6	14	↑	↑	↑	↓	→	→	↓	↓	↑
TYPE II	Laser Cane	$2500	FV FS	L	K H	**2.5/ 5/12	U2.2/3 F6/3	F1.1/3	Hand Held	NC/Alk 1.5V	7	14	→	↑	↓	→	↑	↑	↓	↑	↓
III	Sonicguide	$6000	CS	US	F	13	NA	15/26	Head Worn	NC 12V	2	14	→	↑	↑	↑	→	→	↓	↑	→
IV	Sonic Pathfinder	$2500	U	US	U	13	NA	2.5/6	Head Worn	Perm NC	16	14	↑	↑	↑	↑	→	↑	↓	↑	→

Key:
Output Codes: C = Continuously Variable, D = Discrete Zones, F = Fixed Zone, V = Vibration, S = Sound
Energy Codes: US = Ultrasound, L = Laser Light
Beam Coverage Codes: U = Upper Body, KH = Knee to Head, F = Full Body

Key to Symbols
↑ = Best
→ = Good
↓ = Fair

*Wheelchair Pathfinder vibratory signal is optional
**Laser Cane Ranges: Up Channel = 2.5 feet, Forward Channel = 5 and 12 feet
***Wheelchair Pathfinder: Side Channels = 1 foot, Drop Off Channel = 4 feet, Forward Channels = 4 and 8 feet

Figure 7.14. Summary of ETAs and their characteristics.

Global Positioning Systems

The Global Positioning System (GPS), a technology that has long been used by the military for precision navigation and location information, is now useful and available to travelers with visual impairments. The GPS receivers utilize precisely timed data signals from 3 of 24 available orbiting satellites to determine longitude and latitude. This system becomes useful when the position data is fed into a computerized database and actual street addresses, stored landmarks, and wayfinding points may be relayed to the user at the appropriate time. Within the foreseeable future, the size, weight, and cost of receivers should be within the financial means of some consumers. GPS systems require a clear line of reception from the satellite, thus tall buildings or other obstructing objects may impair or prevent signal reception. GPS devices designed for use by travelers who are visually impaired are on the immediate horizon.

Strider and Atlas Speaks

Arkenstone, a nonprofit corporation, plans to release Strider, a GPS receiving system, in the second half of 1997. Strider, when coupled with Atlas Speaks' "talking map" software and a talking notebook computer, will notify travelers of their current location and help them follow paths plotted ahead of time.

MoBIC Project

The MoBIC (Mobility of Blind and Elderly People Interacting with Computers) Consortium in Europe conducted research field trials in Berlin, Germany, in 1995 and in Birmingham, England, in 1996. The MoBIC device couples GPS signals with an electronic map and synthetic speech. Research and development continues toward the development of a small, lightweight, and less expensive device.

TRAINING ISSUES AND STRATEGIES FOR ETAS

Requirements for Users

It is important for organizations and O&M specialists to assess candidates for the potential use of an ETA and provide students with choices and options. At the present, there is no universally accepted list of requirements for participation, although agencies with ETA programs usually have their own guidelines by which they determine the eligibility of applicants for available programs.

Students should be evaluated based upon their individual needs and characteristics. One guideline that might be considered for candidate selection is whether remaining vision is sufficiently limited as to prevent reliable visual detection of obstacles beyond the ETAs range. When the candidate has more remaining vision, the ETA output may be ignored or distracting or confusing. Another guideline may be the physical ability of the candidate to participate in and complete the training program.

Further guidelines should consider the travel history of the candidate, past and present level of competence, confidence with the primary travel mode, current and future travel needs, and whether travel is in unfamiliar as well as familiar areas. The O&M specialist must consider degree of activity or inactivity and whether the activity is occupational, recreational, civic, or other. If travel is primarily occupational, does the person work in a professional building, factory, office, or on a farm, or perhaps is the person a student?

The O&M specialist must ascertain, in consultation with the student, sensitivity to public reaction, cosmetic acceptability, subtlety of the signal output, and attitudes and reactions of significant others. Careful consideration must be given to the geographical area in which the individual lives and travels, whether the area is urban, rural, residential, or a combination of any of these.

The obvious factors to be considered in

matching a person to a aid are auditory discriminability, visual acuity, motivation, and cost benefit (which ultimately rests with the individual) in terms of time, effort, and money. Two researchers, de Haas and Weisgerber (1978), discussed a series of matching trials that could be utilized to match the proper ETA to a particular user.

Length of Training

The length of training with a device will be influenced by factors including the complexity of the device, the learning speed and needs of the student, staff availability, and financial limitations. The ideal length of training will range from 20 to 120 hours, depending on the student, complexity of the device, and diversity of travel environments in which the device will be used. The Association for Education and Rehabilitation of the Blind and Visually Impaired Division Nine ETA Certification standard recommended minimum training times for ETAs as follows: Sonicguide—40 hours, Laser Cane—20 hours, Pathsounder—8 hours, Mowat Sensor—8 hours. (For further information on training methods and formats on ETAs, see specific training manuals of the devices as well as articles by Farmer [1975], Jackson [1977], and Baird [1977].)

Factors Affecting Use

The majority of ETA users will not utilize the device continuously during all travel (Blasch et al., 1989). Most travelers will choose to use the ETA intermittently, turning the device on when in unfamiliar environments or a crowded environment, and off when in a more familiar, safe, and less crowded environment. When traveling with friends or family, the user may leave the ETA at home. Blasch et al. (1989), in their national survey of ETA use, questioned people on the use of their ETAs in the last 3, 30, and 180 days (see Table 7.1). The reported use of ETAs was much higher than that predicted by O&M specialists.

Table 7.1. Reported Use of Each ETA in the Last 3, 30, and 180 Days

Type of Device	Number of Persons Trained	Respondents Reported Use (percentage) 3 Days	30* Days	180 Days
Mowat Sensor	123	35	59	78
Sonicguide	109	13	25	40
Laser Cane	75	53	65	69
Pathsounder	10	10	20	60

*Definition of user and former user in this study was based on whether or not use was reported in the past 30 days.

ETAs have proven their effectiveness in reducing anxiety through advance knowledge of the presence and location of objects and people in the environment. This preview reduces the possibility of embarrassment through unwanted personal contact with people. Based on recent research (Blasch & De l'Aune, 1992; Blasch et al., 1996), the long cane provides far less coverage than previously believed (see Figure 7.2). The addition of an appropriate ETA could significantly enhance the coverage and preview provided by the long cane. The cosmetic appearance of the device also plays an important role in choice and frequency of utilization. Oftentimes significant others offer their opinions and advice as to the cosmetic acceptability of the device. This impact on device use should be considered during the selection process.

USE AND TRAINING FOR ETAS

The advent of audible signage, digital maps, and global positioning systems (GPS) opens new wayfinding possibilities for persons who are blind or visually impaired. The development of these electronic systems creates a greater degree of psychological comfort and independence for blind people than could be attained with earlier technology. At the same time, however, the new technology poses numerous problems related to the interface of these systems with the blind user. In the future it will be necessary to consider how to provide the most efficient control of the equipment, the most accuracy, the most appropriate level of digital map content, the smallest size and best placement of hardware, and the selection of software that is easy to operate and has enough flexibility to allow for presentation of various levels of information (Blasch & Long, 1994). In addition it is important to consider the type and length of training necessary for effective use of the device.

It is hypothesized that there are at least two different levels of users who are blind, each with different requirements for system interface and orientation information. The first group of users may typically require exact routing and specific directions for navigation. The second group of users may rely more on area overview information and may need fairly general directions. While system requirements are quite clear for the first group of users (a specific route can be provided and—in the case of GPS—the navigating system can control against the deviations from that route), this is not the case for the second group. Creating a mental image of street patterns detailed enough for confident navigation, and providing this geographic image during the trip, is a problem that will require additional study. It appears that different blind users have different requirements for software and data. While the quality of street maps (with information about landmarks, sidewalks, and traffic) is critical for the first group of users, in the second case information needs to be presented that would allow the user to build a mental image of a street pattern based on partial information. In this latter case, information about parallel streets in the distance, connecting streets, and landmarks, may be more important than simple positioning information. These are issues which will need to be studied so that appropriate information can be provided and effective training strategies can be developed.

THE FUTURE OF ELECTRONIC MOBILITY DEVICES AND ELECTRONIC ORIENTATION SYSTEMS

Technological advances offer many possibilities for travelers who are visually impaired. The biggest inhibition to the availability of new technology is cost and market size. Cellular phone technology may be adaptable as a source of location information; this technology is used to track fleets of vehicles but currently lacks the precision afforded by GPSs.

Micropower impulse radar (MIR) is a new technology that uses extremely low power (1 microwatt) radio waves in very rapid randomized pulses (1 million pulses per second) to detect objects and movement. The tiny $1\frac{1}{2}$-inch square circuitboard could be incorporated into a new ETA. A low estimated cost of the technology, due to a large market, may make it an inexpensive choice for future devices (Stover, 1995) These advances notwithstanding, the need for a small, lightweight, inexpensive, situational-use ETA still has not been met.

Entrepreneurs

The entrepreneur who chooses to develop a new electronic travel device is faced with significant challenges. Since the market for new devices is limited, one or two people often perform multifaceted roles in development, testing, marketing, and support. Consultation with experienced researchers, O&M practitioners, and consumers is essential throughout the development process.

There is a concern about the proliferation of devices and misdirected efforts and use of resources. A systematic approach is needed for identification of areas of specific personal needs (e.g., the elderly, and hearing impaired and multiply impaired populations), funding, design, and development of devices to meet those needs, testing of prototypes, and development of training strategies. Too often one or two of these issues are not addressed during the development of new devices, thus resulting in failure. Often there are accompanying news items that offer false hope to consumers and result in shallow promises.

Electrocortical Prosthesis

ETAs now in use are designed to aid in orientation and mobility performance only. Research is in progress to try to develop a substitute for vision that may be useful not only for mobility, but also in education, employment, and leisure activities. An electrocortical prosthesis or a vision substitution system that bypasses the visual pathway is the focus of a few ongoing research projects.

Richard Stone (1990) discussed several research projects at the National Institutes of Health's Neural Prosthesis Program, in which scientists hope to develop a phosphene prosthesis that will enable people who are visually impaired to read and identify objects. A silicon microelectrode array prosthesis in which tiny probes are inserted about 2 millimeters into the brain has been the focus of research.

Problems to be surmounted include corrosion of the electrodes as well as brain tissue growth that results in insulation of the electrodes. Some researchers have experimented with various chemicals and dyes which, when applied to the surface brain tissue, make it possible to stimulate phosphenes without inserting electrodes (De Witt, 1988).

SUMMARY

The impact of ETAs on the rehabilitation of people who are blind has been somewhat disappointing. They do, however, offer advantages and choices to many people with visual impairments, addressing many travel needs. Even though ETAs have not lived up to expectations, research in this area has provided important information relating to the nature of the requirements of the mobility task for individuals with a visual impairment.

An O&M specialist may question the future of electronic travel aids and sensory systems, however, the value and potential for supplementary use of ETAs has been established. It is important to inform individuals who receive instruction in orientation and mobility about ETAs and to help make devices more easily available.

O&M specialists should play an active role in the refinement of the use of these devices. As EOAs continue to evolve and become available, their use should be incorporated into route planning and navigation through the environment. These devices will assist individuals to better plan their travel and identify their location along their travel path. With continued development, devices should become smaller, more reliable, and easier to use. They represent a leap forward in independent travel.

Suggestions/Implications for O&M Specialists

1. There are four types of mobility systems or tools for getting about: human guide, canes, dog guides, and Electronic Travel Aids (ETAs).
2. The function of these mobility systems or tools is to provide information about the travel path in advance of entering the space. With the long cane and ETA, the individual is concerned about the type and amount of coverage the specific device provices.
3. The function of a mobility device such as a cane, is to preview the immediate environment for (a) objects in the path of travel (i.e., object preview), (b) changes in the surface of travel (i.e., surface preview), and (c) the integrity of the surface upon which the foot is to be placed when brought forward (i.e., foot placement preview). Specifically, with the cane, echo location information is functionally available for the traveler.
4. Mobility training focuses on three general areas: devices, skills, and strategies.
5. Several types of canes and walking aids are manufactured to meet the varied needs and demands of persons with visual impairments. Based upon Hoover's pioneering efforts, consumers, engineers, manufacturers, and mobility specialists have since worked in concert toward the continued development of the long cane and refinement of the techniques and strategies employed in its use.
6. Instructors have a responsibility for acquainting students with the various available cane styles.
7. An ETA is a device that emits energy waves to explore the environment within a certain range or distance, processes reflected information, and furnishes the user with certain information about the immediate environment. The device should probe the immediate area and present the detected information to the traveler in an intelligible and useful manner. Blasch, Long, and Griffin-Shirley (1989) state further that ETAs are ". . . devices that transform information about the environment that would normally be relayed through vision into a form that can be conveyed through another sensory modality."
8. Two opposing viewpoints relative to device display and output have been expressed by Russell and Kay. Russell stated that an aid should simply display information indicating to the traveler whether the travel path is or is not clear; a "go-no-go system." Kay's approach has been to display the maximum amount of environmental information that the auditory channel could effectively transmit to enable the user to focus attention on pertinent information (analog system).
9. An ETA can provide a degree of sensory information about the environment which would not be possible using only a long cane or dog guide, such as, range, direction, dimension and height of objects and as with Kay's device character of the environment.
10. Relatively new implementation of technology has researchers introducing or experimenting with use of the Global Positioning System (GPS) and cellular communications systems for orientation and navigation enhancement. The

(*continued on next page*)

Suggestions/Implications for O&M Specialists (continued)

reader will need to evaluate this new technology, as it matures, based upon its true merits for the consumer.

11. Researchers should always keep in mind that consultation with experienced researchers, O&M practitioners, and consumers is essential throughout the development process.
12. Specialists should expect further development in American Deaf Association regulation of signage for potential standardization and possible inclusion of spoken signs or navigational aids.
13. It is important for organizations and O&M specialists to assess candidates for potential use of an ETA and other mobility devices and to provide students with choices and options. Sensitivity to public reaction, cosmetic acceptability, subtlety of the signal output, and attitudes and reactions of significant others play a strong role in the selection of a mobility device.
14. The majority of ETA users will not utilize the device continuously during all travel. Most travelers will use the ETA intermittently, depending on the travel environment.

ACTIVITIES FOR REVIEW

1. Name three key functions of a mobility device.
2. Explain why many travel canes have been coated with materials other than white paint.
3. Discuss the considerations a traveler should take into account when choosing between collapsible/folding or one piece rigid travel canes.
4. What three general components must go hand-in-hand to make an effective travel schema.
5. What factors have prevented high percentage utilization of ETAs by travelers with visual impairments.
6. Name essential sources of information with which the entrepreneur must consult to increase the probability of success in the development of mobility devices.
7. Name potential population groups said to benefit from alternative mobility devices.
8. Name and describe the two functional systems for determination of range mentioned in the text.
9. Identify two potential technology systems (not marketed at press time) for future ETAs.
10. Name the two brands of devices which share the same general infrared light transmission/reception sign system originally developed by the Smith Kettlewell Institute of Visual Sciences.

CHAPTER 8

Dog Guides

Robert H. Whitstock, Lukas Franck, and Rodney Haneline

Humans have long found the instincts, skills, intelligence, and senses of dogs useful in many varied capacities. In exchange for the warmth of the hearth, affection, and food, the speed and protectiveness of the dog has been used to guard the home and flock. Its keen scent and sight has been used in the hunt and to search for the lost. In ancient times the dog was used as a weapon of war. It is also certain that the phenomenon of the dog guide was well known in many cultures of antiquity.

Images of dogs acting as guides to people who were blind are seen in ancient Chinese paintings, on the walls of Pompeii, and in Rembrandt etchings from the 17th century (Coon, 1959). These dogs were probably trained by their owners, but we can only speculate on what tasks they performed and how they fulfilled their functions.

The systematic training of dogs to act as guides for people who are blind did not begin until the end of the First World War. In 1925 and again in 1926, a wealthy American dog fancier, trainer, and breeder of German Shepherds named Dorothy Harrison Eustis (see Figure 8.1) observed one of several German programs in which German Shepherds were trained to guide blinded veterans of the First World War. This program was no doubt in part based on the 19th-century work by Father Johann Klein (Figure 8.2).

At that time the independence, mobility, and social integration of Americans who were blind were severely inhibited. Consequently, in 1927 when Eustis wrote "The Seeing Eye" for *The Saturday Evening Post* describing the German program, it created great interest. One of the many letters she received was from a young Tennessean named Morris Frank, who had been blinded as a teenager (see Figure 8.3).

Frank persuaded Eustis, and her trainer, the geneticist Elliot S. (Jack) Humphrey (Figure 8.4), to train a dog for him at her Fortunate Fields breeding and training center in Vevey, Switzerland (Figure 8.5). It was understood that after training with the dog (a female German Shepherd who came to be named "Buddy") in Switzerland, Frank would return to the United States to test her under American conditions (see Figure 8.6).

This experiment was so successful that Eustis decided to devote her full energies to developing dog guide services for men and women who were blind in both the United States and in other European countries. In January 1929 she and Frank formally established The Seeing Eye, Inc., in Nashville, Frank's hometown; but in June of that year they moved it to Morris County, New Jersey (Putnam, 1979).

In 1938 Donald Schuur and the Detroit Lions Club laid the groundwork for the second organized, nonprofit dog guide school in North America. Leader Dogs for the Blind graduated its first class of four in 1939.

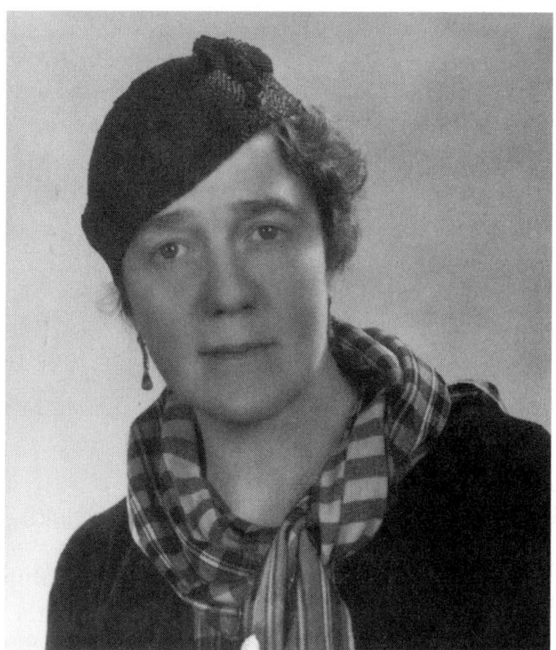

Figure 8.1. Dorothy Harrison Eustis.

Guide Dogs for the Blind in San Rafael, California, was founded in 1942 to try to meet the needs of West Coast veterans of the Second World War who were blind. Its founders were its first two instructors: Chalmers R. (Don) Donaldson and Lois W. Merrihew, and a group of volunteers known as the American Women's Voluntary Services. Many other schools also have their roots in the postwar period.

Guiding Eyes for the Blind in Yorktown Heights, New York, was founded in 1956 by Donald Z. Kauth. It is now one of the four largest schools in the United States, based on yearly graduates. Over the years many other schools have opened their doors.

WHAT DOG GUIDES DO

Dogs guide in response to a specific set of commands given by voice and hand signals. They pull their handlers with the same type of forward motion people use when doing sighted guide technique.

In urban areas a dog guides the person who is visually impaired from the beginning to the end of each block. Once there, the dog stops to indicate the surface change at the juncture of the street and sidewalk. Then the dog waits for the next command, which may be either "Forward," "Left," or "Right." The command tells the dog to

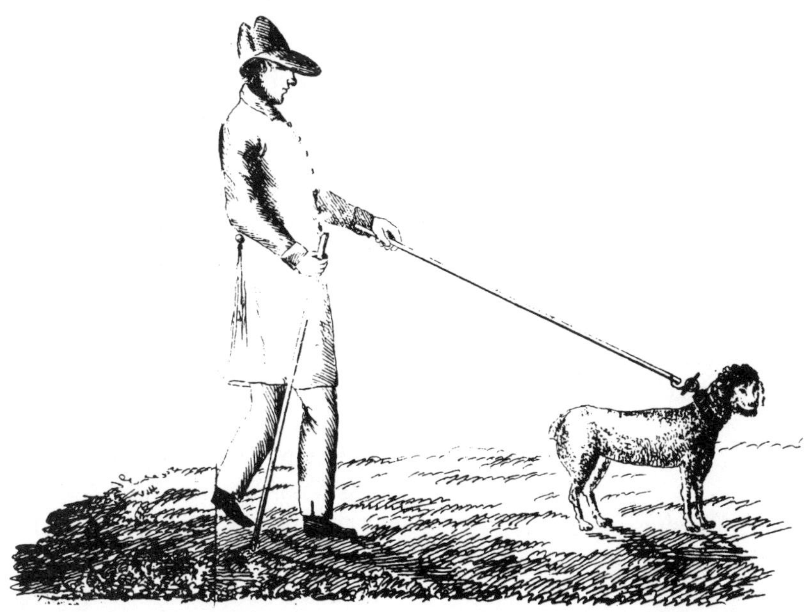

Figure 8.2. Dog guide on a rigid leash as described by Father Johann Wilhelm Klein (1819).

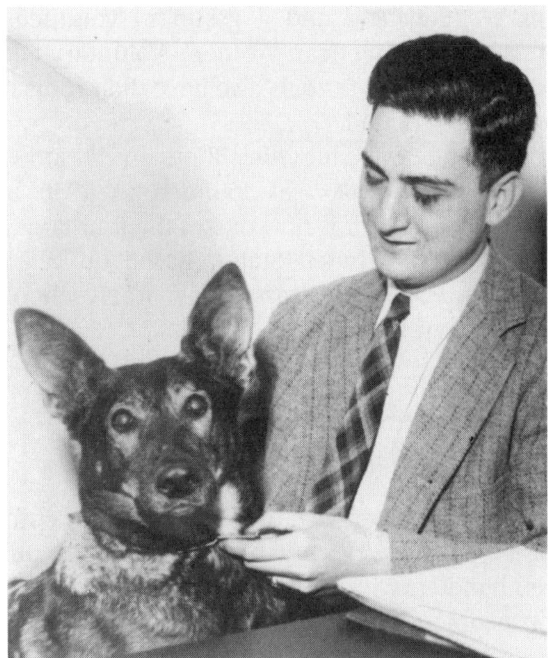

Figure 8.3. Morris Frank and Buddy.

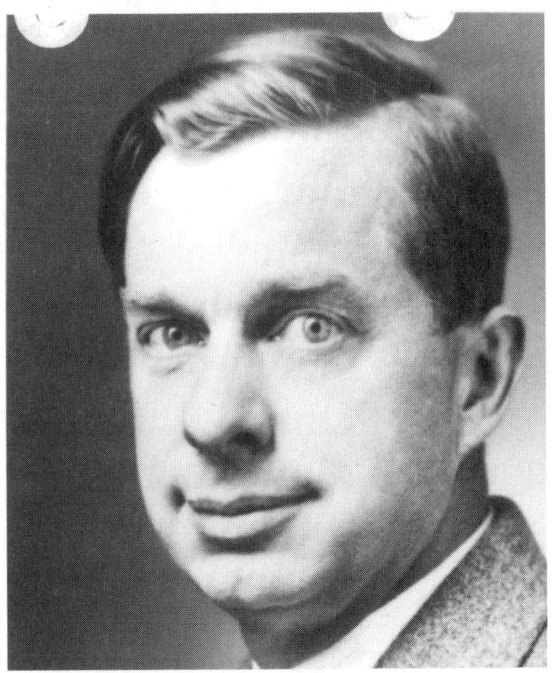

Figure 8.4. Elliot S. (Jack) Humphrey.

turn, if necessary, and begin guiding in the direction indicated. The handler will initiate a street crossing with the "Forward" command.

In areas without sidewalks, dog guides closely shoreline the left edge of the road, working facing

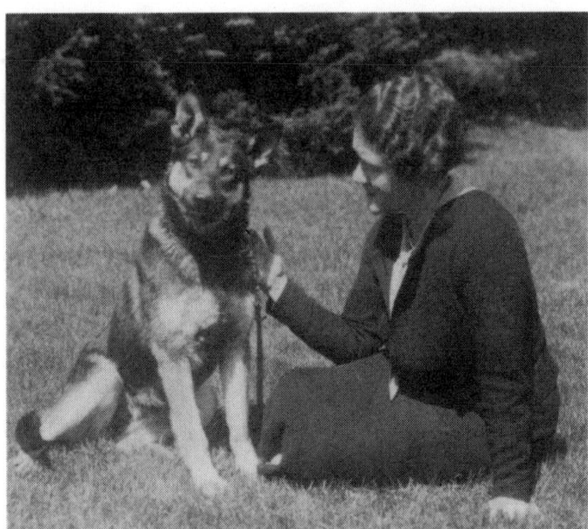

Figure 8.5. Dorothy Eustis at Fortunate Fields.

opposite oncoming traffic. They indicate intersections by following the contour around the corner and stopping. Here again, the traveler who is blind turns, aligns, and initiates the crossing of the road with a "Forward" command.

THE HANDLER'S RESPONSIBILITIES

General Guidelines

Dogs which work in any capacity, such as for the police or customs agencies, are accompanied by humans—called handlers—who direct their dog's efforts. This same terminology is also used with the dog guide. The term *handler* is used to describe the person who is blind who works with the dog guide. This term was chosen to indicate the mutual effort a successful dog guide team requires. Handlers must do what is necessary to get the best possible quality of work from their dogs. They use well-timed commands, praise, encouragement, and the occasional reprimand to reach this goal.

Handlers must give directional commands to direct their dogs in block-by-block increments to their destinations. This presupposes that the handler's general orientation to the environment is sufficient to accurately direct the dog. Moreover,

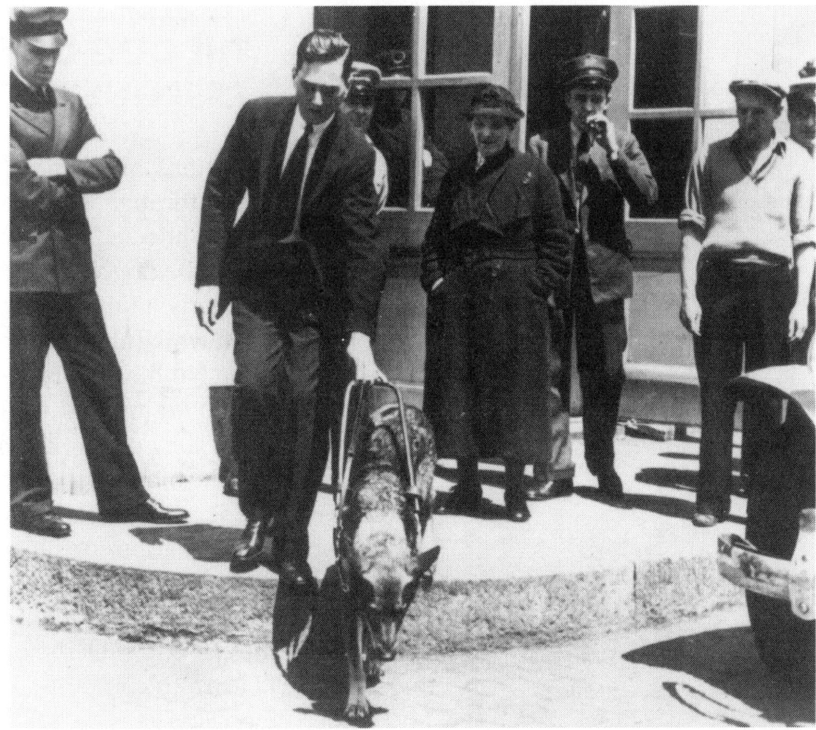

Figure 8.6. Morris Frank follows Buddy as she leads him through the traffic of Vevey, Switzerland, while in training in 1928.

Source: Photo from Seeing Eye.

just as with a cane, it is necessary to use orientation skills, combined with handling skills, to prevent or recover from unplanned detours.

Traffic Judgment and Alignment

Before giving the "Forward" command into the street, the handler must first accurately judge traffic using standard auditory techniques (see Figure 8.7). It is not the dog guide's responsibility to make the initial decision to cross.

Although under normal circumstances they will compensate for a veering tendency, dog guides rely on their handlers for crossing alignment. If the handler's initial direction is wrong by 45 degrees the dog may become confused, with a diagonal crossing or substantial veer being the possible result.

If the command "Left" or "Right" is given at the end of the block or after a crossing, the handler must clearly establish in his or her dog's mind which direction is intended. To accomplish this, handlers use voice and hand signals, but they must also turn properly, using proprioceptive awareness and environmental information to "set" their bodies in the desired direction.

Training Upkeep

Dog guide handlers are taught appropriate techniques to maintain their dogs' training. Accurate work receives warm praise. Praise is the essential component of handling. It is a reinforcement for good work, and also reduces the stress on the dog guide. A dog's error that results in a *misstep* or a *bump* is followed by a reprimand or *correction.* The reason for the correction is then clearly pointed out to the dog, the dog is required to repeat the work, and then praised.

Although highly trained, dog guides are still

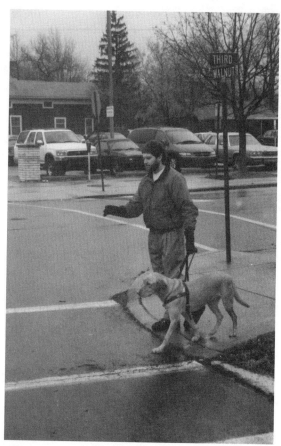

Figure 8.7. An instructor giving a forward command to a dog guide in training.

animals with powerful instincts. From time to time these instincts will surface. Dogs may "sniff" inappropriately, or show an exaggerated level of interest in other animals or people. Handlers must be alert to these behaviors and correct their dogs to refocus their attention on the work at hand. This may require either verbal reprimand or a sharp leash correction, depending on the individual dog and the nature of the distraction.

Dog guides must be socially appropriate. They must be as unobtrusive as possible, and draw no attention to themselves. They must be quiet, well groomed, well behaved, and under good control. Handlers must care for their dogs, and maintain a vigilant watch over their behavior.

THE DOG GUIDE'S RESPONSIBILITIES

The dog's motions are transmitted to the handler's left hand through a stiff, U-shaped handle. The handle is connected to a comfortable beltlike harness which the dog wears and pulls into. The harness handle is an extremely sensitive instrument through which the dog transmits its intentions, and the handler interprets them.

Dog guides are trained to travel in relatively straight lines. They generally will walk from the beginning of the block to the end, unless the handler's desire is to enter a shop, office, or other mid-block destination, or unless there is something preventing progress up the block, requiring a detour. Dogs are also trained to cross streets in straight lines, and to seek the opposite curb. Dog guides will learn to compensate for the handler's tendency to veer.

Dog guides protect their handlers from making contact with obstacles on their way along a block. This includes both stationary objects such as poles and parking meters, and pedestrians. It also includes travel hazards that are over the dog's head such as tree branches or bent poles. In some situations it is necessary for the team to pass, but it is not possible for them to get through side by side due to narrow clearance. Here the dog should pause to let the handler know and either detour around or, in certain situations, following the handler's analysis and acknowledgment, the team may proceed single file with the dog in the lead.

Dog guides pause or stop to alert their handlers to surface changes such as curbs and steps, whether they go up or down, are blended or not. This also extends to anything the handler might trip over such as an oil filler hose across the sidewalk, or a sidewalk lifted by a tree root. Alerted by the dog's stop, the handler should reach forward with a foot to locate the change, praise the dog and then continue with a "Forward" command.

Dog guides are trained to use their own judgment to "intelligently disobey" an inappropriate or unsafe command. This is particularly important in traffic work. Although handlers must decide when to cross the street, their dogs are trained to watch and respect cars. If the handler's judgment is mistaken, the dog guide is trained to intelligently refuse the "Forward" command. If the command has been obeyed, and a crossing vehicle is only apparent when the team is in mid-street, the dog's appropriate response is to slow or stop, continuing only when it is safe to do so.

Dog guides recognize doorways as destinations and will locate probable destinations at their handler's direction. They will also remember destinations previously visited, and will assist in their relocation. Sighted travelers who seek locations they have visited previously will remember the location's appearance. Cane travelers, approaching familiar destinations, will remember the landmarks they used to find the location previously. Dog guide travelers will have the general location in memory, but once in the general area they will put their dog's memory and vision to work to locate the familiar objective.

In adverse weather conditions, especially snow, dog guide travelers often find that their dog's abilities present special advantage. They are not confused by rain or wind, and in addition to providing a good counterbalance in slippery conditions, because dogs travel visually they remain oriented even when the cane traveler's landmarks disappear in snow. They *maintain a line* visually when tactile information is hard to come by, and auditory information confusing.

Additional Functions

Dog guides have a number of additional functions which, although secondary to guide work itself, are highly significant to the dog guide traveler. The most obvious secondary function is, of course, companionship. The dog guide is a companion in travel, and in life as a whole. The bond of affection and mutual respect between handler and dog is a profound one, and frequently is a great source of pleasure and pride to both.

For some individuals who are blind cane travel involves a certain amount of tension, while travel with a sighted guide involves less (Shingledecker, 1983). Many travelers feel that travel with a dog involves less tension than cane travel, in part because of the shared responsibilities, and because the traveler is truly not alone.

The dog guide often serves as social bridge, providing many sighted people with a readily apparent area of common interest with the handler who is blind (Hoyt & Hudson, 1981). The dog may also give the traveler a sense of security from assault. Although dog guides are specifically selected not to be protective, and indeed the overprotective dog is unsuitable for guide work, the dog still may serve as a deterrent to those who might consider the blind traveler easy prey.

THE DOG GUIDE SCHOOL

In the United States and Canada, dog guide schools are private nonprofit institutions. They are supported through private donations and through earnings of their endowments. Schools vary widely in "character" and in many of their policies and philosophies. Most charge nothing for the service they provide, while some charge a fee that represents a small fraction of the true cost of a dog. This fee serves as a means of involving their clients in their own rehabilitation. Most require graduates to sign a contract that allows the school to retain some rights of dog ownership. Some are associated with fraternal organizations, in particular the Lions Clubs; others are not. Some are designed to serve one region of the country, while others are national and even international in approach. Finally, most schools are primarily residential programs. Some exclusively train students in their own homes, while many schools have a home adjustment program for experienced individuals in special circumstances.

THE DEVELOPMENT OF A DOG GUIDE: AN OVERVIEW

Producing dog guide teams is a multistep process. A school must breed or otherwise systematically acquire dogs. The dogs must be raised until they are old enough to begin training. Instructors (after being taught how to train through an apprenticeship process) must train groups of dogs. Once these dogs are ready to be assigned, the instructors must match them with students who are blind and teach the students to care for, control, and work with their dogs.

Once students have graduated or returned home with their new dogs, the school remains in a support role, acting as a knowledgeable resource to answer questions and otherwise provide assistance.

Selecting and Breeding Dogs

Whether they come from the school's own breeding program or from the outside, dog guides must be healthy, intelligent, and of stable and gentle temperament; this latter trait is especially important in a rigorous, stressful, and highly mechanized world. Most dogs selected weigh between 45 and 70 pounds—heavy enough to be felt in harness, but not too large to fit comfortably under a desk, restaurant table, or bus seat. They must have coats that allow for easy maintenance. The breeds that can be used are limited to those that meet these specifications.

Although once synonymous with the term "dog guide," German Shepherds now represent a fraction of the dogs used as guides; Labrador Retrievers are most common. Golden Retrievers also are used frequently. Boxers are useful for people who are allergic to the longer-coated breeds. Many other breeds have been and are used, as are crossbreeds. At several schools a cross between the Labrador and the Golden Retrievers has been bred specifically for use as a guide, and is being used successfully. Some schools specialize in specific breeds. Most schools use both male and female dogs, although the majority are female, and all dogs are neutered before being assigned to handlers who are blind.

Many schools choose to breed at least some of their own dogs. This gives them better quality control of their final product, and an improved ability to predict numbers, health, temperament, and size. Some schools have fairly extensive breeding programs, which may be supplemented by the purchase of litters as pups, or acceptance of donated adults.

Socialization of Puppies

Puppies that are not appropriately socialized to people at the correct developmental stages never form the kinds of bonds to humans that will make them good pets, much less good dog guides. Puppies must also be exposed at a young age to all facets of the human environment if they are to move through this environment as confident, adult guides (Pfaffenberger, Scott, Fuller, Ginsburg, & Biefelt, 1976). Since the 1920s most dog guide schools have therefore placed all potential dog guides in private homes from the ages of about 8 weeks to about 12 to 14 months (Humphrey & Warner, 1934).

Volunteer families raise the dogs and, besides teaching them basic obedience and house manners, introduce their pups to the full range of human activity at a young age. Beginning in 1942 (Putnam, 1979), many dog guide schools developed planned cooperative arrangements with local 4-H clubs. If they are in a 4-H club, children attend club meetings where dogs can be socialized with other dogs. Clubs obtain permission to bring their pups into stores, and there are other group activities. Most puppy raisers are children between 9 and 19 years old, although adults also participate.

Frequently schools have staff members who act as liaisons between the school and the families raising the puppies. The families may keep a journal and records to later assist an instructor during training.

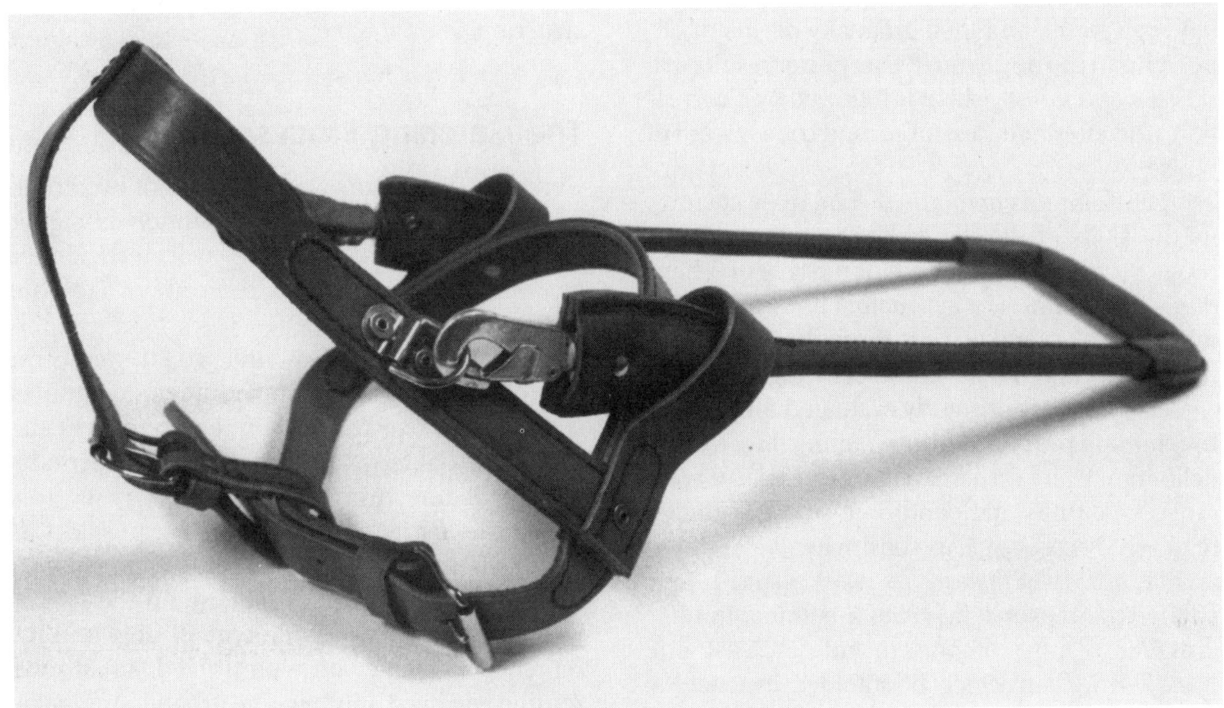

Figure 8.8. Dog guide harness.
Source: Photo by Sally DiMartini

Training Dogs

When the pup is between 13 and 18 months old, physically mature, and emotionally ready to accept the challenge of training, the now-adolescent dog returns to the dog guide school. After a period of adjustment to kennel life, it is assigned to an instructor, along with eight to ten other dogs. The instructor will train this *string* of dogs for 12 to 20 weeks, depending upon the individual school's training cycle.

Training is based on the desire of the dog to please its human companion. This desire allows trainers to use praise as positive reinforcement rather than food rewards, which will not always be available.

The first few weeks of training may take place on the grounds of the dog guide school. The dog either learns, or reviews and refines, the *obedience exercise,* and is introduced to its harness (see Figure 8.8). This comfortable leather girdle encircles its chest, and initially symbolizes "going for a walk." The young dog is taught early to pull consistently against this harness in response to the command "Hup-up," and to lead out.

On the grounds of the school, the dog hears the directional commands for the first time. As it learns, the dog is sometimes reprimanded or *corrected* when it does the wrong thing. Corrections may be verbal scoldings, using the word "No" or "Pfui," or they may be firm jerks on the leash, depending upon the nature of the individual dog and the error the dog made. The dog soon masters the basics and establishes a one-to-one relationship of respect for and trust in the instructor. It then is ready for the next step.

In town, following a sequence of increasing complexity, the dog is taught to stop at curbs and to be aware of clearance alongside and overhead. First obedience, and then *intelligent disobedience,* are encouraged. Traffic awareness begins simply and becomes increasingly sophisticated.

At each step the instructor begins by demonstrating what to do, and then gradually begins to depend upon the dog to do it. Every error results in a *misstep* or a *bump*, which is followed by a correction, and after a successful second try, a reward of praise.

The demands upon the dog increase steadily. As the skills of the dog improve, the instructor progressively assumes more of the role of a handler who is blind. The instructor allows the dog to make mistakes and teaches through them, rather then preventing errors from occurring.

Every dog is constantly evaluated throughout the training process. During training the dogs are deliberately and systematically exposed to a wide range of sounds and conditions and are graded regularly. Factors such as sensitivity to correction and noise, willingness to work, speed and strength, and overall behavior are noted. In their evaluation, most schools include at least one *blindfold test,* in which blindfolded instructors, observed by a supervisor, work each of their dogs on a test route.

The Instructor

Instructors at dog guide schools come from a wide range of backgrounds. Some have experience in dog handling and care, others may come from business or "people-oriented" occupations. Many have college degrees and are often in their mid-20s when they come to the work. Instructors must be in good health, including normal hearing, as the work requires walking 10–15 miles per day in all types of weather. They must also develop good teaching skills. At this time, all of them are sighted.

The dog guide schools develop instructors through apprenticeship programs that last about 3 years. The apprentice may begin working in the kennel, gradually progressing through training a small number of dogs and then a small number of students under constant supervision, to training a full group of ten or more dogs and a full class of about six students. A senior team member then provides direct supervision in a departmental structure.

The Matching Process

Generally instructors work in teams of two, three, or four. Instructors are deliberately assigned more dogs to train than they will need for the students in their next class. There are two reasons for this.

First, not all dogs who go through the rigorous training will complete it as dog guides; some will be rejected for temperament or health problems that crop up during training. Secondly, this procedure provides a large reservoir from which the instructors on the team can select an appropriate dog for each student in the class.

The young, strong, exuberant, on-the-go college student will need one type of dog, and the retired businessperson with a fixed, small-town routine will need another. The urban homemaker needs still another. A test walk (often called the *Juno walk*), in which the instructor simulates the dog by holding one end of the harness handle while the student holds the other, is one assessment tool that the instructor uses to gauge which of the team's dogs is best suited to each individual in the class.

Aside from lifestyle, the instructor assesses the coordination, speed, balance, strength, personality, and breed preference of the student who is blind. Each student will require different clusters of characteristics in their dogs; some dogs are better suited to life in a big city, others to small-town life.

The Student's Experience

Soon after their arrival at the school, students have the first of a series of Juno walks. Aside from the aforementioned evaluative function, these walks also allow instructors to teach the basics of dog handling to new students.

Dogs are assigned early (at many schools on the second or third day). Training begins immediately, sometimes on the school grounds. Training in town starts on quiet residential streets and proceeds through small business sections and into central downtown areas. This follows the same type of sequencing used in orientation and mobility cane training and for the same reasons. Instruction begins one on one, but eventually one instructor may work with two students on the street at the same time, as the distracting presence of the second dog presents a handling challenge to each student.

In the first week, on simple routes, students gradually come to accurately interpret signals coming up to them through the harness handle. New students realize that it is their responsibility to keep their dogs' attention on the work at hand and keep track of the orientation, while it is their dogs' job to keep them out of danger.

By the end of the second week the routes the teams traverse involve complex traffic patterns and pass through the central areas of the town. Teams usually have begun to form the all-important *bond,* which means that the dog has begun to truly care for this new man or woman and is putting its heart into its work on the street. The students, in return, have begun to feel confidence in their dogs.

During the final two weeks of the training process, instructors teach students how to handle their dogs in a wide variety of settings, from department stores to suburban areas without sidewalks, to city buses. Emphasis is placed on situations that the students will encounter in their own unique environments at home.

The Routine

Dog guide schools are unusual residential programs because of their singleness of purpose. At most schools students get *trips* or *workouts* with their dogs twice a day, morning and afternoon. Students rise early to take care of dogs that stay by their sides 24 hours per day. The routines of canine care and guide work develop a rhythm that the students will carry on when they return home.

Again, unlike most rehabilitation programs, dog guide schools include both new students, and those who are described as replacements, in the same classes. A *replacement student* is a visually impaired person who previously had a dog guide and has returned to the school for a new dog because the previous one reached a point where it could no longer give effective service. It is estimated that the average working life of a dog guide is about 8–10 years of actual service, but dogs who serve to the age of 12 are not uncommon. The presence of replacement students in a class is evidence to the new students that dog guides provide independence successfully. Because of their experience with previous dogs, replacements may need less than a full month of training.

Life with a Dog Guide

Life with a dog guide can be divided into two parts: the initial adjustment period after the return home, and the remainder of the dog's working life as a seasoned and settled guide.

When the dog guide first arrives home, it requires a greater amount of attention and thought than it will later on. At first the dog is kept on leash (to facilitate immediate correction of unacceptable behavior) until it learns the rules of the house. Establishing a routine schedule for the dog to relieve itself may also require time and thought during this period until patterns establish themselves. Once the dog is settled, however, and relaxed in its new career, the amount of time and care the dog guide requires is negligible.

The cost of maintaining a healthy dog guide, including its routine veterinary checkups, is about $50 per month. Most dog guides are fed commercial pet foods. Dogs must be given an opportunity to relieve themselves three or four times per day, which with a seasoned dog lasts only a matter of minutes each time. The owner is also asked to maintain, at his convenience, a daily obedience routine, and to groom the dog regularly. These activities take only minutes but pay dividends in good behavior, health, and appearance of the dog. Because of initial careful selection and health maintenance practices, dog guides should require very little medical attention. The seasoned dog is very much a part of its owner's family.

Occasionally, problems develop after a person who is blind has returned home with a dog guide. These may be in the areas of work or behavior. Generally, they occur in the early months of their life together, and the blind person has the skills to deal with most of them. Eventually, however, he or she may turn to the school for advice and even for direct assistance in their home community if needed. All of the schools provide some level of graduate support and assistance, although policies vary among the schools.

DOG GUIDES AND THE ORIENTATION AND MOBILITY SPECIALIST

The orientation and mobility (O&M) specialist typically comes into contact with dog guide handlers at two points in the rehabilitation process. First, he or she advises clients who are blind about mobility choices, and provides them with information about dog guides during mobility training. Results of survey data (The Seeing Eye, 1992) indicate that the O&M specialist is a prime source of motivation behind the blind person's choice to attend a dog guide school. Second, many O&M specialists instructors are asked to provide orientation assistance to a dog guide handler at some point in their careers (The Seeing Eye, 1992).

The O&M specialist is the professional most likely to discuss the possibility of dog guide mobility with visually impaired clients first. To advise a person who is blind in this area, the O&M specialist needs to recognize that the form of mobility which a blind person chooses is highly personal, but that dog guides are not appropriate for all blind people. It has been estimated (Finestone, Lukoff, & Whiteman, 1960) that between 1 and 2 percent of the blind population in the United States use dog guides. A more up-to-date study is not available.

ACCEPTANCE STANDARDS AMONG SCHOOLS

This chapter represents an overview of the dog guide field, but each school sets its own criteria for acceptance of students. This is particularly evident in their consideration of applicants who have hearing losses and residual vision. As of this writing, several schools, among them Leader Dogs and Guiding Eyes, are considering applicants who are deaf–blind. Leader Dogs and some other schools also accept candidates who are legally blind but have a high degree of residual vision.

Some schools apply standards that have been developed internally and are implemented by their field evaluators and admissions staff. Although an O&M instructor's report is very useful and an ophthalmologist's report may contribute valuable information, a functional on-site evaluation by school staff is often necessary before acceptance. Information gathered from such an assessment is also invaluable to the dog guide school in the eventual making of the dog–human match.

There are several factors that a visually impaired client who is considering dog guide training must take into account: personal preference, life circumstances and activity level, amount of remaining vision, age, health and physical condition, and orientation skills.

Personal Preference

Although it is not absolutely essential that the prospective dog guide handler love dogs, a strong dislike or fear of dogs will disqualify some. Dogs must be fed, relieved, and groomed daily, and taken occasionally to visit the veterinarian. These things take time each day. For people who enjoy the companionship of dogs this will be a pleasure. Others may consider it a chore, but soon learn it is not difficult.

The O&M specialist must take care not to discourage those who are unsure on this point, but remind them that this is one aspect of having a dog that should be considered.

Life Circumstances and Activity Level

Dog guides need a certain amount of regular use and attention to be efficient mobility aids. Their work should average out to at least one outdoor mile per day, with more preferred. On some days, the dog might be used for several miles, while on another only sporadically; but likely candidates therefore either are, or desire to be, quite active.

A properly working dog readily accepts the challenge of new situations, so dogs may be particularly valuable to the person who is blind who travels to new situations frequently. The dog's vision and memory, combined with the handler's understanding of sound orientation principles, minimizes the need to memorize many detailed landmarks and information points. Travel therefore becomes less stressful. This may also be true for persons who travel frequently over complex routes that are always in transition, as is often the case in large cities.

Amount of Remaining Vision

Most visually impaired people have too much vision to be able to work effectively with a dog guide. In general, people who travel visually under many conditions while using the cane for identification and as an occasional probe, rather than as a true primary mobility device, will not benefit from dog guide mobility. The traveler will tend to anticipate stops or turns, and "steer" around obstacles when vision is functioning at a high level. Then, when forced by lighting conditions to rely upon the highly skilled and responsible guide, he will find instead a dog that has been unintentionally untrained and is therefore ineffective.

An exception may sometimes be made for people with degenerative eye conditions, who may be able to learn to use a dog to good effect, and establish good working patterns with a dog while they still have relatively effective vision. Usually this transition will be eased through the use of occluders in the training process.

Individual schools vary in their policies concerning acceptance of applicants with residual vision, and some will consider low vision applicants if they meet the standard definition of legal blindness. Schools may also have their own staff assess these applicants.

Age

For many reasons, young people in high school are rarely considered as candidates for dog guides. One reason is that people under the age of 18 years old frequently lack the maturity and responsibility needed to give a dog the level of consistent care and handling that dog guides require. The high-school environment itself has inherent difficulties, with large numbers of adolescents responding to peer pressure and focusing inappropriate attention on the dog and young handler.

The prospective dog guide handler must be in an environment where independent travel is possible. In suburban and rural settings, where school buses pick students up, deliver them to a school and return them in the opposite direction, other options in the student's routine in their home or school neighborhoods must be available if the dog guide is to receive adequate work.

Applicants who satisfy these concerns are not uncommon, but will require careful evaluation by the several schools. The schools also have individual policies concerning high-school age applicants.

There is no upper age limit for dog guide handlers. However, the training is physically strenuous, and many older people will find it too exhausting. Older people who have a strong desire to continue a high level of independent activity, and have maintained good physical condition, may do well with a dog guide. The extension of physical fitness into the senior years due to the cultural emphasis on health and exercise may make more older people who are visually impaired or blind eligible for dog guides.

Hearing

Individuals with hearing loss that prevents them from accurately judging traffic in most situations are generally not good candidates for dog guide training. Their inability to accurately assess traffic leads to repeated incorrect commands, which put undue stress on a dog. However, exceptions may be made if they are willing to seek assistance at crossings, or their living conditions are such as to present a minimum of risk from vehicular traffic.

Individuals with hearing losses in the mild to moderate range can frequently do well with dogs. The dogs provide an additional margin of safety, a sense of security, and, through their behavior, information. Once again, this is an area in which individual schools have different standards for acceptance, and an individual home visit and assessment may be done.

Physical and Mental Health

Potential dog guide handlers should be in good health. Not only is the training rigorous, but once they return home, through their work with their dog, regular exercise will be a part of their life! The average dog guide walks at a brisk pace, although many walk more slowly.

The individual should have good coordination and balance, be of at least average intelligence, and be emotionally stable. Some attempts have been made to train visually impaired people with developmental delays to use dog guides, most notably by Guiding Eyes for the Blind. These attempts have met with very limited success, as the dogs were not used extensively, and the students chose not to replace their original guides.

Dog guides may be especially well suited for clients with diabetic retinopathy. Exercise is an important factor in keeping diabetes under control, and since dog guides need regular attention and exercise, they tend to help keep owners active. Specific conditions such as controlled epilepsy, mild cerebral palsy, heart conditions, or other mild physical problems will not, of themselves, disqualify a person for consideration for a dog guide. The school in question will need to be especially painstaking in the search for a dog appropriate for the person with the additional disability, and this may take time.

Persons with AIDS-related blindness have rarely been considered good candidates for dog guides. This is because the cytomegalovirus responsible for most AIDS vision loss strikes late in the course of the disease, and the person is too weak to consider the use of a dog guide as an option for mobility. However, increased life expectancy and greater stamina for people with AIDS may change the likelihood that such individuals will be considered good candidates for dog guides.

Orientation Skills

As O&M specialists began to have national impact, the dog guide schools quickly saw the increased skills and confidence of applicants who had undergone mobility training. Completion of a mobility training course, and some experience with independent travel, has become increasingly important in selecting new applicants at all the dog guide schools.

It is best for dog guide handlers to have good mobility skills if they are to be effective travelers. It is still possible, however, for some people who have difficulty with spatial concepts to benefit from a dog guide. The dog guide selected must have an especially strong "work ethic" and a lack of distractibility, as distraction would throw the traveler off course. Once again, an independent evaluation by the dog guide school may be necessary.

ASSESSING USER POTENTIAL

Schools take great care in evaluating individuals who apply. The O&M specialist has an important role in the assessment of a client's potential as a dog guide handler. Once a client has applied to a school, the specialist may well be asked to provide a mobility evaluation of the applicant.

The evaluation should include a description of the candidate's coordination, balance, and strength; orientation skills; ability to align with traffic sound; ability to recover when disoriented;

and amount of mobility instruction already received.

Notes on the travel environment in which the client will be functioning and something about his or her routines is helpful, as is information about general abilities, personality, sense of responsibility, and capacity to make mature judgments. If a candidate has vision, a description of how this vision is used in travel is helpful. Best and worst lighting conditions may also be noted. A sample evaluation form is included in this chapter (see Appendix A).

The specialist may be asked to recommend a specific school. If specialists feel uncomfortable with this, they may refer the client to the *Guide to Dog Guide Schools* prepared by Eames and Eames (1994), which lists most of the schools and facts about them.

HOW THE MOBILITY SPECIALIST CAN ASSIST THE DOG GUIDE HANDLER

After the graduate and new dog return home, dog behavior problems and dog work problems are usually best left to the dog guide schools to resolve. Dog guide trainers have specialized training that enables them to attempt to resolve the work and behavior problems which may crop up once a team has left their school. Some problems can be resolved over the phone, and some require on-site assistance.

O&M specialists may play a role in helping handlers who are blind realize that they have a problem with their guide; they should be aware, however, that some handlers may react negatively to criticism because of their close bond with their dogs. When problems occur, O&M specialists may encourage handlers to contact their schools for assistance. If the problem is clearly an issue of safety, and the handler will not contact the school, O&M specialists should consider reporting the problem to the dog guide school on their own. The school should then contact the graduate and offer suggestions or further support.

Travelers who are blind increasingly request orientation assistance from professionals as travel becomes ever more complex. The dog guide handler's needs are somewhat different from those of the cane traveler.

The sound of traffic, and auditory clues and landmarks of every kind are important to both cane and dog travelers. Although the rate of travel is often different for dog guide travelers and cane travelers, all rely heavily upon their sense of distance traveled over time to know they are close to a destination.

Dog guide handlers pay little attention to tactile clues and landmarks, as they are extremely difficult to locate without a cane. Also, since in general dogs view fixed objects as obstacles to clear or avoid, access to such landmarks is limited, although "sound shadows" may still be available. However, landmarks, such as marked surface changes, ramps, and hills, are certainly accessible in many situations, and continue to be essential with a dog guide.

Furthermore, dog guide handlers "read" their dog's behavior for its information value. They use their dog's desire to please, combined with the dog's intelligence and ability to see. In familiar environments dog guides will locate and indicate places they recognize; these indications become landmarks or information points.

The task of the O&M specialist is to help travelers put their dog's abilities and tendencies to work on their behalf. The specialist has two goals: (1) make sure the traveler has an overall orientation to the environment; and (2) if necessary, help travelers teach their dog new goals and intermediate destinations. Later the dog's indication of these goals and destinations will be among the information points and landmarks the traveler uses. A three-step process involving orientation, coaching, and monitoring is useful in whole or in part.

Orientation

An initial orientation to a complex environment is usually best accomplished while the O&M instructor serves as a sighted guide with the dog at

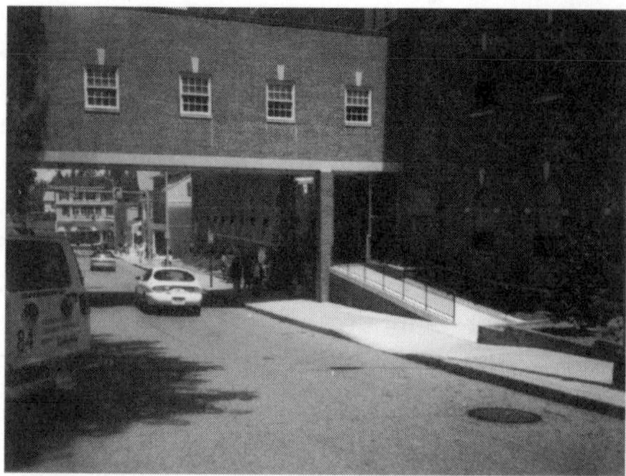

Figure 8.9. The orientation problem to be solved is to locate the ramp leading to the building when approaching from the right. The mid block ramp giving access to the sidewalk may not be available as a clue to the handler as he/she will be at the flatter, top part of the ramp. Sound clues are only available in the form of an echo from the overhead passageway and nearby wall, once past the ramp. A quick 'patterning exercise' might be appropriate.

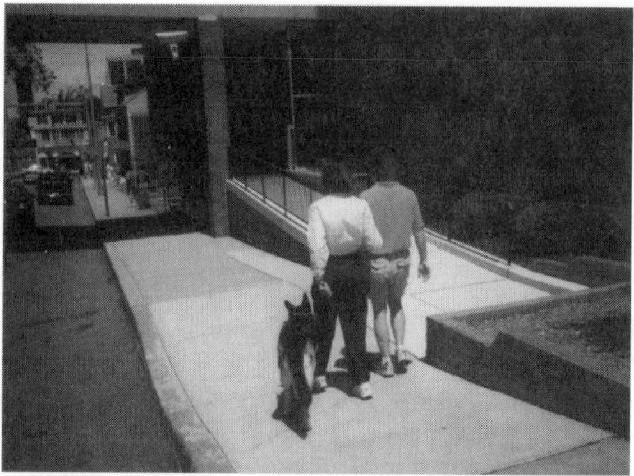

Figure 8.10. As a sighted guide, while the handler heels her dog, walk through the route, explaining the layout, touching upon things which might cause problems. The walk through(s) should allow ample time for the handler to praise her dog at key points, and should end in the building if possible, rather than at the door.

"heel." This allows for thorough and repeated explanations if necessary. If the O&M instructor is unfamiliar with the environment, it is a good idea to leave the team at the starting point, and for the O&M instructor to first explore and develop a route to the destination alone. This avoids confusion when actually teaching the team. Travelers may choose initially to leave their dog at home and to explore an area with a cane.

At specific points which the dog guide must indicate and which are devoid of other environmental clues—for example, the intersection of two pathways on a campus—the handler should put the dog at "sit," and make the point memorable to the dog with lavish praise, then repeat the approach to the spot. If the dog stops successfully, it should be praised. If not, a mild reprimand may be necessary.

Several walks through a complex route may be needed, but take a break at the destination after each walk-through. The handler's praise at the destination will facilitate the dog's learning (see Figures 8.9–8.11).

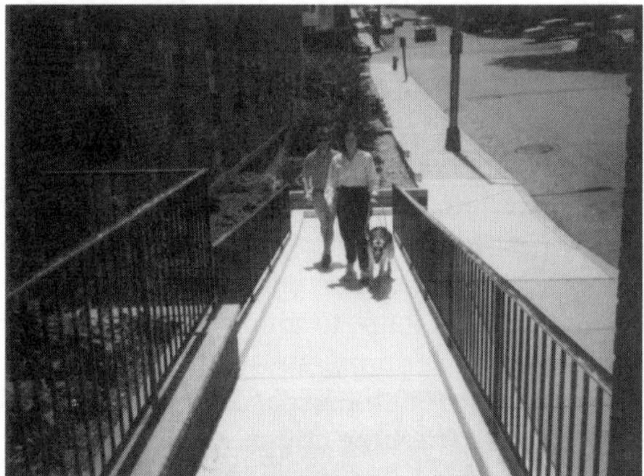

Figure 8.11. Walk through the route a second time in coaching position. Review as you go, and cue the handler in time to allow for a successful route.

Coaching

In this second step the O&M specialist should stay just behind the handler's right shoulder while the team "works" the route. It is a good idea to prompt the handler to let her know she is approaching key points; otherwise mistakes and variation may lead to confusion in the dog's mind. Review and narrate the route as you go, and point out time–distance ratios that become apparent as the team works.

If the dog misses a turn on successive repetitions, take a break and come back later. Also bear in mind that since dogs travel visually, once a dog has a clear destination in mind, the team may skip intermediates and go directly to the final goal. This is natural and acceptable.

Monitoring (or Solo Phase)

When necessary for the traveler's confidence, a monitoring phase may be added. If possible, observation should be conducted from a spot out of the dog's view (this is difficult as dogs are extremely observant). The best way is to have the client begin the trip at a prearranged time, or in response to a phone call. The observer should avoid intervening too quickly, but should it be necessary, the team should calmly be directed to stop and return to the coaching phase.

The three-step process is rarely used in its entirety. It may be necessary in complicated environments, or in situations which are so lacking in environmental information points that the traveler must rely exclusively on the dog's behavior for information. It may also be useful with travelers who have very poor orientation skills or a poor sense of direction. Otherwise, most travelers need little or no assistance. Depending upon the setting, they may sometimes need a verbal orientation to a situation before attempting it on their own. In more difficult situations, a single walk-through either with a sighted guide or with the O&M specialist in a coaching position, may give travelers enough information and experience to make them safe and confident. A few repetitions without a true solo trip may also be just the answer.

It may be difficult to determine what level of assistance, if any, is appropriate. The instructor and the client should establish a partnership from the beginning to determine what the client wants to do, and to review the teaching–learning and travel options that are available.

Self-Familiarization

Typically dog guide handlers will familiarize themselves with an unfamiliar hallway or classroom by initially working the length of the hallway or the perimeter of the room to ascertain that there are no unexpected steps or other hazards. Then the handler will drop the harness, putting the dog off duty, and further explore the room, using standard self-protective hand techniques, and a systematic exploration pattern.

When traveling in a strange neighborhood or town, the ability to solicit quality information is critical. It is the exception to the rules (i.e., the offset crossing with traffic islands, or the major construction site) that causes problems for both dog guide and cane travelers.

To become familiar with the sequence of shops on a block, the handler uses *moving turns,* which are also known as *suggested commands.* Somewhat similar to trailing in function, these commands enlist the dog's vision and initiative to seek out likely looking destinations. If given the command "Right" in the middle of a block, an experienced dog guide will seek out the door of a building or shop. If this turns out to be wrong, another set of commands will bring the traveler to the shop next door.

DOG GUIDES, CANES, AND ELECTRONIC TRAVEL TECHNIQUES

In the early days of The Seeing Eye, students were trained to use a short white cane in the right hand in conjunction with the dog guide in their left. The short cane, while ineffective as a primary mobility device, was recognized as a symbol of blindness, while the dog guide initially was not. It was also felt that a probe might be of some value. It was inconvenient to have both hands occupied and experience proved that the cane was rarely used. Within a decade the cane was phased out in the United States, although it is still used in some European dog guide programs.

Some travelers who are blind may choose to familiarize themselves with new areas using a cane. This may be done either before or after traveling through it with their dog. Leader Dogs encourages their graduates to "heel" their dogs while they explore new indoor environments with their canes and teach destinations to their dogs. All dog guide schools encourage students to keep up their cane skills in order to be prepared for all contingencies. Dogs are inappropriate in certain settings such as sporting events in large arenas, where the handler will in any case likely be accompanied by sighted friends. When waiting for a replacement dog, or if the dog becomes ill, the traveler will need to use the cane to maintain independence. Little research has been conducted into the use of various electronic travel aids (ETAs) in conjunction with dog guides. Experimentation has occurred at the dog guide schools themselves, under the auspice of ETA manufacturers, and by individual blind travelers. Of particular interest are the Sonicguide, Mowat Sensor, and Polaron (Jacobsen, 1979).

The additional information and spatial awareness gained through the proper use of an ETA may enhance travel through the environment (The Seeing Eye 1984). By extending sensory range, an ETA may allow either a cane or dog guide traveler in an unfamiliar environment to accurately locate destinations, and to more effectively interpret clues and landmarks. For this reason it may be useful for teaching potential destinations to a dog in a new environment.

For example, it may initially be easier to locate a recessed entrance using an ETA rather than a cane or dog alone. Once it has been located, the dog guide handler praises her dog. Having learned this door as a potential destination, the dog will likely indicate it by pausing there when next in the area, making future use of the ETA unnecessary.

There are potential problems with ETAs from the point of view of good dog guide use. Dog guide use entails quick motion and rapid mutual responsiveness between dog and handler. Unless additional information provided by the ETA is processed instantaneously, it may disrupt the otherwise smooth functioning of the team (Kay, 1980). The dog guide handler must take care not to use the ETA to do the dog's job and diminish "guide responsibility." The handler must not "steer" or cue the dog when encountering objects detected in or around the travel path. Another common tendency when using the ETA to search for information laterally is to lean away from the dog to extend still further the range of the ETA. This is unsafe and should be avoided.

For this reason training with an ETA should begin separately from work with a dog, and should only be integrated into travel with the dog guide when the traveler has reached a reasonable level of proficiency. As an intermediate step, it may be possible to simulate the effect of dog guide travel through the use of the Juno harness. At the point of integrating the two modes of travel it is essential to involve a dog guide instructor as an advisor.

Dog guide handlers with hearing impairments may benefit from ETA use as a means of receiving additional information from the environment. ETAs that provide tactile feedback are obviously required. The Mowat Sensor and Polaron have been used experimentally, with the Polaron having the advantage of leaving the hands free for communication (Haneline, 1992).

ASSISTANCE AND SERVICE DOGS

Successful dog guide experience has led to the development of techniques for training dogs to be of service to people with other disabilities. This includes people with hearing losses who employ dogs trained to alert them to specific environmental sounds (Hearing Ear Dogs) and dogs trained to assist wheelchair users by pulling their chairs, pulling doors open, retrieving on command, and other functions. There are several organizations around the country doing these types of training, and some have also branched out into dog guide training on a small scale. Two of the largest training organizations are Canine Companions for Independence (founded in 1987) and Paws with a Cause (founded in 1979). Following the experience of people who are blind using dog guides, the Americans with Disabilities Act (ADA) guarantees a person who is disabled the legal right to be accompanied by a service or assistance animal in all areas open to the general public.

THE COUNCIL OF UNITED STATES DOG GUIDE SCHOOLS

The Council of United States Dog Guide Schools was formed in 1987 to foster cooperation among American dog guide schools and develop operational guidelines for the field. Officials of the participating schools meet semiannually to examine application procedures, student services and instruction, graduate services, dog supply, dog training, and kennel facilities. They have developed guidelines that are not mandates, but rather suggestions designed to maintain a high degree of quality services for the consumer.

The Council is currently composed of ten schools in the continental United States. The executive officers and other key staff address issues that affect the field of dog guide training. Selected department heads meet and discuss training procedures, breeding, possible improvements to the training programs, and veterinary issues.

DOG GUIDES AND THE LAW

When Morris Frank first traveled the United States with Buddy in the 1930s, he was frequently refused entrance to restaurants and hotels. He was also denied access to public transportation. This led to a long, and ultimately successful, struggle for which Frank was ideally suited temperamentally. He would not take "no" for an answer. As a result of his efforts and the continued efforts of dog guide handlers since that time, dog guides trained by recognized schools are permitted in all areas to which the public is invited. This right, and the right to housing without discrimination, is protected by laws in all 50 states of United States and in the Canadian provinces. It is also protected at the federal level by the Americans with Disabilities Act.

SUMMARY

The growth of the dog guide movement from one dog guide school in 1929 to at least ten in 1994, and an increase from one dog guide traveler in 1929 to probably more then 8,000 today indicates a healthy and still flourishing phenomenon. The schools have expanded periodically in order to quickly serve their own replacement students as well as to meet the demands of new students. Besides providing mobility instruction, the mobility specialist acts as an informed consultant to the person who is blind who is considering dog guide mobility, and may also be a skilled resource to experienced dog guide travelers.

Suggestions/Implications for O&M Specialists

1. Dog guides have been used by people who are blind in many cultures for at least a thousand years.
2. The systematic training of dog guides began after the First World War, in Germany. That program was observed and described by Dorothy Harrison Eustis, an American breeder and trainer of German Shepherds.
3. Morris Frank pioneered dog guide handling in the United States. The Seeing Eye was founded in January 1929. Many other schools followed, including Leader Dogs For the Blind (Michigan) in 1939, Guide Dogs for the Blind (California) in 1942, and Guiding Eyes (New York) in 1956.
4. Dog guides pull their handlers and respond to commands such as "Left," "Right," and "Forward."
5. Dog guide handlers are responsible for alignment and general orientation, traffic judgment, praise, and training upkeep, as well as the social control of their dogs.
6. Dog guides stop for surface changes that pose hazards, or are significant such as curbs or ramps. They guide their handlers around both stationary objects and pedestrians. They are trained to "intelligently disobey" unsafe or incorrect commands, especially with regard to traffic.
7. Dog guides provide companionship, and may act as a social bridge. Although not protective, they may sometimes act as a deterrent to crime.
8. Dog guide schools vary in policy, and philosophy.
9. Dog guide schools use a multistep process. They must breed (or otherwise acquire) dogs, and raise, train, and match them with students who are blind. They train the "unit" together, and provide follow-up services.
10. The O&M specialist is likely to become involved in the process as an information provider, prior to a student applying or going to a dog guide school.
11. There are several factors that a visually impaired client who is considering a dog guide and the dog guide school they are applying to will take into account. These include: personal preference, life circumstances and activity level, amount of remaining vision, age, health and physical condition, and orientation skills.
12. Usually it is best to let dog guide school personnel resolve dog work and behavior problems, but O&M professionals may be able to help clients realize that they have a problem and should seek assistance.
13. In order to remain oriented, dog guide travelers use acoustic, aromatic, and proprioceptive landmarks and clues as well as time–distance ratios and the sound of traffic.
14. The loss of tactile information is counterbalanced by the information that is contained in the dog's behavior.
15. The O&M specialist may be asked to provide orientation assistance to the dog guide traveler after he returns home. To do so, the specialist should make sure the traveler has an overall orientation to the environment.
16. Teach the handler and the dog a new route together using all or part of a three-step

(*continued on next page*)

Suggestions/Implications for O&M Specialists (continued)

process, including an orientation phase, a coaching phase, and a solo phase.

17. Dog guide handlers frequently familiarize themselves with new environments. Some may choose to use a cane to do so. Dog guide schools encourage handlers to keep up their cane skills.
18. ETAs are infrequently used in conjunction with dog guides, although they may be. Training with an ETA should be done separate from work with a dog guide. The dog guide should be reintegrated into the process after the trainee is proficient with the ETA. A dog guide instructor should be involved as an advisor in the transition.
19. Assistance or Service Dogs for people who are deaf and people in wheelchairs follow the course set by the dog guide movement and are accorded many of the same access rights by the Americans with Disabilities Act.
20. The Council of United States Dog Guide Schools fosters cooperation among the American dog guide schools. It has developed suggested guidelines for the member schools.

ACTIVITIES FOR REVIEW

1. Based on Figure 8.2, speculate on the training and functions of the 19th-century dog guide, and its use in conjunction with the cane the traveler carries in his other hand.
2. O&M training was not a prerequisite for dog guide training prior to the 1970s. Why was it made a virtual requirement after that time.
3. Explain why is it important for a student to have mobility training prior to going to get a dog guide.
4. Discuss the thought process a dog handler must go through before giving the "Forward" command to his or her dog at the downcurb. Keep in mind orientation, safety, and handling requirements. (Is the dog paying attention?)
5. Describe where the instructor should walk when following a dog guide team and why.
6. Discuss if it is always necessary to follow the three-step process outlined in the chapter when orienting someone to a new route.
7. A 30-year-old male, who is diabetic and a former businessman, appears to have low motivation, lost his sight 6 months ago, and has no O&M skills, tells you he does not want your training; he is going to get a dog. What do you tell him and why?
8. A 45-year-old female with RP and cataracts (20/400 10 degrees remaining field) and a mild hearing loss is interested in discussing dog guides with you. She is doing very well with her cane, is employed and very active; in fact, many of her acquaintances do not think she is "really blind." What would you tell her and what would you really think?
9. Make up a hypothetical case study of your own and fill out the mobility evaluation in the appendix.

10. Review several objectives you have traveled to in your blindfold training from the point of view of someone traveling with a dog guide. What landmarks would you lose? How might a dog react? It may be helpful to go with a fellow student as a sighted guide. You may give the commands "Left," "Right," and "Forward." Your "dog" must go to the corners at the end of blocks, and make 90-degree turns at your command. It may wander into parking lots, and you must direct it out by facing the correct direction and using "Left" and "Right" as is appropriate.

APPENDIX A: APPLICATION EVALUATION QUESTIONNAIRE

I. CONCEPT DEVELOPMENT/ LEARNING ABILITY

1. Is the applicant's level of concept development or visual memory sufficient to enable him or her to understand unfamiliar travel areas when they are explained to him or her? ____________
2. Does he or she understand the basic intersection configurations? ____________
3. Are there any deficiencies evident in abstract or motor learning ability? ____________
4. How would you describe his or her rate of learning? ____________

COMMENTS:

II. MOTOR SKILLS/POSTURE & GAIT

1. Does the applicant walk without support, e.g., prosthetic devices, braces, orthopedic cane? ____________
2. Does he or she have full use of both arms and legs? ____________
3. Does he or she demonstrate any gait, postural, or balance abnormalities? ____________
4. Does he or she consistently veer in one direction or another? ____________
5. Does he or she possess enough fine motor coordination to put a collar, leash, and harness on a dog? ____________
6. In an open area where he or she is not concerned about obstacles or drop-offs, how would you describe the applicant's pace? e.g., fast, slow, confident, hesitant, etc. ____________

COMMENTS:

III. PHYSICAL FACTORS/ ENDURANCE

1. Are there any physical problems that adversely affect or limit the applicant's mobility? ____________
2. Does he or she tire easily? ____________

COMMENTS:

IV. TRAVEL SKILLS

1. Does the applicant now travel safely with a long cane? ____________
2. Does he or she demonstrate good cane skills? ____________ Is he or she consistent in his or her use of these skills? ____________
3. Is he or she aware of proprioceptive landmarks when traveling? ____________
4. Is he or she aware of underfooting changes, e.g., brick, asphalt, grass, etc? ____________

5. Does he or she generally make good use of sensory information available to him or her for orientation purposes? ____________

6. Can he or she plan, follow, and reverse a travel route?____________

7. Does he or she use compass directions?

____

COMMENTS:

V. STREET CROSSINGS/TRAFFIC ANALYSIS

1. Can the applicant align himself or herself at downcurbs using traffic sounds?

____

2. Can he or she distinguish between and utilize various traffic control devices?

____

3. Can he or she make decisions as to the appropriate time to cross at most intersections?

____

4. Can he or she recover when he or she reaches upcurbs too far away from the parallel street or misses it on the parallel street side (time–distance judgment)?

____

5. Will he or she seek assistance when necessary? ____________

6. In your opinion, would the applicant, allowed the option, cross most streets on his or her own or wait for assistance?

____

COMMENTS:

VI. PROBLEM-SOLVING SKILLS

1. Does the applicant realize when he or she is off a prescribed route? ____________

   (a) Away from a heavily traveled street onto a side street; ____________

   (b) Diagonal crossings; ____________

   (c) Unwanted turns into recessed store openings; ____________

   (d) Driveways; ____________

   (e) Sidecurbs; ____________

2. Is he or she aware of unwanted turns while traveling, e.g., 90-degree turns around a corner? ____________

3. Does he or she demonstrate good problem-solving skills? ____________

4. What is his or her emotional state when a problem arises? ____________

5. Will he or she seek assistance in a problem situation? ____________
COMMENTS:

VII. TRAVEL ENVIRONMENT

1. Briefly describe the applicant's day-to-day travel environment.

2. Are there any noteworthy travel problems in this area?

3. To what type of travel areas and public transportation has the applicant been exposed?
COMMENTS:

VIII. CONFIDENCE/MOTIVATION/ CHARACTER

1. Is the applicant a confident individual?

   ____

2. Is he or she a confident cane traveler?

   ____

3. Is he or she a stable and responsible individual? ______________
4. Have you found him or her to be cooperative? ______________
5. How would you describe his or her level of motivation with regard to mobility training?

   ____

6. Is the applicant's decision to obtain a guide dog his or her own? ______________
   COMMENTS:

IX. LOW VISION

1. Does the applicant have any residual vision?

   ____

2. Does he or she travel visually?
   ______________ If so, are there times when he or she cannot function visually (e.g., nighttime, in bright light, etc.)?

   ____

3. Have you found that this vision is either useful or a hindrance to him or her while traveling? ______________
   COMMENTS:

X. ORIENTATION AND MOBILITY INSTRUCTOR

1. When did you work with the applicant?

   ____

2. Approximately how many hours of instruction did you give to the applicant?

   ____

3. In your opinion, is the applicant a good candidate for a guide dog?

   ____

4. If the applicant is accepted, would you make any recommendation for special considerations or educational methods?

   ____

   COMMENTS:

APPENDIX B: DOG GUIDE SCHOOLS IN THE UNITED STATES AND CANADA

MEMBERS OF THE COUNCIL OF U.S. DOG GUIDE SCHOOLS

Fidelco Guide Dog Foundation, Inc.
P.O. Box 142
Bloomfield, CT 06002
(203) 243-5200

Guide Dogs For The Blind, Inc.
P.O. Box 1200
San Rafael, CA 94915
(415) 499-4000

Guide Dog Foundations For The Blind, Inc.
371 East Jericho Turnpike
Smithtown, NY 11787
(516) 265-2121

Guide Dogs of The Desert, Inc.
P.O. Box 1692
Palm Springs, CA 92263
(619) 329-6257

Guiding Eyes For The Blind, Inc.
611 Granite Springs Road
Yorktown Heights, NY 10598
(914) 245-4024

Guide Dogs of America
13445 Glenoaks Boulevard
Sylmar, CA 91342
(818) 362-5834

Leader Dogs For The Blind
1039 South Rochester Road
Rochester, MI 48307
(248) 651-9011

Pilot Dogs, Inc.
625 West Town Street
Columbus, OH 43215
(614) 221-6367

Southeastern Guide Dogs
4120 77th Street East
Palmetto, FL 33561
(941) 729-5665

The Seeing Eye, Inc.
P.O. Box 375
Morristown, NJ 07963-0375
(201) 539-4425

CANADIAN DOG GUIDE SCHOOLS AND ADDITIONAL U.S. SCHOOLS

Canadian Guide Dogs for the Blind
P.O. Box 280
4120 Rideau Valley Drive North
Manotick, Ontario
Canada K4M 1A3
(613) 692-7777

Canine Vision Canada
P.O. Box 907
152 Wilson St.
Oakville, Ontario
Canada L6K 3H2
(905) 845-8225

La Fondation Mira Inc (MIRA)
1820 Rang Nord-Ouest
Sante-Madeleine QC
Canada J0H 1S0
(514) 875-6668

Eye Dog Foundation of Arizona (Eye Dog)
8252 South 15 Avenue
Phoenix, AZ 85041
(602) 276-0051
Administrative Office
512 North Larchmont Blvd
Los Angeles, CA 90004

Kansas Specialty Dog Service (KSDS)
P.O. Box 216, Highway 36
Washington, KS 66968
(913) 325-2256

Upstate Guide Dog Association, Inc. (Upstate)
P.O. Box 165
Hamlin, NY 14464
(716) 964-8815

CHAPTER 9

Orientation Aids

Billie Louise Bentzen

Orientation aids such as models and maps can greatly facilitate the learning of spatial concepts and the understanding of complex or extensive spatial layouts. A primary goal of instruction in orientation and mobility (O&M) is that students will have well-developed spatial concepts and detailed knowledge of the spatial layout of areas in which they travel (see Long and Hill, Chapter 2 of this volume). Verbal orientation aids are particularly valuable for route memory, and they can contain much more descriptive information than models or maps. Electronic technology makes it possible to randomly access verbal orientation information such as geographic information systems (GISs), which are electronic databases of spatial information. Coupled with position-tracking technology, GISs could revolutionize the way some persons navigate the environment.

This chapter begins with a discussion of spatial concepts and cognitive maps in order to provide a theoretical framework for understanding the role of orientation aids in instruction in O&M. It then describes the uses of various types of orientation aids, presents key principles to be kept in mind when designing orientation aids, and describes basic methods for making and using these aids. This chapter is primarily intended to help readers understand the excellent opportunities for learning that persons with visual impairments can have by being presented with and using orientation aids. It also gives specialists a conceptual framework and some practical direction to encourage the extensive use of orientation aids in the teaching of O&M.

ORIENTATION AIDS TO TEACH SPATIAL CONCEPTS AND COGNITIVE MAPPING SKILLS

Knowledge of a specific spatial layout is referred to as a *cognitive map*. All travel to a destination that is beyond immediate perceptual experience is based on a traveler's cognitive map, and requires the updating of the traveler's location within that cognitive map in order to arrive at the destination. For travelers who are blind, spatial concepts and cognitive maps come together to form schemas that enable them to travel effectively, even in unfamiliar areas (Foulke, 1971).

Imagine Alice, a kindergartner who has never had any vision. She may have a cognitive map of her classroom which is comprised of a few regularly traveled routes and the landmarks along those routes. For example, she may travel from the door of her classroom to the hook for her jacket by passing a cupboard, then coming to the first hook (her hook) in a row of hooks for the class. If she successfully travels this route, we can infer that Alice has a cognitive map of the route which guides her travel. Her cognitive map has a starting point (the door frame), a landmark (the cupboard) which helps her update her progress—it says "You're going the right way. Your hook comes next."—and it has an end (her hook).

We don't really know what Alice's cognitive map "looks" like, but it is a *route:* it has a beginning, a middle, and an end. It could be a series of sensations—metal doorframe, wooden cupboard, plaster wall where the hooks are—and the actions needed to elicit this series of sensations. It could be something like a verbal list. Or it could be some kind of an egocentric image that includes the information that all of these sensations are on the right side of her body, or it could be some kind of an image that preserves information about the direction and distances between the doorframe, cupboard, and wall.

When Alice enters fourth grade, ideally she would explore her whole classroom, learning where all of its furnishings are in relation to the door, walls, windows, and other furnishings. It will be evident that she has formed an excellent cognitive map of the room when she is able to travel independently throughout the room, no longer needing to learn specific routes in order to move about independently in the classroom.

If Alice has achieved such a high level of competence in moving about her classroom, we will know that she has acquired a *survey level* cognitive map. Unlike the *route level* cognitive maps she was able to form in kindergarten, her cognitive maps now can contain the directions and distances between all (relatively) fixed objects in the room, allowing her to recover from veers or detours, and to plan new routes within areas for which she possesses good survey level cognitive maps.

This high level of spatial orientation is not achieved by all fourth graders who are blind. Indeed, older literature claimed that persons who never had vision were unable to perform such complex spatial tasks (von Senden, 1932/ 1960). However, O&M specialists have regularly observed that some persons who never had vision are exceptionally well oriented, having excellent cognitive mapping abilities coupled with excellent spatial updating skills. Indeed, there is an emerging body of research literature which confirms that although, in general persons who are congenitally totally blind are not able to perform spatial tasks requiring a survey level cognitive map as quickly or accurately as persons who have had sight (Bigelow, 1991; Byrne & Slater, 1983; Casey, 1978; Dodds, Howarth, & Carter, 1982; Herman, Chatman, & Roth, 1983; Rieser, Guth, & Hill, 1982; Rieser, Lockman, & Pick, 1980; Ungar, Blades, Spencer, & Morsley, 1994), there are nonetheless individuals who never had vision who are outstanding in the performance of such tasks (Bentzen, 1991; Landau, Spelke, & Gleitman, 1984; Loomis et al., 1993; Ungar et al., 1994). It may be that although persons who are congenitally blind are typically slower or less accurate in spatial problem-solving than persons who have had sight, they nonetheless use the same abstract spatial framework and are equally capable of abstract spatial thinking (Casals & Valiña, 1991; Easton & Bentzen, 1987; Klatzky, Golledge, Loomis, Cicinelli, & Pellegrino, 1995). Abstract spatial thinking may, however, develop more slowly in congenitally blind children (Juurmaa, 1973; Ochaíta & Huertas, 1993; Potter, 1995).

It has been shown that children who are blind are better able to form a survey level cognitive map, and use it in pointing to objects in the environment, when they study a tactile map (Ungar et al., 1994), or when they use a microcomputer (auditory) simulation (Zimmerman, 1990) than when they explore the environment. This parallels the finding that sighted adults tend to understand spatial relationships better when they learn an environment by studying a map than by traveling through the environment (Golledge, Doherty, & Bell, 1995). However, it appears that although exploration of tactile maps can result in very functional cognitive maps of the general arrangement of objects, they may lack somewhat in precision (Herman, Herman, & Chatman, 1983). Nonetheless, a good, albeit general, cognitive map is often sufficient to enable independent route planning and travel within a known area.

The use of tactile maps, especially with students who never had vision, appears to be an excellent way to familiarize students with new environments and teach spatial concepts.

Although little is known about the form of cognitive maps of persons who are blind, we do know that they sometimes function much like the cognitive maps which persons with normal vision may refer to as "images" or "pictures" in the mind. That is, cognitive maps can be used to determine distances and directions between the self and objects in the environment (Byrne & Slater, 1983; Herman et al., 1983; Ungar et al., 1994), they can be used to plan novel routes in a familiar environment, and they enable blind travelers to update their positions relative to objects in the environment (Bentzen, 1991; Rieser et al., 1982).

These are the kinds of tasks performed by persons with sight, on the basis of information on print maps. The same information can be conveyed to persons who are visually impaired by means of models, or tactile or large-print maps. It can also, but perhaps less efficiently, be conveyed by auditory maps (Blasch, Welsh, & Davidson, 1973). There is evidence that auditory verbal descriptions of a route or a spatial array can result in cognitive images which are similar to those acquired through tactile maps (Casals & Valiña, 1991; Easton & Bentzen, 1987), although the reported research used very simple spatial layouts.

Maps and models provide spatial information that is hard to get by walking about the environment—especially if the environment is larger than a classroom. They preserve the most important spatial relationships of the environment and present these relationships in ways that can be explored relatively quickly, in comfort, and in safety.

Introducing Spatial and Map Concepts

In mainstream education, children typically are taught basic mapping concepts beginning in about the second or third grade. These concepts include the following:

- Symbols represent real objects.
- The location of symbols on a map represents the location of these objects in the mapped space.
- Directions on the map correspond to directions in the mapped space.
- Maps are like a "bird's-eye view."
- Shapes of areas shown on a map show the shapes of areas or objects in the mapped space.

Learning these concepts often involves activities such as mapping an array of objects on a desk using a scale of 1:1 (that is, the size of the map is the same as the size of the desk), and mapping the classroom. These are also excellent activities for children who are visually impaired. In my experience, however, entire classrooms are quite difficult for most children who are visually impaired. Children will best understand maps—and best understand actual spatial layout—if they become mapmakers.

Children who are blind, as young as 4 years of age, have used tactile maps with moveable parts to learn basic spatial concepts, and such mapping concepts as: a symbol represents an object; the location of a symbol on a map represents the location of an object in the environment; symbols which are near (far, opposite, etc.) each other represent objects that are near each other (Franks & Kephart-Cozen, 1982). This research resulted in development of Maps Represent Real Places: Map Study I, a curriculum and materials that are available through the American Printing House for the Blind (APH) (see Figure 9.1).

The child who successfully completes this curriculum is able to independently explore a small room with a few items of furniture and then represent this room on a tactile map. Alternatively, the child is able to look at a map and then go directly to any item in the room. These tasks require a very high level of spatial thinking, and the student who is successful will be well on the way to becoming a proficient navigator as well as a good map reader and mapmaker.

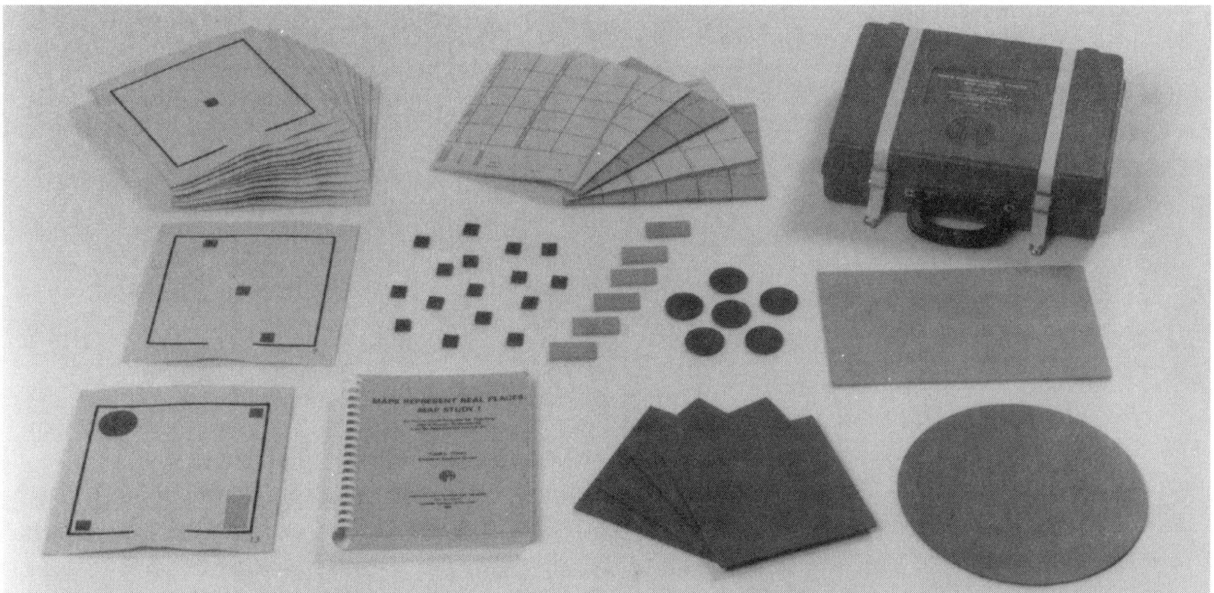

Figure 9.1. The materials in Maps Represent Real Places: Map Study I include large, brightly colored symbols for representing objects in a room; identical smaller-scale symbols; simple 10- × 10-inch maps showing various room arrangements; and sheets for student mapping. A teacher's guide, preliminary screening instrument, lesson plans, and response sheets are also included.

Source: American Printing House for the Blind. Reprinted with permission.

It should be kept in mind that children who are sighted develop the concepts critical for the understanding of models and maps slowly. Young children often fail to make the connection between a symbol and what it represents, even when the symbol is highly realistic (DeLoache & Marzolf, 1992). Two-and-a-half-year-olds typically have difficulty understanding the relationship between a model and the larger space it represents (DeLoache, 1991). Five-year-olds may understand symbols but often do not understand point of view (Liben & Downs, 1993). Map understanding appears to require a child to take alternative and hypothetical viewpoints as well as to understand symbolic relationships (Downs & Liben, 1990). Sighted children do not usually develop the euclidean logic necessary to form survey-level cognitive maps, preserving angles and proportionate distances, until about 9 years of age (Potter, 1995). Children who are blind will typically reach this developmental level somewhat later (Stephens & Grube, 1982).

The curriculum described above may be successfully used at any age because it begins with a small, carefully controlled environment. It uses simple maps with moveable parts to teach students how to perceive spatial relationships and how to form cognitive maps, by observing either the environment or the small, stylized representations of the environment that we call maps. It uses successively smaller and more abstract symbols, which are helpful in teaching the symbol–object association, and it provides repeated experience by going back and forth between large- and small-scale space, which fosters the development of euclidean logic.

CATEGORIES AND CHARACTERISTICS OF ORIENTATION AIDS

There are three primary categories of orientation aids which may be used either separately or in combination.

1. *Models:* three-dimensional representations of objects or spatial layouts
2. *Maps:* two-dimensional, tactile, visual, and tactile–visual representations of spatial layout having information that is perceptible to touch, vision, or to both touch and vision. (Note that while a map may be tactile, it is nonetheless considered two-dimensional because the information conveyed is only two-dimensional.)
3. *Verbal aids:* spoken or written descriptions of spatial layout (survey maps) and/or ways to travel within the environment (route maps)

Special Characteristics of Models

When made to high standards of scale, texture, and color, models are more realistic than maps or verbal aids. They are thus the aids of choice for introducing spatial concepts, or for students who have difficulty with abstractions. Models more closely represent actual three-dimensional space and therefore may be a bridge to the use of maps.

Special Characteristics of Maps

Maps that are perceptible by touch will be referred to as *tactile maps;* those perceptible through vision will be referred to as *visual maps;* and maps perceptible both tactilely and visually will be referred to as *tactile–visual maps.* One distinguishing characteristic of all of these maps is that information access is random; the user can obtain information of different kinds or from different parts of maps in any order. All can be used for such tasks as learning unfamiliar spatial layouts (familiarizations), finding new or alternate routes in a familiar area, and keeping track of one's progress toward a destination (spatial updating). They can also be used to illustrate spatial concepts. Tactile maps excel at representing for touch readers environmental configurations such as intersections, floor plans of buildings, campus layouts, city street patterns, and the relationships between public transportation systems and the areas they serve.

Large-print visual maps may be simultaneously read by persons who have unimpaired vision as well as persons who have low vision. They are less conspicuous than tactile maps because they are similar to maps used by sighted persons. They can be made inexpensively, both for single and multiple copies.

Tactile–visual maps have the characteristics of both tactile and visual maps. They enable persons who can perform some near vision tasks, but who can also profit by tactile input, to make maximum use of both senses, and they permit users to determine which input they will use for the task at hand.

Special Characteristics of Verbal Aids

Tape-recorded (auditory) aids present environmental information, routes to be traveled, and areas in which to travel, in terms which persons who are visually impaired have already learned to recognize. However, there is great variation in ability to understand verbal directions as there is in the ability to understand maps. The tape player itself, although it may be heavier than a map, can be carried by a strap or in a belt-pack, leaving both hands free. The player is inconspicuous, as it is relatively common for sighted persons to carry tape players, and it can operate while the user travels. Auditory maps are the least limited in terms of the amount and detail of information they can convey and still be portable (Blasch et al., 1973). Detailed information about landmarks, suggestions for the use of specific techniques for specific travel situations, and historical, cultural, and aesthetic enrichment information can be included more easily on auditory maps than on tactile maps. Auditory maps can readily contain multiple spatial frames of reference, thus a single map may be suitable for persons having widely different levels of spatial ability. For example, the map may say "Turn left, that is north, so Charles Street is in front of you."

Tape-recorded maps do not require braille skills or sufficient vision to read print, nor indeed do they require literacy. Persons who are blind can themselves make auditory maps of areas or routes by recording those portions of verbal explanations or directions that are necessary to them, or by recording information about a route or an area that is obtained by independent exploration. One distinguishing characteristic of tape-recorded maps is that information access is sequential; there is no easy way for the user to move randomly from one part of the map to another.

Braille provides another medium in which persons who are blind can make verbal maps. They can braille those portions of verbal explanations or directions that are necessary to them, or write down information about a route or an area, which they obtain by independent exploration. If such maps are stored in computer format (particularly using a portable device such as Braille 'n Speak or Braille Mate), they can be retrieved audibly as well as in braille, and users can access different parts of maps randomly.

EXAMPLES OF ORIENTATION AID USE

Models as Aids for Teaching Spatial Concepts

Models are the aids of choice for introducing many concepts and characteristics of the built environment to students who have never had good vision. These students frequently have difficulty forming complete and accurate concepts of components of the environment such as different kinds of buildings, vehicles, and intersections, which are too large for them to see in detail or encompass totally through haptic exploration. Adventitiously visually impaired persons may have incomplete and inaccurate or outdated concepts.

The best models are those that are most like the thing they represent, yet no model conforms totally to the original. Design and construction of a model is always a compromise in which attributes like the original are chosen because they are important to the acquisition of a complete and accurate concept, and attributes unlike the original are chosen because they facilitate observation and understanding. As an example of the former, a little metal car with wheels that turn is better for use with a model of an intersection than a one-piece molded rubber car. An example of the latter is that on a model of an intersection: its vertical scale may be exaggerated, showing curb height to be disproportionate to street width, so that the student can relate going down with a finger on the model to stepping down into the street at a curb. Other unlike attributes may be permitted because they do not present a significant obstacle for the specific learning need.

Wherever possible, scale should be consistent throughout a model. There may be conceptual distortion when relative proportions of parts of a model are not consistent. For example, model cars should be proportional to the width of streets on which they are to be driven. Whenever scale is inconsistent, it is important to be sure that the student understands the inconsistency.

Concepts that are especially well presented using models are those involving *multiple floors*, and ways to go from one floor to another. A child who is blind may race around in her house, upstairs and downstairs, without ever understanding why there are *stairs*—why she needs to go *upstairs* to her bedroom, and come *downstairs* to get to the kitchen. A model house may be used to show her that one floor is above the other, and that stairs are the way to get from one floor to the other. The model can also be used to teach the concept of vertical symmetry.

Models can also be excellent aids to understanding neighborhoods—how houses relate to other features of the residential environment, such as driveways, garages, yards, and sidewalks. Many O&M specialists have models of intersections, some complete with various kinds of shorelines, curb ramps, and crosswalks, which they use when teaching intersection concepts (see Figure 9.2).

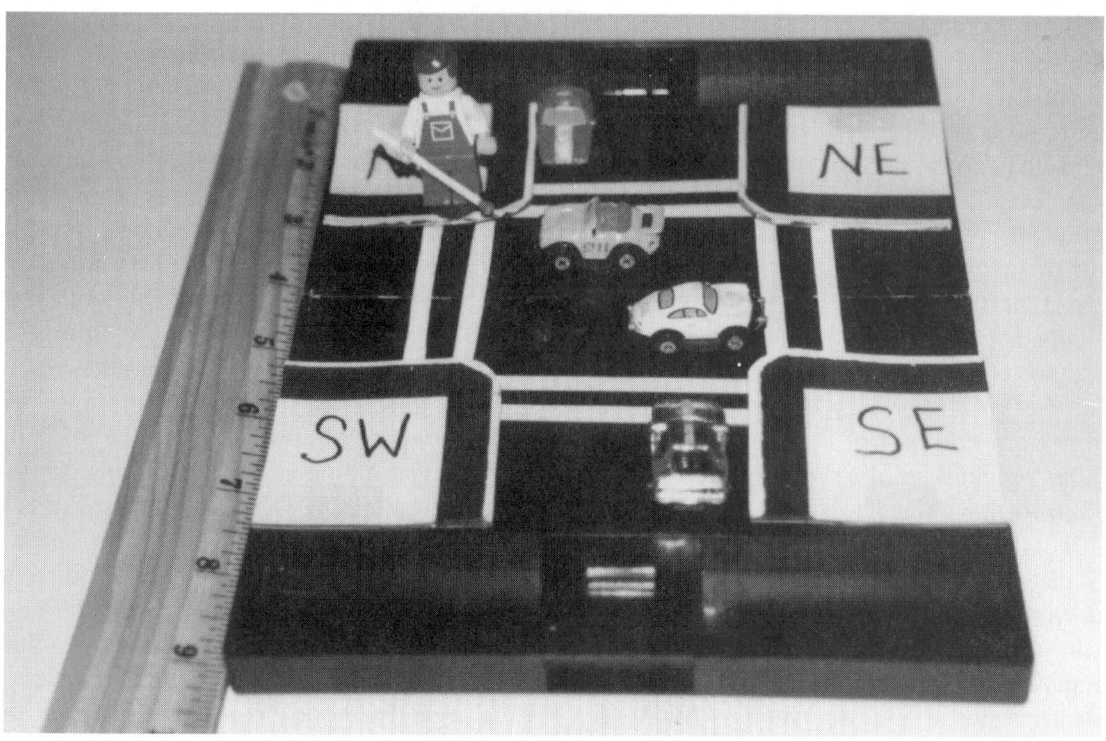

Figure 9.2. This model, which can be carried in a small waist pack, is the creation of an O&M specialist who painted a folding magnetic chessboard to make a base for the model. Raised and high-contrast magnetic shapes are added to the base to show various characteristics of intersections.
Source: Courtesy of Patty Maffei.

Many materials commonly found in the home or classroom can be used to make satisfying models. Students can use Lego bricks to model buildings and neighborhoods, and there are also toy neighborhoods appropriate for the perceptual capabilities of some students, which are complete with such features as stop signs, traffic lights, and railroad crossings.

Tactile, Visual, and Tactile–Visual Maps

Maps are the most commonly used aids for presenting spatial information to persons who are visually impaired as well as to persons who have normal vision. Maps may have visual or tactile information only, or may combine both. They excel in the presentation of information about environmental configurations such as complex intersections or irregular street patterns, even though verbal aids can include greater detail and more varied information.

Some environmental configurations are too complex to be easily described verbally, but they can be constructed and perceived on maps. The configuration of a campus with winding driveways, and walks that are neither parallel nor perpendicular to some of those driveways could be represented on a map. Such a complex configuration, presented as a map, could be supplemented by verbal information about landmarks and other orientation clues.

Extensive environments such as entire cities can be constructed and perceived on small-scale maps more readily than they can be described verbally. Such maps can be supplemented by specific verbal information about features that are helpful or those that are difficult for the visually impaired traveler.

Examples of Map Use

Maps of Intersections

Street crossing is one of the most difficult, but also one of the most essential, skills for independent outdoor travel. Without good concepts of intersection configurations, features, and functions, pedestrians who are visually impaired can safely cross streets only in very limited situations. Maps of intersections can be extremely helpful for teaching these concepts.

One might begin teaching a child who is congenitally blind the concepts associated with intersections by having her first explore one corner of an intersection and discover its key attributes such as the sidewalk, curb, and inside shoreline, all of which define the corner. Then she could create a simple tactile map, by choosing from such preselected materials as narrow cardboard strips, wider sandpaper strips, and fabric squares having good textural contrast, symbols to represent the sidewalk, curb, and inside shoreline. Having the student first observe the relative widths of the curb and the sidewalk, and then choosing narrow strips to represent the curb and wider strips to represent the sidewalk, will emphasize the concept of relative scale. That is, the size and extent of symbols and spaces on maps represent relative size and extent of features and spaces in the environment.

The specialist could continue making this map with the child, always having her observe the environment, then helping her to make the map, until all the corners, as well as the street, are represented. Now an appropriately sized model car can be used to show her how cars can move along the streets. She can listen to a car and then make her map car travel the same way the real car went. She can travel around the intersection and keep track of her position using a symbol for herself that is an appropriate size for the map, and which has a recognizable front. A narrow isosceles triangle is often used, telling the child that the sharp point represents her nose. This front, or "nose," is important because it enables depiction of the student's facing direction as well as location.

Maps are excellent for teaching recovery from veers at intersections. Many students never experience all possible veers at a plus intersection, but in a single lesson using a map (or model), they can consider the consequence of all veers and relate all possible reorientation information to each one. Such model problem-solving experiences should complement the actual experiences that each student has while receiving instruction, both to alleviate emotional stress (Fluharty, McHugh, McHugh, Willits, & Wood, 1976) and to offer the broadest possible range of experiences.

Maps of Routes

Many times maps that have complete spatial layouts of an area (geographic or cartographic maps—see Chapter 2) are unnecessary or undesirable. If the sole objective of a map is to enable users to travel a route between two points, users may not need or be interested in information about locations of other features in the vicinity of the route nor in the relationships between the route and the larger area within which it is to be traveled. Additionally, persons who have cognitive impairments may readily be able to use information presented on a simple route map, although they are unable to understand more complex spatial layout information. The two most common types of route maps are strip maps (which can be tactile, visual, or tactile–visual) and verbal route maps.

Strip Maps. Golledge (1991) conducted research to identify the minimum amount and type of information necessary to enable students who were blind to travel a campus route. He then constructed a series of three tactile strip maps to represent the sequence of straight line segments that constituted a route between two buildings (see Figures 9.3A and 9.3B).

J. W. Wiedel designed and produced a booklet of tactile–visual strip maps, one for each of the rapid-rail lines of the Washington Metropolitan Area Transit Authority (WMATA) (see Figure 9.4). These strip maps accompanied a schematic geographic map of the entire system, which could be used for route planning. The pocket-sized strip maps can easily be carried along for reference en route.

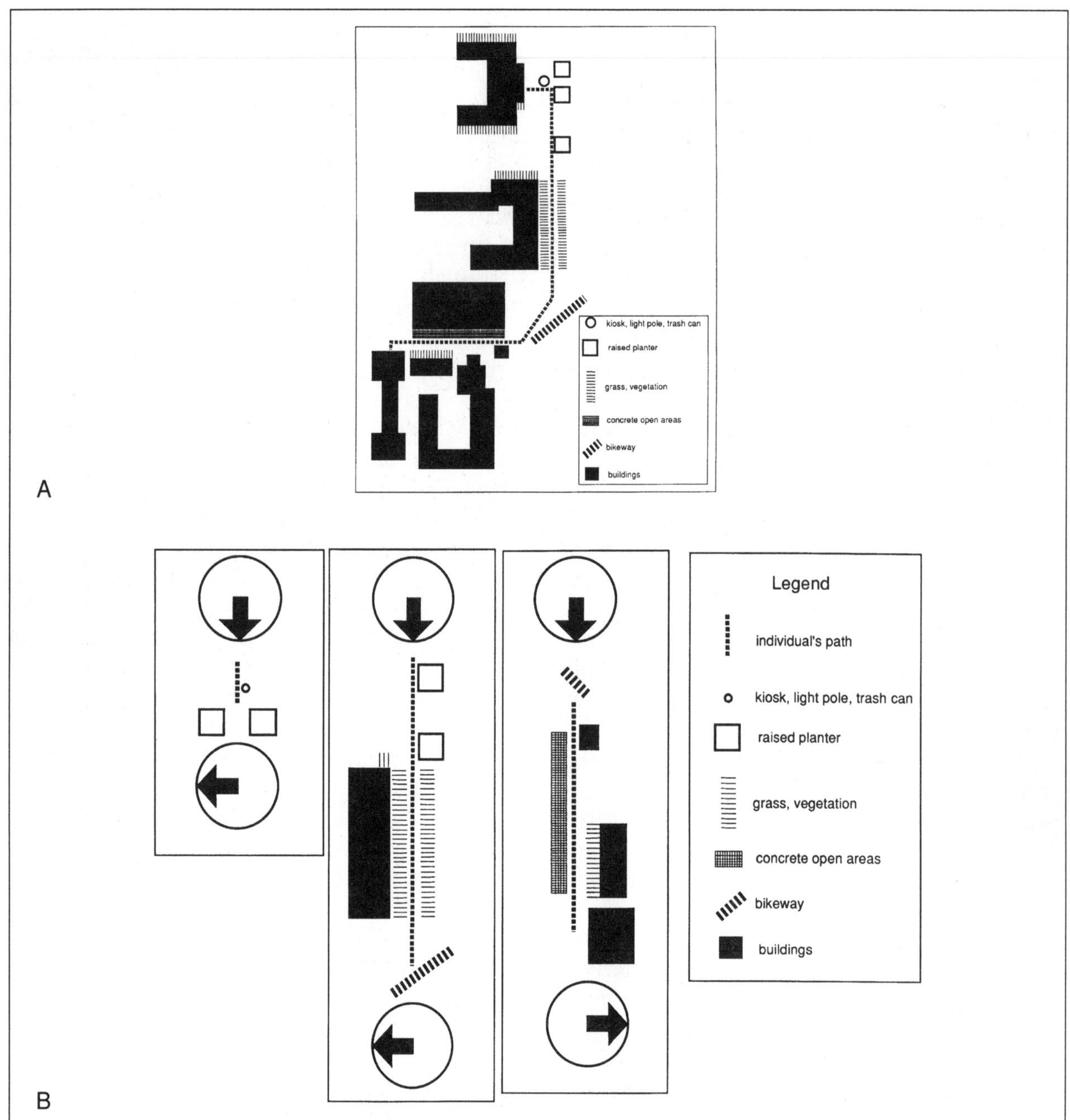

Figure 9.3. (A) A portion of the University of California–Santa Barbara campus, showing a route between two buildings. (B) A series of strip maps that reduces the route shown in Figure 9.3A to three straight segments, and shows significant choice points, changes in travel direction, and selected landmarks to enable updating of one's progress along the route.

Source: *Journal of Visual Impairments & Blindness, 85* (1991), pp. 299–300.

Verbal Route Maps. Verbal route maps can be excellent memory aids for routes that are traveled infrequently or for persons who have memory problems. Tape-recorded maps can be made by travelers who are blind, or by their instructors or friends. Similar verbal maps can, of course, be made in braille or large print. Some blind travelers find that storing route maps on portable computers such as the Braille 'n Speak or Braille Mate enables them to flexibly retrieve informa-

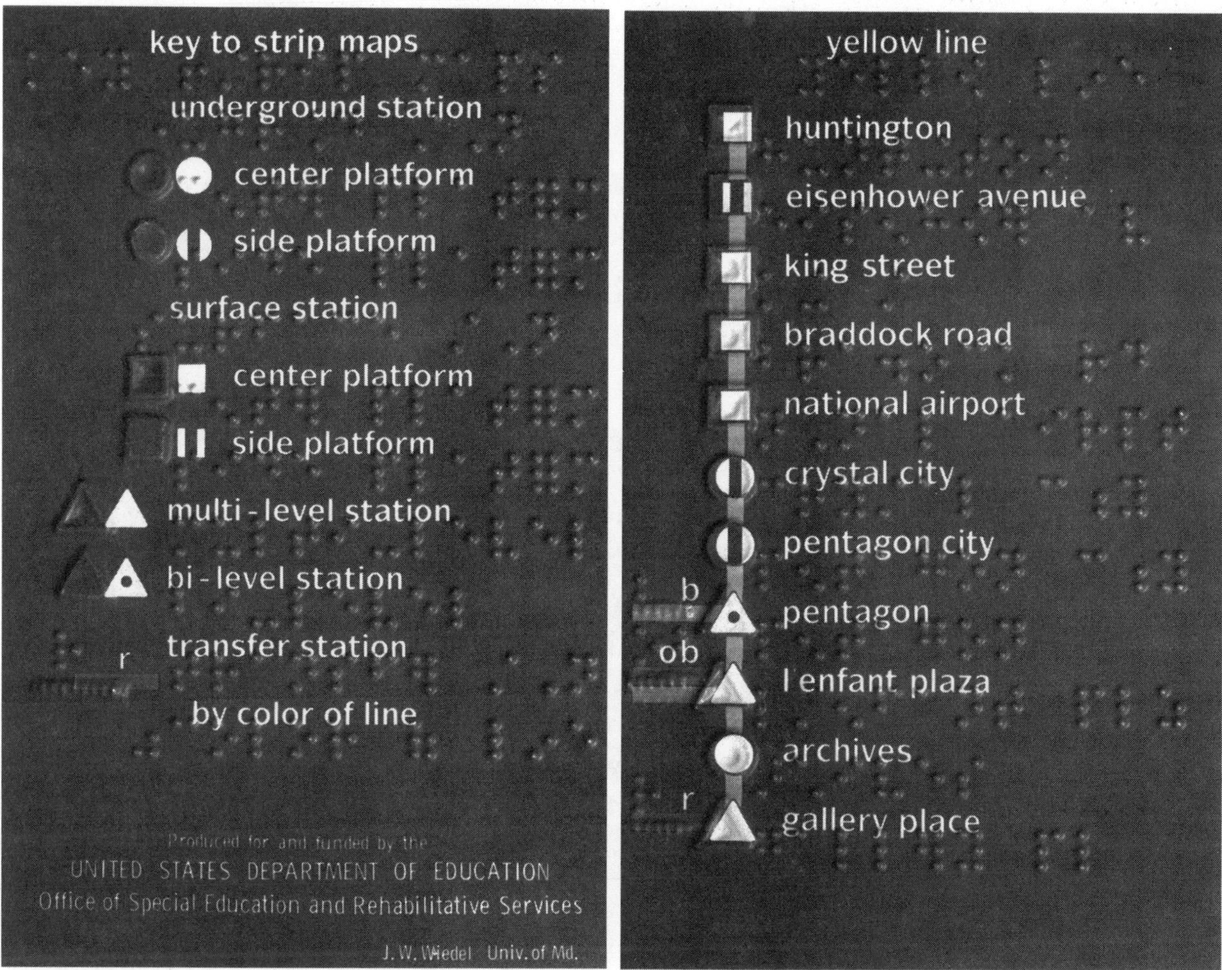

Figure 9.4. Two pages of an eight-page booklet of strip maps. The maps are both tactile and visual.

tion about routes and sections of routes either before traveling or while en route.

Maps of Cities

Although there are few tactile maps of cities in the United States, there are many such maps in some other countries. There have been some national and international efforts to standardize symbols for use on tactile maps of urban areas (First European Symposium on Tactual Town Maps for the Blind, 1984, Brussels, Belgium; National Mapping Council of Australia, 1985; Second European Symposium on Tactual Town Maps for the Blind, 1985, Marburg, Germany). These efforts at standardization have been heavily influenced by James' (1975) Nottingham Kit, now available as the Map and Diagram Making Kit,[1] or Euro-Town kit,[2] which comprises well-researched molded plastic point symbols, soft solder strips of various textures for use as line symbols, and sheets of four different textures to be cut into areal symbols. Figure 9.5 shows the symbols in this kit. (See the section on symbols later in this discussion.)

Americans who are blind are increasingly aware of their rights under the Americans with

[1]Royal National Institute for the Blind, P.O. Box 173, Peterborough PE2 6WS, England; available in the United States from Independent Living Aids, Inc., 27 East Mall, Plainview, NY 11803.

[2]Deutsche Blindenstudienanstalt e.v., Am Schlag 8, P.O. Box 1160, D-3350 Marburg 1, Germany.

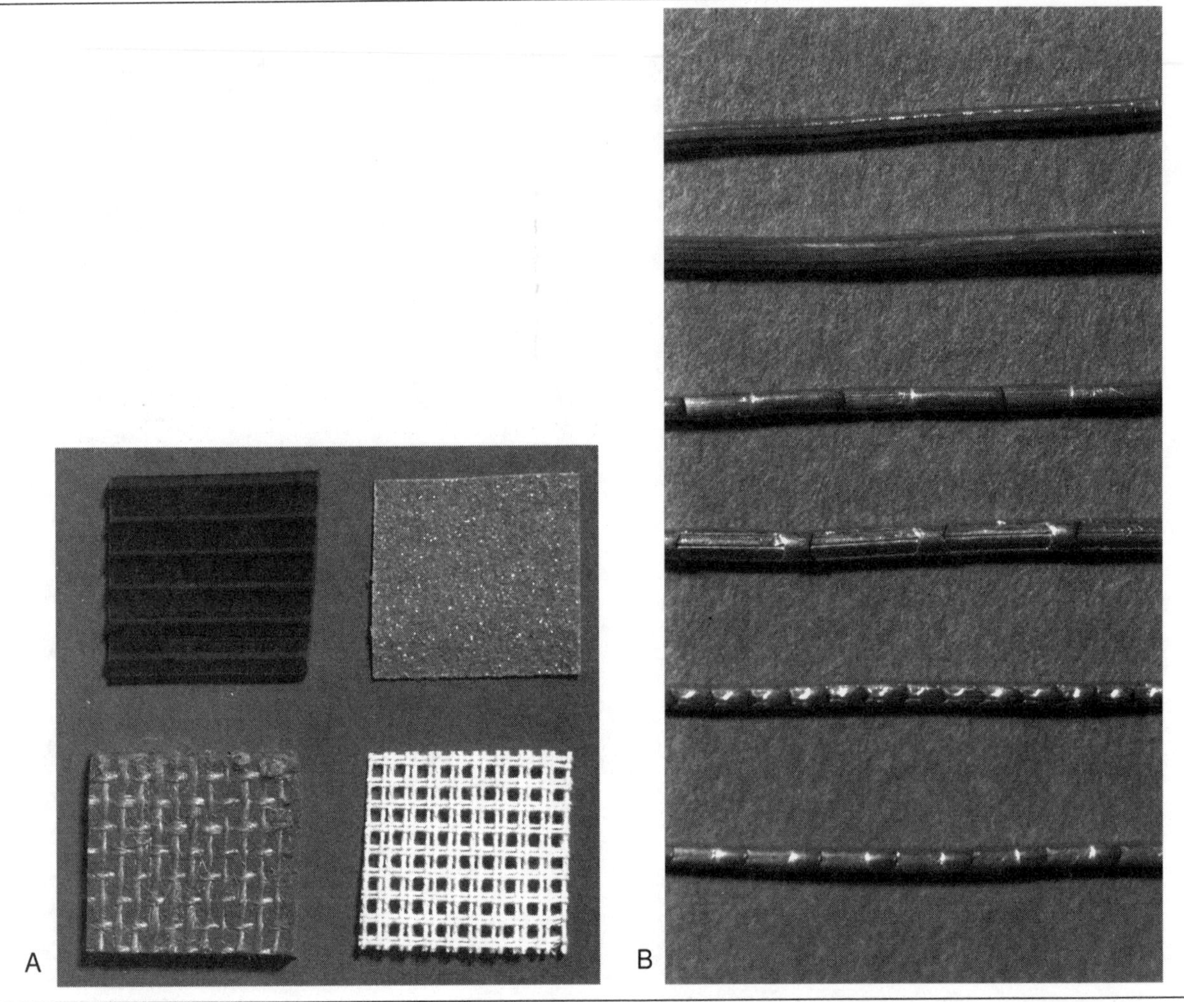

Figure 9.5. Materials for the Map and Diagram Making Kit include 18 point symbols, 6 line symbols, and 4 areal symbols. The symbols are gluded onto a backing such as braille paper or cardboard. The kit includes instructions for using the materials. (A) Areal symbols; (B) line symbols; (C) point symbols; and (D and E) multipurpose symbols.

Source: Figures courtesy of the Graphics Department, Boston College.

Disabilities Act (ADA) to spatial information in the form of tactile maps, and agencies and governments are increasingly investing in the production of such maps.

O&M specialists are encouraged to become involved in projects to design and produce maps of urban areas, and then to incorporate the use of such maps in their instruction of students who are blind. The most useful maps are multicopy maps that can be used at home for route planning, and carried along for reference during travel. Display maps that can only be utilized in one (public) location are much less useful.

Maps of Transit Systems

The ADA requires that transit systems make route (as well as other transit) information available in alternative formats. A number of transit systems are now providing tactile and large-print maps. The independence of persons with visual impairments in using mass transit will be furthered if travelers who are blind are able to use these maps well. O&M specialists should therefore incorporate route planning and updating using maps into their instruction in the use of public transit. At least three projects have documented the usefulness of tactile transit maps (Bentzen, 1977, 1989;

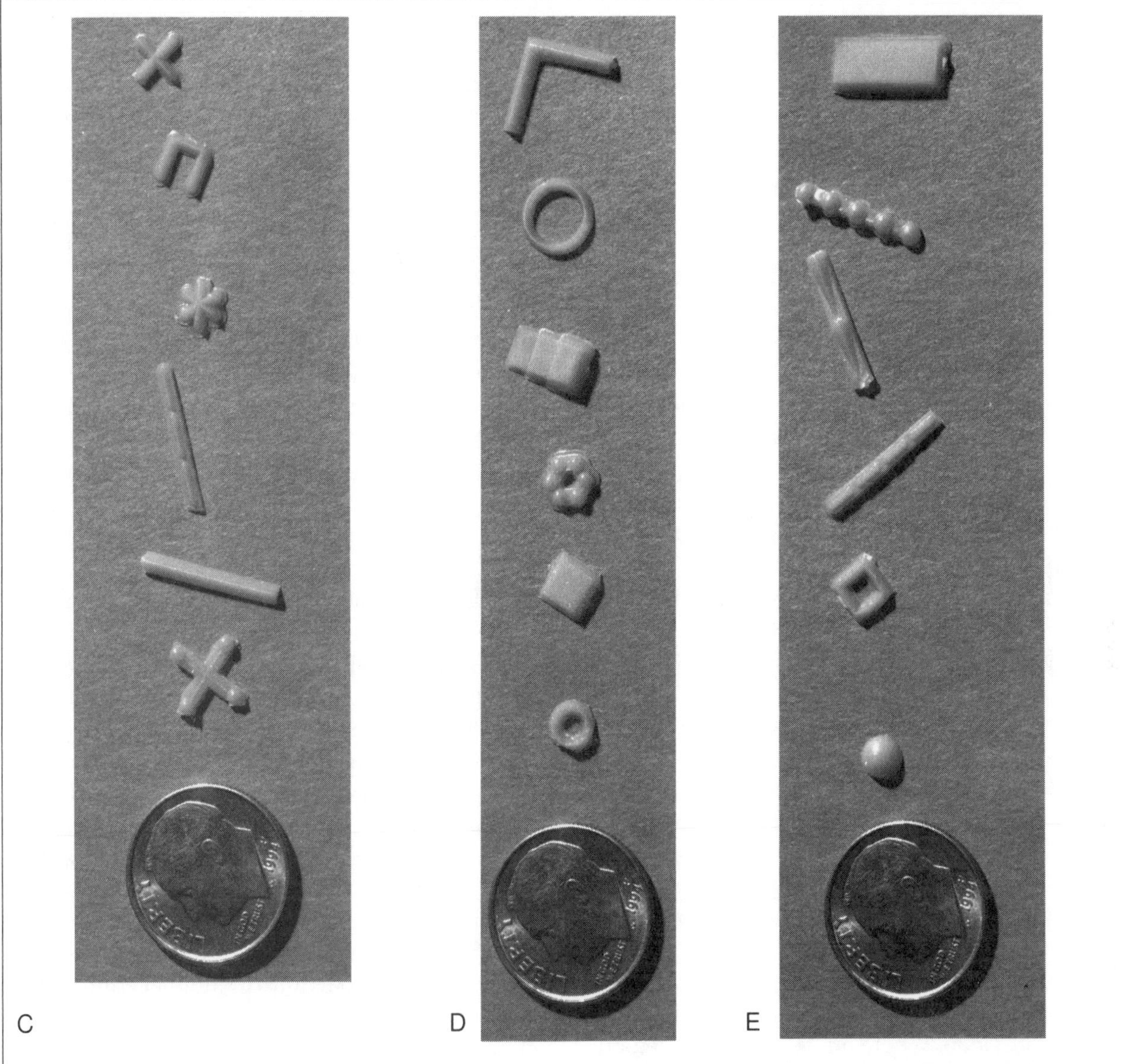

Figure 9.5. ***(continued)***

James & Swain, 1975; Luxton, Banai, & Kuperman, 1994). Verbal (tape-recorded), large-print, and braille (verbal) maps of stations on one rail rapid transit line in Boston are also available.[3] An important aspect of these maps is that they were produced by persons who are blind.

O&M specialists should also be involved in the design of transit maps. For any transit system there will be unique problems, requiring unique decisions regarding information content and display format appropriate to and necessary for travelers who are blind. The same bold graphics used for display maps of transit lines and systems may be made available in paper format and be quite legible to students with low vision.

[3]Massachusetts Bay Transportation Authority (MBTA) Red Line Verbal Map. Massachusetts Association for the Blind, 200 Ivy St., Brookline, MA 02146.

DESIGN PRINCIPLES FOR MAPS

Maps are appropriate for many students and many learning situations. However, whether or not a student benefits by using a map in a particular situation often depends on the creativity and skill of the specialist in designing, making, and using the map. The materials and design of any map must be able to convey the information information needed, and be used in such a manner that students will understand the map itself, and, most importantly, be able to understand the relationship between the map and the environment. This section of this chapter will present principles for designing maps. Subsequent sections will describe some common materials for producing maps, and provide strategies for teaching map reading concepts and skills.

There are a number of issues in the design of maps. The visual acuity and visual efficiency of intended users will determine whether a given map will be most useful if it is tactile, visual, or both tactile and visual. Other issues include: information content, size, scale, choice of symbols, information density, labeling, and provision of supplementary verbal information. Design decisions about each issue impact all the others, so mapmakers need to be aware of the implications of decisions with regard to all these issues. While simply enlarging print maps sometimes makes them usable by persons who have low vision, it is rare that simply raising all information on a print map to make it tactile will result in a map which is very useful to persons who rely on touch for reading; it is likely to have too much information too close together.

In this section of the chapter, map design will be discussed and some guidelines for decision making provided. Where guidelines are based on research, a reference will be given. Other guidelines are based on practice; those given here are drawn from suggestions made by two or more highly experienced mapmakers (specific references will not be given to these). A more comprehensive review of research prior to 1980 can be found in Bentzen (1980). There are several excellent references that provide detailed instructions for mapmaking using one or more techniques (Armstrong, 1973; Edman, 1993; Wiedel & Groves, 1969a, 1969b).

Information Content

Information content is dependent on both what one wants to communicate and to whom. There are two basic rules concerning information content for maps for persons who are visually impaired, regardless of map type (tactile, visual, or tactile–visual).

- Include only information that is absolutely necessary.
- Err on the side of providing too little.

The amount of usable information on a tactile map is less than the total amount that can be recognized (Angwin, 1968a, 1968b). The user may be able to identify all of the symbols on a map, but if much more information is presented than is needed for the user to perform the necessary tasks with the map, relevant information and important relationships may be obscured (Berlá & Murr, 1975). Information to be included should be selected by personal inspection of the area by someone experienced in selecting those elements of the environment that are of greatest significance for travelers who are visually impaired (Wiedel & Groves, 1969a, 1969b).

Map designers should bear in mind that there are a number of environmental features that are not commonly represented on print maps which are either so salient to visually impaired travelers that they are excellent nonvisual landmarks, or so important to the safety of travelers who are blind that they are beneficial when included on tactile maps (or in verbal information accompanying these maps). Examples of such features are slope, changes in walking surface, obstacles, unenclosed stairs, and the nature of traffic controls at intersections—particularly if there is a pedestrian-controlled walk phase.

Size

The overall size of a map is probably best if it is no larger than the span of two hands placed together with the fingers outstretched, about 16–18 inches (400–450 mm). Smaller maps are often better, provided that they are low in information density and the user understands the scale. Perception of both distance and direction on maps is complex. Both the person who reads a map using touch and the person who reads a map using low vision are able to perceive only very limited portions of a map at one time; they must, therefore, integrate over time the spatial relationships that a person with unimpaired vision could see in one glance. Therefore, maps to be used by persons with impaired vision should be as small as possible. Decisions about map size cannot, however, be made independently of decisions about information content and scale; these decisions are always compromises.

Scale

Absolute Scale

Absolute scale on a map expresses the relationship between size of the area mapped and size of the map. It may be expressed in a ratio; for example, the ratio 1:1 means that the map is the same size as the area mapped, and the ratio 1:100 means that one unit on the map corresponds to 100 units in the mapped space. Scale may also be stated verbally, for example, 1 inch = 10 feet. A third way in which scale is commonly indicated on maps is a line divided into equal segments, with a label indicating that, for example, one segment equals 100 feet or 30 meters. Any of these ways of indicating scale can be used on either large-print maps or tactile maps, provided that they are made legible to map users.

Depending on the purposes for which a map is to be used, it is often unnecessary to indicate scale at all. Nonetheless, the map designer has to decide at what scale a map will be made. Decisions about scale will be influenced most by how much information the map is to contain, and how the map is to be used. Secondary considerations will be the actual map space needed for legibility of symbols and labels.

One important determination of scale is the level of graphic abstraction that is meaningful to the map user. Users who are still learning basic environmental concepts may best understand large-scale maps that have rather literal representations of features of the environment. For example, a student who is having difficulty understanding the predictable, useful relationships between streets, curbs, sidewalks, and inside shorelines may benefit greatly by having a large-scale map of an intersection, including sidewalks, curbs, inside shorelines, streets, and crosswalks.

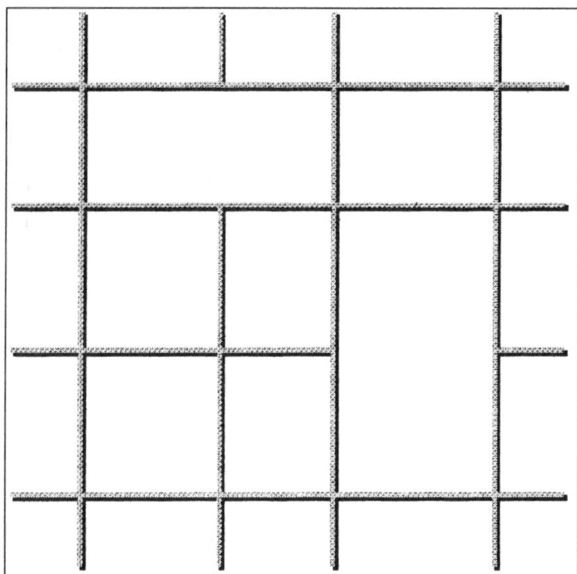

Figure 9.6. If this small-scale map was raised, it would be easy for most users to identify the plus and T intersections.

Source: Drawing courtesy of L. Tabor.

There is, however, a good reason for keeping scale as small as possible to show the needed information and perform the necessary tasks. One of the most difficult map tasks for persons who are visually impaired is shape recognition. This is true regardless of whether these persons read using low vision or touch. Most persons who are visually impaired find shapes easier to recognize in relatively small scale than in relatively large scale. Therefore, if the primary purpose of an aid is to demonstrate a shape, it should be no larger than necessary for good discrimination. It is easy to identify *plus* ("+") and "*T*" intersections in the small-scale map in Figure 9.6. It is much more difficult to understand that the Velcro map shown in Figure 9.11 shows a *plus* ("+") intersection and a "*T*" intersection.

Consistency of Scale

Although persons who are visually impaired can probably acquire the most accurate cognitive maps by use of aids in which every feature is shown at the same scale, it is fortunately not essential for scale to be *absolutely* consistent in all parts of a map for the map to be useful (Armstrong, 1973; Bentzen, 1972; James, 1972; Kidwell & Greer, 1973; Wiedel & Groves, 1969b). There are limitations of the haptic perceptual system, which also apply to perception with impaired vision, which make consistency in scale throughout a map very difficult.

- Symbols that are closer together than $\frac{1}{8}$ inch (3 mm) tend to be perceived as a single symbol. Braille and large print should also be a minimum of $\frac{1}{8}$ inch (3 mm) from the nearest symbol.
- Braille and large print have fixed dimensions that have been determined to result in best legibility. A feature to be labeled may be too small to contain a legible label, and may need to be larger in order to accommodate the label.
- Features must vary from one another in size by at least 25 to 30 percent to be perceived as different in size by most users (Pick, 1980). Larger differences may be better. Inconsistencies in scale may therefore be necessary in order to make differences in the sizes of symbols perceptible.

Symbols

Kinds of Symbols

There are three basic kinds of symbols: point, line, and areal. *Point symbols* show the location of a landmark, clue, or particular travel situation, but say nothing about its shape or dimension. A point symbol may show the location of a certain landmark, such as a specific pedestrian-actuated traffic signal (pushbutton), or it may indicate only that a particular intersection is signalized.

Line symbols convey information that is linear in nature. They indicate both location and direction. A line symbol may represent the location and direction of a specific linear feature such as the Long Island Railway track, or a particular line symbol may be used generically—the same type of line used, for example, to represent the location and direction of all streets in the area shown. Line symbols do not typically convey information about the width or height of what they represent (although they may be modified to do so, especially in situations where a student's conceptual level requires a somewhat literal representation).

Areal symbols convey information about the location of a feature and its shape and size as seen from above. A particular texture or color may be used to show the location, shape, and size of one particular building on a campus; alternatively, the same texture or color may be used in different locations, and in varying shapes and sizes, for all buildings on a campus.

Choice of Symbols

The symbols for a particular map should be ones that are not easily confused with each other, and that are easily perceived and recognized as representing the information they are intended to show. Symbols that are to be used together on a map should differ from each other in as many ways as possible to be most discriminable (Leonard, 1966; Nolan & Morris, 1971; Schiff & Isikow, 1966; Wiedel & Groves, 1969b). A comprehensive illustrated review of symbols in current use is available in Edman (1993). Persons who are engaged in designing multicopy maps of areas, buildings, and facilities are encouraged to base symbol choices on the examples and guidelines available in Edman (1993).

Point symbols can be varied by altering their shape, size, elevation from the background (for tactile maps), and color (for print maps), as well as the nature of their outline (smooth, broken, filled in). Four tactually different circles are visually represented in Figure 9.7. If two circles are to be used as point symbols on the same map, they should differ from one another in two or three characteristics. Other point symbols on the map can also differ in shape. Point symbols should fit under the reader's fingertip, but be large enough

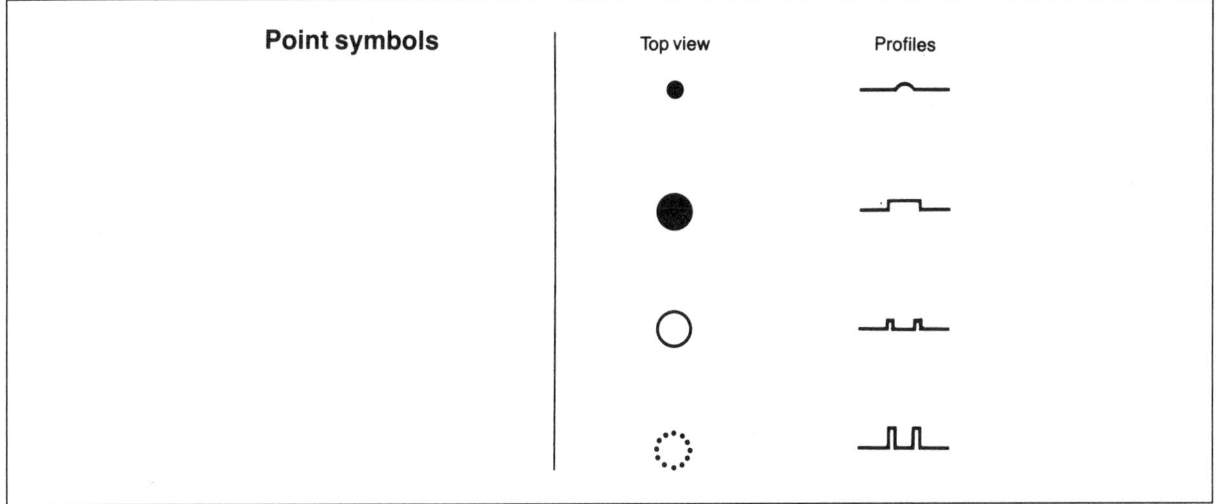

Figure 9.7. Point symbols with the same shape can be varied to make them discriminable.
Source: Drawn by S. Emrich and reprinted from R.L. Welsh and B.B. Blasch (Eds.), *Foundations of Orientation and Mobility* (New York: American Foundation for the Blind, 1980), p. 308.

to be haptically discriminable. If symbols are to be discriminated as different solely on the basis of size or elevation, then the difference in size or elevation should be a minimum of 25 percent (Pick, 1980). Point symbols that are outlined and have straight lines and sharp corners are generally the most legible (Austin & Sleight, 1952; Gill & James, 1973; Lambert & Lederman, 1989).

Symbols that are meaningful, such as a raised shape of a telephone receiver; a sharp, pointed symbol meaning stop or danger; or a miniature staircase are particularly quickly recognized and accurately identified (James & Gill, 1974; Lambert & Lederman, 1989). Use of such meaningful symbols reduces map users' need to refer to a key. On highly schematic maps, two-letter (or two–braille-cell) mnemonic codes may function better than abstract point symbols, whose meaning must be ascertained and remembered (Preiser, 1985).

Line symbols can be varied by making them continuous or interrupted, thick or thin, smooth or rough edged, and single or double (multiple) (see Figure 9.8). Height and profile of lines can also be varied for tactile maps, as can color for visual maps. As with point symbols, line symbols that differ from each other only in width or only in height should differ by a minimum of 25 percent in width or height (Pick, 1980).

In choosing line symbols, it is important to consider the tasks for which they will primarily be used, as well as their discriminability. For example, the line symbol that will be used for the greatest number of tracing tasks on a map should be the one with the best traceability. Narrow, single lines are the easiest to trace by touch, particularly when they are to be traced across intersecting lines (Bentzen, 1983; Bentzen, 1989; Bentzen & Peck, 1979; Easton & Bentzen, 1980). Double raised lines that are more than $\frac{1}{8}$ inch apart are difficult to trace, as both sides of the line are unlikely to be encountered by the fingertip at the same time, and the touch reader must go back and forth to locate both sides. There are, nonetheless, times when it may be desirable to use wider lines—for example, maps of intersections used for teaching recovery from veers at intersections. Double lines also enable the depiction of more detailed information, such as the shapes of curbs or islands. It should be kept in mind, however, that where the width between double lines representing roads is varied, the traceability of the line symbol will vary, and a change in width between the two lines may cause the line to be

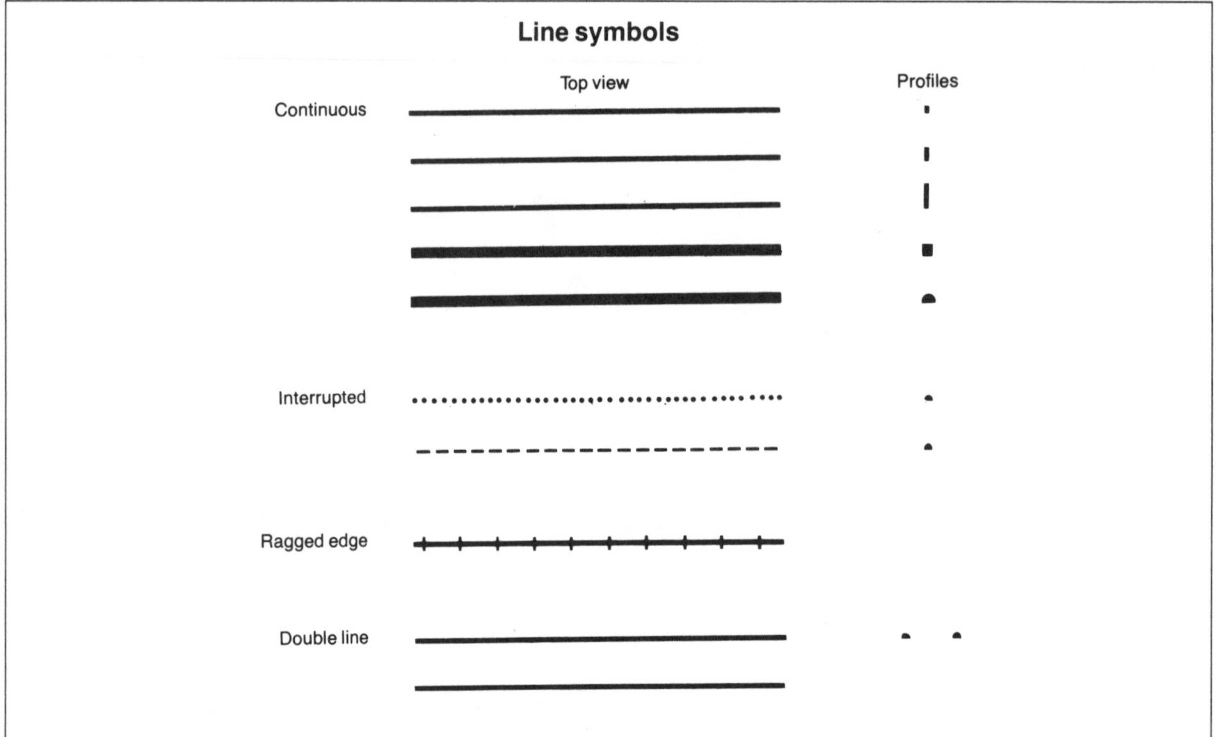

Figure 9.8. Line symbols can be varied to make them discriminable.

Source: Drawn by S. Emrich and reprinted from R.L. Welsh and B.B. Blasch (Eds.), *Foundations of Orientation and Mobility* (New York: American Foundation for the Blind, 1980), p. 309.

perceived and interpreted as an entirely different symbol. Incised lines are very difficult to trace (Nolan, 1971).

Areal symbols should be used to differentiate adjacent areas on a map so that users do not have to trace an outline to determine whether they are "in" or "out of" a particular area. Areal symbols may differ from one another in density of texture elements (spacing between elements), regularity of element spacing, size of elements, shape of elements, and direction of elements (Figure 9.9). On tactile maps they may also differ in intensity or sharpness (rough versus smooth) of the haptic sensation produced, and height in relation to surrounding areas. On print maps they commonly differ in color or gray value.

On tactile maps, differences in *intensity* (or perceived "sharpness") make symbols highly discriminable (Levi & Schiff, 1966), and are easily achieved in some techniques by the use of different grades of sandpaper. Four different grades of standard sandpaper reproduced in vacuum-formed plastic can be readily discriminated in areas as small as $\frac{3}{4}$ square inches (Levi & Schiff, 1966).

Variations in density of texture elements are more distinguishable to touch readers than differences in the shape or orientation of the elements (Levi & Schiff, 1966). Differences in the size of elements can also be a distinguishing characteristic (Nolan & Morris, 1971). However, when an areal symbol is to be used in a small area, it must be a symbol with small elements close together (Levi & Schiff, 1966; Morris & Nolan, 1963).

Areal symbols may obscure line and point symbols on a tactile map (Berlá & Murr, 1975), and should therefore be avoided on areas where line or point symbols are needed to represent significant information or on aids where line tracing

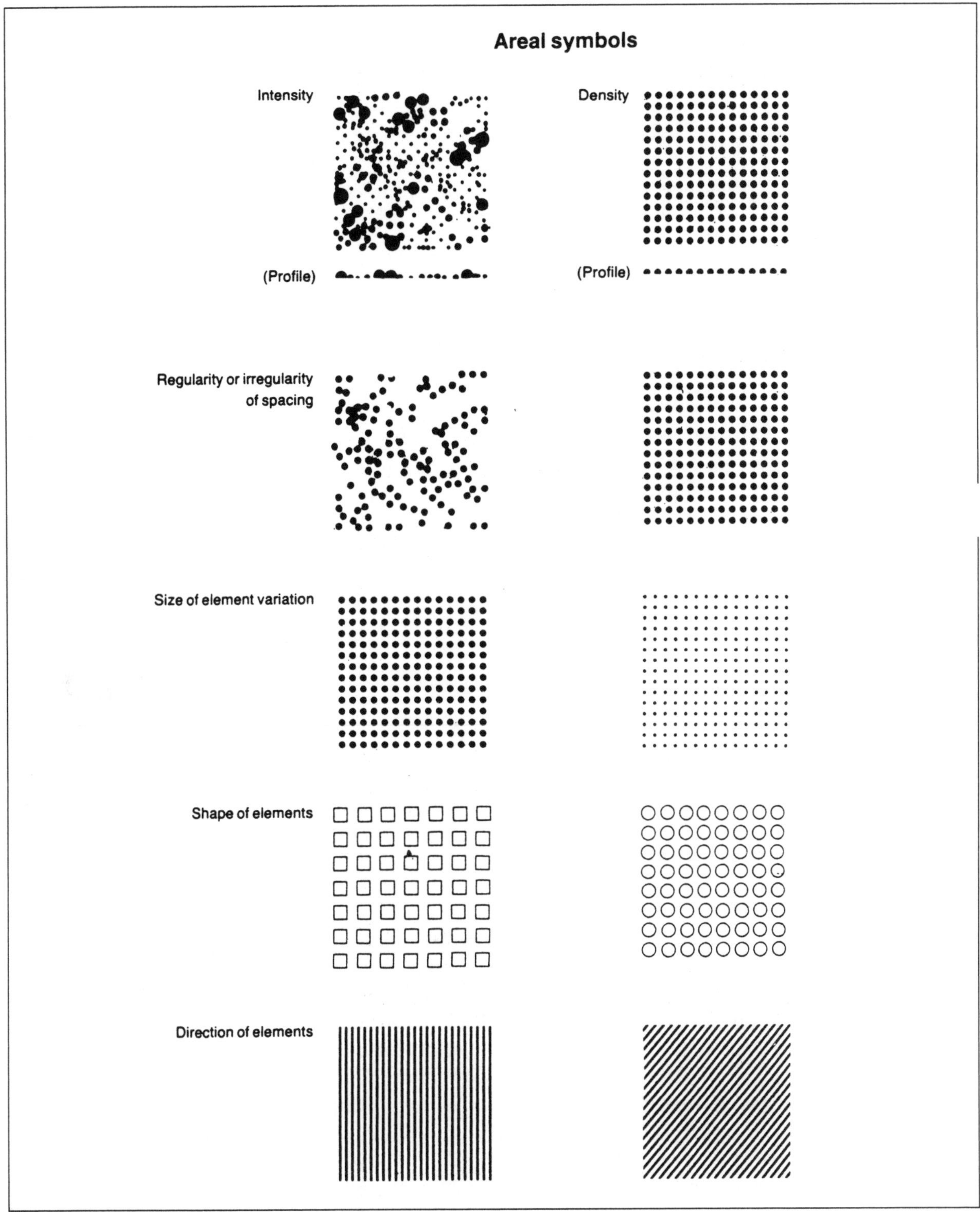

Figure 9.9. Areal symbols can be varied to make them discriminable.

Source: Drawn by S. Emrich and reprinted from R.L. Welsh and B.B. Blasch (Eds.), *Foundations of Orientation and Mobility* (New York: American Foundation for the Blind, 1980), p. 311.

is a major component of the tasks to be performed with the map.

Information Density

Information density for a particular map should be determined by consideration of the user's tactile acuity and haptic perceptual ability. A person whose tactile acuity is reduced by environmental conditions such as cold, or physical conditions such as peripheral neuropathy or calluses, will best be able to use an aid that has maximum spacing between all symbols. A person who has difficulty haptically isolating figure from ground needs maps with minimal information density.

Information density is influenced by other design factors such as information content, scale, size, symbols, and construction materials. There are a number of techniques for reducing information density:

- Use the smallest discriminable symbols.
- Use single-line symbols rather than double lines or a channel.
- Increase the scale.
- Delete unnecessary information, such as borders around maps.
- Place keys on a separate page.
- Place some information on an overlay or underlay.

Overlays and Underlays

A map with an overlay consists of two pages that are hinged together and carefully aligned so that the information on the overlay is directly over related information on the map itself. The reader places one hand on the overlay and the other hand on the page below to read related information. An underlay is made with related information shown on the underside of the same sheet. Underlays are also read with two hands, one on the top and one on the underside.

The drawings in Figure 9.10A–D represent four levels or overlays of a predominantly tactile map of the Perkins School for the Blind campus. Level 1 (Figure 9.10A) contains labels and a marginal grid, bound at the top so it can be used over any of the map pages. It is transparent, and has both print and braille. Level 2 (Figure 9.10B) shows dominant features and configurations of the campus such as paved areas and buildings. Subsequent levels depict more information. Walks are added to Level 3 (Figure 9.10C). Finally, level 4 (Figure 9.10D) contains all information essential for independent route planning to all commonly used destinations on the campus: paved areas, buildings, walks, main entrances, fences or barriers, and the pond. The original tactile maps measured 11 by 11½ inches (28 by 29.5 cm). Proficient travelers who were visually impaired were able to use this map set to plan and travel unfamiliar routes (Bentzen, 1972).

Labels

Adding labels to tactile maps often increases the problems of information density, scale, and choice of symbol size. Braille labels are most legible if they are horizontal, although many users can read labels placed in other directions. Where labels are to be abbreviated, abbreviations should consist of a minimum of two braille cells, and they should be mnemonic; for example, "PS" for Potter Schoolhouse on the map in Figure 9.10A. Labels reduce the need for reference to an index. On any one map, labels should be placed in consistent positions relative to their referents.

A solution to clutter or density added by the use of braille labels is to put them on an overlay or underlay. Overlays and underlays are also suitable for showing multilevel environments such as levels of malls or transit stations.

Grids

On a map of an extended area, it is often desirable to have a *grid* to facilitate locating specific points

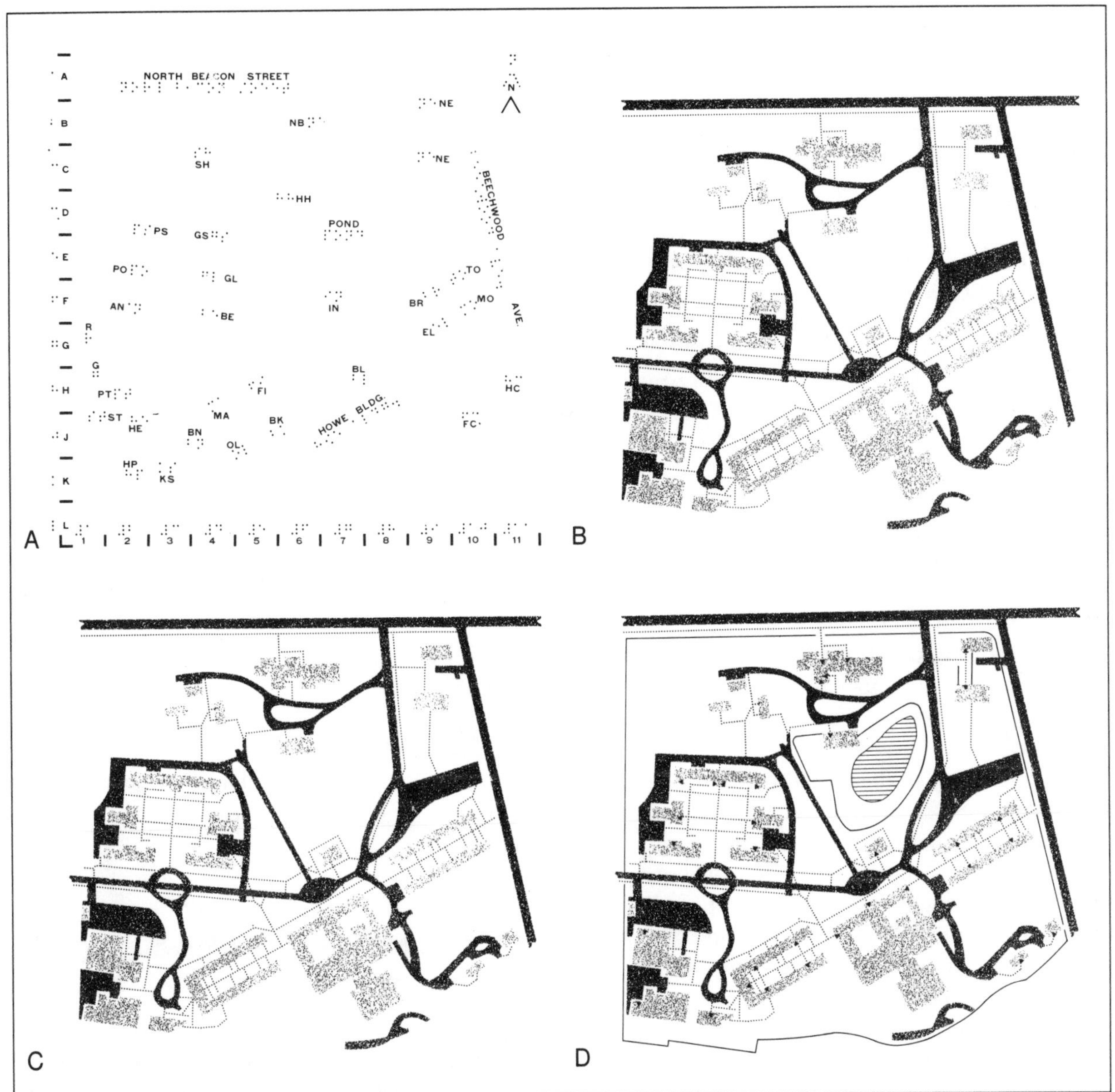

Figure 9.10. (A) Labels and marginal grid of the campus map of the Perkins School for the Blind. (B) Buildings and paved areas (driveways and parking lots). (C) Map in (B) with the addition of walks. (D) Map in (C) with the addition of main entrances (triangles), fences or barriers (solid lines) and the pond.

Source: Drawn by R. Cruedale and reprinted from R.L. Welsh and B.B. Blasch (Eds.), *Foundations of Orientation and Mobility* (New York: American Foundation for the Blind, 1980), pp. 316, 317, 318, 319.

given in a verbal index. This system is commonly used on print maps with indexes and can also be used on tactile maps (Bentzen, 1972). Haptic scanning (or scanning with low vision) is much more time-consuming than scanning with unimpaired vision. A grid system narrows the field that must be searched to find a destination on a map. A tactile or large-print grid can be provided along the margins of a map, or a complete raised or large-print grid can be provided on an overlay or underlay (Armstrong, 1973) (see Figure 9.10A).

MATERIALS AND TECHNIQUES FOR MAKING TACTILE MAPS

Readily Available Craft and Household Materials

Excellent single-copy maps for individual students can be made by gluing commonly available materials onto a base of braille paper or cardboard. Various kinds of string, wire, and even spaghetti can be glued on for line symbols, or lines can be stitched into the base. Buttons, paper fasteners, and staples all make satisfactory point symbols, and various papers, fabrics, and sandpaper make good areal symbols. Maps made of such varied and readily available materials may be both more appealing or interesting to touch than maps made from standardized materials. These maps may also have superior discriminability, because the textures and thermal conductivity of the varied materials will enhance symbol discrimination.

Braille paper or file cards can be used to create maps using either a tracing wheel or chart tape. Tracing wheels with differently spaced teeth can be used to make discriminable lines. Tracing wheels that are small in diameter and have closely spaced teeth, such as the one available from Howe Press, are particularly easy to use. To produce a map using a tracing wheel, you must work in reverse, on the back side of the paper, so that when it is embossed the map will read correctly. Chart tape comes in different widths, textures, and colors, and is still available at some graphics supply stores. (It is becoming less available as computer-aided design [CAD] drawings become more common.) It is excellent for quick production of simple tactile–visual maps. A great advantage of these two systems is that supplies for both can be in a shirt pocket, enabling maps to be made and modified quickly and easily on-site. These materials can be combined on the same map, to create more-discriminable symbols. The materials are not easy for students to use to create their own maps, however.

The above-mentioned materials can also be used to create master copies of maps that will be duplicated in plastic using a vacuum-forming process such as Thermoform. For master copies, care must be taken not to use materials in such a way that they are undercut, or have a top surface that is wider than the base where they are glued to the master; otherwise, good vacuum forming will bring the plastic copies under such symbols, potentially making it impossible to separate the master and a copy without damaging both.

Production of Tactile Maps Using a Brailler

Maps consisting primarily of labels and straight lines that intersect at right angles can be produced by teachers or students on a brailler. Smoothly curved lines cannot be produced on a brailler, but they can be added using a freehand drawing stylus. For individuals who are blind and highly familiar with a brailler, the brailler can be an excellent means for creating simple tactile maps.

Kits and Materials for Producing Single-Copy Maps

There are at least three types of commercially available kits and materials for producing single-copy maps. All can be used by persons who are blind, as well as by their instructors, and they are therefore excellent for teaching cognitive mapping.

Chang Tactual Diagram Kit (Chang Kit)

The Chang Tactual Diagram Kit consists of an 18 × 24 inches black Velcro loop board; 104 yellow, geometric shapes of graduated sizes backed with hook Velcro; and two plastic stick figures. It comes in a carrying case with an instruction manual. The Chang Kit is particularly easy for young children

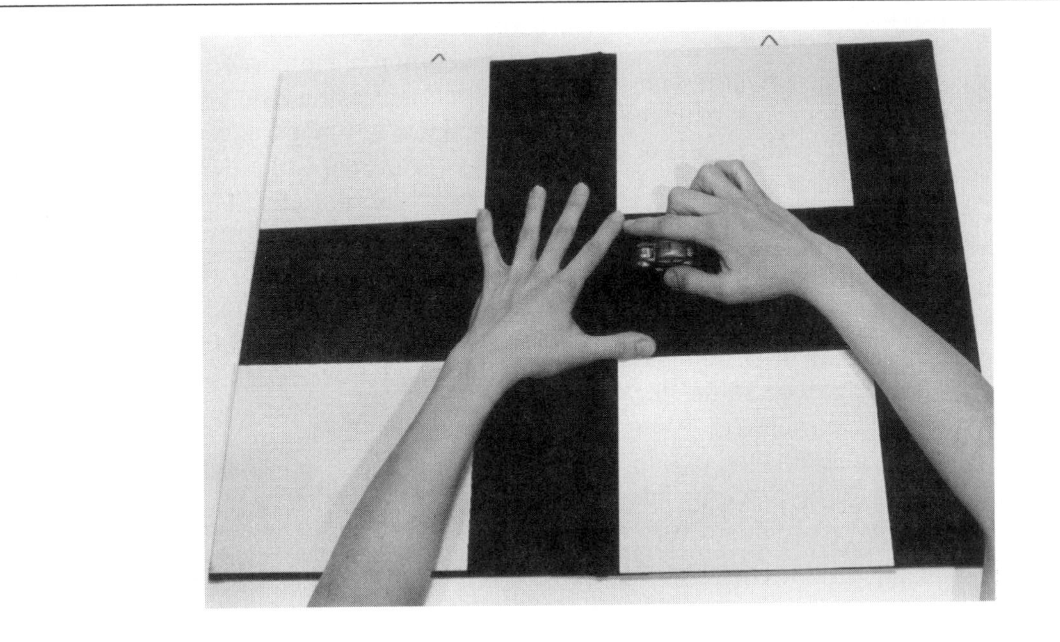

Figure 9.11. Chang Tactual Diagram Kit with a student demonstrating the possible motions of a car at an intersection. The proportion of car to the street width is particularly accurate.

Source: Photo by R. Friedman.

to manipulate, and is pleasing to touch. It is good for showing room arrangements or street layouts. Its large rectangles can be used to represent blocks, and the spaces between them can represent streets; alternatively, long narrow rectangles can represent streets, and the spaces between them can represent blocks (see Figure 9.11).

The kit does not contain small point symbols, but these can be glued onto the smaller plastic shapes, or they can be made by gluing Velcro directly onto items selected for symbols. Braille labels can be glued onto the plastic shapes.

Velcro can also be purchased by the yard or in small shapes, with or without a self-adhesive backing. Teachers can make inexpensive kits that are particularly suited to the needs of their students.

Raised Line Drawing Kit and Raised Line Drawing Board

Both the Raised Line Drawing Kit and the raised line drawing board contain stiff rubber boards to which sheets of Mylar are clamped. Raised graphics are produced by drawing on the Mylar with a ballpoint pen (that preferably has no ink). The pen produces upright raised lines. This is a highly portable system with which teachers and students can communicate their understanding of spatial arrays such as simple room arrangements or complex intersections. It is difficult, however, to produce line, point or area symbols that are discriminable from one another, and there is no visual contrast. Some students find the smooth plastic irritating to read, and young children may lack the control needed to produce legible symbols.

An excellent alternative to the raised-line drawing equipment manufactured in the United States is a Swedish drawing system consisting of textured plastic "sleeves" used over rubber-coated cardboard.[4] The textured plastic is considered more pleasant to touch than Mylar, and because it is in "sleeves" that fit over the drawing board, it is not as difficult to keep in place as separate sheets of Mylar on top of a drawing board.

[4]Available from SIH Laromedel I Solna, Tomtebodavagen 11, S-171 64 Solna, Sweden.

Freund Longhand Writing Kit

The Freund Longhand Writing Kit, sometimes referred to as a "screen board," consists of wire mesh mounted on a $\frac{1}{8}$-inch hardboard. Sheets of newsprint are laid on the mesh, and graphics are produced by drawing with a crayon. Like the raised-line drawing materials described above, this is a simple, useful tool for graphic communication between teachers and students. It is difficult to produce a variety of discriminable symbols using this kit, but it is well suited for quick, nondurable drawings. Drawings can have good visual contrast and can include color. (A satisfactory screen board can also be made by attaching window screening onto hardboard with fabric tape.)

Simple Ways to Make Multicopy Maps

Microcapsule Paper and Flexi-Paper

Microcapsule paper is coated with plastic microcapsules that expand when they are exposed to heat. When a graphic is drawn, photocopied, or laser-printed onto this paper and then exposed to a heat source, the microcapsules expand the most where the paper or plastic is darkest (gets the hottest), which results in a raised image (Andrews, 1985). There are several types of heat sources that may be used.[5]

Flexi-Paper is another product on which a graphic image is raised by passing it through a heat source. It is specifically recommended for use with the Tactile Image Enhancer (TIE), and can also be used with a heat pen.[6] An advantage of Flexi-Paper is that it can be folded or crumpled without affecting the map. It is also weatherproof.

A disadvantage of this technique is that very little variation in symbol height is possible. However, a great advantage is the ease of making the original drawing. Drawings can also be modified with the addition of more information (see Figure 9.12 for an orienteering map produced on microcapsule paper). Digitized atlases (GISs) make it possible to print maps of a desired location in a scale that is appropriate for touch reading. If these maps are printed on microcapsule paper or Flexi-Paper, they can then be readily turned into tactile maps. Extensive editing is sometimes required to delete unnecessary or confusing information or add landmarks of particular interest. CAD systems can also be used to design these maps.

Tactile Graphics Kit

The Tactile Graphics Kit, developed by Barth (1982), contains equipment, supplies, and a guidebook for the creation of aluminum master copies of maps to be duplicated in plastic by vacuum forming. Tools are included to produce seven point symbols, seven line symbols, and four areal symbols, all of which have been demonstrated to be highly discriminable from one another (see Figure 9.13).

Sheet aluminum for making master copies is also available from APH, and a variety of tools available for leather or woodworking, as well as tracing wheels and styli, can be used to make line symbols. Textured materials, point symbols, and labels can be glued onto the aluminum. The maps in Figure 9.10A–D, which predate the Tactile Graphics Kit, were made using this system.

Map and Diagram Making Kit

The well-researched and precisely produced symbols of the Map and Diagram Making Kit are also used to create master copies of maps that are then duplicated in plastic by vacuum forming (see Figure 9.5). Point symbols are injection-molded plastic, line symbols are tooled solder, and areal symbols are sheets of ribbed rubber, linoleum, sandpaper, and tapestry cloth, which are cut to shape. All symbols are glued to a backing such as braille paper. They may be combined with other symbols and techniques, such as placing rolled solder line symbols for streets on top of

[5]Matsumoto Trading Co. 2-14, Nishi Honmachi 1-Chome, Nishi-ku, Osaka, Japan; J. P. Trading, 300 Industrial Way, Brisbane, CA 94005; Reprographics.

[6]Repro-Tronics Inc., 75 Carver Ave., Westwood, NJ 07675.

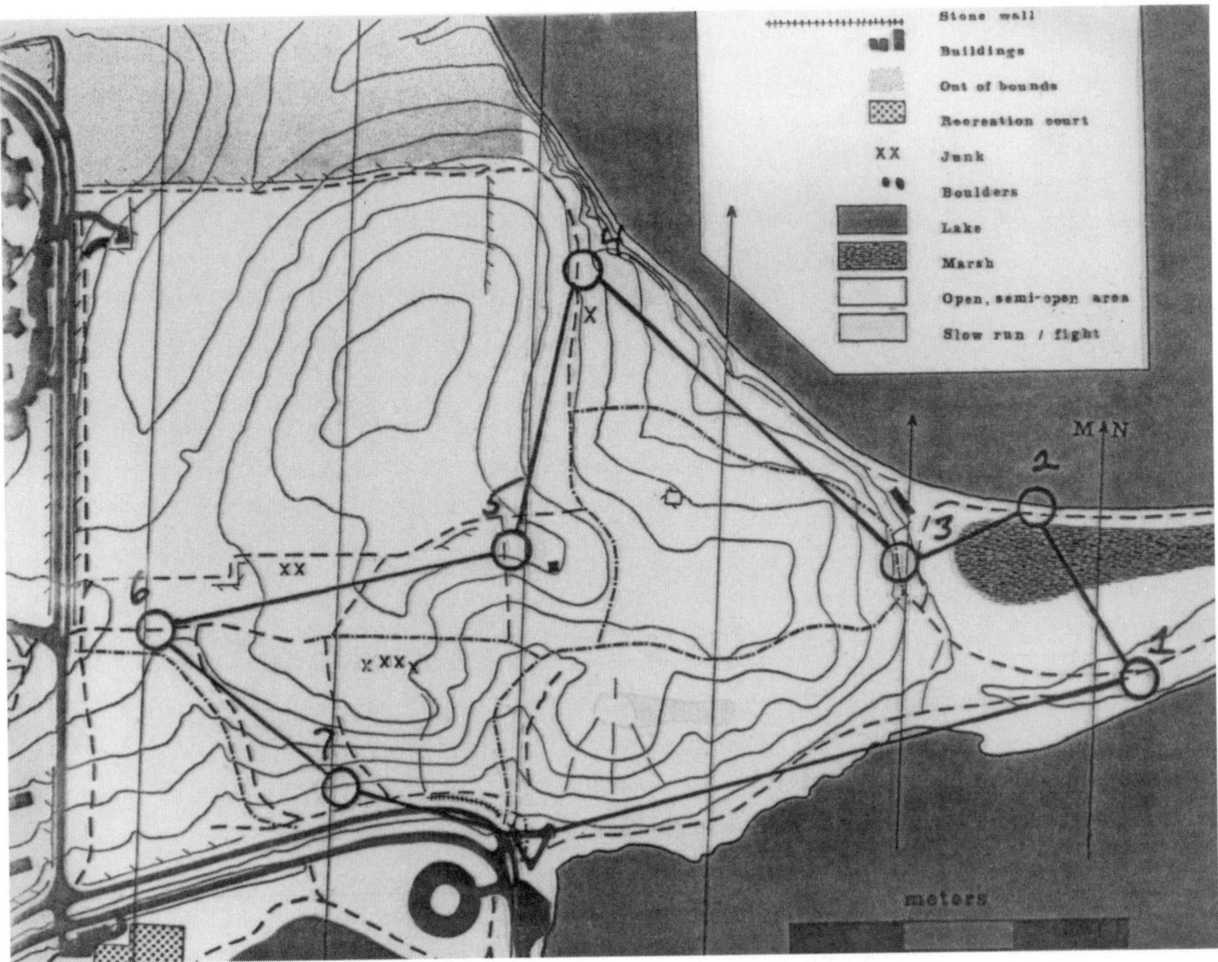

Figure 9.12. Microcapsule map of an orienteering course.

linoleum strips that are cut to show a street layout. The precision of these symbols, coupled-with the fact that they are of multiple heights and have been well researched, enables the production of very detailed maps that are nonetheless quite easy to read by touch. The kit includes easy-to-follow directions for making tactile maps.

Computer-aided Design (CAD) and Production of Tactile–Visual Graphic Maps

CAD design and production of tactile (or tactile–visual) maps, pioneered by Gill (1973a, 1973b) has been further developed at the Computer Center for the Visually Impaired, Baruch College, at the City University of New York. Graphics are designed using CAD software, and are then translated into negative relief by a computer-guided milling machine. A positive master is created by coating the negative created by the milling machine with silicon. Vacuum-formed copies are then produced from the positive master. Maps produced using this process can contain a number of levels of relief as well as braille. The precision in this production process makes symbols particularly discriminable.

CAD systems are also being adapted to produce raised graphics using other technologies, including braille printers and silk screening. Additional information is available in Edman (1993).

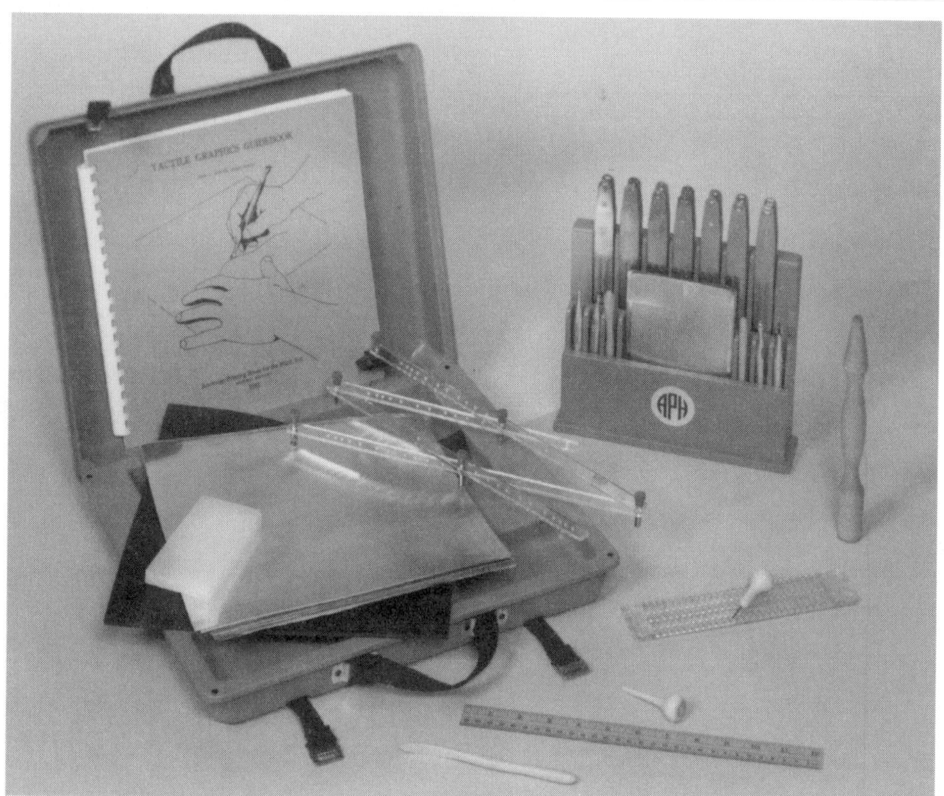

Figure 9.13. The Tactile Graphics Kit includes tools and materials for constructing aluminum foil master maps that can be reproduced on a vacuum-form machine. The tools produce seven point symbols, seven line symbols, and four areal symbols.

Source: American Printing House for the Blind. Reprinted with permission.

It has long been recognized that graphic maps intended to enable independent route planning and travel by persons who are blind function best if they are accompanied by additional verbal information (Bentzen, 1972; Kidwell & Greer, 1973).

An interactive audio-tactile graphics information system called Nomad,[7] developed by Don Parkes (1994; Parkes & Dear, 1991) enables users to independently explore tactile graphics and obtain detailed verbal information as well as recorded environmental sounds associated with particular locations on the graphics. More recently, Parkes (1995) has improved upon Nomad with Tactile Audio Graphics (TAG). These versatile technologies enable persons who are blind to independently discover a wealth of spatial information. More verbal information can be presented by them than on any tactile (or print) aid. Thus, blind users may actually have more information available to them from this map than sighted persons using print maps.

Nomad consists of a specialized electronic touch pad, coupled with a computer. TAG, which is less expensive, more portable and versatile, uses a low cost, conventional, Touch Window. A set of graphics to teach spatial concepts is available from APH, and print or tactile graphics can be made by O&M specialists using any method,

[7]Quantum Technology Pty. Ltd., 5 South St., Rydalmere NSW, 2116, Sydney, Australia; distributed by APH.

and corresponding verbal information easily created using the Nomad program and technology or the TAG system. The TAG system is useable by map-makers who are blind.

TAG and Nomad are promising tools for incorporation into information kiosks that provide graphic spatial layout information in such complex environments as malls, airports, transit stations, and campuses. Many persons who do not consider themselves disabled have difficulty reading maps. An audio-tactile map, incorporated into an information kiosk, would be a particularly user-friendly way for all persons to access spatial layout information. At the simplest level it could name each location touched; at a more complex level it could provide verbal directions for getting from the kiosk to a location; at yet another level it could provide information, such as what's on sale at a shop, flight information, or transit schedules (see Figure 9.14).

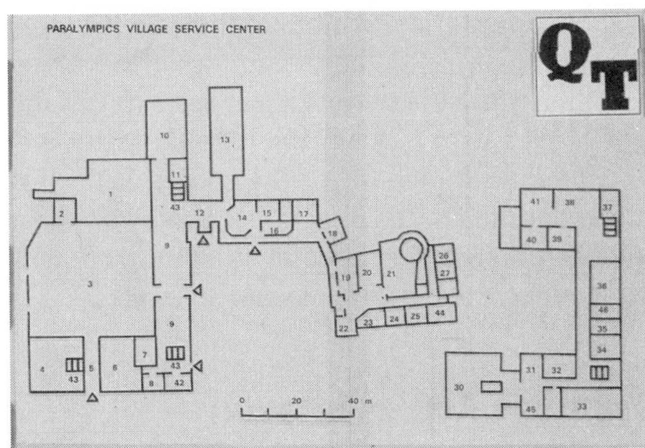

Figure 9.14. Nomad audiotactile map.
Source: Quantum Technology Pty. Ltd., New South Wales, Australia.

TEACHING MAP-READING CONCEPTS

Teaching map-reading concepts and skills to visually impaired persons differs little from teaching the same concepts and skills to persons without visual impairment. In the following section are some general suggestions for teaching these concepts and skills: linear continuity and directionality, symbolic representation, size and scale, shape, and advanced concepts. Materials for each concept should be selected or designed according to the visual and haptic and cognitive abilities of the students. Some specific impairment-related suggestions are made below. Otherwise, it should be assumed that these suggestions apply equally to teaching students who are blind to use tactile maps; teaching low vision students to use specially prepared visual or tactile–visual maps; or teaching low vision students who read regular print to use regular-print maps. In all of these suggested activities the student is asked to draw inferences from a map, travel in the environment to demonstrate the transfer of each concept from a map to the environment, and finally, become a mapmaker. An excellent curriculum for teaching the use of tactile mobility maps is available in Yngström (1991).

Linear Continuity and Directionality

A line conveys linear continuity. To isolate this concept for evaluation or teaching, begin with a map consisting of one straight line. Place the map in front of a student with the line running toward and away from him. Tell the student that the line shows something about where he will be going, and ask the student what he thinks it shows. Many students will be able to generalize that the line means they will go straight ahead, in the direction they are then facing. Another straight line can be connected to the far end of the first line, forming an angle to the left. Students who have good concepts of laterality typically understand that the line means that they will then turn left and walk straight ahead in the new direction. Walk this route in an open space, keeping the map aligned with the environment at all times. When you are at the end of the route, have the student add a line showing a right turn. Then turn right and walk that segment. Continue the lesson by taking turns drawing and walking routes consisting of straight lines and 90-degree turns.

Transfer this concept to a short "L"-shaped route in a bounded space along two sides of a rectangular room. Have the student place on the map an appropriate symbol to indicate his location and bearing at the beginning of the route, and then move the symbol along as he travels the route. Take care to keep the map correctly oriented as the student turns the corner. Later this understanding of the directional quality of linear information will be related to other environmental features, such as streets, and sidewalks.

Symbolic Representation

Symbols represent real objects. Models are a good way to help students who are blind begin to learn this concept, although simple, high-contrast photographs may work better for children with low vision. (Fully sighted children understand photographs before they understand models [DeLoache, 1991].) Students can progress to drawings of objects and to more abstract symbols, through repeated association of the symbol (for example, a red dot for the classroom that has a red door or a square for a square table) with travel to the destination.

Most students can begin by choosing, from preselected materials, symbols to represent objects such as a book, glass, or crayon; tables that are square, round, or rectangular; and placing these on a map. They should talk about why, for example, a circle is a good symbol for a cylindrical glass, or for a round table. Students should also be taught, in an appropriate context, that a graphic symbol may also occasionally be used to represent other kinds of information, such as a place to observe caution, a fixed sound source, or a point at which to solicit aid.

Size and Scale

Size at which information is portrayed on the map is related in an understandable way to object size and distance. Many students use maps very well without ever learning to convert scale to actual distance, but relative distance is a necessary concept for the understanding of nearly all maps—for example, "First I travel a long block, and next, a short block." To relate the concept of scale to mobility in a practical way, the specialist might begin with two lines that point toward and away from students, a short line and a long line. Students may be asked which line is longer, and which line would mean a long walk. Then students might walk different distances in a straight line, and show these distances by making a map.

Ungar, Blades, and Spencer (1996) observed children who were blind who used a particularly effective strategy for judging distances on a tactile map, and subsequently taught the strategy to others. The strategy involved using the number of fingers that could be placed between symbols to estimate distances in terms of fractional relationships with a known distance (i.e., a distance of "two fingers" was half as long as a known distance of "four fingers").

The mathematical concept of scale such as 1 inch = 100 feet (or 1:100 in metric) is taught only after the student has some familiarity with estimating actual distances of travel and has the arithmetical skill necessary to relate the numerical value of scale to the actual distance to be traveled.

Shape

Shapes on maps are related in an understandable way to shapes in the environment mapped. In teaching this concept, it can be helpful to begin by having students match drawings of shapes with corresponding plane shapes. The task is easiest if the drawings and plane shapes are at a scale of 1:1, the shapes fit easily into one hand, and the shapes are presented in the same orientation. Students may then match small drawings with larger plane shapes in different orientations, and next match drawings with objects that have a dominant (top) plane surface in a simple shape, such as jar lids and box tops. Later they can match drawings with larger objects such as tables, which they must walk around in order to understand their shapes.

Now students are ready to make very simple maps using lines (of different lengths) and symbols (at different distances) of objects on a rectangular table. This activity should begin by having students determine the shape of the table and then represent it on the map. The Chang Tactile Diagram Kit can be readily used for this activity, making additional symbols, if needed, from poster board and Velcro.

The next activity could entail mapping a small, simply furnished room. In mapping a room, the following sequence of activities is recommended. The room should first be explored; have students note its shape and the furnishings that will be represented on the map. This exploration should be done from a home base along one wall. When finished, students should sit at home base; facing the opposite wall, and hold a map base (such as a Velcro board or tray) to correspond to the orientation of the room. A symbol should then be placed along the edge of the map closest to the student's body to represent home base. Students should then make tentative selections, from available materials, of symbols to be used to represent furnishings. If necessary, guidance should be given in choosing symbols appropriate in size and shape to what they represent. This is very reinforcing to the learning of the concepts of symbolic representation, size and scale, and shape. Students should arrange the symbols along the opposite wall on their maps, in positions corresponding to their memories of the relative positions of the furnishings. Accuracy can be confirmed by another trip to explore the opposite wall, paying more attention, if necessary, to relative distances between furnishings. The walls to the right and left can be mapped in the same way. Pointing to actual objects as their symbols are placed on the map helps to further connect map location with actual location.

It can be helpful to have students change perspective before they map the wall against which they were originally seated. They should sit against the wall that they were previously facing, so that they now face the original home base. The maps should remain oriented correctly in relation to the room. Students should again point to symbols on the map and the furnishings each represents. They should notice that they point generally to the left for things which are shown on the left side of the map and that previously they pointed generally to the right to point toward these same objects before they changed position. An important generalization to help students at this point: the map did not turn, nor did the room turn; *they* turned. When students have mapped furnishings along the walls, they may add central furnishings.

Concluding tasks can involve planning routes on the map, verbalizing them, and traveling them from various starting points. Each trip will further confirm the relationship between the location of things on the map and things in reality.

A fun activity that can be used in integrated school settings is a game in which students must locate objects hidden by partners in a mapped area; the objects' locations have been marked on the map by the partners. These maps can also be used for drop-off lessons in which students, who have been disoriented, first find their location on the map, and then travel to a destination. They can be challenged to find the shortest route, a new route, or a "funny" route.

Advanced Concepts

Actual location on the Earth of things portrayed on a map can be understood by relating their location on the map to compass directions, and by converting distance on the map to actual distance. The student who has fully grasped the concepts involved in the preceding tasks needs to add an understanding of compass directions as they are shown on a map, and the arithmetic necessary to convert distance on a map to distance on the Earth. This should be taught in conjunction with actual travel in which compass directions are being learned, and it can complement such lessons.

In using the map during actual travel, it is helpful to keep the map oriented so that the northern edge is always facing toward the north (Rossano & Warren, 1989). Whatever is farthest from the student on the map corresponds to the environment in front of him (objects on the left side of the map will be to the student's left, etc.).

Frequent touching of symbols on the map and then pointing to the objects they represent will reinforce this concept as well as the ability to relate the items shown on a map to one's actual body position within the area mapped. It is helpful to use a map that has a number of distinctive landmarks (Ungar et al., in press). Choose some kind of a moveable symbol with a "nose" to represent a student. Have the student stop frequently to place himself or herself on the map, being careful to point the "nose" in the correct direction. When students no longer need to have a symbol for themselves, have them place a finger on each landmark as they come to it.

Many students experience difficulty in transferring what they observe on a map to travel in the environment. The best way to help students transfer map observations to travel is to have them regularly travel with a map, and often a compass, in hand, repeatedly showing their location on the map and pointing toward other locations as well as compass directions. This activity will quickly reveal to a specialist the gaps in the students' knowledge of spatial concepts and the areas mapped; it is a key activity in teaching and diagnosing difficulties in spatial updating. *Orienteering* is an excellent, fun way to promote map use (see Figure 9.12), in combination with other O&M skills and concepts and the use of a compass (Blasch & Brouwer, 1983). Traditionally, orienteering is a timed cross-country race in which the participants use a map and compass to plan the most efficient route between controls (checkpoints) on an unfamiliar course set in a large undeveloped area or any environment appropriate for the skill level of the participants. For O&M, orienteering courses might also be in a city.

TEACHING MAP-READING SKILLS

Scanning Systematically

Scanning in a systematic pattern to locate graphic symbols is, regardless of the type of impairment, essentially the application of organized search procedures to the map. In teaching this skill, maps with few and highly discriminable symbols should be used. First, the student should be shown an isolated sample of a symbol. Then the map should be systematically searched for examples of the symbol, using both hands beside each other in a top-to-bottom pattern, and working from left to right (Berlá, 1972; 1973). This systematic scanning of an entire map (tactile and visual) should give the reader some idea of the size of the map, information density, concentrations of information (if any), and the symbols used. Subsequent haptic or visual scanning for specific symbols may start and go outward from an easily recognized feature on the map.

Ungar, Blades, and Spencer (1995) demonstrated the importance of having effective strategies for learning spatial layouts portrayed by maps. Children whose learning was most accurate frequently related map features to the frame of the map, and also mentioned relationships between features.

Identifying Symbols

When teaching students to identify symbols, the specialist should begin with maps that have just a few, highly discriminable symbols. Students should readily be able to identify each symbol used before they are given tasks requiring the combination of symbol identification with other information-gathering techniques. There is some evidence that haptic readers perform best on discrimination tasks when only the index fingers are used (Berlá & Butterfield, 1977; Foulke, 1964; Hill, 1973; Lappin & Foulke, 1973).

Tracing Line Symbols

Visual or haptic tracing of line symbols may be facilitated by keeping one index finger at a starting point. This will make correction easier if one "gets off the track." The direction of motion of the hand as it explores a tactile line appears to influence the perception of the direction of that line in space (Pick, 1980). Thus, it is important to encourage students to hold maps squarely in front of their bodies, and well aligned with the environment, for the most accurate perception of the directions of lines.

There is some evidence that guiding the finger of a tactile reader along lines results in a more accurate mental image of the shape described by that line than free haptic exploration. The probable reason for this is that haptic line-tracing is not a particularly easy task, and is often accompanied by a good deal of off-line searching, especially if the shape is complex. Touch seems to be poorly suited for the acquisition of two-dimensional information, even when it is raised. Students have difficulty independently experiencing unfamiliar two-dimensional shapes using exploration that is continuous and fluid enough to result in accurate cognitive maps. Thus the preferred strategy for introducing a map to students may be to first guide a preferred finger along the most important lines and then encourage students to retrace the lines until they can do this smoothly without hesitation. When they have done this, they are ready to talk about what those lines mean (Kennedy, 1995).

Recognizing Shapes

The ability to recognize a shape requires the skills of haptically or visually tracing the outline of a shape, recognizing distinctive features of that shape, and comparing the distinctive features with the remembered features. Both haptic readers and persons with reduced visual fields may need practice in combining these skills into shape recognition.

It is of critical importance that such readers have a *system* for shape recognition tasks, as the relationship of distinctive features (hence shape) may appear different if each feature is not perceived, and these features are not perceived in the same order each time the reader looks at the same shape (Gibson, 1966). For example, students may be trained to trace a shape with the index finger of their preferred hand, while using the index finger of their other hand as a reference. Tracing should begin and end at the reference finger. Students should be trained to recognize distinctive features such as "parts that stick out, parts that are pointed, parts that go in, and parts that are curved" (Berlá & Butterfield, 1977). Remember that it is the *outline* of the shape that conveys shape, not any texture that may fill an enclosed shape.

Special Considerations for Persons with Low Vision

Whenever a map is to be read by a person with low vision, lighting should be glare-free. Each kind of map-reading task should be tried with and without any optical aid normally used for near work. The specialist should remember that tasks especially requiring acuity, such as the identification of small symbols, may be easier with an optical aid. Tasks facilitated by a full field—for example, gaining a general idea of the utilization of space or relating widely separated areas of the map to each other—may be easier without an optical aid that magnifies, but also reduces the user's visual field.

Well-designed maps are particularly important when teaching persons with field restrictions, as they are less likely to accurately perceive spatial layout than persons with acuity loss (Rieser, Hill, Talor, Bradfield, & Rosen, 1992).

EMERGING TECHNOLOGIES

There now exist compact disc read-only memory (CD-ROM) databases (GISs) that are atlases of streets and highways throughout the United States. At least one of these GISs can be accessed via home computer to provide verbal directions (in effect, a verbal route map) between any two points in the database.[8] One advantage of a map in the form of a GIS on CD-ROM is that informa-

[8]Atlas Speaks, Arkenstone, 1390 Borregas Avenue, Sunnyvale, CA 94089.

tion can be randomly accessed, unlike verbal tape-recorded maps. Zimmerman (1990) demonstrated that an experimental database of spatial layout information about a 5- by 5-block area could be used by persons who are blind to become familiar with locations of landmarks in that area; he recommended this approach for familiarizing proficient blind travelers with areas that are new to them, such as campuses or public transit routes.

Position tracking systems—including the global positioning system (GPS), to which differential signals are typically added to improve accuracy—are being experimentally coupled with GISs to provide travelers who are blind with real-time information about their location and routes to destinations while they travel (Golledge, Loomis, & Klatzky, 1994). The GPS is an electronic position-sensing technology utilizing orbiting satellites that communicate with portable transmitter/receivers which, in interaction with a GIS, can inform users of their location and relationship to landmarks or coordinates. Some problems that need to be overcome in the application of GPS technology for providing wayfinding information to blind travelers are inaccuracy and its limited applicability (only areas in which a line of sight to at least three GPS satellites can be maintained). Even with the inclusion of an additional differential signal, the accuracy may still be inadequate for telling users which side of a street they are on, and current systems are inoperable indoors, between tall buildings, or under trees. Although these problems may be overcome by the use of other position-tracking technologies, an additional obstacle to implementation of position-tracking technologies is the fact that current GISs (which were mostly developed for vehicular traffic) do not contain information about landmarks and small-scale layouts that may be particularly relevant to blind travelers.

ORIENTATION AIDS AND THE O&M SPECIALIST

Many travel concepts and skills can best be taught using orientation aids, therefore each specialist should be thoroughly familiar with orientation aids, design principles, materials available for production, and techniques for aid use. Specialists should have materials appropriate for their students readily available for use on many lessons.

O&M specialists should also be involved in the design of special-purpose orientation aids for schools, agencies, metropolitan areas, or transit systems that wish to provide mobility maps to visually impaired persons who use their facilities. An informed O&M specialist is the professional most capable of judging which information is most appropriate to promote independent travel in any situation, along with its purpose and the way it is displayed. Any specialist participating in the design of such an aid should be certain that it will be made available in ways which facilitate its optimum use and the best understanding.

Finally, O&M specialists should be alert to the development of new technologies that may speed up familiarization with new areas, or enable travelers who are blind to obtain real-time information about their locations and routes to destinations. The expertise of O&M specialists will be important in the creation of GISs that include information most relevant to and necessary for the independent travel of blind persons.

Suggestions/Implications for O&M Specialists

1. In many instructional situations, survey-level cognitive maps may be acquired more readily from large-print or tactile maps than from exploring an environment.
2. Models more closely represent three-dimensional space and are a good bridge to the use of maps, especially by children who never had sight. The best models are most like the things they represent.
3. Involving students in map-making is an excellent way to teach the skills required for the creation of cognitive maps, especially survey-level cognitive maps.
4. Simple tactile or large-print maps are helpful in teaching basic spatial concepts to children who are visually impaired.
5. Map-reading concepts must be taught to children with visual impairments as they begin to use maps.
   - a. A line conveys linear continuity.
   - b. Symbols represent real objects.
   - c. The size at which information is portrayed on a map is related in an understandable way to real size or distance.
   - d. Shapes on maps are related in an understandable way to shapes in the environment mapped.
6. Map-reading skills must be taught.
   - a. Scanning systematically
   - b. Identifying symbols
   - c. Tracing line symbols
   - d. Recognizing shapes
7. Tactile and visual maps permit random access of information and can convey spatial layout more accurately than verbal aids. They are especially appropriate for layouts such as complex intersections, campuses, transit systems and stations, and urban areas.
8. Verbal aids can contain more descriptive information than tactile maps. Information access is sequential in tape-recorded maps, but it can be random in portable electronic formats. Travelers who are blind can easily make their own verbal maps.
9. Tactile maps should include only the information that is absolutely necessary.
10. Relatively consistent scale should be maintained throughout a map.
11. Map symbols should be easily perceived and recognized. Symbols that are used together on a map should differ in as many ways as possible. The choice of symbols for tactile maps must be based on touch.
12. Complex tactile maps that are to be used independently should be accompanied by additional descriptive information.
13. Electronic databases of geographic information, coupled with position-sensing technology, may revolutionize wayfinding for persons with visual impairments who have access to the technology.
14. O&M specialists need to be involved in the design of tactile and verbal orientation aids for multiple users, such as transit maps and city maps.

ACTIVITIES FOR REVIEW

1. Describe the kinds of information contained in a cognitive map. How would the cognitive maps of rote travelers, route-level travelers, and survey-level travelers differ.
2. Explain why children who are blind should become mapmakers? Is this also important for children who travel using visual information? Is it important for adventitiously blind adults? Why or why not?
3. Describe the orientation aid you would make to help a 10-year-old student who is totally blind and has a severe cognitive disability learn how to get from his or her classroom to the bathroom. What are the advantages of this aid in this situation?
4. Describe three teaching situations in which a model might work better than a map. Give reasons for each.
5. Explain how you might use a map or model of a plus intersection to help an adventitiously blind, adult student anticipate the consequences of veers.
6. Raised-line drawing materials may result in maps that are hard to read and very limited in the types of information available. Nonetheless, they may be excellent materials in some instructional situations. Describe two situations (students and objectives) in which raised-line drawing materials might be excellent tools.
7. Describe how a student's use of a tape-recorded map would differ from the use of a map stored in a Braille 'n Speak. Give examples of situations in which each would be preferred.
8. Explain how you would determine how much information to include in a particular map for an individual student. What information would you include in a map to be used to teach a capable second-grader who is blind how to recover from veers at driveways? Describe two activities that you might do with the student using this map.
9. Describe the limits that the predetermined size of a map places on information content, scale, symbols, and labels. How might you deal with street names in a neighborhood map in order to reduce information density?
10. List the three kinds of map symbols. How must symbols that are to be used together on a tactile map be chosen?
11. Describe the characteristics of tactile line symbols that would function well on transit maps. Why did you choose these characteristics?
12. Describe in some detail an activity you would do with students to help them transfer map skills and concepts to actual travel.

CHAPTER 10

Environmental Accessibility

Billie Louise Bentzen

Accessibility for persons with visual impairments is usually a matter of having the right information at the right time. Having information means having choices and the ability to make the correct choice the first time; it means *not* having to engage in time-consuming deductive reasoning from imprecise clues or frequently having to ask for information or assistance. Having information also means being able to travel more safely: an audible pedestrian signal indicates a safe time to cross a street whose signal phase cannot be judged by listening to traffic; a detectable warning along a transit platform indicates the limit of the safe waiting area.

The primary task of orientation and mobility (O&M) specialists is to provide to persons who are visually impaired appropriate tools and techniques so that they can travel safely, efficiently, and independently in all environments of interest or importance to them. The focus is on travelers, and on what travelers can do for themselves. The firm belief that persons who are visually impaired are capable of safe, efficient, graceful, independent travel is the philosophical foundation on which the profession of O&M rests. It is the philosophy of this author that persons who are blind are able to negotiate virtually any environment; if they have access to the same information as persons who have sight, they can travel in the same way as sighted persons—independently, quickly, efficiently, and with freedom of choice.

Throughout the world there is a growing awareness of and commitment to the rights of all persons, regardless of their abilities, to a built environment that is safe, accessible, and usable. However, it must be recognized at the outset of this chapter that environmental accessibility for persons with visual impairments is a controversial topic. Mettler (1987, p. 481) has articulated a philosophy that opposes environmental design intended to facilitate independent travel by persons who are visually impaired: "Environmental modifications advanced in the name of increasing the independence and integration of blind people, threaten to contribute to their dependence and isolation by reinforcing the belief that blind people are, by nature, inherently incompetent."

However, we live in a society which has long recognized that although most people can travel safely most of the time, there are nonetheless situations which are inherently unsafe for all travelers. Potentially dangerous situations such as construction sites commonly must have barriers around them, while others have various kinds of warning signals, such as audible signals on subway doors that are about to close, or safety yellow warning stripes at the edges of subway platforms. We recognize that nondisabled persons make mistakes and have accidents, so there are numerous requirements and guidelines for making the environment safer for them. Some of these work for persons who are visually impaired and some do not—particularly if they require vision to be effective, such as signs saying "Caution," or flashing warning lights.

It is also recognized that wayfinding in our complex built environment is facilitated for all persons by print information such as numbers on rooms and elevators, street signs at intersections, numbers and destinations on busses, and directional signs in transit stations. Other travel information that we have come to expect includes maps, building directories, and transit schedules. These kinds of information are an important part of what makes the environment accessible to all people.

Many persons who are blind travel with little or no assistance in familiar environments, even ones that contain numerous fixed and moving hazards and few reliable landmarks. These same persons typically must ask for information or assistance in unfamiliar or particularly complex areas, however. They are simply unable to independently obtain the kinds of information, such as street names, building names, and building directories, that persons with sight consider to be essential wayfinding features of the built environment. While all travelers occasionally need to ask for information or assistance in wayfinding, it is known that asking other people is (for people in the United States) the least preferred way to obtain wayfinding information (Battelle Memorial Institute & Ilium Associates, 1976). Because of the lack of wayfinding information in accessible media, persons who are visually impaired are obliged to ask more often, or travel much less. Additionally, asking is made more difficult, sometimes risky, and often embarrassing by the difficulty of judging by nonvisual clues whether the person nearby is likely to be one who knows the answer to the traveler's question, speaks the traveler's language, or is a threatening individual. This chapter assumes that persons who are visually impaired have a right to obtain wayfinding information independently.

Some aspects of the environment have always been difficult for persons who are visually impaired to negotiate safely and efficiently, such as objects that protrude into the path of travel at head height and are not supported by any structure which can reliably be detected by a long cane. Other aspects are becoming more difficult as cues change or are removed, such as the substitution of curb ramps or blended curbs for curbs at corners. This activity chapter will highlight some aspects of the built environment that compromise the safety of travelers with impaired vision, or make orientation difficult. It will also present a number of strategies for making the environment more conducive to safe and well-oriented travel.

The chapter will place environmental accessibility for persons having visual impairments within the historical context of concern for access for all persons, and within the current architectural goal of universal design. The issues presented are ones that must be dealt with worldwide, although particular examples of problems and suggested solutions are drawn primarily from the United States. This is because these are the ones best known to the author, not because they are necessarily the best examples. References to specific standards or guidelines will be minimal, as these vary so widely across time and place. O&M specialists who are committed to fostering independent travel for persons who are visually impaired will seek out those standards, guidelines, and recommendations that are applicable to their country and more immediate locale, in order to be informed, effective advocates for environmental accessibility.

HISTORICAL CONTEXT

In the early 1900s residential schools and rehabilitation facilities for individuals with visual impairments introduced numerous design elements intended to make travel safer and easier for their students or clients. This was long before any general social movement toward architectural accessibility—and also before programs were organized to train people with visual impairments to travel independently. Persons who were blind, as well as the persons responsible for their education and rehabilitation, recognized that the nature of the built environment made a significant difference in their safety and ease of travel. They also recognized that with good training and an aid such as a long cane or dog guide, many blind persons could learn to travel safely and efficiently. Both environmental design and instruction in independent travel skills were pioneered by the field of blindness (Blasch & Stuckey, 1995).

In the United States, the 1970s was a decade of great activism by persons with disabilities, particularly organizations of persons with physical disabilities. This activity culminated in the publication of a landmark industry standard for accessibility known colloquially as the *ANSI Standard (American National Standard for Buildings and Facilities: Providing Accessibility to and Usability for Physically Handicapped People* A117.1, American National Standards Institute, 1980). It was the first accessibility standard in the United States that provided detailed specifications for a number of architectural elements. It was an industry standard, not enforceable by governmental authority, but nonetheless very powerful in guiding product development and the framing of subsequent governmental standards and guidelines that were enforceable.

The *ANSI Standard*'s (1980) emphasis, which reflected the concerns of the major advocates of the 1970s, was on designing an environment that was negotiable by persons using wheelchairs. Thus requirements and specifications for elevators, ramps (including curb ramps), adequate space for maneuvering wheelchairs, and dimensional requirements for reaching or transferring from wheelchairs were particularly well developed.

The concept of an accessible route was articulated and a symbol of accessibility was standardized. An accessible route, broadly speaking, is one that is negotiable by persons using wheelchairs. Such accessible routes are to be provided to link all features in the built environment—for example, providing a route without curbs linking a parking space for persons with disabilities to the facility the parking lot serves. Accessible routes may not include stairs. However, curbs and stairs are not only negotiable by persons with visual impairments, they may be important cues used by travelers who are blind to determine just where they are in an environment. An accessible route, as defined in the United States, is one that may not be desired by or even particularly safe for persons who are visually impaired!

The standard wheelchair access symbol which identifies an accessible space such as a building or restroom can logically be interpreted as indicating that the building can be negotiated without using stairs and the rest rooms have adequate space and appropriately designed facilities to be managed by persons using wheelchairs. There is, however, no logical association of this symbol with access features such as braille signs for identifying rooms in a hotel or braille menus in a restaurant. Thus the whole approach to architectural accessibility, at least in the United States, was initially guided by, and remains somewhat limited by, concern for providing environments negotiable by persons using wheelchairs.

There is, however—even in the landmark *ANSI Standard* (1980)—some concern for persons with other disabilities, including persons who are visually impaired. For example, tactile characters (but not braille) were required in elevators; objects were permitted to intrude in the path of travel only by amounts that were presumably detectable by users of long canes; tactile warning surfaces were to be included in designs for curb ramps and preceding some staircases; and signs were to be high in contrast and have particular font characteristics to assure high legibility. There was not much research on which to base these particular requirements, and some of them did not really improve access, but it is at least reassuring that in this landmark document some attention was paid to the fact that how the environment is built affects the ability of visually impaired persons to travel safely and efficiently.

It was already recognized that compromises were needed if environments were to be accessible to all people. For example, people who used wheelchairs needed curb ramps; replacing curbs with curb ramps would result in the removal of the primary cue used by persons who were blind to inform them that they had arrived at a street.

Therefore curb ramps needed to have surfaces that were detectable by blind travelers. Some research preceded this standard which indicated that a ridged rubber mat was highly detectable (Aiello & Steinfeld, 1980). The resulting standard loosely described a number of surfaces that could be used. Curiously, the ridged rubber mat was not included, but grooved concrete was—and no testing had indicated that it was detectable!

Another major milestone in the disability rights movement in the United States was the passage in 1990 of the Americans with Disabilities Act (ADA), a civil rights law providing for nondiscrimination on the basis of disability in such areas as employment, public accommodations, and government services. In 1991, the Architectural and Transportation Barriers Compliance Board (commonly called the Access Board) published *The Americans with Disabilities Act (ADA) Accessibility Guidelines for Buildings and Facilities* (or *ADAAG*), which provides specifications intended to make the built environment accessible to all people with disabilities, specifically including those with sensory and cognitive disabilities. A summary of the sections of *ADAAG* specifically applicable to persons with visual impairments may be found in Wiener (1992).

ADAAG does not require that the United States be made accessible overnight; standards are to be applied to new construction and alterations, and only to existing construction when this is "readily achievable"—a concept that takes into account the cost and difficulty of modifications. For public transit there are various extended timetables for bringing all properties into compliance.

At the time of this writing, *ADAAG* has been in existence for about six years, and signs of its implementation abound. Since the concept of providing accessibility for persons using wheelchairs has been well established for more than a decade, and architects, planners, and builders understand this concept, we are seeing a rapid proliferation of such costly features as ramps, elevators, and accessible rest rooms. Accessibility features that are particularly beneficial to persons with visual impairments, while often less costly, are slower in coming, less well understood, and some are so controversial as to have been temporarily suspended.

UNIVERSAL DESIGN

Leading architects, designers, and planners who are particularly well informed about and sensitive to the needs of persons with disabilities (many of them have disabilities themselves), are proposing that instead of promoting architectural accessibility by stipulating design specifications for particular elements, all architectural elements should be accessible to (or adaptable for the use of) all persons, including those with disabilities. This emphasis provides for a more usable environment over time in a society in which an increasing proportion of the population is living longer and consequently developing disabilities—in fact, there are now few of us who will not experience one or more disabling conditions at some time in our lives.

The concept of universal design recognizes that design which facilitates getting about by persons with disabilities typically benefits most other people. For example, signs that can be read by persons with low vision are easier for all persons to read (Bentzen, Nolin, Easton, & Mitchell, 1995c; Bentzen, 1996; Bentzen & Easton, 1995). Detectable warning surfaces installed at the edges of transit platforms to provide the same kind of advance warning for travelers who are blind about the presence of a hazardous drop as is provided for sighted travelers by a visually contrasting edge have resulted in decreased falls from transit platforms for all riders (BART). In one study in which persons who were not visually impaired were asked to rate the effect on their travel of particular design characteristics intended to make transit stations and vehicles more accessible for visually impaired persons, the result was that a majority of persons thought that these design characteristics would make their own travel easier (Bentzen, Jackson, & Peck, 1981a).

In their excellent book on design that accommodates the needs of persons with visual impairments, Barker, Barrick, and Wilson (1995, p. 16) emphasize that "good architecture and design will empower and integrate all people." They provide three key design concepts:

- *Logical layout.* Layouts in which users can anticipate locations of facilities, such as stairs located next to elevators, or men's and women's rest rooms being adjacent to one another, help all users solve wayfinding problems.
- *Visibility.* Environments in which key features such as handrails, stair nosings, and doors have high visual contrast with their surroundings are safer and more negotiable for all sighted persons, including those with low vision.
- *Lighting.* Good lighting enhances visibility of signs and architectural features and does not cause glare or heavy shadows. Although optimal lighting for individuals varies, in general persons with low vision are thought to need 50–100 percent more light than persons with unimpaired vision. Persons who are 60 years of age also need approximately twice as much light as persons who are 40.

PARTICULAR PROBLEMS AND SUGGESTED SOLUTIONS

This section is intended to help readers perceive in the built environment particular characteristics that make travel difficult for some persons with visual impairments. It is not a comprehensive list of all the environmental access problems experienced by persons with visual impairments. It is biased toward those problems characteristic of cities in the United States. The intent is to sharpen the perception of readers, not to teach them about specific problems.

This section also provides suggested solutions to many problems. Where the solutions are based on empirical research, this will be mentioned. The reader should bear in mind that suggested solutions are also typically those used or proposed in the United States at the time of this writing. A rationale is presented for each suggested solution, but the reader should always assume that other options may exist that are better. Many solutions are based on rapidly changing technologies that are likely to have advanced by the time this book is published.

Environmental Design Affects Wayfinding

Researchers interested in the effects of environmental design on spatial orientation typically use the term *wayfinding* to encompass all of the perceptual and cognitive tasks that enable travelers to find their way to destinations—wayfinding may also be considered to be synonymous with the "orientation" component of O&M. It has been found that, in general, complex environments cause disorientation, as do environments with repeated symmetrical designs. Areas lacking distinctive landmarks are also confusing (Weisman, 1981; O'Neil, 1992; Appleyard, 1976; Peponis, Zimring, & Choi, 1990). While signage is universally used by architects to aid orientation, some researchers doubt that signage is actually able to effectively direct users of environments that are architecturally illegible (Arthur & Passini, 1992)—for example, environments in which functional spaces are not clearly defined and logically linked, in which circulation systems are not clearly discernible, or in which entrances and exits are not conspicuous and recognizable. Good visual access, or the degree to which one part of a facility can be seen from another, aids in navigation (Garling, Lindberg, & Mantyla, 1983), and the presence of distinctive landmarks such as color coding and conspicuous, unique decorative features is also helpful (Evans, Fellows, Zorn, & Doty, 1980).

This research is still in its infancy, and comparable research has not been conducted with persons who are visually impaired, but it helps us understand why even the most accomplished travelers who are blind may have difficulty in some environments. Universal design should certainly pay attention at the outset to creating layouts in which spatial orientation is easy. This is particularly important in environments used by many people who have little or no prior familiarity with them, such as hotels, malls, airports, and transit stations. Environments that facilitate orientation by sighted persons are likely to be easier for blind persons to navigate than environments which are more difficult for sighted persons. Conversely, facilities designed for ease of wayfinding by visually impaired persons are likely to be exemplary with regard to wayfinding by persons with unimpaired vision. O&M specialists who are skilled in analyzing available wayfinding information in an environment from the perspective of persons with visual impairments have much to offer architects, urban planners, and environmental graphic designers.

O&M specialists who grapple daily and consciously with orientation problems caused by poor design might think the design of environments that facilitate wayfinding would be a major emphasis in the education of architects. However, wayfinding is more conventionally considered to be the province of graphic designers, who are expected to provide whatever assistance (in the form of signs and other graphic elements) may be necessary to enable people to use a building *after* the major architectural decisions are made. An excellent resource on designing environments that facilitate wayfinding is *Wayfinding: People, Signs and Architecture* by Arthur and Passini (1992). The authors' stance is that wayfinding should be as easy as possible for all users of built environments, and they suggest a number of strategies that are particularly helpful for persons with visual impairments.

Accessibility of Buildings

Some aspects of buildings that may affect the ability of persons who are visually impaired to travel independently, safely, and efficiently include: protruding objects; stairs and handrails; elevators; and printed information on signs, maps, and directories.

Protruding Objects

It is generally recognized that objects which protrude into travel paths can endanger persons who have visual impairments; U.S. standards therefore limit the amount by which objects can protrude. The current *ADAAG* (4.4.1) says that

> objects protruding from walls (for example, telephones) with their leading edges between 27 in and 80 in (685 mm and 2030 mm) above the finished floor shall protrude no more than 4 in (100 mm) into walks, halls, corridors, passageways, or aisles. Objects mounted with their leading edges at or below 27 in (685 mm) above the finished floor may protrude any amount. Free standing objects mounted on posts or pylons may overhang 12 in (305 mm) maximum from 27 in to 80 in (685 mm to 2030 mm) above the ground or finished floor.

The reference to the leading edge being 27 inches attempts to give architects ways to design facilities such as drinking fountains and telephones that are both accessible to persons who use wheelchairs and would likely be picked up by travelers who are blind and use a long cane. (A proficient adult long-cane user was expected to encounter the obstacle with the shaft of the cane in time to avoid bodily contact.) However, Karnes, Schiedeck, and Postello (1994), in a pilot project, found that proficient adult blind travelers using long canes had frequent body contacts with wall-mounted objects protruding 4 inches (100 mm) at heights of 27–70 inches (685–1855 mm), and even more frequent body contacts with pole-mounted objects protruding 12 inches (305 mm) (see Figures 10.1A and 10.1B).

In new construction, particularly in medical facilities and facilities for children, it is better to recess wall-mounted objects such as drinking

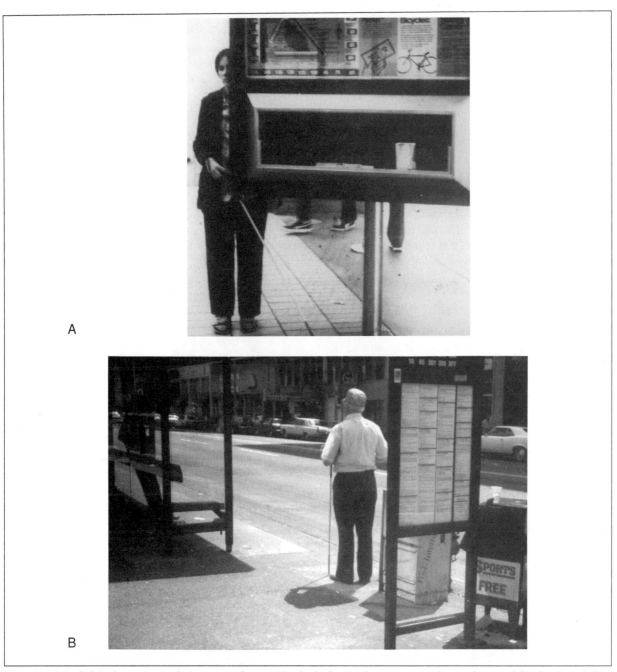

Figure 10.1. (A) Pole-mounted signs can be particularly hazardous to travelers who are blind, especially persons of short stature or those who do not extend the hand that holds the long cane out in front of their body. This sign in a BART station in San Francisco would be much less hazardous if it was mounted on two poles at the sides of the sign, and those two poles were connected by a horizontal bar 12 inches above the floor. (B) This pole-mounted sign in Seattle is a safer design.

Source: *Journal of Visual Impairment & Blindness, 11* (1983), p. 471.

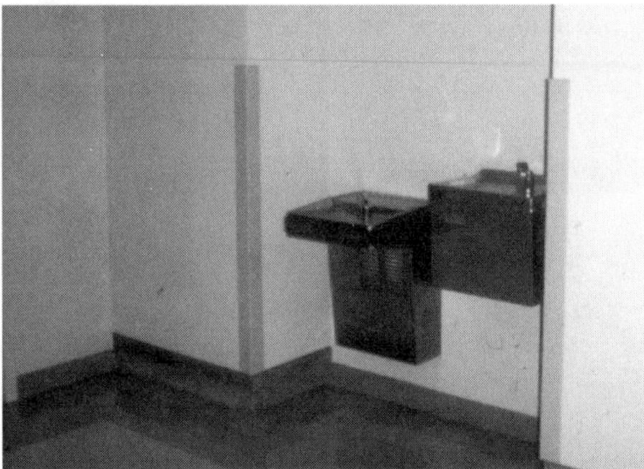

Figure 10.2. This pair of drinking fountains that are recessed into the wall are completely out of the line of travel, yet fully accessible to all travelers.

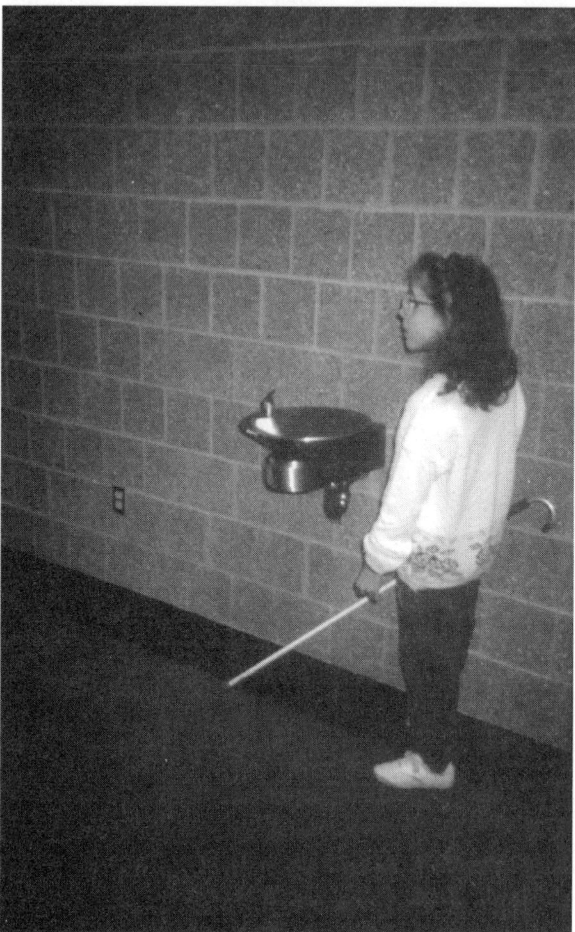

Figure 10.3. This drinking fountain is hazardous to young travelers who are blind, even those with excellent cane technique. Children need to be able to trail the walls of their school corridors safely as they develop protective techniques.

fountains and fire extinguishers (see Figures 10.2 and 10.3). In all environments pole-mounted objects should protrude no more than 4 inches (100 mm). Where there is no alternative to mounting a large sign on a pole, the sign should be mounted on two poles placed at both sides of the sign, and a cross bar should connect the two poles at a height of about 12 inches (100 mm). The cross bar will readily be detected by a traveler using a long cane.

Stairs and Handrails

Stairs are an especially common cause of accidents for all persons, hence considerable attention has been paid to making them safe and easy to negotiate (Templer, 1992). Some of the specifications for stairs and handrails are also helpful to many travelers who are blind. In general, stairs are considered to be safest and easiest to negotiate when treads and risers are at a moderate width and height, and the dimensions are the same for the full width of each stair and for the entire length of a staircase; when stair nosings protrude slightly beyond the base of the riser below; when risers are closed; when handrails are continuous on both the inside and outside of a staircase; and when the ends of handrails protrude horizontally about 1 foot (305 mm) beyond the top and bottom of the stairs (see Figure 10.4). The ends of handrails must, of course, be rounded and returned to the wall, floor, or a post in such a way that they do not become protruding objects (see Figures 10.5 and 10.6).

For persons with low vision, it is often difficult to see where stairs begin and end. It is extremely helpful if the nosings of stairs, particularly the top and bottom stairs, contrast visually with the treads and risers. It is also helpful if stringers contrast visually with adjoining treads and risers (see Figure 10.7).

A protruding structure that can be particu-

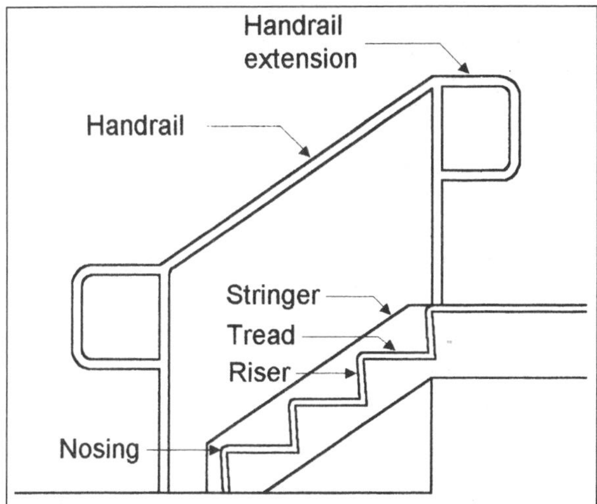

Figure 10.4. Stairs should have closed risers; treads and risers of consistent and moderate dimensions; handrails that are continuous on both the inside and outside of the stairs and extend horizontally beyond the top and bottom of the stairs; and nosings and stringers that contrast with treads and risers.

Source: Drawing courtesy of L. Tabor.

larly hazardous is a staircase or escalator which is not enclosed from the underside. Travelers who are blind may run headfirst into such structures, having not previously encountered any part of the structure with the long cane (Figure 10.8). Such construction is prohibited by some standards (*ADAAG* 4.4.1). To make existing unprotected stairs or escalators less hazardous, a rail can be added, as in Figure 10.8, or benches, planters, or other furnishings can be used—all relatively inexpensive solutions.

Elevators

Unfamiliar elevators can be particularly challenging for persons who are visually impaired. Questions that must be answered by elevator users are: Where is the elevator? Where is the elevator call button? Has the elevator call button been pressed? Has an elevator arrived? Is the arriving elevator going up or down? Where is the elevator control panel? Where is the correct button for my floor? Which button identifies the street level? How do I access safety features of the elevator

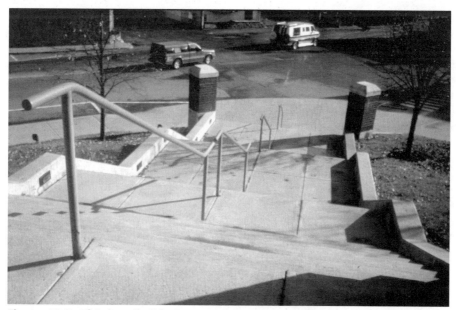

Figure 10.5. This handrail in Portsmouth, New Hampshire, extends beyond the top of this staircase, but is it safe? Can the location of each step be seen?

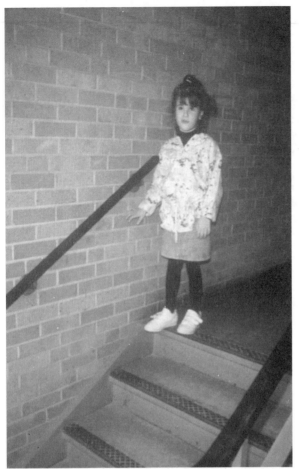

Figure 10.6. The sharp-cornered handrail shown here ends at the top riser. This child, who is frightened of stairs and has poor balance, cannot find and grasp the handrail until she has arrived at the riser. The end of the handrail is much higher than her moderately extended trailing hand. The stair nosings do contrast with the treads and risers, however, and the stringer (light blue) contrasts with the (tan) brick wall.

such as the "Door open," "Stop," and "Bell" buttons? Which floor is the elevator stopping on now? All of these questions are normally answerable by using visual information; all can be made answerable by using either auditory or tactile information.

Locations of elevator call buttons and of elevator control panels are somewhat standardized, and this aids in their location.

> *ADAAG* 4.10.3: Call buttons in elevator lobbies and halls shall be centered at 42 inches (1065 mm) above the floor. . . . The button designating the up direction shall be on top.
>
> *ADAAG* 4.10.12(3): All floor buttons shall be no higher than 54 inches (1370 mm) above the finish floor for side approach and 48 inches (1220 mm) for front approach. Emergency controls, including the emergency alarm and emergency stop, shall be grouped at the bottom of the panel and shall have their centerlines no less than 35 inches (890 mm) above the finish floor.

It is difficult, however, to have standard locations that work in all situations or for all people. Lower elevator control panels are more accessible to persons in wheelchairs or persons of short stature, but they are more difficult to read using touch or low vision.

Auditory solutions are recommended for providing information about whether an elevator has arrived, whether it is going up or down, and what floor the elevator is stopping on. Tones coming from the location of arriving elevators alert users who have hearing that an elevator has arrived and inform them of the travel direction of the elevator, one tone for up, and two tones for down. Information about which floor the elevator is on may be in the form of tones that sound as each floor is passed (this necessitates counting tones to know which floor the elevator is stopping on), or verbal announcements.

Tactile characters and symbols, and braille are also recommended for identifying buttons on elevator panels and for identifying each floor. Research indicates that tactile characters (numbers and capital letters) in fonts that are not extreme in any dimension, do not have serifs, are $\frac{5}{8}$ inch (16 mm) high, and are raised $\frac{1}{32}$ inch (8 mm) from a base surface are highly legible to persons with unimpaired tactile sensitivity. They are most legible if the strokes constituting the characters are somewhat rounded or trapezoidal in cross section; rectangular strokes are less legible and may be quite uncomfortable to read (Bentzen, 1989).

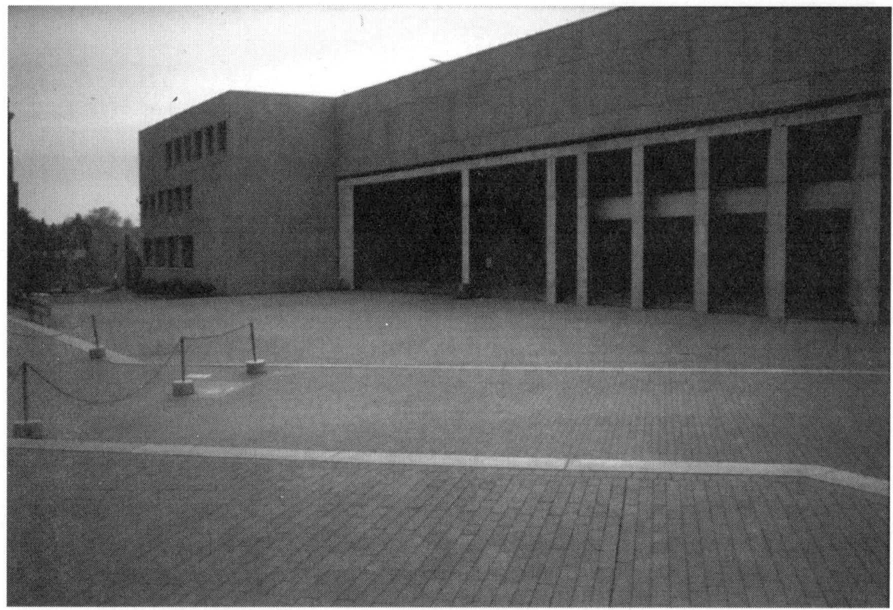

Figure 10.7. So-called monumental stairs present many difficulties. These stairs are about 100 feet long and zigzag across a plaza at Boston College. To the traveler with low vision, they may simply appear to be a decoration on a level walking surface.

The same principle is true for braille (Bürklen, 1932).

The elevator industry in the United States has standardized symbols to identify the special buttons on elevator control panels (ASME A17.1 1990). These symbols are shown in the left panel of Figure 10.9, and in the right panel of Figure 10.9 are symbols that research has shown to be more quickly identifiable (Liddicoat, Meyers, & Lozano, 1982).

Raised characters 2 inches (50 mm) high, with a stroke width of $\frac{1}{4}$ inch (7 mm) are also highly legible, and are required, together with braille, on elevator casings in the United States; this makes it possible to tactilely determine the floor at which an elevator has stopped. Incised characters $\frac{5}{8}$ inch (16 mm) high are nearly impossible to read by touch, and incised characters 2 inches (50 mm) high are much more difficult to read than similar raised characters (Bentzen, 1989).

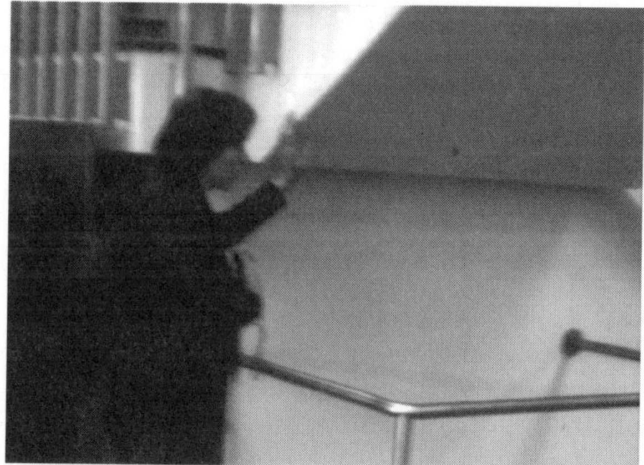

Figure 10.8. Hanging stairs create head-high obstacles. In this BART station in San Francisco, a railing is used as a barrier. The railing would be improved by the addition of a lower bar.

Signs

In order for travelers to benefit from information provided on signs, signs must first be located, then read, and finally understood. This is true whether the signs are conventional print or electronic signs, whether they are tactile, or whether they are audible. Locating and reading (or hearing) print, tactile, and audible signs will be discussed below, followed by some suggestions for making signs understandable, which apply to all three kinds of signs.

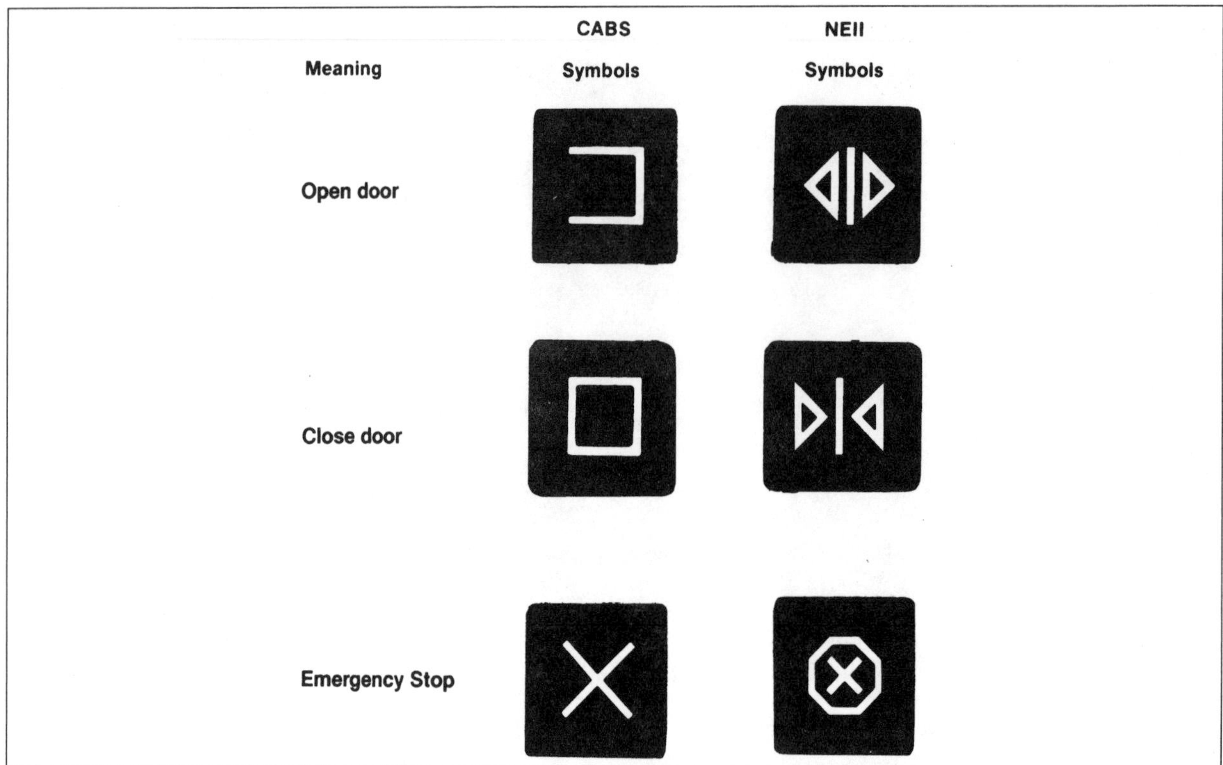

Figure 10.9. Research sponsored by the California Alliance of Blind Students (CABS) found that the tactile elevator symbols on the left were discriminated more quickly and accurately than were those on the right, which are standardized by the National Elevator Industry, Inc., and are required by the Americans with Disabilities Act Accessibility Guidelines.

Source: C.M. Liddicoat, L.S. Meyers, and E. Lozano, Jr., "A Comparison of Two Sets of Nonbraille Elevator Symbols," *Journal of Visual Impairment & Blindness, 76* (1982), p. 194.

Print Signs. Print signs that are poorly designed, poor in contrast, poorly placed, poorly illuminated, affected by glare, or simply dirty are difficult for all persons to read—particularly persons with visual impairments. Signs are easy to locate when they are in consistent locations. Arthur and Passini (1992) recommend that a horizontal band on walls, 16 inches (400 mm) deep, placed with its bottom edge 47 inches (1200 mm) above the floor, be devoted exclusively to wayfinding information. Such consistency would particularly benefit persons with peripheral visual field defects. Barker et al. (1995) emphasize that a sign board must contrast with its background. They recommend that where this is not possible, a contrasting border 10 percent of the width of the sign should be put around the sign.

There is a limited amount of information on design criteria that enhance sign legibility for persons who are visually impaired. Based on clinical measures of visual acuity, the character heights in Table 10.1 have been recommended for signs that are to be read at particular distances (Bentzen et al., 1981a). These recommendations are intended to enable persons with as little as 20/400 acuity to read the signs at the given distances, and these assume that the signs have a very legible font, and are high in contrast, low in glare, and well illuminated.

As anyone who has worked with persons who have low vision knows well, clinical measures of visual acuity do not give a very good idea of how any one person will actually be able to use visual information. The best we can say about the

Table 10.1. Sign Legibility Recommendations

Minimum Character Size	Maximum Viewing Distance
8 in (200 mm)	20 ft (6 m)
6 in (150 mm)	15 ft (4.5 m)
4 in (100 mm)	10 ft (3 m)
3 in (75 mm)	7.5 ft (2.5 m)
2 in (50 mm)	5 ft (1.5 m)

character heights recommended in the above table is that they will make signs more legible than smaller heights, but we cannot guarantee that such signs will be legible to all persons having no less than 20/200 acuity in all situations (Georgia Institute of Technology, 1985; Peter Muller-Munk Associates, 1986). Changeable message signs such as flip-dot, light-emitting diode (LED), or liquid crystal display (LCD) signs are particularly difficult for persons with low vision (Bentzen, 1996; Bentzen et al., 1995c; Garvey, 1994).

There are many overlapping issues in sign design. Legibility of signs that have characters at a given height is also a function of the following font aspects: character proportion, stroke width to height ratio, presence or absence of serifs, and intercharacter spacing. The limited research on the legibility of signs or fonts that have different characteristics differs somewhat in results. These differing results are possibly due to differences in the population investigated, the research design, and the precise nature of the font characteristics examined. However, these results generally indicate that fonts in which characters have little or no serif, character proportions (as measured using an uppercase letter X) are between 3:5 and 1:1, stroke width is between 1:5 and 1:10, and intercharacter spacing is wide (by industry standards) are highly legible even for persons with visual acuity as low as 20/200 (Georgia Institute of Technology, 1985; Peter Muller-Munk Associates, 1986).

The effect of case on legibility of signs is not well understood despite a moderate amount of research on the subject. While it is clear that for reading continuous text, mixed upper- and lowercase characters promote legibility for print readers (because we recognize words in context partly by perceiving their "footprints"), research results on the effect of case on sign legibility are less clear. Apparently, for persons with low vision who read brief signs whose messages are not anticipated, all uppercase characters result in better legibility simply because the critical details of each character are larger than for lowercase characters with the same character (stem) height (Bentzen, 1996; Bentzen et al., 1995c). However, it is possible that if persons with low vision were looking for a particular (anticipated) sign such as "Information," mixed cases might result in greater legibility.

High visual contrast is an essential ingredient of legibility. In general, light lettering on a dark background is more legible than dark lettering on a light background (Barker et al., 1995), and the best contrast for persons with low vision is provided by white characters on a black background (Rand Corporation, 1975). This is probably due to the phenomenon called *halation* or irradiation, in which the perceived size of a light figure on a dark background is 10–12 percent larger, bolder, or fatter than the perceived size of the same figure when it is dark on a light background (Arthur & Passini, 1992). However, for persons with low vision, halation may be exaggerated, and perception of critically informative dark spaces within and between characters may be compromised. This is particularly noticeable for signs that have interior illumination or LED or LCD displays. Therefore fonts with narrow intercharacter spacing should be avoided (Bentzen, 1996; Bentzen et al., 1995c).

While it is sometimes assumed that symbols or pictograms are a good approach to providing universally readable signs, there are few that are universally understandable even to persons who have no difficulty seeing them (Arthur & Passini, 1992). Even arrows may be ambiguous (Figure 10.10). For persons with low vision, critical details of pictograms may not be perceptible. *ADAAG*

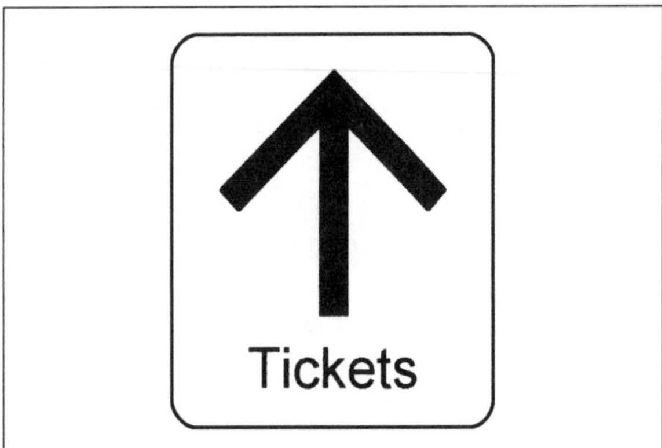

Figure 10.10. Arrows are often ambiguous. According to this sign, are tickets straight ahead, or up one level?

Source: Drawing courtesy of L. Tabor.

(4.30.4) requires that pictograms be accompanied by print. If the print is large enough to be legible to persons with low vision, saving space is not a rationale for using pictograms. At any rate, it can never be assumed that pictograms alone, no matter how large or high in contrast they are, will communicate the same message to all viewers.

Tactile Signs. Since the landmark *ANSI Standard* (1980), it has been taken for granted in the United States that at least some information on signs could and should be available to persons who read by touch. As only a small portion of touch readers read braille, it was commonly considered adequate for tactile signs to consist of raised characters only, as these were considered to be legible to all touch readers.

However, braille can be read so much faster than raised print, and is so much easier for those persons who read it, that more recent standards in the United States (including *ADAAG* 4.30.4) require standard-size grade 2 braille in addition to raised characters. These tactile signs are required, however, only where permanent signs identify rooms or spaces (such as room numbers, rest rooms, and special purpose rooms such as "Auditorium"), not for more general wayfinding information. In fact, reading more than a number or name in raised characters is so time-consuming (and hence may be quite conspicuous) that few touch readers are likely to take the time to gain wayfinding information in this way. Tactile pictograms generally do not work very well, therefore they should not be expected to provide critical wayfinding information to persons who are visually impaired.

The problem of finding signs is much greater for touch readers than for print readers, which makes tactile signage somewhat limited in its use. In this author's opinion, tactile signage is appropriate only for labeling doorways or entrances, and it works well only when it is in standard locations. *ADAAG* (4.30.6) requires that tactile signs be placed 60 inches (1525 mm) above the floor to the centerline of the sign, and to the latch side of doors (so that they will not be obscured by opened doors), or to the right of double doors, and out of the swing of those doors.

Handrails are being used as locations for tactile (particularly braille) signs in some few locations. Some people believe this has little merit. Where one expects to find handrails—that is, at stairs and ramps—it is particularly important for the safety of all persons that there be no obstructions. A person reading a tactile sign inevitably becomes a temporary obstruction—particularly so because, if users travel on the right-hand side of stairs, they will have to move forward to the beginning of the messages and then back up to read them to the end. Where handrails are added to an environment to provide locations for tactile signs, these handrails may not be found by travelers who are blind, and the handrails may not provide optimal travel paths from one location to another.

Tactile signs at doors that label entrances, exits, and interior rooms and spaces are useful and used, and appear to be the only current practical means of providing this information to persons who are deaf–blind. Tactile signs inevitably have a drawback for all readers, however—they cannot be read until touched by the reader. Thus they cannot provide wayfinding information from a distance.

Tactile signs are not very effective for providing directional information such as "Information desk to the right. Elevators to the left." There is simply no way the location of signs with general wayfinding information can be standard enough for such signs to be effective. (See the section "Transit Stations," below, for more discussion about tactile signs for wayfinding.)

Audible Signs. Several technologies now exist or are in development for presenting via speech, information that is typically found on print signs. These technologies utilize infrared, inductive loop, or AM or FM transmission, or they may be recorded speech messages that are activated by a push button located near the sign. In some technologies the message comes to the user via a speaker or earpiece from a personal receiver; in others, the message is broadcast for all passersby to hear.

From the user's perspective, the ideal audible signs might be audible when needed, but silent when unnecessary; audible to the user only, not to all passersby; capable of being picked up from a distance and not require that users first find a push button; and cognitively simple, not requiring comprehension of and memory for verbal directions. They should also precisely provide the information desired by the individual user, be free, be minuscule, weigh nothing, and not require use of the hands. No existing or proposed technology meets all these criteria. The one that comes closest to meeting these criteria is the infrared remote signage system developed by engineers (who are blind) at the Rehabilitation Engineering Research Center of The Smith-Kettlewell Eye Research Institute in San Francisco.

This system (now available as Talking Signs®) consists of infrared transmitters that most typically label landmarks such as "Information desk," "Elevators," and "Public telephone," and less commonly provide directional information such as "Hallway to the right for rooms 100 to 120." A recorded speech message is picked up by a handheld receiver in the vicinity of and oriented toward a transmitter, and the message is heard either through a speaker incorporated into the receiver or an earpiece. The distance

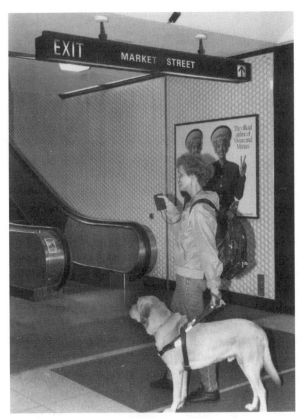

Figure 10.11. A traveler locating an exit using the Talking Signs® system in the Powell Station, San Francisco.

Source: Courtesy of Gretchen Hildner/S.F. MUNI.

and direction at which messages can be picked up can be adjusted from approximately 4–400 feet and approximately 5–360 degrees (see Figure 10.11).

What may at first seem to be a disadvantage—infrared transmitters are directional, therefore the user must scan around with the receiver to pick up a message—turns out to be a great advantage. When users pick up a message, they simply home in on it; as long as they hear a loud, clear message, they are getting closer to the transmitter or what it labels. There are no directions to understand or remember. Using the infrared system is thus more of a perceptual motor rather than a cognitive process, unlike systems that rely on inductive loop, or AM or FM transmission, which are inherently nondirectional and can therefore only give guidance by providing verbal directions (Bentzen & Mitchell, 1995).

The infrared system is also useful for persons with cognitive disabilities (Bentzen, Crandall, & Myers, in press), and persons with mild to moderate hearing loss are able to use the system (Bentzen & Mitchell, 1995; Crandall, Bentzen, Myers, & Mitchell, 1995b). Persons who are deaf–blind are able to use the system (by feeling speaker vibrations) to determine when they are facing a transmitter, although they are not able to decipher the message.

Making Signs Understandable. For signs to be understood, they must be in plain language—that is, the common language of users in that geographic area, not the language of the staff or planners. Even wording label signs in an understandable way requires extensive interviewing of people who will use a building. For instance, "X ray" is usually preferable to "Radiology" and the fare barrier in San Francisco transit stations is referred to as a "faregate," whether it goes back and forth, or round and round. Similar facilities in Philadelphia, however, are commonly referred to as "turnstiles." For persons with visual impairments, brief signs usually work best, but they must also clearly communicate the information that is needed. Signs that simply label destinations are usually clear, so long as they are in plain language. When signs contain directional information, however, there is great possibility for confusion.

It is much easier to make print signs unambiguous than either tactile or audible signs. Print signs can only be seen from predictable and controllable directions and, in well-designed environments, circulation routes are usually visible. There is often no surface to which a tactile sign can be attached at the locations travelers need information. For instance, travelers typically need wayfinding information when entering a space, such as when they come into a building or step off an escalator. In any well-designed public building there is never a wall or surface suitable for mounting a tactile sign directly in front of users who are entering a building or stepping off of an escalator, and for good reason; it would impair the flow of traffic for all building users. Placing tactile signposts in such locations would be very ill-advised for the same reasons.

Nondirectional audible signage (such as may be provided by inductive loop, or AM or FM technology) has a similar problem. Because it can potentially be picked up from any direction, a nondirectional message that says the traveler should go to the right, left, or straight ahead can always potentially be understood, acted upon correctly, and result in the traveler heading away from the destination! One manufacturer of audible signage tried substituting compass directions for such egocentric directions when creating a prototype signage system for a hotel. However, it was found to be uncommon for users who were blind to know which way was east, for example, when they were indoors (Bentzen & Mitchell, 1995).

Persons developing tactile and nondirectional audible signage systems sometimes need to provide distance information because users can't scan the environment, perceive signs from a distance, and simply head for them as they can when using print or directional audible signs. Complete verbal directions must be given. Developers have tried to provide distance information to users in at least two ways—steps or paces, and feet (Bentzen & Mitchell, 1995; B. L. Bentzen, personal observation in Philadelphia, July 1995). The number of steps is clearly inappropriate, as users hastened to point out, and although travelers who are blind can learn to estimate walking distance, most are not very good at it (Bentzen, 1991).

Remote infrared signage, because it is inherently directional, functions somewhat like print signs. A message is picked up from a predictable, controllable direction, and as long as users can still pick up the message clearly, they are headed in its direction—there is thus no need for distance information.

Maps

Display maps are a common way to provide wayfinding information in buildings. They may even be required in some situations, such as providing emergency egress information. However, tactile display maps that generally work the best are those which can be interrogated using a system such as Nomad or TAG (see Chapter 9). This is both because of the additional verbal information available from such maps and because the verbal information can be accessed interactively.

Some persons who are blind are capable of getting about using information provided by tactile maps (Bentzen, 1977; see also Chapter 9), but many are not. Furthermore, reading tactile maps requires more time and effort than reading print maps. Blind travelers are typically uncomfortable spending the time it takes to use tactile display maps in public places. Maps that are distributed to blind travelers, however, are an excellent aid to persons who desire them.

Tactile maps are not advisable for emergency egress information because it is unlikely that in emergency situations blind occupants of a building will be able to locate and effectively use them. It has been demonstrated that sighted persons who are elderly have great difficulty comprehending and using spatial information displayed on a map (Blasch, 1994). In addition, sighted university students solved wayfinding problems much more slowly using "you-are-here" maps of a complex area than using signs (Butler, Acquino, Hissong, & Scott, 1993).

Another approach to providing emergency egress information is by means of solid-state voice recordings activated by uniquely shaped push buttons at predictable locations, such as above elevator call buttons, just inside the doors of hotel rooms, and above tactile signs labeling exits. This verbal wayfinding information would be useful for all persons who, for many reasons, are unable to or choose not to use print maps or signs.

Building Directories

There are a number of ways to provide directory information to persons who are visually impaired. Ideally a building directory should be easy to locate and easy to get information from, and provides information that is easy to follow. Few systems meet all these criteria. Raised and braille display directories may be difficult to locate; if they contain more than a few entries, finding and reading the desired entry can be very time consuming and embarrassingly conspicuous, and the size of the directory may be prohibitive. Where there is a staffed information desk that is easy to locate, staff members may be trained to provide good verbal directions to persons requesting them, and to offer a large-print or braille directory. In a large building, a telephone handset on or near the entrance or a security desk may enable users to query a service person.

Information kiosks that provide directory information to users on a video display, and which may be interrogated by a touch screen, place travelers who are blind at a particular disadvantage. There are, however, several approaches to making such kiosks accessible to persons with visual impairments. Location of the kiosks is the first step. This may be facilitated by the use of audible signs as discussed previously. Once located, accessibility may be possible if the kiosks are able to give speech output, and keyboard or keypad input is possible in addition to a touch screen.

Vanderheiden, at the University of Wisconsin (1995), has pioneered the development of a prototype accessibility system for touch-screen kiosks he calls Talking Fingertip, which has implications for individuals with low vision, blindness, cognitive impairments, and language and reading problems. In this system, speech output is enabled by touching the top of the screen. Users can then tactilely explore screen contents, obtaining speech output describing all graphics as well as text. When the speech output is activated, the interactive capability of the kiosk is altered to require users to press a key to indicate that the last screen position touched contains the information selected by the user.

Another approach to making information kiosks accessible is the use of interactive speech, in which speech recognition technology that is speaker-independent, has a large vocabulary, and recognizes continuous speech responds in speech, using information from a database of wayfinding information. The user of such a kiosk might, for example, pick up a handset on the kiosk and say, "Where is Mr. Jones' office?" The kiosk might ask the user, "Do you want Mr. Henry Jones or Mr. Samuel Jones?" When the user replies, "Mr. Samuel Jones," the kiosk might reply, "Take the elevator on the opposite side of the lobby to the twelfth floor. Turn left when you leave the elevator, and Mr. Samuel Jones' office will be the third door on the right hand side of the hall." (The feasibility of such a system has been developed for providing wayfinding information for transit routes [Bentzen, Crandall, Chigier, Warden, & Carosella, 1995a].)

Accessibility of Intersections

In order to cross streets independently, travelers must be able to recognize that they have arrived at an intersecting street; determine the configuration of the intersection so that they can establish an optimal location, heading, and procedure for crossing; and identify the type of traffic control so that they can determine a safe time to initiate a crossing. It is also helpful to be able to determine or confirm the name of the intersecting street. When intersections are familiar, some of this information may already be known. Much of this information is typically obtained by listening to traffic patterns and sounds of individual vehicles (Jacobson, 1993; Hill & Ponder, 1976).

That most travelers who are blind cross streets safely most of the time attests to their ability to apply principles and skills for street crossing which have continued to evolve with the growth of the field of O&M. These principles and skills are based on acquiring the necessary information through limited vision or other sensory modalities. (It is also attributable to the fact that blind travelers, like sighted travelers, cross familiar streets much more frequently than they cross unfamiliar streets.) Nonetheless, there are many intersections that blind individuals consider to be unsafe for crossing without the assistance of a human guide. Individual differences in impairments, skills, abilities, and personality determine which streets any individual will choose to cross independently.

Since the beginning of organized instruction in independent travel for individuals who are blind, there have been many changes in intersection configurations, traffic control systems and technology, and in vehicular traffic; some have made crossing streets more difficult for persons with visual impairments.

Detecting Streets

The presence of a drop-off in the line of travel, which could be tactilely and kinesthetically identified as a curb, used to be the only information needed to tell travelers in urban and suburban areas that they had arrived at intersecting streets. Since the 1960s, however, increasing attention to sidewalk accessibility for persons who cannot negotiate curbs has resulted in the disappearance of drop-offs at many intersections. Curbs are replaced by clearly defined curb ramps at some intersections and what persons who are blind commonly call *blended curbs* at others (traffic engineers may refer to blended curbs as depressed corners or raised intersections). (See Figure 10.12.)

As the primary cue alerting travelers who were blind to the presence of streets disappeared, it was recognized that curb ramps—which enabled some persons to use sidewalks—could handicap blind travelers, who would, in some cases, be unable to detect intersecting streets. Japan was the first country to make up for the information lost by the removal of curbs, by adding, beginning in the 1960s, a warning surface detectable both under foot and by a person using a long cane. While neither the surface configuration nor its placement were standardized, most of the Japanese surfaces that were intended to be warnings had a surface configuration of domes, which might be somewhat flattened or truncated on top, and were about 2.5 inches (66 mm) apart (measured from center to center of diagonally opposite domes in any square arrangement). Most warning surfaces were placed on the lower

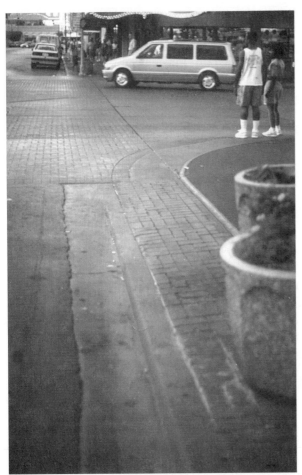

Figure 10.12. At this street corner in Las Vegas, there is little to indicate to the traveler without vision just where the pedestrian way ends and the vehicular way begins.

end of curb ramps, or along the former curb line where there were blended curbs; warning widths varied from about 12 inches (305 mm) to about 36 inches (950 mm). Materials used included rubber, stainless steel, cast pavers, and tiles. Although they still are not standardized, warning surfaces at curb ramps and blended curbs are now commonplace throughout Japan.

In England, a warning surface with a standardized pattern of truncated domes (referred to as modified blister paving) has been recommended for use in specified locations and dimensions on curb ramps and blended curbs since 1983 (Department of Transport, 1991; Gallon, Oxley, & Simms, 1991; Transport and Road Research Laboratory, 1983). These warnings can now be found throughout England. Most are cast pavers.

With publication of the 1980 *ANSI Standard* (A117.1), there was recognition in the United States that the removal of curbs at intersections could handicap persons with visual impairments. What were then referred to as tactile warnings were specified for the entire surface of curb ramps and a 36-inch (915 mm) wide strip was specified along the entire edge of blended curbs, which were referred to as hazardous vehicular ways. *ADAAG* 4.29, adopted as a U.S. standard in 1991, required the placement of a particular surface (now called a *detectable warning*) that is similar to the truncated domes already in use in Japan (Murakami, Aoke, Taniai, & Muranaka, 1982), England (Transport and Road Research Laboratory, 1983), and Australia (Peck, Tauchi, Shimizu, Murakami, & Okhura, 1991), and that it be in the same locations and have the dimensions specified in the *ANSI Standards* (1980). The surface specification was based on extensive research sponsored by the U.S. Department of Transportation (Peck & Bentzen, 1987; Templer & Wineman, 1980; Templer, Wineman, & Zimring, 1982). The *ADAAG* specification (4.29.2) for the detectable warning surface is as follows (see Figure 10.13):

> Detectable warnings shall consist of raised truncated domes with a diameter of nominal 0.9 in (23 mm), a height of nominal 0.2 in (5 mm) and a center-to-center spacing of nominal 2.35 in (60 mm) and shall contrast visually with adjoining surfaces, either light-on-dark or dark-on-light.

This surface, and others much like it, have repeatedly been demonstrated to be highly detectable when used in association with a wide variety of adjoining surfaces (Bentzen, Nolin, Easton, Desmarais, & Mitchell, 1993; Mitchell, 1988; Murakami, Ohkura, Tauchi, Shimizu, & Ikegami, 1991; Peck et al., 1991; Tijerina, Jackson, & Tornow, 1994; Toronto Transit Commission, 1990). Many other surfaces that were anticipated to be highly detectable have not proved to be so.

The requirement for detectable warnings

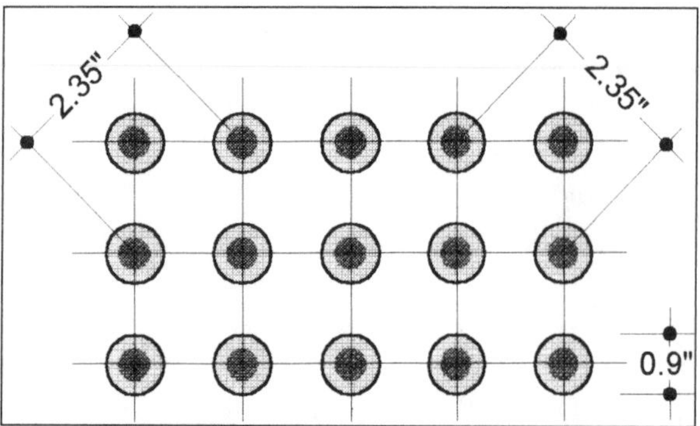

Figure 10.13. The detectable warning pattern specified by Americans with Disabilities Act Accessibility Guidelines. The truncated domes can be aligned in either a square or diagonal grid. Both appear to be equally detectable, but the square alignment appears to be easier for persons with wheelchairs to negotiate, especially when it is used on sloping surfaces such as curb ramps.

Source: Drawing courtesy of L. Tabor.

quickly became one of the most controversial provisions of *ADAAG*, strongly advocated by some travelers who were blind and the O&M profession, and strongly opposed by other blind travelers and some individuals and organizations concerned with safety of persons with physical disabilities. Blind persons opposing detectable warnings at intersections claimed that they were unnecessary and that no research demonstrated that the remaining, nonvisual clues were insufficient to enable blind travelers to detect streets reliably when they were approached via curb ramps or blended curbs. Two subsequent research projects (Bentzen & Barlow, 1995; Hauger, Safewright, Rigby, & McAuley, 1994) confirmed that, not surprisingly, the removal of the single reliable cue to the presence of an intersecting street (that is, the downcurb) did result in the inability of even skilled, frequent travelers who were blind to detect some streets. Bentzen and Barlow found that on 35 percent of approaches to unfamiliar streets, blind travelers who used a long cane failed to detect the presence of an intersecting street before stepping into it; this was true even when there was traffic on the intersecting street.

Bentzen and Barlow also found that the failure to detect streets was highly correlated with the slope of the curb ramp and the abruptness of change in angle between the approaching sidewalk and the curb ramp. Both projects (Barlow & Bentzen, 1995; Hauger et al., 1994) found that street detection was more likely when curb ramps were at the apex of a corner than when they were in the line of travel. Hauger et al. also found that apex curb ramps were more likely to lead to unsuccessful street crossings.

Bentzen (1994; also Bentzen et al., 1993; Bentzen, Nolin, Easton, Desmarais, & Mitchell, 1994b) and Hauger et al. (1994) found that truncated dome detectable warnings on slopes or curb ramps had little effect on safety and negotiability for persons with physical disabilities in comparison with concrete curb ramps. In fact, Hauger et al. found that persons with physical disabilities generally considered curb ramps with detectable warnings to be safer, more slip resistant, and more stable, and require less effort to negotiate than concrete curb ramps. Both teams of investigators found, however, that a small minority of persons with physical disabilities were adversely affected by detectable warnings. Barlow and Bentzen (1995) concluded by recommending that, as a compromise solution, only 24 inches (610 mm) of truncated dome detectable warning be installed along the bottom of curb ramps, as that amount had previously been demonstrated to be sufficient to enable detection and stopping on most approaches.

Intersection Configuration

It is often possible to determine the configuration of intersections by listening to traffic (Hill & Ponder, 1976; Jacobson, 1993). However, as cars become quieter, this is becoming more difficult (see the section "Quiet Vehicles," below). There are also particular types of intersections for which it is particularly difficult to determine configuration, including the location and direction of the crosswalk. These include intersection configurations where any street enters at other than a 90-degree angle, where there is a special turning lane, where corners are especially rounded, and where the corner is built out. These also include intersections where most of the traffic turns, and/or where (or when) there is little traffic. It is particularly difficult to detect, and hence to plan, for negotiating traffic islands or median strips.

Some configurations are simply difficult to negotiate even if the traveler is able to determine them. Exceedingly wide streets are difficult because even a slight veer while crossing can result in missing the opposite corner entirely (Guth & LaDuke, 1994; Willoughby & Duffy, 1989). Intersections having entirely blended curbs or curb ramps at the apex have been shown to be associated with unsuccessful street crossings (Hauger et al., 1994).

There are several solutions that either help travelers determine the configuration of an intersection or guide them across a street, whether or not they have been able to determine the intersection configuration. In some countries large raised arrows on pedestrian-activated audible pedestrian signals help travelers know the direction of the opposite corner. In Denmark, crossing direction is indicated by the orientation of a raised bar on the pedestrian signal housing (Figure 10.14). The bar has raised bumps to indicate the presence and number of traffic islands or median strips that may be encountered while crossing.

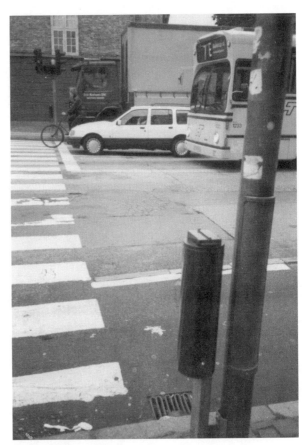

Figure 10.14. The audible traffic signal system in Copenhagen incorporates a raised bar that shows the direction of the crosswalk. The bar has a single bump at the end closest to the street, indicating that there is no traffic island; the first upcurb is at the far side of the street. Traffic islands are indicated by an additional bump or bumps on the bar. This is not a pedestrian-activated signal.

Audible pedestrian signals that can be heard across the street also help travelers establish and maintain a bearing toward the opposite corner, whether they understand the configuration of the intersection or not. An audible traffic signal that is particularly effective in helping travelers establish and maintain a correct bearing features a brief melody which alternates from one side of the street to the other (Hall, Rabelle, & Zibihaylo, 1994).

Particularly difficult intersections to deal with are those that are irregular or especially wide, or in which the crosswalk is not straight. Tactile guide strips have been demonstrated to be effective in such situations (Elias, 1974; Herms, Elias, & Robbins, 1974) (see Figures 10.15 A and B). Tactile guide strips are typically raised about $\frac{1}{4}$ inch (7 mm) above the road surface, and are installed in the center of crosswalks. A person who uses a long cane uses a guide strip by following it using constant contact technique. Because the guide strip runs down the center of the crosswalk, it allows blind pedestrians to avoid idling cars on one side of the crosswalk as well as parallel traffic on the other side. Other materials and configurations are used in other countries (Gómez, 1991; Murakami et al., 1982; Shimizu, Murakami, Ohkura, Tanaka, & Tauchi, 1991).

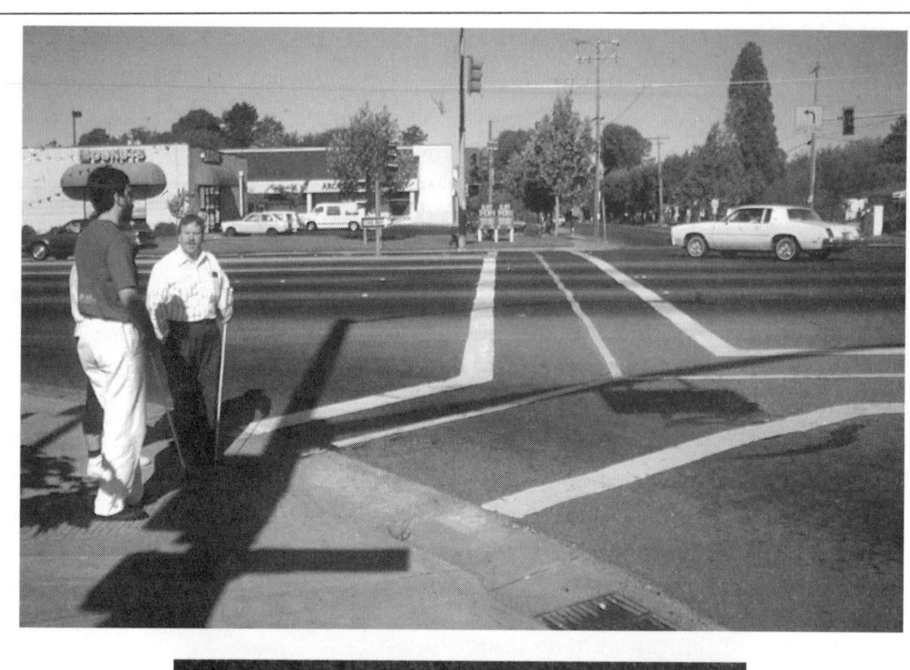

A

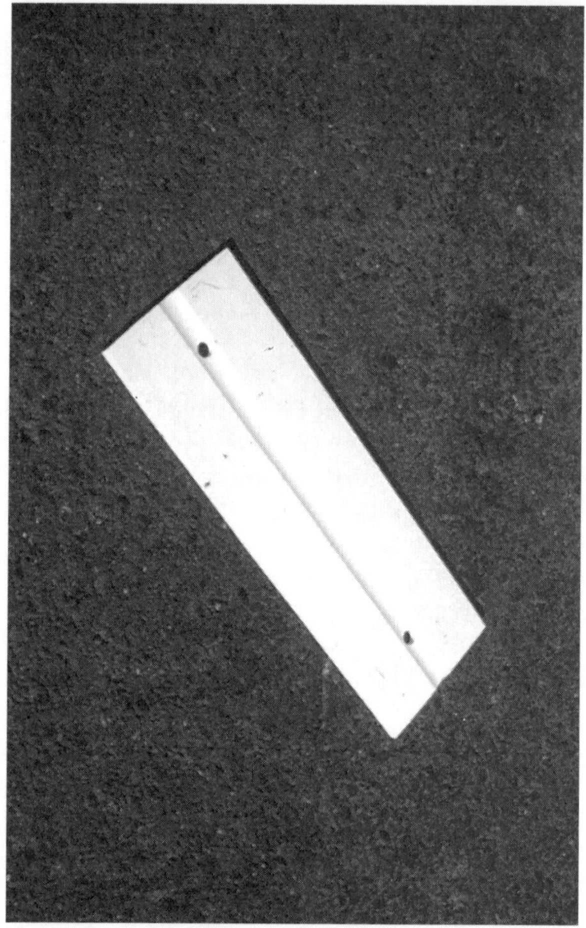

B

Figure 10.15. (A) Tactile guide strips are used in the center of the crosswalk at this intersection in Sacramento, California, where the crosswalks change direction in the intersection. (B) A close-up of one section of the guide strip material.

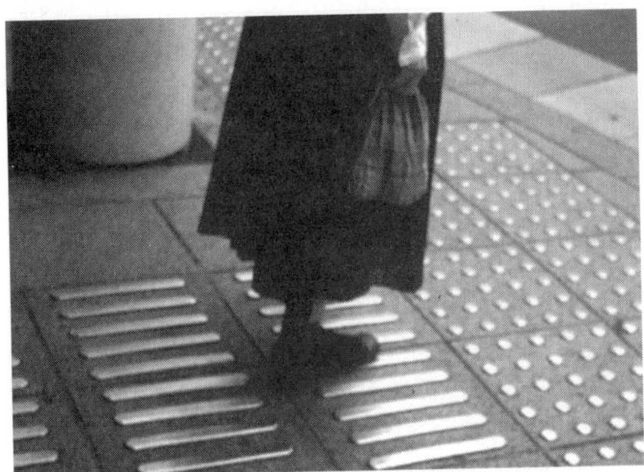

Figure 10.16. The raised linear surface at a street corner in Japan indicates the direction of the crosswalk. The truncated dome surfaces indicates the limit of the pedestrian way.

Both the location and bearing of crosswalks are sometimes indicated by tactile surfaces with a raised linear pattern that is aligned in the intended direction of travel and placed between an inside shoreline and a detectable warning. Such raised linear surfaces are currently used in Japan (Figure 10.16) and Sacramento, California.

Traffic Control

Where traffic is abundant on all streets at an intersection, it is usually possible for travelers who are blind to determine whether vehicular traffic on streets is controlled by stop signs or traffic lights. Where intersections are light controlled, it is often easy to determine which street has the right of way. Nonetheless, delayed or prolonged green lights, separate turning signals, and permitted right turns on red lights after stopping make it difficult to determine traffic control patterns at many intersections. Even if one understands the traffic control at an intersection, it may still be difficult to determine a safe time to initiate a crossing. Particularly difficult and hazardous are intersections with fast but intermittent traffic, in which it is difficult to determine the onset of parallel traffic.

Intersections in which there is a designated walk phase present particular challenges, especially if all traffic is stopped during the walk phase. Although such signals often provide the only safe time for any pedestrian to cross, in any situation when there is no audibly idling traffic on all the streets at an intersection, there is insufficient auditory information for travelers who are blind to know whether there is simply no traffic on one street (for what could be a very short moment), or whether the walk phase has begun. Where walk phases are pedestrian actuated, it may be difficult for persons who are visually impaired to locate the pushbutton (Peck & Uslan, 1990). Where all traffic is stopped during a walk phase, it may be not only difficult to determine the onset of the walk phase, but also to maintain a straight line of travel toward an opposite upcurb because of the unpredictability of pedestrian travel directions. Traffic signals that are dynamically adjusted by the volume of traffic flow are particularly difficult for blind travelers, because it is not possible to determine with any certainty when and for how long walk phases or parallel traffic phases will occur.

A common solution to the problem of knowing when it is safe to cross at light-controlled intersections is the use of audible pedestrian signals (APS). APSs have been common in some countries for many years, and there are many types. (A review of the use of audible pedestrian signals in the United States may be found in Peck & Uslan, 1990.)

A number of issues regarding whether APSs should be used in any situation, and which type, are as follows:

- APSs should be standard throughout a country or region.
- APS technology should be selected to meet the requirements of specific users or intersections.
- APSs should only be on pedestrian actuated signals so that their use will minimally disturb other people.
- APSs should both inform users about the onset of the crossing phase and serve as

audible beacons that provide guidance to the opposite corner.

- APSs should inform users about the onset of the crossing phase, but should not be loud enough to function as audible beacons.
- APSs should provide both audible and vibrotactile information so that they are usable by persons who are deaf–blind as well as persons who are blind.
- During the wait phase, APSs should emit a sound audible only from very nearby, to help users locate the button to actuate the signal.
- Pedestrian-controlled APSs should always be positioned at the crosswalk, so that it is safe to cross from the location of the control button.
- Pairs of APSs indicating the walk phases of two streets at an intersection should emit different sounds, so users can know by the sound which street has the walk phase.
- Only one street at any intersection requires an APS.
- All light-controlled intersections should have APSs, so that travelers who are blind will always know they are available.
- APSs should only be placed at intersections where there is insufficient auditory information to reliably determine the onset of the walk phase.
- APSs should be audible to users only.
- APSs should not require that users have particular personal equipment to use them.

APS technologies and applications exist to satisfy all of these requirements, but the reader will note that some requirements are mutually exclusive. The choice of APS technology and decisions about where and how it is to be installed should be based on careful consideration by all stakeholders of all possible requirements, as all decisions will have both advantages and disadvantages. Stakeholders must include pedestrians who are blind, O&M specialists, and traffic engineers.

Most APSs sound like some kind of bell, buzz, bird call, or melody, and most can be heard by anyone in the vicinity. The remote infrared signage technology Talking Signs® takes a different approach. This system, as used at a number of intersections in San Francisco as this volume went to press, uses recorded speech to tell users "Walk sign," or "Wait." Messages that are audible only to users, and only when users are standing at a crosswalk, are heard by means of small receivers when they are activated by users. As users approach corners, they can also receive messages that tell them the name of the intersecting street, the parallel street, which block they are on (for example, 100 block), and which direction they are traveling. Messages could also be used to describe intersection configuration and/or the traffic control system.

Quiet Vehicles

A goal of vehicle designers is the elimination of unnecessary noise. Internal combustion engines are becoming quieter, and electric vehicles are also very quiet (see Wiener & Lawson, Chapter 4 of this volume). Tire noise is a major component of the sound made by moving vehicles, but it is minimized in some vehicles and under certain road conditions, and is absent when vehicles are idling. There is increasing concern among pedestrians who are blind (American Council of the Blind, 1991) that quiet vehicles make the determination of intersection configuration, intersection control, and safe crossing time difficult, thereby decreasing both the orientation and safety of blind pedestrians, and increasing their need for assistance.

There are several technological approaches to these problems, none of which was implemented or available as this book went to press. These include the following:

- Require vehicles to make no less than a particular amount of noise, which has particular spectral characteristics that make vehicles highly localizable, make vehicular speed easy to judge, can be heard from a particular minimum distance under the worst listening conditions, and are not easily masked by other common environmental sounds.
- Make available to persons who are blind a device that can inform them about the direction and speed of vehicles approaching from any direction.
- Make available to persons who are blind a device that would activate sound-emitters on all vehicles within a certain distance.

Vehicle manufacturers and the general public are predictably opposed to increasing vehicular sounds. The task of developing a technology that can give persons who are blind, and particularly those who are deaf–blind, information about the direction and speed of vehicles approaching from any distance is daunting. Excellent technology exists for determining speed and distance of an approaching vehicle if one points the device toward the vehicle. However, it is very difficult to communicate this information to blind pedestrians, in a form sufficiently analogous to auditory perception of direction and distance of moving vehicles to enable split-second decision making.

Any device that indicates the direction of approaching vehicles only in relation to its own orientation is of somewhat limited value. While such a device perhaps could provide information analogous to visual information available to persons who are deaf but who have normal vision, it would be impossible for users to simultaneously pick up and follow the motions of all vehicles that define the configuration of an intersection or may suddenly turn across one's path of travel. The great advantage of hearing traffic, as opposed to seeing it, is that while we may listen somewhat selectively, persons with unimpaired hearing have an auditory field of 360 degrees and are normally able to simultaneously judge the general direction as well as the speed and distance of vehicles in all directions at once. In fact, persons with normal vision and hearing, when crossing streets, frequently first hear and localize approaching vehicles and then look at them. Thus if vehicles are not heard, they may not be seen.

Accessibility of Transportation

Persons who are visually impaired are especially dependent on various forms of public transport. While all forms of public transport are regularly used by individuals with visual impairments and can be used quite independently by persons traveling familiar routes, traveling unfamiliar routes by public transportation typically requires asking for information and assistance (Hill & Ponder, 1976; Jacobson, 1993; LaGrow & Weessies, 1994). Golledge, Costanzo, and Marston (1995) found that the greatest need for improving accessibility of mass transit for persons with visual impairments is improved access to information.

Public transportation also presents many opportunities for accident or injury to all travelers; for travelers who are blind, the lack of the opportunity to assess dangerous situations before moving into them may result in greater likelihood of accident or injury. For the Bay Area Rapid Transit (BART) in San Francisco, during the ten years before detectable warnings were installed along platform edges, approximately one-fourth of all accidents along the edges of raised platforms involved persons who were visually impaired (McGean, 1991). Because of their great reliance on public transportation, it is especially important that public transportation terminals and vehicles of all kinds are safe for persons with visual impairments, and provide wayfinding information in accessible formats. Fear can be a major obstacle to the use of transit, expecially for rapid rail systems (Hines, 1990).

Transit Stations

Transit stations present some challenges to safety and wayfinding for persons with visual impair-

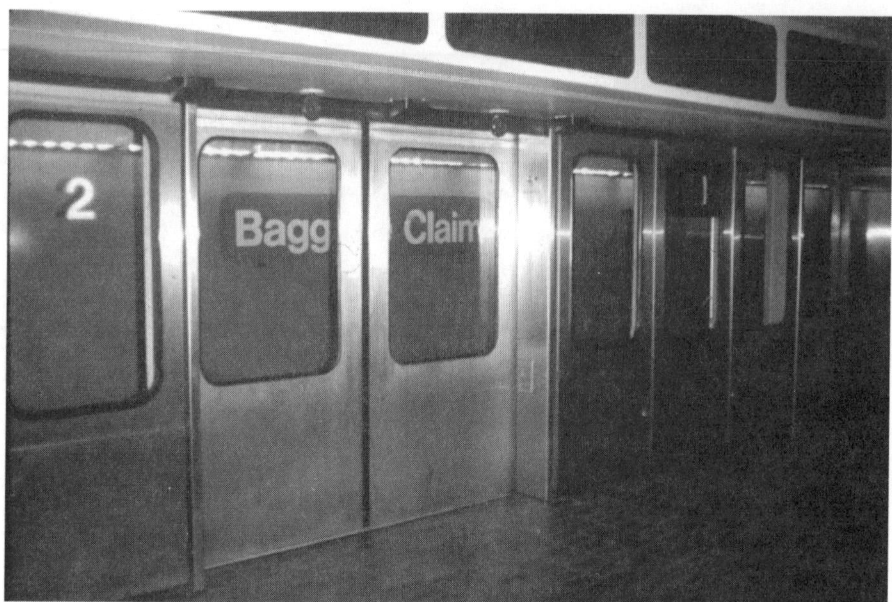

Figure 10.17. In people-movers such as this one at the Atlanta airport, transit platforms are considered so unsafe that they are bordered by wall instead of exposed edges.

ments, that are not present in other buildings or at intersections. These unique challenges will be discussed in this section. Fare payment is a unique requirement of public transit; therefore a number of problems and potential solutions regarding fare payment will also be presented in this section.

Safety. One element common to some light, heavy, rapid, or mono rail transit stations is a waiting platform that is raised above the track-bed, and therefore has a drop-off. In all other environments, raised pedestrian ways are commonly required to have guard rails or barriers along edges where there is a drop-off. In the people-mover industry, all riders are prevented from inadvertently stepping off platform edges by the presence of barrier walls with doors that open only when and where vehicle doors open (Figure 10.17). In rapid rail, the track bed includes an electrified rail. Thus all persons on transit platforms where there is a drop-off are at risk for falling, vehicular, and sometimes electrical accidents. Travel techniques are often modified for travel along platforms with a drop-off, and even minor deviations from perfect cane technique can result in failure to detect the edge with the cane (Uslan, Wiener, & Newcomer, 1990). The frequently severe consequences of falls onto track-beds have resulted in a variety of measures to reduce risks for all transit riders. These include guard rails (Figure 10.18), safety yellow warning stripes (Figure 10.19), textured warning surfaces (Figure 10.20), and lights (Figure 10.21) along platform edges.

In the United States, *ADAAG* requires that the detectable warning surface illustrated in Figure 10.13 be placed along the leading 24 inches (610 mm) of all transit platforms undergoing new construction and alterations; eventually this will be required for all stations. This warning surface must visually contrast with the adjoining platform surface, either light on dark or dark on light, and, when used indoors, must also contrast with the adjoining surface in resiliency or the sound it makes when a long cane is used on the surface (*ADAAG* 4.29.2). During the seven years following the installation of such a surface on all platform edges in the BART system, platform edge accidents decreased for all riders, but especially for

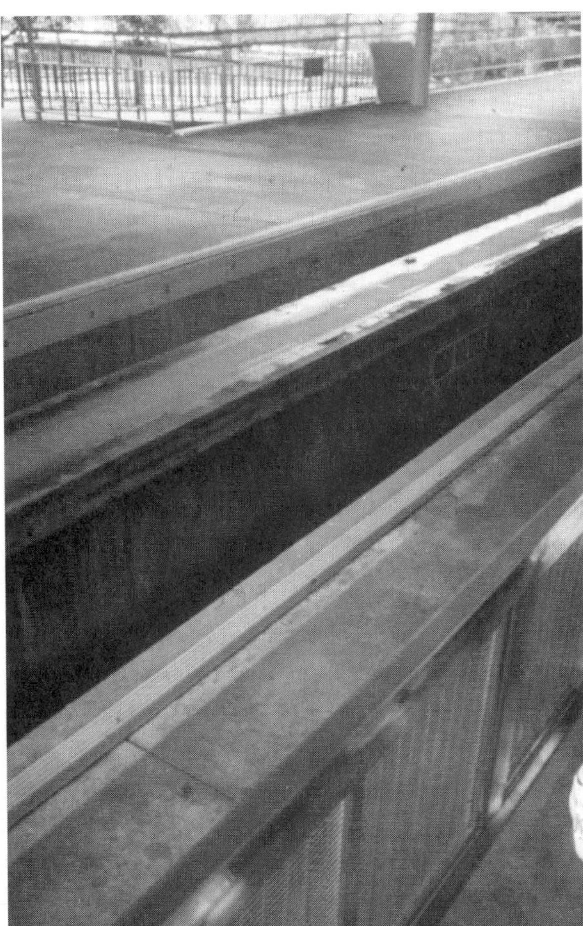

Figure 10.18. Railings protect monorail users from falls along platform edges at Disney World.

riders with visual impairments (McGean, 1991). This warning surface had not resulted in any accidents to or adverse comments from individuals or groups of BART riders as this book went to press. Prior to the installation of this surface, research conducted at BART indicated that the surface was likely to have little effect on persons with physical disabilities and might, in some cases, be beneficial (Peck & Bentzen, 1987).

The rationale for the width of detectable warnings required by *ADAAG* was the following: First, 24 inches (610 mm) has repeatedly been demonstrated as a sufficient width for a surface that is highly detectable both under foot and by use of a long cane, for enabling most travelers who are blind to detect and stop on that surface (Peck & Bentzen, 1987; Templer & Wineman, 1980; Templer et al., 1982). Second, transit managers wanted the warning to be as narrow as possible. They did not want riders to either stand and wait on the warning, or travel on it when there were not any trains at a platform. Therefore a warning surface needed to reduce the effective standing capacity of platforms as little as possible, while both enabling blind passengers to stop at a safe distance from the platform edge without having to contact the edge to determine its location, and demarcating the limit of the safe waiting area for all passengers. Additionally, transit managers reasoned that while most passengers would wait behind the warning most of the time, there would nonetheless be a small minority of passengers who would choose to walk along the warning, between the edge and waiting passengers, if the warning was wider than 24 inches (610 mm) (R. Weule, personal communication, 1986).

The rationale for the placement of detectable warnings as required by *ADAAG* was as follows: Advocates wanted the warning to be at or very near the platform edge to prevent the possibility that a traveler could interpret a width of platform between the warning and the edge as a safe place to stand. Transit managers wanted the warning to be at the edge so that on *retrofitted* platforms with detectable warnings, there would be sufficient platform width away from the edge to accommodate a typical number of rush hour riders without causing riders to stand on the warning due to crowded conditions.

Another contributor to the rationale for *ADAAG* specifications regarding both the width and placement of detectable warnings on transit platform edges was a decrease in accidents for all riders on BART (McGean, 1991) and Metro Dade (A. Hartkorn, personal communication, 1994). In San Francisco, riders in stations with different platforms that served both BART and Muni (San Francisco Municipal Railway) were observed standing at different distances from the platform edge. On BART platforms, which had 24-inch (610 mm) detectable warnings along the edges, passengers tended to wait behind the warning—that

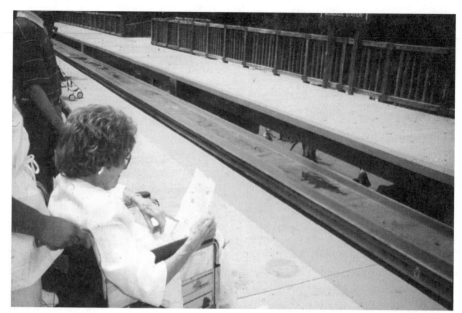

Figure 10.19. A safety yellow stripe alerts sighted passengers to the exact location of this platform edge at the Miami Zoo.

is, at least 2 feet (610 mm) from the edge, while on Muni platforms, which did not have detectable warnings, passengers waited closer to the edge (McGean, 1991).

A 70 percent contrast in light reflectance between a detectable warning and an adjoining platform surface is recommended by *ADAAG* (A4.29.2). Warnings may be either dark on a light platform or light on a dark platform. Many advocates wanted all detectable warnings to be safety yellow, a color that is standardized both in the United States (ANSI Z535.1–1991, 6.3) and internationally (ISO 3864–1984(E)) for use as a warning. Other persons argued that safety yellow might not contrast enough with some platform colors to be highly detectable, therefore designers should have the option of using various colors. Recent research indicates the color safety yellow is so salient, even to most persons with very low vision, that it is highly visible even when used on platforms with light reflectance value differences as little as 40 percent (new, gray–white concrete) (Bentzen, Nolin, and Easton, 1994a). This finding, coupled with the fact that safety yellow is standardized for warnings and thus readily brings to mind a need for caution, is a strong argument for the use of safety yellow warnings at transit platform edges. An additional advantage to using safety yellow is its high contrast with the normally dark trackbed beyond the platform edge. (Travelers with low vision may interpret the junction between a light platform and a dark detectable warning as an edge of a platform that does not have a warning.)

Lights embedded in platform edges may not provide any extra measure of safety to travelers with low vision. Recent laboratory research by Tijerina et al. (1994) suggests that the lights in the platform edges at the Washington Metropolitan Area Transit Authority (WMATA) stations probably do not enable travelers with low vision to detect these platform edges from greater distances than the distances for similar edges without embedded lights (see Figure 10.21). An additional feature of the lighting design of WMATA stations is a center strip of rather bright lights located between adjacent center tracks that serve side platforms and low down against the walls along tracks served by center platforms. These bright lights are reported to be very confusing to

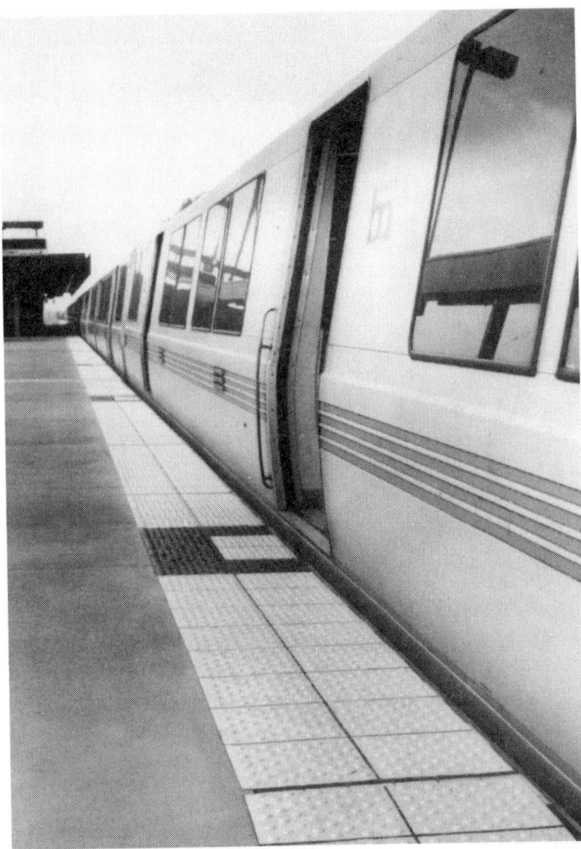

Figure 10.20. This detectable warning (complying with Americans with Disabilities Act Accessibility Guidelines) along the edges of all BART platforms resulted in a decrease in platform edge accidents for all riders.

Source: T. K. McKean, *Innovative Solutions for Disabled Transit Accessibility* (Washington, DC: U.S. Department of Transportation, Urban Mass Transit Administration, 1991).

travelers with low vision, who may mistake them for the dimmer lights along the platform edge and believe that they can safely procede up to the bright lights (Beattie, 1995). Such ambiguous perceptual information must be carefully avoided.

Wayfinding. There are numerous wayfinding challenges involved in the use of public transportation. Individuals traveling unfamiliar routes need to know what transit line or lines to take, where to get on, where and how to change lines if necessary, and where to get off. They need to know how to get to the starting point, and how to get from the final transit stop to their actual destination. Thus they need information about neighborhood layout as well as information about the transit system itself (Bentzen et al., 1981a; Golledge et al., 1995). Travelers with unimpaired vision can usually negotiate unfamiliar routes to and from and within transit stations without assistance, even ones that are long or complex.

Travelers who are visually impaired often have insufficient perceptually available information to enable them to travel to and from unfamiliar transit stations, and within transit stations, without assistance. However, spatial layout information that enables them to independently travel to and from and within unfamiliar stations can be provided by either verbal maps or route descriptions, or tactile or large-print maps (see Bentzen, Chapter 9 of this volume).

The feasibility of using an interactive speech system to provide transit information, including routes between stations, transit lines, transfer information, detailed descriptions (verbal maps) of the areas around station entrances, and detailed transit station descriptions, was demonstrated in 1994 by Integrated Speech Solutions, Inc.* (Bentzen et al., 1995a). Information of particular interest to travelers with visual impairments included whether stations were underground or above ground, how to get from the entrance to the fare barrier, how to get from the fare barrier to the platform for a train going in the desired direction, which part of the train would be nearest the location where the traveler reached the platform, and which way to turn when exiting the train in order to reach particular station exits. Participants who were blind and had no explicit training in using the system interrogated the system to find out how to travel between two stations, how to enter the first station, and how to exit at the destination. The system is speaker-independent, and recognizes continuous speech with a large vocabulary. It is intended to be used via a telephone handset, either a typical telephone or a dedicated telephone handset at an information

*Now known as Pure Speech, Inc., Cambridge, MA.

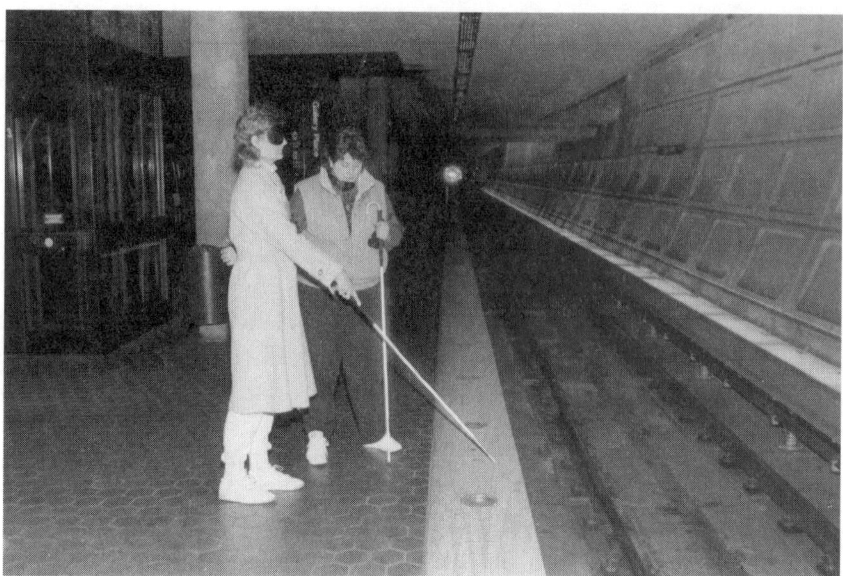

Figure 10.21. Travelers with low vision sometimes confuse the bright lights in the trackbed of the Washington Metropolitan Area Transit Authority with the dimmer embedded lights along the granite platform edge. If they believe that they can safely walk up to the lights, they may fall to the trackbed.

kiosk. Users may ask questions at any level of the information hierarchy at any time in the discourse; they are not constrained to a particular hierarchical sequence, as in the more common menu-driven telephone information systems.

Spatial layout of even very complex transit stations is predictable enough that, if a station is thoroughly labeled with remote infrared audible signs, travelers may not need additional information to independently travel even complex unfamiliar routes (Crandall et al., 1995b). A remote infrared audible signage system (Talking Signs®) in the Powell station in San Francisco provides the information needed by travelers, at the time and place they need it. For example, when travelers enter the station from any entrance, they are able to pick up a directional message or label that enables them to locate the fare barriers for both BART and Muni; once they have negotiated the correct fare barrier they are able to pick up information that enables them to get to the platform; once they reach the platform they are able to pick up information about the location of the main boarding area for the train they wish to take. Other labels and directional signs enable independent location of fare machines, station agents, exits, public telephones, restrooms, and retail facilities (see Figure 10.11).

Persons with visual impairments do not require individual instruction in order to use the signage system, although efficiency for most is greater after either individual instruction or personal practice (Crandall et al., 1995b). Persons with cognitive disabilities as well as persons who have visual impairments benefit from the system (Bentzen et al., in press). A similar remote infrared audible signage system is being developed by a European consortium specifically for use in transit stations. It is planned that this system will transmit in several languages on different frequencies (Stephens & Longley, 1995). It will be integrated with the passenger information system in transit stations, so that it not only labels key landmarks, but also presents variable information such as the destination or time of the next train arriving on a platform.

Bus Stops. For persons who are blind, the task of locating an unfamiliar bus stop and confirming that it is the correct stop, without very explicit directions or a map, is nearly impossible without personal assistance in locations where bus stops may or may not be marked by shelters or distinctive poles, and where they may be located anywhere along a block. Standard stop location, and distinctive stop features such as shelters, special poles, and special pavers are the most common solutions to this problem (Chen, 1990). The use of personal navigation technology could make independent location of unfamiliar bus stops possible for users if it is sufficiently precise and uses databases containing bus stop locations (see Bentzen, Chapter 9 of this volume). Other aids to the location of bus stops are tactile signs, remote infrared audible signs, and remotely activated audible signs.

The Talking Signs® system as well as tactile (raised print and braille) signs were used in a pilot project to label several bus stops in San Francisco (Crandall, Bentzen, & Myers, 1995a). Travelers who are blind were more successful at locating unfamiliar bus stops using remote infrared signage alone than using tactile signs alone. While participants generally preferred audible signage to tactile signs, most liked the idea of having tactile as well as audible signs because the former were absolutely definitive, and using them did not require that the user carry any technological devices.

When using only tactile signs, persons using dog guides resorted to leashing their dogs as they haptically explored to find poles or shelters that might be bus stops; they were unable to use their dogs for guidance or safety because the dogs guided them away from poles and shelters. A great advantage of the remote infrared signage system was that messages were directional and could be picked up from a distance, thus travelers could know whether they were headed in the correct direction.

Another approach to making bus stops distinguishable from other locations along a sidewalk is the use of distinctively shaped poles, or attaching raised signs at standard heights on bus stop poles.

Fare Payment. Paying one's fare in a modern transit system frequently requires interaction with one or more kinds of ticket purchase machines or ticket validating or canceling machines. Many technologies exist; ticket purchase equipment typically requires the user to follow a particular sequence to insert money, locate and press a number of buttons, and remove a ticket. In order to know the value of a ticket, they may require that users read electronic messages. Turnstiles typically require that tickets be inserted in a particular orientation.

In some locations, in order to purchase a ticket with the correct value for a specific trip, riders must locate their origin and destination on a map to determine the number of fare zones between them, or they must refer to a table of fares for different destinations (see Figures 10.22 A and B). *ADAAG* recognizes that such fare equipment presents obstacles to independent use by persons who are visually impaired. Such equipment is required to be independently usable by travelers who are blind, but *ADAAG* does not specify a particular way in which it is to be made accessible. The primary way in which fare equipment is being adapted in the United States, as this book goes to press, is the addition of instructions and labels in braille and raised characters. When the equipment is complex and the instructions long (see Figure 10.22B), it is unlikely that many riders will choose to spend the time required to tactilely read them. Tactile labels, however, can be very helpful to touch readers who are familiar with operation of the equipment. Currently no satisfactory method for presenting changeable electronic messages in an accessible format has been implemented in the United States, although speech output is technologically feasible.

A system in which infrared transmitters with very low power and a narrow beam width (Talking Signs®) are used to make public terminals, including ticket machines, accessible to persons who are blind, is under development at The Smith-Kettlewell Eye Research Institute in San Francisco (W. Crandall, personal communication, 1995). The technology is first being developed for automated teller machines (ATMs), and will then be modified for fare machines and other point-of-sale machines. Users will receive messages through Talking Signs® system receivers when the receivers are held up to buttons and screens. As implemented for ATMs, this infrared signage provides three levels of information: (1) a label for the terminal, enabling prospective users to locate it from a distance; (2)

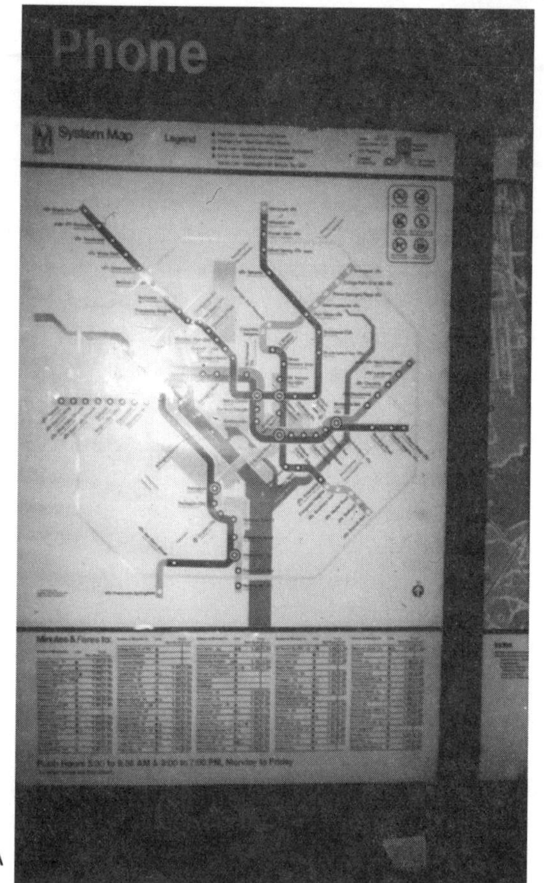

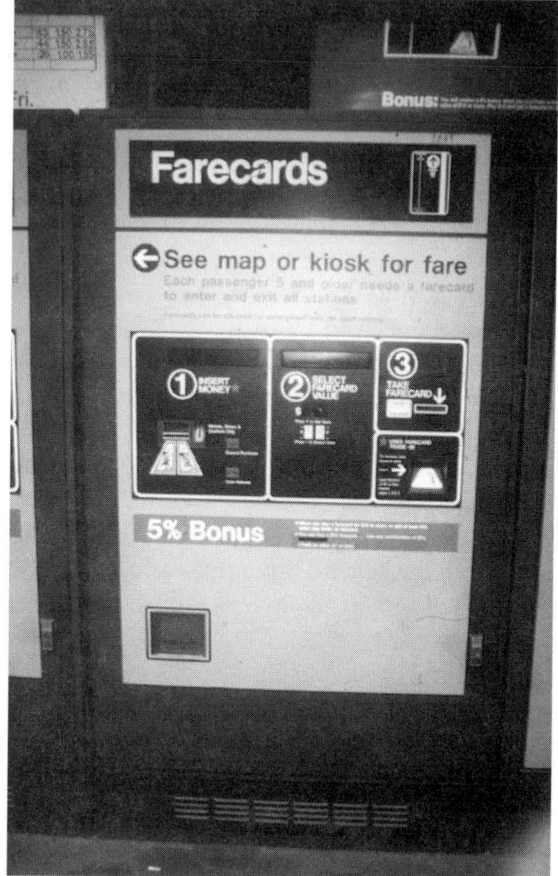

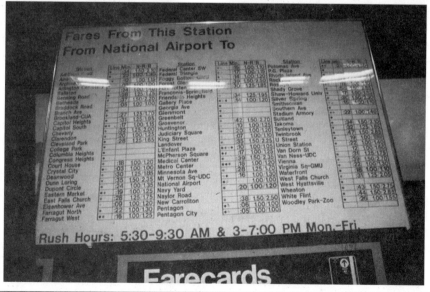

Figure 10.22. (A) Travelers using the Washington Metropolitan Area Transportation Authority must read a map to determine how to reach their destination. The glare makes map reading difficult. (B) Travelers must consult a table of fares applicable to different categories of passengers. (C) After consulting a map and a table of fares, passengers are ready to purchase a fare card for (at least) the appropriate value. One fare machine in each bank of machines at a station entrance now has braille labels.

"screen equivalent" information to allow the terminal functions to be interactive; (3) labels for input and output slots and controls. At the third level, dynamic labeling of controls whose function changes in the course of a transaction will be provided. Such a well-integrated system would provide users with a high degree of interactivity.

Another approach is the use of "smart cards" that would indicate to fare machines that temporary modifications in machine function are desired by a user. Such modifications might include speech output, large print, and a slower operating rate. Contactless smart cards could activate an audible signal to guide users to a fare transaction machine (Gill, 1994, 1996).

Simply orienting fare cards correctly can be time-consuming for travelers who are visually impaired, making their travel inefficient, and delaying other passengers. A simple tactile indicator on one corner of a fare card, such as a cut-off corner or a notch, can greatly increase the efficiency of fare card orientation for all users (Bentzen, Jackson, & Peck, 1981b; Gill, 1996). In transit systems where tokens are used for payment, it may be difficult to distinguish tokens from coins using touch alone. In the United States, a token with a hole in it is readily distinguished from coins (Bentzen et al., 1981b). This speeds fare payment for all riders who reach into pockets or purses to find tokens.

Smart cards are being used and considered for improving access to many services for all users. A smart card is a credit card-sized plastic card incorporating an integrated microcircuit. There are a number of types of smart cards in use for particular purposes in various parts of the world; the most common type is a prepaid card that may be used for a variety of applications, including transit fares and telephone calls. Contactless smart cards are being developed that allow functions to be performed without direct contact between the card and the terminal. Use of contactless cards in transit can speed movement of all passengers through fare barriers. For persons with visual impairments, the advantages are that no card reader or slot must be located, and the card does not have to be taken out of a purse or wallet and correctly oriented and inserted (see Hill, 1994, for a comprehensive discussion of the use of smart cards in public transit and Gill, 1994, for a review of the entire smart card industry with regard to its potential for increasing accessibility for persons with disabilities).

Transit Vehicles

There are a number of challenges in the use of transit vehicles by travelers who are visually impaired. Most are regularly met by asking drivers or other passengers for information. However, it may be difficult and time-consuming to locate an individual to ask, and that individual may not have the information, may not speak the same language, may give wrong information, or may be rude or threatening. Thus, it is desirable to provide information in formats that enable independent use of transit vehicles by persons who are visually impaired. Travelers must identify the correct vehicle, locate the door to that vehicle, determine when to get off, and locate the correct exit from the vehicle. At times all of this information is self-evident, and travelers may need no assistance; visually impaired travelers who are traveling highly familiar routes on familiar equipment, particularly when only one vehicle serves that route, frequently require no additional information. However, unanticipated changes are typical of transit environments, so cautious travelers nonetheless like to be reassured that they are boarding the correct vehicle and getting off at the correct stop.

Identifying Vehicles. Travelers with normal vision identify vehicles approaching stops, or those that are stationary at stops by reading vehicle identification signs, which are typically on the fronts and sides of vehicles. Vehicle identification signs must have highly legible fonts, and large enough characters to be read at a distance, and they must be high in contrast, well illuminated, and free from glare and dirt. All of these factors affect the readability of signs for all transit riders, but they are particularly important to persons with low vision (Figure 10.23 A, B, C, and D).

Until the last decade, the most common vehicle identification signs in the United States were

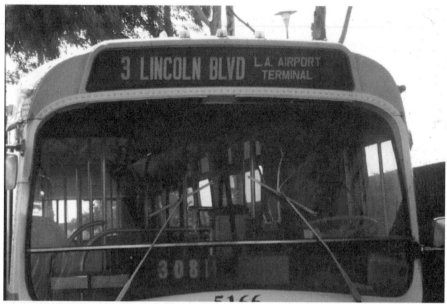

(A) This bus in Los Angeles has a conventional "curtain sign." Although the sign has good contrast, even the largest letters are too tall in proportion to their width and too close together to be read easily.

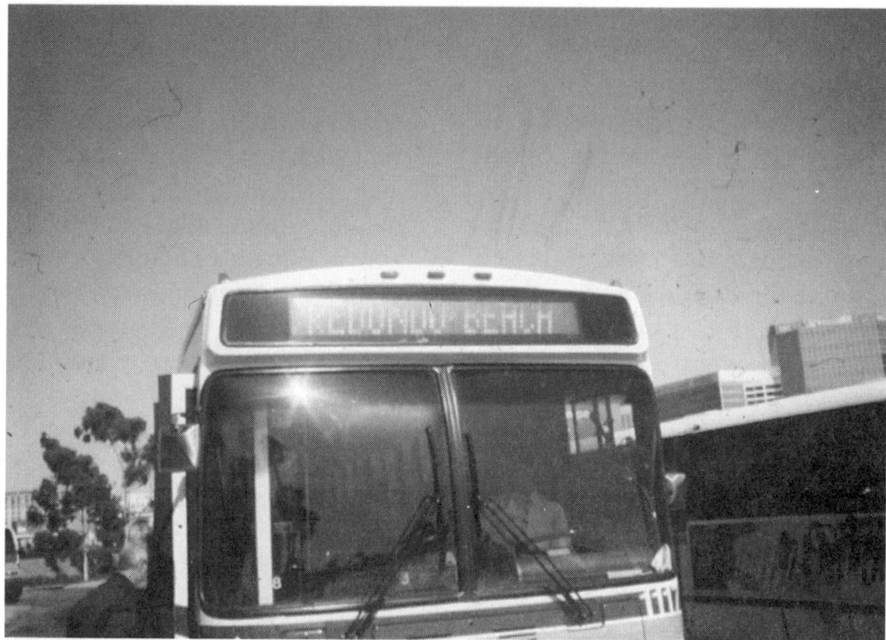

(B) The electronic sign on this bus in Los Angeles is difficult for all riders to read because of the glare on its surface.

(continued on next page)

Figure 10.23.

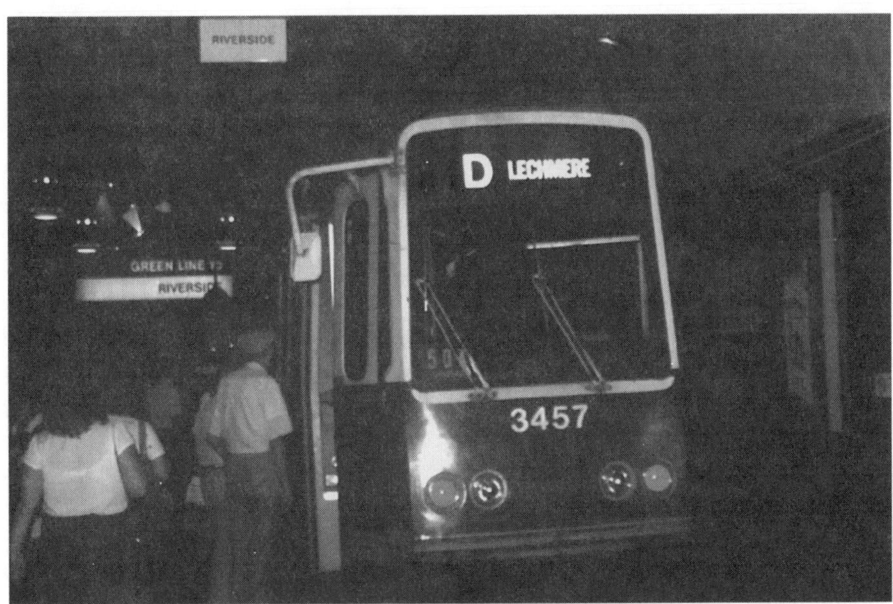

(C) The single big letter on the curtain sign of this light rail vehicle in Boston is highly legible, although the destination is difficult to read.

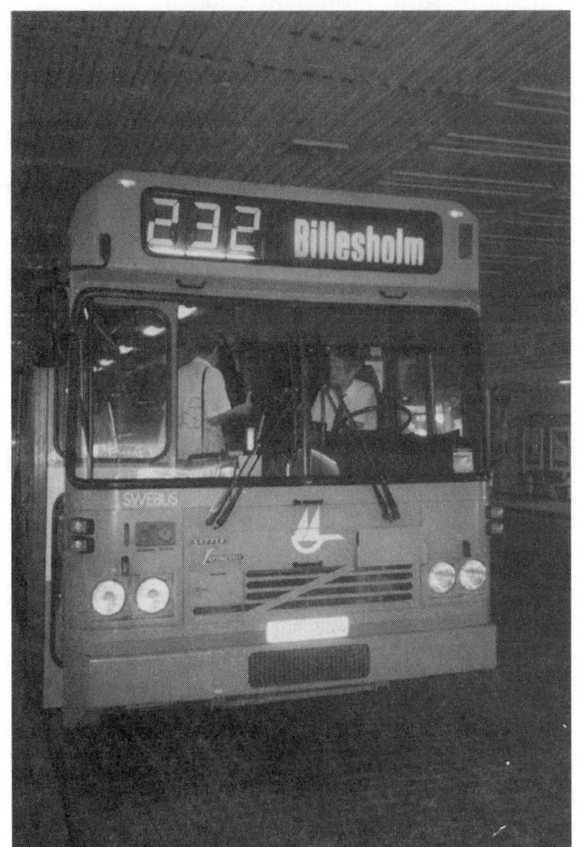

(D) Electronic signs can be made more legible. The number of this bus in Denmark is quite legible; the destination is less so.

"curtain signs," signs printed on coated fabric and rolled up like window shades. These are expensive to manufacture, unlikely to last for the life of the vehicle, and not easy to modify. With the advent of technologies for changeable message signs (CMSs), initial costs have increased, but maintenance may be less costly, less operator time and effort are required to change messages, and the signs are easy to modify. Three technologies are being used: flip-dot, an electromagnetic system in which a matrix of dots that are dark on one side and light on the other are flipped in patterns forming letters and numbers; light-emitting diodes (LED); and liquid crystal displays (LCD). The three technologies have different characteristics that make each one the most suitable for a particular application. A discussion of these characteristics is beyond the scope of this chapter; however, all of these technologies produce characters that are based on a matrix of dots or lights, resulting in character strokes which are not continuous. In general, such matrix signs tend to be less legible than conventional signs in which characters have continuous strokes (Garvey, 1994; Bentzen et al., 1995c).

One research project on the readability of signs by persons with varying amounts of vision, specifically dynamic situations in which the sign approaches a person (as on an approaching bus), looked at both conventional print signs and CMS flip-dot signs (Bentzen, 1996; Bentzen et al., 1995c). The best readability for persons with normal vision (acuity . 20/70), persons with low vision (20/80–20/180), and persons who are legally blind (20/200–20/400), was achieved by conventional print signs consisting of all capital letters. Conventional print signs on the front of vehicles that approached and came to a stop were read from approximately 30 feet per inch (9.2 m per 25.6 mm) of character height by persons with normal vision. Persons with low vision read the same signs from approximately 6 feet per inch (1.84 m per 25.6 mm), and persons who were legally blind could read the signs from approximately 2 feet per inch (0.61 m per 25.6 mm) of character height. Thus it was only when vehicles were very close to a stop that persons who are legally blind were able to read the signs in daytime conditions, even though those signs had excellent contrast (white on black), had a highly legible font (Helvetica bold), and were free from glare and dirt.

When similar groups of participants read flip-dot signs consisting of all capital letters under the same dynamic conditions, the best readability was achieved for all groups when spacing between characters was 1.5 to 2.0 times the width of strokes, and the characters had wide character width-to-height proportions (7:10 versus 9:14) and wide stroke width-to-height proportions (2:10 versus 2:14). Legibility distances for these CMSs were less than for conventional print signs, 19 feet per inch (5.83 m per 2.56 mm) for persons with normal vision, and 3 feet per inch (0.9 m per 2.56 mm) for persons with low vision. Persons who are legally blind correctly read less than 25 percent of signs 8 inches (200 mm) high from any distance, up to and including the moment at which the bus stopped.

Other approaches to making vehicle identification accessible to all persons who for any reason are unable to read print vehicle identification signs involve presenting vehicle information in spoken form. An operational solution is to have drivers identify vehicles with a route number and name or destination when they open vehicle doors. This rarely works well, at least in the United States, so automated methods are being developed for presenting speech messages. At the simplest level, annunciators can automatically identify vehicles each time a boarding door opens. Neither of these approaches enables waiting passengers to identify vehicles from a distance, which is sometimes essential if passengers must hail vehicles for them to stop.

Two other approaches have remote capability, however. In one, automated vehicle-locating systems communicate the identity of approaching buses to fixed receivers located at stops; the vehicle identification information is then heard from a loudspeaker at the stop. In another approach, remote infrared transmitters are placed in the front and side sign cavities of buses, and individuals hear bus identification information from handheld receivers when vehicles are at a distance of 50–400 feet (15–120 m), as well as when they are stationary at a stop, platform, or bus terminal (Crandall et al., 1995a).

A very different approach is to have travelers who cannot read vehicle identification signs hold up a placard with a very large number that corresponds to the route number of the bus they wish to board. Bus drivers are then required to stop in front of passengers holding these placards.

Locating Vehicle Doors. In most situations travelers who are blind are able to localize open vehicle doors from at least a short distance away by listening for the sound of a door that is opening, or by listening to the sounds of other passengers. On some light rail vehicles, however, doors do not open to admit passengers unless they push a button. Passengers who are visually impaired, when they are alone on a platform, typically locate the push button by contacting the side of the vehicle with a long cane or hand and then trailing it until they find the button. This is time-consuming, and it can be unsafe because a driver may not see an approaching passenger and may move the vehicle while the individual is in contact with the vehicle side. If the buttons emitted a highly localizable sound that was audible from only 5–10 feet (1.5–3 m) away, blind travelers could locate these buttons by listening.

In some transit systems where rail vehicles are automatically stopped at predetermined locations along platforms, the location of vehicle doors has been indicated by raised, directional floor surfaces. Such surfaces are required by the California Title 24 Accessibility Standards (Section 3325(d)); they are to be placed directly behind detectable warnings that indicate the platform edge, with the linear surface aligned perpendicular to the platform edge.

Knowing When to Get Off. On fixed-stop systems, riders often count stops to know when to get off. When vehicles do not necessarily stop at each potential stop, however, travelers who are blind have traditionally relied on drivers and/or fellow passengers to let them know when they have arrived at their stop. One thing that must always be learned by riders on such routes, however, is what to do if the driver fails to announce the stop (Jacobson, 1993; LaGrow & Weessies, 1994).

Obtaining next-stop information from drivers, at least in the United States, is not a particularly reliable system. When there are automated vehicle-locating systems, this technology can be integrated with both CMSs and annunciators in vehicles to announce upcoming stops in both visual and audible formats. In some cases the next-stop CMSs are used for advertising and/or entertainment as well as next-stop announcements. Where this is the case, CMS next-stop signs are most legible if they are separated at least 3 inches (76.8 mm) from CMSs with other messages. It is desirable to precede next-stop messages with an alert tone, and to display "NEXT STOP" on the CMS prior to the name of the stop. CMS next-stop signs are most legible if the characters have only moderately wide width-to-height ratios (5:7 is more legible than 6:7), if character strokes are narrow (1 pixel wide is more legible than 2 pixels wide), and if intercharacter spacing is wide (spacing two times the stroke width makes signs more legible than spacing equal to stroke width) (Bentzen & Easton, 1995).

In some localities the general ridership seems to like having all stops announced audibly, while in other places only main stop announcements are desired (Rochester-Genesee Regional Transportation Authority, 1995). One way to make next-stop announcements audible only to persons who want to hear them is to transmit next-stop messages using remote infrared signage technology. In whatever way the electronic message system for CMSs acquires its information about the next stop, this same system can communicate with an infrared transmitter on the vehicle, which then announces each stop—only to those passengers who have receivers, and only when they want to hear the messages.

Knowing which Door to Exit. Passengers who have vision are able to perceive at a distance the side of a vehicle on which exit doors are opening. Persons who are blind do not have this information at a distance to help them plan how to make their way to the exit. They must rely on haptic exploration, and sounds of doors as well as other exiting passengers. On many systems next-stop messages include which side of the vehicle to exit.

RESPONSIBILITIES OF O&M SPECIALISTS

In all situations involving safety and wayfinding for persons who are visually impaired, O&M specialists are important consultants, together with local persons who have visual impairments. Persons who are experts in environmental accessibility for persons with other disabilities typically do not have a sufficient understanding of what makes travel safe and independent wayfinding possible for visually impaired persons, to enable them to provide adequate guidance to architects and planners. It is particularly important for O&M specialists and blind travelers to be involved in the development and implementation of specialized wayfinding systems for visually impaired persons, as appropriate technology and placement and wording of signs require a high level of sophistication regarding the wayfinding strategies and capabilities of visually impaired persons.

O&M specialists need to take a proactive role in the expanding field of architectural accessibility (Bentzen, 1984). In the United States, particularly, accessibility is still only commonly understood to be an issue that is relevant to persons with physical disabilities, although the ADA explicitly applies to persons with sensory and cognitive disabilities as well. Planners, architects, graphic designers, and local building officials typically have little understanding of the accessibility needs of persons with visual impairments. Even well-respected consulting groups specializing in accessibility have made serious errors in planning accommodations for persons with visual impairments.

O&M specialists need to be active, together with persons with visual impairments, in setting standards and monitoring environments to be sure that they comply with standards as well as are truly beneficial to visually impaired persons. They also need to be well informed about all relevant standards for accessibility so that they can be effective advocates and consultants for new building projects or projects in which modifications are made to make environments more accessible (Wiener, 1992).

Suggestions/Implications for O&M Specialists

1. O&M specialists need to be informed, effective advocates for environmental access at local, state, and federal levels. Environmental access for persons with visual impairments is primarily a matter of having the right information at the right time.
2. If persons with visual impairments have access to the same information for wayfinding and safety that is routinely provided for persons with sight, they can travel in the same way as sighted persons—independently, quickly, efficiently, and with freedom of choice.
3. Universal design, including logical spatial layout, highly visible key architectural features, and good lighting, benefits persons who do not have disabilities as well as persons with disabilities, including most persons with visual impairments.
4. O&M specialists who are skilled in analyzing environments from a wayfinding information perspective have much to offer architects and urban planners, who do not typically have academic training in environmental analysis for wayfinding.
5. The ADA recognizes the right of persons with visual impairments to information for safety and wayfinding. When students in O&M do not have the information they need, it is the responsibility of the O&M specialist to be proactive in helping the relevant building owner, transit system, or community to provide the needed information.
6. Information for safety and wayfinding that is often unavailable to persons with visual impairments includes, but is not limited to, the names of streets and landmarks; room numbers; bus numbers and destinations; directional information in transit stations; intersection configuration and type of traffic control; and the status of traffic-light cycles.

(continued on next page)

Suggestions/Implications for O&M Specialists (continued)

7. Intersection design and traffic control systems are increasingly varied, and increasingly require pedestrian actuation of walk phases. Visually impaired pedestrians may be unaware that there is no safe crossing time unless they push a button; they may be unable to locate the button; and they may have insufficient auditory information to determine the onset of the "walk" phase.

8. Audible pedestrian signals can often solve the above problems. Numerous types exist, all with advantages and disadvantages. There is currently a lack of consensus in the O&M profession regarding the desired characteristics of audible pedestrian signals. Different types may be needed in different situations.

9. Vehicle manufacturers work hard to make vehicles as quiet as possible. The increasing presence of electric and other very quiet vehicles increases the likelihood that visually impaired travelers will have insufficient auditory information to reliably determine safe crossing times.

10. As persons wtih visual impairments are especially dependent on public transportation, it is incumbent upon O&M specialists to ensure that public transportation systems serving their students provide sufficient information for safe, independent travel, even on unfamiliar routes.

ACTIVITIES FOR REVIEW

1. Obtain copies of the *Americans with Disabilities Act Accessibility Guidelines* (*ADAAG*) and your state accessibility regulations. Highlight those sections that affect independent travel of persons with visual impairments.
2. Assess a government building in terms of its compliance with *ADAAG* sections that affect independent travel of persons with visual impairments. Are there ways in which the building is out of compliance? What suggestions would you have for this building to facilitate or improve independent travel of persons with visual impairments?
3. Analyze a building in which it is particularly easy to become disoriented. What is it about the layout of the building that causes way-finding problems? Is it possible to make way-finding in the building easier? If so, describe what would be required.
4. In your locale, how do travelers who are blind obtain the following information needed for traveling on buses? (a) route and schedule information; (b) location of bus stops; (c) the number and destination of buses; (d) where to get off?
5. Describe how your local bus company could make information more readily available to persons who are visually impaired.
6. Analyze an intersection that you would not recommend for some persons who are blind to cross unassisted. Is there a type of audible pedestrian signal (APS) which would make this intersection easier and safer to negotiate? What characteristics would you like the APS to have?
7. As a traffic-calming measure, some communities are raising the street level at

intersections to form speed tables. This typically results in totally blended curbs. How may this affect the information available at such an intersection to pedestrians who are blind?

8. Explain how the advent of quiet cars may negatively impact the information used by pedestrians who are blind to analyze intersections and cross streets safely?

9. Describe environmental designs particularly intended to increase access for persons with visual impairments that are likely to increase safety, ease, or confidence in travel for persons who do not have visual impairments.

PART THREE
The Learner

CHAPTER 11

Learning Theory and Teaching Methodologies

William H. Jacobson and Robert H. Bradley

People are constantly changing. Some of these changes are called learning; specifically, learning involves changes that result from experience. Learning has definitely taken place if the information received through one or more sensory modalities results in a change in a person's behavior or understanding.

Learning takes many forms. It can be as simple as learning the name of some common object, or it can be as complex as learning to familiarize oneself to a novel environment or learning to make judgments regarding how to reorient oneself when lost. There are theories that attempt to explain how the process of learning occurs, and there are principles of learning designed to help facilitate acquisition of particular classes of competencies or skills. This chapter discusses some of the major theories and principles of learning and their potential applicability to some of the learning goals for orientation and mobility (O&M) instruction.

APPLYING THEORIES OF LEARNING TO THE MOBILITY PROCESS

This chapter does not identify the major shortcomings of any particular learning theory, but rather identifies those learning principles which can assist with the practical decisions one needs to make when actually designing an instructional mobility strategy aimed at a particular learning goal. The purpose of a learning theory is to explain how individuals learn. Most learning theories can be categorized into two major types: behavioral and cognitive. *Behavioral learning* theories, in general, attempt to explain learning in terms of observable changes in the behavior of a person. In contrast, *cognitive learning* theories attempt to explain learning in terms of the mental processes that a person uses to more fully understand some concept or strategy.

Behavioral Learning Theory

Behavioral learning theories can be further subdivided into two major categories: classical conditioning and operant conditioning. Both have applicability to the mobility learning processes.

Classical Conditioning

Classical conditioning involves reflexive actions (Baldwin & Baldwin, 1986). That is, human beings are born with a large number of *reflexes*. These reflexes are essentially action responses to certain specific sets of external conditions; they are designed to occur automatically whenever a person encounters a particular set of circumstances.

For instance, people start salivating when they can smell or taste food. In the terminology of classical conditioning, salivation is an *unconditioned response* that occurs naturally in the presence of certain particular unconditioned stimuli (e.g., the smell of food). These responses are innate, not learned. Many reflexive responses, such as salivation and the knee-jerk reaction, are well known. But human beings also have a large number of less well-known reflexive responses that typically occur under circumstances of threat or harm. Such reflexes (e.g., the eye-blink response) are designed to help us avoid harm or exercise vigilance in the face of some threatening circumstance. Reflexes are simply preparatory actions that enable us to better take care of basic biological needs.

However, human beings may learn to make reflexive responses in circumstances other than those for which they are biologically designed. Biologically, people do not start salivating when they hear the sound of a bell; but if it is their mother's practice to ring a dinner bell in order to call them for dinner, the association of that dinner bell with what comes immediately after may cause them to salivate prior to actually smelling or seeing any food. Making a reflexive response to something that normally would not produce that response is called a *conditioned* (or learned) *response.*

Those events in the environment (stimuli) that automatically cause a reflex to occur (e.g., a puff of air to the eye causes an eye to blink or the smell of food causes salivation) are called *unconditioned stimuli.* They evoke the reflexive (or unconditioned) response merely because human beings are biologically geared to react in that way. No learning has to occur in order for the response to occur automatically in the presence of the unconditioned stimuli. For all human reflexive responses, most stimuli in the environment are neutral; that is, they do not automatically evoke the reflexive response.

Conditioning can be used to change behavior by pairing a neutral stimulus that typically would not elicit a response with an unconditioned stimulus that naturally elicits a response. With repeated pairing the neutral stimulus alone will produce the desired response. For example, if a dog is presented with a neutral stimulus such as the sound of a bell that is consistently paired with the presentation of food, eventually the conditioned response of salivation will occur at the sound of the bell.

Primary and Secondary Conditioned Stimuli as Reinforcers. The principles of classical conditioning, which involve repeated pairings of an unconditioned stimulus with a conditioned stimulus, can be useful in certain areas of O&M instruction. Pavlov hypothesized that biologically meaningful stimuli that elicit survival-promoting reflexes can be powerful primary reinforcers. These include innate pleasurable stimuli such as food and water. For behaviorists (Barker, 1994), food functions as a *primary reinforcer*; that is, the receipt of food appears to be naturally pleasurable and motivating in that people will act to obtain food without being prompted or rewarded for doing so. Because certain food items (as the unconditioned stimuli) provoke unconditioned pleasure responses, an O&M instructor can condition any other stimulus (e.g., praise) so that it also excites the pleasure responses. By associating praise (or any other stimulus for that matter) with food, the praise becomes what behaviorists call a *secondary reinforcer*—it becomes so well associated with food or a primary reinforcer that students will become motivated to act to get praise itself.

Establishing, then using, secondary reinforcers is very important for O&M instruction. Using primary reinforcers such as food to promote certain behavior (learning) from low-functioning students may well be effective in the early stages of instruction, but it becomes counterproductive when the long-term desired goal for a student is to behave in the appropriate way in the real world (a world where food rewards are not likely to be offered constantly by family, friends, teachers, and acquaintances). Establishing a variety of secondary reinforcers by means of classical conditioning can help the O&M instructor gradually associate desired behavior patterns with reinforcement modalities and schedules that are more likely to be found in the actual environment of the student.

What is more important to understand is that classical conditioning principles are often involved in natural human learning circumstances. Because of people's own history of personal experiences, many have learned to respond positively to secondary reinforcers. It is important for the O&M specialist to identify the secondary reinforcers that are important to the student. Typical secondary reinforcers can be classified into the five categories of (1) commodities, (2) activities, (3) social reinforcers, (4) feedback, and (5) token reinforcers (Spiegler, 1983). Commodities include such items as toys, books, clothes, jewelry, compact discs, and recreational equipment. Activities might include listening to music, shopping, playing games, reading, resting, partying, talking, cooking, dancing, and traveling. Social reinforcers include various forms of interactions that result in praise, approval of others, friendly gestures, physical contact, and personal attention. Feedback or gaining information about one's own behavior can be reinforcing. For example, learning that one is performing a skill correctly may often lead to a further increase in proficiency. Token or symbolic reinforcers, such as money, grades, or passes to go out at night or on weekends can also be used as effective secondary reinforcers. The O&M specialist should observe the student carefully to determine which stimuli are valued by the student. These reinforcers, if used properly, can be used to strengthen desired behaviors.

Deconditioning and Desensitization. There is substantial evidence that numerous fears and phobias result from classical conditioning processes (Davey, 1992). Unintentional pairings oftentimes may lead to maladjustive behaviors. A student, as one example, who was constantly jostled and bumped by passersby in a particular crowded hallway may tend to stop moving or freeze up when traveling through that hallway, even when there is no one present. Another student who stumbled previously on a stairway may lock her knees when trying to walk up or down steps—or refuse to use stairs at all while under instruction on a mobility lesson.

Two points are important in this regard. First, there are some procedures developed for deconditioning people so that they do not feel anxious and display the reflexive internal actions during the types of situations where previously they were conditioned to do so. The process is called *systematic desensitization* (Wolpe, Salter, & Reyna, 1964). Second, even if an instructor does not have the time to engage in designed deconditioning procedures, it is important to bear in mind that a lot of students are blocked from learning because they have learned anxiety responses that are very hard for them to control or overcome. Systematic desensitization is a multistage process that begins by extinguishing conditioned fear responses to stimuli far removed from the target situation. The target behavior is systematically approached in small steps with time allowed to extinguish the conditioned fear response at each step. For example, in the first situation described above the student is taken to another, quieter hallway for instruction, and another after that until the skills are learned and practiced without the threat of being jostled by passersby. The other student with a fear of stairs might be shown how to walk up and down one step (e.g., a balance beam sitting on the floor), then two steps, and then three, etc., until a whole stairwaylike situation is gradually introduced. This exercise might be done in a gymnasium or auditorium, which generally is not associated with stairs or stairwells.

In still another example, suppose a student becomes highly agitated when approaching a major intersection. Before placing the student in such situations where classically conditioned fear responses would emerge, the O&M instructor might begin in a place far removed from any traffic—perhaps in an office where the student is asked to imagine a street with no traffic or listen to an audiotape of a quiet engine motor running. Only gradually, and by small degrees, does the student begin imagining situations more like a real major intersection or experiencing circumstances that are more like a busy intersection.

When the student is taken to an actual intersection, the instructor might at first take him across the street using the sighted guide technique to further minimize the fear or threat of traffic. A further step might be for the two to walk side by side, brushing shoulders and, later, for the instructor to walk in front of the student while having him come toward the sound of his voice. All the while throughout this process the O&M instructor is at hand using a soft, reassuring voice, gentle touches, and related techniques to engender a calm state in the student. The instructor must make certain that the student is not showing signs of the conditioned fear response before moving to the next step. Systematic desensitization may take a long time to complete; plateaus and even reversals are quite common. Using desensitization procedures to help a person unhook the reflexive actions (e.g., a knot in the stomach) from the conditions in which they have learned to display them could be very important in enabling students to learn more productively and comfortably in new learning situations.

Deconditioning classically conditioned reflexive responses to threat involves two principles: (1) demonstrating to the student that the new learning situation, in fact, contains no negative consequences in a threatening situation. (By repeating this experience, e.g., walking up and down stairs, and talking a person through the experience, the classically conditioned response may gradually become extinguished since the elements that initially produced it are no longer present in the new circumstance); and (2) actually producing in the student contradictory biological impulses, impulses associated with supportive and nonthreatening circumstances. Mobility lessons can help to modulate anxiety responses if they are designed with a calm and soothing atmosphere or if they teach a student the means to control how close a threatening stimulus may get. Any teaching technique that would produce the physiological responses associated with dread and anxiety (even including highly energetic teaching styles by teachers) should generally be avoided in instructional circumstances where a student is known to be anxious about the learning situation.

Operant Conditioning

Whereas the principles of classical conditioning are infrequently used to assist students in learning particular new mobility skills or knowledge, the principles of operant conditioning are frequently used for such purposes. *Operant conditioning* involves the use of pleasant and unpleasant consequences to change behavior (Walker & Shea, 1980). It is based on the premise (called the *law of effect*) that if an act is followed by a satisfying change in the environment, the likelihood of that act being repeated in similar situations is reinforced or increased (Barker, 1994). However, if a behavior is followed by an unsatisfying change in the environment, the likelihood of that behavior being repeated is decreased. In effect, in operant conditioning the environment operates on the individual to change behavior by providing consequences for the individual's behavior.

The Principles of Reinforcement and Punishment. A *reinforcer* is defined as any consequence that strengthens or increases the frequency of a behavior. Human beings are diverse and complex creatures. What functions as a reinforcer for some may not be a reinforcer for others. And certainly the extent to which something operates as a reinforcer for one person may be very different from the extent to which it can operate as a reinforcer for another person. We can determine whether something is reinforcing for a person and how powerful it is as a reinforcer only if we examine its effect on a particular individual. Similarly, a punisher can be viewed as such only if it reduces a specific behavior. For example, removing a child from the classroom can be considered a punishment for some children, while for others it may serve as a reinforcer. If remaining in the classroom is desired by the child, then removing her from the classroom is a punishment. However, if the classroom is considered an unpleasant place, removing the child may actually turn out to be a reward. Choosing the right reinforcer or punisher is one of the most significant decisions an O&M instructor has to make in using the principles of operant conditioning to assist students in learning new skills and knowledge.

Behavior Change. The environment operates in two basic ways to change behavior. As stated earlier, when the environment is reinforcing, it strengthens or increases the likelihood that a behavior will be repeated. However, when the environment is punishing, it weakens or decreases the likelihood that a behavior will occur (Table 11.1). When using operant conditioning, the term "positive" is used not as a value judgment, but instead to indicate that a stimulus has been applied. Similarly the term "negative" is not used as a value statement, but as an indicator that a stimulus has been removed.

Reinforcers. Reinforcers are those stimuli that result in increasing the frequency of the desired behavior. Reinforcement can be of two varieties: positive reinforcement and negative reinforcement. In *positive reinforcement* the environment provides a valued stimulus so as to strengthen a behavior. Praising a child for using the upper hand and forearm in the correct position or for walking in step with the cane serve as positive reinforcements. Another example might include providing a hall pass as a reward for consistently safe indoor travel. In *negative reinforcement* behavior is strengthened by removing an aversive stimulus. Allowing a student to bump into an obstacle because he does not hold his cane in the correct diagonal position is an example. The behavior of holding the cane in the proper diagonal position removes the aversive stimulus of bumping into objects. Another example of negative reinforcement might include allowing a person to experience the consequence of stepping off the curb on his side and into the street because he is using a cane arc that is too narrow. In this situation the student learns that in order to avoid the unpleasant stimulus of stepping off the curb, he must use a wider arc.

Punishers. *Punishers* are those stimuli that result in decreasing the frequency of the behavior. Punishment can be of two varieties: positive punishment and negative punishment. In *positive punishment* an aversive stimulus is provided to weaken a behavior. When a parent yells at a young child for running into the street, this is considered positive punishment because the aversive stimulus of yelling decreases the likelihood of the child repeating the behavior. When an O&M instructor voices displeasure to a student because he decides not to use a cane in school, this is an example of positive punishment. Hopefully this weakens the behavior of walking without protection. In *negative punishment* a valued or prized stimulus is removed to weaken the occurrence of a particular behavior. Sending a child to his room when he is screaming instead of allowing him to play is an example of negative punishment. In this case it takes away the valued activity of play in order to weaken the behavior of screaming. In O&M a traveler who exhibits acting-out behavior in a favorite public restaurant may be removed from that restaurant in order to weaken the acting-out behavior.

Thus the consequences a person encounters in a mobility situation are likely to play a crucial role in determining that person's future behavior in similar situations; and, more specifically, they will play a crucial role in whether the person learns the skill that is the target of the lesson.

The Selection of Reinforcers and Punishers. As mentioned earlier, reinforcers fall into two broad classes, primary reinforcers and secondary reinforcers (Barker, 1994). Primary reinforcers are not commonly used in instructional situations. There are occasions, however, when the systematic use of primary reinforcers is a good idea. For example, instructors may find it useful to employ food items for individuals whose cognitive abilities are quite limited or who are highly uncooperative in responding to reinforcers that might typically be

Table 11.1. Behavior Change: An Overview

Type of Stimulus	Reinforcers	Punishers
Positive	**Providing a positive stimulus to strengthen a behavior.** Example: A hall pass is given to reward a student for safe indoor travel.	**Adding aversive stimulus to weaken a behavior.** Example: An O&M instructor chastizes a student for not using a cane at school in order to encourage him or her to do so in the future.
Negative	**Removing aversive stimulus to strengthen a behavior.** Example: Too narrow an arc width causes stepping off a curb on side, but a wider arc width corrects this situation.	**Removing a valued stimulus to weaken a behavior.** Example: A student is removed from a favorite restaurant when he or she exhibits acting out behavior.

used—that is, someone for whom commonly used secondary reinforcers like praise (or opportunities to engage in other pleasurable activities) have not been fully learned. In order to engage a severely retarded student in following a specific route from the door of the bedroom to the bathroom, it may require the careful use of primary reinforcers.

It is much more common for instructors to use secondary reinforcers to increase some desired behavior on the part of the learner. Secondary reinforcers are things that acquire their value by being associated with primary reinforcers or other well-established secondary reinforcers.

Which kind of reinforcer to use to increase the probability that a student will learn some new skill or knowledge depends on several factors of the characteristics of the person being reinforced. First, a symbolic or token reinforcer is more likely to be satisfying to mature persons, for example, because they understand its ultimate value to them; second, the context of instruction is limited in terms of the kinds of social reinforcers that one would consider appropriate to give (e.g., one would not necessarily give a hug to an immature adult who could confuse that form of praise with affection); and third, the types of reinforcers the instructor has the ability to offer may be limited (in some instances an instructor may simply not have the ability to offer access to some fun activity).

The choice of reinforcer also depends on one's short-term and long-term goals for the student. Most instructors have as a goal that students will become self-motivating, and self-sufficient, and will develop a sense of self-efficacy. In the natural environment students will often not have access to a consistent supply of reinforcers such as they might be offered in an instructional setting. Therefore it is important that instructors be aware of the needs for the transition from the instructional setting to the more natural environment. For this reason it is important that instructional strategies be designed so that the student will ultimately not remain dependent upon the kinds of reinforcers that may often be unavailable in the natural environment (e.g., constant praise for remaining in step while swinging the cane). Thus, while certain types of social or activity or token reinforcers may be quite useful in initial stages of instruction, it is often important that the type of reinforcer be adjusted so that it becomes more and more like the actual environmental settings (Walker & Shea, 1980).

How frequently and regularly reinforcers are used must also be considered (the concept of schedules of reinforcement is discussed at greater length later in this chapter). When skills are just beginning to be inculcated, it may be useful to reinforce a student after every successful behavior. As a student walks in a hallway using the sighted guide techniques with the instructor, as an example, the instructor continually praises the student after each aspect of the skill is successfully demonstrated (e.g., after going from basic sighted guide into transferring sides, and after transferring sides to narrow spaces). However, once the behavior is more stable, less frequent and less regular reinforcement may be better as a student is not likely to continue to be reinforced after each desired behavior once he is in the natural environment.

So far our discussion has focused on positive reinforcers (things or conditions that a person would find pleasurable). As mentioned earlier, one can also decrease the likelihood of persons displaying a particular set of behaviors by considering stimuli that people dislike or by removing them from pleasurable stimuli. If the practicing of keeping the hand centered when swinging the cane is considered by an individual to be an unpleasant task, then just being allowed to stop and relax might be considered quite reinforcing. The purpose of a negative reinforcer (that is, an opportunity to escape an unpleasant situation) is the same as the goal of positive reinforcers: namely, to strengthen a behavior or to increase its frequency of occurrence.

A negative reinforcer is very different from a punishment, however. The purpose of punishment is to weaken a behavior or to decrease its likelihood of occurrence. Punishment involves the use of unpleasant consequences to weaken a behavior whereas negative reinforcers involve releasing a person from an unpleasant situation to strengthen a behavior. Although punishment is a rapid way of changing behaviors, it is rarely recommended as a means of helping students to learn because of the high probability of negative side effects from its use, as well as a tendency toward quick extinction. The use of negative reinforcers, on the other hand, is a different matter. Escaping an unpleasant circumstance is viewed by most people in a very different manner than actually experiencing the unpleasant circumstance.

Shaping of Behaviors. The use of behavioral learning theory typically involves the process of *shaping* (Hill & Horton, 1985). The instructor begins by determining precisely what it is that the student needs to learn; that is, the ultimate goal or end state of the instructional process. Then the instructor determines the student's current abilities or set of behaviors with respect to the goal. For example, if the goal of instruction is to enable a person to be able to use the diagonal cane technique, it is important to recognize that effective use of the technique requires a number of more specific prerequisite capabilities. For instance, can the person position his arm or is the person not even capable of using a proper grasp? One looks at the student's current set of capabilities and behaviors at the desired end state for the instruction, and then tries to imagine all the steps that would be necessary to move the student from the current state of capability to the desired end state. Reinforcement techniques are used to gradually mold the student's behavior (e.g., shaping the behavior) so that the behavior gradually comes to approximate the desired end state. Most often this process involves making tiny improvements in the direction of the goal.

To be successful in shaping behavior so that it gradually comes to look like the desired end state, the instructor depends on two functions: (1) task analysis, or carefully breaking down the desired terminal behavior into sufficiently small subtasks so that each increment in performance toward the final goal is readily achievable; and (2) proper sequencing of subtasks so that the ultimate end state is achieved with an acceptable level of efficiency. Reinforcement is given at first to reward any behavior that approximates the desired goal. Later, rewards are given only as the behavior more closely meets the criterion. Small, incremental improvements and performance should typically be the targets of reinforcement. Requiring improvement in too-large steps may be frustrating and may actually stop progress. Careful monitoring of the student's actual progress through the stages of instruction is imperative. It may be necessary that one of the steps along the route be further broken down into substeps so that the student can make continued progress toward the ultimate goal. An example of breaking the task into its components and then teaching each component through shaping can be seen in the touch technique. First, instruction is given on how to grasp the cane, then how to position the hand and arm, and then how to move the cane hand. As the student masters one skill, another is added to the chain.

In summary, the initial task analysis (or break down) of the desired terminal behavior into subgoals is not likely to be the final task analysis necessary to ultimately achieve the final goal of instruction. This rule applies to social behavior and communicative behavior as well as for knowledge and skills. For example, if a goal for a student is to have her complete all aspects of a route in a specific sequence, it may be necessary in some cases to simply travel part of the route, even if it is not completed. Requiring that the final goal (i.e., the complete route) be successfully achieved before any reinforcement is offered is likely to be counterproductive. A *backward-chain procedure* may at times solve this problem by teaching the last substep (or link in the chain of substeps) first. The last link always requires the learner to reach the final goal. After it is learned, the next-to-last substep or link is then introduced and learned. It is then linked to the final substep so that the two links become chained together. The other substeps are linked to the chain in this manner until, in this case, the entire route is learned (Jacobson, 1993). Usually the end of a complex route is the most difficult substep to learn and remember. Backward-chaining makes this easier by providing more practice with the final segments. This approach is most often useful for students with cognitive disabilities.

Extinction of Behaviors. The purpose of any reinforcer is to strengthen behavior. What happens when a reinforcer is no longer present? Eventually many behaviors that have been reinforced will be weakened and ultimately they may disappear altogether. This process is called extinction. This natural process should be a serious concern for an instructor. The instructor must realize that all the hard work which was employed to reinforce a behavior until it was completely learned might well be for naught once the instructional process is over and the student returns to situations where the reinforcement is not continued. For example, O&M specialists might continually remind their students to keep their hand centered while using two-point touch cane technique, only to find that the cane hand often drifts away from midline to the dominant side of the body when the reinforcement, the instructor's feedback, is no longer present.

There are circumstances where the process of extinction is not likely to be of great concern, however. There are things that once learned are unlikely ever to be unlearned or forgotten. Once a particular level of skill, for example, is attained, there may be no need to worry that a person will essentially lose this skill. There are other situations where the development of a skill or knowledge is sufficiently rewarding for its own sake and once a person is in the actual environment, there will be sufficient reinforcers of the new skill or knowledge so that the process of extinction is unlikely to occur. However, there are circumstances where the process of extinction can be more serious. If a behavior is a difficult one for the student to engage in (if it is particularly onerous) or if the skill is one not likely to provide its own rewards, then even though it was well mastered during the time of instruction, it may eventually be lost. The extinction of the skill may be due to disuse since there are no reinforcers that are continuously present in the natural environment. The student who is constantly being reminded by the instructor to keep being in step or in rhythm while swinging the cane is a good example of this. Once the reminders are no longer present, students oftentimes no longer detect when they are out of step or out of rhythm and, as a result, may trip off of curbs or stairs.

In these cases the instructor may need to consider two options. First, the instructor will need to be very thoughtful in the choice of reinforcers and the process used to reinforce during the time of instruction so that the transition to the natural environment is one in which the process of extinction is likely to be slow. Instruction may need to go on somewhat longer and the reinforcement process used may need to gradually change to resemble what the student will face after leaving the instructional setting. This may well include helping the student learn how to reinforce himself for engaging in the desired behavior by recognizing the effectiveness of the technique. Solo and independent lessons are two good examples of methods of helping students develop independent skills in semicontrolled yet transitional settings.

The second option the instructor may need to consider is making arrangements for what will occur after the instructional program is completed. That is, the instructor may need to try to arrange for situations, activities, or encounters, in the student's most immediate environment that may be useful follow-ups (which actually contain some reinforcement).

Schedules of Reinforcement. To use the principles of behavioral learning theories successfully (i.e., in the process of shaping behavior), it is generally not necessary—and often not wise—to reinforce each successful attempt at displaying the behavior that one is trying to reinforce. The effects of reinforcement on behavior depends upon many things, including the schedule of reinforcement that one uses to establish and maintain the behavior. The term *schedule of reinforcement* refers to the frequency with which reinforcers are administered, the amount of time that elapses between opportunities for reinforcement, and the predictability of the reinforcement.

Generally speaking, schedules of reinforcement are classified into four major groups: (1) a fixed ratio schedule—the reinforcer is administered after a fixed number of successful behaviors; (2) a variable ratio schedule—the number of behaviors required for reinforcement is unpredictable, although it is certain that the behavior will eventually be reinforced, and this rate of reinforcement will average out to a certain number per so many correct behaviors; (3) a fixed interval schedule—the behavior is reinforced on a set time schedule so long as the behavior that is to be strengthened is performed correctly when the time for the reward occurs; and (4) a variable interval ratio—the reinforcement is available at some times, but not at others and the person being reinforced has no idea when the behavior will be reinforced; this averages out to a certain time per correct behavior.

The *fixed ratio schedule* of reinforcement is probably the most commonly used schedule in an instructional setting. One example: each time students answer a question on a travel route they are told whether the answer is correct. Sometimes the fixed ratio involves the completion of a set number of behaviors before the reinforcement is given (e.g., it may be necessary to walk the entire distance down a hallway using proper cane skills five separate times before one is given praise). In working with students it is often useful to begin with a fixed ratio reinforcement schedule that initially reinforces them every time they display the desired behavior, and then to gradually increase the number of successful behaviors that need to be made before a reinforcement is given. In other words, first the instructor reinforces them every time they do the skill correctly, but gradually the requirements are increased so that they have to do it several times before the instructor reinforces them.

Continuous reinforcement (i.e., a reinforcement after every successful behavior) is frequently useful as a motivating device to get people to work hard in the beginning. However, since any given reinforcer is likely to lose part of its value if it is offered frequently, it is then helpful to move to a reinforcement schedule that requires more successful behaviors before the reinforcer is given. This adjusted fixed ratio leads to continued high levels of effort on the part of the student. Perhaps the best example in this area is the use of praise as a reinforcer for successful behavior. It is nice to hear lots of praise early on, but most people do not want to hear "Good job" time and time again after each successful effort. Praise might be saved to every fifth time or every tenth time down the hallway, or whatever other fixed ratio ultimately can sustain the high level of performance. The environment itself can be self-reinforcing. This is particularly true when the desired behavior removes an aversive stimulus. For example, when traveling in a hallway without using a cane, the learner may constantly bump into objects (benches or chairs, drinking fountains, etc.). However, by using the cane correctly, the learner no longer bumps into objects with the body, but does so with the cane, which acts as a bumper guard for the traveler.

Real life more often operates on what is called a *variable ratio* of reinforcement, in that one rarely knows how often one will have to perform a desired behavior before one receives reinforcement. However, even though the timing of the reinforcement is somewhat unpredictable, it works because one believes that sooner or later reinforcement is almost certain to come. The fact is, most people are not praised every time they do something right, and certainly they are not praised every fifth or tenth time they do something right. But most people believe that if they continue to do something right, they are likely to get a sufficient number of "Attaboys" or "That's good" so that it sustains them in maintaining a reasonably high level of appropriate behavior.

What makes a variable ratio schedule of reinforcements so powerful is that is it is highly resistant to extinction. Since the actual rate at which people are going to be reinforced is somewhat unpredictable, they are likely to continue executing the behavior over a long period of time without a reinforcer, just with the general belief that sooner or later the reinforcement will in fact be forthcoming.

The variable ratio schedule is generally not a good way to start the process of utilizing behavioral principles, but it is one that sooner or later might be valuable in situations where extinction is likely to be a major factor once a student gets into the authentic situation. In fact, *fixed interval schedules* of reinforcement are all too common in most instructional settings. For example, a test may be given once a week every Friday, a book report due at the end of every month, and so forth. The problem with this schedule of reinforcement is that it encourages a differential level of effort across the time period in which the behavior is supposed to occur. Students tend to cram the night before an exam, which they know is to occur on Friday, or they tend to stay up all night and work feverishly to finish the book report on the day before it is due.

A method that is much more effective in producing a continued level of effort is a *variable interval schedule.* If students are unaware of when a test will be given or when they will be called upon to provide an update on their book report, then they are likely to spend the effort to keep up-to-date with assignments. If students value the reinforcer (whether it be a good grade or praise from the instructor or relief from being given even more onerous assignments, etc.), then they are inclined to keep a fairly steady pace in their efforts to produce the desired behavior. Variable ratio schedules and variable interval schedules are very effective in maintaining a high rate of behavior and are highly resistant to extinction.

The principles of operant conditioning can be applied to a wide array of instructional tasks, from learning concepts and rules to learning motor skills. However, the instructor has one great advantage when applying these principles to motor skills: every motor movement provides kinesthetic feedback to the person engaged in the act. In effect, the person has instantaneous and continuous knowledge of what is happening during the motor movement. This knowledge of what is happening (learning theorists call it *knowledge of results*) can function as a very powerful reinforcer of motor acts that are part of a motor chain.

This natural kinesthetic feedback has three distinct advantages for instruction in motor skills. First, it is self-reinforcing. It is pleasing to people when they "feel" or "sense" that a motor movement is going correctly. By observing the face of an infant as its first wobbly steps turn into smoother walking movements, one notices the pleasure of doing it right for the first time. An athlete knows the precise moment a motor act is completed correctly—whether it be a good shot at the basket (even before the ball swishes through the net) or when the golf ball falls close to the pin. Second, well-learned motor acts are highly resistant to extinction because the kinesthetic feedback is always there to serve as a kind of reinforcer (one never forgets how to ride a bike!). Third, the instructor can use kinesthetic feedback to plan and execute effective lessons. The instructor can tell the student what he or she will feel in the muscles at various stages during the motor movement, and constantly remind him or her of what the right kind of movement should feel like. The instructor can position the student so that the student is more likely to experience what the correct (or incorrect) movement will feel like. Similarly, the instructor can also ask the student what he or she is sensing about a motor movement so that appropriate corrections in the movement can be made. In summary, the self-reinforcing quality of kinesthetic feedback can be used to great effect in both planning and executing lessons aimed at improving motor skills.

As students learn a motor skill, they may need to *overlearn* it in order to maintain a level of proficiency (and efficiency), especially in situations that are novel or produce high anxiety (Croce & Jacobson, 1986; Jacobson, 1993). Motor learning occurs through conscious responses in which the student practices the activity over and over again (Kottke, Halpern, Easton, Ozel, & Burrell, 1978). Kottke et.al. (1978) estimated the number of repetitions needed to perform a skill in a coordinated fashion, as follows: walking required 3 million steps; a baseball throw required 1.6 million throws; and, playing a violin required 2.5 million notes! Should a kinesthetic memory of a skill—that is, the ability to reproduce a movement in a coordinated fashion at will—not be ingrained in an individual, then when situations are stressful or novel the likelihood of that skill being performed efficiently is minimal.

For some students cane skills should be overlearned before an instructor can expect the student to use them during unanticipated situations. To overlearn a skill, the instructors set criteria for skill acquisition. For example, they may decide that to demonstrate the ability to walk in a straight line, students must travel five complete routes up and down a hallway without making contact with a wall to either side. To ensure overlearning, the criterion may be raised to ten round-trips in the hallways (Jacobson, 1993).

Researchers have found that several factors affect the acquisition of complex motor behaviors (Herman, 1982; Croce & Jacobson, 1986; Kottke et al., 1978; Martinuik, 1979; McClenaghan, 1983; Turnbull, 1982). Many of these factors that affect the acquisition of motor behaviors can be learned, including: physical fitness (muscular strength and endurance, flexibility, and cardiovascular endurance); motor fitness (agility, coordination, balance, reaction time); mental image and rehearsal; and various psychological factors (emotion, self-confidence, arousal level, intelligence, and motivation). When developing instructional strategies, O&M instructors must consider the following factors: verbal directions should include a multisensory approach, although some learners prefer one modality over another; initial lessons should include short practice sessions, but longer, less frequent sessions may occur after learning has taken place; the early lessons should stress accuracy, not speed; and the skill should be broken down into its component parts and built upon until the whole is achieved (Croce & Jacobson, 1986).

The principles of behavioral learning theory have been well developed over the last 70 years. We have touched only on the highlights. There are many good sources for describing in much greater detail the actual application of these principles for any number of instructional settings. Those who are interested in employing behavioral techniques are advised to consult all of these detailed explanations of the actual utilization of behavioral techniques prior to attempting to use them for the purposes of instruction.

Cognitive Learning Theory

The behavior approach to human learning offers a wide array of principles and techniques useful for instruction. It is an approach to learning with a rich history. Over the past three decades a substantial amount of work has been produced by cognitive psychologists which offers a new array of instructional techniques that can be used to complement behaviorist approaches (Gardner, 1985). Cognitivists are concerned with phenomena such as memory, attention, problem solving, and language, and they are particularly interested in conceptual learning, or learning in which meaningful associations are made between a class of elements that may be grouped together based upon some shared characteristic (Slavin, 1991). There are some relatively simple concepts that students can learn, mostly by the process of observation with perhaps only a small amount of verbal input (the concept of a long cane, for instance). However, many concepts, especially complex concepts, require a different instructional process.

There are essentially two ways that concepts can be taught (Tennyson & Park, 1980): either the learner can be given instances and non-instances of a concept and then asked to derive the definition for the concept, or a student can first be given the definition and then asked to identify correct instances and non-instances representative of the concept. For most concepts it typically makes sense to first give the definition, then present several carefully selected instances and non-instances, and finally restate the definition. One can carefully point out how instances typify a definition, and how non-instances have certain attributes that do not allow them to be identified as instances. To summarize, the instructor must first give the rule that specifies the definition of the concept, then provide examples of the concept, and then restate the rule so that students understand clearly why certain instances of the concept satisfy the rule.

For cognitivists, helping students make sense of information is the central issue for instruction (Ausubel, 1963; Bransford, Sherwood, Vye, & Rieser, 1986a). For cognitivists the most important consideration is to design instruction so that "meaningful" (nonarbitrary) connections are made between ideas and events (Wittrock, 1986). Meaningful learning involves making nonarbitrary associations between that which is to be learned and the information an individual already has. Cognitivists believe that as human beings, we try to make sense of our experiences. We all do not derive the same meaning from similar experiences, but we all try to make some sense of those experiences by organizing them into *schema* or *scripts* (Anderson & Bower, 1983). For example, some individuals may understand the concept of a block by focusing in on the four sides while others may pay more attention to the four corners.

Gestalt Learning Theory

Gestalt theory was originated by Max Wertheimer and his two cofounders, Wolfgang Kohler and Kurt Koffka. The Gestalt movement was launched by Wertheimer's 1912 article on apparent motion. Within the article he stated that if the eye sees stimuli in a certain way, it gives the illusion of motion. He found, for example, that two lights flashing on and off in sequence would be perceived as a movement of the light. Wertheimer named this apparent motion the *phi phenomenon.* He recognized that simply analyzing each of the two lights separately could not explain the phenomena. He concluded that the experience is different from the parts which make it up and that the person adds an organization to the experience which goes beyond the sensory information. *Gestalt* is a German term that means configuration or organization. Gestalt theory therefore defines the world into meaningful wholes rather than isolated stimuli. For example, we perceive buildings, fences, trees, and cars instead of just recognizing lines, color, and sounds. The theme of Gestalt theory is therefore that the whole is greater than the sum of its parts. Early in this century Gestalt psychologists tried to demonstrate the inherent capacity for making sense out of one's environment in their studies of insight and closure (i.e., the tendency of human beings to "fill in the gaps" when perceptual stimulus was incomplete) (Slavin, 1991). In studying how human beings (and even animals) process sensory information that is recorded in the sensory register, Gestalt psychologists soon became aware that the information initially received in memory was not stored or dealt with in the same form that it was received by the senses. Experiments were conducted in which a person was shown a representation of a common figure such as a square or a cube in which some of the lines had gaps in them. The individuals viewing these partial representations were then asked to state what the figure represented. Almost all were able to correctly identify the square or cube or whatever figure was presented, even though parts of the figure were missing or slightly irregular in their presentation to the senses. When applied to motor learning, this concept helps explain how an individual is able to go from learning small parts of a task to performing the entire task. The intangible components of a task finally come together to form a whole. As an example, a person being taught how to swim learns rhythmic breathing, proper stroking, and kicking, but may still sink when trying to swim. Once a gestalt is reached a new awareness occurs and the components are integrated in a way that is greater than the sum of its parts, and the individual can keep afloat and swim. A similar situation can occur with touch technique as all of the components finally come together and smooth movement is possible.

This illustrates the *principle of closure*, which states that people organize their perception so that they are as simple and logical as possible. They fill in gaps in perceptions as necessary to make sense of the total presentation. The distinction between a perception (or how a person interprets stimuli and organizes them) and a sensation (or how the information is actually received by the sensory apparatus) is an important one in the field of psychology and has great significance for instruction.

In their many studies of human perception Gestalt psychologists also demonstrated that human beings (again, just as with other animals) attempt to discriminate among the figures in complex figural presentations. As humans we are able to separate figures from the background in which the figures are embedded. Since we often encounter circumstances in which the thing we wish to identify is enmeshed within a complex context, it is important that we are able to separate figure from ground. From the standpoint of learning, however, the ability to do complex processing of sensory information is a mixed blessing, because not all human beings make the same separations of figure from ground when confronted with the same sensory information. When several people look into a crowd, it is not uncommon for one person to be able to identify an individual for whom they are searching while the person standing behind is not able to spot that individual against the sea of other individuals. Sometimes it is important for the instructor to assist a learner in the process of scanning a complex stimulus array so that the learner can identify the key figure within a matrix of sensory information upon which she needs to focus. Learning to separate key features of a stimulus array is critical to the analysis of art objects or musical performances, for instance.

Cognitive Theory

Cognitivists believe that over time human beings build up a network of connected facts and concepts called *schemes* (Anderson, 1985). What is not known at this point is precisely how human beings construct and store these networks of connected facts and concepts in long-term memory. Are they most often stored hierarchically, with less inclusive ideas or concepts stored beneath more inclusive or broader concepts? We do not fully know. However these schemes of facts and concepts are constructed and stored, it appears they are useful to the individual in terms of making sense of new information as it is encountered.

Not every idea or fact in a network is equally strongly anchored to the other facts and ideas in that network (Ausubel, 1963). In the developing network of understandings about animals, a child may not be so sure of exactly how insects fit into an understanding of what animals are all about compared to his understanding about how mammals fit. On a related subject, cognitive theorists also believe that one concept or fact may be part of several schemes or networks of connected facts and concepts. Part of one's idea of what a dog is all about might be connected to an understanding about mammals in general, and another part connected to an understanding of house pets. Concepts about mammals and concepts about house pets represent different networks of ideas, but each helps us to understand a bit about dogs.

For the cognitivist, the learner is a very active participant in the process of learning (Pressley & Levin, 1983). Indeed, most of the learning that any individual undergoes is viewed as a function of what cognitivists call *generative* or *constructed learning.* That is, all learners are presumed to be actively involved in a process of trying to integrate new information into their existing understandings or schemes. In our effort to "make sense of our experiences," we are constantly in the process of discovering and generating new information.

The challenge to the instructor who wishes to utilize cognitive strategies for assisting learners is to connect new understandings and new facts to the learner's current network of facts and concepts (Pressley, Goodchild, Fleet, Zajchowski, & Evans, 1989). How can an instructor organize information so that the learner comes to understand it (i.e., connects it to the learner's current set of understandings)? Put another way, how can an instructor organize and present the material to be learned so that the learner engages the new information in a way which promotes the kinds of understanding the instructor is trying to establish—how can the new be connected with the old?

The instructor has a number of strategies that might be considered. For example, providing the proper orientation or set to any new information can often assist the learner in making connections with existing schemata. Ausubel (1960) developed a method called advance organizers to orient students to material they are about to learn and help them recall related information that can be used to assist in incorporating the new information. An *advance organizer* is essentially an initial statement or visual presentation about the subject to be learned that provides a structure for the new information and relates it to information the student already possesses. In one of the classic studies on the use of advance organizers for the purposes of instruction, Ausubel and Yousser (1963) presented students some written information comparing Buddhism with Christianity, with the idea that since most of the students were Christian, the process of understanding Buddhism could begin with an orientation that anchored new ideas about Buddhism to old ideas the students already possessed about Christianity. This organizing framework was presented prior to having the students read detailed information about Buddhism itself. If there is a clear structure to the information that a student is to learn or if the material to be learned has distinct similarities to something the student is already likely to know, then the use of an advance organizer might very well assist the student in deriving meaning from (therefore, learning) the new information. The student can actively utilize the existing store of information to help discover the new information that the instructor hopes will be learned. In O&M the presentation of a tactile, auditory, or print map of an indoor area may serve a similar function of providing a framework for the later placements of landmarks and clues. Later the structure of the hallways may serve to prepare the traveler to understand the similar structure of outdoor street patterns, landmarks, and clues.

The use of *analogies* can also be helpful in some cases to help provide a kind of meaningful structure for students to learn something new (Gentner, 1989). It is common for people to use sports analogies and military analogies or analogies based on common experiences, such as going to the doctor, eating dinner, or going to school for the purposes of helping a person learn information about new circumstances. Instructors, then, relate the teaching exercises to real-life situations the students may one day encounter. For example, when learning to think ahead while walking along a route, the learner might be asked to remember what it was like to drive a car (if he had that experience). When driving a car, it is necessary to look several blocks ahead in order to plan for upcoming events (a possible traffic light change, a traffic jam, a detour, etc.). The same is true for the traveler with a visual impairment to look ahead (if she has residual vision) or listen ahead for traffic or other ambient sounds that might cue her as to the upcoming traffic control at the next intersection or any other unusual events—the individual must always plan ahead while traveling.

Another effective strategy used to help students learn is the insertion of questions during instruction so that students stop to assess their own understanding of a particular concept or situation (Rothkope, 1965; Jacobson, 1993). Proper use of questions enables the students to become more active in utilizing their current stores of information in the service of learning new information. Simple strategies such as repeating back the route description before traveling the route or repeating back information received about a travel environment can be helpful in getting students to attend to information that is presented.

More involved strategies, such as pointing to a landmark, listening for a sound cue, or mapping out an area, can assist the learners in actually processing information. For example, if mapping an area involves relating objects in space to one another, then it requires the learner to do some processing of the information before the map can be created. The effectiveness of a particular strategy is likely to depend not only on the ability of the learner to engage in these instructional practices, but also on the goal of the lesson and the extent to which the new information is connectable to the student's previous cache of information.

MEMORY AND INFORMATION PROCESSING

Important elements in O&M are the use of memory and the processing of information. Students are required to learn landmarks, clues, and street patterns. Once they have this information in mind they must identify their position in the environment based upon this information. The ability to travel from one position to another depends upon the ability to put together pieces of information in sequential order. Memory is extremely important as the student attempts to retain route instructions provided by the specialist.

During the last 20 years of this century our society has moved from the Industrial Age to the Information Age. With advances in communication and computer technologies, information has become a dominant theme of postindustrial life. In this context, it is not surprising our society has interest in how human beings process information. Because of some obvious similarities of how computers process information and how the brain appears to process information, information processing has become prominent in the area of cognitive psychology. No area of learning theory has received more attention or made more advances in the past 20 years than information processing theories. Critical to these theories is how information is stored in the memory, how it is organized among the various components of the human memory system, how it is recalled from memory, and how it is used for the solution of various problems and in the learning of new information.

To understand information processing theories of learning, it is critical to understand how human memory operates. Most experts in memory believe that the memory system essentially consists of three major components: the sensory register, short-term memory, and long-term memory (Bransford, 1979). All information from the external world comes from the senses and is held for a very brief period of time in the first component of human memory, called the sensory register. The *sensory register* holds information only for 1 to 2 seconds. If nothing happens to this information, it is rapidly lost. In fact, most of the stimuli that actually impact our senses are soon forgotten; they never go into long-term memory for use later on as information.

To move from the sensory register into *short-term memory,* any stimuli or information must undergo an initial level of processing (Atkinson & Shiffrin, 1968). A person must pay attention to stimuli as they impact the sensory register if the stimuli are to be processed and ultimately retained in memory. It is also essential that a person not be so overwhelmed with external stimuli that it is difficult to attend to critical stimuli. If the information is not moved from the sensory register into short-term memory, it gets lost. From the viewpoint of information processing theory, the importance of an instructional situation that facilitates attending to important stimuli and controls the amount and type of competing stimuli is very critical. This is why mobility instructors attempt to control the learning environment at the earliest stages of training by teaching in quiet hallways, rooms, and buildings. As students develop skills and integrate sensory information, they are able to process incoming stimuli and weed out the extraneous stimuli of ambient sounds and noises.

Gaining and maintaining attention to the material to be learned is critical if the information is ever to be stored in *long-term memory,* where it can be retrieved for action or future learning. There are a number of things that instructors can do to help gain students' attention on the instructional task (Olson & Pau, 1966). One thing that O&M instructors frequently do is to make clear to students that the material presented is important or that the learning activity is important. This is sometimes done directly by stating the importance of the lesson, and it is sometimes done more indirectly through the use of various kinds of cues, or through highlighting the objectives of the lesson in some way. A lesson usually begins, for example, with an explanation of the objectives of the tasks, why the lesson is important, why the student is being asked to do the skills in a particular fashion, and what the ramifications are for not doing the skills a certain way.

O&M instructors can also gain the attention of students by making the lesson interesting in some way. They may attempt to heighten the emotional content of the material, try an unusual or novel way of presenting the material, or accompany the material with a teaching strategy that is especially engaging. When working with children, instructors may pair the lesson with a trip to the store to purchase something the child wants, thus combining the lesson objectives with the desire to translate those objectives into a real-life travel situation—all the while fulfilling the child's needs. Good instructors, like good performers, have numerous ways of trying to gain the attention of students.

Figure 11.1 displays a diagram depicting the sequence of information processing from the sensory register through short-term memory to long-term memory. As the diagram shows, after information impacts the sensory register, it must immediately be processed before it can be moved into short-term memory. Short-term memory is a storage system that can hold a limited amount of information for a few seconds. Any thought a person is actually conscious of having at a given moment is being held in her short-term memory. In effect, to be conscious of a thought involves some processing of the information. It means that the information has moved beyond the sensory register to at least the second component of the memory system, short-term memory. Once a person stops thinking about something, it disappears from short-term memory.

What the diagram of memory storage does not depict is the relative size of short-term versus long-term memory. There is very little room in short-term memory. If something is not done to information to move it into long-term memory, it will last no more than about 30 seconds. One of the ways of maintaining an item in short-term memory is the process of *rehearsal.* If people say something over and over again for a period of time, they can keep it for the time in short-term memory.

The problem is, short-term memory has such a limited capacity that information which is put into short-term memory can easily be crowded out by new information just coming into short-term memory. Most people have experienced the embarrassing situation of being introduced to several people, one right after the other. It is quite difficult to remember every person's name. Just when people think they have learned one per-

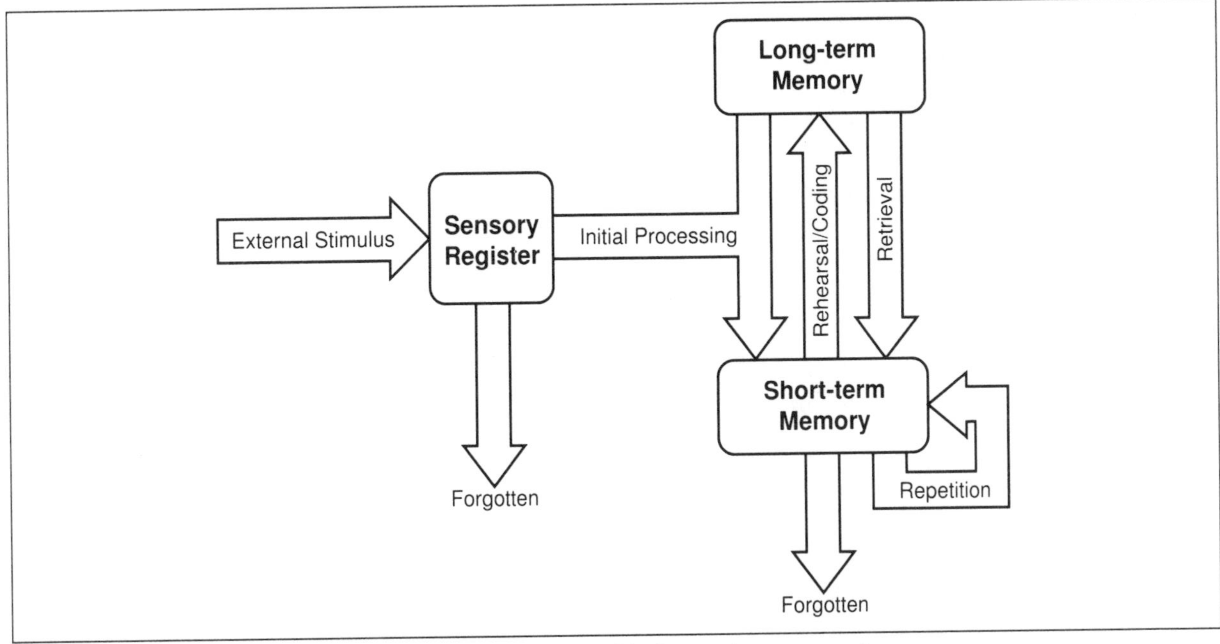

Figure 11.1. Sequence of information processing.

son's name, they hear another person's name and the conflict between those two names drives one or even both out of short-term memory. In order to be successful, teachers must allocate time for rehearsal during instructional activities. Trying to present too much information in too little time tends to be ineffective because students simply do not have the time to rehearse each piece of information sufficiently so that it can be moved into long-term memory. It is very often effective for teachers to break up an instructional lesson to give students time to rehearse information so that they can move it into long-term memory storage. The more difficult the material to be learned, the more complex it is, and the more important it is to allow such time for rehearsal of new information.

Moving information from short-term memory to long-term memory usually entails more than simply rehearsing it (Slavin, 1991). Most often people have to organize or code the information so that it is retainable in long-term memory. For example, as people meet someone new and hear his name, they might try associating the name with a particular attribute (e.g., carrot-red hair) of that person so that the name can be recalled. Since visual images are often easier to recall than words, associating the person's name with a visual image can be helpful. For a person with a visual impairment, it may be necessary to associate some other feature with a name, such as the sound of the voice or the smell of a particular perfume.

Long-term memory is that part of the memory system where information can be kept for long periods of time. The capacity of the long-term memory storage system is not really known. However, it is believed to be quite large. Some memory theorists believe that all the information ever transferred to long-term memory is retained in long-term memory. In other words, we never exceed our capacity in the area of long-term memory.

As best as can be determined, information in memory is stored in three fundamentally different ways: as episodes, procedures, or semantic categories (Tulving, 1985). *Episodic memory* is an individual's memory of personal experiences, a kind of mental videotape of things seen or heard. If asked, people can very often recall what they had for dinner last night or where they went last weekend. This information is stored very much like a script for a movie. People sometimes amaze themselves with how many details of a previous experience can actually be recalled upon being asked, or which just seem to burst into their consciousness. Some of the events stored in episodic memory are quite easily recalled because people have essentially the same experience of a similar circumstance quite frequently. For example, most people can probably describe their bedroom in great detail because they spend so much time in that room. They can describe how it is laid out, the furniture, the decorations, and so forth. Other things are relatively easy to recall because they have high salience due to a high emotional value that is attached to them. Many people, for instance, say they can recall precisely where they were and what they were doing when they first heard the news of President Kennedy's death.

Most of the episodes of people's lives, however, are nowhere near that easy to recall. Few episodes are charged with the kind of emotion that makes them easy to recall. Too many episodes contain experiences that are a bit too similar to many other experiences, making it difficult to sort out what happened in one particular circumstance versus what happened in the others. Was it Amsterdam or Rotterdam where we visited that Gothic cathedral? Was it three Christmases ago, or five, when Uncle Louie sang "Rudolph the Red Nosed Reindeer" after dinner? Was it Inkster or Creston that had the mailbox on the corner? In effect, after having met numerous people, visited numerous different places, or eaten in numerous restaurants, it becomes difficult to remember precisely what each was like and what occurred during the time of the encounter.

From an instructional standpoint the nice thing about episodic memory is that it is memory which comes attached to a story (it has a beginning, a middle, and an end with a cast of characters and/or schemes). It also tends to come with lots of texture (colors, shapes, sounds, smells, etc.). Its linear organization and substantial texture makes it easier to recall. The fact is, sometimes when a person is confronted with just a small bit from a total episode in memory (a snippet of song, part of a scene), suddenly the full episode comes flooding back. However, it is critical to remember that no memory has a solid boundary. Everything stored in long-term memory is subject to change over time with the receipt of new information (i.e., the boundaries of each memory cache are permeable). The memory of the third grade classroom may begin to bleed into the memory of the second-grade classroom, etc. The details of events or places can become different or distorted with the passage of time.

The majority of things people must learn in school-like situations need to be stored in either semantic or procedural memory. *Procedural memory* is the ability to recall how to do something, especially a physical task. This type of memory appears to be stored as a kind of series of stimulus response pairings. For example, there is a certain set of actions that occur in the process of swinging a long cane. It is a fluid set of actions composed of a long sequence of small movements together with kinesthetic feedback that tells a person about those movements as they are in progress. After practicing swinging the cane for a long time, students seem to instinctively know what to do and seem unconsciously able to go through the act of cane swinging.

If these memory events were not stored so well in memory, it would be impossible for people to engage in any kind of complex physical activity; they would forever be clumsy in their efforts to execute even mundane everyday tasks. Like episodic memory, the information in procedural memory has the advantage of being stored as a very prescribed sequence of actions. Procedures, like episodes, have a beginning, middle, and end. Instructors can help students learn to execute procedures smoothly and efficiently by providing the right kind of setup and guidance for the execution of these procedures. Good instruction also involves providing consistent feedback on the effectiveness or the success of executing a procedure. Procedures must always be taught with the understanding that they must ultimately move from the beginning through the middle to the end, to be executed in their entirety and with full success. However, procedures can be broken into smaller sections. Each section can be taught from its beginning through the middle to the end, then the sections can be connected so that the full movement can be executed properly. In other words, even in the task of swinging the cane it is not necessary that the complete execution of the task be taught from the outset. Some smaller component of it can be used and then taken from memory and connected to other components so that the full act can ultimately be executed with precision.

For most of the information learned in school, semantic memory is the primary type of memory that is used. *Semantic memory* is organized in a very different way from either episodic or procedural memory (Anderson, 1985; Chang, 1986); there is no natural beginning, middle, and end to items stored in semantic memory. In fact, many different kinds of organizations might be used in an effort to hold information that is in semantic memory. Things are mentally organized into networks of connected ideas or relationships called *schemes*. The way facts and ideas and relationships are organized in semantic memory varies enormously from person to person and even within persons across time and concepts. Some of the ideas stored in long-term memory are associated with a vast number of other ideas and facts. Such large networks of ideas have advantages and disadvantages for learning and recalling information.

The key for successful movement of information into long-term memory storage is to try to facilitate associations with (a) high salience, (b) common experience, (c) vivid sensory imagery, and (d) multiple potential paths for making connections (Anderson, 1985). At the same time, the instructor must try to make clear how new information is different from information that a learner already possesses. Most people can recall the experience of feeling that they understood something as it was being presented by a teacher during class, only to start having difficulty remembering precisely what was said moments or days after the class is over.

For both student and instructor the most difficult task one faces in learning new information is to move the information from short-term to long-term memory in such a way that it is retrievable later on. Just how this might be done most efficiently is subject to much speculation and a great deal of research. One of the most widely accepted approaches is called *levels of processing theory*. Essentially what this theory stipulates is that the more thoroughly one can process information, the more likely it is that one can move the information from short-term to long-term memory.

According to the levels of processing theory, the more people attends to the details of the new information and the more mental processing they do with the new information, the more likely they are to remember it (Craik, 1979). For example, almost everyone has difficulty remembering the details of history lessons. Students are often asked to recall the leading characters of history and what they are famous for. If in the process of trying to learn about an important historical figure they go beyond trying to remember the person's name and their position, such as recalling specific details about what they did, who they were with, the circumstances that surrounded them, and even little details about the clothes they wore, the name of the horse they rode, or any other element about their life, the more likely it is the students will be able to store the information about the person in long-term memory so that they can ultimately recall it. A student may even imagine whether a famous person from the past might be able to accomplish the same things today, or the student may think about the difference between the past and the present and how the famous person could have lived differently. All of this effort to try to connect the historical character with other events, times, and places involves processing the information at deeper levels. With regards to mobility, paying attention to detail may also enable the traveler to better remember important information. For example, the traveler who wants to remember the location of the courthouse may have greater success if she associates the courthouse with its various features such as the three tiers of stairs, the plaza used as a waiting area, and the pillars that represent the classical architecture.

Our understanding is that the more often this can be done, the more likely information can be successfully moved from short-term to long-term memory. The trick for the mobility instructor is to encourage the learner to engage at this level of processing and to set up activities during instruction that increase the likelihood of it happening. Asking the student to repeat or paraphrase what was said in the lesson, state its implications for some other situation, imagine what it would be like in a different place or time, or describe how it is related to something else can all be of potential value in this effort.

GUIDED vs. DISCOVERY LEARNING

The task of the O&M instructor, then, nis to determine how the student would best learn the material to be taught, develop strategies to teach the material, and provide a nonthreatening atmosphere for instruction that is conducive to learning. The teaching strategies employed by the instructor are determined in part by the type of material to be learned—a motor skill may best be learned by using a behavioral approach, while an orientation skill may best be learned by employing a cognitive approach to learning.

When the same type of solutions are needed to solve similar problems, a *guided learning model* is most effective. The teaching tends to be more regimented and more passive, but it is an efficient way to provide knowledge and skills. In one type of guided learning model the instructor presents the information in final form, and the student merely receives the information (Ausubel, Novak, & Hanesian, 1978; Mettler, 1994). For example, the teaching of cane techniques and procedures to solve particular problems—such as grasping and swinging the cane for shorelining to locate a landmark, or recovering from an errant street crossing to relocate the street corner—both require certain step-by-step procedures provided by the instructor. Guided learning is useful, then, to handle situations where the same response is needed over and over again and where the environment is predictable.

In contrast, in *discovery learning* the material to be learned is not taught by the instructor, but is discovered by the learner while working through a problem. The task given by the instructor is given as a problem to be solved by the learner. Some information is provided as to the approach to be taken to solve it. One example of discovery learning is the presentation of a shape to a young child, who is then asked to determine its salient characteristics. In another example, the student is lost and is asked to work his or her way out of the problem independently, while some ideas of how to approach the problem may be presented. In other situations where discovery learning is provided, special routes may be developed that force the student to solve problems: sidewalks that dead-end or end prematurely; barriers or hazards that block the desired route; or alleys and streets that are not anticipated. The pace of learning may be dictated by how well a student integrates the material (from short-term to long-term memory) and executes the skill in both familiar and novel situations and environments.

Guided learning procedures, then, should be removed once the learner is just capable of learning the task (Schmidt, 1991). At that time "the instructor merely hints at ways the learner can acquire information to solve the problem . . . or point[s] out that the learner has all the information necessary to solve the problem" (Mettler, 1994, p. 340). Guided learning, with the burden of responsibility placed on the instructor's shoulders, shifts quickly to discovery learning, where the burden of responsibility is on the student. The learning that takes place can be transferred to other tasks in the future. Ausubel states that discovery learning can enhance learning, retention, and transfer but requires increased time and effort.

Among learning theorists there is a debate as

to whether the guided or discovery approach is better. Some believe that the best learning takes place when only the correct responses are presented. Others argue that learning from mistakes is best because the learner appreciates the variety of responses that are possible in an unpredictable environment; this builds flexibility and results in a repertoire of useful strategies. It is suggested by Schmidt (1991) that learning takes place at first through the guided method for some of the fundamental skills. Strategies and tactics, however, may be best learned through discovery learning.

When the learner knows the fundamental skills, the following self-discovery techniques can be used: (1) hinting at ways the learner can resolve the problem but without being specific and removing the challenge; 2) suggesting that the learner has all the knowledge to solve the problem but has not put it together correctly, and then hinting at other ways of interpreting the situation; and (3) providing no information at all and leaving the solution totally up to the student.

The approach that is eventually chosen depends upon the readiness of the student (Welsh, 1980). The new student may require more help from in the instructor in the form of partial information and encouragement. As the student becomes more self-assured, more independent discovery can be expected.

SUMMARY

It is clear that there are various approaches to understanding learning. The behavioral approach requires that new habits are learned while the cognitive approach depends upon changes in cognitive structures. When using a behavioral model, an instructor tries to arrange the environment and the instruction in a way that rewards the individual for correct behavior. The cognitive model allows the individual to experience the situation and discover strategies to solve the present problem and generalize to similar future problems. The O&M specialist must be familiar with both approaches and the various tools that make teaching effective with each model. The O&M specialist must select the specific learning tools that best meet the learning needs of the individual student in the specific environment. Only with an integration of the two models will the most effective learning take place.

Learning evolves over time through peaks, valleys, and plateaus. However one views it, teaching orientation skills and mobility skills to individuals with visual impairments can be a challenging endeavor, as no two students will learn the same skills in the same way. Although they cannot always offer a precise prescription of what to do for each student, the principles of learning can nonetheless help guide the process to a more productive conclusion.

Suggestions/Implications for O&M Specialists

1. The purpose of a learning theory is to explain how individuals learn. There are two major types of learning theories: behavioral and cognitive.
2. Behavioral learning theories attempt to explain learning in terms of observable changes in the behavior of a person.
3. Cognitive learning theories attempt to explain learning in terms of the mental processes that a person uses to more fully understand some concept or strategy.
4. Classical conditioning is a behavioral theory involving reflexive actions. Conditioning can be used to change behavior by pairing a neutral stimulus that typically would not elicit a response with an unconditioned stimulus that naturally elicits a response.
5. Systemic desensitization is a procedure developed for deconditioning people so that they do not feel anxious and display reflexive internal actions during the types of situations where they were previously conditioned to react.
6. Mobility lessons can help to modulate anxiety responses if they are designed with a calm and soothing atmosphere or if they teach a student the means to control how close a threatening stimulus may get. Any teaching technique that would produce the physiological responses associated with dread and anxiety should generally be avoided in instructional circumstances where a student is known to be anxious about the learning situation.
7. Operant conditioning involves the use of pleasant and unpleasant consequences to change behavior. It is based on the law of effect which states that if an act is followed by a satisfying change in the environment, the likelihood of the act being repeated in similar situations is reinforced or increased. If, on the other hand, the behavior is followed by an unsatisfying change in the environment, the likelihood that the behavior will be repeated is decreased.
8. Positive reinforcers indicate that a stimulus has been applied, whereas negative reinforcers indicate that a stimulus has been removed. In positive reinforcement, the environment provides a valued stimulus so as to strengthen a behavior. In negative reinforcment, behavior is strengthened by removing an aversive stimulus.
9. Punishers are those stimuli that result in decreasing the frequency of the behavior. In positive punishment an aversive stimulus is provided to weaken a behavior. In negative punishment a valued or prized stimulus is removed to weaken the occurrence of a behavior.
10. Shaping behavior involves assessing the student's current set of capabilities and behaviors at the desired end state for instruction, and trying to imagine all the steps that would be necessary to move the student from the current state of capability to the desired end state.
11. Shaping behaviors depends on both a careful task analysis so that each increment in performance toward the final goal is readily achievable, and a proper sequencing of the subtasks so that the end state is achieved with an acceptable level of efficiency.

(continued on next page)

Suggestions/Implications for O&M Specialists (continued)

12. Meaningful learning involves making nonarbitrary associations between the material to be learned and the information that an individual already has absorbed.
13. Gestalt learning theory defines the world into meaningful wholes rather than isolated stimuli. The whole is greater than the sum of its parts.
14. In cognitive theories, the learner is an active participant in the process of learning. It is presumed that all learners are constantly in the process of discovering and generating new information. The challenge to the O&M instructor is to connect new understandings and new facts to the learner's current network of facts and concepts.
15. Advance organizers, analogies, and questioning are three strategies to help students learn new concepts and process new information.
16. Information must move from the sensory register into short-term memory, and go very quickly into long-term memory in order for it to be maintained. In order to retain something in memory, rehearsal and association are necessary for later recall. Successful movement into long-term memory storage should offer associations that have high salience, are part of a common experience, have vivid sensory imagery, and provide multiple paths for making connections.
17. The levels of processing theory explains how information is moved from short-term to long-term memory in such a way that it is retrievable later on. It stipulates that the more thoroughly one can process information, the more likely one can move the information from short-term to long-term memory. The more a person attends to the details of new information, the more likely she are to remember it.
18. How the student will best learn the material to be taught is a challenge for the O&M instructor. When the same types of solutions are needed to solve similar problems, a guided learning model is most effective. In contrast, in discovery learning the material to be learned is discovered by the learner, and not taught by the instructor.

ACTIVITIES FOR REVIEW

1. Explain the differences between the two types of learning theories, and how each applies to the O&M process.
2. Explain the difference between a conditioned response and an unconditioned response using as an example an O&M skill.
3. List the five categories of secondary reinforcers, and explain why they are so important for O&M instruction.
4. Explain the process of systematic desensitization as it can be applied to the O&M process.
5. What is the difference between positive and negative reinforcement, and how can each be applied to the O&M process?
6. Explain the differences between positive and negative punishers, and how they may be applied to the O&M learning process.
7. Why is negative reinforcement a better tool than negative punishment in the teaching and learning of O&M?

8. Discuss the different situations when the extinction of a mobility skill is unimportant and other times when it is critically important.
9. Explain the four different schedules of reinforcement with an example of each in the learning and teaching of an O&M skill.
10. What is overlearning and how is it applied to a motor skill?
11. How do the different memory theories impact on one's ability to teach O&M?
12. Give examples of mobility tasks that would best be learned through a guided learning approach, and some that would best be learned through a discovery learning approach.

CHAPTER 12

Services for Children and Adults: Standard Program Design

George J. Zimmerman and Christine A. Roman

Imagine your first day on the job as the new orientation and mobility (O&M) specialist in an agency that serves a large geographical area. The agency serves adults and children with visual disabilities, individuals who are totally blind and have low vision. You are the first O&M specialist ever hired. Your caseload includes children from 6 years of age up to 55-year-old adults. Most of your students have low vision; the remainder are totally blind. Many are adventitiously visually disabled while others are congenitally visually disabled. You are anxious about whether you are able to plan age-appropriate O&M programs for such a diverse population. As diverse as your caseload is, so are the needs and goals of the students you will teach. You will need to be flexible in your approach, creative in your thinking, and willing to adapt your instructional style to meet the needs of the individuals you will serve.

This chapter will discuss the typical ways in which a program of O&M assessment and instruction are designed. It will focus on learners who possess average intelligence and ability. Other chapters in this book focus on learners who are younger or older, and who have additional disabilities. This chapter will cover issues related to assessment and program planning, and present examples of how the O&M specialist integrates assessment results into program goals.

ASSESSMENT

In the development of an appropriate O&M program for a student between 6 and 55 years of age, the goals should emerge directly from the information obtained through an O&M assessment. *Assessment* in this context refers to the gathering of information and initial decisions that are made prior to the delivery of service (LaDuke & Welsh, 1980). Through informal interviews and discussions with the student and family, review of the student's records, observation of the student's travel, and criterion-referenced testing, the O&M specialist will be able to make appropriate recommendations regarding O&M program needs. When delivering O&M services to children, the specialist may also need to administer formal assessment instruments in order to design a broader program of O&M that includes systematic instruction in concept development.

Referral

O&M services are initiated through referrals by counselors, social workers, teachers, eye care providers, or the students themselves. After interviewing an adult who is visually disabled, the counselor or social worker may recommend that the student be seen by the O&M specialist for an O&M assessment. Children are referred for services through the school district personnel, a teacher of the visually disabled, or a parent. Upon receipt of the referral, the informal assessment process begins and consists of an interview with the student and family, a review of pertinent records, and direct observations of the student's current level of travel skills.

Initial Visit and O&M Interview

The first step in the informal assessment process begins with an initial visit and O&M interview with the student and family members. The setting may be the student's home or it may be the work site, school, or agency, depending upon the needs or wishes of the student. The purpose is to gather information regarding the student's current educational or employment status, and the student's previous O&M experiences; to learn about the environments in which the student travels most often; and to determine the student's short- and long-term O&M needs and goals. If the student is of school age, then a parent should be available to participate in the discussion. The initial visit and interview also provides an opportunity for the specialist to learn about the student's family, culture, and support for O&M services. Although this section is entitled "Initial Visit and Interview," it may be necessary for various reasons (e.g., time limitations, illness) to schedule additional visits to complete the assessment.

The following student interview assessment items are designed to facilitate discussion regarding the student's travel experiences and potential outcomes. Each of the six items contains O&M questions commonly asked during an interview. This is only a sample list of selected items and questions and is not meant to be exhaustive.

Student Interview Assessment Items

1. *Student's current educational and employment status.* The interview begins with the collection of background information related to age and school or employment status. Through identification of a student's work or school setting, the O&M specialist is able to gather pertinent cues regarding the student's level of independence. For example, work settings can vary from a sheltered work environment to supported employment in a fast food restaurant to employment in a high-rise office building within a complex urban setting. If the student is seeking employment, it is useful to learn about the way in which the student is arranging and traveling to interviews. In schools, some students with visual disabilities may spend the majority of their school day in a single classroom while others follow schedules that require them to travel to numerous classrooms or buildings.

2. *Previous travel experiences.* In order to design an inclusive program of O&M instruction, it is important to gather information about the variety and complexity of the individual's prior travel experiences during the assessment interview. The specialist who serves the needs of the school age learner should be familiar with the range and variety of travel skills incorporated into the routines of the learner's peers and family. For example, if it is typical for students in a seventh-grade class to move from classroom to classroom throughout the school day, it is important to ask whether the student with visual disabilities follows the same routine. Questions related to whether the individual feels confident when traveling around the home, neighborhood, school, or employment setting, and in familiar or unfamiliar small and complex business environments can provide the specialist vital information for future planning.

3. *Previous formal or informal O&M instruction.* In the next phase of the interview, information regarding type and extent of previous O&M instruction is obtained. What formal O&M instruction was provided and by whom? What was the length of the program? Was instruction provided indoors or outdoors or both? In familiar or unfamiliar environments or both? What systems of travel were taught (sighted guide, cane, optical or nonoptical devices or both, electronic travel device, dog guide)? Was any informal O&M train-

ing provided, and if so, by whom (family members, teachers)?

Formal O&M instruction occurs when the student receives instruction in the methods of safe and efficient travel by a professional O&M specialist. Instruction typically follows a designated set of standards of practice and ethics that have been established in the profession. Informal experiences in O&M may include advice from friends, family members, or individuals who may or may not be familiar with the principles of education or rehabilitation for individuals with visual disabilities. The student's ability to utilize appropriate O&M techniques may not be exclusively dependent upon the formal versus informal instruction previously received, but it does provide a framework from which to begin to plan. The following scenario may be useful in understanding how previous information about O&M instruction is used in assessing a student's current O&M needs.

Barbara is a 28-year-old woman who was born with congenital low vision. Barbara was educated in a public school; five years after graduating from high school, she began work in an office building within a mile of her apartment. Barbara's job consists of telephone communication to arrange and confirm appointments for a business. Barbara depends on paratransit for travel to and from work. She rarely leaves the building, even for lunch, and reports that she does not feel confident about her ability to cross the streets of the small business area in which her office is located. When asked to report on her previous O&M training, Barbara described receiving mobility assistance throughout her public school years from friends, family members, and school teachers. She described this assistance as learning routes inside her elementary and high school buildings. She never learned to travel in her home neighborhood independently. Barbara's formal O&M assessment did not begin until years after graduating from high school. A friend who is also visually disabled encouraged Barbara to contact the vocational rehabilitation agency to describe her situation. A home visit with the O&M specialist was scheduled.

The example above illustrates how the collection of information regarding previous O&M instructional experiences can provide insights into factors that influence an individual's ability to utilize independent travel techniques. In Barbara's case the O&M specialist is able to determine that a lack of formal O&M assessment and instruction early in Barbara's school years probably contributed to her lack of travel confidence and ability.

4. *Current travel experiences.* To determine the student's current travel competence, questions regarding whether the student presently travels independently within the home, school, neighborhood, shopping, or employment setting should be asked. Information pertaining to whether the student's amount or complexity of travel has been altered because of recent changes in visual, physical, or emotional status will need to addressed. During this phase of the interview it will be necessary to examine and compare the student's present travel skills with the desired outcomes or personal travel goals. For example, a student may currently be comfortable traveling independently only within the neighborhood, but desires to travel independently to the local small business district to shop, fulfill appointments, or meet friends for lunch. In this situation the student is able to provide essential information to assist in the integration of present skills with further skills to meet the student's aspiration for increased independent travel.

The information regarding current travel competence should also be considered in terms of age appropriateness and the student's living or learning settings. For example, students who live in urban settings may typically learn to use various modes of public transportation to participate in social events at a younger age than students from a rural environment whose social activities may not lend themselves to public transportation, or for whom public transportation is not readily available.

5. *Utilization of residual vision.* One of the more important aspects of the interview is to determine whether the student has and utilizes residual vision, and if so, how useful or dependable

that vision is for O&M purposes. Many of the students served by the O&M specialist will possess vision which, although limited, may be useful for obtaining spatial orientation information to indoor or outdoors environments. The O&M specialist will want to know whether the student uses residual vision to identify locations within a space to remain oriented while traveling. The O&M specialist will also need to determine whether the student is capable of using residual vision to avoid obstacles and locate important environmental features (i.e., curbs and stairs) in the environment. Interview questions that solicit information about the types and size of objects viewed, the distance the objects or obstacles are from the student when viewed, and the lighting conditions under which the object or obstacles are detected will increase the O&M specialist's understanding of the student's level of independence.

6. *Identification of O&M needs and goals.* Identification of O&M needs and goals is the final and most important phase of the interview assessment. In this phase the O&M specialist encourages the student to discuss anticipated outcomes from the delivery of service. The high school student who is totally blind, for example, may want to become more familiar with the layout of the mall to socialize and meet friends. An adult who has low vision may decide that learning to travel using sunfilters and a visor will facilitate independent travel in brightly lighted areas. Identification of needs and goals are highly personal and unique with each individual (LaGrow & Weessies, 1994).

In this final phase of the O&M interview, questions that relate to whether the student is satisfied with the degree of independence afforded at school or work should be discussed. A list of activities which the student would like to participate in but cannot because of travel difficulties would help in the formation of the eventual program of instruction. Similarly, a list of places the student would like to visit (e.g., friends' homes) and the modes of transportation the student would like to become more confident in using would further assist the O&M specialist when designing a program of instruction.

The initial visit and interview affords an opportunity to learn about the family support and cultural perspectives that impact the student's motivation for travel and opportunities for independence. Understanding how "independence" is defined by the family and what if any limitation will be placed on the student's independence once instruction has begun will be critical to the development and implementation of the O&M program. Although discussed separately in the next section of this chapter, issues relating to family assessment cannot in reality be separated from the assessment material presented above. The information presented below on family and cultural aspects needs to be infused throughout the various sections of the O&M interview.

Family Assessment

Because this chapter includes O&M assessment and instruction for both the school-age student and the adult student, family assessment considerations will include factors that examine the child and the adult within the context of family and community. Specifically, this section discusses the importance of integrating family and cultural perspectives into the assessment report and formulation of an O&M plan. It also provides questions that can be used to create a Family Questionnaire that can be used when discussing needs and goals with family members.

Family Aspects. O&M specialists engage in assessment and instruction with children or adults who are members of family systems. For an adult student the family comprises members including spouses, children, or extended family relatives. Each of these members makes a unique contribution to the social context of the family and has a perspective that impacts the family as a whole and the adult with visual disabilities as an individual. When planning assessment and instruction with an adult student, the O&M specialist is obligated to consider the travel needs of the student as well as the needs of the family with whom the student resides. The family viewpoint regarding the O&M assessment and potential instruction can be influenced by a variety of factors including the age of onset of the student's visual disability, the student's medical status, family ethnicity, socioeconomic status, religious attitudes, or family dynamics. Although the specialist must maintain primary concern for the travel needs of the student, these needs cannot be fully understood without considering the perspectives of the family.

Meshelda is a 35-year-old woman who became visually disabled due to diabetic retinopathy. Because her medical status had been unstable, Meshelda's husband encouraged her to take a leave of absence from her management position at a large retail company. It has been 6 months since Meshelda's last hospitalization and her condition is presently stable. Meshelda contacted an agency for the visually disabled requesting O&M training so that she could return to work and contribute to the family's income. Meshelda's husband and her 12-year-old son however, are fearful for her health and safety. Meshelda's husband told the agency caseworker that he would rather get a second job than worry about his wife being so vulnerable in public. Meshelda responded by stating that perhaps she would wait a little longer before returning to work.

This scenario helps illustrate the complexity of how a family member's visual disability may impact a family. Although Meshelda was ready to face the challenges of returning to work as an individual with visual disabilities, her husband and son's conflicts interfered with her ability to meet this goal. It is clear that in order to successfully meet Meshelda's O&M needs, the emotional needs of the other family members will also have to be addressed. Such family factors are not unexpected, and it is critical that the O&M assessment and instruction be designed appropriately and consider the student as well as the family system.

When serving the child, the specialist must be sensitive to the differences in perspectives between the professional's opinion about service and the perspectives held by the family. It is critical for O&M professionals to remain astute to the fact that many parents who pursue O&M instruction for their child only have the experience of their own child to consider. Parents may not be able to readily project images of their visually disabled son or daughter being able to become successful and independent as they mature to adulthood. The professional must respect the strong emotional impact the student with visual disability may have on a family; families are entitled to revisit feelings of sadness, guilt, anger, denial, and resolution throughout their lives.

According to Ferrell (1985) with regard to the education of children with visual disabilities, "Working with parents is no longer an ideal—it is a mandate" (p. 3). In the Council for Exceptional Children's position paper, *Parent/Educator Cooperative Efforts in Education of the Visually Handicapped* (Hart & Ferrell, 1985), it is recognized that professionals who work directly in accordance with the needs of the family enable greater educational gains for the child. This position is therefore germane when considering the development of an O&M program for a school age learner who is visually disabled.

Family Questionnaire. As part of the student's interview, it is important to examine the perspectives of the family's anticipated O&M goals and expectations for the student. One method is through the use of a family questionnaire. The questionnaire can serve as a method to promote dialogue regarding the formation of mutual goal planning.

The following questions represent a sample of the questions an O&M specialist may consider in gathering family perspectives regarding O&M for their family member. What is the typical number of miles your family travels together each week? How would you characterize your family outings and shopping events? Do you travel in large city areas? What is your primary mode of travel (e.g., car, public transportation)? Are there methods or modes of travel that your family member is not currently employing that you would like to see be used? In what settings or situations do you feel that your family member travels most comfortably and competently? Do you feel that your family member's social skills are restricted because of O&M limitations? Are you comfortable with your family member's current ability to request assistance from others? Are you satisfied with your family member's ability to locate common areas within public facilities such as elevators, stairways, and rest rooms? Do you believe that you, your family member, and family have an adequate understanding of your family member's visual disability and how it affects safe and efficient travel?

The use of a questionnaire provides one technique for soliciting input from families. There are many routes that can be followed in creating a partnership with families who have a family member with a visual disability. Each time O&M specialists begin instruction with a new student, they enter into the lives of the student's parents, siblings, spouses, children, and frequently extended family members. The effectiveness of the O&M instruction may largely depend upon the ability of the professional to understand and respect and integrate into instruction the unique needs of each family.

The application of O&M also presents unique external symbols of disability that may cause conflict for some families. Materials such as low vision devices and canes are external representations clearly associated with low vision and total blindness. Some families welcome the incorporation of these devices into instruction as a means to increased independence, while other families experience reluctance at the use of a device that publicizes their child's or spouse's disability. Neither perspective is inherently right or wrong. The following example may help illustrate this circumstance.

Jack, a second-grade student who is totally blind, rides the public school bus with his fourth-grade brother Alex every day. Alex has never discussed his brother's visual disability with his friends. He has followed his parents' instructions to "keep it in the family." Jack's O&M instruction has recently incorporated the use of a cane for independent travel to and from the bus, and Alex has since noticed that classmates are now asking questions about his brother. One day after Alex overheard students on the bus whispering comments about Jack, Alex asked his parents if Jack could please stop using his cane at bus time.

Knowing the emotional position of the student's family members can assist the professional in remaining sensitive to the families' current beliefs and aid in the identification of appropriate instructional goals and outcomes.

Cultural Aspects. There are currently more than 19 million people in the United States who speak languages other than English as their native language (Baca & Cervantes, 1989). The cultural influences of African Americans, Hispanics, Asian Americans, and Native Americans impact the behavior of the individuals of these groups in unique ways. If instruction in O&M is delivered by an individual whose ethnic and cultural background differ from the ethnic and cultural background of the student, the instructor has the responsibility to learn more about the values derived from the student's cultural experience. Without the ability to consider a variety of cultural perspectives, the instructor's expectations may clash with the expectations placed on the student by the family and possibly the student's own expectations. This clash in beliefs places the student in unnecessary social conflict and may significantly affect the outcomes of instruction. The following example may illustrate this situation.

Anna is a fourth-grade public school student who has received vision and O&M services since kindergarten. Her parents have lived in the United States since their immigration from Taiwan 10 years ago. Chinese is the dominant language in Anna's home. Anna's parents have instructed their daughter in the social traditions of Taiwan. Anna is expected to be quiet and obedient in class; teachers are not to be challenged. She has been told not to take the initiative in class, but to expect to be told what to do by the adults. In fact, Anna has been instructed not to attempt to creatively solve problems, but rather to follow the steps provided by teachers in problems she encounters.

Anna receives O&M instruction from a specialist whose cultural descent is middle-class European. The instructor is concerned about Anna's progress. He has asked Anna to help plan simple routes and discuss alternate routes to specific destinations; however, he notes that Anna always waits for recommendations from the instructor. He has unsuccessfully attempted to encourage Anna to solicit assistance from adults in both indoor or outdoor settings. The instructor has prodded Anna to advocate for herself when she cannot read material presented on the chalkboard, but thus far Anna has not voiced her needs to the classroom teacher. The O&M specialist states that Anna is not making progress like the other students he works with.

The value system of Anna's Asian culture appears to be in conflict with the expectations of the school. The Asian cultural view holds beliefs that a person should not do anything that would make the individual stand out from the group. More indirect subtle means of communication are acceptable over assertive direct interaction. The family structure considers males more in authority than females, and children are generally to remain passive and obedient (Kitano, 1973). Given the powerful influence of culture in the lives of individuals, O&M specialists will find it necessary to consider the cultural perspectives of their students and their own competence in cultural awareness.

Upon completion of the O&M interview with the student and family, the O&M specialist is now ready to begin the second phase of the informal assessment, review of the student's records. Before leaving, the O&M specialist should discuss with the student the process of reviewing the records and how that will be helpful to the development of the O&M program plan.

Review of Records

Before a program of instruction begins, the O&M specialist may need to receive the student's or the family's approval to review any clinical records necessary to assist in program planning. Information gathered pertaining to the student's medical and ocular history, clinical low vision assessments, physical and occupational therapy assessments, speech and language assessments, psychosocial assessments, educational assessments, or employment status should be reviewed to determine the student's potential for travel. A review of the records from previous O&M instruction may include additional assessment information, such as a functional vision evaluation.

The availability of information through clinical reports may vary widely from individual to individual. Although the ophthalmological and low vision evaluations are considered to be most critical, there are a number of additional clinical assessments and records pertinent to the planning and implementation of O&M instruction. Medical histories, physical therapy assessments, occupational therapy assessments, audiological assessments, speech and language assessments, and psychological assessments contribute to better understanding the student's capabilities. Once the histories and assessments identified above are reviewed, it will be necessary to integrate the essential information regarding, for example, potential medication effects, degree of hearing loss, or orthopedic considerations into the student's profile. Not only is the information contained in these records important in O&M program development, but the professionals from the various related fields may serve as valuable resource.

Table 12.1 may serve as a reference when considering information useful for planning and conducting an O&M assessment. Each section of the table lists a type of clinical and functional assessment, information typically contained in each type of assessment, and the application of the particular assessment information to O&M instruction.

The information gained from the student interview and review of the student's records will help form the basis for the next phase of the informal O&M assessment: observation of the student's O&M skills.

Table 12.1. Information for an O&M Assessment

Type of Evaluation	Information Contained	Application to O&M Instruction
Ophthalmologic/medical optometric low vision Conducted by: Ophthalmologist Physician Optometrist Low vision specialist	Ocular health Etiology of condition Stability/progression of condition Medications, side effects Near and distance acuity Visual fields Binocularity Visual motility Color vision Contrast sensitivity Photosensitivity Recommended low vision devices, optical and nonoptical Physical restrictions	Understanding of student's visual status Instructor may be alerted to student's potential fluctuations in visual performance Acuity information assists instructor in student's near and distance capabilities (e.g., detail identification at near or landmarks at distance) Instructor may utilize sun shields for photosensitive students Instructor designs lessons based on physical limitations, levels of endurance Day versus night travel considerations Application of optical and nonoptical devices in travel Instructor considers the appropriate use of color in selection of cues, landmarks in travel Instructor considers monocular or binocular function; implications for visual scanning and laterality
*Functional vision evaluation/ ecological assessment** Conducted by: O&M specialist Teacher of children with visual disabilities Rehabilitation teacher of adults with visual disabilities Low vision rehabilitation training specialist	Student observed in tasks within natural contexts to assess functional use of: Distance vision Near vision Visual fields Visual motility Color/contrast Bonocularity Effects of lighting (natural, incandescent, fluorescent)	Determination of students' ability to visually detect: Landmarks Drop-offs Vehicles Pedestrians Signs, addresses Determination of student's ability to gather visual information in central and peripheral fields (i.e., pedestrian or vehicular traffic) Determination of student's ability to avoid obstacles Determination of student's ability to maintain a straight line of travel

(*continued on next page*)

Table 12.1—*Continued*

Type of Evaluation	Information Contained	Application to O&M Instruction
		Determination of student's ability to adapt to sudden shifts in illumination levels Determination of student's ability to visually scan for information
Physical therapy Conducted by: Physical therapist	Evaluation of movement, muscle tone, range of motion Evaluation of strength, endurance Identification of typical/atypical motor patterns Evaluation and prescription of orthopedic and mobility equipment (i.e., orthosis, wheelchairs)	Determination of student's normal, increased, or decreased muscle tone and its relationship to posture & gait patterns Determine methodology of instruction in self-protective techniques, type/length of cane based on restrictions in range of motion Determination of adaptive forms of mobility devices for students who have motor impairments Determination of activities, length/duration of routes in accordance with student's strength & endurace
Occupational therapy/recreation therapy Conducted by: Occupational therapist Recreational therapist Rehabilitation teacher (recreation and leisure)	Evaluation of fine motor function including tactile abilities: Awareness Discrimiation Object identification Sensitivity Dexterity and coordination Strength and endurance Evaluation of typical vs. atypical fine motor patterns Assessment of fine motor manipulations in the development of self-help routines Assessment of appropriate leisure and recreation skills and interests	Determination of ability to derive information through textual cues in the environment Determination of levels of assistance necessary in tasks of independent living (i.e., handling money, dressing) Determination of appropriate hand for cane use, type of cane tip in transmission of vibratory inforamtion Suggestion of lessons that integrate recreation and leisure interests with O&M skills
Audiological speech and language evaluation Conducted by: Audiologist Speech & language clinician	Evaluation of presence/absence/type of hearing loss Identification of threshold hearing frequencies and appropriate decibel levels Identification of outer ear, middle ear, or sensorineural pathology	Determination of the ability to utilize spoken or environmental cues in indoor or outdoor travel Determination of type/complexity of language prompts or directions used in O&M instruction

(*continued on next page*)

Table 12.1—*Continued*

Tye of Evaluation	Information Contained	Application to O&M Instruction
	Evaluation of monaural/binaural auditory function Evaluation of auditory perceptual differences Evaluation of hearing amplification equipment Evaluation of expressive and receptive language Evaluation of voice disorders	Determination of selection of auditory cues used in O&M instruction for: Traffic sounds, both vehicular and pedestrian Direction/location of sound cue Distance a student can first perceive a sound cue Ability to determine foreground and background auditory cues Determination of the student's ability to express needs and solicit assistance Use of alternative communicaton devices

*Conducted within living, learning, work environments

Direct Observation

As part of the O&M assessment plan it is necessary to directly observe the student's functional travel skills in the environment. During these observations it is important to monitor the student's motor skills (gait, use of cane), sensory skills (visual, auditory, tactile) and spatial orientation skills (use of landmarks and clues, cardinal directions), noting the student's safety and confidence. On occasion there is discrepancy between the performance of the individual in the environment and the information obtained by interviews (LaDuke & Welsh, 1980). The following example illustrates this scenario.

Raul is a seventh-grade student in public school. He has been diagnosed with glaucoma and reports that he rarely experiences difficulty in moving through high-activity areas of the school such as hallways, gym class, and the cafeteria. The O&M specialist learns through observations that Raul has been accomplishing these movement tasks through the unsolicited assistance of a classmate. The classroom teacher has typically directed a student to "make sure Raul gets there safely." Upon request Raul attempts to find the school office, but is frequently disoriented and cannot describe the route or formulate a plan to accomplish the task. In order to assess whether the student's travel skills are commensurate with the goals identified, direct observation of the student traveling in a variety of environments must be a part of the O&M assessment.

Familiar Environments

To begin the observation session, the specialist might ask the student to "show the O&M specialist around" a familiar area. The student selects the area and while traveling demonstrates their current O&M skill level. A familiar environment consists of settings in which the student typically lives, works, learns, and engages in social activities. It is crucial to learn about and analyze the multiple settings in which the student travels in order to determine which aspects of the familiar setting present potential instructional opportunities and challenges. Observing the student travel in those settings will provide insight into specific tasks that cause the most difficulty in terms of environment and skill. For example, the specialist may observe the student's typical method for crossing a traffic–light controlled intersection while en route to work. The student, who has low vision and uses a telescopic device, indicates that she finds the intersection confusing and difficult to cross. Through observation the specialist has determined that the student's unsystematic use of the telescopic device, combined with the recent installation of street signs has resulted in the student's inability to locate the walk/don't walk light. Observations and analysis of the everyday travel routines in the familiar setting can provide key assessment information critical to program development.

Unfamiliar Environments

Depending upon the student's stated needs and goals, it may also be necessary to observe the student traveling in an unfamiliar environment. An unfamiliar environment will probably contain typical landmark and information points (e.g., corner mailboxes, drinking fountains, lamp posts), but they are settings in which the student does not usually travel. Sometimes travel in familiar environments may be considered the same as travel in unfamiliar environments when the environments are constantly changing. Observation in unfamiliar environments may be necessary for the individual who has a need to generalize travel over numerous settings (LaGrow & Weessies, 1994). For example, the O&M skills of a student who demonstrates the ability to successfully utilize room familiarization techniques in the familiar classroom may be verified by demonstrating the skills in a novel classroom within the same building. Observations of travel in novel settings enables the specialist to assess how well the student competently utilizes motor, sensory, and spatial orientation skills and techniques to remain safe in environments that are not as predictable as the environments previously traveled. For example, the specialist may observe that the student's cane techniques or orientation skills degrade as the level of complexity in the unfamiliar environment increases. Observation of travel in novel settings permits monitoring of the student's ability to solve problems related to recovery and modify techniques to match the demands of the environment, and assess the student's level of anxiety and willingness to solicit assistance for reorientation purposes.

Up to this point in the informal assessment process, the specialist has interviewed the student, reviewed the student's records, and completed an observation of the student's functional travel skills, including functional visual abilities. This process assists with identifying the program goals for instruction. Before writing the O&M program plan, the specialist who works with children may also need to conduct one last assessment procedure, formal assessment and observation of the child's conceptual understanding of body, positions in space, and the environment. The administration of these instruments should take place only after the child and family interview and the child's records have been reviewed. This may mean that administration of the instrument(s) is done in conjunction with the direct observation phase of the informal assessment process. In this final section on assessment, a description of these formal assessment instruments is presented.

Formal Assessment Instruments

Norm-Referenced Testing

Formal assessment generally refers to norm-referenced tests that are used to compare one group or individual to another group. An intelligence quotient (IQ) test is one example of a norm-referenced test. In mobility the use of norm-referenced tests is limited to development of concepts in children. The Hill Performance Test of Selected Positional Concepts (HPTSPC) (1981) is one example of a formal assessment instrument available to the O&M specialist, which uses normative data to compare acquisition of positional concepts of children who are visually disabled between 6 and 10 years of age. Another example of a formal assessment instrument is the Body Image of Blind Children (BIBC) (Cratty & Sams, 1968) which assesses the child's ability to identify body parts and their movement; laterality of body parts (right and left); body planes (front, back, up, down); and directionality (projection of right and left on another individual or object). This instrument is useful when assessing body image concepts of children between 5 and 16 years of age. A third instrument used to assess the O&M skills of children who are blind and possess multiple disabilities is the Peabody Mobility Scale (PMS) (Harley, Merbler, & Wood, 1975). The Orientation and Mobility Scale for Young Blind Children–Short Form (MSYBC) (Lord, 1969) is useful for assessing movement behaviors of children between 3 and 12 years of age. However, the PMS, BIBC, and the MSYBC lack adequate reliability and validity data, which are necessary to make comparative conclusions. The HPTSPC demonstrates a high degree of reliability and validity, and comparisons between child and group performance can be made.

Criterion-Referenced Testing

Each of the above instruments may also be used informally to know and document how well an individual student performs over time. This approach is referred to as *criterion-referenced testing*. Unlike the use of percentiles with a norm-referenced test, the individual's performance over time becomes the comparative measure. Criterion-referenced testing is an essential element of teaching. If after initially evaluating the individual's acquisition or performance of a skill(s) the performance of the skill(s) is inadequate, or if the student has never been taught the skill(s), remedial instruction would begin. Initially the specialist decides whether the student needs to demonstrate skill acquisition or proficiency at a criterion level of 100 percent of the time with 100 percent accuracy or less. Some skills, such as making the decision to cross a busy street at a safe time without assistance, may predetermine the level of criterion which should be set (100 percent accuracy all of the time), while others (transferring sides) may have lower criterion levels established. The student is then retested following instruction to determine whether the criterion level has been achieved and skills have been acquired.

The use of criterion-referenced testing is common for establishing baseline performance and comparing performance at the midpoint and final evaluations. Although criterion-referenced testing is usually referred to as an assessment protocol, it is equally valuable as a teaching tool. It is also useful when developing lesson plans and task analysis during the program planning and implementation process.

The use of these formal or informal assessment instruments, the observation of the student's functional travel skills a review of the student's records, and an interview with the student and family all provide the basis for the next phase of the program design and implementation, the development of the program plan. In the next section a brief review of writing program goals and outcomes is presented. Vignettes are used to demonstrate how information obtained from the student interview, review of the student's records, and observation of the student's travel skills can be used when designing individual program goals and outcomes. A plan for instruction is also presented for each vignette.

PROGRAM PLANNING

The implementation of an O&M program designed to appropriately meet the needs of a child or adult is dependent upon a qualitative plan of instruction. Traditionally, a plan of instruction consisted of broad instructional units with more detailed individual lesson plans (Mager, 1967). For example, an O&M unit may be labeled "Outdoor Residential Travel," with specific lessons, such as residential house numbering systems, included in the unit. With the more traditional approach, the design of the unit and lesson plans would focus on actions the instructor would implement in order to accomplish the lesson. Phrases such as "take the student" and "give the student" indicate performance of the O&M specialist, but do not describe the behavior or action taken by the student in completing the task.

In contrast to the traditional unit and lesson-plan approach is an alternative approach which implements instructional plans that are student-centered. This approach is in part influenced by federal guidelines for the development of educational instructional goals and objectives. The student-centered approach has now been adopted more broadly to include both children and adults who require specialized services and instruction. The fundamental difference in this more recent methodology for program planning is that the instruction is specifically written to describe the behaviors and actions performed by the student in accomplishing the task. Previously used phrases such as "take the student . . ." are replaced with terminology such as "the student will travel . . ." or "the student will arrive . . ." Although some specialists may be more familiar with the traditional methods for unit and lesson planning, shifting the focus of instructional planning to observable student behaviors promotes increased benefits for the student.

The O&M plan may be written in the form of an Individualized Education Program (IEP) for children and youths up to 21 years of age; an Individualized Transition Plan (ITP) for children 16 years of age through high-school graduation; or an Individualized Written Rehabilitation Plan (IWRP) for the adult student. The information contained within each plan will differ, depending upon the type of plan. For example, most IEPs include all of the specific components of an instructional plan, including outcomes, long-range goals, and short-term objectives. The ITP is similar in content and structure to the IEP, but the demands for the IWRP for an adult are less content-specific. Only a statement of O&M goals and a recommendation for a time to reach the stated goals is sufficient for implementing an O&M program with an adult. Regardless of the type of plan, the proposed O&M program should reflect the combined experience and expertise of the student, the student's family when appropriate, the O&M specialist, and related educational or rehabilitation members of the team. Each member of the planning team contributes a unique and integral viewpoint; no plan of O&M instruction can be adequately developed in isolation from the other contributing members of the educational or rehabilitation team.

Table 12.2 is a Behavioral Objectives Chart that lists the components or categories included in a standard education or rehabilitation plan. As indicated above, there are many variations to the standard plan. In the example in Table 12.2, an instructional outcome, long-range goal, short-term objective, task analysis, and performance criteria are included to demonstrate how each component is used to guide the instructional process. It should be remembered that the use of the program plan is required for children (e.g., IEP) and youths in transition (e.g., ITP). It is also required when working with adults, but with much more flexibility.

Instructional Outcomes

Each O&M plan should be directed toward an overall result, or outcome, that enables the student to have greater access to school, home, work, or social community. The identification of the instructional outcome is the first step in the process of program planning. In some cases the outcome may be easy to identify. For example, an individual who is visually disabled and entering college may readily identify the O&M instructional outcome as the ability to independently travel to classes. In other situations the student and specialist may have to engage in discussions to identify an appropriate outcome. Such discussions integrate information related to age; personal interests; present and future travel needs; physical, medical, and cognitive status; and previous O&M instruction. In the Behavioral Objectives Chart (see Table 12.2) the outcome "to travel independently in the school setting" provides an instructional endpoint for the student and O&M specialist to focus upon and is the foundation for establishing program goals, objectives, and criteria for success. Outcomes are both the beginning

Table 12.2. Behavioral Objectives Chart

Outcome: To travel independently in the school setting			
Long-Range Goal	*Short-Term Objectives*	*Task Analysis*	*Performance Criteria*
To increase self-advocacy skills and the ability to solicit assistance.	The client will request assistance from familiar individuals in appropriate instances within the school building or on the school grounds.	Following discussion with the instructor, the student will identify questions that when answered will provide information necessary to reach travel goal.	In the classroom the student will identify four of five questions within two O&M sessions.
		When prompted, the student will role-play and ask the instructor questions.	The student will ask four of five questions of the instructor within 5 mintues of being verbally prompted.
		After role-playing and when prompted, the student will approach other students in class and ask questions regarding assistance	The student will ask four of the five questions of each of the five students within three O&M sessions.
		On successive days the student will ask appropriate questions of a student in the hall and locate an unfamiliar travel objective using that information.	Through correct solicitation, the student will successfully locate the required objective each time in an unfamiliar environment.

point of the program planning and the endpoint of the instructional goals.

Long-Range Goals

In order to achieve an O&M outcome, individual sets of instruction are designed. The instructional sets are organized into the long-range goals, which together constitute the necessary components to accomplish the outcome. The long-range goals are designed as instructional building blocks that broadly define the major sets of instruction, from introductory lessons to the final stages of the training. As in previous stages of program development, the long-range goals should be designed in conjunction with the student, family members, and additional members of the educational or rehabilitation team. It is the O&M specialist who will synthesize the team input and will ultimately be responsible for the selection of the most appropriate long-range O&M goals.

In selecting long-range goals, or sets of instruction, the O&M specialist should consider beginning instruction by building on O&M strengths the student presently has. The long-range goal in the example in Table 12.2 is "to increase self-advocacy skills and the ability to solicit assistance." Initial instruction in environments familiar or comfortable to the student may reduce anxiety about O&M instruction while also building rapport with the instructor (see chapter 6). As instructional units become more advanced and incorporate increased levels of complexity, the student and instructor will have adequate time to develop the necessary trust intrinsic to successful O&M instruction.

Although there is no predetermined set of long-range goals intended to accomplish a single outcome, the general principle is to begin planning instruction with foundational skills and progress toward increased instructional and environmental complexity. It is also important to recognize that while there is no general rule regarding the amount of time necessary for a child in a school setting to accomplish the long-range goal, there are program time limits placed upon adults who receive O&M services through residential or community based agencies. Long-range goals must be selected based on the instructor's assessment of the student's ability to reach proficiency within a preset time frame. For example, the specialist who works with school-age students will be held accountable for completion of the long-range goals and short-term objectives written in a student's annual IEP. In cases where the completion of the long-range goals for a unit of O&M training require instruction beyond an annual IEP, the O&M specialist must be prepared to provide documentation for the continuation of the instruction. Similarly, when working with adults the specialist must submit a proposal for instructional time in which the student is expected to attain the long-range goals. This time frame is included in the IWRP. If additional time is needed beyond the initial proposal, then documentation explaining the rationale for the continuation must be included in the revised IWRP.

Short-Term Objectives

Properly written long-range goals lead to a set of short-term objectives. The short-term objectives are the individual plans of action that, when accomplished by the student, are intended to systematically guide the student toward the long-term goal, and ultimately to the accomplishment of the O&M instructional outcome. Short-term objectives are generally intended to be observable, measurable statements that are written to describe a course of skill development necessary to complete the long-range goal. The short-term objectives are student-centered and should be written to describe student's expected performance.

Similar to the long-range goals, the short-term objectives should be written for sequential instruction, adding new skills to previously accomplished foundational skills. Although not strictly hierarchical, new objectives within a long-term goal unit are generally not attempted until antecedent skills are demonstrated according to established criteria. The short-term objectives example in the Behavioral Objectives Chart is "the client will request assistance from familiar individuals in appropriate instances within the school building or on the school grounds" (see Table 12.2). A third level of program planning that further delineates O&M instruction is the use of task analysis in lesson planning.

Task Analysis in Lesson Planning

Task analysis is a method in which skill areas are broken down and sequenced into a series of subskills. The use of task analysis is intended to break an objective into small, easy-to-instruct subtasks. The subtasks are sequenced from the easiest to the most difficult and are generally organized in the natural order in which they must be performed. Using task analysis assists in pinpointing exactly where each session of instruction should begin, and it becomes the framework for planning individual sessions. Task analysis benefits the student by enabling the student to realize success as each subtask of the objective is accomplished. The specialist may choose to write individual lesson plans without task analysis because some agencies or school districts may specify a methodology that best fulfills local IEP compliance.

Using the instructional outcome and long-range goal identified in the Behavioral Objectives Chart (see Table 12.2) as the basis for the O&M program, a task analysis of the specific short-term objective will need to developed. Each task analysis progression or each lesson plan will be designed and restructured regularly based on the instructional performance of the student. Task analyses and daily lesson plans are intended to provide a fluid plan that is not only student-centered, but also enables the specialist to fine-tune instruction.

Performance Criteria

Determining successful acquisition of a skill is contingent upon the student's ability to demonstrate successful performance of the skill in multiple settings, under various conditions, a multiple number of times. Each task analysis component of the short-term objective should include a performance item that is both observable and measurable. The conditions of the performance may define the settings or environments in which the skill is to be demonstrated. In a Behavioral Objectives Chart the condition describes the actual setting (e.g., school hallway). Additionally, the frequency or number of times the skill is to be performed should also be included (e.g., twice). Finally, the accuracy with which the skill is to be demonstrated is also to be stated (e.g., only in school hallway during initial phases of instruction or 100 percent of the time). Each of these variables should be included following each task analysis.

To implement an individualized program of instruction when working with a school-age learner, the O&M specialist must plan specific outcomes, long-range goals, short-term objectives, and analysis of the tasks or subtasks, and maintain accurate records of progress. Although the specialist may devote a substantial period of time in designing individual instruction, the planning should not be viewed as time spent developing a rigid set of technical procedures. Systematic planning of O&M instruction does not hinder the potential for creativity in lessons; rather, it assists in insuring effective instruction that in turn facilitates a successful and broadening experience for the student.

Vignettes

The following vignettes provide examples of how an O&M program can be implemented from referral to the beginning of instruction. The first vignette describes the process of planning an O&M program of instruction for a school-age individual, and the second example describes the process of program planning for an adult.

School-Focused Vignette

Jane is a new student in the fifth grade of a public school. Jane's family recently relocated from a neighboring town; it is the middle of the school year and Jane has had to make many adjustments. Jane was diagnosed with optic atrophy when she was 10 months old and has been receiving vision support services and O&M instruction since preschool.

Referral. Because Jane previously received vision support and O&M services, Jane's new school district was immediately alerted to the presence of a student with visual disabilities. For a period of 30 days in the new educational setting, Jane's current IEP is considered valid. The teacher of children with visual disabilities and the O&M specialist in the new district are contacted to begin assessment procedures and to plan an appropriate instructional program for Jane. Appropriate consent forms to review records and to assess Jane are in place.

Assessment. The assessment begins with an informal visit and interview with Jane and with her classroom teacher. The O&M specialist will also interview Jane's parents and then will plan a series of direct observations of Jane's current O&M skills.

In a conversation about the school and Jane's new home, Jane and her teacher are both provided an opportunity to describe the school and neighborhood environments in which Jane travels most often. Questions which relate to Jane's current educational status, previous travel experience, and her current travel experience are asked. The specialist learns that the classroom teacher does not have concerns regarding Jane's academic performance; Jane is working at her grade level in academic subjects. The classroom teacher reports, however, that Jane seems to have difficulty finding some of the classrooms in the building. Jane is often late for class in the morning or between classes. The teacher further states that Jane is reluctant to join in extracurricular activities. The classroom teacher reports concern regarding Jane's safety to travel outside the classroom independently.

In the initial informal interview with Jane the information reported is somewhat different than that of the classroom teacher. Jane reports that she likes her new school but that she is not sure where in the hallway her locker is located. The identification numbers on the lockers and above some of the classroom doors are "hard to read." Jane further reports that she has never used a cane and never felt as though she needed one. She received O&M instruction once a month in her previous school and feels as though she knew the layout of that school "like the back of her hand." Jane states that she may enjoy participating in after school activities, but she has had so many headaches that she is usually anxious to get home and rest after school.

The final informal interview is concluded at Jane's home where her parents provide input regarding Jane's O&M skills. Jane's parents discuss their concerns about Jane's headaches and her confusion about bus numbers, locker numbers, and classroom numbers. They report confidence about Jane's ability to compete academically; however, they state concern over Jane's confusion about where things are in her new school environment. Jane's O&M skills in her new neighborhood remain unknown; her parents report that Jane engages primarily in indoor activities since the move.

The review of Jane's previous records includes ophthalmologic records, low vision evaluations records, educational records, previous vision and O&M IEPs. Information from these records provides information such as: a diagnosis of congenital optic nerve atrophy, a recommendation for the use of a CCTV for near work in the classroom, achievement test scores and cumulative grades, and a chronicle of vision and O&M services. Jane's previous O&M goals included orientation in space, self-protective techniques, trailing, and use of a human guide in novel settings.

After the review of records the O&M specialist uses information from Jane, her classroom teacher, and Jane's parents to begin the direct observations of Jane's O&M skills in familiar and novel environments. Jane is asked to "show the O&M specialist around" indoor and outdoor settings Jane has described as comfortable or familiar. It is during the direct observation phase that the O&M specialist notices Jane's difficulty with orientation cues in settings with high degrees of illumination or with highly reflective surfaces. These areas include the concrete, unshaded recreation area of the school yard and the high gloss floors and walls of the school corridors and some of the classrooms. The school lockers are high-gloss painted metal that also reflect light and the identification numbers are located above the lockers on low-contrast metal plates.

The direct observation in Jane's neighborhood also provides important information. Jane' s new house is located in a new housing development. The housing plan was cleared of trees, and new concrete sidewalks and driveways were constructed. Jane moves through the winding path of sidewalks with her head down. The street signs have low-contrast beige lettering on a light green background; when asked to identify the street name Jane squints and incorrectly guesses the street name. After complaining of a headache, Jane travels with the sighted guide back to her house.

Observation of Jane's O&M skills is also conducted in an unfamiliar setting in a shopping center in Jane's community. Jane is observed indoors and outdoors and is asked to perform a number of age-appropriate O&M tasks. Jane is able to locate items in stores when the label is high contrast or when it is within arm's reach. When the lighting is incandescent, filtered, or indirect, Jane is able to locate items more readily than when the light is natural, intense, or direct. In areas with carpeted floors and light-absorbing walls, Jane remains oriented and maintains a upright head position. The results of the interviews and the direct observations have enabled the O&M specialist to understand the impact contrast, illumination, and distance have on Jane's O&M performance. Because Jane's new home and school environments have higher amounts of reflective and uncomfortable glare, Jane's ability to become oriented and move safely and efficiently have been compromised.

Identification of Program Goals. The task now focuses on using the assessment findings to determine program priorities, identify the outcomes and long- and short-term goals, and write these goals into Jane's IEP. The educational team responsible for the development of an appropriate IEP for Jane consists of Jane, her parents, the O&M specialist, the teacher of children with visual disabilities, Jane's classroom teacher(s), the school psychologist, and a school district representative. Jane and her parents will be provided with the opportunity to state their goals and priorities for O&M instruction.

Together the team members will discuss the assessment findings and develop specific outcomes for Jane's O&M instruction. The team also considers Jane's age, her cognitive level, the appropriate settings for instruction, and her visual status. The following behavioral charts identify the instructional outcomes, long-range goals, short-term objectives, task analysis, and performance criteria for Jane's IEP (Tables 12.3 and 12.4).

As in the previous example, each of the IEP long-range goals is broken down into short-term objectives. Using the short-term objectives, the O&M specialist is able to systematically provide instruction toward the accomplishment of the goal. After the outcomes, the long-range goals and the short-term objectives are developed and approved by the team, the IEP is signed and Jane's O&M instruction can begin. Using the IEP as an instructional guide, the O&M specialist begins planning individual lessons. The lesson plans describe the activities of each session and contains a task analysis of a skill to be mastered. An example of the task analysis and the performance criteria for Jane's short-term objectives is provided in Tables 12.3 and 12.4. Carefully designed lesson plans and task analysis are the individual pieces of the puzzle that ultimately complete the picture for Jane's O&M needs. In the next example an adult who is experiencing more specific travel difficulties is presented.

Adult or Community-Focused Vignette

Alphonse is a 40-year-old Internal Revenue Service (IRS) employee who is diagnosed with advanced retinitis pigmentosa (RP). He has worked for the IRS for eight years and is being relocated to a new office in another part of the city. He lives with his wife and three children in a suburban community outside of the city, and he rides public transportation to and from his work. Alphonse previously received O&M services when he first began working for the IRS, but has not received additional services since then. Table 12.5 is an example of an IWRP written for Alphonse.

Referral. Alphonse noticed a change in his vision approximately 1 year ago and wanted to make contact with the state office at that time, but delayed calling. His office relocation, which requires learning a whole new commuter train and bus transportation system and schedule, was the impetus for the self-referral. He will be moving to the new office in 1 month. The rehabilitation counselor indicated that she would arrange to meet with Alphonse at his office. After meeting

Table 12.3. Jane's Individualized Education Program Chart (#1)

Outcome: To travel independently in school and neighborhood

Long-Range Goal #1	*Short-Term Objectives*	*Task Analysis*	*Performance Criteria*
Jane will utilize a system to identify symbols at a distance.	Jane will correctly identify 8–10 street signs, room numbers, locker numbers, bus numbers, or other symbols that Jane describes as "too far away" to read.	Jane will meet with the O&M specialist to discuss her class schedule and which classes she is typically "late" for.	In large print, Jane will write out her weekly class schedule and verbally identify which classes she is typicall "late" for.
		Jane will review her class schedule with the O&M specialist and will be asked to identify the location of classroom numbers.	In large print, Jane will be asked to write the classroom numbers.
		Jane will devise a list of classrooms with "can read" and "cannot read" room numbers.	From the weekly class schedule, Jane will make two lists in large print; one for classroom numbers she can read easily, and a second for classroom numbers she cannot read easily.
		Jane and the O&M specialist will discuss the relationship between her ability to read classroom numbers and her ability to be on time for class.	Jane will utilize an optical device which will allow her to verify classroom numbers from a distance.

with Alphonse the counselor recommended that he receive immediate O&M services.

Initial Visit and Interview. The O&M specialist contacts Alphonse and agrees to meet with him and his family at their home in the evening. During the interview Alphonse reports that his initial reason for calling was based on the change of transportation needs from his home to the new office. He is not sure how to get to the new office. He admits that he was recently seen by the low vision specialist and his belief about further loss of peripheral vision was confirmed by the results of the peripheral field test. During the interview Alphonse is asked about a typical day of travel. He describes his current travel routine of walking to the bus stop at the end of his block, riding the bus one-half mile to the train station and traveling into the city where he rides the subway and walks the two blocks to his current office location. He then verbally describes the reverse route home. He reports having difficulty traveling when entering and exiting his office building in the morning and evening, and when entering and

Table 12.4. Jane's Individualized Education Program Chart (#2)

Outcome: To travel independently in school and neighborhood

Long-Range Goal #2	*Short-Term Objectives*	*Task Analysis*	*Performance Criteria*
Jane will utilize a telescopic device to identify symbols at a distance.	While using a 2.8X telescope, Jane will demonstrate the ability to scan an area for a target, focus, and identify the letters, numbers, or symbols.	While positioned in front of a blackboard, Jane will spot the equivalent-sized letters, numbers, symbols written on the board using the 2.8X telescope.	While seated in a chair and with both arms resting on a table while holding the telescope in her right hand, Jane will verbally identify five of the ten letters, numbers, or symbols written on the blackboard.
		When presented with letters, numbers, or symbols of varying sizes, Jane will focus the 2.8X telescope to locate and identify them.	While seated in a chair and with both arms resting on a table while holding the telescope in her right hand, Jane will focus the telescope and correctly identify five of ten letters, numbers, or symbols in 2 mintues.
		From a stationary position while using the 2.8X telescope, Jane will move her upper body to scan for and identify letters, numbers, and symbols.	While standing and holding the telescope in her right hand, Jane will locate five of ten letters, numbers, or symbols in 2 minutes by moving her upper body from left to right.
		Using the 2.8X telescope, Jane will locate the fire extinguisher and locker numbers in the school corridor.	Jane will locate the fire extinguisher unaided, then use the telescope to identify five of five locker numbers.

exiting the subway station. He does not report having any difficulties traveling in or around his home.

Alphonse's spouse is asked about aspects of his travels that cause concern to her. She states that she has noticed Alphonse having more problems traveling when moving from a well-lighted area (e.g., the mall) to a more dimly lighted area (e.g., outdoors at night), but that she is usually with him when this occurs.

Questions pertaining to Alphonse's previous O&M experiences are then reviewed. He reports that his first and only exposure to O&M services was 8 years ago when he received itinerant O&M services from the state office of blindness and visual services. His instructor at that time taught Alphonse how to use a folding cane for street crossing identification.

Before the O&M specialist leaves, an observation of Alphonse traveling from his current of-

Table 12.5. Alphonse's Individualized Written Rehabilitation Program Chart

Outcome: To travel independently to and from home and new office			
Long-Range Goal	*Short-Term Objectives*	*Task Analysis*	*Performance Criteria*
Alphonse will use his folding cane while traveling in higher density populated areas.	While traveling downtown, Alphonse will use his folding cane for identification and protection.	Alphonse will unfold his cane upon exiting his office building.	After stepping onto the pavement outside the main entrance of the office building, Alphonse will unfold his cane five out of five trials.
		Alphonse will use the unfolded cane in a modified technique while traveling on downtown sidewalks and for crossing streets.	While traveling downtown, Alphonse will use his folding cane in a modified two-point touch technique to locate up- and downcurbs at each corner.
	When entering a subway or train station, Alphonse will use his folding cane to locate the turnstile.	Alphonse will slow his pace and use a modified touch technique upon entering the subway and train station.	Alphonse will shorten his grip on the cane, slow his pace, and use a modified two-point touch technique to locate the turnstile, deposit the fare, and pass through the turnstile correctly five out of five trials.
	While walking on a subway and train platform, Alphonse will use his folding cane to locate the platform edge or train car.	Alphonse will locate the platform edge, turn 180 degrees, and reposition himself three steps away from the edge, facing the rails.	Alphonse will locate the platform edge and reposition himself correctly five out of five trials.

fice location to his home is scheduled. Also permission to review Alphonse's ophthalmologic and optometric records, medical records, and previous O&M report is requested and granted.

Review of Records. As a part of the intake process, the rehabilitation counselor for the state agency obtained the ophthalmological and clinical low vision evaluation records. She also was able to obtain a copy of the original IWRP and previous O&M records. Information obtained from these records includes: a diagnosis of advanced retinitis pigmentosa and developing cataracts, the recent clinical low vision report depicting the 5-degree central field, a recommendation for the use of a reverse telescopic device, and a chronicle of IWRP and O&M goals from 8 years ago. Alphonse's previous O&M goals included instruction in the use of the folding cane for street crossings and identification and familiarization to the routes between his home and office.

Direct Observations. The O&M specialist completes the review of the records and combines that information with the information obtained from the interview with Alphonse and his family. He contacts Alphonse and schedules a time when he can meet Alphonse at his office at the end of a work day. His purpose is to observe Alphonse traveling the entire route from his current office location to his home. A meeting time of 5:15 P.M. outside the office building is arranged. The lateness of the meeting time is intentional, to observe Alphonse traveling after the sun has set. Alphonse is observed traveling outdoors, crossing busy lighted intersections, traveling on a subway, traveling on a commuter train, and walking in a suburban neighborhood to his home.

During this time the O&M specialist observes Alphonse's ability to travel a familiar route. He is also interested in how well Alphonse travels when leaving and entering dark and light areas. He noticed Alphonse slowing his pace and becoming more hesitant at the light/dark situations. Because of his familiarity with the route, Alphonse knew where to stand at the subway and train platforms and bus stop locations. Alphonse used his folding cane, but only at intersections.

Identification of Program Goals. Based upon the interview, review of records, and observation of Alphonse traveling in a familiar environment, it is recommended that program priorities should be written and immediate O&M services should be provided. The specialist will identify the program outcomes and write these goals into Alphonse's new IWRP. In the following example, the instructional outcomes, long-range goals, short-term objectives, task analysis, and performance criteria are specified (Table 12.5). Unlike the requirements of the IEP or the ITP, the IWRP does not need to include all goals, objectives, analysis, and performance criteria. The IWRP does require that a recommended time frame for goal attainment be included in the original program. Adjustments to this proposed time frame generally occur at the midpoint of the program, which is about the time when the first evaluation report is due. Submission of the final evaluation report to the rehabilitation counselor or case manager occurs when O&M services are completed.

Alphonse's IWRP team consists of the O&M specialist, the case manager or rehabilitation counselor, and the rehabilitation supervisor. The goals include the needs expressed by Alphonse and his family.

Developing functional student-centered instructional outcomes and goals based upon the information gathered during the informal assessment is pivotal to the success of the O&M program of instruction. In the example above, informal assessment information was used to develop specific instructional goals and objectives. These in turn were used to guide the instructional process.

CONCLUSION

Developing an appropriate program in O&M, whether working with children or adults, requires knowledge and skills in many areas. The O&M specialist who serves students across this age range must be familiar with factors of human growth and development; have a sound understanding of the psychosocial impact of visual disabilities; be informed about the education and rehabilitation process; be proactive in the areas of career education, transition, and employment; be acquainted with the effect of culture and the family system; have a handle on how to be an effective member of a team; be conversant in advocacy; be adept at listening and interviewing; and most of all, she must be sensitive to the needs and lives of the students and families being served. Using the knowledge acquired from these areas, along with the skills of assessment and teaching, the O&M specialist is better able to design an individualized program of instruction that will assure success and independence.

Suggestions/Implications for O&M Specialists

1. The goals of any O&M program should emerge directly from the information obtained through the O&M assessment.
2. There are no standard assessment instruments available to the O&M specialist to use when assessing an adult's O&M skills.
3. The O&M specialist uses informal assessment instruments in conjunction with norm-referenced spatial and positional concept assessment instruments when assessing the O&M skills of young children.
4. The O&M specialist uses the initial visit and interview as a method for learning about the student, as well as learning about the student's family and its culture and support for O&M services.
5. Combining the information obtained during the initial visit with a review of the student's clinical records (i.e., ophthalmologic, occupational therapy, speech and language) will provide the O&M specialist with additional information necessary for the development of appropriate O&M goals.
6. Direct observations of the student moving about her familiar and unfamiliar environment provides the O&M specialist with information about the student's motor, sensory, and spatial orientation skills.
7. Measuring a student's performance over time is known as criterion-referenced testing.
8. Criterion-referenced testing is useful for establishing baseline performance and comparing performance at the midpoint and final evaluations.
9. An Individualized Education Program, Individualized Transition Plan, and Individualized Written Rehabilitation Plan are various forms that identify instructional goals and outcomes for children and adults.
10. Outcomes are both the beginning point of program planning and the endpoint of the instructional goals.
11. Task analysis is a method in which skill areas are broken down and sequenced into a series of subskills.
12. Systematic planning of O&M instruction does not hinder the potential for creativity in lessons; rather, it assists in ensuring effective instruction, which in turn facilitates successful and broadening experiences for the student.

ACTIVITIES FOR REVIEW

1. Design a hypothetical scenario of an initial visit and O&M interview. Incorporate information regarding the student's family, culture, educational status, and previous educational experience. Using the "interview" information, identify four O&M needs.
2. Discuss the factors that influence parents readiness for the initiation of O&M services.
3. Interview three adults who are currently cane travelers. Compare their statements regarding family or spouse support in the planning phases of instruction.

4. Explain how an O&M instructor can recognize signs of cultural "mismatch" between the instructor and student. Describe possible methods an instructor can use to facilitate cultural sensitivity.
5. Using Table 12.1, select an evaluation category (physical therapy, occupational therapy, etc.) and list five examples of how the assessment information in that category pertains to an elementary student, secondary student, and adult client's O&M instruction.
6. Compare the broad purposes of both informal and formal assessment methods.
7. Videotape an indoor living or learning environment and compile informal assessment interview questions based on your analysis of the environment.
8. Describe the elements common to the O&M section of an IEP, ITP, and an IWRP.
9. Identify a hypothetical O&M program need. Develop a long-range goal, short-term objectives, task analyses, and criterion for success to address the identified need.
10. Review three to four annual O&M IEPs for an individual student. Note the evaluation techniques used and comment on the progression of the long-range goals over the 3- to 4-year period.

CHAPTER 13

The Preschool Learner

Annette C. Skellenger and Everett W. Hill

Amazing and complex changes occur within the first 5 to 6 years of an individual's life. Much of what the individual will become is rooted in the experiences and learning that occur in the early years of life. It is believed that more learning occurs in this 5-year period than in any other. Physical, emotional, and cognitive development in this phase is rapid and convoluted. Learning results in algorithmic development, with each learned item not only affecting the next step within a particular domain, but also affecting learning in many other domains. For the most part, the wealth of information attained in the first 5 years is learned through activities that bear little resemblence to formal instruction. This chapter discusses the developmental nature of the preschool learner with a visual impairment and focuses on the necessity of preserving as closely as possible the informal, incidental nature of learning when providing orientation and mobility (O&M) instruction with learners of this age.

Because of the complexity of early development, the O&M process with preschool children is very different from that faced by O&M specialists who work with the elderly, adventitiously impaired adults, or even school-age children who did not receive specific input related to O&M in their early years. For these individuals, O&M is primarily a process of building onto the O&M-related strengths and needs the individual already has. With preschool children, the process is entirely the opposite. With these children the process is the initial *development* of skills both directly and indirectly related to O&M and the interweaving of these skills into the overall latticework of development. For example, an 8-year-old child knows how to move her body in a variety of ways. The O&M process will consist of teaching her a specific way to move her hand so that she gets adequate coverage with the long-cane touch technique. In contrast, the O&M process with an infant will consist of being sure that the child includes the practice of lateral wrist movement among the earliest hand movements so that it is an internal component of the child's movement repertoire once he is ready to begin specific cane skills instruction. The educational process is different in these two instances, and it is important that O&M with preschoolers not become a "down-sizing" of processes which have been employed with adult learners. As it will be shown, much of the *content* of O&M will remain the same, but it is imperative that processes for instilling that content be form-fitted to the all-encompassing developmental nature of learners in the first 5 to 6 years of their lives.

The process of O&M with preschool learners is in fact so different because little of it consists of "formal instruction." Because the child is "under construction" in this phase, much of the O&M consists of making sure the child is aware of, and can use, the building blocks on which to build later more typical skills. Much of the learning in O&M will occur through the practice of activities that bear little resemblance to "formal" O&M. For example, the O&M specialist may take advantage of a "teachable moment" to explore the concept of *shoreline* when the child begins making a long path with large plastic waffle blocks during play time. Much that may be learned to facilitate O&M will also include activities to facilitate skills such as reading . . . or face-washing. In addition to emphasizing functional use of skills, O&M with preschool learners will focus on the developmental practice of subskills so that the child will later be ready to integrate their use in more formal O&M instructional activities. While the definition of O&M includes instruction to facilitate travel in any environment, the process of O&M with preschool learners may be thought of as the arranging for the facilitation of travel both in current and in *next* environments. These differences in process are so considerable that the term *O&M development* will be used here to describe the process with young preschool learners rather than *O&M instruction,* which is used with 4- and 5-year-olds as well as with older learners.

Despite the fact that a major portion of learning occurs before a child is 5 years of age, until recently children in this age range have not typically been included in formalized schools. This fact has been so predominant that it has led to the label commonly used to describe the group of children under the age of 6 years: *preschoolers.* The mandates of P.L. 99–457 (passed in 1986), however, now require that children at risk or with disabilities from the age of 3 years (or from birth at the discretion of individual states) receive the educational support necessary to allow them the opportunities of their peers who are developing without disabilities. Because learning in the preschool years normally occurs in a manner different from that commonly used in formalized education, it is important that O&M specialists, as well as other professionals working with children in the early years, become familiar with development and the developmental needs of children in the preschool years. Intervention programs and processes should duplicate as closely as possible the learning that typically occurs in normally developing children without formal intervention.

CHARACTERISTICS OF THE PRESCHOOL LEARNER

Learning and development during the early childhood years are extremely complex—much too complex to be discussed in detail here. Table 13.1, however, presents some of the major theories that have been proposed to explain growth and development; Allen and Marotz (1994) provide one possible resource that describes the many milestones which are used to mark the progress of development in more detail. Some of the characteristics of children of preschool age that should be considered by O&M specialists include

1. The dependence and interrelationship between the child and other family members is especially strong and important in the early years.
2. Children of this age are in the sensorimotor phase of development, which includes much exploration and experimentation, often in the form of play.
3. It is a period of extreme creativity and imagination. Through play and other self-propelled exploration, the child is, in effect, creating knowledge.
4. The desire to explore often results in short attention spans.
5. Much that is learned during this period is understood as isolated parts. The child has not yet fully learned to integrate isolated parts into a whole.

O&M development should be built on an understanding of the above characteristics, as described further in later sections of this chapter. In addition, a major overriding role of O&M specialists working with preschool learners will be the facilitation of the child's typically innate enjoyment of exploration, which is so often

Table 13.1. Selected Theories of Child Development

Ages	Psychosexual: Freud	Psychosocial: Erikson (1963)	Developmental Tasks: Havighurst (1972)	Cognitive Development: Piaget	Moral Development: Kohlberg (1981)
0	*Oral stage* Successful feeding leads to security	*Basic trust vs. basic mistrust* Dependence on caregivers	*Stage 1* Learning to take solid foods Learning to walk Learning to talk	*Early sensorimotor stage* Modification of reflexes	*Completely egocentric* No moral concepts Fear of punishment
1	*Anal stage* Toilet training leads to conflicts about compliance with external demands	*Autonomy vs. shame, doubt* Need to adjust to socialization demands		*Later sensorimotor stage* Tertiary circular reactions Invention of new meanings through mental combinations	
2			*Stage 2* Learning to control the elimination of body wastes Learning sex differences Sexual modesty Forming concepts and learning Langauge to describe social and physical reality Getting ready to read Learning to distinguish right and wrong and beginning to develop a conscience	*Peroperational period* Semantic function (using signifiers, i.e., symbols and signs) Egocentrism Rigidity of thought Semilogical reasoning	
3	*Phallic stage* Pride on body and skills Oedipal conflict	*Initiative vs. guilt* Need to adjust to rules Desire to explore Developing sense of right and wrong			

(continued on next page)

Table 13.1. *Continued*

Ages	Psychosexual: Freud	Psychosocial: Erikson (1963)	Developmental Tasks: Havighurst (1972)	Cognitive Development: Piaget	Moral Development: Kohlberg (1981)
4					*Preconventional* Punishment and obedience orientation Instrumental relativist orientation
5	*Latency stage* Repression of childhood sexuality Free to concentrate on developmental tasks of childhood	*Industry vs. inferiority* Facing and meeting expectations of others Coping with frustration and failure			
6			*Stage 3* Learning physical skills necessary for ordinary games Building wholesome attitudes toward oneself as a growing organism Learning to get along with agemates Learning an appropriate masculine or feminine role Developing concepts necessary for everyday living Developing conscience, morality, and a scale of values Achieving personal independence	*Concrete operational period* Concept of conservation Relations Temporal–spatial representations	

(continued on next page)

Table 13.1. ***Continued***

Ages	Psychosexual: Freud	Psychosocial: Erikson (1963)	Developmental Tasks: Havighurst (1972)	Cognitive Development: Piaget	Moral Development: Kohlberg (1981)
			Developing attitudes toward social groups and institutions		
7					
8					
9					*Conventional level* Interpersonal concordance or "Good Boy–Nice Girl" orientation Social system and conscience maintenance
10					
11					
12	*Genital stage* New, more mature personality begins to develop More mature sexual and intimacy relationships	*Identity vs. role diffusion* Need to question old values, to achieve mature sense of identity	*Stage 4* Achieving new and more mature relations with age-mates of both sexes Achieving a masculine or feminine social role Accepting one's physique and using the body effectively Achieving emotional independence of parents and other adults Preparing for marriage and family life Preparing for an economic career	*Formal operational period* Advanced logical and mathematical schema Comprehension of abstract or symbolic content Reduced need for objects for thinking	

(*continued on next page*)

Table 13.1. *Continued*

Ages	Psychosexual: Freud	Psychosocial: Erikson (1963)	Developmental Tasks: Havighurst (1972)	Cognitive Development: Piaget	Moral Development: Kohlberg (1981)
			Acquiring a set of values and an ethical system as a guide to behavior		
			Desiring and achieving socially responsible behavior		
13					
14					
15					*Postconventional*
					Autonomous or principled level
					Social contract orientation
					Universal ethical principle orientation

thwarted by absent or impaired vision. Through creative adaptations, the child should be motivated and assisted to explore his total environment. With an attitude of discovering enjoyment through exploration in the preschool years, individuals will be more likely to reach toward independence and find a similar joy in its attainment.

IMPACT OF THE FAMILY

The family, as described by family systems theory, is both made up of its individual members and is much more than only the sum of the members (Minuchin, 1974). Actions of each individual within the family system affect the actions of each of the other members, and both individual members and the system itself constantly strive to achieve balance within the system. If one member acts out or has unique needs, the family system must react in such a way as to balance the action or need.

Each individual is tied explicitly and enduringly to his or her family. The human infant requires a relatively long period after birth to achieve physical stability for independence, and therefore the tie between the individual and family is particularly strong in the early years to allow the child protection while he learns the skills necessary for self-sufficiency. As the child matures and moves into greater contact with others outside the family system, the direct effect of the family often lessens, but emotional and indirect effects remain strong throughout the life span.

Family systems whose members include a child with visual impairments share the same characteristics of all families. The impact of the family on an infant or preschooler with visual impairments is as strong as that of other families. It is critical that O&M specialists who work with preschool learners understand the integral relationship that exists between the learner and the family and include components in the intervention package which acknowledge this critical relationship.

The O&M specialist who works with preschool learners will fill two major roles in relation to the family. One role entails supporting the family (as well as individual members) as it strives for balance in reaction to the addition of a member with a visual impairment. Another role entails the provision of O&M-specific information and collaboration to support the education of the preschool learner.

Support for the Family and Family Members

As mentioned earlier, family systems are constantly acting to achieve balance as members act outside normal limits or have unique needs. Especially when a child is very young, families with a child with a visual impairment may spend a great deal of energy attempting to cope with the additional stresses of having a child with unique needs. Such stresses include the difficulty of coping with other family members' reactions to visual impairment, possible feelings of guilt, stress of long periods of hospitalization, and stress of additional financial considerations that may be required of families of some young children with visual impairments. It is important to point out that not all families experience levels of stress beyond the normal; however, those who do often are especially vulnerable during the period when they are trying to find ways to balance the needs of the preschool learner with the needs of the rest of the family. It is imperative that all professionals who have contact with the family during this time understand the stresses being faced and provide whatever support is called for.

Support may come in the form of direct support by the professional—a "shoulder to cry on," or through assistance in locating other systems of support. In studies of families with children with disabilities, it was found that those families which appear to be coping most effectively are the ones with strong social support networks beyond those provided by the professional community (Dunst & Trivette, 1988). These systems can take the form of extended families, church groups, or neighborhood communities. One very critical support the professional can give is to help the family realize and strengthen the social supports available to it. When the family is ready, this can include adding to their network other families with children with a visual impairment and successful adults who are visually impaired. Many resources currently exist that offer suggestions for interacting with and supporting families. Among these are *Enabling and Empowering Families*, by Dunst, Trivette, and Deal (1988).

O&M Information and Collaboration

As important as emotional support can be, most family members and professionals agree that concrete, action-oriented information is the most valuable resource professionals can provide. The act of parenting is typically learned incidentally through watching one's own parents and the parents of others. Typical experience, however, does not include information on ways to assist the child to initiate and maintain movement through the environment without, or with limited, sight. The O&M specialist working with preschool learners will need to provide information both to (1) help the family acquaint themselves with the O&M process and the all-encompassing impact it can have on the development of the child, and (2) help the family members learn ways to support and facilitate skills that will eventually allow the child with a visual impairment to safely negotiate the environment.

First, it is important that the O&M specialist provide information to the family about the process of O&M development in which their child will be involved. As discussed earlier, the family system reacts to individual differences of its members and works to achieve its own balance. Balance may be attained by either accepting or rejecting the problem or difference. If the family system does not accept O&M development, the child will be continually in conflict with the family system or with the O&M specialist, and will most likely receive little benefit from O&M development. Support of the family will result in increased benefit from O&M service. In addition, understanding of the process and impact of O&M in the early years is likely to positively benefit the child by reducing parents' tendency toward overprotection. Parents will also be more likely to assist and reinforce instruction if they understand and support the reasons behind it. Finally, the positive impact of support of the O&M process in the early years will have a cyclical and increasingly positive impact on development throughout the child's life. Examples of methods for helping the family to understand the O&M process include:

1. Provide information pertaining to development as it relates to O&M. Include information pertaining to the interconnectedness of motor development and development in other domains, as well as realistic expectations for the sequence of attainment of specific skills.
2. Provide opportunities for family members to meet and become familiar with individuals with visual impairments of a variety of ages, especially with regard to their travel skills. Help the family understand the continuum of O&M and provide realistic examples of how they might expect their child to travel at various ages.
3. Provide written and recorded resources pertaining to O&M, especially in the early years, for the family to refer to when needed. Some resources include *An Orientation and Mobility Primer for Families and Young Children* (Dodson-Burk & Hill, 1989a), *Pathways to Independence* (O'Mara, 1989), and *Move with Me* (Blind Childrens Center, 1986).

The second major way O&M specialists can provide O&M-related information to families is help them learn specific ways in which they can facilitate O&M skill development. It is true that the family is the child's first teacher, and as such, likely the most effective of all teachers. Many advantages exist when parents act as teachers, including: (1) direct and constant access to behavior as it occurs naturally, therefore (2) an increase in the likelihood that behaviors will generalize and be maintained; (3) parents can act as natural reinforcers for the child; (4) instruction can be most effectively individualized to their child's needs; (5) all family members can assist with learning, thereby increasing the amount of intervention that can be provided (Shearer & Shearer, 1976). It is the role of the O&M specialist and other professionals to assist the parents in their natural teaching role. Some parents will need only the content specific to the skills they are working on. Others may require input regarding their general patterns of interacting with the child as they facilitate O&M skills. Excellent advice regarding general patterns of interaction between children with visual impairments and their families can be found in *Reach Out and Teach* (Ferrell, 1985).

As the child develops, the O&M specialist, parents, and other professionals will share varying responsibilities for teaching and integrating O&M skills. It is imperative that the O&M specialist support the family members while ensuring that O&M-specific skills are included from the earliest possible point in each child's life. The following sections discuss the form and content that O&M development might include in the early years. The responsibility for this content should and will shift between a variety of individuals. Suggestions are meant to be used by all significant individuals in the child's life.

Empowering the Family

Two overriding considerations when working with families require mention. One is that assistance, whether emotional or content-oriented, should be given in such a way that the family will eventually require little or no assistance from outside sources and have the means for dealing with future events. As Barber, Turnbull, Behr, and Kerns (1988) suggest, "A critical aspect of supporting families during the early years is to empower them with coping strategies that can help them to run the full course with their son or daughter and to avoid the trap of investing their energies heavily for a short period of time and then burning out" (pp. 197).

The second, and ultimately primary, consideration is that the assistance and means for providing assistance be "family driven." The addition of a family member with a disability does not take away the family's right, and indeed necessity, to chart its own course or make its own decisions. The Division for Early Childhood of the Council for Exceptional Children has time and again—in its mission statement, statement of best practices, and organizational strategic planning—emphasized the overriding right of families to decide how and what assistance they wish to receive. Professionals can and should make suggestions, provide rationale, and explain processes. Families will ultimately make the decisions.

INFUSION OF VISION USE INTO O&M DEVELOPMENTAL ACTIVITIES

The vast majority of young children with visual impairments retain some visual ability that can be used to assist in O&M functioning. Since vision is learned, early experiences help children develop visual skills. Visual ability is difficult to accurately test, especially when the child is very young. Except for ennucleations and clear cases of total blindness, children should at all times be facilitated to use their vision and activities should be incorporated to help the child to function most effectively visually. Many excellent resources exist. *Look at Me* (Smith & Cote, 1982), *More than a Flashlight* (Harrell & Akeson, 1987), *Project IVEY* (State of Florida, 1983), and *Program to Develop Efficiency in Visual Functioning* (Barraga & Morris, 1980), offer general suggestions. *Beyond Arm's Reach* (Smith & O'Donnell, 1991) gives specific suggestions for facilitating vision relative to O&M, including many skills and activities that can be used with young children. Although they are not specifically mentioned in each section, strategies for facilitating vision should be subsumed under all of the following suggestions.

O&M DEVELOPMENT AND INSTRUCTION

In addition to the direct involvement of significant others into the O&M process, the form O&M development will take with preschool learners will differ significantly from the process followed in more "formal" instruction. This difference is even apparent during assessment, which should be the initial level of all structured learning.

Assessment

The unique characteristics of learners in the preschool years will impact the form of assessment used with these children. The assessment process will be less structured and require much more subjective decisions than more typical assessment procedures with older learners. The actual format of the assessment will vary depending on the age of the child, but whatever the age, a major portion of assessment information will be obtained through unstructured, incidental observation of the child during naturally occurring activities. Young children do not understand the testing process, are not used to complying on command, are not capable of consistent response, or may comply on command even though it may not be indicative of their actual functioning. In addition, for most of the preschool years, especially before the child has mastered verbal language, the child's responses are very individualized and therefore difficult to read, especially by individuals unfamiliar with the child. For these reasons and others, assessment procedures with preschool learners may include the following:

1. Reliance primarily on information obtained through observation of the child during day-to-day activities. Inference may need to be made regarding O&M-related skills from observation of different yet related skill areas. For example: picking up a block using a pincer grasp may indicate the child's probable ability to isolate the index finger to place it along the cane in the normal grip.
2. Indication of the child's functioning as based on a parent or teacher's report.
3. Planned inclusion of the parent or teacher in the assessment process. This may include asking the parent to ask for a specific behavior from the child and watching the response, or it may consist of giving the teacher a list of behaviors one would like to see and asking her to include them in some way during play time.
4. The taking of time to develop rapport and shared understanding (including specifying what is meant by the specialist's termonology) before the O&M specialist attempts to solicit behavior from the child directly. This is very important.
5. The probable necessity for multiple observations and assessment sessions to ensure the accuracy of the information obtained. Direct assessment sessions, when they are possible, should be of short duration, often no more than 5 to 10 minutes at a time.
6. Inclusion of behaviors other than those directly related to O&M skills. Assessment of infants may include behaviors such as object permanence, cause and effect, bringing hands to midline, strength of attachment to caregivers, and clarity of nonverbal communications. A similar range of behaviors may be observed at each of the sublevels within the preschool years, with more "typical" O&M behaviors included with children of increasing ages. See Table 13.2 for suggestions of skills to be included.
7. Requests for behavior structured through playful activities rather than through direct request.
8. Individualization of the actual assessment tool, which is often designed by teachers. The *Preschool Orientation and Mobility Screening* (Dodson-Burk & Hill, 1989b) can be used with many children and can act as a guideline for the development of more individualized testing tools.

Structure of Lessons

O&M development and instruction with preschoolers will vary along a number of dimensions, particularly depending on an individual child's age and severity of impairment. Many individuals (including physical therapists, occupational therapists, classroom teachers, adapted physical education teachers, parents, and others) will share responsibility for facilitating O&M development. In addition, the process of facilitating development might occur in a variety of settings that range from the home-based to center-based (Joffee, 1988), and may incorporate different service delivery systems, from parent and teacher collaborations to typical pull-out instruction. The overall format of O&M development will be jointly decided by the family and significant professionals working with each child. The overall format will influence many of the specific details of the process, but as much as possible, O&M development and instruction should include components such as those discussed below.

Following the Child's Lead

All components of instruction need to be flexible to take advantage of "teachable moments" and to follow the child's lead (MacDonald & Gillette, 1984; Monighan-Nourot, Scales, VanHoorn, & Al-

Table 13.2. Possible Items to Include in O&M Assessments of Preschool Learners

What is the child's temperament type?

What objects, activities, or people are particularly motivating to the child?

How does the child demonstrate reactions to negative stimuli?

Which attachment behaviors are demonstrated by the child (including reaction to separation from significant adults, or using caregiver as a "secure base" from which to explore)?

Does the child demonstrate social referencing (i.e., look to parent or other individuals for indication of what is safe and appropriate behavior in a given situation)?

How does the child initiate social contact with (1) adults, (2) peers?

What play behaviors are demonstrated by the child?

Which home or school responsibilities does the child demonstrate on a regular basis?

How does the child express emotions (verbally, facially, physically, etc.)?

Which stereotypic behaviors are demonstrated by the child?

Evaluate the child's self-control behaviors, including: Does the child respond consistently to "No"? Is the child able to be redirected?

What familiarization behaviors are demonstrated by the child? Specifically, how does the child familiarize himself or herself to (1) space, (2) objects?

Does the child reach for sound (in what directions and to what distances)?

What level of grasp does the child demonstrate?
Does the child demonstrate trunk rotation?

Does the child cross his or her midline (visually, physically)?

Does the child demonstrate an understanding of object permanence?

Does the child demonstrate turns and facing movements (describe)?

Is the child familiar with and able to use a variety of "tools"?

Source: Adapted from Kay Clarke, *Orientation and Mobility Assessment for Young Children* (Worthington, OH: VisAbility Services).

may, 1987). While an overall plan of instruction is needed, typical learning in the preschool years occurs incidentally and the real value of learning at this stage seems to come from the opportunity for the child to discover and "create" knowledge for him- or herself. To simulate these types of situations as closely as possible for preschool learners with visual impairments, it is important to allow them to direct their own learning as much as possible. However, because vision often limits the ability of children with visual impairments to totally learn incidentally, the role of the O&M specialist will be to watch very carefully for signs that the child is interested (or not) in a topic and be ready to supply just enough support, modeling, and content information to facilitate learning. The proverbial "bag of tricks," both teaching ideas and materials to facilitate learning, becomes an actuality when teaching O&M to preschool learners (Table 13.3).

Table 13.3. Possible Items to Include in the O&M "Bag of Tricks"

Item	Potential Use
Index card sets with one goal, game, or activity per card	1. Rotating "lesson planning" and data collection system, i.e., each day's lesson can be planned by selecting those objectives included in the day's lesson and notes taken on the child's success
Kitchen timer with winding knob	1. Sound source to find or follow 2. Reinforcer for child to make the timer "ding" when he or she reaches his or her objective
Large, uncluttered pictures of animals	1. Stimuli for various visual training activities 2. Prompts for stimulating gross motor movements, i.e., "Hop to the picture of the bunny"
Brightly colored stuffed animal	1. Stimulus for various visual training activities 2. Reinforcer—waiting at the objective to receive a hug

This is not to say, however, that O&M development will be unplanned or random, or that the O&M specialist will never take total control of the learning situation. Especially as the child gets older and reaches the age to enter more typical learning situations, the O&M specialist will need to carefully balance following the child's lead with the attainment of developmentally selected objectives. With practice and genuine rapport between the teacher and learner, the two goals usually can fit together very nicely. When structuring learning, the O&M specialist should take as many of the following principles into consideration as possible:

Daily Scheduling of Sessions

As mandated by P.L. 94–142, decisions regarding the amount and type of duration of service should be made on an individual basis by team decision, and should be reflected in each learner's Individualized Family Service Plan (IFSP) or Individualized Education Program (IEP). The following guidelines, however, may be considered when scheduling for O&M. Sessions devoted to O&M development with preschool learners should be of short duration, typically no more than 20 minutes at a time. In addition, sessions should be scheduled at least on a daily basis, and when possible skills should be practiced more than one time every day. Even when the child is 4 or 5 years old and receiving some typical, direct pull-out instruction from the O&M specialist, it is important that all efforts be made to offer this instruction 5 days a week. The more consistent the scheduling and model of instruction, the more likely the child will internalize the skills being practiced. Skills can be further facilitated and practiced through effective collaboration of instructional assistants, teachers, mobility assistants, and family members to allow repeated practice throughout the day.

Inclusion of Numerous Activities

Sessions consist of several short, varied activities, each usually focusing on the practice of isolated skills. Because the child is at the experimental stage, he is not yet able to integrate parts into the whole. Attention spans are typically very short. In one instruction period activities might jump from quick practice discriminating between walking "backward" and "forward" to auditorily localizing and reaching for a sound source, to practicing ten jumps, to tactilely following a line "across" the mapboard. Activities often will be planned, not to achieve one overall goal or complete one overall functional route, as is typically done with older children. Intead, the goal with preschool children is the opportunity to experience as many different activities as possible that can *later* be integrated into a whole.

Use of Play in Sessions

Sessions will often look more like play than work. Play is the typical learning medium for preschool learners and therefore should be encouraged. Many early childhood educators have discussed ways to assess and allow learning to occur through actual self-initiated play (Linder, 1990, 1993; Musslewhite, 1986; Parsons, 1986; Tait, 1972), and this is one medium that should be explored by classroom teachers and O&M specialists. In addition, learning can be structured through play*ful* activities such as games and songs. With creativity, virtually all O&M concepts can be packaged into playful form. Examples of games which have been devised to facilitate O&M can be found in *Simon Says Is not the Only Game* (Leary & von Schneden, 1982).

Flexible Lesson Planning

Lesson planning will be a delicate balance between planning specific objectives as well as having many activities in reserve that can be called upon when the child indicates an interest in something. Objectives for the session, teaching strategies, and activities and materials should all be thought out in advance and the lesson sequence should be described. Planning and evaluation formats should also include, however, a system for planning and recording activities that may have occurred by following the child's indication of interest.

Inclusion of Teaching Components

Because the experience children have during O&M lessons is often the very first time they have come into contact with a particular idea or concept, it is crucial that lessons include a teaching component. The teaching component will introduce the child to the concept and allow him to completely explore it before asking her to do anything with the concept. This will require breaking all skills down to their most basic level and providing teaching at this level. For example, before the child is taught how to open or close doors or trail across openings, it is necessary for the child to have many experiences with doors, the components of door, different types of doors, and their movements, etc. In addition, the concept of "door" needs to be broken down to the point where the door and the way it feels is separated from the door*way* and the way it feels (i.e., the way the "door" will feel when the door is open when the child is trailing). The two entities will need to be learned separately and their relationship examined.

Inclusion of Receptive and Expressive Learning

As soon as it is possible, teaching should include both a receptive and expressive component. Generally educators of children with visual impairments are good at verbally identifying items in the child's environment—giving the child receptive content. For learning to be complete, it is important that the child, whenever capable, also be able to expressively identify a label when she is in contact with the item. In the example above, after the door and door*way* are identified for the child, the O&M specialist would guide the child along a hallway and ask the child to verbally (or through other communication systems when and if necessary) discriminate when in contact with one or the other. Only after learning is demonstrated at this level can techniques be taught for going across door*ways* or for going to the "second door" (when all the child feels is the door*way* because the door happens to be open).

Use of Adult Attention and Behavior Strategies to Assist Motivation

Because learning and motivation often do not come from the completion of a route or objective as they do for older learners, motivation will often need to come from the attention and interaction with the adult, and from behavioral strategies used to facilitate learning.

Prompting. Especially in the early years when attention spans are short, children require the assistance of prompts from the teacher to help them understand or remember what behavior is required next. Prompts, or short reminders of what is expected, can be verbal or physical, and the type of prompt used will often change as the child progresses through a learning sequence (see Jacobson and Bradley, chapter 11 of this volume). A sequence of "most-to-least" prompting is often used to facilitate the initial learning of behaviors. This sequence is (1) full physical prompt or modeling, (2) partial physical prompt, (3) full verbal prompt, or (4) partial verbal prompt. An example of the stages that might be used to help a child learn to walk faster might include:

1. Patterning the child through full physical assistance by holding both of the child's hands and walking fast,
2. Having the child trail the wall with one hand while the other is held by an adult,
3. Having the child trail the wall and an adult occasionally touch the child's free hand to give a feeling of pulling away (forward),
4. Having the child occasionally touch the wall,
5. Having the child walk down the middle of the hall with an adult who gives an occasional physical touch,
6. Having the child walk the child down the hall with an adult providing continual verbal reminders to walk fast,
7. Having the child walk along the hall with an adult giving an occasional verbal reminder.

Reinforcement. Individuals learn most efficiently when the learning is followed by, or is part of, an item or activity that provides positive reinforcement. Categories of secondary reinforcers include (1) natural consequences, (2) social activities, (3) privileges of activities, and (4) tokens. Both the choice of reinforcers and the schedule on which they are distributed will affect the learning that occurs. Schedules for distribution can range from continuous reinforcement, where every response is reinforced, to variable reinforcement, where reinforcement is offered on a random schedule (see Jacobson and Bradley, chapter 11 of this volume). As the child progresses through the learning sequence, both the type of reinforcer and the schedule will change. Whenever possible, this change should include the use of less-intrusive reinforcers, such as praise or natural consequences, and these should be offered on the least frequent schedule possible.

For young children positive reinforcement can often be provided through the natural reinforcement of an activity that is fun or playful. With creativity, most objectives can be "packaged" in the form of a game or made into a song or paired with a favorite activity or sound. Young learners also often respond very well to the use of praise. Many children receive reinforcement simply from the attention they receive from the O&M specialist during lessons. The use of gamelike activities in a playful interaction with the O&M specialist often provides all the reinforcement necessary for most young learners.

MATERIALS

The number and variety of materials used to facilitate O&M development in the preschool years are limited only by the limitation in the creativity of the instructor and/or the budget available. The wide range of materials and equipment used to support instruction can be broken down into two main categories: toys and other items that enhance learning activities, and canes and other devices that facilitate and enhance independent movement.

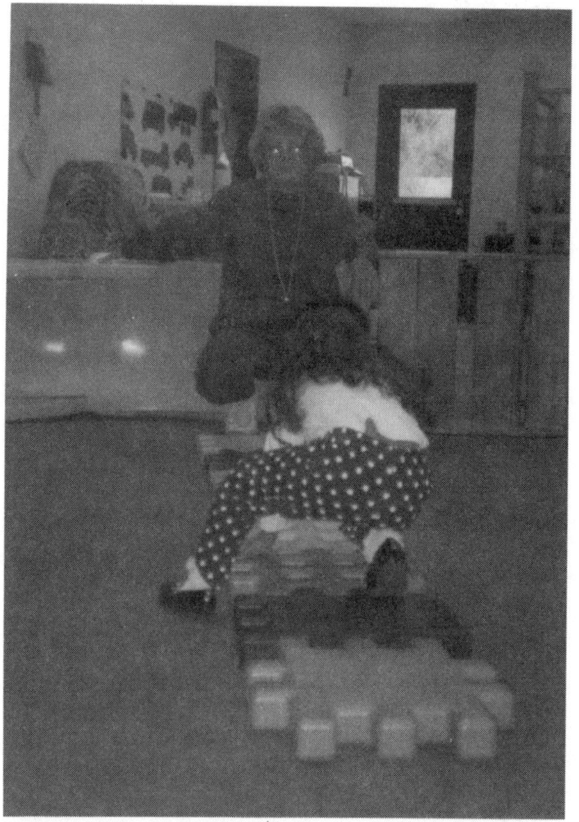

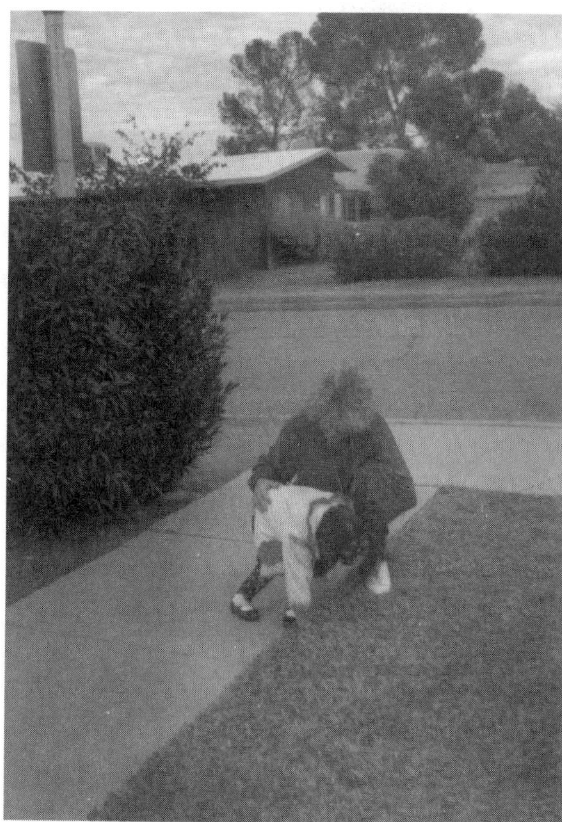

Figure 13.1. O&M concepts can be learned during playtimes and later transferred to other environments.

Materials That Enhance Learning Activities

Virtually every activity can be made more motivating and enjoyable through the use of interesting, playful materials. There are nearly endless numbers of toys and records that can be adapted or used directly to teach O&M development. A few examples are included in the following paragraphs.

A large set of 1-foot-square waffle blocks can be fit together to make a long "track." The child can practice balance while walking "along" the track, then she can be a car and go "across" the tracks by walking from one "side" to the other. This same set can be used to explore and learn the meaning of "shoreline," and all of these concepts can later be transferred to learning about hallways, sidewalks, and streets (Figure 13.1).

A ticking kitchen timer can act both as a sound stimulus to be followed and a self-reinforcer as the child practices wrist movements to turn the knob to make the timer ring once he or she has reached the end of the route. A feather duster can be used to practice flexion and extension of the wrist as for later cane use as the child pretends to "dust off" the instructor or himself. Records can be used to motivate movement and learn the functional use of concepts (see Table 13.4).

Even early mapping skills can be practiced through the use of motivating mapboards made of magnets or Velcro and felt (photos). In addition to practicing concepts such as "across" and "parallel," the use of these boards can also facilitate the tracking skills needed for mapping and braille reading as well, and it requires the use of a fine

Table 13.4. Records to Teach Body Image and Contents

Emphasis	Concept	Song	Record	Activity
Rhythmic movement	Slow	Friendly Giant Big	Pretend	Moving slowly to music
		Big Heavy Box		
	Fast	Rushing Little Ants		Moving fast to music
	Kinds of movements		These Are Me	Carrying out simple movements with music
	Tip toes, jogging high stepping			
	Combined movements			Carrying out combinations of simple movements to music
	Leaps and runs jump, run, bend			
Body parts	Face	These Are Baby Baby's Eyes	Music for 1's and 2's	Finding face part
	Fingers and hands	Dance Thumbkin	Folk Song	Finding different fingers
		Clapping Hands	Carnival	Doing hand movements
		Finger song	Building a City	Doing hand movements
	Whole body	My Little Hands Are Moving	Visit to My Friend	Moving each body part separately and together
		Head, Shoulder	Little Johnny Brown	Touching body parts
		Beautiful	Everybody Cries Sometimes	Moving body parts
		Arms Arm Song	Everybody Cries Sometimes	
			Sesame Street Live	Making up dances with body parts
		Legs & Arms	Building a City	Moving body parts up and down
Spatial relations	Up/down	Put Your Finger in the Air	Songs to Grow	Finding body parts

(*continued on next page*)

Table 13.4. *Continued*

Emphasis	Concept	Song	Record	Activity
		Little Birds	Learning Basic Skills Thru Music	Following directions in bird song
		Once there Was a King	My Street Begins at My House	Following directions in song
		People on Bus	Activity & Game Songs	Hands act out peo- ple going up/down
		Monkey Song	Train to the Zoo	Jump up high like a monkey
	Left/Right	Put Your Hand in the Air	Learning Basic Skills Thru Music (1)	Put left & right hands in different places
		Left & Right	What Can the Difference Be	Listen to the song
	Left/Right	Looby Zoo	We All Live Together	Put left and right body parts into circle
	Above/Below	Play	Homemade Bread	Play instruments above and below
	In front/Behind	Play	Homemade Bread	Play instruments in front and behind
	Big/Little	Bit & Small	What Can the Difference Be	Listen to the song
		Big & Little	Music for 1's & 2's	Listen to sounds from big and little things
	In/Out	In & Out	What Can the Difference Be	Listen to the song
	Top/Bottom	Top & Bottom	What Can the Difference Be	Listen to the song
	Front/Back	Jolly Is the Miller	American Game & Activity Songs	Follow the dance directions
	Over/Under	Los Is Blue	Mod Marches	Crawl over & under chairs/tables with music
	To/From	Penny Lane	Mod Marches	March to and from door, window in time to music

(*continued on next page*)

Table 13.4. *Continued*

Emphasis	Concept	Song	Record	Activity
Spatial Relations (cont'd)	On/off	Yellow Submarine	Mod Marches	Walk on/off rug pattern made of rag strips in time to music
	Into/out of	Lodi Dancing song	Mod Marches	Crawl into/out of tunnel in time to music
	Following directions in space and using sound cues	Dancing song	I'm Not Small	Follow directions in song
		Pretty Sound	Homemade Band	
		Wildwood	Homemade Band	Stop/start with sound cues
		Skip to My Lou	We'll Live Together	Follow directions in song
		Creepy the Crawly Caterpillar	Visit to My Little Friend	Follow directions in song
		Visit to My Little Friend	Visit to My Little Friend	Follow directions in song
		It's a Small World	Mod Marches	Have races to the record player at one end of room
Solving problems in space		Making a Bridge	Ideas Thoughts & Feelings	Use body to make different kinds of bridges
		Move Around the Room	Ideas Thoughts & Feelings	Use body to move on 1–4 legs
		Can You Guess What I Am?	Ideas Thoughts & Feelings	Use body to represent different things
		Follow Along	Ideas Thoughts & Feelings	See if partner can imitate movement

Selected Suggested Records for O&M
Educational Activities, Box 392, Freeport, NY 11520
(Homemade Band, Mod Marches, Ideas Thoughts & Feelings, Learning Basic Skills Thru Music, Pretend, Folk Song, Carnival, Everybody Cries Sometimes)
Children's Record Guild, 100 6th Ave., New York, NY 10013
(Visit to My Little Friend, Train to the Zoo, Building a City)
CMS Records, Inc., 14 Warren St., New York, NY 10007
(Activity and Tune song, Music for 1's & 2's)
Folkways, 906 Sylvan Avenue, Englewood Cliffs, NJ 07632
(Songs to Grow On, American Games & Activity Songs for Children, Little Johnny Brown, My Street Begins at My House)

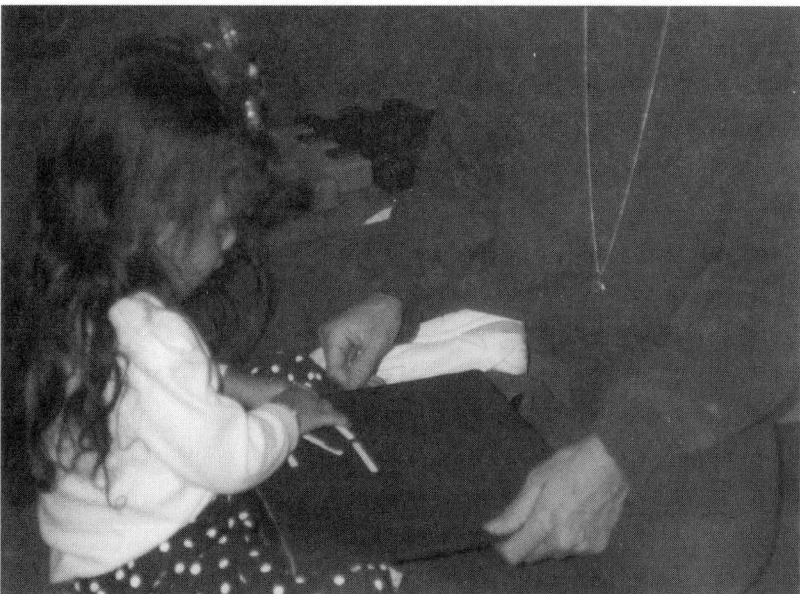

Figure 13.2. Beginning mapping skills can be learned using a variety of interesting materials.

pincer grasp (and isolation of the index finger) to remove the magnet or Velcro piece from the board. Introduced correctly, mapping boards can allow the child to both learn to read maps and make his or her own map of a route or simple area (Figure 13.2).

The variety of materials for use in O&M is nearly endless. Virtually any activity can be made more fun, and therefore increase possible learning, through the imaginative selection of materials (Figure 13.3).

Devices that Enhance Independent Movement

Much of the early discussion related to O&M instruction with preschool children focused on questions regarding long-cane instruction. Strong arguments have been made both against (Ferrell, 1979) and for (Dykes, 1992; Pogrund & Rosen, 1989; Pogrund et al., 1993) long-cane instruction with young children. The use of items, such as toy shopping carts and hula hoops, have been suggested for use as "bumpers" (Bobach, 1988; Clarke, 1988), and special construction of adaptive mobility devices were widely discussed (Foy, Kirchner, & Waple, 1991; Foy, Von Scheden, & Waiculonis, 1992). Many options exist and the majority of O&M Specialists who work with preschool children appear to include some type of "long cane" instruction (including alternatives) in their instruction with preschool learners (Dykes, 1992; Skellenger & Hill, 1991; see also Farmer and Smith, chapter 7, and Rosen, chapter 5 in this volume). Much research is still needed regarding the process of instruction to be followed once a device has been selected, and the factors influencing the decision of which device to use with which child. Clarke (1988), however, has offered many excellent suggestions to begin the discussion regarding the selection of devices. Cane readiness and cane instruction, through the use of adapted items, adaptive mobility devices (AMDs), and long canes will all play an important role in the development and instruction of preschool learners.

Adaptive Mobility Devices

Preschool learners often do not have the gross motor control to adequately demonstrate and

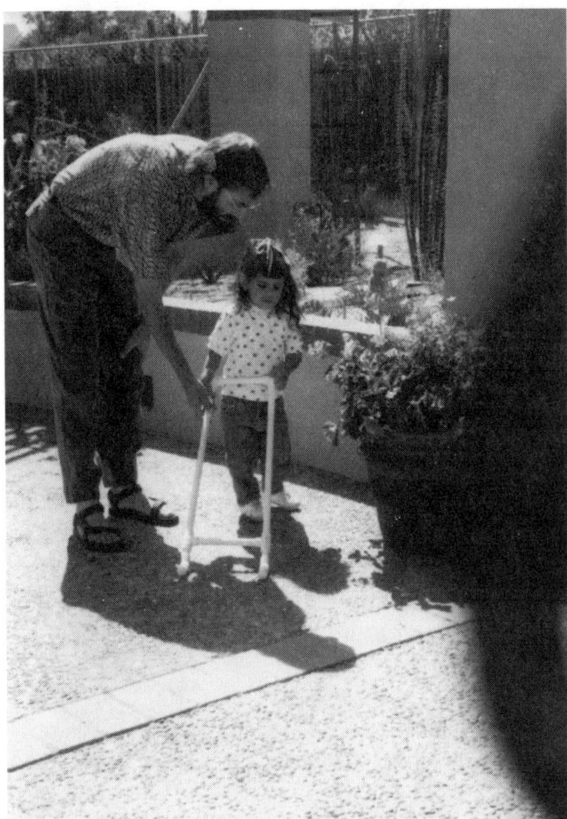

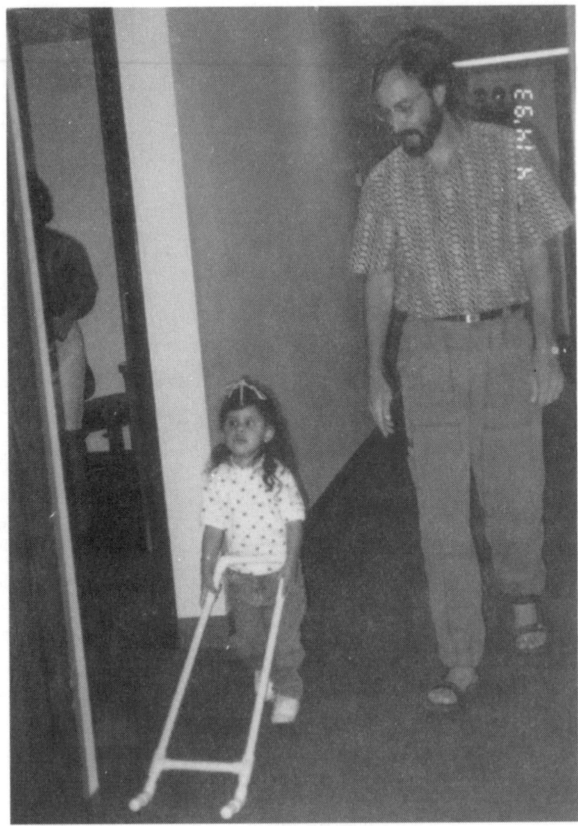

Figure 13.3. Many travel environments, situations, and skills can be made available to preschool learners using adaptive mobility devices.

maintain protective techniques (lower hand and forearm, upper hand and forearm) as are typically taught to older learners. These children, however, can greatly benefit from feelings of protection, which will most likely increase their willingness to move about independently. As suggested by Clarke (1988), a wide variety of devices may be used by preschool learners to provide protection from, and give information about, the environment and therefore increase the amount and type of movement independently practiced by the child. These include the use of devices such as toy shopping carts or "popcorn poppers," as well as adaptive canes designed specifically for use by individuals who lack some of the precursory fine-motor and cognitive skills for typical long-cane use.

AMDs will fill a number of roles with preschool learners. For some children, primarily those with severe, multiple impairments, the AMD will be the sole mobility device when the learner appears unable to learn the skills for long-cane use. For other children, the AMD will provide primary support to facilitate movement until the child demonstrates higher developmental skills that indicate readiness to begin long-cane instruction. For the majority of preschool learners, however, instruction may best include simultaneous instruction and use of *both* an AMD and the long cane. Because the child is at such a young age, it may be difficult to determine whether he will have the ability to eventually use a long cane. For this reason, it may be best to include opportunities to use both types of devices. The child may use an AMD to facilitate day-to-day, functional movement such as movement with his class between the classroom and the lunchroom, or in the backyard at home. At the same time more formal O&M lessons may focus on beginning instruction in long-cane use. Sim-

Table 13.5 Possible Skills to Include in Instruction with Adaptive Canes

Maintain cane tip on the ground.

Maintain both hands on the cane.

Maintain the cane in front of the body.

When the cane goes off the sidewalk, return cane to sidewalk before foot goes off the sidewalk.

When contacting persons or objects (a) stop and pull cane toward self, (b) locate a clear area to the right or left, (c) go around object.

Trail wall or edge of sidewalk on the right with the tip of the cane.

When going through doorways, (a) make contact with the door, walk up to the door while maintaining cane in front of body, (b) open door, (c) put cane through the doorway, then (d) walk through the doorway, closing the door behind.

When traveling up stairs, position the cane parallel to the body and lift it up about 1 inch from the ground. The tip of the cane should touch each step as the student moves forward.

When traveling down stairs, the cane should be held at a 45-degree angle from the body with the tip on the lower stair. The motion of the student's body should keep the cane moving. When the bottom of the steps is reached, the cane tip will contact the floor first.

When reaching the destination, park cane in designated area.

When using a sighted guide, the child should carry the cane, resting the top parallel bar on his or her shoulder with the cane (from top to bottom) parallel with the body. One hand should hold on to the cane.

Source: Eileen Siffermann.

ple readiness activities can range from drills and practice in using constant contact, to games of "reach and find" to help the child learn to discriminate different textures through the cane tip, to learning of the names of the parts of the cane in a song (Pogrund et al., 1993).

Suggestions regarding the construction of and instruction in the use of AMDs can be found in Clarke (1992), Foy et al., (1991), Foy et al., (1992) and Pogrund et al. (1993). (See Table 13.5 for a list of possible skills to include.)

Long Canes

Despite earlier questions regarding the applicability of long canes with young learners, long-cane instruction is included, to varying degrees, within the instructional sequence of many preschool learners. In addition to dual instruction in the use of the AMD and long cane for many learners as suggested above, other learners may show sufficient development for use of the long cane as their primary mobility device. The use of a specially designed "kiddy cane" has been suggested by Pogrund, Fazzi, and Schreier (1993). The long cane may be used for day-to-day activities and/or during more formalized O&M lessons, and a range of techniques, from the adapted diagonal (keeping the cane still and roughly across the front of the child) to constant contact, may be included.

LESSON CONTENT

The majority of learning that occurs in the first 5 to 6 years of life focuses on experimentation in the use of the senses and the motoric system. The child learns about the information that he receives through the sensory systems and learns motoric patterns to act on this information. The child then begins to learn to organize information into categories. For this reason, much of the content of O&M lessons involves the areas of sensory awareness, body image and concept, gross and fine motor activities, and conceptual awareness. In addition, however, the child in this phase is also laying the groundwork for eventual learning in all areas of O&M. While the majority of the content focuses on the skill areas listed above, the content of O&M development should include in some manner activities that focus on all areas of typical O&M instruction.

Sensory Awareness

Very young children, and children with severe multiple impairments, may need to be assisted to become aware of, tolerate, and discriminate the sensory messages they receive before they will be able to make cognitive use of this information to assist travel. It is important that sensory information be verbally pointed out to the child and that the child be actively involved with visual, tactile, auditory, and olfactory information which they will later experience and utilize during independent travel. Resources offering suggestions for facilitating sensory awareness include *Look at Me* (Smith & Cote, 1982), *A Curriculum Guide for the Development of Body & Sensory Awareness for the Visually Impaired* (Illinois Office of Education, 1973), and *Teaching Age Appropriate Purposeful Skills: An Orientation and Mobility Curriculum for Students with Visual Impairments* (Pogrund et al., 1993).

Body Concept

Our individual bodies act both as the receptors of learning and the reference point for understanding the relationships between all significant objects in the environment. It is critical that preschool learners develop a clear body concept on which to base future learning. Body concept is the abstraction in the mind that represents the body to us through input from the senses. Cratty identified four phases in the development of the body concept, which also overlaps the domain of spatial concepts:

Phase 1: body planes, parts, and movements (developed at the mental age [MA] of 2 to 5 years in children without disabilities).

Phase 2: right–left discrimination (MA 5 to 7 years). This includes planes, or sides of objects in same plane as the child.

Phase 3: complex judgments of the body and body–object relationships (MA 6 to 8 years).

Phase 4: identification of parts and relationships through another person's reference system (MA 8 to 9 years).

Others who have discussed the development of body image include Anthony, Fazzi, Lampert, and Pogrund (1992), Hill and Blasch (1980), and Pogrund et al. (1993).

Motor Development, Gait, and Posture

Much that is learned about the body and body image is learned through gross motor movements and repetitive motor patterns. Preschool learners need to be encouraged, and facilitated if necessary, to practice a wide variety of gross motor activities. Practice should be made enjoyable and should focus on quality of movement in addition to providing as much repetitive practice as possible. Because a basic assumption of all independent travel includes the ability to control and maintain gross motor activity, early gross motor practice is critical for later success.

A number of general characteristics of motor development should impact the choice and sequence of motor activities with preschool learners. These include

1. Motor skills apparently cannot be learned until the child is developmentally ready. Even well-structured, rigourous attempts to teach walking will be unsuccessful unless the child is developmentally ready to learn walking.
2. Motor development proceeds from general or mass movement patterns to specific or fine motor patterns.
3. Motor development progresses in head-to-foot (cephalo/caudal) progression and from central to distant (proximal/distal) progression. Activities involving the head and shoulders should be practiced and mastered before attempting activities that require foot control. Likewise, activities involving hand or finger control should not be emphasized until control of the shoulders and upper arms has been mastered.
4. Skills that are overlearned will be retained longer.
5. Motor behavior is specific. Learning one motor skill does not necessarily improve the learning of other motor skills.

Preschool learners will benefit from engagement in virtually any and all functional motor activities. Among the types of skills to be included are those focusing on (1) movement across the midline (reaching with the right hand for object on the left), (2) trunk rotation and segmentation ("log-rolling" so that the hips roll before the shoulders), (3) isolated movement of small body parts (picking up objects with the forefinger and thumb rather than the whole palm), (4) upper body strength (pushing or pulling heaving objects), (5) full extension of joints (holding arms out to the side with elbows straight rather than bent slightly), and (6) increasing stamina. In addition to the selection of activities from the wide variety of resources pertaining to physical education and adapted physical education, Brown and Bour (1986) and Pogrund et al. (1993) offer suggestions of activities specifically selected for children with visual impairments.

Auditory Development

Use of the auditory sense provides a major portion of information for many individuals with visual impairments, and many advanced O&M skills are facilitated by its use. As with other sensory modalities, young learners may need to be stimulated through repeated exposure to be aware of the existance and usefulness of sound. Preschool learners should be provided with as many opportunities to experience as wide a variety of sound sources as possible; from those that normally occur in their environment, such as the sound of the refrigerator motor, to those that are less familiar, such as the sound of cars moving through a tunnel or overpass. In addition to experiential activities, the preschool learner can be involved in the active use or identification of sound. Preschool learners can learn to use sound in many ways, such as (1) reaching for sound (this appears to be an indicator of object permanence as well as an intregral component for providing motivation for locomotion), (2) following a continuous sound source, (3) following a discontinuous sound source, (4) walking to a continuous, then discontinuous sound source and bending over to find it before contacting it with the feet, and (5) moving in a specified pattern in relation to a stationary sound source (i.e. away from it, toward it, parallel to it). Other activities and suggestions for factilitating the use of sound can be found in Brothers, and Huff (1972).

Concept Development

Concept development is crucial for all individuals. The *understanding* of any entity is difficult without the ability to form concepts, and the functional use of an entity requires understanding of the concept on which it is based. The individual with limitations in concept development may also experience limitations in the ability to function in relation to that concept.

Concepts are mental representations, images, or ideas of what something should be (Hill & Blasch, 1980). They are perceptions resulting from synthesis of sense impressions and the integration of the diverse data on a phenomenon in an orderly way. Concepts are formed by classifying or grouping objects or events with similar properties. The ability to perceive and discriminate similarities, therefore, is fundamental for concept development. Formation of concepts can occur at many different levels, including (a) concrete understanding—identification of specific characteristics of an object or action, (b) functional understanding—identification of what the object does or what one can do with it, and (c) abstract understanding—summarization of all major characteristics of the object (Zweibelson & Barg, 1967). Concept development typically occurs incidentally through day-to-day inspection or interaction with the object or entity.

Because a major source of sense impression (vision) is limited or absent for children with visual impairments, concept formation must often be taught more directly than through the more incidental means available to children without disabilities. For the individual with a visual impairment, concept development is a continual, conscious process that requires the individual to learn to relate to objects on many different levels. For example, it is not enough for the child with visual impairments to learn to identify the parts of a car by touch. She must also come to understand the sound a car makes as it passes her on her parallel side, the way it feels when she rides inside it, and the multitude of paths one can take in relation to the path of a pedestrian (Baird & Goldie, 1979).

One of the first steps in assisting children with visual impairments with concept development is an assessment of the concepts possessed by a child. A number of assessment tools are available including *The Body Image of Blind Children* (Cratty & Sams, 1968), *Stanford Multi-Modality Imagery Test* (Dauterman, 1972), Kephart Scale (Kephart, Kephart, & Schwarz, 1974), and *The Hill Performance Test of Selected Positional Concepts* (Hill, 1981). It is important during any assessment of concept understanding that differentiation be made between the ability to verbally describe the concept and a concrete, functional understanding of the concept. Children with visual impairments often demonstrate inadequate understanding of the world around them and use verbalisms rather than actual understanding. Verbalisms may be the result of inaccurate or vague concepts resulting from insufficient sensory experience (Harley, 1963). It is important, therefore, to assess not only verbal understanding of a concept but also to require a physical demonstration of functional understanding of the concept.

Development of understanding of a concept begins with the reception of sensory information about the entity. Instruction to increase concept development will begin with a multitude of sensory experiences. Kind and amount of sensory experience appears to be crucial to the adequacy and variety of concepts formed by an individual, especially for children with visual impairments. Even before the child is capable of cognitive synthesis of information into an organized concept, he should be exposed to as large a variety of sensory experiences as possible. This may include taking the infant to the grocery store, helping him hold and haptically explore a wide variety of items, riding on a city bus, crawling outside on a variety of surfaces with the smell of flowers around him, and accompanying the family to a symphonic concert.

A further step in the development of concepts is the systematic exploration of an entity. Three premises appear to be imperative for adequate concept development at this level. The first is that concrete *experience* with the concept appears crucial. Rather than only reading about bus travel or even passively riding a bus with an adult, the preschool learner should be allowed to tactilely and physically explore the bus layout, carry the money for the fare, and be assisted to deposit the fare in the box. The second premise for complete concept development is that the breadth of experience appears to be more important than quantity. For example, in addition to the above experiences, the process should be verbally described to the child while doing it, bus riding should be compared (physically experienced) with riding in a car, and the sound of buses should be compared with other sounds while standing at an intersection. The third premise involves the necessity for the individual to internalize the concept by being able to apply a label to it. This will be necessary to facilitate generalization. In addition to the above premises, it also appears important that the length of exposure to the concept be long enough to allow the child to fully differentiate it from other concepts. Further information regarding concept development for O&M can be found in Hapeman (1967) and Hill (1986). Examples of activities that will facilitate concept development can be found in Baird and Goldie (1979).

The list of concepts that a child will need to assist travel is nearly endless (see Hill & Blasch, 1980, for one listing). They can be roughly grouped, however, into a number of subgroups that include (a) spatial and positional concepts such as "in front," "along," "next," and "end," (b) environmental concepts such as "block," "corner," "camber," and "shoreline," (c) concepts relating to the nature of objects such as "objects remain in the same place unless moved by someone" and "objects that move (such as cars) will change their relative location to you even if you are standing still," (d) concepts that facilitate orientation, such as numbering systems and cardinal directions, and (e) concepts that facilitate mobility, such as time and distance.

The development of functional concepts to assist travel is a crucial component of instruction with preschool learners. The attainment of concrete, functional concepts will require nearly endless hours of systematic involvement. The responsibility for this involvement should be shared by all the significant individuals in a preschool learner's life. Concept development will be most complete if adults team together to provide as wide a variety of experiences in as systematic a process as possible.

Formalized Mobility Techniques

O&M development with preschool learners should include experience and practice in formal mobility techniques such as sighted guide and self-protective techniques (Figure 13.4). Because many very young children do not demonstrate the motor control necessary to replicate exact

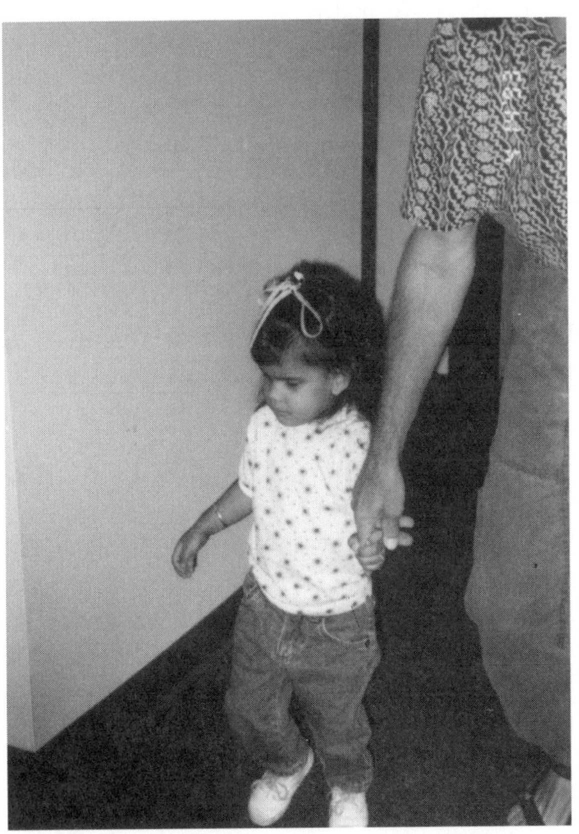

Figure 13.4. Adaptations in formal mobility techniques may benefit the preschool learner.

technique, activities in this area may fit into "readiness" activities, or may involve adaptation of the techniques. Readiness activities might include playing statues to help the child learn muscle control to later hold her arm in a protective position. Adaptations may include teaching the child to grasp the guide's index and forefinger rather than the wrist or elbow (Anthony et al., 1992).

Continuum of O&M Skills

In addition to the areas of sensory awareness, body image, gross motor skills, and concept development, O&M instruction with preschool learners can include components of more advanced, "traditional" O&M instruction such as residential travel, basic skills, and downtown travel. With creativity, virtually every component of O&M instruction can be introduced in some form during the preschool years. The appendix to this chapter provides examples of activities for use with preschool learners that will act as readiness activities to support later acquisition of advanced skills.

CONCLUSION

The preschool years provide young learners with exciting opportunities for self-directed learning. O&M services in these years attend to the developmental nature of the child and should be based on the interests of the child. It is the role of the O&M specialist to assist learners of this age, and their family members, to develop positive attitudes toward exploration and independence, and to begin to explore the myriad of skills and activities upon which more typical O&M instruction will later be based. Through the creative use of materials, including adaptive mobility devices and long canes, playful activities can be incorporated into both the day-to-day activities of the child and more structured O&M lessons. The multiple "significant others" in the child's world can work together to provide a wide variety of experiences that will allow the child to begin learning in all of the multiple skills which will later constitute more formal O&M instruction. Through the creativity of O&M specialists and others, the child can begin to experience the independence provided by learning.

Suggestions to Include Advanced O&M Skills into Preschool Lessons

O&M Skill	Age of Learner		
	Infant[a]	Toddler[b]	Preschooler[c]
Concept of turns/accurate turns	Make distinct turns (not curves) when carrying or walking with infant.	Continue making distinct turns when walking together.	Continue with previous activities.
		When walking together, have a word or signal that you say or do whenever you make a turn to help the child clue into the fact that a difference in the movement is occurring.	Play a game where the child is the "driver" and you are the "car," and you turn whenever the child tells you to (or makes motion as if turning the steering wheel).
		Show child the difference between "turn" (90°), "turn around" (180°), and "turn all the way around" (360°). Try to be consistent in your use of these terms.	Talk about how turning changes the direction you are traveling—put items in front of the child and to the side she will be turning, and show how the relative location changes.
		Play (modified) "Mother May I" by asking the child to make one of the above turns (gross approximations), and if done correctly they will "find" you in front of them—reward with hugs, tickles, etc.	
Analyzing traffic sounds and patterns	Take infant to a variety of areas with different levels of traffic. Be sure to include areas with high levels of traffic. Provide time to listen to the traffic and become used to it.	Continue with previous activities.	On a quiet street, talk about how the sound of the car is quiet, then gets louder as it approaches, then gets quiet again.
	Help child to localize and reach for sounds—start with hand-over-hand, then physical assistance from elbow, physical assistance from shoulder, etc.	Help child to learn to turn to face sounds.	As child demonstrates ability to localize sound, help him to point to and follow movement of car along the street. Do this first on a quiet street, then on busier streets.

(*continued on next page*)

Suggestions to Include Advanced O&M Skills into Preschool Lessons (*Continued*)

O&M Skill	Age of Learner: Infant[a]	Toddler[b]	Preschooler[c]
	Use a sound maker that can be activated by hitting it and encourage child to make it sound each time he or she is correct.	While standing next to a street, talk about "loud"- and "quiet"-sounding cars.	As child demonstrates understanding of spatial concepts, show child how traffic moves from in front to behind you when you are standing with the street beside you, and how traffic moves from side to side when you are facing the street.
		While standing next to different types of streets, ask the child to tell when there are cars on the street and when there are no cars.	
		Talk about the different sounds made by "fast" cars and "slow" cars—play games with cars and act out going fast and slow, read stories about vehicles that go fast or slow.	
Compass orientation	Begin to incorporate compass terms into your daily vocabulary—if possible, use them when giving directions to others or to describe locations of items in the house, etc.	Identify three or four key locations in the house (or school) and refer to them with labels in compass terms—i.e., call the front door the "east door" (or whichever direction it faces), talk about the clothesrack being on the north wall.	Continue with previous activities.
			Play a game of "detective"—take the child to locations in the house that you have been identifying with compass labels and see if he or she can tell what it is (what direction it is associated with).

(*continued on next page*)

Suggestions to Include Advanced O&M Skills into Preschool Lessons (*Continued*)

O&M Skill	Age of Learner		
	Infant[a]	Toddler[b]	Preschooler[c]
			When walking between labeled compass locations, talk about how you need to turn to get from one to the other.
		Play games to teach and practice basic spatial concepts, specifically "in front" and "behind."	As child demonstrates understanding of spatial concepts of "in front" and "behind," talk about north being in front of you when you are walking toward the north clothesrack.
		Teach child about opposites—use physical movements as much as possible, i.e., the opposite of "stop" is "go," the opposite of "up" is "down," etc.	As child demonstrates understanding of opposites, talk about north and south being opposites and "when north is in front of you, south is behind you."
Public transportation	Plan periodic family "field trips"—instead of driving downtown to go to the library, park at the outskirts and take a city bus, or take a cab to the grocery store occasionally.	Continue family "field trips"—talk with student about what transportation you will take, read a story about the type of transportation, play games with toy models of the type of transportation.	Continue family "field trips"—give the child responsibility for portions of the trip, i.e., have him or her hold the money and hand it to the bus driver as you get on, have her ask the bus driver to tell when you are at your stop.
Mapping skills	Accustom child to wide variety of tactual materials—help him or her to explore/scan the entire item.	Provide child with a magnetic or Velcro mapboard—encourage him or her to make designs with the pieces.	Play a game with the child where you place a magnet on the board and he or she tactually searches for it using appropriate search patterns.
			As child is able, play the above game and have the child tell where he or she found the magnet on the board (i.e., "near the top and near the right side").

(*continued on next page*)

Suggestions to Include Advanced O&M Skills into Preschool Lessons (*Continued*)

	Age of Learner		
O&M Skill	**Infant**[a]	**Toddler**[b]	**Preschooler**[c]
			Help to child learn to make magnet lines that go all the way "across" the board or "from top to bottom."
		Walk in a hallway carrying mapboard and as you walk from one end of the hall to the other, place magnets in a longer and longer line going away from child's body.	
			As child is able, continue as above, but also examine an intersecting hallway and place magnets to show the intersection.

[a]Approximately in the range of 6–18 months old.
[b]Approximately in the range of 12–36 months old.
[c]Approximately in the range of 3–6 years old.

Suggestions/Implications for O&M Specialists

1. O&M services with preschool learners include both typical "formalized" learning activities as well as learning that occurs on a more incidental basis.
2. Children of this age are in the sensorimotor phase of development, which includes much exploration and experimentation, often in the form of play.
3. Close collaboration with the preschool learner's family is especially important during this age. The O&M specialist should fill two major roles in this relationship: providing emotional support and providing O&M-specific information.
4. O&M assessments of preschool learners primarily include observations of the child in day-to-day activities and actively involve significant others to elicit both formalized O&M skills and skills not directly associated with O&M.
5. To allow the repeated practice that is so necesary at this age, O&M services should be provided as often as possible and should be reinforced on a daily basis by the "significant others" in the child's environment.
6. O&M specialists serving preschool learners need to become proficient at following the child's lead to take advantage of teachable moments in addition to following more formalized lesson planning.
7. For many preschool learners, O&M services include practice in the use of both an AMD and a long cane. AMDs may be used primarily for day-to-day travel, with more advanced long-cane skills being practiced during O&M lessons.
8. The focus of much of the instruction with preschool learners should be in the following important areas: sensory awareness, body concept, motor development, auditory development, and concept development.
9. Curricula for preschool learners should also focus on providing "readiness skills" for all of the more advanced travel skills, such as downtown travel and the use of transportation.

ACTIVITIES FOR REVIEW

1. What are some of the ways in which the O&M process differs for preschoolers as compared with other populations?
2. As described in this chapter, what is the difference between O&M instruction and O&M development?
3. Describe some of the key characteristics of preschool learners that affect the O&M process.
4. Describe the O&M specialist's role when working with families of preschool learners with visual impairment.
5. Explain why it is important for the O&M specialist to help the family understand the O&M process.
6. List some of the components of the assessment process with preschool learners. In what ways are these the same or different from those used with older learners?
7. Describe the major consideration in implementing O&M with preschool learners.

8. Explain the characteristics that describe O&M development or instruction with preschool learners.
9. Give an example of a teaching component to implement for a preschool learner with visual impairments (not given in this chapter) and a playful means to provide practice.
10. Describe the sequence to utilize for prompting a preschool learner through trailing technique.
11. List the major areas that should be incorporated into an O&M program for the preschool years
12. Choose a toy or play material typically found in a preschool classroom and describe its use in teaching O&M-related concepts.
13. Describe at least two ways long canes can be incorporated into O&M process with preschool learners.
14. List four or five skills that can be taught to children who are learning the use of adaptive canes.
15. List the four levels of body concept development as described by Cratty & Sams (1968).
16. Explain the three considerations that appear to be important in successful concept development with preschool learners.
17. Define the five major types of concepts that should be included in the O&M process.

CHAPTER 14

Orientation and Mobility for the Older Person

John E. Crews and Harvey C. Clark

Providing orientation and mobility (O&M) training to people who are older and visually impaired presents a series of challenges both to the new and seasoned instructor. The circumstances of older people are often different from those of younger individuals, insofar that elders may experience multiple social and health changes. Retirement, death of a spouse, or increased disability of a spouse may create significant demands upon an older person. Moreover, increasing levels of disability and decreased stamina may compromise the ability to travel independently. Although these deficits are not limited to older people experiencing visual impairments, these changes do manifest themselves in very different ways for elders experiencing vision loss. The vision problems that force an older person to cease driving a car have consequences for mobility and self-esteem. The absence of mass transportation and sidewalks, the safety issues of the neighborhood, and the impact of a climate's severely hot summers or severely cold winters can further limit the options of an older traveler.

Although it is important not to overstate or understate the condition of older people experiencing visual impairment, it is imperative that the O&M instructor recognizes the combined effects of changes brought on by age in combination with diminished vision. For example, managing a flight of steps may prove difficult, but when those steps are snow covered and when the older person fears falling, travel choices may be severely compromised; perhaps more importantly, the older person may have less control over his or her travel options.

While the travel goal for younger people may be independent O&M in a variety of environments, many older people may prefer to be accompanied by another person, and that choice would be unaffected by vision. In addition, older travelers may have a fairly modest array of places where they wish to go: the grocery, pharmacy, some places of recreation, and homes of friends and family may pretty much define an individual's travel destinations. Many older people are less likely to travel in unfamiliar places on a regular basis. In addition to reaching particular destinations, an older person may wish to travel for exercise or the independence that a walk around the neighborhood might provide. O&M training must respect these individual circumstances.

Of the estimated 4,293,000 noninstitutionalized civilians in the United States experiencing severe visual impairment in 1990, 82 percent were over the age of 55 (Nelson & Dimitrova, 1993). About 2.7 million individuals experiencing visual impairment are over the age of 65, and that number may grow to nearly 6 million by the year 2030, when all the baby boomers have joined the ranks of elders (Crews, 1994). As a consequence, elders experiencing vision loss constitute a group that is both increasing in absolute size and as a proportion of the visually impaired population.

Vision loss and aging are inextricably related to larger issues of the general aging of the population and the changes in social support, economic well-being, and psychosocial concerns that these changes imply. Moreover, vision loss and aging are inescapably related to larger issues of disability among older people. And, finally, elders who experience vision loss represent a group of individuals whose circumstances are both complex and fluid. Within the group of elders who are visually impaired, the population is remarkably heterogeneous. Knowing that someone is older and visually impaired says little about the rehabilitation expectations and outcomes for that person, and it says absolutely nothing about the human capacity and desire of the individual. Therefore, we must appreciate the complexity of the circumstances of older people who have lost vision, and in addition, we must be sensitive to the needs of those who care for and about elders.

This chapter is divided into two sections. The first section provides an overview of various contexts of aging and vision loss. The discussion focuses particularly upon aging trends, aging and disability, and the characteristics and circumstances of elders experiencing vision loss. The second section employs a series of case studies to present practice issues and solutions related to O&M instruction for older people who have lost their vision.

THE CONTEXTS OF AGING AND VISION LOSS

The Aging of America

In 1989, of the 249 million citizens in the United States, 12 percent were over the age of 65. In the coming decades, elders will increase in absolute numbers and as a proportion of the population. The number of elders will more than double from 31 million to nearly 66 million between the years 1990 and 2030. At the beginning of the 20th century, only 1 person in 25 was over the age of 65; in 1989, 1 person in 8 was over 65, and by 2030, the over-65 population will represent 1 of every 5 citizens (U.S. Select Committee on Aging, 1991).

Many factors are leading to these dramatic demographic shifts, and the consequences of these changes will ripple through every aspect of the nation's social fabric. Increased longevity accounts for only a portion of these changes. For example, the average life span in 1900 was 47; in 1990, the average life span had increased to 75, a 28-year increase in less than 100 years. Moreover, the over-85 age group is the fastest growing segment of the population, a phenomenon that will be sustained well into the next century.

Declining mortality rates and declining birth rates are, moreover, changing the balance of the distribution of the population in the United States. As a consequence, the proportion of older people and younger people will continue to shift. For example, in 1900, older people represented 4 percent of the population, and those under 18 represented 40 percent of the population. By 1980, those over 65 constituted 11 percent of the population while the percentage of younger people had declined to 28 percent. By 2030, those over 65 will represent over 22 percent of the population, while those under 18 will constitute 21 percent. One consequence of this change in population distribution is that the number of working-age people will continue to decline in relation to the number of older people. In 1900, there were 7 older people for every 100 working-age people. In 1990, the ratio was 20 older people for every 100 working-age people. By 2020, the ratio will increase to 29 per 100, and by 2030, it will increase to 38 older people per 100 working-age people. These demographic shifts have implications for caregiving as the pool of caregivers continues to decline, and it has equal economic implications for costs of retirement programs and health care.

In addition, the ratio of men and women varies dramatically with age. While men slightly outnumber women in all age groups under age 35, women outnumber men by 3 to 2 for those over age 65. For those over age 85, there are 2 men for every 5 women. Therefore, women can generally expect to live many years as widows, and they can expect to experience a longer period of retirement.

These demographic changes will drive the economic circumstances of older people. For example, in 1900, the average man could expect to live 1.2 years in retirement. Today, the average older man can expect to live 13.6 years in retirement.

Aging and Disability

Age does not cause blindness, but age certainly predicts vision loss. Age alone does not cause other impairments, but it marks a time when impairments and activity limitations increase dramatically. For many people who lose vision, other health conditions may compromise independence. The loss of vision may represent the inability to function in a number of areas, but the loss of hearing, for example, in addition to a loss of vision, may have a profound impact upon the capacity of an individual to sustain independence (LaForge, Spector, & Sternberg, 1992).

Although there is some evidence to indicate that the prevalence of disability is decreasing slightly among older people (Manton, Corder, & Stallard, 1993), the absolute increase in the number of elders means that many more people will experience disability (Pope & Tarlov, 1991).

One way to understand disablement among older people is to consider an individual's activity limitation. The National Health Interview Survey (NHIS) provides a representative survey of the civilian, noninstitutionalized population. Activity limitation is classified into three categories: (1) limited, but not in major activity; (2) limited in the kind or amount of major activity, and (3) unable to carry out major activity. The numbers cited in this survey undercount the number of older people because it does not take into account institutionalized populations, those who are older, and those whose disability limits independent function. Activity limitation increases with age, from 2.2 percent for children under age 5 to 37.6 percent for those over age 70. While

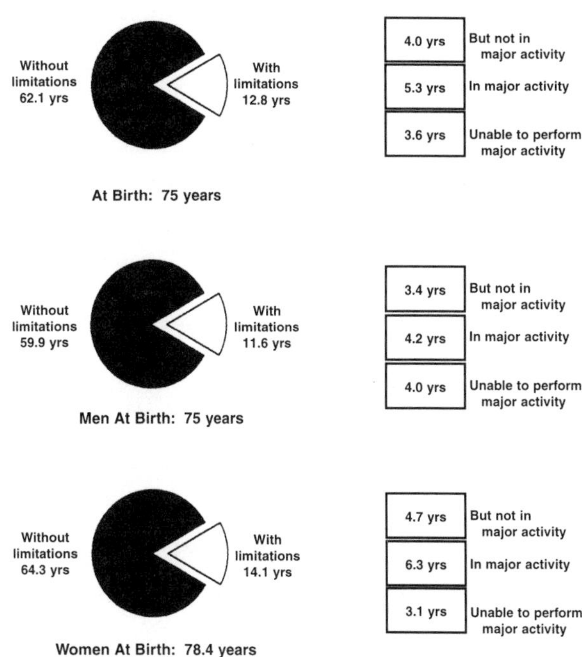

Figure 14.1. Expected years of life with activity limitation at birth, by sex.

Source: Reprinted, by permission of the publisher, from A. M. Pope and A. R. Tarlov, *Disability in America: Toward a National Agenda for Prevention* (Washington, DC: National Academy Press, 1991), p. 63.

women have slightly lower rates of limitation, the large number of older women means that women account for 53 percent of those with activity limitation. African-Americans and families with lower incomes tend to report higher rates of activity limitation (Pope & Tarlov, 1991).

Of the current anticipated life expectancy of 75 years, 12.8 years will be spent with some degree of limitation—4.0 years with limitation but not in major activity, 5.3 years with limitation in major activity, and 3.6 years unable to perform major activity (Figure 14.1). Women can expect to live more years with activity limitation (14.1 years) than men (11.6 years).

Recent strides in life expectancy have led to increased years of activity limitation. From 1970 to 1987, life expectancy increased 4.7 years. Of those years, activity limitation increased from

Table 14.1. Life Expectancy, Active Life Expectancy, and Dependent Life Expectancy, Massachusetts

Age Group	Life Expectancy	Active Life Expectancy	Dependent Life Expectancy	Age Beginning Dependency	Age Ending Dependency
65–69	16.5	10.0	6.5	75.0	81.5
70–74	14.1	8.1	6.0	78.1	84.1
75–79	11.6	6.8	4.8	81.8	86.6
80–84	8.9	4.7	4.2	84.7	88.9
85+	7.3	2.9	4.4	87.9	92.0

Source: Reprinted, by permission of the publisher, from J. P. Fulton and S. Katz, "Characteristics of the Disabled Elderly and Implicaton for Rehabilitation," in S. J. Brody and G. E. Ruff (Eds.) *Aging and Rehabilitation: Advances in the State of the Art,* (New York: Springer, 1986), p. 38.

10.4 years to 12.8. In other words, more than half of the increase in life expectancy is in years with activity limitation. When men and women are compared, a remarkable pattern emerges. From 1970 to 1987, men experienced an increase of 4.4 years of life expectancy. Of those years, two-thirds (2.8 years) was without activity limitation; by contrast, women added 3.6 years of additional life expectancy, and nearly all of it (3.3 years) was with activity limitation (Pope & Tarlov, 1991).

Activity limitation does not begin with one cause and end with one consequence. For example, vision impairment among older people may lead to the inability to avoid hazards, and consequently, poor vision may result in a fall that precipitates a cascade of health crises.

A study by Fulton and Katz (1986) illustrates the potential value of rehabilitation interventions among older people. In this study, Fulton and Katz calculated the number of years of life expectancy among 1,625 people, and then they calculated the years of active life and years of dependent life (see Table 14.1). "Dependent" was defined as being dependent in one of the daily living activities of bathing, toileting, dressing, transferring, eating, personal grooming, and walking across a room. The study notes that someone age 65 to 69 can expect to live an additional 16.5 years; of those years, 10.0 will be years of active life, and 6.5 years will be dependent. Indeed, an 85-year-old can expect to live 7.3 years, and of those years, 2.9 will be active, and 4.4 will be dependent.

In many respects, the role of rehabilitation is to preserve years of active life for as long as possible, even though age-related impairments may threaten continued independence. While the first goal of rehabilitation may be to restore function, for many people an equally desirable goal may be to sustain function. Brody (1986) notes that the role of rehabilitation is to "achieve maximum physical and mental restoration and/or maintenance of functional skills for independent living and the prevention of institutionalization" (p. xvii). Moreover, Williams (1984) underlines the importance of realistic expectations in rehabilitation outcomes. He asserts the importance of the concept of "small gains" and cites the example of transferring from chair to wheelchair as an example of small gains that may prevent institutionalization and increase quality of life. A broad array of rehabilitative, community, and family supports may contribute to an older person's ability to sustain active life. In the Fulton and Katz study, for example, it is not known to what degree older people who are visually impaired would be classified as "dependent." However, rehabilitation "training" for individuals who are blind should reduce dependency and thus contribute to years of active life.

Brummel-Smith (1990) asserts that geriatric rehabilitation is complicated by changes that are both age-related and disease-related. Age-related and disease-related changes can be classified as biological, psychological, and social. *Age-related biological* changes include changes in muscle strength and cardiac and pulmonary function. Exercise capacity may be diminished because of deconditioning, and muscle mass may decrease with age. Normal *age-related psychological changes* may lead to a slower pace of learning and negative views regarding the ability to recover from physical losses. *Social age-related changes* include ageism that may affect the decision of health care professionals to encourage or refer to rehabilitation services.

In addition, Brummel-Smith notes biological, psychological, and social disease-related changes. Disease-related biological changes imply that older people experience multiple diseases that are interactive; consequently, the older person may be treated with multiple medications that may further complicate recovery and rehabilitation. Brummel-Smith notes that "It is a rare patient in geriatric rehabilitation that has only his or her disabling disease with which to contend" (p. 13). Disease-related psychological changes include cognitive and affective problems that are undetected, misdiagnosed, or ignored. In particular, low motivation may be of particular concern (Kemp, 1990). Finally, Brummel-Smith observes that disease-related social changes prevent the older person with a disability from being integrated into society. While, Brummel-Smith says, "Much of the physical and psychologic adaptation to disability is accomplished in the first 2 years after the disabling problem begins. . . . social adaptation must continue throughout a person's lifetime" (p. 14).

In recent years, increased scholarly attention has been given to the issue of geriatric rehabilitation, and that body of knowledge has clear application to the rehabilitation needs of older people experiencing vision impairments (Williams, 1984; Brody & Ruff, 1986; Kemp, Brummel-Smith, & Ramsdell, 1990).

Aging and Vision Loss

Just as the aging population will continue to surge in the coming decades, the number of older people experiencing vision loss will likewise continue to grow. Although the leading causes of blindness among older people—macular degeneration, cataracts, glaucoma, and diabetic retinopathy—are well documented (Rosenbloom, 1992), accurate predictions regarding the extent of this growth is confused because of the variety of studies conducted regarding the prevalence of vision problems. State registers, small-sample studies, and large-sample studies all appear to have undercounted the number of older people experiencing vision loss (Tielsch, Sommer, Witt, & Royall, 1990). The task of acquiring useful data is compounded by problems with definition of vision impairment and the conflict between self-report and clinical data. Nevertheless, two recent studies are promising. Estimates regarding the number and characteristics of older people experiencing vision impairment have been scant until a recent study by the National Center for Health Statistics (NCHS) NHIS 1984 Supplement on Aging (Havlik, 1986) and the Baltimore Eye Study (Tielsch et al., 1990). The NCHS study is characterized by a large sample of self-report functional data on a noninstitutionalized civilian population. The 1984 Supplement on Aging relied on a series of questions to address near, intermediate, and distance vision tasks. Table 14.2 (adapted from Nelson, 1987) reveals reported visual function among age cohorts over the age of 65. Each task becomes increasingly difficult with age. Severe vision impairment, defined as the inability to read newspaper print with best correction, increases from 4.7 percent of the population ages 65–74, to 9.9 percent in the age group 75–84, to 25 percent over the age of 85. Overall, those individuals over the age of 65 reported a severe vision loss prevalence rate of 7.8 percent. This prevalence rate stands in stark contrast to the prevalence rate for younger age groups.

The increasing number of older people experiencing vision loss is driven by the same factors

Table 14.2. Estimated Population of Noninstitutionalized Severely Visually Impaired Persons: United States, 1990

Age	Rate per 1,000 Persons	Number in United States
0–17	1.5	95,410
18–44	3.2	349,350
45–54	13.5	340,510
55–64	28.4	600,600
65–74	59.0	1,068,290
75–84	118.4	1,190,520
85 & over	210.6	648,680
Totals	17.3	4,292,360

Source: Adapted from K. A. Nelson and G. Dimitrova, "Statistical Brief #36: Severe Visual Impairment in the United States and in Each State, 1990," *Journal of Visual Impairment & Blindness,* 87(3) (1993), p. 82.

dictating increases in other age-related disabilities: the number of elders is increasing rapidly, and the most rapid growth is in the ranks of the older old. The combined effect is a surging population.

The most striking observation about vision impairment is the strong correlation to age. Nelson and Dimitrova (1993) recently analyzed the 1977 and CHS and 1984 Supplement on Aging to create age-specific estimates for all age groups in each state. Table 14.3 is adapted from her study, and it reveals that the prevalence of severe vision impairment among children ages 0 to 17 is 1.5 per 1,000; the prevalence increases dramatically with each cohort, and among those over the age of 85, the prevalence rate is 210.6 per 1,000. In other words, out of 2,000 children, 3 would be visually impaired, and out of 2,000 people over age 85, 421 would be severely visually impaired. Other Supplement of Aging studies, as noted before, report slightly higher prevalence rates.

Nelson and Dimitrova's (1993) study reveals that elders over the age of 65 constitute 68 percent of the severely visually impaired population (see also Nelson, 1987). These numbers would increase perhaps by 500,000 if those individuals residing in institutional settings (principally nursing homes) were included in these estimates (Kirchner, 1989, cited in Nelson & Dimitrova, 1993; Kirchner & Peterson, 1980).

Table 14.3 estimates the population of visually impaired elders from 1950 to 2030. These projections are valid to the extent that they do not anticipate medical advances that may reduce vision problems. Nevertheless, in 1950 vision impairment among elders was simply not recognized as a significant public policy issue, in part because of the relatively small numbers involved. Prior to 1970 the largest age cohort was the 65–74 age group. However, by 1980, the 75–84 age group became the largest group experiencing vision impairment, and by 2010, the largest group will be those over the age of 85. By 2030, the population of elders experiencing severe vision impairment is likely to exceed 5.8 million. These demographic shifts become significant because of the increasing likelihood of the onset of other age-related disabilities, need for caregiving, and increasing likelihood of institutionalization.

The Baltimore Eye Study revealed that among younger cohorts, the rates of blindness and visual impairments among African-Americans was twice that of whites, but among older age groups, blindness rates among whites were the same or exceeded those of African-Americans. The study found no difference between blindness and visual impairment by sex (Tielsch et al., 1990).

Moreover, the 1984 Supplement on Aging underscores the grave impact of multiple disabilities among older people experiencing vision impairments. Data from the 1986 preliminary report (see Table 14.4) reveal that people who are visually impaired ages 65–74 are three times more likely to have difficulty walking than their sighted peers. In addition, they are three times more likely to have difficulty getting out of bed or a chair, and they are more than four times more likely to have difficulty getting outside. Although it is understandable that vision impairment may create activity limitations, the NCHS study also shows that among those who are visually impaired, arthritis/

Table 14.3. Prevalence of Severe Vision Impairment for Persons Aged 65 and Over, United States, 1950–2030

Age	1950	1960	1970	1980	1990	2000	2010	2020	2030
65–74	395,500	516,900	585,000	732,300	863,500	857,400	988,800	1,455,700	1,691,400
75–84	324,500	458,700	606,300	765,200	983,400	1,189,700	1,208,600	1,429,900	2,127,200
85+	144,300	232,300	353,300	560,000	813,500	1,155,500	1,528,800	1,662,800	2,032,300
Total	864,300	1,207,900	1,544,600	2,057,500	2,660,400	3,202,600	3,726,200	4,548,400	5,850,900

Sources: Data from U.S. Select Committee on Aging, *Aging America: Trends and Projections, 1991 Edition* (Washington, DC: U.S. Select Committee on Aging, 1991), p. 7. K. A. Nelson, "Statistical Brief #35: Visual Impairment Among Elderly Americans: Statistics in Transition," *Journal of Visual Impairment & Blindness,* 81 (1987), pp. 81–82. J. E. Crews, "The Demographic, Social and Conceptual Contexts of Aging and Vision Loss," *Journal of the American Optometric Association,* 65 (1994), p. 64.

Table 14.4. Limitations and Conditions Reported for Individuals Ages 65–74 and Over Age 85 Who Experience Visual Impairments

	65–74 Years		85+ Years	
	No Visual Impairment	Visual Impairment	No Visual Impairment	Visual Impairment
Difficulty walking	12.3	33.1	39.0	52.9
Difficulty getting outside	4.4	18.4	28.9	46.2
Difficulty getting in & out of bed or chair	5.8	17.8	19.3	24.4
Arthritis or rheumatism	49.2	66.8	53.3	57.1
Cardiovascular disease	11.3	27.9	25.0	45.0
Hypertension	42.6	55.1	39.7	54.6

Source: Reprinted, by permission of the publisher, from R. J. Havlik, "Aging in the Eighties, Impaired Senses for Sound and Light in Persons Age 65 and over: Preliminary Data from the Supplement on Aging to the National Health Interview Survey: United States, January–June, 1984," *Advance Data, 125* (1986), p. 4.

rheumatism, cardiovascular disease, and hypertension demonstrate significantly greater prevalence. Those elders over the age of 85 experiencing vision loss also report greater activity limitations and a greater prevalence of rates of arthritis/rheumatism, cardiovascular disease, and hypertension than their sighted peers.

Normal aging and disability among elders create important frames for the issue of vision loss among elders. As people get older, various social changes typically characterize aging; that is, widowhood, decreased economic status, and shifts in caregiving roles are relatively normal changes. Disability is not a normal part of aging, but disability becomes increasingly common. Normal changes to the eye, including the cornea, lens, and vitreous are to be expected, and they have the effect of degrading vision, but severe vision loss cannot be dismissed as normal (see Mancil & Owsley, 1988).

For the most part, people who are older and visually impaired are people who have grown up, reared their children, worked, and retired as sighted people. It is in or near retirement that they have lost their vision. The circumstances of an older person experiencing vision impairment becomes increasingly complex if vision loss is accompanied by other age-related physical and psychosocial changes. The combined effect of these changes have the potential to dramatically complicate the rehabilitation process.

THE PRACTICE OF O&M AMONG ELDERS

Very little rigorous research has addressed travel habits among older people who are visually impaired. Generally, the available research confirms that older people experience travel restrictions (Ponchillia & Kaarlela, 1986) and are less likely to travel independently than their sighted peers (Havlik, 1986). Often these travel restrictions appear correlated with other psychosocial limitations (Branch, Horowitz, & Carr, 1989; Gillman, Simmel, & Simon, 1986), as one would probably expect. Straw, Harley, and Zimmerman (1991) noted the lack of valid and reliable testing instruments for older people who are visually impaired, and they proposed the development of a more standardized curriculum that recognized the great variability of the population. Of particular concern to the older student and the O&M specialist is the increased likelihood of falls that older people often experience (LaGrow & Blasch, 1992). Although considerable attention has been given to falls in the literature on aging (see Connell, 1987), research among older visually impaired individuals is sparse. Researchers recognize that falls are a complex phenomenon resulting from the potential interaction of biological (Connell, 1987; Gerson, Jarjoura, & McCord, 1989) and environmental (Long, 1992) characteristics.

A recent study by Long, Boyette, and Griffin-Shirley (1996) compared a small group ($n = 32$) of older visually impaired people with a small group ($n = 28$) of older sighted people living in the community. These two groups were compared on demographic characteristics and travel habits. The group of visually impaired older people reported higher levels of depression than their sighted peers (see Horowitz, 1995), and they demonstrated significantly different travel patterns than the older sighted group. While 14 percent of older sighted people reported that they never traveled outside of their house or yard during the past year, 44 percent of older visually impaired people reported *no* such travel. Moreover, while 79 percent of older people reported they were somewhat or very satisfied with their ability to travel independently, only 42 percent of older visually impaired people reported similar levels of satisfaction. Finally, 86 percent of older sighted people reported they were somewhat or very satisfied with "the number of opportunities to leave home alone or accompanied," and only 50 percent of older visually impaired people provided the same response.

The most dramatic findings of this study revealed the powerful effect of the presence of sidewalks on travel: of the visually impaired group, those "individuals with access to sidewalks were 13 times mores likely to travel than those without sidewalks" (p. 319). In addition, the duration of vision loss also presented a powerful effect: the researchers noted that those having a "longer than median duration of loss" reported more frequent travel than individuals with "shorter duration of loss" (p. 319). This small sample study also revealed that older visually impaired people traveled alone infrequently, and although the "number of destinations in the week prior to the interview" did not differ between the visually impaired group and the sighted group, those with visual impairments reported they "were significantly less satisfied with the number of opportunities they had to leave their home."

Just as the goals and circumstances among elders may differ widely, teaching methods are likely to differ as well. The O&M objectives of the vital, independent, highly motivated 65-year-old may not differ significantly from the objectives of a 35-year-old, and in fact the methods of instruction may not differ at all. Similarly, the objectives and instructional methods of teaching someone who is 80, is experiencing multiple impairments, and has modest travel goals would be very different.

Adapting O&M instruction for older people involves paying attention to the following four broad issues:

- assessment of function
- collaboration with the student and the rehabilitation team
- relevance of instruction to the student's needs
- modification of instruction in response to the individual's health and circumstances

Assessment addresses the following areas: review of available medical or rehabilitation information, quality and size of social networks, an interview with the client regarding travel objectives and interest, and observation of ambulation in representative environments (indoors, residential, and small business). Assessment should result in a plan encompassing content, sequence, pace, and length of training. It may be advisable to conduct assessment activities along routes the older person intends to travel following training in order to build interest in the training process.

Client self-report is not always reliable, and therefore the practitioner may need to place more weight on observation than the interview. Some clients may underestimate their ability to perform specific tasks, or they may be surprised that O&M training deals with a broad range of travel activities. It is helpful to discuss the results of the assessment process in order to continue with the collaborative approach to individualization.

The responsibility of the O&M practitioner is to assess each student's personal characteristics, needs, and desires in order to create a relevant educational experience. In order to establish individualized services, the instructor must work in collaboration with the student and family members to create relevant, jointly identified goals. The assessment process reveals areas for modification and defines the emphasis, pace, and sequence of instruction. As the student increases competence as a traveler, significant others can be involved to support and encourage implementation of new skills.

Collaboration refers to instituting a routine of sharing information and making joint decisions with the student. The goal of collaboration is to provide both instructor and student an opportunity to influence the other. Approaching older students in this manner indicates the practitioner is intent upon demonstrating respect, understanding, and empathy throughout the teaching process.

Collaboration also refers to the teamwork approach existing between the O&M instructor and other professionals involved in treating other health or psychosocial concerns. Collaboration may determine the effects of medications on the student's alertness, coordination, balance, or reasoning ability. Collaboration may also address social support and social integration concerns. Potential collaborators include physicians, nurses, social service providers, spouse, or family members.

Attention to *relevance* is necessary to ensure that training provides solutions for practical problems experienced in daily life. Adjustments can be made in presentation, emphasis, pace, and sequencing of instruction to ensure that suitability for individual circumstances is maintained. Relevance should be a natural outgrowth of the collaborative approach.

Modification, defined as tailoring the instruction to meet the unique needs of individuals, is at the heart of the individualized instructional process. Deficits in health, balance, coordination, physical strength or endurance, psychosocial or emotional well-being, or cognitive performance are examples of factors that lead to modifying training. Other factors to be considered include amount and type of vision, living situation (alone or with family), and type of home environment.

CASE HISTORIES

Mrs. Q

Mrs. Q was a 63-year-old widow living alone in a mobile home on her property in a rural area 25 miles from the nearest metropolitan area. She cared for her disabled mother, who lived next door. Mrs. Q's vision impairment was caused by age-related macular degeneration. Her visual acuity was 20/200 in the right eye and "count fingers at face" in the left eye.

In addition to her vision problems, Mrs. Q experienced multiple impairments, including bilateral hearing loss with a hearing aid for the right ear, hypertension, hypothyroidism, occasional dizziness and headaches, a 30-year history of hypoglycemia, chronic abdominal pain with history of surgery for intestinal obstructions, and cardiac tachycardia and dysrhythmia. In addition, clinical reports indicated she had fallen several times; she had experienced a vertebral disk problem 3 months prior to the beginning of training as a result of a fall from her porch steps. During the interview, she explained that she had a broken toe on her left foot, and she was on medication for pain. Mrs. Q reported difficulties with arthritis, mainly in her right knee and hand.

During the assessment interview, Mrs. Q reported the following mobility problems: falls, contacts with objects while moving, problems maintaining straight-line travel, difficulties with level-change detection and step-edge detection, unreliable depth perception, variations in visual acuity in the presence of rapid lighting changes, disorientation in unfamiliar areas, and uncertainty regarding timing and safety of street crossings. She described regular use of NoIR 40 percent amber shades for outdoor travel. Transportation was provided by her mother and occasionally by a sister-in-law.

Mrs. Q stated the following mobility goals: attainment of independent movement on her own property; recreational walking in her home rural area; access to an alternate form of transportation; independent travel in residential; semibusiness, and business areas; and independent travel at her church. She was especially concerned about negotiating the steep steps to her church basement. She was highly motivated for training, and she realized she needed to improve the safety and effectiveness of her ambulation in order to maintain her independence at home. Mrs. Q expressed concern about the possibility of institutionalization if she could not do her own shopping and housekeeping.

Collaboration involved the O&M specialist and the client, as well as the primary physician. Mrs. Q's doctor recommended exercise, especially walking, in order to maintain control of her cardiac and hypoglycemic problems. Assurances were given to the O&M instructor that Mrs. Q's medical treatment would be enhanced by the opportunity for exercise on a regular basis. Drug interactions were ruled out. Mrs. Q and the O&M specialist carried hard candy on all lessons; the O&M instructor also carried a tube of glucose gel.

Relevance of training was addressed by the referral source; Mrs. Q and her rehabilitation counselor both agreed that comprehensive O&M training was required for her to remain in her home and continue to care for her mother. Mrs. Q recognized that O&M training was relevant to her well-being.

Assessment took the form of an extensive interview, conducted during the first visit. Observational portions of the assessment were conducted in small increments at subsequent meetings to limit physical exertion. Assessment revealed both need and capacity for a comprehensive O&M training program.

Modification involved adjustments primarily in presentation, pace, and sequence. Fairly equal emphasis was placed on all outdoor skills because of the comprehensive nature of Mrs. Q's stated goals. Skills modifications included extensive use of a modified (constant contact) touch technique combined with support cane use during all outdoor travel.

Presentation was enhanced by modeling techniques demonstrated by the instructor. Mrs. Q acknowledged the need to use two canes because of her difficulties with ambulation, and she expressed misgivings about the appearance of using two canes at once. Following description and demonstration of techniques, the O&M specialist continued to model use of a support cane and long cane while observing and correcting Mrs. Q's performance, providing a positive role model and decreasing feelings of self-consciousness. Presenting the same appearance as the client during training proved to be a successful teaching technique.

In addition, lessons were scheduled during temperate weather. In spring, midday lessons were appropriate, in order to avoid the coolness of early morning. As the training program continued into mid- to late summer, lesson times in the early morning or evening became necessary, in order to avoid exposure to extreme heat. The best time for lessons changed again in the early fall.

Pace was dictated by the client's variable strength and endurance. Due to Mrs. Q's health problems, lesson times were variable in length, according to her physical capabilities on a given day. Relatively more time was spent developing safe and effective travel techniques on her difficult-to-negotiate graded gravel country lane than on technique development on smoother nearby county roads where ambulation was less difficult. As Mrs. Q gained physical strength and endurance, the pace of instruction expanded to approximate that of a normal lesson.

Sequence was initially dictated by the demands of Mrs. Q's home environment. The skills required for her to negotiate her front steps, her home property, and the narrow gravel lane leading to her mother's house were covered first. Travel to the end of the country lane to her mailbox came next. After that, travel techniques appropriate for negotiating and crossing paved county roads were presented. Residential sidewalk travel, residential street crossings, and traffic-light–controlled street crossings were presented in a series of lessons conducted in the nearest metropolitan area. Shopping-area lessons were provided in malls and in retail stores. Finally, several night lessons were conducted both in the student's home area and in the nearest urban area.

Mrs. Q's family remained unsupportive of her desire to remain independent; therefore, she took steps to build a nonfamily support network from the community. Involvement of significant others was limited to coaching Mrs. Q on how to educate members of her primary support group, her local church. Mrs. Q learned to enlist the assistance of sighted guides when necessary and to instruct them in proper guiding behaviors. She also learned how to solicit information using a combination of open and closed questions and how to direct others to assist her. Mrs. Q used her increased independence to seek out referral sources for additional services. Access to a rural transportation service and the skills to safely and successfully take advantage of transportation resources were the keys to maintaining independence on her own terms.

Mrs. R

Mrs. R was a 73-year-old woman who lived with her husband in a quiet rural residential area approximately six blocks from the business district of her small hometown. Her O&M training program was remarkable for a repeated pattern of increased independence followed by adverse health events, reassessment, and further training under more limiting circumstances. Although instruction involved fewer than 50 sessions, O&M training played a significant role in maintaining her quality of life.

File information, confirmed at the initial interview, revealed the following: Mrs. R's original visual diagnosis was age-related macular degeneration affecting both eyes. In addition, the right eye had been enucleated following an acute episode of closed-angle glaucoma. She had suffered one stroke; 21 transient ischemic attacks were documented over the previous 2 years, putting her at risk for some dementia-like symptoms. Hearing loss was present, as well as spinal arthritis. Slow blood clotting due to blood thinners was indicated in her records, and she experienced occasional dizziness upon rising from a stationary sitting position. Telephone consultation with Mrs. R's physician confirmed Mrs. R's ability to participation in rehabilitation activities, as long as she did not overtire.

Relevance was established through a collaborative approach to assessment and goal setting. During the initial interview, Mrs. R indicated she was afraid of falling, especially on her front steps, and she frequently experienced problems with object contacts indoors on her blind side. Although Mrs. R had a collapsible long cane, she displayed no effective or systematic techniques for negotiating steps and stairs or for protection from bumping into objects; therefore an immediate introduction to appropriate techniques was initiated. Diagonal cane technique was recommended to address difficulties with object contacts in her home, and Mrs. R was informed that a variant of diagonal technique would help with the negotiation of steps and stairs.

Orientation was not a problem indoors, but outdoors, Mrs. R had difficulty maintaining orientation because of ineffective scanning and general anxiety regarding ambulation. She displayed no systematic method for using the long cane to clear outdoor walking surfaces or maintain proper rural travel positioning. A brief demonstration of the modified, constant contact, touch technique ended assessment activities on a positive note.

As a result of the demonstration of using two canes, Mrs. R expressed optimism regarding her ability to learn long cane techniques for indoor and outdoor travel. Her stated mobility goals included accompanied but physically independent travel in unfamiliar places, rural residential travel, sidewalk travel, travel in the nearby small business area of her hometown, and home neighborhood walking for exercise and recreation.

Mrs. R's primary caregiver, her husband, was present during the interview portion of assessment. He expressed reservations about her ability to learn, based upon his observation of her decreased memory. Because Mr. R frequently answered questions directed to his wife, he was asked to remain in the home during the outdoor portion of the assessment. His absence gave Mrs. R an opportunity to speak more freely; she regarded Mr. R's behavior as well-intentioned but overprotective. She acknowledged experiencing decreased memory after her strokes, but asserted she was confident that with repetition and practice, she could learn techniques for safe and independent travel in her home area. Her high motivation made her an excellent candidate for rehabilitation.

The instructor modified the training program to adjust presentation including a deliberate attempt to build structure and repetition into the training program. Skills, with an obvious application in the home area, were emphasized in a carefully planned sequence. Training began inside the home and progressed to walking on the home property, then to accompanied travel in Mrs. R's quiet, rural residential neighborhood. Training culminated in sidewalk travel to and alongside a nearby busy county road. Pace was leisurely and established by client, and the pace increased as Mrs. R expressed a willingness to apply independent application of skills. She was eventually able to travel six blocks to her neighborhood grocery store while the instructor and her husband followed behind. Mrs. R and her husband were both surprised to find that she was able to hear well enough to make parallel traffic street crossings alongside a busy county road leading to the grocery store.

Involvement of Mrs. R's significant others played a key role in the success of her training program. Her husband was clearly overprotective at the beginning of training, but Mrs. R had a daughter living in town and a son living out of town who were supportive and telephoned encouragement to her frequently. After Mrs. R demonstrated her ability to travel safely and effectively in her home neighborhoods, Mr. R became enthusiastic about her progress and participated willingly in subsequent phases of training.

Soon after mastering the residential and semibusiness travel skills required to travel to the grocery store, Mrs. R suffered another acute glaucoma episode, resulting in total blindness. Following a brief reassessment demonstrating that further training could lead to increased independence, work on indoor techniques began again. A careful review of sighted guide procedures was followed by practice with hand trailing, protective techniques, and familiarization and self-familiarization procedures.

While regaining confidence in her ability to move about, Mrs. R needed a slower pace and opportunities for much repetition. Continuing outdoor travel became irrelevant until confidence regarding indoor travel was regained.

Because diagonal cane technique was not displayed in a consistent, accurate, and disciplined manner in this phase of training, constant contact touch technique and touch trailing were used for travel within the home. In addition, much time was dedicated to instructing Mr. R as an appropriate guide. Within a shorter period of time than Mrs. R or her family expected, she was once again ready to begin outdoor rural residential training.

However, Mrs. R suffered yet another stroke, resulting in severe memory problems and spatial disorientation in her home. Assessment took the form of room-by-room examination, in order to find any area of the home where rudimentary spatial orientation existed. At the beginning of this cycle of training, Mrs. R was best oriented in her kitchen. Training was highly structured and highly repetitive, with familiarization to the entire house carefully linked to the success experienced in the kitchen. During this sequence of lessons, the O&M instructor taught Mr. R to serve as his wife's mobility coach to maintain gains in function. A significant amount of time was devoted to teaching Mr. R how to evaluate Mrs. R's performance in the home, especially in deciding when and how to intervene during her attempts to orient and walk about the home independently.

Transfer of responsibility from the instructor to the primary caregiver was accomplished in small increments over an extended period of time; the effectiveness with which Mr. R directed Mrs. R's travel steadily increased throughout these training sessions. Mr. R's training initially took the form of observing how to supervise safe movement, progressed through a sequence of lessons in which the instructor actively supervised Mr. R's direction of movement activities, and culminated in observation of a few sessions in which Mr. R demonstrated his comfort in directing Mrs. R's movement along familiar routes inside the home. Factors that were emphasized included the use of positive reinforcement, the advantages of establishing a structured routine, the necessity of approaching recognizable landmarks from the same direction, and the need for persistence in daily practice sessions. Mr. R became quite proficient in his role of mobility coach. A variant of the sighted guide procedure allowed Mr. R to give both physical support and guidance to his wife .

Some supervised use of the long cane during walks up and down the R family driveway helped to increase physical strength and stamina. Throughout this stage of training Mrs. R's physician had continued to advise an appropriate level of activity to aid in health maintenance.

Just as Mr. and Mrs. R were beginning to feel comfortable with their new routine, Mrs. R experienced a final catastrophic setback. One evening while Mr. R was reading in an adjacent room, Mrs. R fell from her bed, breaking her hip and setting in motion a cascade of events that resulted in her death less than 3 weeks after the fall.

Mrs. R's case serves to illustrate the necessity of successive training opportunities for people who experience decreasing function. In order to effectively provide services, the professional must reassess on a case-by-case basis, set relevant goals, involve significant others, and maintain as much independent functioning as possible. Providing additional services is a much more attractive option than defaulting to further loss of function, which may eventually result in institutionalization.

Mrs. R's case also illustrates one approach to dealing with elders with dementia who require O&M training. A careful assessment may indicate capabilities for limited or supervised independent movement in specific environments even if a great deal of independence is impossible. Caregivers may be trained to give the kind of support that Mr. R gave to his wife. In these cases, painstaking care should be given to assessment, and the practitioner should introduce O&M skills that the older person experiencing dementia is capable of learning or of practicing under supervision. The O&M specialist should teach applicable techniques to the student's greatest level of capacity, then transfer responsibility for maintaining those skills to the primary caregivers. As with Mr. R, this circumstance may involve teaching how to maintain skills, followed by observation of the mobility coach interacting with the client. Because dementia is typically a progressive disorder, the O&M professional should anticipate the necessity for several sequences of training and should expect to be available for consultation with caregivers.

Mr. T

Mr. T was a 74-year-old man with no significant medical problems other than a moderate hearing loss in the right ear. His visual impairment was caused by age-related macular degeneration. Mr. T lived with his wife in a single-family dwelling in a quiet, completely sidewalked 20-block residential area containing many four-way stops. Mr. T's wife served as his primary transportation, with occasional rides available from friends or from a son who lived 115 miles away. City bus transportation was unavailable in Mr. T's hometown.

Mr. T participated in a comprehensive residential blind rehabilitation program. Assessment began with discussions regarding problems encountered during ambulation. Mr. T reported difficulties with below-the-knee object contacts, negotiation of unexpected steps and gradients, level change (upcurb and downcurb) detection, depth perception, orientation in unfamiliar areas, and safe timing of street crossings.

Observation of the client's travel along unfamiliar routes in indoor, residential, and business areas confirmed Mr. T's concerns, and helped ensure the creation of relevant goals for training. Through further discussion, Mr. T elected to participate in a complete O&M training program. He chose to include bus travel and independent travel lessons in order to build confidence.

Mr. T required no significant modifications to his O&M training in the areas of presentation, emphasis, or pace. Because Mr. T was a physically active man whose main concern was outdoor travel, sequence was modified in order to present business-area travel skills as early as possible in the training sequence, followed by residential, rural residential, small business, and bus travel training. This arrangement enabled Mr. T to travel safely and effectively to nearby restaurants in the urban environment surrounding the training facility. The modifications had more to do with individualizing the educational program according to special interests and preferences than with accommodating age-related needs.

Near the end of training, Mr. T's wife came to the rehabilitation center to observe Mr. T in all areas of his rehabilitation training. She observed Mr. T travel via city bus to an incorrect destination in a busy urban business district, realize his mistake, reorient, and locate the selected destination, all while maintaining effective environmental awareness and safety skills. In addition, Mrs. T received training in sighted guide technique and in direction-giving, as well as acquiring information about the functional implications of her husband's eye condition.

Mr. T's O&M program did not differ appreciably from the way in which training would be offered any reasonably healthy adult. He participated in 9 weeks of training, 2 hours per day, 5 days per week. The level of skills attainment achieved by Mr. T indicated that he had reached the O&M training goals outlined in his rehabilitation plan; more important, however, he expressed his satisfaction with his increased ability to travel in familiar and unfamiliar environments.

PRESENTATION AND PACE OF INSTRUCTION

Presentation of instruction should be sensitive to educational and cultural factors. Presentation encompasses specific teaching techniques, such as description, demonstration, shaping, or modeling of skills. In addition, particular requirements of individual learners, such as the need for rest breaks, structure, or repetition, should be addressed as well as attention to the best time of day for lessons and the need for slow and distinctive speech.

Pace refers to matching the tempo of instruction to the client's speed of learning. Specific lessons may be divided into "mini-courses" in order to achieve the goal of consistent, accurate, and disciplined level of performance.

The sequence of instruction may be altered to address areas of extreme interest first, even if this strategy is not completely congruent with the traditional approach of progressing from simple to complex environments. It is possible to progress in an orderly fashion from familiar to unfamiliar areas, from simple skills to more complex skills, from active familiarization to self-familiarization, and from accompanied to independent travel, even in areas of moderate to high complexity. When the training program is viewed as a process, rather than as a rigidly sequenced experience, opportunities occur to be flexible without sacrificing quality. A valid approach begins training in areas of high interest, even if initial attempts to travel effectively are not entirely successful. These experiences, given proper follow-up, can lead to interest in developing the underlying skills required to complete the process.

For example, consider the mature student who lives in an urban area and has a keen interest in learning to walk two blocks and crossing busy streets at traffic-light–controlled intersections in order to shop for groceries. This student might be well served by a training sequence that introduces the particular skills required to accomplish this route, encourages practice of those skills until they are mastered, and then extends the application of those skills into new, perhaps unfamiliar, areas. Aspects of traveling the route that present problems indicate areas requiring skills development and practice. Development, generalization, and transfer of a relatively complete subset of skills can therefore be initiated as an organized instructional unit. The student gains valuable skills, accomplishes a specific, relevant, and high-interest task, and becomes encouraged to invest in further training, thus creating a pattern of success.

The practitioner must also assess the older student's social environment to identify appropriate friends and family to involve in the training program. In supportive cases, involvement may be productive in the early stages of training. For situations in which significant others may discourage risk taking, involvement may occur after rehabilitation gains have been achieved. In any case, it is necessary that family members understand the importance of encouraging and supporting behaviors to maintain independence.

Activities that can promote effective involvement of significant others include training in basic skills, observation of the O&M student's independent functioning in various environments, use of low vision simulation experiences, and observation of other students at beginning, intermediate, and advanced stages of training.

CONCLUSION

It is likely that O&M professionals will encounter greater numbers of older people as rehabilitation organizations respond to increases in the numbers of elders experiencing vision loss. This increased exposure will expand and perhaps test the capacity of O&M instructors to respond to the complex, fluid needs of older people.

In all probability, as the population of older people increases, there will be increasing demands from consumers for organizations and professionals to respond to their particular needs. The consumer of the new millennium will be different from, and probably more demanding than, previous generations. Therefore, it is important to recognize and embrace the changes in consumer expectations.

Older consumers as a group present great variability in terms of health, social and economic circumstances, and expectations for rehabilitation outcomes. Age alone is not a reliable predictor of rehabilitation services or rehabilitation outcomes. Much of the hallmark of rehabilitation services—the individualized rehabilitation plan—remains applicable to older people. While elders may report multiple age-related health conditions, most will continue to remain productive and generally report positive health well into their 70s. For others, their health may decline or caregiving responsibilities may take a toll.

Rehabilitation professionals need to respond to the great variety presented by older people. For some, travel goals and training techniques will be much like those for young travelers. These individuals may have ambitious goals for independent travel in the community and unfamiliar environments. For others, travel goals will be more modest. The neighborhood and familiar environments will define their travel objectives to a large extent. Others may have very limited goals that may be defined by the home or institution.

Each student in each of these circumstances is worthy, and each student benefits from the therapeutic effect that increased travel skills produce. The aim of O&M instructors for serving older people is the same as for any consumer—to recognize the strengths and goals of each individual, and respond to those needs in a way that enhances choice, dignity, control, and quality of life.

Suggestions/Implications for O&M Specialists

1. The O&M specialist must recognize that older people who experience visual impairments represent a heterogeneous population, and age and etiology does not predict their rehabilitation needs.
2. The overwhelming majority of people experiencing vision impairments are older people. Some 2.7 million older people experience severe vision impairment; this population will grow to nearly 6 million by the year 2030. Rehabilitation agencies and consequently O&M specialists will be increasingly called upon to serve older people.
3. Because of the composition of the older population, there will be increasing demands to provide rehabilitation services to older women. Because the support systems for older people are so fragile, achieving meaningful rehabilitation outcomes becomes increasingly important since other support systems may not be available.
4. The study by Fulton and Katz (1986) makes a powerful case for the importance of preserving years of productivity. It is important for the O&M professional to be actively engaged in achieving rehabilitation outcomes that preserve these years of productivity.
5. The 1986 Havlik study demonstrates the increased limitation and greater numbers of health conditions associated with vision loss. The O&M specialist must be aware of these potential implications as rehabilitation programs are designed for older people.
6. It is important for O&M specialists to recognize the important value of individualized planning that responds to the particular needs of the consumer, rather than standard lesson plans that may have no meaning to the consumer's circumstances.
7. The concept of small gains remains critical in rehabilitation services among older people. Modest gains in capacity may create great gains in self-esteem and a sense of control. The O&M specialist must champion the concept of small gains in the presentation of instruction.

ACTIVITIES FOR REVIEW

1. As an O&M instructor, you receive a referral for a 78-year-old man who lives with his wife and is diagnosed with macular degeneration. What do you believe these pieces of information tell you about the rehabilitation program you might wish to provide?
2. Increasingly, consumers direct their own rehabilitation programs. How might you go about convincing an older person to undertake the risks of learning new skills, if the individual were not particularly inclined to take risks?
3. Beyond the obvious functional implications associated with vision loss among older people, what policy issues do you believe are likely to become increasingly important in the coming decades?
4. Review Table 14.4 (Havlik, 1986). Given the pattern of multiple health conditions and secondary health conditions associated with aging and vision loss, how might you alter your approaches to providing O&M instruction when serving older people with visual impairments?
5. Given the circumstances of older people, what special consideration might you suggest for providing instruction when it particularly hot or cold outside?
6. Describe the potential strategies for involving family members in a rehabilitation program. What happens when family members are controlling or too pessimistic?
7. For many older people, the loss of vision leads to a severe attack upon self-esteem. What strategies might you employ to address this concern?
8. In the case histories, the account of Mrs. R ends with her death. Given the goals of rehabilitation and the expectation of independence, how would you justify the effort involved in providing O&M services?
9. Given what you have read in this chapter, describe the potential benefits of rehabilitation teams working with older people.
10. Many residents of nursing homes experience vision loss as well as other health problems. What are some potential changes in the environment (light, glare, color) that might be made to a nursing home to make it more accessible for an older person with vision loss?

CHAPTER 15

Learners with Visual and Physical Impairments

Sandra Rosen

Many people with visual impairments have medical conditions, either related or unrelated to their visual impairment, that limit their ability to walk or to walk without assistance. These conditions fall into three categories: (1) chronic health impairments (e.g., heart conditions, respiratory conditions, circulatory conditions), (2) neurological impairments (e.g., brain injury, spinal cord injury), and (3) orthopedic impairments (e.g., arthritis, amputations).

CHRONIC HEALTH IMPAIRMENTS

In general, chronic health impairments do not affect one's ability to walk, but can affect one's endurance in walking. For this reason, some people with chronic health impairments may use a wheelchair in situations that involve a lot of walking (e.g., traveling in shopping malls, going to the corner post office).

Chronic health impairments include heart diseases commonly seen in the elderly, such as angina pectoris (a condition characterized by decreased circulation to the heart muscle and episodes of chest pains during overexertion), and congestive heart disease (weakening of the heart muscle and the heart's ability to pump blood). These conditions often impair the heart's ability keep up with the increased circulatory demands of exercise. People with these conditions generally limit their physical activity; some may use a wheelchair if they need to travel long distances. In the latter instance, the wheelchair is generally pushed by another person, because manually propelling a wheelchair actually places even greater physical demands on the heart than does walking.

Common lung diseases such as emphysema (which causes shortness of breath when overexerting) also limit a person's ability to exercise. People with severe emphysema may also use a wheelchair (again, propelled by another person) for traveling long distances.

An example of a circulatory problem that can limit a person's ability to walk long distances is one called intermittent claudication. This condition is characterized by an inability of the circulatory system to pump sufficient blood (into the legs, for example) to keep up with the muscles' metabolic needs when exercising. With this condition, a person may experience leg pain when walking long distances; therefore a person who is subject to intermittent claudication might not need an ambulatory aid when walking short distances, but would perhaps use a wheelchair to travel longer distances.

NEUROLOGICAL IMPAIRMENTS

Neurological impairments are those that affect the brain or spinal cord or both. Two common neurological conditions that involve the brain include cerebral palsy and acquired brain injury. Cerebral palsy generally occurs prenatally, at birth, or during the first few years of life and is caused by damage to the motor areas of the brain. Depending on the parts of the brain involved, it can be characterized by a wide variety of motor problems including impaired coordination; impaired balance; excessively high, low, or fluctuating muscle tone; and in some cases, impaired sensation. Acquired brain injury can have the same motor effects as cerebral palsy and generally occurs as a result of trauma (e.g., auto accident, gunshot wounds), or medical conditions (e.g., stroke, meningitis, tumor). In addition, people with cerebral palsy or acquired brain injury may have additional impairments in vision, speech, language, and learning ability. When balance is impaired due to neurological impairment, people will often use ambulatory aids for assistance in getting around.

Common conditions affecting the spinal cord include spina bifida (a failure of the spinal cord to form completely at birth) and spinal cord injury due to trauma (e.g., accidents) or medical conditions (e.g., polio, tumors). When the spinal cord is injured, the muscles normally controlled by the injured portion of the spinal cord can be either significantly weakened or paralyzed. Sensation below the level of injury is also affected in some conditions. Many people with spinal cord injuries use ambulatory aids when their balance is impaired due to weakened or paralyzed muscles.

ORTHOPEDIC IMPAIRMENTS

Common orthopedic impairments include arthritis and amputations. With regard to arthritis, there are two general categories—rheumatoid arthritis and osteoarthritis. Rheumatoid arthritis is an autoimmune process that can affect children as well as adults, causing pain and damage to affected joints. Osteoarthritis is more commonly seen in adults and generally results from long-term wear and tear on the joints (most often the hips and knees). People with arthritis may use ambulatory aids to either reduce the stress of weight bearing on affected joints, or to assist with balance when muscle strength or joint stability or both are decreased due to the long-term effects of the disease.

Amputations are sometimes performed on people whose limbs have been irreparably damaged as a result of trauma (e.g., auto accident), or who suffer medical conditions that would threaten their lives if the affected limb is not amputated. Such medical conditions include diabetes mellitus, in which a pressure sore that fails to heal can potentially cause blood poisoning, and bone cancer, in which the cancer might spread to other parts of the body if the affected limb is not amputated. Following a partial or complete leg amputation, people are often fitted with prostheses and many are able to walk without ambulatory aids. Others may use aids if they are unable to walk with sufficient balance using the prosthesis, or if they need to limit stress on the remaining portion of the limb while walking.

AMBULATORY AIDS

Some people with the conditions just described rely on ambulatory aids for physical support to move in their environments. Ambulatory aids include wheelchairs, orthopedic canes, crutches, and walkers. While a wheelchair may not be an "ambulatory" aid in the strictest sense of the word, it does provide some people with ambulation difficulties a means of mobility, and in that regard it can also be considered an ambulatory aid.

While the term *ambulatory aids,* in its broadest sense, can be used to include a number of devices that are prescribed for very specific purposes, such as scooters and medically prescribed strollers, most devices fall into four common categories: wheelchairs, walkers, crutches, and canes. Although this chapter cannot provide a comprehensive treatment of the topic of ambulatory aids, it provides an overview of devices that are commonly used by people who, because of physical impairments, require physical support for mobility. It also provides information on the proper use and care of these aids, as well as on the use of ambulatory aids in conjunction with orientation and mobility (O&M) skills for people with visual impairments. In general, people use wheelchairs when they are unable to walk or when they have limited endurance in walking. Others, who need physical support to walk, may use walkers, crutches, or canes. The choice of aids depends upon several factors such as the person's medical condition, the terrain to be traversed, social situations, or even the person's level of fatigue on a given day. Some people may even use a variety of aids over time if their physical condition is such that they either experience an improvement as a result of healing or the benefits of therapy, or experience a decrease in function due to the effects of a progressive disorder.

There are three basic elements of travel for all people, whether sighted or visually impaired, ambulatory or not. They are orientation, the negotiation of obstacles in the travel path, and the detection and avoidance of hazards. Inherent in these elements are factors such as safety, quality, and efficiency of movement. However, for the individual who is visually impaired in addition to needing an ambulatory aid, there are special and unique considerations for support as well as environmental preview. In reviewing each type of mobility aid, the author will focus on the standard uses of each aid as well as modifications to the aid, or its use, to enable the user to safely and efficiently negotiate the environment when vision is impaired. Although the approaches presented by no means represent the entire spectrum of possibilities or even mobility skills, it is hoped that they will stimulate thought and creative approaches to mobility for users of ambulatory aids who have visual impairments.

Wheelchairs

There are many different types of wheelchairs, from standard models to models especially designed for extra physical support, to "sport" models designed for speed. There are even wheelchairs specifically designed for racing. Some wheelchairs are manually propelled (commonly referred to as "manual" wheelchairs), others are motorized (commonly called "electric" wheelchairs) (see Figure 15.1). All wheelchairs should be individually measured and prescribed for the user in order to provide proper support and maximum efficiency of movement. In addition, depending on the user's physical abilities and needs, wheelchairs can be equipped with special features such as extended headrests (for people who require head support), extended footrests (for people who must keep one or both legs elevated), anti-tip bars that prevent the wheelchair from tipping over backwards, removable armrests, and wheel adaptations (for people who can use only one arm or who are unable to grasp the hand rim easily when propelling a manual wheelchair). In addition, there are a number of accessories that can be special ordered to make the use of wheelchairs safer and easier. Such accessories include wheelchair trays and baskets to hold items, specially designed brakes that prevent wheelchairs from rolling backward unexpectedly on inclines, and anti-tip bars. Accessories and aids can generally be purchased at medical supply stores.

Manual wheelchairs are propelled when the user pushes forward or pulls backward on the metal rims attached to the big wheels. By grasping both left and right rims simultaneously and pushing forward or pulling backward an equal amount, one moves in a straight line. By pushing more on one rim than the other, or pushing one forward while pulling the other backward, one can turn the wheelchair. Manual wheelchairs can also be maneuvered easily by another person over level ground and curbs. Procedures for maneuvering a manual wheelchair in various environments are outlined in Sidebar 15.1.

Motorized wheelchairs are most commonly used by people who lack the endurance or upper arm strength to propel a wheelchair manually or for those who travel long distances. Some people also prefer them because they require almost no physical effort to propel. Motorized wheelchairs consist of a sturdy wheelchair frame with a

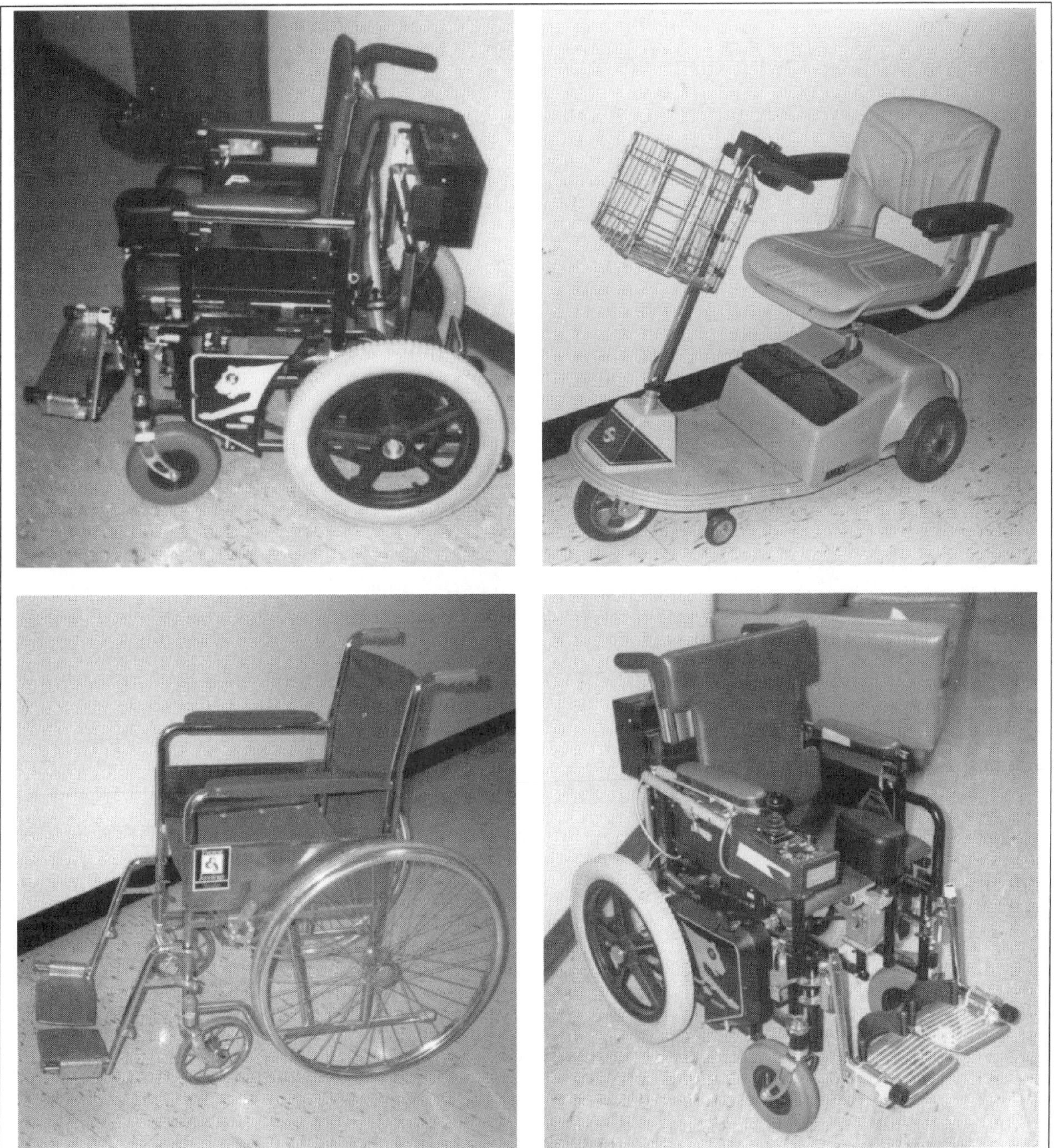

Figure 15.1. Examples of manual and motorized wheelchairs and scooters.

battery-operated motor enclosed in a case housed in the back of the wheelchair between the large wheels. The user propels the wheelchair forward or backward, or turns it by using a joystick mounted on the frame next to the armrest. For users who lack sufficient arm use to operate a joystick, motorized wheelchairs can be operated using controls that are activated by head movement, eye control, or even by mouth. The speed of the wheelchair can be preset at slow, medium, or fast, or can be set to allow the user to accelerate to any desired speed within an available range

SIDEBAR 15.1

Procedures for Maneuvering a Manual Wheelchair

Sighted Guide Technique

A. Participating in Basic Travel

1. Guide pushes wheelchair, providing information about the route as necessary.
2. Alternately, guide gives verbal directions while walking beside the chair as traveler wheels himself or herself.

B. Negotiating Doorways

1. Guide holds door open as traveler maneuvers wheelchair through doorway.
2. Alternatively, traveler holds door open with appropriate hand while guide pushes wheelchair through doorway. (Note: In certain situations, going through backwards may be more efficient.)

C. Negotiating Curbs

1. Upcurb
   - **a.** Guide pushes wheelchair so that front wheels are directly in front of curb.
   - **b.** Guide tilts chair backward by stepping down on tilt bar (located between big wheels) and moves forward until front wheels pass over top of curb and rear wheels contact curb.
   - **c.** Guide gently lowers front of chair so that front wheels contact ground; guide then pushes chair forward until big wheels contact the side of the curb.
   - **d.** Guide leans forward and lifts or rolls the chair up and over the curb.
2. Downcurb
   Method #1:
   - **a.** Guide pushes wheelchair so that front wheels are directly in front of curb.
   - **b.** Guide tilts chair backward by stepping down on tilt bar (located between big wheels).
   - **c.** Guide moves forward until front wheels pass over top of curb, gently lowering chair down the curb, making sure that both rear wheels contact pavement at same time.
   - **d.** Guide gently lowers front of chair so that front wheels contact ground.

   Method #2:
   - **a.** Guide turns wheelchair around to face away from the curb.
   - **b.** Guide lowers big wheels down the curb, making sure that both rear wheels contact pavement at same time.
   - **c.** Guide pulls wheelchair backward, gently lowering front wheels down the curb.

Independent Travel

A. Negotiating Doorways

1. Doors That Push Open
   - **a.** Traveler maneuvers wheelchair up to door and positions it at a slight angle to allow one hand to contact the door.
   - **b.** Traveler leans slightly forward in the chair and pushes door open, using the other hand to propel the wheelchair through the doorway.
   - **c.** As soon as footrests clear the door, the traveler releases the door and uses both hands to propel the wheelchair forward out of the doorway.
     Note: If the door is not heavy, traveler can push it open with the footrests.
2. Doors That Pull Open
   - **a.** Traveler positions wheelchair in front of, and at a slight angle to, the door, but far enough away so that door will not contact footrests as it opens.
   - **b.** Using one hand to pull the door open, the traveler propels the wheelchair through the doorway with the other hand.
     Note: Sometimes it helps to pull the door open quickly so that it has a slight swing. This allows the traveler to move the wheelchair into the doorway while the door swings closed. The traveler can then continue through the doorway without needing to hold the door open.

(up to 7 mph) depending upon the user's preference and ability to efficiently control the chair's direction of movement. The motor works in part on a gear system to also prevent runaways when on an incline or decline.

Despite the ease of movement they provide, motorized wheelchairs do have their disadvantages. First of all, they are very expensive, costing $4,000 to $20,000. Second, they may carry with them hidden expenses, such as the need to have specially equipped vans for transporting the user when in the wheelchair, and the need to replace batteries every year or two. Third, motorized wheelchairs require careful maintenance and regular recharging of the battery. This battery generally allows an average of 20 miles (ranging from 15–25 miles) of continuous use depending upon such factors as the kind of motorized wheelchair, the weight of the user, and the type of terrain being traversed. Also, extremes of hot and cold temperatures will reduce the amount of time the battery will remain charged. Active wheelchair users may need to recharge the battery each night. A common indication that the battery power is running low is an undesired decrease in speed. Some wheelchairs are equipped with a gauge or panel displaying a series of lights that light up in succession, indicating the amount of charge remaining in a battery. These lights will often flash when the battery needs to be recharged. If the battery loses power, the wheelchair can be pushed manually by another person, although it will be necessary to disconnect the gears in the motor, and the wheelchair may still be physically difficult to push. Fourth, motorized wheelchairs are very heavy and therefore difficult to load into a car for transport. They also cannot be taken up or down curbs, but must be taken over curb ramps, driveways, blended curbs, or curb cuts.

Mobility for People with Visual Impairments Who Use Wheelchairs

One of the great challenges in travel encountered by wheelchair users who are visually impaired is the quick avoidance of obstacles, hazards, and drop-offs in the travel path. If users do not have sufficient warning of obstacles, hazards, or drop-offs, or reaction time for stopping the wheelchair safely, they can inadvertently contact these things—with the potential for injury. In such a case, it may be necessary to recommend a decrease in available speed of the wheelchair. Such a change can be done at any medical supply store with a simple adjustment. A possible additional alternative would be to provide the user with an electronic travel aid (ETA), or a long cane or both to enable him to be aware of such things sooner.

For obstacle or hazard detection, the list of innovative solutions is endless. To warn a person of an approaching downstep, raised or colored strips (often rubber, metal or vinyl tape) can be placed on the floor sufficiently in advance of the down step to allow the wheelchair user time to stop safely. In order to avoid unexpected and potentially painful contacts with walls, upsteps, garbage cans, furniture, and other objects, one can purchase footrests that are longer than the user's foot. Longer footrests can avoid many stubbed toes. These footrests can be purchased from dealers who sell wheelchairs. To detect obstacles at waist height, a lap tray provides an effective bumper.

Collisions with objects on the side such as walls, doors, counters, etc., can cause scrapes, bruises, and painful bumps when a hand is unexpectedly caught between the metal pushing rim of the wheel and the object. One solution is to place flexible curb feelers (available at auto supply stores) on the post of the front wheel or on the vertical post at the front of the armrest (see Figure 15.2). The feeler will gently scrape an obstacle alongside the wheelchair before the user is close enough to contact it with his hand. The curb feeler also makes an audible signal as it contacts an object, letting people know that they are very close to it. Curb feelers, when positioned at a 45-degree angle backward (rather than perpendicular to the traveler's path) will gently slide along a surface without scratching it and will bend backward when traversing doorways, thereby not blocking passage.

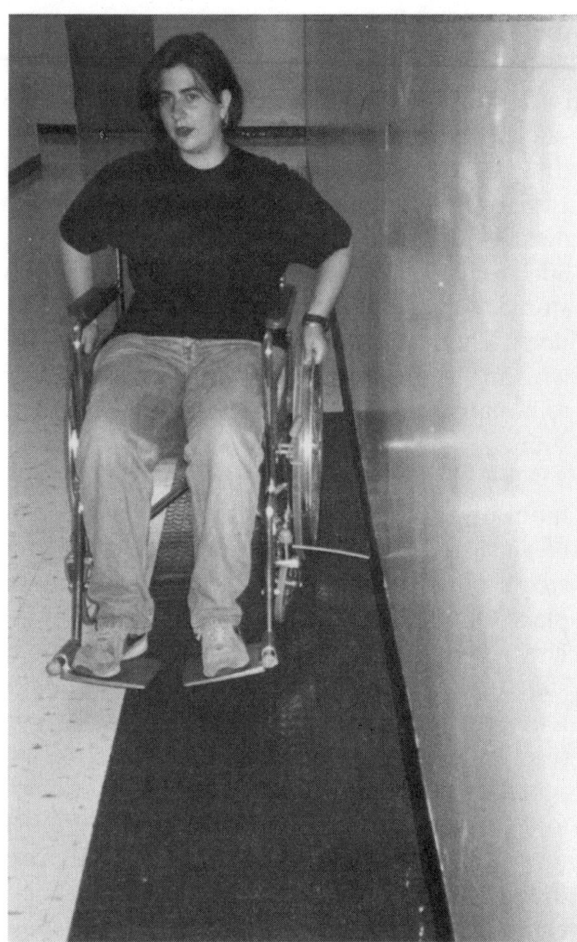

Figure 15.2. Curb feelers attached to a wheelchair.

ETAs provide another means of travel without unwanted encounters with obstacles or hazards. Although the use of ETAs is a relatively expensive proposition compared to longer footrests and curb feelers, they are quite effective. The Mowat Sensor, placed on its side and clamped to a wheelchair tray, or otherwise secured in a position at the user's midline, provides an arc of ultrasound that covers body and wheelchair width quite well (Coleman & Weinstock, 1984). The Mowat Sensor may also be placed on a swivel bracket for scanning.

The Sonicguide and Sonic Pathfinder provide similar coverage. The use of these devices, however, requires the user to keep his head up at all times so the device will not detect the user's lap unintentionally. This can be difficult in the presence of certain physical impairments. Other ETAs such as the Russell Pathsounder, Sensory 6, and the Polaron, will similarly provide an arc of protection (see Chapter 9 for more detailed descriptions of ETAs). The one disadvantage of each of the above systems, both electronic and nonelectronic, however, is that they will not detect downcurbs or descending stairs. Two solutions to this problem are the use of the Wheelchair Pathfinder by Nurion and the use of a long cane. The Wheelchair Pathfinder detects objects at waist-to-head height using ultrasound in a fashion similar to that used by the Mowat Sensor and other aids. The ultrasound emitter can also be configured to enable one to trail a wall. The Wheelchair Pathfinder also emits a laser beam, pointed downward, to detect downsteps and other drop-offs that the wheelchair user is approaching. While the Wheelchair Pathfinder has been used with some success by wheelchair users, it does not, however, reliably detect drop-offs alongside the wheelchair, such as a sidewalk curb.

The second solution, the use of the long cane by the wheelchair user, is really not as complicated and formidable a task as one might imagine. It may require the use of a motorized wheelchair, scooter, or a means of propelling a manual wheelchair with one arm. One method of propelling a wheelchair with one arm is often used by people who have hemiplegia (paralysis on one side of the body). They propel forward (and consequently to the opposite side) by pushing on the rim of the large wheel with their stronger arm, and then correct their direction by pushing against the ground with their foot, much as one does when sitting on a scooter or wheeled office chair and turning or rolling from one desk to another. For people who are able to use one foot for steering, this method frees one hand to use a cane or ETA, or to trail.

Another option for propelling a wheelchair using only one arm is to use a wheelchair equipped with a one-arm drive mechanism or to use a monodrive wheelchair. The one-arm drive mechanism consists of two concentric rims on one of the large wheels. To turn left, one rim is pushed; to turn right, the other rim is pushed. To move forward or backward, both rims are pushed or pulled simultaneously. Use of the one-arm drive, however, requires a high level of strength and motor control to use and it is difficult to move forward in a perfectly straight line without periodic veer correction.

Similarly, the monodrive wheelchair is one that is manually propelled by pumping a hand lever back and forth. To turn, the user turns the hand grip of the lever left or right. To brake, the user pushes the lever fully forward. Although the monodrive wheelchair has been shown to maneuver fairly easily over rough terrain, its pump mechanism can make it difficult to identify veering.

Last, it should be mentioned that while motorized scooters are comfortable and easy to use when people can visually negotiate around obstacles and hazards, they are difficult to use when people use a long cane. This is because the steering bar is generally located directly in front of the body at midline, and the scooter often requires two hands to steer. Also, it should be noted that the three-wheeled scooter models can tip over more easily than a wheelchair when encountering uneven terrain.

When using a long cane to travel in a wheelchair, it may be necessary to use a cane that is longer than the standard length if additional reaction time is needed to stop the wheelchair. Also, because broken sidewalks, sudden slopes, sewers and grates, and curbs can pose hazards for the wheelchair, the user will need advance warning of these objects. Folding canes are excellent for this purpose because they can be folded easily and stored out of the way when not needed. It is recommended that the wheelchair user not use a telescoping cane, or use it with caution, because the added momentum often present in the movement of the wheelchair may cause some canes to collapse rather than remain extended when contacting obstacles in front of the user.

In using the long cane, one holds it either with the hand centered or to the side with one's arm supported on the armrest. This choice generally depends upon physical ability, need, and personal preference. Similarly, one can choose to use either the handshake or pencil grip, depending on personal preference. The tip remains in contact with the ground at all times. This is done to increase detection of even subtle terrain changes such as slight drop-offs, bumps, slopes, or grass, which can impact the stability or maneuverability of the wheelchair. A marshmallow tip, ball tip, or a glide tip are recommended to minimize chances of the cane tip sticking in sidewalk cracks or rough surfaces. Marshmallow and ball tips also do not wear down as readily as standard nylon tips. Using a constant-contact technique minimizes the physical effort of using a cane for people with limited arm strength. The user will also make a wider than normal arc with the cane, because it is important to cover the width of the wheelchair rather than just the body width (an additional 4–8 inches). Also, just as it is important to clear the area in front of the user before proceeding forward, it is important to carefully clear to the side before turning in order to detect any obstacles, hazards, or level changes that the front casters of the wheelchair or footrests might encounter during the turning process.

Orientation

Two other challenges facing wheelchair users who are visually impaired are maintaining orientation to the environment and following a straight line of travel. Orientation to the environment, use of landmarks, and, when necessary, assistance with travel in a straight line can be accomplished through trailing. Straight-line travel is especially problematic for many wheelchair users who do not have sufficient vision to aid them in this task. When using a wheelchair, one does not have the degree of proprioceptive feedback of direction that is available when walking, and it is much harder to monitor one's movement through space. Also, many neurological conditions such as a stroke, cerebral palsy, and traumatic brain injury can impair the proprioceptive sensory system, making it even harder for a person to monitor his or her position in space. For some students, practice in pushing equally with both arms can be helpful in increasing proprioceptive awareness of straight-line travel. Otherwise, trailing the wall or other parallel surfaces is an excellent means of monitoring direction of travel, as is counting doorways or using other landmarks along the wall to navigate. Trailing can be done in a quiet environment by listening to the sound of a curb feeler gently scraping across the parallel surface. When contacting surfaces of different materials, the sound made will change. In this way a student in school, for example, can differentiate between tile walls, metal lockers, wood or brick, or glass surfaces. Similarly, the number of openings, whether doorways or intersecting hallways, can be identified by the cessation of sound from the curb feeler. For the user who wishes to trail at hand height (to locate a landmark that will not be detected by the curb feeler, or who just wishes to have this type of contact with the environment), standard trailing can be done with the hand nearest the wall while the wheelchair is propelled using the opposite hand (the procedure here is similar to that used by people with hemiplegia: propel with the hand rim and steer by pushing the hand against the wall as one trails, instead of pushing off with the foot). This is a slow and often cumbersome procedure, but it can be very effective.

Negotiating a curb ramp at a street corner can also be a challenge for the wheelchair user with a visual impairment. The following safety tips can make the trip easier. First, before entering the ramp, she must identify the direction of the downward slope. She must enter the downward slope of the ramp slowly, and stop the wheelchair before the front wheels cross the lip of the ramp and go into the street. It is also important to enter the downward slope of the ramp straight-on with the wheelchair centered on the ramp. If the wheelchair is not centered between the beveled sides of the ramp (where the ramp rises to the height of the curb), the wheelchair could list sideways on the ramp or come down with an uncomfortable and potentially dangerous bump when the wheelchair rolls forward over the beveled ramp edge onto the street. Using the cane in constant-contact technique is one way to monitor the location of the wheelchair relative to the street edge of the ramp and the beveled sides. Once positioned at the edge of the ramp, the wheelchair user positions the cane in the waiting position and crosses at the appropriate time. She then positions the wheelchair to go up the center of the wheelchair ramp on the other side of the street. If she veers during the crossing, she can locate the upward ramp on the other side of the street using the standard street-crossing recovery skills, including using the cane (if present) along the curb edge to locate the ramp.

It is also important to note that a downward slope of a wheelchair ramp may be angled kitty-corner rather than directly across the street. Because it may be necessary to enter the street on an angle rather than aligned for a straight crossing, independent crossings at such intersections may not be appropriate for all people to attempt, and may be difficult even for the most adept traveler to attempt at all intersections. The safety and effectiveness with which a person can negotiate curb ramps should be determined by the wheelchair user and the O&M specialist on a case-by-case basis.

Visibility

One additional problem commonly faced by wheelchair users is visibility. Because a wheelchair can be quieter than a cane, it may be a silent moving obstacle to other travelers who are blind. Some wheelchair users place a playing card in the spokes of the large wheel to give an auditory indicator of their movement. As the card wears and softens, the sound becomes quieter, so users replace the card periodically. If users wish to begin with a quieter sound, they can soften the card

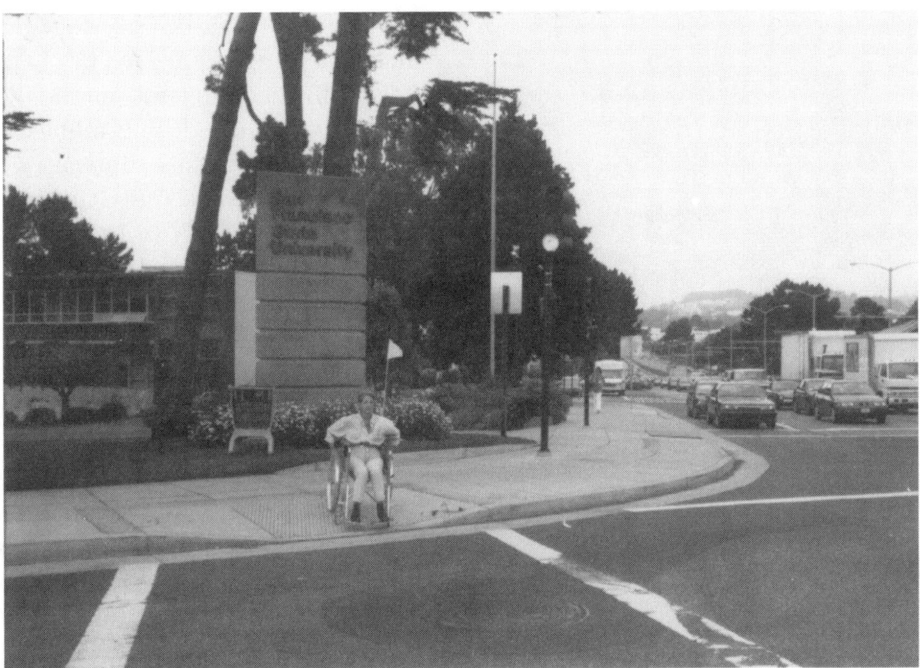

Figure 15.3. This traveler has attached a bicycle flag to his wheelchair to enable drivers to see him more easily in traffic.

slightly before use. Visibility to traffic is another concern of wheelchair users. Because they are lower to the ground than people who are standing and because they might show up in unexpected places (e.g., moving along a road edge, or entering a road from a driveway in areas where there are no curb ramps), there is the concern that they will not be seen readily by drivers. This is critical in street crossings and areas without sidewalks where the wheelchair user might need to travel on the road edge. In response to this concern, some wheelchair users attach a red bicycle flag on a tall pole to the handle of their wheelchair to draw drivers' attention to them (see Figure 15.3). Bicycle dealers can often provide custom brackets to attach flags to the wheelchair.

A special consideration in providing O&M instruction to people who use wheelchairs is that of transferring from a manual wheelchair to another sitting surface, such as a car seat. Depending on the person's medical condition, strength, and weight; model of wheelchair used; environmental considerations; and personal preference, this transfer can be accomplished in one of several ways. Sometimes wheelchair users are able to transfer in and out of the wheelchair without assistance. Sometimes they will use special equipment such as a sliding board (see Figure 15.4). At times, the O&M specialist may need to provide assistance during the transfer process. If the planned program of O&M instruction requires that the student transfer in or out of the wheelchair, the O&M specialist should become familiar with the technique(s) used by that student and how to safely and effectively assist, if necessary. The specialist can do this by simply asking the student and a family member for information (or even a demonstration, if appropriate). Additionally, physical therapists, occupational therapists, and other medical personnel can provide general information and guidelines on safe and effective transfer techniques.

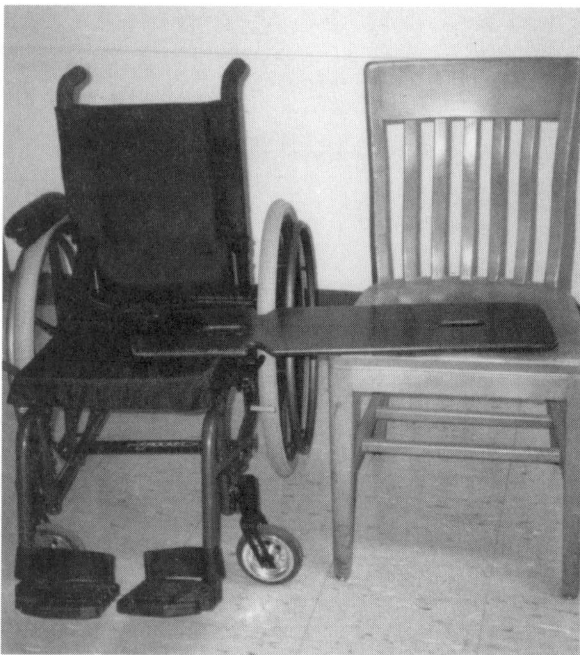

Figure 15.4. Sliding boards are sometimes positioned for a transfer to a chair.

Walkers

Of all the ambulatory aids (exclusive of wheelchairs), walkers provide the most physical support to the user. While there are many different types of walkers, they all consist of four legs and a handle (or two) with which the user maneuvers them. Most walkers will fit into the back of a car or a large trunk, and some are designed to fold for easier transport. Most are equipped with tips especially designed to grip the ground securely with suction-cup action when weight is placed on the walker. Some walkers are held in front of the person; some are held on the side; others are placed behind the person, and pulled forward with each step (see Figure 15.5). These latter walkers are often used by children who need support from behind to maintain an erect posture while walking. Some walkers are designed for use with one hand, some for use on stairs, and others for use by people who lack the strength or coordination to lift the walker with each step. There is also a variety of wheeled walkers. Some have wheels only on the front two legs, and others have wheels on all four legs. They are used by people who do not have sufficient strength, coordination, or balance to lift the walker during ambulation. The user simply rolls the walker forward or lifts the two back legs and rolls the walker forward on the front two wheels. With the latter model, if the user places any weight on the walker, the back legs contact the ground automatically and provide a stable support. Some walkers even come with fold-down seats for people who may have limited endurance and need to travel distances longer than their endurance allows. In addition to these basic types of walkers, there are a variety of modifications for children depending on age, physical size, and physical impairment. Last, there is a variety of accessories available such as carrying baskets that fit on the front or sides of walkers.

When using a walker (without wheels) on level ground, the method used remains fairly constant regardless of the type of walker used. The user should first pick the walker up and place it down, touching all four legs to the ground at the same time. Some users find that if they place the back legs down first and then lower the front legs while they step forward, they can walk faster. This can be dangerous, however, because if the person should begin to lose his or her balance and lean on the walker while only the back two legs are resting on the floor, the walker can slip out of position, allowing the person to fall. Similarly, after placing all four feet on the ground, the user should never walk more than halfway into the walker (for walkers held in front). Stepping forward too close to the front bar can also cause the walker to unexpectedly tilt forward, and the user can fall.

The typical gait or walking pattern when using a walker is as follows: walker, weaker leg, stronger leg. If the person is unable to bear weight on the weaker leg, then the gait pattern is: walker, followed by the stronger leg. In this situation, the person generally holds the weak leg forward, off the ground. (Bending the knee and allowing the weight of the lower leg to fall behind the body line

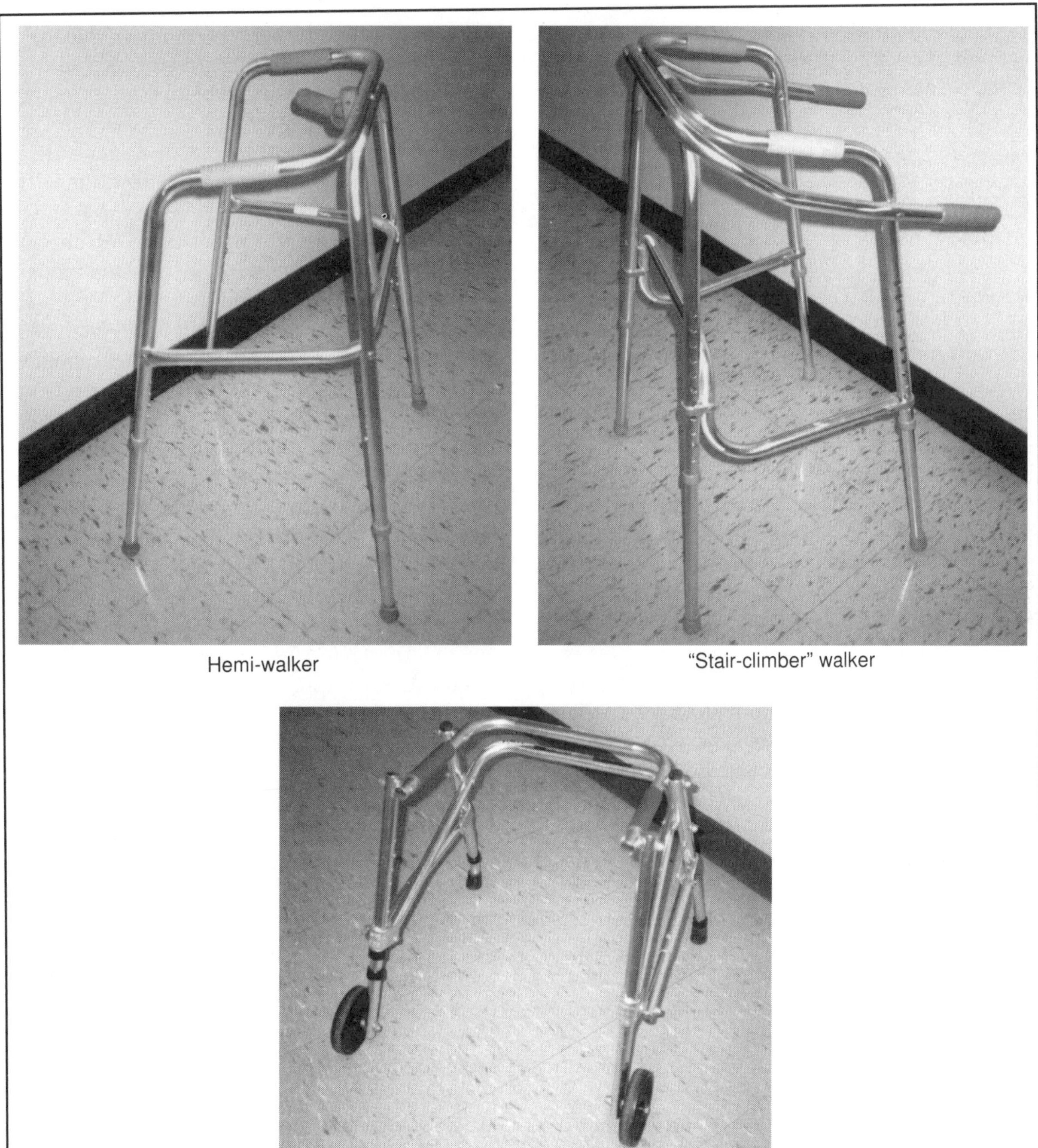

Hemi-walker

"Stair-climber" walker

Child's walker with two wheels

Figure 15.5. Examples of walkers.

can cause an unexpected loss of balance in some people). If there is to be an exception to this rule, it will be determined by a physical therapist.

Mobility for People with Visual Impairments Who use Walkers

Adapted mobility for those who use a walker follows many of the same principles as for those who use a wheelchair. With regard to orientation, straight-line travel can be difficult for people who use walkers as it is for those who use wheelchairs. Practice in extending both arms forward equidistantly with each step may help some people to improve proprioceptive awareness of straight-line travel. While walkers do not safely detect drop-offs, some walkers provide obstacle detection. Those which are held in front of the user provide a ready-made forward bumper to indicate contact with an obstacle in the traveler's path. Walkers held on the side will detect obstacles on the side. Walkers held behind the user, however, provide no obstacle detection. In this situation, it may be possible to adapt the walker by placing a removable bar or strap across the opening to detect obstacles in front before the user contacts them with his or her body. Homemade devices can be easily fabricated to serve this function; however, such devices must be attached so they do not interfere with foot placement during ambulation or become a hazard to a person when getting into and out of the walker. A physical therapist can be of assistance in determining the best type and location of such a device for a specific user.

Similarly, one can trail a wall on the side by sliding the near legs of the walker along it. Alternatively, curb feelers mounted on the front leg of the walker (about 2 inches off the ground, and facing backward at a 45-degree angle) provide information about objects on the user's side before any unwanted contact with the hand. Mounting the feelers at about 2 inches off the ground is recommended, because at this height they will be low enough to detect steps, curbs, or similar low objects.

Early obstacle detection is extremely important for people who use walkers. Due to the effects of impaired balance, sudden changes in terrain can sometimes present serious challenges to balance, even when one is using an ambulatory aid. As with wheelchairs, ETAs and the long cane provide excellent means of obstacle detection. The difficulty arises, however, when both hands are needed to maneuver the walker. One solution to this is the use of a walker designed specifically for use with one hand. One model is held on a person's side. It may provide slightly less support than a front model, but it will free the use of one hand for the long cane. Another model is a front model with a small handle that protrudes from the center bar of the walker (see Figure 15.6). The handle is angled slightly to the right for right-handed users, and to the left for left-handed users. The walker can be lifted by the handle and moved into position for each succeeding step with only one hand. Although designed for use by people with only one functional hand, it can be successfully used by people who have two hands but need one hand free to trail a wall or use a long cane without sacrificing the support of a walker.

Crutches

Crutches provide slightly less physical support than walkers, but more than canes. There are two basic types of crutches: underarm and lofstrand (also called forearm or Canadian crutches) (see Figure 15.6), and people may use either one or two crutches depending on their need for support. Lofstrand crutches, made of metal, provide slightly less support than underarm crutches, but require less coordination to use and allow users much greater flexibility. The metal forearm cuff allows people to lift their arm up or forward to open doors or handle objects (such as money when paying for items at a store) without the crutch falling away. The gait patterns for both types of crutches are the same and are determined by a physical therapist based upon a person's strength, coordination, and stamina. There are three basic gait patterns, named for the number of contacts by foot or crutch with the ground in a cycle (see Figure 15.7). A two-point gait is perhaps the most efficient and allows the

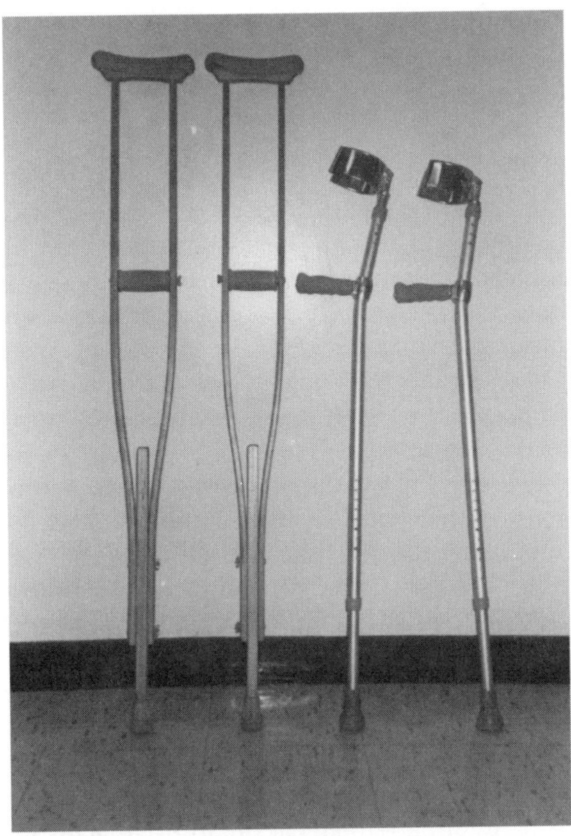
Figure 15.6. Underarm crutches and forearm crutches.

fastest movement. In the two-point gait, the user moves both crutches forward simultaneously, then steps forward with the stronger leg while holding the weaker leg in the air (if unable to bear weight on it). Another version of the two-point gait for people who are able to bear weight on the weaker leg is to move both crutches and the weaker leg forward simultaneously, place them on the ground, and then step forward with the stronger leg. In each case, there are only two points of contact with the ground in each cycle. The three-point gait is similar, with only one additional point of contact during the cycle. In the three-point gait, the user moves both crutches forward simultaneously, then steps forward with the weaker leg, followed by the stronger leg. As in using the walker, the weaker leg always precedes the stronger leg because this affords greater stability. The four-point gait involves moving each crutch and each leg forward separately, and in order. Basically, the user moves the right crutch ahead, followed by the left leg, then the left crutch followed by the right leg. As the user becomes

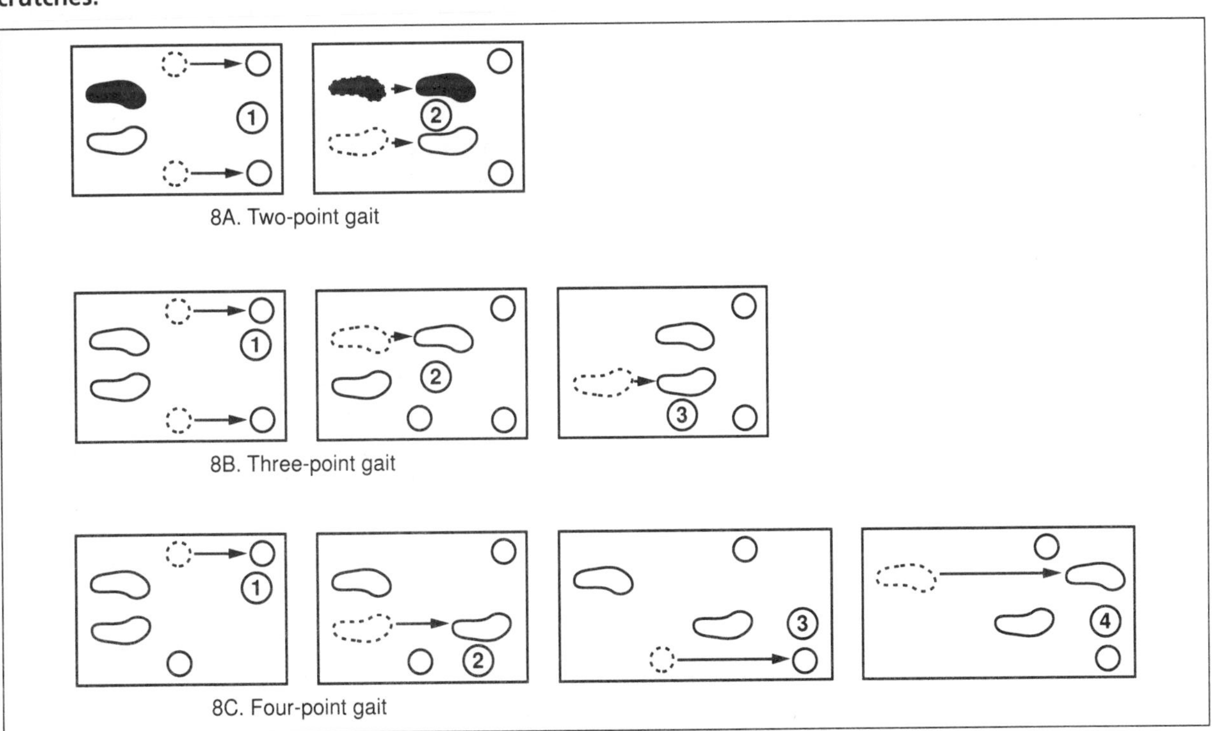

Figure 15.7. Diagrams of typical gait patterns with two crutches.

more skilled, and when sufficient balance and coordination are present, the user may speed up the process by moving one crutch and the opposite leg forward at the same time. This most closely resembles the reciprocal gait pattern of normal walking where a leg and the opposite arm move forward at the same time. An important rule for the traveler without sufficient vision to preview the area ahead is to always step only up to where the crutches have cleared, never beyond.

To ascend stairs, people can walk up to the first riser, so that their toes are 2–3 inches away from it. They then step up onto the first step with their stronger leg, followed by the weaker leg and the crutches. To descend stairs, people can walk up to the edge of the first step, place both crutches down one step, then step down with the weaker leg first. If they have sufficient balance to stand on one leg, they can lower the crutches and the weaker leg to the next step at the same time (see Figure 15.8). They then repeat the process for each successive step. Travel on stairs takes a lot of strength and coordination. For people who do not have sufficient strength or coordination to do this, they may choose to use the hand railing. To do this, they place the crutch nearest the railing in their other hand and hold it sideways (see Figure 15.9) by grasping the shaft of the crutch just below the hand grip. The procedure for ascending or descending stairs is then performed as above.

Support Canes

Canes provide the least support of all ambulatory aids. There are several kinds: quad canes, tripods, and straight, named by the number of points of contact the base makes with the ground (see Figure 15.10). Quad canes provide the greatest amount of support due to their relatively large base of support, followed by the tripod cane and the standard cane. The basic gait patterns on both level ground and stairs are the same as for using crutches.

Mobility for People with Visual Impairments Who Use Crutches or Support Canes

As was seen for those who use walkers, people who use two crutches or canes can be faced with the difficult challenge of detecting obstacles with sufficient warning to avoid collisions (and sometimes a subsequent loss of balance). There are some solutions, however, each with varying degrees of effectiveness and ease of use, depending upon the person's physical abilities and travel needs. One solution is to use ETAs to obtain advance warning of obstacles (other than downsteps) in one's path. Another solution is to use the ambulatory aid(s)to trail and clear the path in front. This latter solution can be used by those who possess sufficient strength, coordination, and balance to support themselves on one crutch or cane while using the other as a probe. As shown in Figure 15.11, the person can place their weight on one crutch while placing the tip of the other crutch across their body, then sliding it in an arc in front of them back to its original resting point. This clears a one-step distance ahead. To trail, the user simply taps the tip of the aid against the wall or vertical surface being trailed, then places the aid forward, in position for the next step. Teaching a student with a visual impairment to use an ambulatory aid to clear a path and to trail should be done with the advice of, or in conjunction with, a physical therapist to ensure that this procedure can be done safely without causing excessive physical strain or potentially aggravating an existing medical condition.

Another method of clearing a path and trailing is to use a long cane. If people only use one crutch or support cane for walking, they can often use a long cane easily. In this situation, they hold and use the crutch or support cane in the hand dictated by their support needs (generally on the side opposite the weaker leg) and hold the long cane in the other hand. This is true whether or not they are left- or right-handed. The gait pattern for using the crutch or support cane remains the same—the aid, followed by the weaker leg,

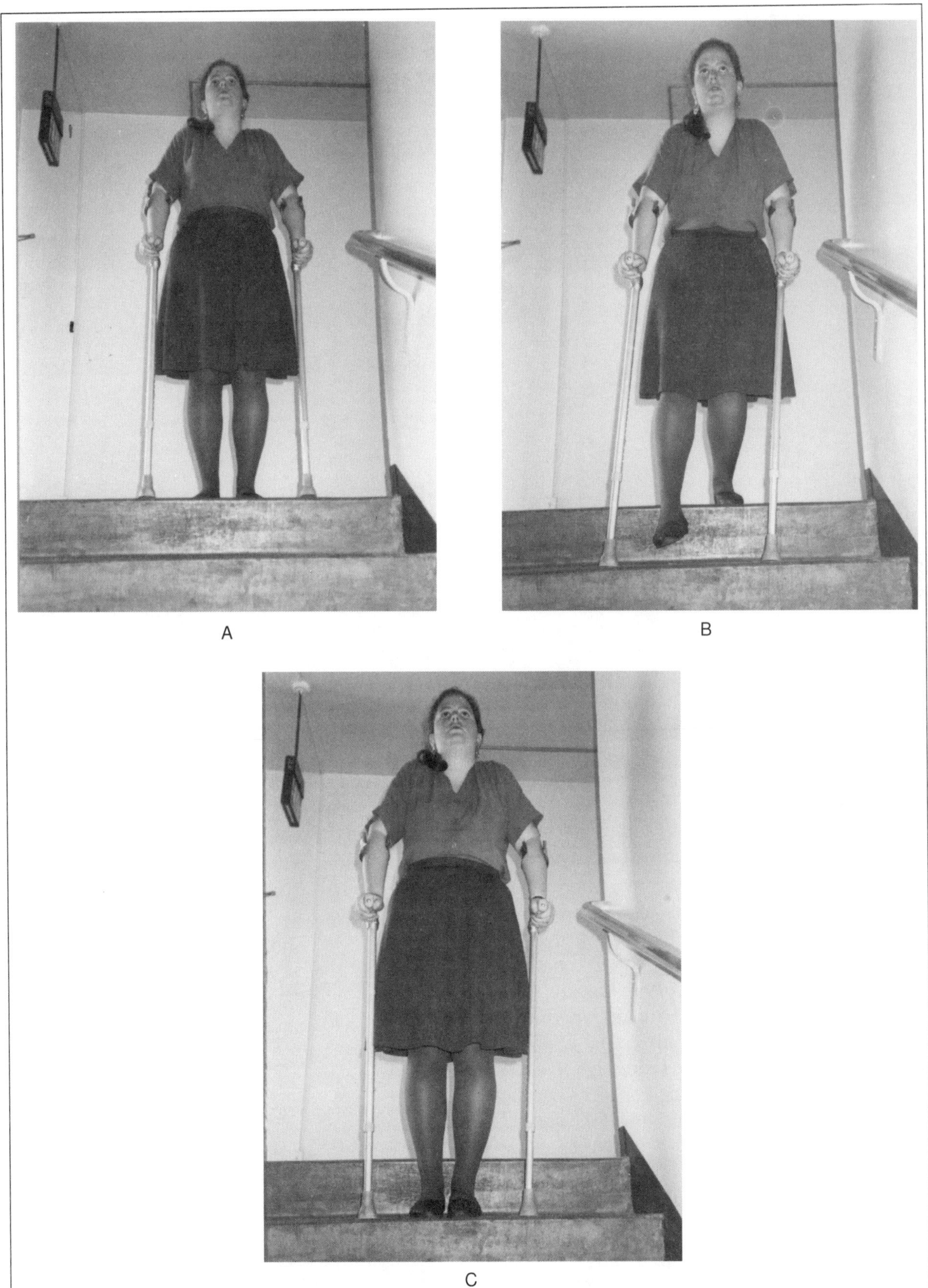

Figure 15.8. Descending stairs when using crutches.

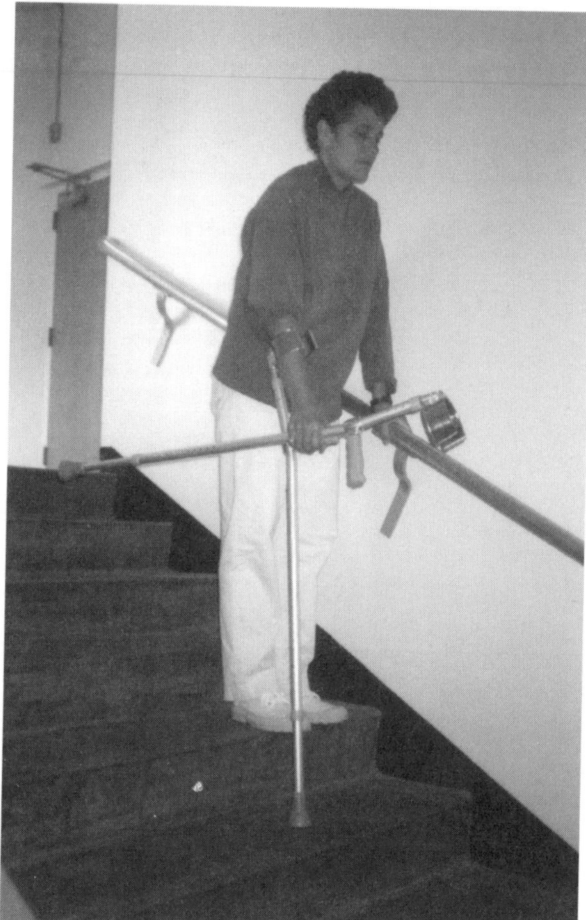

Figure 15.9. Holding crutches when descending stairs and using a railing.

then the stronger leg. Some people will move the aid and the weaker leg forward together for increased speed. The long cane is also used in a traditional manner, with the hand and arm position remaining the same as when using it alone. The users keep "in step" with the long cane as they walk, contacting the cane tip to the ground on one side as the foot on the opposite side steps down. In this way (assuming the aid is held in the left hand), the crutch or support cane and the tip of the long cane will touch the ground on the left as the right heel steps down. Then the long cane will touch down on the right as the person steps forward with her left foot. The process is then repeated. To ascend or descend stairs, the person again combines the standard procedures for using the ambulatory aid and the long

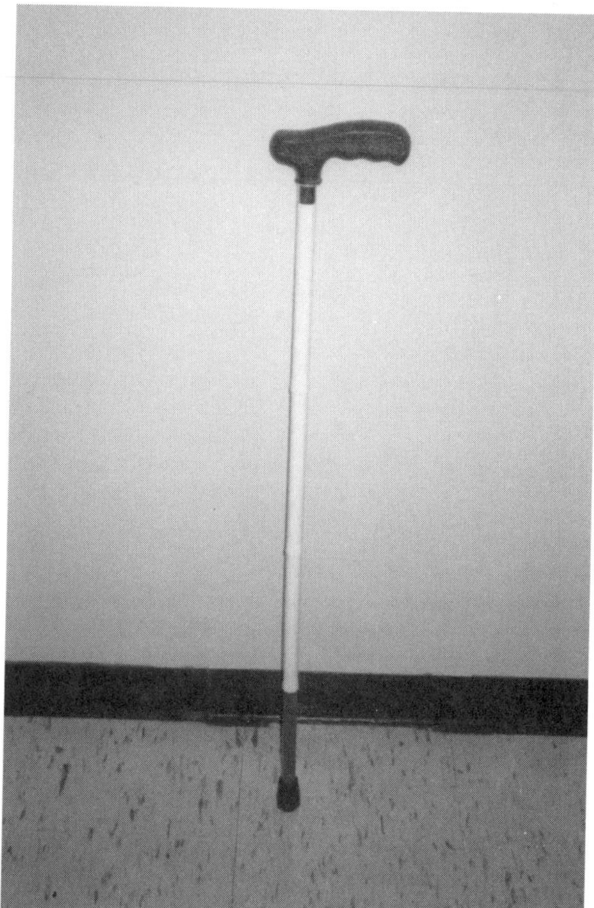

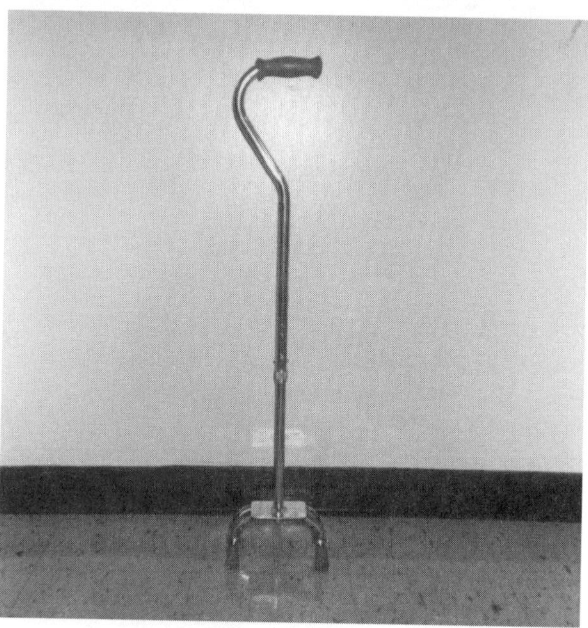

Figure 15.10. Examples of canes: Straight Cane (above) and Quad Cane (below).

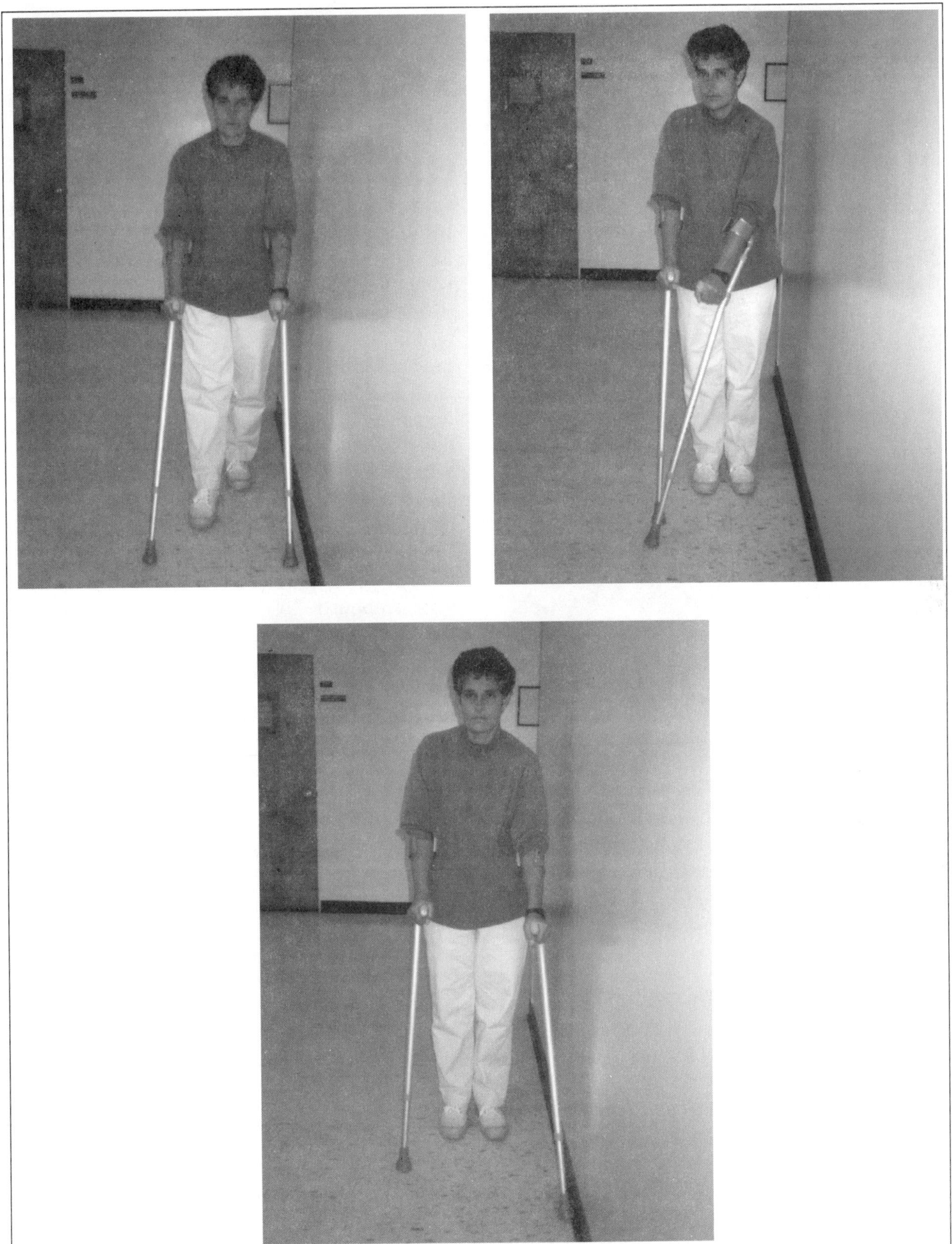

Figure 15.11. Using a crutch as a long cane.

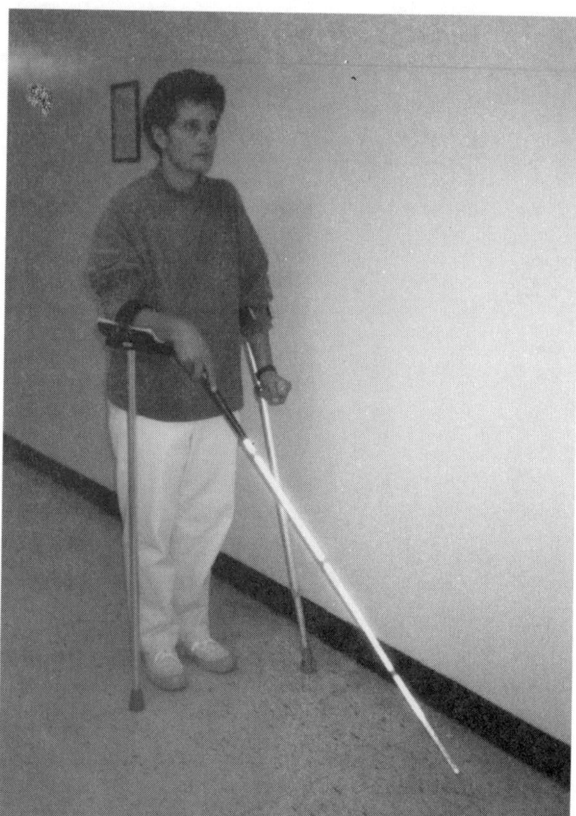

Figure 15.12. Forearm trough crutch attachment.

cane on stairs. Again, a longer cane than usual may be helpful if additional reaction time is needed when balance is impaired. Using an ambulatory aid and a long cane together takes coordination and practice, but it is an effective and efficient means of independent travel for people who need to use both.

For those who use two crutches and still need or wish to use a long cane, it is possible to attach a "forearm trough" to one crutch (see Figure 15.12).The trough is generally used by people who lack sufficient hand strength to grasp a crutch handle. When used by people with visual impairments, however, it enables them to manipulate the crutch with arm motion alone, leaving the hand free to hold a long cane, handle doors, and manipulate objects in the environment. Although use of a forearm trough can be awkward, it provides some travelers with an effective means of mobility without sacrificing stability.

SPOTTING BY THE O&M SPECIALIST

No discussion of ambulatory aids used by people with visual impairments would be complete without addressing techniques the O&M specialist can use to ensure students' physical safety while they learn independent travel skills. When people using ambulatory aids walk on uneven terrain, ice, wet or slippery surfaces; or ascend or descend stairs or curbs; or become fatigued, balance can become much more precarious than under ordinary circumstances. In these situations, careful spotting is necessary to assist students to maintain balance, or avoid serious injury should they lose balance and fall. *Spotting* refers to the procedure by which an O&M specialist carefully positions himself or herself next to a student, watches for signs indicating that the student is about to lose balance, and responds instantly in order to provide physical support or to break a fall. The best position for spotting is to stand slightly behind and to the side of the student on level ground. When ascending stairs, it is important to stand behind and below the student. When descending stairs, the O&M specialist should stand in front of and below the student. A trick used by physical therapists to enable them to most effectively and safely stabilize a person who has started to fall, or to lessen the impact of the fall, is to hold onto the person's belt when walking down stairs, or in other situations where balance may be unsure. The O&M instructor holds onto the belt in a palm-up position for greatest leverage (see Figure 15.13). Holding onto a student's belt needs to be done with the student's permission; it provides an excellent means of spotting when there is a possibility that the student will lose balance. The O&M instructor may also wish to carry a spare belt with him for students who do not have their own. For this purpose, a man's leather belt, at least 2 inches wide, works well. Women's belts, elastic or cloth belts, or narrower belts are generally not strong enough for spotting purposes. By purchasing a man's belt (the largest size possible), and drilling holes in the

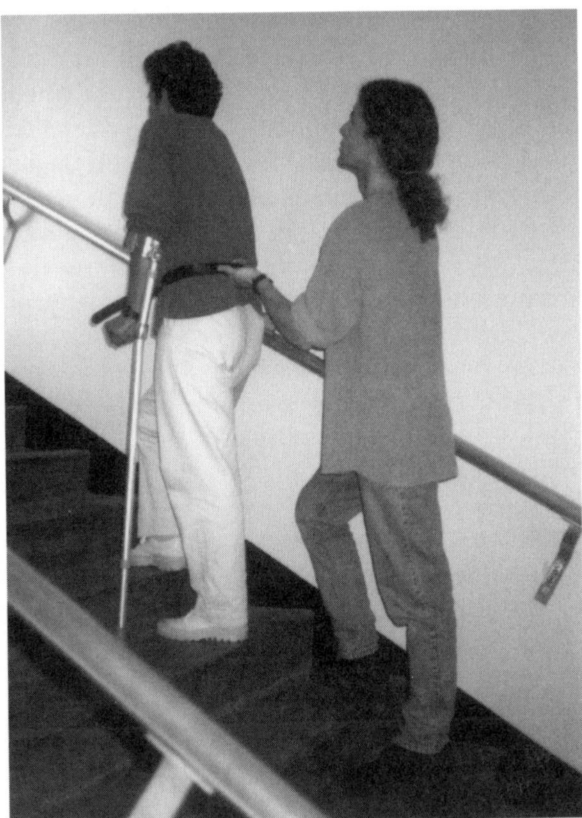

Figure 15.13. Using belt in spotting.

belt at 1 inch intervals (done inexpensively at shoe repair shops), the O&M specialist will have a belt available that fits all students. The belt should be as snug a fit as the student can comfortably tolerate in order to provide maximum leverage for the instructor to prevent a fall should the situation arise.

USING AMBULATORY AIDS ON MASS TRANSIT

With regard to the use of public transportation, there are several considerations. Most cities equip buses with lifts that raise wheelchair users in and out of the bus. To use a lift, the user generally backs onto it, facing the curb. It is important that he or she move completely onto the lift so that the gate can close on the sidewalk side. If using a manual wheelchair, the person locks the brakes (motorized wheelchairs lock automatically when the joystick is not in the "drive" position). Wheelchair users who are unable to look behind them will often attach mirrors to the sides of the wheelchair to assist them in backing up. When the lift is raised to the height of the bus floor, the wheelchair user rolls backward and takes a place alongside the window at the front of the bus. While some bus aisles are large enough for a person to enter in a forward direction and then turn around, this is not always the case. Once in place, the brakes of manual wheelchairs should then be locked to keep the wheelchair from rolling as the bus starts, stops, and turns. Some buses are equipped with special clamps or tie-downs to secure the wheels and prevent rolling when the bus is in motion. Not all buses are so equipped, however, and the clamps do not fit all wheelchairs. For added protection against rolling during a sudden stop, some wheelchair users choose to hold onto a nearby vertical pole. To exit the bus, the wheelchair user will move forward onto the lift, which is then lowered to the curb. Lifts generally have railings that wheelchair users can hold for extra stability during the raising and lowering process. In keeping with the mandates of the Americans with Disabilities Act (ADA), the Architectural and Transportation Barriers Compliance Board issued guidelines (1991) to ensure access for the disabled on public transportation. Public transportation agencies across the country are in the process of making buses and trains wheelchair accessible. As of this writing, most cities have been able to equip their entire fleet with lifts; other cities have only been able to equip a few of their buses so far. It may therefore be necessary to contact the bus company for information on the times or routes such buses run or request that an accessible bus be used on a given route at a given time.

Subways are generally accessible to people using wheelchairs or ambulatory aids as the floor of the subway car is level with the platform. It is important to be very careful of the gap between the subway car and platform when boarding or exiting, however, as the tips of walkers, crutches, or support canes can catch in the gap, as can some very small wheels on wheelchairs. Most wheelchairs have front wheels that are large enough to move smoothly over the gap, but if the wheels are small, users will generally move quickly over the gap to "bridge it" before the wheel can slip down. Users also can make a point of entering the door from a "straight-on" direction in order to minimize the chances of a wheel catching in the gap.

Buses and subways generally have seating next to the door for people with mobility problems. In some cases, seats are removed immediately next to the door to leave space for wheelchairs, or the front seats fold away to allow room for them. Crutches and support canes, as well as long canes, are held vertically, out of the aisle when the user is seated, to avoid tripping nearby passengers.

Some cities have discount fares for people with disabilities, senior citizens, and even young children. Many cities also have paratransit services available for people who are unable to take public transportation.

CHOICE OF EQUIPMENT

It is the role of the physical or occupational therapist to determine the type of wheelchair (including accessories) that a person will use. Therapists are also responsible for fitting the wheelchair to the user to ensure that it is the proper size, and teaching the person how to use it. Physical therapists additionally prescribe, fit, and teach people how to use other ambulatory aids. This instruction includes use of the aid on level ground such as a tile floor, on uneven ground such as grass, up- and downcurbs, and when possible, on stairs (however, some aids cannot be used on stairs).

The choice of aids for a given person is made based on several interrelated factors such as the person's age, balance, coordination, muscle tone, need for postural support, presence of sensory impairment, diagnosis or prognosis of medical situation, endurance, level of activity, and sometimes even financial considerations, such as insurance coverage. This decision can often be based on factors that are not always apparent to the lay person. For example, a person who appears to be able to walk with fair balance when not using a cane at all might actually be given two canes. Such a case might be a person with fragile bones who has impaired balance and can be seriously hurt if she steps down hard on one foot when catching her balance. Furthermore, the aids prescribed can change as a person's medical situation improves or worsens, or as children mature or people age. For this reason it is important that the aids used by a person are prescribed by a physical therapist or physician, and that no changes are made without consulting a physical therapist or physician.

At the same time, however, the requirements of O&M, such as reaction time when encountering obstacles, the effect on balance of unexpected collisions with objects, and early detection of steps and changes in terrain may not be factors that physical therapists consider when prescribing ambulatory aids. It is therefore important for O&M specialists and physical therapists to work in concert, whenever possible, to prescribe aids or revise a system to meet both the physical support and independent mobility needs of the person with a visual impairment.

MAINTENANCE OF EQUIPMENT

The need for regular maintenance of wheelchairs can range from minimal to significant. Wheelchairs must be kept clean, dry, and rust-free. They should be inspected periodically for loose and worn parts. Pneumatic tires must be properly inflated at all times. The motor of a motorized wheelchair will need regular maintenance to adjust drive belt tensions, inspect wires for worn insulation, and maintain battery terminals free from corrosion.

Very little maintenance is required of walkers, crutches, and canes. Basically it consists of inspecting the crutch or cane tips for signs of wear and cracking. Over time, the rubber may dry through exposure to heat and sun, and may crack. When this occurs, it is best to replace the

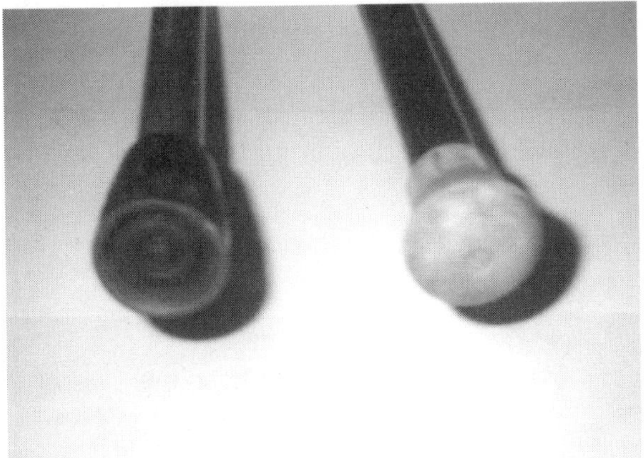

Figure 15.14. Crutch and cane tips, in good condition (left) and worn (right).

tips before they crack completely open and fall off. Similarly, the bottoms of the tips need regular inspection. When new, the bottom of the tip has a series of concentric rings that form a ridged suction cup (see Figure 15.14). This provides a mild suction with the ground when weight is applied to the aid, providing increased traction and increased stability. When the tip begins to wear, the ridges wear down and the bottom of the tip becomes smoother, much the same way that the tread on a tire wears through use. When this happens, traction is decreased for the cane tip, just as it is for automobile tires. The cane tip is then more likely to slip on wet or slippery surfaces such as wet pavement or a waxed floor. When the ridges are worn, it is time to replace the tip. Replacement tips can be purchased inexpensively from any medical supply store.

RESOURCES

When serving persons who use ambulatory aids, the O&M specialist can confer with other professionals as resources. Working together, the O&M specialist and physical therapist can determine the proper aids for a student, given the combination of physical and visual travel needs. Physical therapists can answer questions about the proper fit and use of aids. In addition to physical therapists, occupational therapists can provide information on the proper fit and use of wheelchairs. Rehabilitation engineers (specialists in developing equipment to meet unique needs of people with physical disabilities) are also excellent resources when questions arise concerning the need to adapt equipment for more efficient or safer use.

SUMMARY

Independent mobility for people with visual impairments who use ambulatory aids is an achievable goal. The number of people with visual impairments who use ambulatory aids is increasing and will continue to increase in the future. This increase provides an exciting challenge and opportunity for O&M specialists to teach safe and effective travel skills to people who may once have thought they could never travel because they could not hold a long cane, or to whom services had been denied because of the "limitations" of their physical impairment.

Suggestions/Implications for O&M Specialists

1. The number of people with visual impairments who use ambulatory aids is increasing and will continue to increase in the future. As a result, O&M specialists are increasingly being called upon to serve not only visually impaired people who are physically able, but also a variety of those who have physical disabilities.
2. There are two basic reasons that people use ambulatory aid(s): (a) they lack sufficient strength or balance to walk without the aid(s), or (b) for medical reasons they must limit the amount of weight or stress placed on their legs.
3. *Travelers Who Use Wheelchairs:*
   - **a.** Some of the greater challenges in travel encountered by wheelchair users who are visually impaired are the quick-avoidance obstacles, hazards, and drop-offs in the travel path. Possible ways in which to address this challenge include:
     - Decreasing the available speed of a motorized wheelchair.:
     - Using an ETA or a long cane that enable the traveler to be aware of obstacles and hazards sooner.:
     - Placing raised or colored strips (often metal or vinyl tape) on the floor sufficiently in advance of a downstep to allow the wheelchair user time to stop safely.:
     - Using footrests that are longer than the user's foot to avoid stubbing toes when objects are contacted. These footrests can be purchased from dealers who sell wheelchairs. Some people secure a foam pad to the front of each footrest to cushion impact with objects.:
     - Using a lap tray to detect obstacles at waist height.:
     - Placing flexible curb feelers on the post of the front wheel or on the vertical post at the front of the armrest to detect obstacles or hazards on the side of the travel path. The curb feeler makes an audible signal as it contacts objects, letting travelers know that they are very close to an object.:
     - Using ETAs.:
     - Using a long cane. Users of manually propelled wheelchairs can free one hand to hold the cane by equipping the wheelchair with a one-arm drive mechanism, using a monodrive wheelchair, or propelling a standard wheelchair with one hand while steering with one foot.
   - **b.** When using a long cane while traveling in a wheelchair, it may be necessary for the user to use a cane that is longer than the standard length if additional reaction time is needed to stop the wheelchair. Folding canes are excellent for this purpose; it is recommended that the wheelchair user not use a telescoping cane, or use it with caution, because the added momentum often present in the movement of the wheelchair may cause some canes to collapse rather than remain extended when contacting obstacles in front of the user.
   - **c.** In using the long cane while traveling in a wheelchair, the user must ensure that the tip remains in contact with the ground at

(*continued on next page*)

Suggestions/Implications for O&M Specialists (continued)

all times. A marshmallow tip or ball tip on an aluminum cane, or a glide tip on a fiberglass cane are recommended to minimize chances of the cane tip sticking in sidewalk cracks or rough surfaces. The user needs to also make a wider than normal arc with the cane in order to cover the width of the wheelchair.

d. Trailing a wall or other parallel surface can be done when using a wheelchair by:

- Listening to the sound of the curb feeler gently scraping across the parallel surface when traveling in a quiet environment.:
- Performing standard trailing with the hand nearest the wall while propelling the manual wheelchair using the opposite rim.

e. To most safely negotiate a wheelchair ramp when using a wheelchair, one should slowly enter the center of downward slope of the ramp straight on. This prevents the front casters of the wheelchair from lining up with either the left or right upward slope of the beveled ramp, which in turn could cause the wheelchair to list sideways on the ramp, or come down with an uncomfortable and potentially dangerous bump when the wheelchair rolls forward over the beveled ramp edge onto the street. It is also important to stop the wheelchair before the front casters cross the lip of the ramp and go into the street.

f. Because wheelchair users are lower to the ground than people who are standing, their visibility to traffic is a concern. To increase visibility, the user can attach a red bicycle flag on a tall pole to the back of the wheelchair to draw drivers' attention to the traveler.

g. If the planned program of O&M instruction requires that the student transfer in or out of the wheelchair, the O&M specialist should become familiar with the technique(s) used by that student and how to safely and effectively assist if necessary. The traveler and/or family member, physical therapists, occupational therapists, and other medical personnel can provide general information and guidelines on safe and effective transfer techniques.

4. *Travelers Who Use Walkers:*

a. When using the walker on level ground, the user should pick the walker up and place it down, touching all four legs to the ground at the same time. Similarly, after placing all four feet on the ground, the user should only walk halfway into the walker to prevent it from unexpectedly tilting forward.

b. The typical gait (walking) pattern when using a walker is: walker, followed by the weaker leg, and then by the stronger leg.

c. To detect obstacles in the travel path:

- Walkers that are held in front of the user provide a ready-made forward bumper to indicate contact with an obstacle in the traveler's path. Walkers held on the side will detect obstacles on the side.:
- Walkers held behind the user provide no obstacle detection. In this situation,

(*continued on next page*)

Suggestions/Implications for O&M Specialists (continued)

it may be possible to adapt the walker by placing a removable bar or strap across the opening to detect obstacles in front before the user contacts them with her body. A physical therapist can be of assistance in determining the best type and location of such a device for a specific user.:

- The traveler can trail a wall on the side by sliding the near legs of the walker along the wall. Alternatively, curb feelers mounted on the front leg of the walker provide information about objects on the user's side. Mounting the feelers at about 2 inches off the ground is recommended because at this height they will be low enough to detect steps, curbs, or similar low objects.:
- Using ETAs:
- Using the long cane. In order to free one hand for holding the cane, many travelers use a walker designed specifically for use with one hand.

5. *Travelers Who Use Crutches or Canes:*
   a. It is the physical therapist who determines the type of crutches or canes a person will use, as well as the gait pattern. These determinations are based upon a person's strength, coordination, and stamina.
   b. To detect obstacles and hazards in the travel path:
      - One can use ETAs to obtain advance warning of obstacles (other than downsteps) in one's path.:
      - One can use a crutch or cane to trail and to clear the path in front. This latter solution requires that one possess sufficient strength, coordination, and balance to support oneself on one crutch or cane while using the other as a probe. An important rule for the traveler without sufficient vision for previewing the area ahead is to always step only up to where the crutch or cane has cleared, never beyond. Teaching a student with a visual impairment to use an ambulatory aid to clear a path and trail should be done with the advice of, or in conjunction with, a physical therapist to ensure that this procedure can be done safely without causing excessive physical strain or potentially aggravating an existing medical condition.:
      - One can use a long cane. If a traveler only uses one crutch or support cane for walking, they can easily use a long cane by holding and using the crutch or support cane in the hand dictated by their support needs (generally on the side opposite the weaker leg) and holding the long cane in the other hand (the gait pattern for using the crutch or support cane remains the same as does the manner for using the long cane). A longer cane than usual may be needed to allow any additional reaction time needed when balance is impaired.
6. *Spotting by the O&M Specialist:*
   a. When people using ambulatory aids walk on uneven terrain, ice, or wet or slippery

(*continued on next page*)

Suggestions/Implications for O&M Specialists (continued)

surfaces; ascend or descend stairs or curbs; or become fatigued, balance can become much more precarious than normal.

b. The best position for the O&M specialist to stand when spotting a student is slightly behind and to the side of the student on level ground. When ascending stairs, it is important to stand behind (below) the student. When descending stairs, stand in front of (below) the student.

c. A trick to most effectively and safely stabilize a person who has started to fall, or to lessen the impact of the fall, is to hold onto the person's belt (with the person's permission) when walking down stairs, or in other situations where balance may be unsure.

7. *Use of Mass Transit by People who Use Ambulatory Aids*

   a. Most cities equip buses with lifts that raise wheelchair users in and out of the bus.

   b. The brakes of manual wheelchairs should be locked to keep the wheelchair from rolling as the bus starts, stops, and turns. Some buses are equipped with special clamps or tie-downs to secure the wheels and prevent rolling when the bus is in motion.

   c. For added protection against rolling during a sudden stop, some wheelchair users choose to hold onto a nearby vertical pole.

   d. Subways are generally accessible to people using wheelchairs or ambulatory aids as the floor of the subway car is level with the platform. It is important to be very careful of the gap between the subway car and the platform when boarding or exiting, however, as the tips of walkers, crutches, or support canes can catch in the gap, as can some very small wheels on wheelchairs. Users also can make a point of entering the door from a "straight-on" direction in order to minimize the chances of a wheel catching in the gap.

   e. Buses and subways generally have seating next to the door for people with mobility problems. Crutches and support canes, as well as long canes, are held vertically, out of the aisle when the user is seated, to avoid tripping nearby passengers.

   f. Some cities have discount fares for people with disabilities, senior citizens, and even young children. Many cities also have paratransit services available for people who are unable to take public transportation.

8. *Choice and Maintenance of Equipment:*

   a. It is the role of the physical or occupational therapist to determine the type of wheelchair (including accessories) that a person will use, fit it to the user, and teach the person how to use it. Physical therapists additionally prescribe, fit, and teach people how to use other ambulatory aids.

   b. Physical and occupational therapists may not be prepared to consider the special requirements of mobility for a visually impaired person, such as reaction time when encountering obstacles, the effect on balance of unexpected collisions with

(*continued on next page*)

Suggestions/Implications for O&M Specialists (continued)

objects, and early detection of steps and changes in terrain. It is therefore important for O&M specialists and physical or occupational therapists to work together whenever possible, to prescribe ambulatory aid(s) or revise a system to meet both the physical support and independent mobility needs of the person with a visual impairment.

c. Wheelchairs must be kept clean, dry, and rust-free, and should be inspected periodically for loose and worn parts. Pneumatic tires must be properly inflated at all times.

d. Maintenance of walkers, crutches, and canes consists of inspecting the tips for signs of wear and cracking. Replacement tips can be purchased inexpensively from any medical supply store.

9. When serving students who use ambulatory aids, the O&M specialist is never alone. Physical therapists can answer questions about the proper fit and use of aid(s). In addition to physical therapists, occupational therapists can provide information on the proper fit and use of wheelchairs. Rehabilitation engineers (specialists in developing equipment to meet unique needs of people with physical disabilities) are excellent resources when questions arise concerning the need to adapt equipment for more efficient or safer use.

ACTIVITIES FOR REVIEW

1. Visit the physical therapy department at a local hospital to observe people being fit with ambulatory devices and instructed in their use.
2. Contact medical equipment specialists to find out what kinds of equipment and accessories might be available for your student. Sales representatives are generally happy to talk to people.
3. Talk to people who use ambulatory aids to learn about tips for use in specific environments, as well as the pros and cons of each type of device and accessories.
4. Rent or borrow a wheelchair or other ambulatory aid(s) and spend a day using them. The experience will give you an excellent sense of what students experience and how the use of aid(s) impacts mobility.

CHAPTER 16

Learners with Visual and Cognitive Impairments

Elga Joffee and Paul Ehresman

Instructors of orientation and mobility (O&M) teach a diverse population of learners who have unique needs for mastering the skills and techniques necessary for traveling. This diversity of students reflects differences in age, cultural background, personality, learning style, lifestyle and setting, health situation, and other physical, sensory, or cognitive impairments that may exist in addition to visual impairments. Students with vision and cognitive impairments may experience difficulties in a number of areas including sensorimotor skills, communication and language, or vision and hearing, as well as behavioral or intellectual functioning. It is important to consider each individual's unique set of skills and interests, and recognize that the manner in which people with visual and cognitive impairments learn and use O&M skills and techniques is highly individualized.

This chapter covers general information about teaching O&M to learners with visual and cognitive impairments, and specifically addresses topics related to mental retardation and traumatic brain injury. It is important to maintain a perspective of the combined effects of multiple impairments on learning and performance. The combined effects do not represent an additive approach (e.g., visual impairments and mental retardation) but rather a compounding of effects (i.e., the combined impact on learning when a person who is mentally retarded is visually impaired as well). Educational and rehabilitation programs that provide services to individuals with visual and cognitive impairments need to consider these combined effects, rather than approach intervention from the perspective of addressing a series of specialized service needs related to isolated disabling conditions. The conditions described in this chapter are those whose prevalence make it especially probable that O&M instructors will encounter them in practice.

VISUAL AND COGNITIVE IMPAIRMENTS: DEMOGRAPHIC INFORMATION

Individuals with multiple impairments, including those with visual and cognitive impairments, constitute a segment of the population that utilizes O&M. Like most incidence and prevalence demographic information, precise data about these and other multiple impairments (e.g., vision and physical impairments) within the population of persons who are visually impaired is not available (Uslan, Hill, & Peck, 1989). However, based on data collected in 1980 (Kirchner & Peterson, 1980), it is likely that visually impaired persons with multiple impairments outnumber those who have visual impairments alone. As reported by Uslan et al. (1989), a 1983 survey of O&M practitioners found that approximately 51 percent of their clients during the previous 12 months were multiply impaired. However, the nature or the severity of the multiple impairments was not reported. Scholl (1986) reports that vision problems are found in an estimated 30 percent of the population of students with multiple impairments whose primary diagnosis does not involve vision. Kirchner (1990), based on a study conducted in Virginia, estimated that over 60 percent of children with visual impairments had multiple disabilities. A Colorado study suggests that O&M specialists actually serve three times more school-age students who are visually impaired than are reported as visually impaired by counts maintained by the federal government (Ferrell & Suvak, 1996). These students are classified with a disability other than visual impairments (Corn, Ferrell, Spungin, & Zimmerman, 1996).

It is important, therefore, to incorporate accurate visual examinations in the routine health care and educational management of persons with severe and profound mental retardation, other cognitive impairments, and related health disorders. In addition, further research into the prevalence of visual impairments in otherwise disabled populations is necessary to identify current needs for O&M services, and to estimate more accurately future personnel and training needs.

In the 1950s, many premature babies who were treated with oxygen administered in incubators developed retinal disorders, originally called retrolental fibroplasia—now called retinopathy of prematurity—that resulted in severe visual impairment or total blindness. Changes in the medical management of prematurity have since improved the prognosis for premature infants whose birth weight exceeds 3 pounds; however, this same improved medical technology has enabled infants with birth weights as low as 1 pound to survive (Lyon, 1985). These low-birth-weight infants often experience a succession of medical challenges during the neonatal period that can result in severe sensorimotor and cognitive disabilities, as well as blindness. Continued increases in the population of children and youth with severe visual and multiple impairments can be anticipated. Powerful social forces that emerged during the 1970s and 1980s, associated with poverty, changing patterns of sexual behavior, limited access to primary health care, poor maternal and child health, as well as maternal substance abuse contribute to this anticipated steady growth (Joffee & Rikhye, 1991).

TEACHING O&M TO PERSONS WITH VISUAL AND COGNITIVE IMPAIRMENTS

History

The development and research of O&M skills and techniques started in the late 1940s and continue to the present day. The initial emphasis was primarily in relation to adults whose only disability was visual impairment. However, O&M instructors have provided services to individuals with visual and multiple impairments since the profession's inception. The individualized approach to services, including the involvement of learners and their families in assessment, program development, and implementation, has characterized O&M instruction. This approach has enabled O&M specialists to address the needs of a wide range of learners, including individuals of all ages who have blindness as a single disability as well as those who have cognitive impairments and other disabilities.

During the late 1960s Eichorn and McDade (1969) carried out a demonstration project at the Greene Blind Unit of the Walter E. Fernald State School in Massachusetts. This project investigated the feasibility of systematically teaching O&M to residents who were blind and living in a state institution for persons with mental retardation. The researchers also wanted to evaluate if established methods used for teaching blind persons who are not mentally retarded are suited to those with mental retardation. Eichorn and McDade (1969) demonstrated that for individuals whose intelligence quotients ranged from 30–81, the established O&M instructional model was effective for teaching travel skills when certain adaptations were made, including

- breaking tasks down into their simplest components, and teaching each task separately, when feasible;
- providing abundant repetition and verbal reinforcement;
- increasing the amount of instructional time devoted to orientation skills, such as utilizing compass directions and applying directional and positional concepts;
- teaching concrete and practical applications of O&M techniques; and
- building in opportunities for students to experience progress and success in each O&M lesson.

Eichorn and McDade (1969) concluded that "afforded enough instruction with special modifications of methods and procedure, a large number of blind residents of institutions for the mentally retarded can profit from a program of orientation and mobility (p. 71)." Eichorn and McDade also observed that an O&M instructor working with this population should have specific knowledge related to the procedures used for teaching individuals who are mentally retarded, and should have personal attributes that permit them to work comfortably with nonprofessional as well as professional personnel from other disciplines.

Eichorn and McDade (1969) noted that very few people with mental retardation were receiving O&M and rehabilitation services. There may have been several explanations and contributing factors for that observation, such as a lack of personnel with either the interest or the knowledge to work with the population of visually impaired individuals with mental retardation. Also, the professional preparation of O&M instructors had only been in existence since 1960, and limited numbers of O&M specialists were available. These new professionals were primarily recruited by rehabilitation agencies and, to a lesser extent, educational programs. When O&M instructors were employed by educational programs, the general administrative policy regarding who received O&M services gave preference to visually impaired high-school students first. Because of the limited O&M services, visually impaired individuals with additional impairments were often a very low priority. In a similar fashion, the administrators of educational and rehabilitation programs questioned the value, including the cost of the extensive number of instructional hours, of providing O&M services to the visually impaired individual with mental retardation. Moreover, the possible lack of an articulated model for teaching O&M to students with severe multiple impairments (Joffee & Rikhye, 1991) may have resulted in many special education and rehabilitation programs either omitting O&M service or using strategies that were ineffective. In addition, there was a question whether many students with severe and profound mental retardation were capable of benefiting from O&M services because they were unable to build from prerequisites to more advanced techniques (Bailey & Head, 1993; Gee, Harrell, & Rosenberg, 1987; Joffee & Rikhye, 1991). Typically, more capable students received O&M instruction more frequently than students with multiple impairments (Chen & Smith, 1992).

In 1976 Hill and Ponder (1976) introduced their guide for O&M practitioners stating that the ultimate goal of O&M is to enable the student to enter any environment, familiar or unfamiliar, and function safely and independently. O&M instructor preparation stressed the unique nature and body of knowledge of the O&M profession, the special relationship between the learner and the instructor, and one-on-one instruction.

Hill and Ponder (1976) cautioned that neither the terminology nor the ordering and format of skills presented in their work was "sacred," and that they did not intend to write a lesson sequence or curriculum guide. They discussed functional understanding and assimilation of prerequisite skills such as walking a straight line, executing turns, and divergent thinking, and stated that those skills would influence a student's level of proficiency in O&M and the degree of independence acquired. With regard to teaching learners with multiple disabilities, they noted that the instructor must be flexible enough to adapt or modify the appropriate mobility skill to meet the student's individual needs.

Bryant and Jansen (1980) asserted that the steps involved in designing and implementing O&M programming for multiply impaired persons were not significantly different from those required for any good instructional program: instruction should be realistically designed, creatively implemented, and periodically evaluated for its effectiveness; and the instructor will most often have to rely on resourcefulness to achieve success. Harley, Wood, and Merbler (1980) and Harley, Long, Merbler, & Wood (1987) determined that families and teachers with systematic training in basic O&M skills—such as the sighted guide and trailing techniques—can provide effective instruction and support for learners with visual and multiple impairments. Hill, Dodson-Burk, and Smith (1989) identified the need to provide O&M instruction that is integrated across daily routines, people, and environments, using a method of instruction that requires the O&M specialist to provide direct service to learners and to consult with staff and families.

In 1985 Gee and Goetz (Gee et al., 1987) examined the premise that prerequisite skill mastery influences the level of proficiency in O&M and the degree of independence that can be acquired by students with severe multiple impairments. They demonstrated that visually impaired students with severe mental retardation who failed to demonstrate conceptual and sensory prerequisites when evaluated according to the Peabody Mobility Scale were successful in learning and generalizing mobility tasks carried out in the students' daily living environments. These students were taught using a modified instructional approach for functional skill development in response to the demands of the students' daily travel environments.

Beginning in the late 1960s, change in special education policy had a major impact on the field of O&M. This change in policy resulted from several acts including the 1970 Education of the Handicapped Act (EHA), amended in 1975 with the Education for All Handicapped Children Act (P.L.94–142), and the 1988 Individuals with Disabilities Education Act (IDEA). This legislation moved the educational emphasis from institutionalization to mainstreaming patients out of large institutions and into community facilities. The practice of mainstreaming schools and rehabilitation agencies examined issues of curriculum, content, instructional methods, and placement, and increased numbers of individuals with multiple impairments receiving services in community-based educational and rehabilitation programs. In addition to prompting the development of innovative instructional approaches and strategies, these trends facilitated the collaboration of O&M instructors who worked with students who were severely multiply impaired with colleagues in related fields. The resulting collaboration provided the opportunity to share and glean new approaches for assessment, instruction, and follow-up. Multidisciplinary and transdisciplinary teaming, ecological assessments, individualized and augmentative communication systems and modes became integrated into instructional models for teaching learners with multiple impairments (Bailey & Head, 1993; Chen & Smith, 1992; Joffee in Huebner, Prickett, Welch, & Joffee, 1995).

In many educational settings, O&M instructional models for students with severe multiple impairments, including students with vision and cognitive impairments, are now based on instruction in natural settings—in other words, instruction that takes place in the settings where students are naturally required to use travel skills at the time when they need to use them. This model is focused on teaching skills for daily living needs and not necessarily for generalizability or according to a predetermined sequence of prerequisite techniques. Early work (Bentzen, 1973) in this area demonstrated that skill and concepts learned in a structured teaching situation are not automatically transferred to performing daily activities. The traditional "pull-out" service model for teaching O&M in many cases, therefore, was modified or supplemented with O&M instruction that took place while students were engaged in their daily travel, for example, while they moved from one class to another or participated in daily school activities that occurred in outdoor environments (Bailey & Head, 1993). In rehabilitation programs for adults and elders, approaches such as the andragogical approach discussed by Welsh (1980) focused on teaching O&M skills for meeting immediate life needs. The teaching of critical skills for meeting immediate life needs has also been used in the treatment plans developed for individuals with Acquired Immunodeficiency Syndrome (AIDS) (Keister, 1990).

The O&M program's instructional model is based on principles including individualized instruction, teaching in real environments, environmental problem solving, lessons of graduated difficulty and responsibility, and the synthesis of skills (see Blasch, LaGrow, & Peterson, chapter 19) that can be supplemented by curricula, techniques, and methodologies to meet the diverse individual needs of learners with a wide range of multiple impairments, including those who have visual impairments, mental retardation, and other cognitive impairments (Bailey & Head, 1993; Joffee, & Rikhye, 1991; Lolli & Joffee, 1995; Uslan et al., 1989).

O&M professionals now possess expanded resources to individualize their instructional programs to address the unique needs of learners with a wide range of multiple impairments. It is likely that the instructional models and curricula that O&M instructors use to teach individuals with visual and cognitive impairments will continue to evolve through ongoing examination and modification as O&M professionals respond to changing demographics, the needs of individuals who have visual and cognitive impairments, and emerging innovative practices in the field of blindness and related disciplines.

The material that follows presents basic information about visual and cognitive impairments frequently encountered by O&M instructors, and explores principles and techniques for teaching O&M to learners with these impairments in both educational and rehabilitation programs. Topics specifically addressed in this chapter are visual impairments and mental retardation, and visual impairments and traumatic brain injury.

Visual Impairments and Mental Retardation

Learners with mental retardation constitute a diverse group, ranging from those with mild developmental delays to those with moderate to severe and profound mental retardation. Graham (1966) found a high prevalence of mental retardation in his study of multiply impaired children who were blind. It is likely that the combination of visual impairment and mental retardation is the most frequently encountered by O&M specialists.

Various classifications of the levels of mental retardation have been offered in the professional literature. These are often numerically defined categories that convey little information about an individual's potential for learning and utilizing travel skills. Functional performance groupings for describing three levels of learners with mental retardation have been developed by the travel training professionals at the Arc (Pinedo, 1995), and have been modified by the authors so they are relevant for teaching O&M to learners with mental retardation. These levels consider functional skills that are related to travel tasks and describe the travel that is typically achieved by persons functioning at these levels. However, some individuals with mental retardation have been able to achieve greater independence than suggested by these levels.

1. *Functional Level One*
   Learners possess the cognitive, communication, judgment, and social skills to achieve rote travel in most daily indoor and outdoor travel environments, including public transportation. They can utilize the routes they have mastered safely, effectively, and independently. These travelers require specific instruction for travel on routes that are new to

them or to make changes in the routes they use regularly.

2. *Functional Level Two*
Learners have limited but functional cognitive, expressive, and receptive communication skills, and exhibit limited judgment and social skills to achieve rote travel in their daily indoor and outdoor travel environments. Learners can utilize most indoor routes they have mastered safely, effectively, and independently. They can travel a specified but limited number of outdoor routes, including simple trips on mass transit or special van service. These travelers require specific instruction to master routes that are new to them or to make changes in the travel routes they use regularly.

3. *Functional Level Three*
Learners have severely limited cognitive, expressive, and receptive verbal communication skills, communicating primarily through the use of nonverbal strategies, and have limited interactive social skills. These learners travel purposefully in indoor and outdoor environments making use of the sighted guide technique and basic indoor mobility skills and may use an adaptive mobility device or possibly the standard cane. Their travel is typically supervised, and can include the use of continuous tactile landmarks, such as railings or tactile guide strips.

The functional levels described above illustrate the diverse and complex goals of individuals with mental retardation who are learning to travel. As with all learners, these individuals need to develop safe and purposeful movement to build self-esteem and confidence, have opportunities for learning, and acquire the skills to manage their daily living needs. Learners with mental retardation require additional time to acquire O&M skills, and they need repeated experiences to develop a sense of anticipation and master skills (Chen & Smith, 1992). In addition to the conventional elements of the O&M curriculum, their instructional needs include instruction that integrates specialized communication, judgment, and social skill-building as part of the O&M program. Consistent with the model identified by Eichorn and McDade (1969), students at the Functional Level One often do very well acquiring travel skills through a program that progresses slowly, breaks learning experiences down into small manageable tasks, makes realistic demands on verbal skills, builds in opportunity for abundant practice and successes in a range of environments, involves home and family, and is task specific. The instructional picture, however, is more complex for learners who perform in a manner consistent with Functional Levels Two and Three.

Team Approach

The notion of teaming is critical for teaching learners with mental retardation to travel since students require a constant environment with continual reinforcement. Interdisciplinary, intradisciplinary, multidisciplinary, and transdisciplinary approaches allow related professionals to participate in assessment and reinforce the skills taught by the O&M instructor. The need for and the level of involvement and reinforcement by the learners' caregivers and professionals from related disciplines becomes more pronounced as the complexity of the student's needs increases.

Frequently these individuals have an extensive history of medical treatment. In addition to the visual condition, other medical conditions and medications may have a major impact and present a greater challenge to the team and the O&M specialist.

The evaluation process required prior to the development of the Individualized Education Program (IEP) or an Individualized Written Rehabilitation Plan (IWRP) involves observational assessment over a period of days and possibly weeks by the team of professionals, and includes participation by parents, family members, and the student, when appropriate. The most efficient team of professional evaluators works together frequently and has repeated team-building opportunities.

One approach to the assessment process can be center-based. This assessment approach requires students to be removed from their current educational or rehabilitation placement. The student is presented assessment activities that are individualized and functional, and have a high interest value. The evaluators, representing different disciplines, come together to observe the student. For example: the communication specialist interacts with the student while performing a cooking activity. The communication specialist records the student's communicative interactions and the pragmatics of such communication. The occupational therapist observes the student's fine motor skills. The O&M specialist observes the students' movement, noting skills in areas such as spatial awareness, audition, and negotiating environments and objects within environments. After a period of time, the evaluators meet to review their observations, report on their findings, and develop strategies to enhance learning for this student. A multidisciplinary team conference and a written evaluation report of the student's skills across all disciplines is prepared. The report contains recommendations for instructional modifications and strategies.

Immediately following the multidisciplinary team conference, the evaluation enters an implementation phase, which allows evaluators the opportunity to assess the effectiveness of the instructional approaches and strategies that were identified. As a member of the evaluation team, O&M specialists have the opportunity during this time to document the manner in which O&M skills and techniques are infused into students' instructional programs and the manner in which skills and techniques are reinforced by all persons involved in the students' daily activities.

Another approach to evaluation involves assessments that are carried out within familiar daily environments. In this approach, the student does not need to be removed to a center for evaluation, and is often based on a team approach as well. When students' skills are evaluated in the context of familiar daily environments at home, school, rehabilitation programs, vocational settings, or in the community, it is often possible to identify the specific areas and situations where students need to build skills to carry out their daily activities, and discover naturally occurring stimuli, cues, and reinforcers for learning.

Each approach to assessment has advantages and disadvantages that need to be considered with respect to students' individual needs and circumstances. In familiar settings, students' routine behavior can be so reinforced that students might not be challenged to perform, or the familiar setting may be so structured that students do not have the opportunity to encounter situations which can promote future skill development. Conversely, in a center-based assessment model, students may be challenged by the newness of the environment, the change in personnel, and environmental stimuli, making it difficult for the student to focus behavior on the skills that are being evaluated.

O&M Program Planning and Implementation

O&M program planning and implementation derive directly from the assessment process. For an O&M specialist providing services to mentally retarded and visually impaired students, the model of instruction requires flexibility and creativity. Mentally retarded individuals typically learn within a functional and time-appropriate activity, that is to say, concrete learning rather than abstract generalizability. Therefore the route to the lunch room is taught at the time when the student is going to lunch. This model is referred to as *infused instruction,* which is different from a *pull-out* model of instruction.

Within a weekly schedule of activities, the O&M specialist reviews with the classroom staff the student's schedule. Opportune times for O&M instruction are identified and scheduled. Following the assessment period, the student's objectives for learning daily travel skills are established. For example, the student's objectives may include learning to travel independently from the

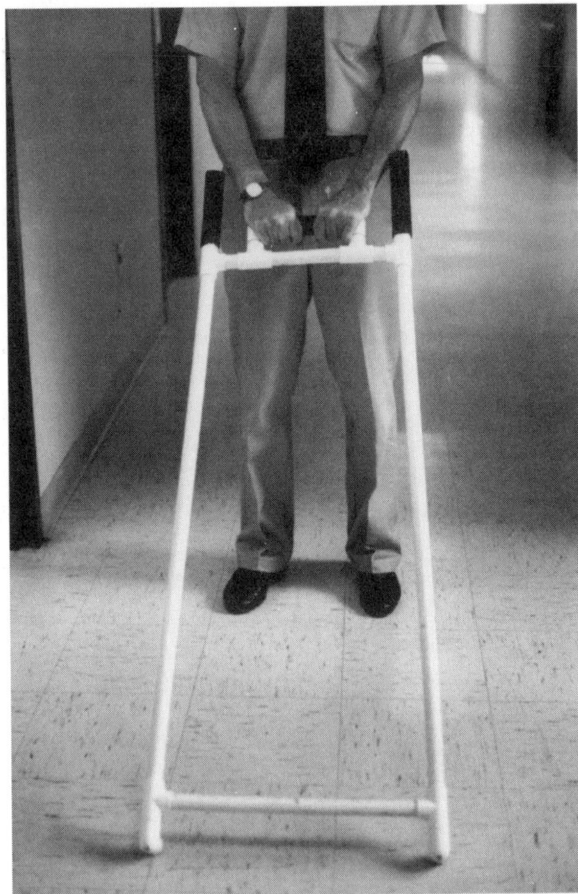

Figure 16.1. Adaptive mobility devices such as the one shown here are made by O&M instructors to meet the individual needs of students.

Source: Reprinted by permission from K. M. Huebner, J. G. Prickett, T. R. Welch, & E. Joffee (Eds.). *Hand in Hand: Essentials of Communication and Orientation and Mobility for Your Students Who Are Deaf-Blind* (New York: AFB Press, 1995), p. 608.

classroom to the lunch room using an adaptive mobility device (AMD) (Figure 16.1). To accommodate the student's needs, the recommended instructional frequency and duration is set at two times a week for 30-minute sessions. The student's lunch is scheduled for 11:30 A.M., and the O&M specialist identifies two days within the week to work with the student, from 11:15 to 11:45 A.M. During that time the O&M specialist teaches the student the skills related to the effective use of the adaptive mobility device to travel from the classroom to the lunch room. The pace and content of the instruction is very important, and the instructional time is rich with opportunities for learning. The O&M specialist prepares a written instructional plan identifying the manner in which techniques are introduced, reviewed, reinforced, and applied throughout the day; and establishes and maintains a monitoring system to observe and document the student's progress with respect to goals and objectives. The O&M specialist's instructional plan incorporates and utilizes the recommendations from the other disciplines, such as communication, occupational, and physical therapy. Learning strategies identified and utilized by the O&M specialist are utilized by other members of the team, as appropriate.

When establishing O&M goals and developing and implementing O&M programs, it is generally worthwhile to make detailed lists or inventories of all the movement activities learners need to engage in during the course of the day for each domain or setting—home school, community, rehabilitation center, work—covered in the assessment. O&M instructors working independently or with team members then identify how learners presently accomplish this movement, and decide which movement tasks should be targeted for instruction, the mobility skills and techniques to be taught, the sequence of instructional activities, and the level of independence the learner will seek to achieve. O&M instructors can create a mobility planning worksheet for this purpose (see Figure 16.2).

Once the O&M instructor has completed the mobility planning worksheet, either independently or with the team, strategies are selected for instructional approaches, integrating communication skill development, efficient sensorimotor functioning, sensory or cognitive training, and social skill development, as appropriate. Considerations for specialized instructional strategies include

- utilizing hand-over-hand instruction and physical positioning to introduce and monitor indoor mobility and cane techniques, gradually fading this support as learners progress.

MOBILITY PLANNING WORKSHEET

Student's name ____

School ____

Date of planning meeting ____

Completed by ____

STARTING POINT	DESTINATION	PRESENT METHOD OF TRAVEL	MOBILITY GOAL

Figure 16.2. An example of a mobility planning worksheet used to develop a mobility program for a student's daily travel.

Source: Reprinted by permission from K. M. Huebner, J. G. Prickett, T. R. Welch, & E. Joffee (Eds.). *Hand in Hand: Essentials of Communication and Orientation and Mobility for Your Students Who Are Deaf-Blind.* (New York: AFB Press, 1995).

- creating a system of prompts, with time frames and milestones for fading prompts.
- providing instruction using communication strategies (verbal and/or nonverbal) that are appropriate for the student's learning needs.
- providing abundant opportunities for repetition and successful experiences during lessons, and opportunities to practice and utilize skills between lessons.
- providing several shortened periods of instruction throughout the school day.
- providing O&M instruction in natural settings at the time when movement skills are utilized.
- breaking down instructional activities related to teaching travel routes using a task analysis approach.
- modifying mobility devices or techniques to meet the unique needs of the learner.
- team-teaching certain skills, such as introducing cane technique to a student who has cerebral palsy together with the physical and/or occupational therapist, at times when collaboration with other team members will enhance instruction.
- working with an orientation and mobility assistant (OMA) who is prepared to teach sighted guide technique for indoor and outdoor travel, and monitor and practice indoor O&M activities.
- participating with the learner in the activity just prior to and immediately following an O&M lesson, to help the learner make the transition to and from an O&M lesson that is integrated in daily routines.
- beginning O&M lessons at a learner's favorite place or in a very familiar location, and building to lessons that address travel needs in other locations.
- breaking a long daily travel route into segments and introducing learners to portions of the route, gradually piecing together the full route.
- introducing new O&M skills with the cooperation of a significant person in the learner's life, who has a good rapport with the student.

There are instances when it may be impractical to conduct some or all O&M instruction within the context of the learner's regular schedule. In these situations, instructors may find it feasible to teach O&M skills in a simulated context that recreates the regular travel situation, using appropriate cues, stimuli, communication techniques, etc. One example of this pull-out instruction would be to follow a student's scheduled daily travel routine in the normal daily order during each lesson. Depending on the student's level of understanding, the instructor may need to perform appropriate activities relative to each route—reading aloud from a book at the library, letting the student play maracas briefly in the band room, or pausing for a snack in the dining room. For learners with very limited receptive language skills, the instructor in the above case might provide object cues at the beginning of each route to indicate the student's intended destinations. Object cues for this student may be a book, maracas, or a spoon. (O&M instructors interested in additional information about the use of object cues and other individualized communication systems in O&M instruction can refer to the self-study text, *Hand in Hand: Essentials of Communication and Orientation and Mobility for Your Students Who Are Deaf–Blind* [Huebner et al., 1995] and the video, *We Can Do It Together* [Joffee, n.d.]).

Adaptive Mobility Devices

When teaching learners with mental retardation, O&M instructors have sometimes found it helpful to use commercially available AMDs, modified walkers, T-bar–handled or based devices, and various types of handmade devices fabricated from polyvinyl chloride piping (Bosbach, 1988; Foy, Kirchner, & Waple, 1991; Ehresman, 1995).

Often O&M instructors select these devices when students are unable to control the long cane's arc or have behavior problems or motor difficulties (Chen & Smith, 1992). Issues surrounding the use of such devices have often been concerned with transition to a regular cane, detection of drop-offs, and acceptance of the devices by the general public. Transition questions should be addressed by the O&M instructor and other members of the transdisciplinary team when the decision is made to use an AMD. Sometimes avoiding the term "pre-cane device," a common manner of identifying AMDs, is an important way to focus on the present travel needs of the individual. If transition to a long cane is anticipated, the behaviors that will need to be established or extinguished before then need to be determined.

Using an AMD that takes the form of a modified wheeled walker design can facilitate the detection of drop-offs for learners with moderate and severe mental retardation. These designs may be more efficient than a regular cane since they check at once both sides of the user's path. Flat-bottomed AMD designs can be subtly modified to provide similarly useful tactile feedback.

Placing a red strip along the bottom few inches of each side or support shaft of a white or light-colored AMD can convey the message that the device is one for use by persons who are blind. This design consideration can help ease its acceptance by the general public.

Teaching the AMD or the Long Cane

It is important for O&M instructors to apply the principle of teaching functional skills in natural contexts to facilitate the introduction and teaching of long cane skills and techniques. Some of the following guidelines have been successful with either the AMD or the long cane:

- Select a route that is functional in the context of daily travel. This strategy will enhance motivation to learn cane technique by enabling the learner to acquire new skills that are relevant to accomplishing travel.
- Identify each mobility task necessary to travel along the route.
- Teach the appropriate cane skill to complete each task along the route as the learner travels the route.
- Use hand-over-hand and physical positioning assistance to introduce cane skills and techniques (e.g., cane manipulation, cane placement, constant contact technique, two-point touch technique, trailing, clearing doorways, cane techniques for stairs, etc.) and to practice these skills with the student.
- Fade hand-over-hand and positioning assistance as the learner gains experience with the techniques by gradually withdrawing physical support.
- For the long cane, provide a rhythmic beat to assist the learner to achieve even timing and walk with a steady cadence when swinging the cane. Simple songs in common time or beats provided by hand clapping or rhythm instruments have been effective.
- Create an obstacle course along a wall or a travel path. Ask the learner to travel the path and either locate and remove the obstacles or clear a path around the obstacles.
- Gradually incorporate long-cane use for travel along additional routes in the learner's daily travel environment, working up to the application of cane techniques to routes in the school and the

community that the learner has been negotiating with the use of a sighted guide.

Utilizing Specialized Instructional Strategies

Implementing the strategy of teaching indoor mobility and cane techniques by providing hand-over-hand instruction and physical positioning can be accomplished with the instructor positioned behind the learner so that the instructor's arms and hands are placed in direct contact with the student. The learner and the instructor are then positioned together for using the technique. In this position, the instructor and the learner move forward, for example, to trail a wall, manipulate the cane in constant contact technique, etc. Instructors gradually fade support by providing less physical positioning and tactile assistance and allowing sufficient time to elapse after initiating physical contact for the learner to respond. This waiting is critical because many learners with moderate to severe mental retardation may need extra time to process and respond to stimulation, or they have learned to expect things to be done for them and need to develop the sense that they are expected to perform on their own.

Using language or communication techniques that are consistent with the learner's level of functioning is also important. Concrete language cues or other communication uses such as touch, object, or picture cues are an important part of a successful O&M program—for example, a learner functioning on the concrete level of cognitive development can more easily understand the concrete directions, "Walk to the end of this sidewalk, put your cane tip in the street, stop, and wait for me," than the more abstract directions, "Go to the corner and wait to be met."

Readers interested in further information about ecological assessment, task analysis, the transdisciplinary team, and instructional strategies for working with learners who are mentally retarded are urged to consult Sailor and Guess (1983), Snell (1983), or Goetz, Guess, and Stremel-Campbell (1987).

Traumatic Brain Injury and Organic Brain Dysfunction

When learners with visual impairments who have traumatic brain injury (TBI)—also referred to as internal head injury or organic brain dysfunction—receive special education or rehabilitation services, O&M instructors are part of the service team, playing an important role in planning effective and safe strategies for travel. The O&M specialist works closely with families, physicians, occupational and physical therapists, communication specialists, neuropsychologists, and other related health service providers. The service team is likely to follow an interdisciplinary or transdisciplinary model, especially if the student also has severe multiple disabilities. TBI is often associated with accidents, such as automobile and motorcycle collisions, and gunshot wounds. Sometimes similar symptoms are found with organic brain damage that is not caused by trauma, but rather is a result of pathologies related to tumors, stroke, elevated intracranial pressure, anoxia (lack of oxygen to the brain), systemic disease, brain deformity present at birth, or cerebral bleeding associated with prematurity. Functional limitation of traumatic brain injury and organic brain injury may be similar, depending on the location of the damage. The visual symptoms of a person with these pathologies are a function of the etiology, and the behavioral manifestations are often related to the etiology as well as individual characteristics such as motivation, personality, and intelligence. Visual disorders include field losses and degraded acuity. Symptoms may include double vision, field anomalies, cortical blindness, low vision, or total blindness. Functional visual loss may also be imposed by perceptual deficits. For both cortical blindness and functional visual loss, the eyes and the optic nerves may function normally; however, the brain may not be able to process or interpret visual information.

Depending on the nature and etiology of the pathology, O&M instructors may be called upon to provide services in hospitals, extended health care facilities, cognitive rehabilitation centers, nursing homes, general vocational rehabilitation programs, or blindness service rehabilitation programs. Service delivery may be center- or home-based, or in transition from the center-based health care or rehabilitation setting to home services.

Behavioral Difficulties

Behavioral symptoms related to brain trauma or organic dysfunction are highly individualized, depending on etiology or location of injury. Some individuals are severely affected by a cluster of behavioral symptoms, and others experience mild behavioral symptoms for which they can readily compensate. The behavioral manifestations that can affect how students learn O&M and travel include short- or long-term memory deficits, reduced ability to process and use information, diminished cognitive ability, inconsistent cognitive skills (e.g., individual can read but cannot write, or can match shapes but cannot name them), reduced ability to concentrate on cognitive tasks, language processing problems, reduced alertness, distraction by internal thoughts and external events, tendency to fatigue, confusion in crowds, verboseness, low tolerance for frustration, restlessness, impatience, inappropriate social behavior, slow acquisition of skills and routes, inability to carryover new learning, and inability to attend to multiple stimuli. Confabulation, or inventing information to fill in memory gaps, a general sense of disorientation even when travel is proceeding correctly, and a lack of insight or awareness of the manner in which the brain damage is affecting performance have been observed by instructors teaching students who have organic brain damage.

Typical Challenges

There are many common O&M challenges experienced by persons with brain injury. Difficulty with spatial relationships and sequencing causes the individual to become confused. Some individuals have difficulty maintaining self-to-object relationships and thus become disoriented in rooms or buildings, and during outdoor travel. Individuals may also have trouble understanding object-to-object relationships and thus not be able to plan travel routes. Inability to follow a sequence may also result in trouble following a travel route and later reversing that route. The individual may not be able to remember and follow a sequence of landmarks. Similarly, an individual may have trouble following a sequence of room numbers or addresses. The traveler may also be unable to establish primary landmarks. For example, a traveler may select a garbage can on the sidewalk or people sitting in front of a store as landmarks. The traveler fails to realize that a landmark must be permanent and easily recognizable. Other difficulties with landmarks may be perceptual in nature. The traveler might recognize a visual landmark when viewed from one direction, but may not recognize the same landmark when approaching it from another direction. When using tactile information, the traveler might not understand what is being touched. Auditory information can also be distorted. A traveler might be aware of the presence of traffic sounds but not understand where the car is coming from.

Some individuals experience short-term memory loss that interferes with travel. Directions provided by the O&M specialist may be forgotten, as may be travel routes, the names of stores, bus routes, and bus schedules. An individual may even forget an objective while en route to that objective.

Some individuals with traumatic or organic brain dysfunction experience diminished cognitive ability. An individual may experience difficulty with problem-solving activities. Instead of looking for alternative solutions to a problem, the traveler may be fixed on only one possible approach, even in the face of failure. For example, when asked to find evaporated milk in the grocery store, the traveler may reach an impasse when it is not found among cartons of milk in the cooler. The individual may have difficulty thinking of alternative locations for the canned milk. In a similar fashion, when disoriented outdoors, the traveler may not be able to generate hypotheses about what went wrong or what to try next. Those individuals with language difficulties may take the instructor too literally. One student with traumatic brain injury was upset when the O&M specialist said that he had let the "cat out of the bag." The student said that he had not remembered releasing a cat. Another student started to leave the building after the O&M specialist jokingly said "get out of here."

For some individuals behavioral problems become a major obstacle. They may need to talk continually and therefore not be able to function independently. Others, because of low frustration tolerance, may act out by yelling, arguing, swearing, and exhibiting a short temper. Some individuals may not be able to inhibit their actions. They might exhibit inappropriate social behavior such as making offensive remarks in public, exposing themselves, or blurting out whatever comes to mind. Many are unaware of the inappropriateness of their behavior or its affect on others.

Some students who are distracted by internal and external events may not be able to concentrate during travel. For example, if a student is thirsty or is experiencing pain, he may not be able to pay attention to directions given by the O&M specialist. Other students may be overwhelmed by crowds of people they encounter in shopping malls or on downtown sidewalks.

Planning and Providing Services

To plan O&M services for learners with traumatic or organic brain damage, O&M instructors evaluate the learner's orientation, judgment, and safety skills. Careful attention is directed to assessing the learner's ability to recognize and use landmarks, make judgments about safety, establish and maintain orientation to time and place, understand and follow a series of directions, read and understand print or braille signs, reverse routes, communicate effectively, and interact in a socially appropriate manner. Effective strategies for teaching learners with traumatic or organic brain damage include the following:

General Strategies

- Build O&M skills on areas of strength and interest which remain from before the trauma incident that caused the individual's brain damage.
- Teach O&M techniques and their applications in naturally occurring, daily living environments.
- Provide exercises in interpreting sensory information.
- When distractions occur, refocus the student by restating the directions.
- Facilitate cognitive tasks by assisting the student to develop alternative solutions to problems.
- When frustration becomes too high, provide assistance before the tolerance level is reached.
- Above all else, be consistent.

Communication Strategies

- Use language that is specific, clearly communicate each action step, and don't rely upon colloquial expressions.
- Present a series of instructions that are exact, but do not overwhelm the student with too much information.
- Present information in a calm and organized manner to avoid triggering emotional reactions. Use age-appropriate levels—don't talk down to adults; most individuals are aware of their deficits.
- Leave nothing vague at the beginning of a lesson.

Lesson Strategies

- Use structured, uncluttered, and simple environments to introduce O&M skills and techniques.
- Noises, crowds, and music may interfere with focusing on a task. Control this as

much as possible until the student is ready for them.

- Divide complex tasks into a series of small ones, and have the student repeat each of the landmarks before starting a route.
- Teach small segments of a route and chain them together, either in a forward or backward manner.
- Plan lessons that follow a specific order of activities.
- Provide repetition from one lesson to the next.
- Plan rest periods during lessons to avoid fatigue.
- Create environmental redundancy to facilitate instruction by selecting a point of orientation for each environment and route that is used, relating travel routes to daily living routines, and teaching learners to follow routes consistently for all daily travel tasks.
- Reserve time prior to and after the lesson for talking about issues important to the student.
- Use a student's interests to determine lesson travel objectives.

To facilitate safe and effective travel, O&M instructors have found it beneficial to teach compensatory techniques—techniques that compensate for cognitive deficits associated with organic brain damage. These techniques assist persons with traumatic or organic brain damage to structure their travel agendas, plan and follow routes, and maintain their personal safety during travel. Examples of compensatory techniques are colored cue cards with word prompts; picture or object cues that represent destinations; labels along indoor routes that contain print signs, arrows, or picture cues; written or taped routes; and cards with emergency procedures for dealing with disorientation and transit breakdowns or service disruptions. Encourage students to keep a journal (print, braille, or tape) to document information that they will need, such as appointment times, routes, landmarks, schedules, and materials to bring (umbrella, bus money).

The unique nature of safe and independent travel for individuals with traumatic or organic brain dysfunction is a challenge for the O&M instructor, the learner, and the special education or rehabilitation team. Close and open communication between the learner and the O&M instructor during all phases of the O&M program—from planning O&M services to making determinations about how an individual will ultimately travel—are critical to the safety and well-being of the learner.

Suggestions/Implications for O&M Specialists

1. Assessment and instruction models and strategies used in the field of special education can be helpful in providing O&M instruction to individuals who have a combination of cognitive impairments.
2. It is necessary for members of various disciplines (e.g., O&M, physical therapy, occupational therapy, speech and language therapy) to share information when devising and implementing instructional objectives to facilitate consistent service delivery to students with visual and cognitive impairments.
3. O&M specialists should present instructional material in a context and manner consistent with each learner's needs. Some students with visual and cognitive impairments may benefit from instruction provided according to a pull-out model, whereas others may need immersed instruction provided while students are performing the actual travel routes they use each day.
4. O&M instructors can work in consultation with other members of the learner's instructional team when determining appropriate language or communication cues, behavior interventions, and reinforcers.
5. Choosing the appropriate mobility device for students with visual and cognitive impairments and teaching students to use the device for daily travel should be initiated and carried out by the O&M specialist in cooperation with other members of the instructional team. For example, when an O&M specialist evaluates a student to determine the suitability of a "wheeled walker" AMD, the O&M specialist should consult with the physical therapist on the instructional team.
6. Long-term goals for persons with visual and cognitive impairments may range from using an AMD under supervision along specified indoor routes, to independent travel along certain routes or in a certain area of the community. O&M specialists should enter each new instructional situation with a willingness to create a curriculum designed to help the student achieve the highest appropriate level of independence.
7. Visual impairments caused by traumatic brain injury or organic brain dysfunction range from low vision to total blindness, and are often accompanied by difficulties in behavior, memory, and various thought processes. Careful and thorough assessment of the student's strengths and weaknesses, and a methodical and consistent approach during instruction are keys to successful instruction.
8. Of special importance when teaching O&M to persons with traumatic or organic brain injury: determining that students accurately analyze available sensory input. Provide a backup system to use when students become disoriented, or nonstandard events such as transit delays, rerouting, or other emergencies occur during travel. Compensatory strategies such as cue cards and cards with emergency procedures are among the backup systems O&M specialists have found particularly useful.

ACTIVITIES FOR REVIEW

1. Discuss the meaning of the compounding effects of multiple impairments on the educational and rehabilitation needs of an O&M student who has cortical blindness, severe mental retardation, and cerebral palsy.
2. Describe the kinds of skills instructors of O&M acquire to become effective teachers of students with visual and cognitive impairments. Relate these skills to the assessment, goal setting, program planning, and program implementation phases of O&M instruction.
3. Identify and discuss the approaches to providing O&M services and the legislative changes which have occurred since the inception of the profession of O&M that have influenced current practice for teaching students with visual and cognitive impairments.
4. This chapter presents a discussion of three functional levels of mental retardation with respect to O&M. Discuss an effective way for O&M instructors to draw on these levels of functioning when designing a student's O&M program.
5. Identify and define the teaming strategies that may be used in the instruction of students with visual and cognitive impairments. Evaluate the strengths and limitations of each strategy for a student with a visual and cognitive impairment receiving services in: (1) a center-base rehabilitation program; (2) a community-based public day school; (3) a home-based rehabilitation program; (4) a special school.
6. What are two approaches for conducting assessments for learners with visual and cognitive impairments, and in which critical areas do these approaches differ? What criteria do you believe are important when selecting an assessment approach?
7. Explain how O&M program planning, implementation, and ongoing evaluation are related to assessment for students with visual and cognitive impairments. Discuss the "Mobility Planning Worksheet" in this context.
8. Describe the specialized instructional strategies that you believe will be most relevant for teaching indoor mobility to a 10-year-old student who lacks apparent expressive and receptive verbal communication skills and has had no prior instruction in O&M.
9. In which ways do AMDs have certain advantages for students with visual and cognitive impairments?
10. Describe the typical behaviors and learning challenges that are characteristic of O&M students who have traumatic brain injury or organic brain dysfunction. What are the instructional strategies that O&M instructors use to address these challenges?

CHAPTER 17

Learners with Visual and Health Impairments

Elga Joffee and Deborah Rower

Orientation and mobility (O&M) specialists provide services to individuals of all ages who are blind or visually impaired. These individuals, as do all people, experience a variety of systemic and other health conditions that may have an impact on their need for O&M programs and services. It is incumbent on the O&M specialists to have a thorough understanding of an individual's state of health and related health considerations. Two health conditions are addressed in great detail in this chapter: diabetes mellitus and human immunodeficiency virus/acquired immunodeficiency syndrome (AIDS), whose occurrence among persons who are blind or visually impaired makes it probable that O&M specialists will encounter them in practice.

DEMOGRAPHIC BACKGROUND

Visual impairment caused by complications of diabetes mellitus is a leading cause of new cases of blindness among adults in the United States (Van Sohn, 1985). There are approximately 5,000 new cases of blindness related to diabetes reported annually (State of New York, 1986). Individuals with diabetes-related vision loss are heavily represented in vocational rehabilitation programs for adults.

Visual impairments are associated with AIDS, especially with the later stages of the disease (Kiester, 1990). Although most people who are infected with human immunodeficiency virus (HIV) (that is, people who are HIV-positive) develop AIDS, some do not. The increasing numbers of persons who are HIV-positive and persons living with AIDS (PLWA), as well as the ongoing evolution of life-prolonging treatments, can be expected to contribute to the increasing incidence of AIDS-related visual impairment. Nationally, as of June 1994, the total number of PLWAs over the age of 5 reported to the Centers for Disease Control was 401,749 (Centers for Disease Control, 1994). The total number of HIV-positive cases from states with confidential HIV reporting through June 1994 was 62,443, with the greatest prevalence of HIV-positive cases reported for males between the ages of 25–34, and the largest growing segment of AIDS cases reported among women in this age group (Centers for Disease Control, 1994). Therefore O&M instructors can expect to provide services to individuals of all ages who have AIDS.

DIABETES

Diabetes mellitus is a serious metabolic disease that affects many systems of the body. It can cause visual impairment, and in some instances total blindness. Retinal degeneration related to diabetes, diabetic retinopathy, is one of the leading causes of adult visual impairment in the United States. O&M specialists often encounter students with diabetes in rehabilitation programs, although some older adolescents and young adults with diabetes experience visual disability during the school years. It is important for O&M specialists to understand the basic nature of diabetes, its primary and secondary complications, and how the disease affects behavior and functioning in order to develop and carry out effective O&M programs for students with diabetes that safeguard the well-being of this unique group.

Diabetes is a disease that prevents the body from metabolizing carbohydrates because of a lack of the hormone insulin, which is produced in the pancreas. There are several types of diabetes, which some believe may actually be a collection of discrete metabolic disorders manifesting similar symptoms. An individual with diabetes is not able to use sugars and starches properly, and must treat this condition by special diet, insulin injections, or orally administered insulin to control the amount of sugar in the blood. Not all diabetics require oral or injected insulin to control their diabetes. Regardless of the treatment regimen, diabetic control requires diligent adherence to the prescribed medical management plan, and for those taking insulin, includes balancing a combination of diet control, insulin medications, and activity level. Each individual's diabetic control is unique and may change throughout the course of the disease.

The primary complications of diabetes include ketosis, which can lead to diabetic coma; and hypoglycemia, which can induce insulin shock. Ketosis and diabetic coma occur when the body, deprived of insulin, fails to metabolize sugars and starches and begins to metabolize body protein for nourishment and energy. In ketosis, an individual experiences excessive thirst; deep, labored breathing; and vomiting. The skin may appear very flushed and dry, the breath may have a fruity odor, and the individual may become weak, drowsy, and lethargic. Ketosis and diabetic coma occur when diabetes goes untreated. Often ketosis or coma is the critical event that leads to an initial diagnosis of diabetes. Ketosis or coma also occur when individuals who are diabetic neglect to take their insulin properly and according to schedule, fail to adhere to their diets, or experience a condition known as "brittle diabetes," where diabetic control is difficult to achieve and maintain. O&M specialists must learn to recognize the symptoms of ketosis, poor diabetic management, or brittle diabetes and be prepared to address medical emergencies that may arise during lessons. They must also work in cooperation with the other members of the rehabilitation team, such as nurses, counselors, or social workers when providing services to diabetic students who are neglecting good management, to assure safe and effective rehabilitation. O&M specialists who are working with brittle diabetics must set goals and pace lessons in a manner that the learner can tolerate.

Hypoglycemia, the other primary complication of diabetes, is a low level of blood sugar that results when injected or orally administered insulin exceeds the amount required by the body. This can occur because an individual's activity level is now greater than when the insulin dose was first established, because of an elevation in metabolism related to stress, a result of poor eating habits, a delayed meal, or incorrect administration of insulin. Taking an overdose of insulin can occur when a person who is diabetic and severely visually impaired confuses premeasured doses, misreads a syringe, or self-administers insulin when confused because of hypoglycemia. Hypoglycemia is manifested in one or many ways; the most likely is pronounced perspiration. A diabetic in early hypoglycemia may appear pale and breathe rapidly. As the condition progresses, the individual may begin to tremble and appear to lack coordination. Speech and clear thought may be impaired temporarily. Often individuals experiencing hypoglycemia vigorously deny that they are having a problem, and some resist assistance when it is offered.

The symptoms of hypoglycemia are remedied by the immediate ingestion of sugar, preferably in liquid form. Orange juice, fruit juices, soft drinks, glucose tubes and tablets, cake icing, or sugar and water solutions are effective. However, it is important to advise against hard candy or tablets to avoid choking. If a hypoglycemic reaction is anticipated, eating a candy bar will forestall a severe reaction. O&M specialists must be alert for signs of hypoglycemia whenever they teach individuals who are diabetic, and be prepared to administer sugar when necessary. Persons who have experienced a severe hypoglycemic reaction may be temporarily disoriented and fatigued. It may be necessary to discontinue a lesson and make arrangements for transporting a student back home or to the rehabilitation center. O&M specialists should request that their students be in contact with the primary health care provider on the rehabilitation team when hypoglycemia occurs. It may be necessary for a physician to adjust insulin dosages. Hypoglycemic reactions often occur immediately after students with diabetes begin their O&M programs or when they achieve a level of skill that allows them to increase their level of activity. It is good practice for O&M specialists to ascertain that diabetic students eat properly prior to each O&M lesson.

The secondary complications of diabetes are also of major importance to O&M specialists. These complications include small blood vessel disease, peripheral neuropathy, nephropathy, and retinopathy. Diabetic small blood vessel disease causes the degeneration of capillaries in the body. Especially vulnerable to the effects of capillary degeneration are the retinas, peripheral nerves, heart, and kidneys. Diabetic retinopathy causes the blindness and visual impairments associated with diabetes and is related to diabetic small blood vessel disease, which affects the capillaries in the retina. Diabetic retinopathy occurs when tiny blood vessels in the retina break and cause small hemorrhages on or in the retina. This results in a loss of vision at the site of the hemorrhage, and causes generally blurred vision because blood clouds the vitreous humor, the clear fluid that fills the globe of the eye. Blurred vision usually resolves to some degree as the blood is absorbed by the body and the vitreous clears. For this and other reasons, O&M specialists can expect students who are diabetic to experience fluctuating vision and must teach students strategies for dealing with this situation.

A more severe form of diabetic retinopathy, diabetic proliferans, causes the formation of additional blood vessels at sites where hemorrhages occurred. These proliferating blood vessels are weak, can burst, create retinal tears and scar tissue, and may eventually cause retinal detachment. Laser treatments have proven to be effective in managing proliferating diabetic retinopathy by destroying proliferating blood vessels before they hemorrhage, and in sealing retinal tears. Laser treatments damage treated areas, and do not guarantee against further hemorrhaging. They do not restore vision. O&M instructors often find the need to explain this to students who mistakenly believe that their vision will improve as a result of laser treatments, and who sometimes attribute the clearing of blurred vision from the absorption of blood in the vitreous to cures related to laser care. O&M instructors need to be alert for diabetic students who report an acute change for the worse in their vision during an O&M lesson. Because of the possibility of retinal detachment, they should treat this as a medical emergency if it occurs.

O&M specialists also need to understand the effects of peripheral neuropathy, which is a reduction in sensation in the extremities experienced by diabetics. Peripheral neuropathy occurs when the peripheral nerves die as the capillaries that nourish them degenerate from diabetic small blood vessel disease. O&M specialists are especially concerned about peripheral neuropathy because they must teach students with reduced sensation in their hands and feet to grip and use the long cane, interpret tactile information conveyed through the cane's shaft and grip, and detect tactile information underfoot. O&M instructors devise strategies for utilizing multisensory cues, modified cane techniques, or electronic travel aids that can assist in the detection of elements such as stair rails, street signs, or other objects that project into the path of travel.

Another major concern for O&M instructors which is related to small blood vessel disease and peripheral neuropathy is the serious risk of infection faced by diabetic students. Physical injury to any degree is dangerous for persons with diabetes. A small bruise or bump may develop into serious complications, with sores becoming gangrenous because of poor circulation and elevated blood sugar, which provides a rich medium upon which infection can thrive. It is not unusual for diabetics to have a foot or leg amputation which was originally caused by a sore that did not heal and became gangrenous. Diabetics with peripheral neuropathy who are also blind may not see or feel a simple injury to their legs or feet, such as a blister or a mild skin abrasion, that may occur during travel. Consequently, essential immediate medical treatment may be delayed, causing potentially serious results. O&M instructors must be extremely alert to even the slightest change in a student's gait that could indicate an improperly fitting shoe, a blister, or an ingrown toenail. Additionally, O&M instructors should routinely, with the consent of the student, examine the diabetic student's extremities after lessons, especially if the student is wearing new shoes, the weather is unusually severe, or the instructor observes the student walking with a gait pattern that is unusual. Diabetic students should be encouraged to examine their own extremities carefully after taking walks, and a member of their family should be encouraged to do so as well on a regular basis.

Advanced peripheral neuropathy sometimes is associated with a condition called "dropped foot," where the individual experiences difficulty flexing the foot upward and downward. Orthopedic braces and shoes are prescribed for this condition. O&M instructors should be vigilant for diabetic students who trip often, and refer these individuals for medical evaluation. Tripping may be associated with reduced sensation in the lower extremities caused by peripheral neuropathy, or it may be a sign of the onset of more serious problems that require medical management.

Nephropathy, or degeneration of the small blood vessels in the kidneys, is another complication of diabetes that is important to O&M specialists. Diabetic students who have nephropathy often experience severely elevated blood pressure or undergo regular kidney dialysis. Regardless of the severity of a learner's nephropathy, O&M instructors must be aware that they are instructing an individual whose strength and stamina are seriously compromised. Realistic time frames for instruction and practice are of critical importance.

Students who are diabetic benefit significantly from mastering independent travel skills. It is important for O&M instructors, however, to accommodate the special health needs of these students by setting realistic goals, planning lessons that are paced to meet the learner's physical condition, teaching students basic self-care skills, and devising strategies for dealing with health emergencies that may arise during instruction or independent travel.

ACQUIRED IMMUNODEFICIENCY SYNDROME

O&M instructors are increasingly called upon to teach students who are HIV-positive or have AIDS. There are specific eye diseases related to AIDS that are frequently manifested in the later stages of the disease. However, a person of any age with a visual impairment may be HIV-positive or may live with AIDS and have a visual impairment that is not related to AIDS.

Often O&M instructors may be unaware or unsure if the individuals they are teaching are HIV-positive or are living with AIDS. Organizational, local, and federal policies and statutes ensuring nondiscrimination and confidentiality prohibit certain clinical and educational records and personnel files from including potentially discriminatory information about HIV and AIDS (Joffee, 1995). Consequently, instructors may be teaching persons who are HIV-positive or have AIDS and find no information about this condition in school or rehabilitation center records. Currently there is no reliable way to identify all those who have been exposed to or have become infected with HIV. HIV can have an incubation period of between 5 and 9 years, and it can take up to 6 months for the HIV antibody to be produced and thus detected once an individual has been infected. O&M instructors should be vigilant in following current public health practices and organizational infection control procedures, which will be discussed in greater detail later in this section.

Information about the incidence and prevalence of HIV and AIDS, methods for their detection and treatment, and the characteristics of persons who are HIV-positive or are living with AIDS is constantly changing. The material covered in this discussion is the most current information at the time of writing. However, O&M instructors are advised to stay abreast of evolving medical findings, treatments, and public health policies.

Definitions

AIDS is a condition that compromises the body's ability to fight off disease because of the deterioration of the immune system. Human immunodeficiency virus (or HIV), the proposed cause of AIDS, is a virus that attacks the body's immune system. Persons who are infected with HIV may incubate the virus for several years before becoming symptomatic—that is, exhibit symptoms of AIDS—or they may be infected immediately. When HIV antibodies are detected, persons with HIV are considered to be HIV-positive. Although most people who are HIV-positive develop AIDS, some do not.

PLWAs are at serious risk from a host of infections, known as opportunistic infections, many of which would not pose a threat to a person with a normal immune system. Certain types of cancers and bacterial and viral infections, as well as parasite and fungal infections are characteristic of the infections that threaten and afflict PLWAs. Breaking down the acronym AIDS offers some insight into the disease:

- Acquired: The condition is not hereditary or caused by medication;
- Immuno: The condition relates to the body's defense against disease;
- Deficiency: The condition relates to a lack of cellular immunity; and
- Syndrome: The condition involves a set of symptoms that signal a diagnosis (New York City Board of Education, 1986).

Persons infected with HIV may develop systemic illness or AIDS-related complex (ARC). ARC describes non–life-threatening infections caused by infectious agents the body cannot ward off because of the HIV infection. Symptoms experienced by persons with ARC include night sweats, swollen glands, chronic diarrhea, and weight loss. When an individual with HIV-related systemic illness develops symptoms that meet the criteria set up by the Centers for Disease Control (CDC) to define AIDS, they are then reclassified as having AIDS.

Transmission of HIV

HIV is transmitted in body fluids, specifically blood, semen, vaginal secretions, and breast milk. Other body fluids, such as urine, saliva, and vomit do not pose the risk of transmitting HIV unless blood is visibly present in these fluids. HIV is spread by direct contact with infected body fluids that enter an individual's bloodstream by direct entry into a vein, or through a break in the skin or mucous linings in the eyes, mouth, nose, vagina, rectum or urethra. HIV is a fragile virus that does not survive long outside of body fluids, or in body fluids that have left the body and are no longer at body temperature. Therefore HIV cannot be transmitted through casual contact, shaking hands, or hugging. Sharing air, water, food, a bathroom, or a water fountain with individuals who are HIV-positive will not transmit this virus (Kiester, 1990).

Treatment

Drug treatment regimens for individuals who are HIV-positive or have AIDS are continually evolving. Often these treatments can be highly toxic and result in side effects that may impact on an individual's capacity to participate in daily living activities, including O&M instruction. PLWAs frequently weigh the anticipated medical benefits of treatments and the side effects of available drugs when working with their physician to establish their course of treatment.

Eye Diseases Associated with AIDS

There are numerous AIDS-related opportunistic infections that affect the eye. Some are external and do not seriously impair visual function, while others affect the visual system or are systemic and can severely affect visual functioning. The infections that are external or affect the visual system are as follows:

- Kaposi's sarcoma, a vascular tumor that appears as a bruised area. When it affects the eyes, the tumor may be present on the eyelid or conjunctiva. Although the tumor has no affect on visual function, it may cause discomfort and therefore be treated with cryotherapy, surgical excision, radiation, or chemotherapy.
- Uveitis, an infection in the uveal tract of the eye that affects visual function by degrading or compromising acuity. This visual complication may be the first sign of several chronic infections for HIV-positive individuals. These infections may include tuberculosis, syphilis, histoplasmosis, coccidiomycosis, and toxoplasmosis.
- HIV retinopathy, a noninfectious microvascular disorder that is characterized by the presence of "cotton-wool spots," microaneurysms, retinal hemorrhages, telangiectatic vascular changes, and areas of capillary nonperfusion. These changes are found in approximately 70 percent of persons with advanced HIV disease, and approximately 40 percent of those persons with ARC (Ai & Luckie, 1994). Functionally, these individuals can suffer from field losses. Retinal detachments, commonly found in the periphery, occur in 17 to 34 percent of the population with HIV retinitis (Ai & Luckie, 1994). This may occur during an active infection or after the retinitis has been stabilized.

A number of systemic infectious diseases can affect the visual function of PLWAs. The most prevalent systemic disease is cytomegalovirus (CMV), a member of the herpes group of viruses. Studies show that 50 percent of the urban dwelling population in the United States and Europe have been infected with CMV; however, CMV disease affecting the eye tends to occur only in the developing fetus or individuals whose immune system is compromised (Ai & Luckie, 1994). Visual changes associated with CMV affect approximately 20 percent of PLWAs. Often the diagnosis of CMV as the cause of blindness for an adventitiously blind adult may be the only clue in a medical record that an individual may have AIDS.

Clinically, CMV appears as lesions on the retina with varying amounts of hemorrhage. Swelling of the optic nerve and vessel closure may also occur. Changes can occur on one or both eyes. CMV may cause blurry vision or visual field loss, and also has been known to cause total blindness related to damage to the retina.

Toxoplasmosis, a protozoan parasite that causes a retinochoriod infection, is another infection that can affect the vision of PLWAs, resulting in decreased visual acuity. It is important to note that this protozoan parasite affects the central nervous system, and that neurological symptoms are present in 10 to 40 percent of the cases of toxoplasmosis retinochoroiditis (Ai & Luckie, 1994).

Persons who have AIDS may also have syphilis, and the visual disorders associated with syphilis including a form of uveitis, chorioretinitis, retinal perivasculitis, intraretinal hemorrhage, papillitis, and panuvetis. The clinical management of syphilis by administration of intravenous penicillin to treat the systemic infection can improve visual function.

Universal Precautions for O&M Instructors

Universal precautions are steps that human service providers take to prevent the spread of infection (Kiester, 1990). O&M instructors should establish and carry out universal precautions, such as hand washing, when working directly with students. This is important for the welfare of the instructor, as well as for the learner living with AIDS, who has a compromised immune system and may be at risk of contracting an infection from the instructor. Simple hand washing prior to working with a learner and immediately after the session is completed is the first and best line of protection against spreading communicable diseases. The following is suggested with respect to hand washing:

- Hands should be washed vigorously with soap and water, keeping fingers pointed downward into the sink.
- Hands should be rinsed and dried completely using a fresh disposable towel that is discarded immediately after use. Fingers and hands should point upward during rinsing.
- The water faucet should be turned off using a fresh dry paper towel that is discarded immediately after use.
- In situations where running water is not available, hands should be washed thoroughly with antiseptic skin-cleansing tissue, such as Zephiran towelettes. Carrying a sealable disposable plastic bag for discarding used towels is recommended.

O&M instructors who work in educational, institutional, or rehabilitation settings where students exhibit "challenging behaviors," for example, biting or scratching, can wear protective latex gloves when providing instruction. They may be required to do so by the facility providing care. Protective latex gloves must be worn whenever there is a blood spill, or when the O&M instructor is working with a learner who has open lesions or bleeding wounds. Knowledge and experience about putting on and removing latex gloves are important. These guidelines should be followed:

- If possible, before putting on gloves, wash hands thoroughly (see above).
- Remove gloves, one at a time. The first glove is removed by grasping the edge of the outside of the glove with the thumb and forefinger of the other hand. Gently pull the glove down over the hand so that it comes off inside-out. Dispose of the glove. The second glove is removed with the thumb and forefinger of the ungloved hand by grasping the inside of the cuff of the glove so that the ungloved hand is between the glove and the hand. Carefully remove the glove so that it comes off inside out. Dispose of the glove.
- If there is no place to immediately dispose of used gloves, place them inside a sealable disposable plastic bag to discard at a later time.

In most cases PLWAs will be able to clean their own blood spills in the event of an injury; however, O&M instructors should be prepared to do the following in the case of an emergency:

- The area where blood has spilled should be cleaned with detergent and then with a bleach solution of 1:10 parts.
- All materials used to clean up blood spills should be disposed of as infectious waste. (Contact an organization's nurse or building/facility manager for information

about disposing of infectious waste materials.)

Prior to working with a PLWA, O&M instructors should be tested for tuberculosis (TB). This test is required at many public and private human service organizations at the initiation of employment and regular intervals thereafter. TB is communicable to others through droplets emitted from the nose and mouth, and spreads rapidly in crowded conditions where there is poor sanitation. Healthy persons with intact immune systems who observe good personal hygiene habits are not at high risk for contracting TB; however, persons with AIDS are extremely vulnerable because of their compromised immune systems.

O&M Services

Initiating Contact and Planning Services

Referrals for O&M services for PLWAs may originate from conventional sources, as well as those that are relatively new to O&M instructors, including a school district's committee on special education, a hospital social worker, a case manager from an agency that deals with consumers who have AIDS, or an organization serving the needs of the gay community. O&M instructors should become familiar with the national and local services and service networks available to PLWAs.

Administratively, priority should to be given to initiating services to PLWAs once a referral is completed, because of the speed with which their health can change. This rapid initiation of services is important for addressing quality of life concerns related to safe, purposeful mobility.

When establishing initial contact and arranging the first meeting between a PLWA and an O&M instructor, the instructor should make all attempts communicate directly with the PLWA to gather background information from the individual, rather than from an intermediary. This will enable the instructor to obtain firsthand information regarding the individual's health situation and personal health-related needs, for example, the most suitable time of day to schedule O&M assessments and instruction, with the consideration that a PLWA's medical regimen may affect the times when outdoor activities are possible.

O&M instructors providing services to PLWAS should plan to confirm all meetings with the learner several hours before scheduled appointments, because the PLWA's health and capacity to participate in an O&M session can change significantly from lesson to lesson.

In-service education regarding blindness and visual impairments, as well as the nature of O&M instruction for PLWAs, their families, and other service providers in the AIDS-support network is an integral part of O&M services to PLWAs. Accurate information about the capabilities and needs of persons who are blind or visually impaired serves to dispel myths about blindness and visual impairment, and conveys practical knowledge to those involved in caring for PLWAs.

Assessment and Goal Setting

O&M assessments for PLWAs include the conventional assessment considerations, with special emphasis on establishing a clear picture of the PLWA's physical and emotional health. The aim is to develop O&M programs that set realistic goals and respect the individual's physical capacity and motivation. An important consideration is establishing lesson time frames (time of day and duration), locations, and activities that are appropriate. Assessments for this purpose focus on the following:

- the current nature of visual functioning
- the stability of the visual status
- the speed at which visual functioning is deteriorating
- a self-reported description of the PLWA's physical stamina

- physical, cognitive, or sensorimotor symptoms
- motivation to participate in an O&M program.

Motivation to participate in an O&M program varies widely from one individual to the next. The onset of vision loss often coincides with a PLWA's experiencing his or her own mortality. The effect of this experience is highly personal and individual, and has an impact on motivation. Frequently PLWAs' level of motivation is reflected by their perception of "time." Highly motivated PLWAs express the feeling that time is of the essence and training should be provided immediately so they can resume their normal level of mobility for daily living needs. Others may see their vision loss as the beginning of the end. Perceiving that time is not on their side, they may exhibit a low level of motivation to learn O&M skills.

Gathering input from family members, significant others, and health professionals involved in the lives of PLWAs—that is provided with the consent of the learner—can help the O&M instructor clarify the nature of the PLWA's status. This process also facilitates a dialogue with other caregivers about the concerns that these individuals may have regarding the PLWA's vision loss.

When O&M instructors provide services to PLWAs as part of a multidisciplinary team, O&M assessment information is shared with other members of the rehabilitation or educational team, including the rehabilitation teacher, social worker, teacher of the visually impaired, and other health care providers.

Instructional Programs

O&M program development derives directly from assessment—from the needs and interests identified by the instructor and the learner during the assessment process. To be successful in enabling PLWAs to address these needs, O&M instructors should establish realistic instructional goals with their students and allow the PLWA to remain in control of the course and pace of the O&M program. For example, appropriate and realistic O&M instructional goals for a severely ill PLWA may simply be demonstrating sighted guide skills to family members or significant others, providing guidance about the importance of speaking precisely to persons with visual impairments, and assuring caregivers that they are providing the best possible care for the PLWA.

In the early years of the AIDS epidemic, individuals diagnosed with AIDS experienced rapid physical deterioration, and because of their fragile health and limited longevity, they were only able to benefit from limited O&M instructional services in areas related to indoor and basic cane techniques, for example, sighted guide, trailing, direction taking, indoor diagonal cane technique, and the use of the cane for identification.

Advances in the treatment of AIDS have prolonged the lives and stamina of PLWAs. Consequently, those who experience vision loss have the capacity to learn and use a wide range of O&M skills and techniques. Instructors increasingly have been teaching skills for outdoor travel, including the use of long-cane techniques and optical devices for home, neighborhood, and business travel, and travel on public transportation. Trips accomplished by PLWAs, for example, can be as simple as the route to the mailbox or as complex as the route from a suburban community to the city to enjoy a cultural event. It is important to keep in mind, however, that because a PLWA's condition can deteriorate quickly and unpredictably, basic indoor techniques should be included in the instructional program and reviewed periodically.

Revising Goals

As for all consumers, evaluation is an ongoing component of the instructional program for PLWAs. Instructional goals should be reviewed by the instructor and the learner at regular intervals to measure the learner's progress and assess the continued suitability of the original instructional goals. This is particularly important for students who may be experiencing physical debilitation and severe pain, or cognitive deterioration associated with AIDS-related dementia. In this instance, the O&M instructor may observe that the PLWA is suddenly having a difficult time learning new skills, forgets skills that were mastered, or is confusing the past with present experiences.

O&M instructors need to assess O&M goals with students who have AIDS-related dementia and exhibit disorientation with respect to time and place. For example, a student with AIDS-related dementia who is learning O&M skills for home travel during a summer month and comments about the beautiful Christmas tree in the corner of the living room may need to assess the suitability of future independent O&M goals for travel in unsupervised environments. Goals may need to be refocused so that indoor travel tasks are achieved using compensatory strategies, such as those suitable for persons with a head injury (see chapter 16 of the this volume), or increased reliance on the sighted guide technique.

The critical element for successfully refocusing the O&M goals for students with AIDS is to involve the learner in all phases of the process and provide information about the elements that need to be considered, especially regarding safety. In this manner, students are able to make informed decisions about their progress and maintain control of their situation. This is especially important should it become necessary to decide to terminate O&M services.

Terminating O&M services because of the learner's failing health, or refocusing the learner's goals so that travel is facilitated by the use of guides can be a difficult step for the instructor and the learner. This situation is facilitated when the instructor actively supports the learner's choices, and reviews with the learner the skills that have been mastered, thus providing the learner with a sense of accomplishment.

Support for the O&M Instructor

Providing O&M services to PLWAs is a challenging and rewarding experience; nevertheless certain aspects of this work that an O&M instructor may experience for the first time include

- working with a person who is terminally ill;
- dealing with the reactions of family, friends, and other professionals;
- working with a member of the gay community or an IV drug user; and
- resolving personal concerns about contracting AIDS.

It is helpful for O&M instructors to address these concerns and others they may have by learning as much about AIDs and PLWAs as is possible, and to hold each learner's value and dignity in high regard. AIDS is a medical issue not a moral one. It is also important for O&M service providers to maintain a rational perspective about the types of behaviors associated with the spread of AIDS, and bear in mind that health care providers regularly take effective and reasonable precautions when treating patients ill with AIDS that can be used by O&M instructors.

A strong support network for O&M instructors providing services to PLWAs is important. Teams, in-service education programs, networking with AIDS service and support groups, and the instructor's family and friends are all important sources of support.

Allaying rational and irrational anxiety about contracting AIDS can be facilitated through networking with established AIDS support groups. Talking with others can and does help. After many years of working with PLWAs, an instructor was scratched by a cat in the home of a PLWA. Rationally, it was clear that there was no way to contract AIDS from a cat, but nevertheless, there was a definite sense of relief when the instructor and the support group members shared their irrational fears about contracting AIDS, and discussed their strategies for dealing with these fears.

Learning to deal with the feeling of helplessness, as well as developing a sense of appreciation for what the human spirit can accomplish can be achieved with input from other professionals working with PLWAs. The professionals on teams involved in the care of PLWAs should meet at regularly scheduled times to share new medical information, establish formal procedures for care, and offer support and insights to one and other. In addition, inviting professionals who regularly work with persons who are terminally ill or are part of the AIDS network of services to address staff at blindness service organizations and schools will help O&M instructors develop coping skills and insights. The American Cancer Society is an excellent resource in this area.

O&M instructors seeking additional resources and information are encouraged to contact their local Department of Health, Visiting Nurse Association, or AIDS treatment hotlines. Reference librarians may refer O&M instructors to newsletters such as *GMHC Treatment Issues—The Gay Men's Health Crisis Newsletter of Experimental AIDS Therapies,* or medical and public health updates for current information. *Understanding AIDS,* a pamphlet available in print or in braille, is another useful resource (available from the U.S. Department of Health and Human Services, Public Health Service, Centers for Disease Control, National AIDS Information Clearing House, P.O. Box 6003, Rockville, MD 20850).

SUMMARY

The advances in health care have had a significant impact on the demographics of consumers of special education and rehabilitation services. The changing demographics include many more individuals born with multiple impairments and who are surviving longer and leading more productive lives.

The specific causes and etiologies that result in individuals with multiple impairments discussed in this chapter will continue to change even more. Therefore, adapting O&M and programs to visually impaired people with additional special needs will have to continue to respond to ever-changing consumers. The instructional models and curricula that O&M instructors use to teach individuals with visual and multiple impairments will continue to evolve through ongoing examination, communication, and modification by O&M professionals and related disciplines to develop innovative practices in the field of blindness.

Suggestions/Implications for O&M Specialists

1. Diabetic retinopathy is one of the leading causes of adult visual impairment. Therefore, O&M specialists need to know how to recognize and respond to symptoms such as insulin reaction and ketosis when teaching students who have diabetes.
2. O&M specialists need to recognize that students with diabetes must eat properly prior to and following O&M lessons, and they should be prepared to administer an appropriate form of sugar if students become verbally disoriented, sweaty, or have "sweet" breath during lessons. Avoid administering sugar in the form of hard candy to prevent choking.
3. Students who are diabetic are at high risk of serious infection, even from small lesions. Therefore, O&M specialists need to monitor students for injuries, such as cuts, bruises, or blisters that may occur during lessons, and note whether students' footwear or prosthetic devices fit properly.
4. Individuals with diabetic retinopathy experience fluctuations in vision often related to diabetic small blood vessel disease or laser treatments, which can be misinterpreted as a reversal of the disease or cure. These experiences can affect adjustment to vision impairment and motivation to learn O&M skills, and should be addressed by O&M instructors as part of the O&M program.
5. O&M specialists may be unaware or unsure if individuals they are teaching are HIV-positive or have AIDS. Therefore, O&M instructors should follow current public health practices and appropriate infection control procedures when providing services.
6. O&M specialists can obtain reliable information about HIV and AIDS from health care professionals at local departments of health, visiting nurse associations, or AIDS hotlines.
7. HIV is a fragile virus that does not survive long outside of body fluids, or in fluids that have left the body and are no longer at body temperature. Therefore, HIV cannot be transmitted through casual contact such as sharing air, water, food, a bathroom, or a water fountain that may take place between the student and instructor during lessons.
8. O&M specialists should become knowledgeable about "universal precautions" and integrate these precautions into their service delivery procedures.
9. Persons living with AIDS are extremely susceptible to communicable diseases because of their compromised immune systems. Therefore, O&M specialists should reschedule lessons with these students if the specialist has a contagious illness, such as an upper respiratory infection (a cold), which would otherwise not preclude working.
10. O&M instructors need to initiate O&M services, schedule, and pace lessons with students who have AIDS, while considering the fluctuating and sometimes fragile state of the student's health. It may be necessary to reevaluate and change instructional goals and strategies during the instructional period.

(continued on next page)

Suggestions/Implications for O&M Specialists (continued)

11. O&M specialists who teach students with AIDS-related vision loss may find it helpful to participate in or network with support groups for health care practitioners who work with persons living with AIDS.
12. O&M specialists who work in educational, residential, rehabilitation, or institutional facilities may be required to wear protective latex gloves when providing instruction. It is important to have knowledge and experience about putting on and removing latex gloves. The nurse or infection control officer in a facility are resources for O&M specialists for this purpose.

ACTIVITIES FOR REVIEW

1. Discuss the primary and secondary complications of diabetes mellitus and the manner in which they can affect an O&M student's adjustment to visual impairment and progress in the O&M program.
2. Describe how an O&M specialist might respond when a student who recently became blind with diabetic retinopathy reports that ophthalmologic treatment is restoring their vision.
3. Identify the health emergencies that a learner with diabetes may experience during O&M lessons, and the appropriate ways for the O&M specialist to respond.
4. Explain the circumstances under which the O&M specialist should be particularly vigilant when working with a student who has diabetes.
5. Describe the precautions O&M specialists should discuss with students who are diabetic regarding the prevention of infections at the site of minor lesions on their extremities, particularly the feet.
6. Discuss the manner in which organizational, local, and federal policies and statutes assuring nondiscrimination and confidentiality affect the practice of O&M, particularly with respect to record-keeping and reporting procedures for learners who have AIDS or other communicative diseases.
7. The body of knowledge regarding HIV and AIDS is continually evolving. Explain why it is important for O&M specialists to stay abreast of new information about AIDS treatment and public health policy, and the manner in which O&M specialists can monitor these changes.
8. Define the term "universal precautions." Describe two precautionary measures O&M specialists need to know, and provide examples of situations when these precautions may be necessary during O&M lessons. Would you consider using these techniques for learners who are not identified as having HIV or AIDS? Why?
9. Describe the manner in which O&M specialists assess a learner who is referred for AIDS-related vision loss, and the considerations for using assessment outcomes for program planning and implementation.
10. Describe the potential benefits of AIDS support groups for O&M instructors who provide services to learners with AIDS-related vision loss.

CHAPTER 18

Learners with Visual and Hearing Impairments

Dennis Lolli and Dona Sauerburger

Most orientation and mobility (O&M) specialists who teach visually impaired people will, at one time or another, teach people who also have a hearing impairment. There are approximately 8,000 children and youth who are both deaf and blind in the United States and its territories (Baldwin, 1992), and a growing number of adults who are deaf-blind, estimated to be between 30,000 to 40,000 (Watson & Watson, 1993).

As one might imagine, individuals with hearing and visual impairments encompass a range of personal characteristics, with no common qualities relating to physical disabilities, cognitive abilities, personality, or potential for independent travel. People who are both blind and deaf use many of the same techniques to travel as do blind people who have hearing. They often achieve a high level of independence; many use public transportation, commute to work, shop and run errands, and travel alone across the country. The deaf-blind population is heterogeneous. There are variations in time, degree, and mode of occurrence of the disabilities, which may suggest ways to approach the client's O&M needs. The mobility specialist should determine the adventitious versus congenital nature of the sensory loss, whether there is a syndrome, and the extent of remaining sensory abilities.

The O&M specialist should not be overwhelmed by the thought of working with a person who is deaf-blind, but instead focus on the person's distinct qualities. In most respects, teaching O&M to people who have a hearing impairment is similar to teaching people who have normal hearing. With the exception of street-crossing strategies, the mobility techniques are predominately the same. Although deaf people with visual impairments cannot rely on sounds for orientation, their other orientation strategies, such as the use of spatial memory and kinesthetic and tactile senses, are identical to those of hearing people. The primary distinctions, which must be considered throughout the program of the deaf-blind client, are the communication methods used by the client, the need to correct any deficits in conceptual understanding caused by the limited sensory input, and the issues of interaction and communication of the client with the public.

Generally, as with individuals who are blind, the nature of how and when the disability occurred should be considered. Hearing children normally acquire the spoken language of their culture; those who are born deaf will also acquire language if they are exposed to communication in a modality that they can perceive, such as sign language. Often, however, this environment is not provided, resulting in impaired development of language, conceptual understanding, and interpersonal relationships. This potentially profound impact of congenital deafness is multiplied when the person is blind as well. Conversely, people who have good language skills and conceptual understanding and who lose their hearing and vision adventitiously must usually learn new ways to communicate and learn about the world around them. For example, people who had relied on spoken language may need to learn such skills as signing, lipreading, or having words spelled to them when they become deaf. Those who had relied on lipreading or sign language may need to learn to perceive language and learn new concepts by tactile methods when they become blind. Even after learning these skills, difficulties may continue because their friends, family, colleagues, and others are not willing or able to accommodate to their new methods of communication.

When people's sensory input is limited, their ability to know what is happening around them is also limited. It is understood how this affects the concept development and environmental awareness of children and adults who are blind, but this effect is multiplied exponentially for blind people who also have a hearing impairment.

> "The disconnection of the deaf-blind person with his/her environment is present in all of his/her movements: i.e., although he/she may be well trained, there is always a risk that something may happen which he/she may be incapable of grasping or controlling. Things happen around one in which one feels implicated but will never know exactly how they happened. One needs to have a great sense of self-control and a sense of calm, the ability to deduce and resolve problems and a strong practical sense." (Alvarez Reyes, 1993)

A great deal of the incidental learning that takes place during everyday experiences by children and adults who have either a hearing or a visual impairment is not possible for those who have both. Thus it is critical that O&M specialists provide information about and discuss the events and qualities within environments for their deaf-blind students. Without this opportunity to discuss things with others, even those who have a variety of experiences can be experientially deprived because they are not aware of, or do not understand, what is happening.

Often, decisions are made for people who are deaf-blind, without their even being aware of or involved with the choices, because of their dual sensory impairment. Frequently, they will need to learn how to assert themselves, make decisions, and gather the information needed to do so. The instructor facilitates this development, and does not make decisions for students or assume that because they are deaf-blind they should use certain procedures. Students can make informed decisions about which procedure to use when the instructor provides them with information and feedback about the effectiveness of their strategies and techniques. The instructor should also be flexible, and adapt techniques when needed for the specific needs of the student. The goals of O&M instruction must be developed with the student and, when appropriate, with rehabilitation or education team members, including parents or care providers; teachers and involved staff members; communication specialists; and occupational and physical therapists.

Those who cannot see or hear sufficiently must communicate and learn about their world primarily through touch, resulting in a need for physical contact, which makes some people uncomfortable. It can be difficult for clients and instructors to attend to learning when there is discomfort or uncertainty about what is acceptable, and others may take advantage of clients who don't know what is appropriate. The instructor and the client can reduce the uncertainty by discussing this issue frankly and clarifying each of their levels of comfort with touching, and consider what kinds of physical contact are appropriate and acceptable with others. Interaction with the public can also be difficult because of the reluctance of some people to touch or be touched by others. Some methods of communication that are effective with the public require less physical contact than others, and clients should choose those with which they are comfortable. By being aware that some people are uneasy about touching, clients can be patient when the public seems reluctant or unable to communicate with them, and flexible about trying alternative methods.

When people have diminished communication, regardless of the cause, they may be insulated from their environment and isolated from others. Their ability to express themselves, be aware of what is happening around them or understand what they experience, comprehend which options are available, and make choices can be severely restricted. In some cases, what may be perceived as inappropriate behavior, lack of cooperation, or even an apparent inability to benefit from O&M instruction may be the result of a person being unable to anticipate or even understand what is occurring in the environment, control his or her own life by making choices, or express himself or herself adequately.

Thus, when working with students who are deaf-blind whose communication skills are minimal, the O&M specialist should help develop strategies to enable them to anticipate what is happening, understand the intent of their O&M sessions, and make choices. For example, signs or symbols can be developed with the service team to indicate destinations (see "Signals and Symbols" in the Communications section of this chapter). These students can best learn to anticipate each activity if activities are scheduled consistently and regularly. Instruction of O&M techniques ideally should occur when students normally would use those techniques to travel from one location to another. When appropriate, the O&M instructor should work with the communication specialist and team to develop communication (or, if needed, language) that is appropriate to the client's needs, and encourage others to communicate as fully as possible with the client. An excellent resource about enhancing communication with clients whose language is undeveloped is Baumgart, Johnson, and Helmstetter (1990).

COMMUNICATION

Because it is crucial that the instructor and client have clear, meaningful communication, the instructor's first priority is to determine the most effective ways to communicate by talking with and observing the client or by gathering information from those who know him or her, and to arrange for that communication to be provided. The instructor is encouraged to learn as much of the client's language and mode of communication as is practical, and arrange for whatever consultation, assistance, and interpretation are required to achieve comfortable, comprehensive communication.

There is not only a considerable variety of communication methods and systems that are used by people who are deaf-blind in the United States and Canada, there are also several languages, the most prominent of which are American Sign Language (ASL) and English. In general, ASL is the native language of people who were born deaf in the United States and Canada. It is conveyed with signs and facial and body movements (the signs and some body movements can be perceived tactilely by those who are blind). ASL does not convey English with visual signs; like any language, it has a grammar and structure of its own. The common language and shared experiences of deaf people who use ASL has generated a deaf culture that unites them.

Most people who lost their hearing after they learned to speak or have remaining functional hearing continue to use the language that is spoken in their community, such as English. English is also preferred by some people who are congenitally deaf who were raised using the "oral" method of communication. With people whose hearing is impaired, English is usually conveyed through a combination of (1) residual hearing; (2) lipreading, which is sometimes augmented with "cued speech," in which sounds that cannot be discerned by lipreading are conveyed by the hands; (3) signs that are created or adapted from ASL and used in the same order as English syntax ("Signed English"); or (4) the spelling out of words, for example with fingerspelling or braille devices. (These methods are discussed later in this chapter.)

The term "total communication" traditionally means using a combination of modes to communicate, such as speaking while using Signed English or cued speech. This simultaneous use of several modes cannot be done when using ASL because ASL is another language. One cannot speak English at the same time as signing ASL any more than one can speak English while writing Spanish. Since it is as difficult to become fluent in ASL as it is to learn any language, what most English-speaking people who are learning "sign language" use is Signed English or a combination of ASL and English (often referred to as "Pidgin Signed English"). For many people who are congenitally deaf, English (even if conveyed with signs) is a second language which some understand, and some do not. Thus, if the client understands ASL, but not English, fluently, an ASL interpreter is required even if the O&M specialist can sign in English or spell to him or her.

If the student will receive messages visually, the hand movements, print, or objects being used to convey the communication should be the appropriate size, contrast, and distance from the student. Suitable lighting conditions are also very important. For example, if the O&M specialist is signing to the student, the light should be in front of the specialist (bright light from behind should be avoided); the specialist should wear clothes of a solid color that contrasts with the color of his or her skin; and the signs should be made from a distance that is comfortable for the student. For students with restricted visual fields, the signs should fit within the area that they can see, which increases the farther the specialist is from the student. When writing notes, the specialist should use letters of the size, thickness, and contrast that the student can see easily, perhaps using magnifiers, lights, or other equipment. When using objects as symbols, the O&M specialist should choose and position them so that the student can see them readily.

When O&M specialists approach clients who receive communication tactilely, they should touch them on the hand, arm, or shoulder to avoid startling them, and establish a signal or "name-sign" with which they can identify themselves. A specialist's fingernails should be smooth and short to avoid scratching the client. In hot conditions, powder can be sprinkled onto the hands to make the contact less sticky, and to communicate in cold weather, the specialist and the client can each put their hands into a muff to keep warm.

Some people who are deaf or deaf-blind have minimal language skills. This is because either they were not sufficiently exposed to any language in a mode that they could perceive, or they have cognitive impairments which interfere with their ability to process language, or both. These people might communicate with gestures and body language, facial and vocal expressions, and symbols or signs, most of which can be conveyed tactilely with those who cannot see. Techniques that may be effective for communicating with them are gestures, expressions, and demonstrations, and using signs and symbols to represent objects, destinations, or concepts. The authors have observed deaf-blind adults with minimal communication improve their ability to express themselves, make choices, and understand others after they were exposed to consistent, frequent communication in a mode that they could perceive (tactile, visual, auditory, or a combination).

Many people who are deaf-blind use various modes of communication because their vision or hearing fluctuates or is deteriorating. For instance, some people need to switch to a different mode when circumstances are noisy or poorly lit, such as those who normally can see signs or symbols well, but need to perceive by touch in certain lighting conditions. Others who are blind and losing their hearing may be in the process of changing from communicating auditorily to learning to use signs or braille devices. Some deaf people who are losing their vision adjust to communicating tactilely by feeling others' signs. It is important to be flexible and use whichever mode is most effective in that situation for the client.

During O&M training, people who are deaf-blind learn to use taxis and call for directions and bus information. This can be done using technology that enables deaf-blind people to use a telephone and recognize when someone is at their door. A variety of pagers that are developed and sold to deaf people will alert them to such sounds as telephones, doorbells, alarm clocks, and smoke alarms; some are installed or wired at the source, and others are portable and can be used when visiting hotels or other places. These pagers or "alerting devices" can provide output that deaf-blind people can use, such as flashing lights, loud buzzers, air from fans, or vibrating receivers that can be carried, worn, placed under pillows, or attached to beds. Telephones are accessible to deaf and deaf-blind people with TTYs. They connect the TTY to a telephone, dial the number of someone who has another TTY, and then use their TTY keyboard to type messages that appear on the other person's TTY screen. Some TTYs have enlarged print. Braille output is available for TTYs with computer technology, and with such devices as the Telebraille II and the Infotouch, which provide a braille screen or printer connected to special TTYs. By using these TTY devices and calling the "relay services" that are now available throughout the United States, deaf and deaf-blind people can communicate over the phone with people who do not have TTYs. They give the number of the other person to the relay operator, who then reads their TTY messages to the other person and types the other person's message back to them.

COMMUNICATION TECHNIQUES

Many of the techniques listed here can be adapted to the needs of the student and used visually or tactilely. Details of their use, as well as other methods of communication that might be useful, are in Kates and Schein (1980) and Sauerburger (1993).

Use of Interpreters

Instructors who are not proficient in the language, mode, or system that the client uses need to use interpreters who are proficient in that communication. Traditionally, that means professional interpreters of sign language, but some clients use other modes. For example, braillists sometimes interpret for clients who are blind who have become deaf; to help understand and convey information to students who use specific nonverbal or symbolic communication systems, the best interpreters may be staff members who are familiar with those systems.

Professional, impartial interpreters convey each person's message and expression accurately in the language or method that the other uses. They do not summarize, clarify, or explain what each person is saying, or interject their opinions. Problems that arise with interpreting are usually the result of using interpreters who are not professional and impartial, or the failure to establish each person's role beforehand. For example, when the interpreter explains for the instructor instead of interpreting the message accurately, the client must be content with the interpreter's understanding of what the instructor is teaching, rather than the instructor's intended meaning. Before starting a mobility lesson with the interpreter, the mobility specialist should explain that if the need for intervention arises, he or she will initiate how and when it occurs.

When using an interpreter with students who cannot see or hear the O&M specialist, establishing rapport and having them get to know the O&M specialist can be a challenge. The O&M specialist may discuss how he or she and the client would prefer that this be done. For example, it might be decided that the O&M specialist will have physical contact such as shaking hands or hugging when greeting or leaving; or the O&M specialist (rather than the interpreter) will guide the client when needed and provide hands-on demonstrations, and so forth.

To find out how to contact qualified interpreters, the O&M specialist might ask clients or the agency that referred them, or contact agencies that serve deaf people in the O&M specialist's area. The United States and Canada each have professional organizations for interpreters that can help find local contacts: The Registry of Interpreters for the Deaf in Silver Spring, Maryland, and the Association of Visual Language Interpreters of Canada in Edmonton, Alberta.

ASL and Signs

Complete communication can be achieved by signing or having an interpreter sign with those clients who understand ASL or an English version of signs, and it is never too late for clients to learn signs. Those who cannot see the signs can feel them, but information that is normally conveyed in facial movements must then be conveyed through the hands. People who are deaf-blind and experienced can recognize most signs by placing one hand on the instructor's dominant hand as he or she signs, and others will place both hands on the instructor's hands.

Spoken English

Most people who became deaf after learning to speak, as well as a few people who are congenitally deaf and had extensive training, can speak well enough to be understood readily. To communicate verbally with the public, some deaf-blind people play prerecorded messages using a device such as the Attention-Getter or a tape recorder.

Many people who are deaf-blind retain enough vision or hearing to understand spoken English by reading lips or listening or both. Those who rely on hearing should be asked whether they prefer high or low tones and at what distance the instructor should speak, and background noises should be avoided. An assistive listening device can enable the O&M specialist to speak into a microphone that transmits the voice (by wire or broadcast) to the listener's receiver or hearing device, reducing interference from other sounds. If the student is reading the instructor's lips, he or she should speak clearly without exaggerating and have good lighting on his or her face.

Spelled-Out Words

There are numerous ways that the O&M specialist and the client can spell to each other, which can be effective if the client understands English well. The alphabets and devices mentioned below, as well as additional spelling methods such as the alphabet glove and finger braille, are described in Kates and Schein (1980) and Sauerburger (1993).

Printed, Typewritten, or Braille Notes

Some students can read written notes if the letters are legible enough, and some use braille notes. Many people who are deaf-blind can write notes to others as needed, or the notes can be typed ahead of time or written with assistance. Cards with messages that are used repeatedly may be prepared or purchased and laminated.

Fingerspelling

Each letter of the American Manual Alphabet is made by forming a distinct shape of the hand, called fingerspelling. People who cannot see the hand shapes can feel them by either holding up their hand while the letters are formed into their cupped palm, or placing their hand over the instructor's while he or she fingerspells.

Print on Palm

The O&M specialist can use a finger to draw capital letters onto the palm of the person who is deaf-blind, making each letter large enough to fill the palm, and pausing or tapping the palm between words. Some people who are blind may need to learn or review the shapes of the letters to use this technique. To discern the letters more easily as they are printed on the palm, a deaf-blind person can put his or her free hand over the instructor's to feel the hand movement. Clients who cannot readily perceive letters printed on their palm may perceive them better on their arm or back, or the instructor can use the client's own finger to print letters on his or her own palm or on a table or wall.

Mechanical Devices

Several devices, including the Alva Braille Carrier, Telebraille II, Teletouch, TTYs, Infotouch, and computers and modems, can be used in person, over the phone, or both, to send or receive messages using braille, print (sometimes enlarged), or both.

Alphabet Cards and Plates

With plates or cards that have print letters along with raised or braille letters, such as the Brailtalk (which has both), people can spell messages to the person who is deaf-blind by placing his or her finger on the letters, and the deaf-blind person can point to the letters to spell to them.

Demonstrations and Gestures

Often the easiest way to explain a technique, whether the student has hearing or is deaf, is to demonstrate it, either by having the student see or feel the instructor use the technique, or by positioning the student and giving feedback while he or she tries it. For example, while the student tries to use the cane correctly, the instructor can place a hand over the student's hand and move the cane; the instructor can position the student's arm in upper hand and forearm technique while the student approaches an overhanging obstacle, and so forth.

Concepts and techniques can be explained using representative models and tactile maps and graphics, as well as by drawing shapes on the client's hand or back, or using the instructor's hands (preferably in standard ASL handshapes, such as the ASL signs that represent "vehicle," "chair," "person," and "wall") to represent the position or movement of objects or people. For example, a person can be represented by a raised index finger or by the entire hand with two fingers pointing down to represent the legs. One of the instructor's hands can represent a chair, a wall, or the landing of a stair, while the other hand represents the person moving toward the chair or parallel to the wall, or leaning back while standing at the edge of the landing, and so forth. The instructor's finger could also represent a cane moving in the technique being described, the instructor's hands can represent vehicles moving to illustrate traffic patterns, and so on. The instructor's hand movements can be observed by clients either visually, or tactilely by placing their hands on the instructor's.

People who are deaf-blind can also use gestures and demonstrations to communicate with others, such as pointing to what they want, or gesturing to a salesperson that they want to buy an item that they found. To explain to another person how to communicate with them, for example, they might demonstrate how to print on their palm.

Signals and Symbols

Communication can often be expedited by signals that are universally understood, such as a "yes" or "no" shake of the head. Signals can also be established as needed, such as by tapping students a certain way to indicate corrections needed in their technique ("two taps on your elbow means you're out of step"), or by making up a signal to indicate that they are approaching a door when the instructor is guiding them. When people who are deaf-blind ask others a question, they can show a note or say, "Please tap me twice to signal 'yes' and once for 'no'" or vice versa. O&M specialists should also use a signal to identify themselves each time they approach students who cannot see or hear them. Each deaf-blind person should learn the signal to indicate an emergency, made by using a finger to trace an "X" on his or her back or arm.

Symbols or "object cues," which are often used with people with limited language skills, can indicate specific things (such as juice or a coat), destinations (such as the client's desk, playground, or woodworking shop), or concepts (such as time to prepare for bed, feelings and desires such as anger or happiness, or wanting to rest or take a walk, and so forth). For example, clients with limited language skills may request juice by showing the instructor a certain cup, and the instructor might ask them to get their coat by handing them a symbolic square of fabric. Because it is so important for clients to understand the purpose of O&M lessons and strategies, destinations should be consistently and clearly explained to them each time a route is initiated, and this can also be done with symbols or object cues. For example, they might be given a spoon whenever they are going to the cafeteria, a seat-belt buckle each time they go to the car, and a piece of sandpaper to indicate that they are going to the woodworking shop.

Photographs or pictures may be used for such purposes as to provide students with a way to indicate their frustration, boredom, or satisfaction, or to order food. These communication tools would require tactile labeling, such as "hamburger" and "french fries with ketchup," and so forth. Some clients may learn best if the symbols initially are actual items, such as a Cheerio "o" to represent breakfast, a glass to represent drink, or scissors to represent crafts class. Once understood, these symbols are then paired with and eventually replaced by increasingly abstract symbols, such as ASL signs, textured squares or forms, or drawings. Other clients may be able to learn abstract symbols or signs without first learning concrete symbols.

Unless the signal or symbol that the instructor teaches the student is intended for limited use between them, it should be as universally understood as possible, such as ASL signs—which many people recognize—or symbols which are labeled so that people who are new to the student, as well as salespeople and other strangers, can understand them. According to Baumgart et al. (1990), whatever is chosen to augment communication should be appropriate for the student's age and social interaction and, most important, meet the student's needs to communicate and understand.

A "calendar box," which usually consists of a row of boxes, or a long box with dividers forming separate cubicles into which symbols are placed, can be used to convey a client's schedule, using a symbol for each activity. The client reaches into the first box to retrieve, for example, a cup to signify that it is time for a snack; after snack time he or she returns the cup to the empty bin and checks the next bin to find perhaps a ball, which is understood by that client to symbolize time for gym. The symbol can be carried, perhaps in a waist pack, to the activity, then returned to indicate that the activity is completed, or it can be placed in a "finished" box designated to receive object cues from completed activities. The next bin is then checked for the next object.

CONSIDERATIONS FOR O&M TRAINING

While most of the O&M techniques for people who are deaf-blind are the same as those for hearing blind people, there are a few modifications and considerations which relate to communication issues or inability to hear. In addition, some deaf people have balance difficulty because of vestibular system impairments that were often unnoticed until they lost their vision or used a blindfold. With practice, they usually learn to react more quickly to proprioceptive information, and develop compensatory strategies (see Chapter 5 of this volume, which deals with balance difficulty).

For orientation, people who are deaf-blind may rely on the information from their kinesthetic experiences rather than auditory information. The O&M specialist should build in sufficient experiences for students to gain an accurate spatial representation of their environment. Students may also pay particular attention to vibrations, air movements, and smells. For example, the student might know that the instructor is nearby from the slight vibration of the instructor's feet hitting the floor or stair, or the air the instructor stirs as he or she walks by. A large percentage of deaf-blind individuals also have useful residual vision or hearing or both, which should be assessed and utilized fully (see Chapters 3 and 4).

Communication and learning styles need to be considered when planning the O&M program. The length of the program or individual sessions for people with whom communication is slow or cumbersome will need to be longer than it is for other people. Individuals who are deaf-blind and multiply impaired often require an approach that allows for skills and concepts to first be presented in a descriptive way, then presented experientially, and finally presented and reviewed descriptively. Throughout this process, the instructor should keep in mind whether the student is conceptualizing either by sequential memorization of landmarks, understanding the interrelationship among the parts of the route, or understanding the spatial layout and the relationship of objects and landmarks within the area, and thereby being able to plan multiple routes through it.

Because they cannot hear environmental sounds or the cane on the surface of the ground, some travelers who are deaf-blind may prefer such adaptations as a longer cane or a wider than normal arc. This modification provides the traveler with a little more environmental information but, unless the cane tip touches the ground as it passes in front of him or her, it may not provide sufficient warning of upcoming drop-offs. Using the constant-contact cane technique also provides ongoing tactile information and is preferred by many deaf-blind travelers.

TRAVELING IN THE COMMUNITY

In order to travel independently in the community, people must know how to communicate and interact with the public, be able to make decisions, and be aware of the environment and safety issues. Although these are important to include in O&M programs for people who are blind, their importance is multiplied for blind people who are also deaf.

Because it is virtually impossible for any person to travel within a community without interacting with people, travelers need to consider how to do so effectively, and be aware of their effect on the public. Although this is somewhat difficult for people who cannot see others, the difficulty is magnified for people who also cannot hear, which makes this one of the most crucial issues for the O&M specialist to address. Many people with visual and hearing impairments assume that others recognize that they can not hear or that others know how to communicate with them. Yet, not only is the public typically unaware of their disability, even when people who are deaf-blind write or say that they are deaf-blind and explain how to communicate, people usually do not understand or are too shocked to respond appropriately. The deaf-blind person often misconstrues their reaction and assumes that they are calloused, intentionally rude, afraid of, or have an aversion to deaf-blind people. When this happens repeatedly, it can lead to a vicious cycle, and the deaf-blind person becomes reluctant to interact with the public further. To alleviate this situation, the O&M instructor can (1) prepare the client with successful strategies to communicate with the public; (2) help the client realize that people will be mystified and uninformed, and will require patience and repeated explanations of exactly how to communicate with or help him or her; and (3) describe how others reacted when they interacted with the client. When providing this feedback, the instructor must give details and be honest.

Because access to pedestrians may be difficult or undependable for travelers who are deaf-blind once they are in the community, it is usually best if they gather relevant information and plan their trip as much as possible ahead of time. For example, they will want to know about community characteristics, general business hours, locations that are likely to have pedestrian traffic, how safe or dangerous the area is, whether there are particular areas within the community that should be avoided, and so forth.

Communication Strategies with the Public

Travelers who are deaf-blind should be able to communicate with the public, not only to solicit aid to cross streets, but also for such tasks as finding a salesperson and making a purchase, or getting information or assistance when they are lost or need to plan alternative routes because of construction or bus changes. Because people often do not respond to the first approach or explanation, the deaf-blind traveler should be skilled at several communication methods that can be used with the public. For example, one person may use gestures, prepared cards, and pictures labeled tactilely; another uses spoken English, printing on the palm, and gestures. Travelers whose communication skills are limited must learn to recognize when they need assistance and be familiar with strategies to get it.

To communicate with others, the traveler must first get their attention using such strategies as the following:

- gestures, such as tapping the cane or appearing to look around for help;
- sounds, such as spoken voice, prerecorded messages, or a whistle;
- notes, cards, or signs held where others can see them. These should be legible and, if being held up for others to see, with key words visible from a distance. To avoid showing the wrong message or holding it upside down, the notes and cards should be organized, and easily identifiable to the traveler using such tactics as clipped corners, staples, hole punches, color coding, special notations in large print or braille, and so forth.

Regardless of the method used, the traveler's message should provide information in the following order:

- First: The assistance being requested;
- Second: How others can offer assistance or communicate;
- Last: The traveler's visual and hearing impairment.

For example, an effective message might be, "Can you please tell me if this is the 90 bus? Please nod your head 'yes' or 'no' because I am deaf and can't see well." Typical cards may be worded,

> Please help me to
> CROSS STREET.
> TAP ME if you can help because
> I am DEAF and BLIND.
> Thank you!

> Please HELP ME get some
> INFORMATION
> so I can find where I am going.
> TAP ME if you can help because
> I am both DEAF and BLIND
> You can print letters in my palm
> with your finger. THANK YOU.

The traveler must specify to others exactly how they can communicate or assist; the method chosen will depend on the situation and the traveler's skills. Some suggestions are for the traveler to ask the public to

- tap the traveler to indicate their presence or willingness to help (the traveler might then give more specific instructions);
- write or spell to the traveler in a specified manner, such as print in large letters with a marker that the traveler provides, type into a Teletouch, print on the traveler's palm, and so forth;
- speak to the traveler in a specified manner, such as in a place where the traveler can lipread well, or into the microphone of the traveler's assistive listening device, or close to the traveler's ear, or with an interpreter to translate the message, and so forth;
- signal "yes" or "no" by nodding their head, or tapping twice for "yes" and once for "no," and so forth;
- do something specific, such as point to (or turn the traveler to face toward) the destination or guide him or her to it, make a phone call, draw a map, and so forth. A traveler who wants to expedite communication or whose limited understanding of English makes it difficult to understand statements written by others might instead plan the communication to structure their response. For example, the traveler might ask others to check items from a multiple-choice list or fill in blanks in a form prepared ahead of time (with assistance if needed), or point (with

their own or the traveler's finger) to the appropriate place on a tactile, braille, or large-print list, map, or form, and so on.

Some examples of using these principles effectively to get people's attention, communicate the traveler's need, and explain how the public should respond are as follows:

A traveler enters an unfamiliar store and stands near the door while tapping his white cane and holding up a card saying, "Please help me find a salesperson. Tap me if you understand. You can print letters on my palm—I am deaf and blind" (the key words are enlarged). Someone touches him hesitantly, and he shows the person how to print on his palm. The person doesn't respond, so he writes another note saying, "Please use your finger to print on my palm; I am looking for a salesperson," again shows how to print, then extends his palm and waits. The person prints, "I am a saleslady. Can I help you?" The traveler hands her a typewritten note with a list of items and the message, "I would like to buy these items. Please get them while I wait here, and print in my palm the names of any items which you do not have. Thank you." The woman goes and fills a basket with the items, shows them to him, and he nods in approval. He takes out his wallet and again demonstrates that he wants her to print the price in his palm. She does so, he pays, and she places the items in a bag. He thanks her with a smile and a nod, and turns to leave with the bag. When he doesn't find the door immediately, she pulls him towards it. He takes her arm and follows her outside, thanks her again, and walks back to his bus stop.

A traveler stands near a corner, and whenever she sees movement of people passing by she says, "Excuse me—please tell me where Matthew's Drug Store is." She finally notices that one person has stopped, and says, "Please write on this paper whether it is on this block or across the street—use very large letters because I am deaf and can't see well." She hands the person the paper and a thick marker; after he hands it back to her, she holds it close to her face and reads, "It is on this block." She asks him how many doors from the corner it is, hands him the paper and marker, and he writes "6 doors." She points first to her right and says, "Is it this way . . . " then to her left " . . . or that way? Please move my hand to point toward the store." He doesn't comply, but she can see he is moving his arms. "I can't see you," she explains, "please either point my hand toward the store, or guide me to it." He takes her by the arm, she uses the Hines break to take his arm, and they walk toward the store. When he stops, she thanks him, finds the door, and enters.

Public Transportation

Because communication with the public is difficult for many travelers who are deaf-blind, it is essential that they plan ahead as much as possible when using public transportation. Accurate background information will be needed relating to schedules, route numbers or names, and fares. When using buses, trains, or taxis, there should be an awareness of the form of assistance that will be needed. A plan should include how to communicate to obtain assistance and then prepare whatever notes, cards, recorded messages, equipment, maps, or drawings will be needed. To get some of this information by telephone, travelers may use amplifiers, TTY with relay service, or an interpreter.

Travelers who cannot see, hear, or reliably feel the air movement when the bus or train approaches can use an electronic travel aid (ETA) or vibrotactile device to detect it, or solicit aid using strategies already described. If there are usually no other people where the traveler waits for the bus, he or she can hold up a card or sign informing drivers which bus is desired, asking to be guided to it when it arrives, and explaining that he or she is deaf and blind. Taxi passengers need to inform the dispatcher how the driver should announce and identify himself or herself (for example, ring the doorbell and hand the traveler his or her identification when the door opens; look in the lobby for a tall man with blond hair and a white cane and tap him on the shoulder; ask the dispatcher to call the traveler and inform him or her that the taxi is in front of the house; and so forth). When the driver arrives, the traveler should inform him or her how to communicate, and repeat the explanation if needed (especially when the driver needs to inform the traveler of the fare).

Travelers should use an appropriate communication method to inform the bus or taxi driver where they want to get off. Giving the driver a note, even if the communication is verbal, helps avoid misunderstandings as well as awkward situations when the driver forgets the destination and tries to ask the traveler to repeat it. Travelers who cannot recognize when they have arrived at their destination should ask the driver to inform them by a specified method (tap or wave at them, hand them their note back, or whatever is most appropriate). Bus drivers may see the travelers and be less likely to forget about them if they sit near the door. Holding a note with the name of their stop on their lap also helps others remember to inform them when to get off.

Train passengers often can recognize their station by counting how many times the train stops and opens its doors (the vibrations can sometimes be felt in the wall next to the doors as they open) or noting such cues as which stations are far apart, crowded, above ground or below, and so forth.

CROSSING STREETS AND DRIVEWAYS

Travelers who are deaf-blind need to know when they can detect vehicles or traffic signals well enough to recognize the appropriate time to cross a given intersection, and when they must use other strategies. At intersections with no traffic control, this is determined not only by the degree of the traveler's residual vision and hearing (as augmented by visual and hearing aids, if needed), but also by the width of the street, the speed of the traveler and traffic, and factors that affect visibility and sounds, such as heavy rain or fog, lighting conditions, obstructions from construction, bends in the road, noise, and so forth. Students with functional vision or hearing or both should learn how various conditions affect their abilities, and how to judge when they can or cannot detect vehicles sufficiently to know when it is safe to cross. This can be done by providing practice sessions facilitated by using the timing methods for assessing the detection of traffic, which take each of these factors into consideration (Sauerburger, 1989). In addition, students whose visual field is severely restricted will need to learn to scan more slowly for cars.

At intersections with traffic signals, travelers who are deaf who cannot reliably see the traffic light but can see the vehicles need to learn how to watch the traffic to analyze its pattern and recognize the appropriate time to cross, just as hearing blind travelers need to analyze by listening. Often, those whose vision has changed need to learn how to scan effectively and when to look in which direction. For example, many clients who could readily see cars turning in front of them before their visual fields became severely restricted do not realize that they now need to turn their eyes to look toward the sources of turning cars at the appropriate times during their crossing.

Travelers who are deaf and visually impaired who cross with crowds may be tempted to follow from behind where they can see the crowd easily, or may keep walking without realizing the crowd has stopped to let a car pass. They must learn to cross with the crowd, not behind or ahead of it, so they will not be in danger from vehicles that the crowd is avoiding.

CROSSING WITHOUT SUFFICIENT HEARING OR VISION

There are a variety of situations where people who have visual and hearing impairments cannot reliably recognize the appropriate time to cross a given intersection, including driveways and entrances, alleys, residential streets, and busy urban intersections. In these situations, they must decide whether or not to accept the risk of crossing there independently without using assistance or alternative strategies. These decisions will vary from individual to individual. Most independent travelers who are deaf-blind consider the danger of crossing driveways and entrances by themselves to be negligible, and consider that busy streets are too dangerous to cross alone. Some feel safe crossing short dead-end residential streets alone, and others consider those streets too dangerous. Each traveler needs to decide whether he or she feels that the danger is small enough or too great at a given intersection or entrance at a particular time of day to risk crossing alone.

To make these decisions, travelers need information about each intersection being considered. If they cannot hear or see the situation well enough, the instructor or a friend can stand with them at the intersection of the street or driveway at the times of day they are likely to cross, and describe the situation and how well the drivers can see and react to them. Any moving vehicles can be depicted by pointing to them as they pass, or setting up a signal, such as moving a finger along the student's back, to indicate passing vehicles and their speed. In addition, people who are not knowledgeable about streets or about the concepts of danger and safety (for example, some people who are congenitally deaf-blind or developmentally disabled) will first need to develop an understanding of the relative danger of intersections and moving vehicles.

If travelers who are deaf-blind decide to cross particular driveways, entrances, or streets alone even though they cannot see or hear the vehicles sufficiently to know when it is clear to cross, they accept the risk that they might cross there when vehicles are approaching, and trust that drivers will avoid them. It may help to warn drivers by such tactics as raising their cane forward and then down again before crossing, or having signs saying "deaf-blind pedestrian" installed nearby. Vibrotactile devices such as the Tactaid II+ or 7, which convert sounds into vibrations that can be felt, may also be helpful for such crossings, as well as providing an awareness of environmental sounds. Even at quiet streets, however, these devices cannot detect the sounds of most cars until they are only 3–6 seconds away, which usually is not enough time to get safely to the other side of the street, but which may be enough warning to avoid stepping unexpectedly in front of or walking into moving vehicles. Before crossing entrances or streets where drivers' attention may be diverted with trying to pull into heavy traffic, the traveler may try to get their attention by such tactics as tapping the cane or blowing a whistle.

Soliciting Aid

When the traveler who is deaf-blind decides not to cross the intersection or entrance alone, he or she can get assistance from passersby, drivers, neighbors, and shopkeepers. Passersby can usually be used if, at the time when the traveler needs to cross, someone normally walks by at least every five minutes. The traveler should stand at the curb facing the street and get people's attention, show his or her need for assistance, and indicate how they can help. This can be done by either holding up an explanatory card, asking for assistance verbally or with prerecorded messages, using body language such as tapping the cane and appearing to look around for help, or a combination of these tactics. If the traveler cannot recognize when people stop to help, the card or voice should explain that they need to tap him or her to offer assistance.

When help is offered, the traveler should indicate which street he or she wants to cross, then reach out to take the helper's arm, using the Hines break if necessary. By taking the helper's arm rather than vice versa, the traveler can avoid being left in the middle of the street or maneuvered after crossing by an oversolicitous guide. Once on the other side, the traveler thanks the helper and continues on his or her way, appearing confident.

At intersections where pedestrians are rare, some travelers who are deaf-blind make arrangements with such people as neighbors, shopkeepers, and office workers. Travelers who need to cross a street at the same time every day often ask the helper to watch for them at that time, others call ahead to let the helper know they are coming, and some get the helper's attention (for example, by blowing a whistle) when they arrive or, when possible, they go to the helper's door.

In isolated areas where there is frequent traffic but no pedestrians or buildings, travelers who are deaf-blind have been able to obtain assistance from drivers if they can get their attention and if the driver can safely pull over. The traveler holds up a conveniently sized sign where the drivers can see it, saying "Please help me to CROSS STREET" (the words "cross street" are written large enough to be seen across the street), then "Please TAP ME if you can help because I am DEAF and BLIND." This is especially effective at intersections where drivers normally stop for a traffic signal or stop sign; one traveler who used this technique usually waited no more than five minutes for a driver to pull over and guide him across when the weather was good. As before, when help is offered the traveler indicates which street he or she wants to cross.

Alternative Strategies

When there is no way to get assistance and the traveler has decided it is too risky to cross alone, alternate routes should be considered, or perhaps paratransit, taxis, or carpools. If the street must be crossed to use a bus, travelers might take the bus to the end of the line to get on or off on their side of the street and avoid the crossing altogether. Sometimes the installation of a vibrating or audible traffic signal can provide enough information for the traveler who is deaf-blind to cross safely, but the risks from cars turning into the traveler's path must be considered. In certain situations a dog guide may be a solution; according to a 1992 survey (Sauerburger, 1993), some dog guide schools that have experience with deaf-blind clients say that at intersections where the likelihood is minimal that the client will start to cross at the wrong time (such as at entrances and quiet streets or where the client can detect most vehicles), dogs which are specially chosen and trained can be responsible for determining whether it is safe to proceed. However, dog guides should not be given this responsibility where the client is likely to initiate a crossing at the wrong time, such as at busy or complex intersections.

DOG GUIDES

Some people who are deaf-blind choose to use dog guides for many of the same reasons as do people who are blind and can hear, and they can utilize the dog guide just as effectively. Like any dog guide user, deaf-blind travelers must know where they are going, which, as already explained in this chapter, many deaf-blind people can do well. They must also recognize when the dog needs correction (for example, when it is distracted and reaches to sniff something or veers the wrong way), which is normally accomplished by noting the dog's movement, not by hearing. Those who are unable to give the dog appropriate verbal commands can use a dog guide trained to recognize hand signals or gestures.

There are increasing numbers of dog guide schools that accept applicants who are deaf-blind. At least one school is now also experimenting with incorporating certain responsibilities of hearing ear dogs (which alert their deaf owners to such sounds as doorbells, telephones, and alarms) with those of a dog guide.

SUMMARY

Any attempt to present a total picture of O&M for persons who are deaf-blind will be incomplete. When the novice to deaf-blindness finds himself or herself with a deaf-blind student, he or she should not hesitate to get involved. Meet the prospective student through the assistance of an interpreter, if needed. Get to know the person and resist the fear of the unknown. Later on, the O&M specialist may seek to consult articles, others who have experience, and family members. The purpose of this chapter is to encourage O&M specialists to become knowledgeably and professionally involved.

Suggestions/Implications for O&M Specialists

1. The O&M specialist should not be intimidated about working with people who are deaf-blind because, with the exception of communication, most of the training and mobility strategies will be the same as they are for hearing blind people.
2. Because limited sensory input results in limited incidental learning and knowledge of what is happening, it is critical that O&M specialists provide information about and discuss the events and qualities within environments for their students who are deaf-blind. Without this opportunity to discuss things with others, even those who have a variety of experiences can be experientially deprived because they aren't aware of or don't understand what is happening.
3. For people whose communication is minimal, one of the priorities of the O&M specialist is to help develop strategies to enable them to anticipate what is happening, understand the intent of their O&M sessions, and make choices.
4. Because people who cannot see or hear must communicate and learn about their world primarily through touch, there is a need for physical contact, which makes some people uncomfortable, and this can make it difficult for them to attend to learning. The instructor and the client can reduce the uncertainty by discussing this issue frankly; clarifying each of their levels of comfort with touching; and considering what kinds of physical contact are appropriate and acceptable with others.
5. Clear, comfortable communication is necessary for learning to take place, so an O&M specialist's first priority is to determine how he or she can communicate most proficiently with students and arrange for whatever interpreters or communication systems are needed. The O&M specialist should be aware of the common communication techniques and tips for using them, which are explained in this chapter, but should also realize that each person who is deaf-blind is unique, and, in order to learn effectively, he or she will need to use communication methods that are appropriate and comfortable for that person.
6. American Sign Language (ASL) is a distinct language, and not the English language conveyed with signs. Thus when the O&M specialist is working with students whose language is ASL, it would be inappropriate and ineffective to teach by using English, even if it is spelled out or signed for the student. If the O&M specialist is not fluent in ASL, an interpreter is needed to teach these students.
7. The O&M specialist should establish a way to quickly identify himself or herself, such as creating a special signal or sign, and use it whenever approaching the student who is deaf-blind.
8. The O&M specialist can teach students who are deaf-blind how to phone for directions, bus information, and taxis, just as he or she does with hearing-blind students, because there are devices and relay services by which deaf-blind people can use the telephone to call other people. They can also be alerted to the ringing telephone, doorbell, and smoke alarm by using pagers that are marketed for deaf people.

(continued on next page)

Suggestions/Implications for O&M Specialists (continued)

9. Individuals who are deaf-blind and multiply impaired often require an approach which allows for skills and concepts to first be presented in a descriptive way, then presented experientially, and finally presented and reviewed descriptively again.
10. Although it is important that O&M programs include learning how to communicate and interact with the public, be able to make decisions, and be aware of the environment and safety issues, these issues are even more important for students who are deaf-blind.
11. One of the crucial issues for the O&M specialist to address when teaching people who are deaf-blind is how to interact with the public. The O&M instructor should (a) prepare the client with successful strategies to communicate with the public; (b) help the client realize that people will need to be informed (often repeatedly) exactly how to communicate with or help the deaf-blind person, and (c) describe how others reacted when they interacted with the client.
12. Because the public often does not respond to the first approach or explanation of the person who is deaf-blind, the deaf-blind traveler should be skilled at several communication methods that can be used with the public. Regardless of the method used, the traveler's message should provide information in the following order: what assistance is being requested; how others can offer assistance or communicate; and the traveler's visual and hearing impairment.
13. O&M specialists teach students who are deaf-blind who have functional vision or hearing how to use it most effectively to cross streets, including where and how to scan for vehicles that might cross their path. They also teach them how to recognize those situations in which they are unable to detect vehicles or traffic signals well enough to know when is the appropriate time to cross a given intersection or driveway, and to make decisions concerning which of these situations are too risky to cross independently. The O&M specialist provides them with enough information to make these decisions (such as frequency of moving vehicles, the likelihood that drivers will see and stop for them, and so forth), and alternative strategies such as how to solicit assistance and plan alternative routes.

ACTIVITIES FOR REVIEW

1. It is possible for students who are deaf-blind who have a variety of experiences to be experientially deprived. How can this happen and how can it be avoided?
2. Explain the O&M instructor's first priority when meeting a student who is deaf-blind.
3. Describe how an O&M instructor who is not fluent in American Sign Language (ASL) should communicate with a student whose primary language is ASL.
4. Discuss whether O&M instructors rely on spelling (fingerspelling, writing notes, Teletouch, and so forth) to communicate with students who are deaf-blind whose language is ASL.

5. Describe how people who are deaf-blind should communicate with the public. What information should their message convey, and in what order?
6. When people who are deaf-blind communicate with the public, they should explain how the other person can respond. What are some ways that the public can respond to deaf-blind people?
7. Without proper intervention and training, many people who are deaf-blind become reluctant to interact with the public. Why does this happen, and what can the O&M specialist do to prevent it?
8. Explain how people who are deaf-blind can call bus companies for information.
9. Explain how people who are deaf-blind can use taxis.
10. Describe how people who are deaf with functional vision can cross at intersections with traffic signals when they cannot see the signal.
11. Explain the choices available to people in situations where their hearing and vision is insufficient to identify the appropriate time to cross a street.

CHAPTER 19

Other Learners with Mobility Limitations

Bruce B. Blasch, Steven J. LaGrow, and Lydia Peterson

There are approximately 46 million Americans with disabilities and 13 million with functional mobility limitations, of whom only about 20 percent have sensory impairments that affect their level of activity (Axelson, Thomas, Chesney, Coveny, & Eve-Anchassi, 1994). The rest have other disabilities or health problems that lead to restrictions in independent mobility as they interact with the environment (Blasch, 1994). Many would benefit from mobility services, yet there has been a tendency to disregard the mobility instruction needs of this population, perhaps on the assumption that they are able to teach themselves to travel, or the belief that ambulation is all that is required for one to be mobile.

This is not to say that the mobility needs of this population have been totally ignored. There are professionally staffed programs available to assist persons with certain physical impairments to learn to use prosthetic devices or other equipment such as wheelchairs and orthopedic canes, to assist in locomotion, or to relearn the use of muscles needed for ambulation (Blasch & Welsh, 1980). There are also programs to teach cognitively impaired individuals specific routes, methods for crossing streets, or bus riding skills (LaGrow, Wiener, & LaDuke, 1990). These programs, however, are generally limited in focus and thus fail to recognize the comprehensive nature of mobility as a skill area and the myriad of subtle factors involved in independent travel (Blasch & Welsh, 1980).

The Wisconsin Council of Developmental Disabilities funded a project (Blasch, 1982) to employ an orientation and mobility (O&M) specialist to provide mobility instruction to individuals with a broad range of disabilities. The individuals served had the following disabilities and diseases: intellectual, communication, hearing, behavioral, and learning disabilities, and specific physical disabilities such as cerebral palsy, cardiopulmonary pathology, muscular dystrophy, emphysema, and epilepsy. In 7 percent of the students, visual impairment was listed as a secondary impairment. While there are many reasons for providing this service, one of the outcome measures used in this study was cost saving. Cost savings reflected the difference between the costs for specialized transportation provided prior to the implementation of this program and the costs for public transportation required after instruction in its use had been provided. This figure was determined for 36 participants. A cost savings of $117,540 was realized in its first year of operation (Blasch, 1982). An even more telling measure of the perceived value of this program, however, may be the fact that Milwaukee County (Wisconsin) Department of Public works hired the O&M instructor involved, at the end of the project, to continue providing mobility instruction for this population. Similar programs have been carried out by Pittsburgh Public Schools (Laus, 1974, 1977). Montgomery County (Norristown, PA) Intermediate Unit No. 23 (Williams, Hoff, Millaway, & Cassidy, 1982), and Wayne County (Dearborn Heights, MI) Associations for the Retarded (Brambila-Hickman & Denniston, 1984). These programs have demonstrated the effectiveness of providing mobility instruction to individuals with disabilities other than visual impairment, and that the O&M specialist who has had additional preparation is the professional prepared to offer this service. This chapter presents the principles and some specific techniques for teaching O&M to individuals with functional mobility limitations.

INDEPENDENT TRAVEL

Independence in mobility involves a number of skills including those required for ambulation or movement, environmental negotiation, and effective social interaction (Blasch & Welsh, 1980). Independent movement refers to the act of moving through the environment in a safe and efficient manner (LaGrow & Weessies, 1994), while environmental negotiation, or wayfinding, refers to the act of moving through the environment with purpose (i.e., to reach a destination) (Passini, Dupré, & Langlois, 1986). Social interaction is essential to the cooperative act of travel required by complex environments (e.g., acquiring assistance or directions, using public transportation, interacting with others during travel) and is generally a part of the ultimate reason for traveling (i.e., interacting with those at the destination of travel). Deficiency in any of these aspects of independent travel may result in a functional mobility limitation.

FUNCTIONAL LIMITATIONS

Any number of conditions may affect mobility. Visual impairment and blindness are among the more obvious of these conditions. The field of blindness and visual impairment has developed the most systematic and comprehensive programs of mobility instruction. The specific mobility consequences of these conditions are well known (Long, McNeal, & Griffin-Shirley, 1990; Smith, De l'Aune, & Geruschat, 1992; Uslan, 1990; Hill & Ponder, 1976; Jacobson, 1993; LaGrow & Weessies, 1994; Welsh & Blasch, 1980). Other conditions are less obvious and often have more subtle effects on one's ability to travel. A hearing impairment, for example, would not necessarily restrict one's ability to get about in an environment. Yet, like a visual impairment, it results in a reduction in the amount and range of information available to the traveler. Those with significant hearing impairments may not benefit from auditory signals, warnings, and environmental or route descriptors, nor may they rely upon public address announcements concerning the arrival, departure, location, destination, or upcoming stop when using public transportation. Most significant, however, they may have difficulty interacting with others throughout every stage of the travel process.

Others encounter problems when planning or carrying out routes of travel for different reasons. Mobility skills require the traveler to possess accurate spatial, directional, and environmental concepts; store and recall information from memory; make decisions; and solve problems (Hill & Blasch, 1980). Problems may arise as the result of a number of conditions, including mental retardation, specific learning disabilities, attention deficits, brain damage, mental illness, dementia and experiential deficits (Welsh, 1972; Hughes, Smith, & Benitz, 1977; Blasch & Welsh, 1980).

The person with mental retardation may, like the person who is hearing impaired, experience communication problems and, like the person who is congenitally blind, lack certain basic concepts about the environment (Laus, 1977). He is likely to be unable to understand the general layout of the environment sufficiently to solve orientation problems and take alternative routes. He may be stigmatized by certain visible aspects of his disability or inappropriate behaviors in public. Many mentally retarded persons also have basic posture and gait deficiencies and lack basic skills such as those necessary in money exchanges and safety procedures in negotiating street crossings. All of these difficulties can create interaction problems for the person and make his family strongly resist his traveling alone.

A person who has severe emotional problems may also have travel difficulties. She may lack confidence in her ability to handle the complexity and confusion of large city environments. In some cases distinctive postures and gait patterns result from institutionalization, while in others an individual's abnormal gait may be modeled by other individuals. Therefore, the individual may have developed what has been referred to as an "institutional gait" or pacing behavior that may stigmatize the individual on the street (Haring & Schiefelbusch, 1967). She may exhibit inappropriate and stigmatizing behaviors that cause interaction problems with others. Difficulties with crowded areas and crowds in general may produce great anxiety. Orientation problems and crossing busy streets can cause stress and discourage travel. She may have difficulty planning trips and allowing sufficient time to get to appointments, or may allow too much time and arrive inappropriately early for job interviews or work.

Individuals with certain learning disabilities also may have travel problems. Some are unable to sort out the complex stimuli of the urban environment and become disoriented, particularly if they are away from a frequently traveled route. They may be unable to read street signs and the names of stores or businesses and therefore have to develop other strategies to maintain orientation and locate objectives. Some persons with learning disabilities are unable to use the numbering systems in large buildings and thus have orientation difficulties. They may have other difficulties, such as time and money concepts, and coordination deficiencies that make driving difficult or impossible.

Vestibular defects, physical disabilities, heart disease, impairments of the central nervous system, arthritis, emphysema, obesity, and frailty or poor health may reduce one's ability to travel any distance and even the range or speed of movement within an environment. Problems with gait and stability make it difficult to deal with uneven terrain, steps and stairs without railings, and deep curbs and obstacles in the path of travel that must be stepped over. Orthopedic and other mobility aids used to counter these difficulties (i.e., canes, walkers, wheelchairs, electric scooters, and so forth) may not fit through tight spaces, remain stable on lateral tilts, be capable of traversing curbs and steps, or fit on public transport. Furthermore, the speed at which the individual travels, with or without aids, may not be sufficient to allow for safe crossings at some intersections. Similar problems may be faced by elderly or frail travelers as well.

Elderly persons have a number of mobility problems associated with diseases and disabilities that frequently accompany the aging process. They may be unable to pass a driver's test or they may have a restricted driver's license. If the elderly person can no longer drive, they may become a "passive passenger" and consequently pay less attention to the environment and their orientation. They also may not be able to walk long distances and have difficulty on stairs and inclines. They may fear falling and the complications that come with injury, and they may not be able to cross streets quickly enough to guarantee their safety. Some older persons have their mobility further limited by their environment, especially where they feel vulnerable to attacks and muggings.

Functional mobility limitations can arise for a number of reasons. One cannot predict the difficulties an individual may face with travel by simply identifying a disorder or diagnostic category (Blasch & Welsh, 1980). An analysis of a number of factors is necessary (Blasch, 1994).

FACTORS AFFECTING INDEPENDENT MOBILITY

The potential for independent mobility is affected by the interaction between one's personal abilities (Pa), which is in turn affected by impairment, illness and age, and the environmental demands of travel (Ed). As the environmental demand increases, the potential for independence decreases. This interaction may be mediated or modified through an intervention (I). This intervention may be designed to reduce environmental demand or provide the traveler with the skills needed to deal with the environment, or both. Thus, one's potential for mobility independence (Mi) can be conceptualized using the following formula: Mi = (Pa − Ed) + I. The following sections, "Personal Abilities" and "Environmental Demands," are presented in relation to factors that limit functional abilities. The sections "Intervention" and "Providing Mobility Instruction to Sighted Individuals with Disabilities," present some of the positive approaches to enhance mobility independence.

PERSONAL ABILITIES

Personal abilities are affected by the presence of impairments, illnesses, and other conditions affecting one's sensory, cognitive, motor, and psychosocial ability. These functional limitations may interact in a manner or degree that subsequently affects the individual's ability to gather, process, or act upon environmental information for the purpose of travel. The degree, type, and number of disabilities affecting the individual interact with other personal variables, including self-concept, motivation, experience, and knowledge, to affect one's overall performance (Blasch & Welsh, 1980). The range of disabilities that have affected independent mobility and have been successfully addressed by an O&M specialist include intellectual, communication, hearing, behavioral, and learning disabilities; cerebral palsy; cardiopulmonary pathology; muscular dystrophy; emphysema; epilepsy; and mental illness (Blasch, 1982). This listing of disabilities served by an O&M specialist is certainly not exhaustive, but serves as a sample of impairments affecting independent mobility. The following represents a more comprehensive listing of personal abilities that relate to one's independent mobility:

- **I.** Sensory:
  - **A.** Visual
  - **B.** Auditory
  - **C.** Vestibular
  - **D.** Tactile
  - **E.** Proprioceptive
  - **F.** Olfactory
  - **G.** Gustatory
- **II.** Cognitive:
  - **A.** Concept development
  - **B.** Problem-solving and decision-making abilities
  - **C.** Information-gathering and processing abilities
  - **D.** Short- and long-term memory
- **III.** Motor/Psychomotor:
  - **A.** Perceptual abilities
  - **B.** Body awareness
  - **C.** Posture
  - **D.** Balance and gait
  - **E.** Speed
  - **F.** Endurance/Stamina
  - **G.** Strength
  - **H.** Flexibility
  - **I.** Agility
  - **J.** Perceptual/Motor coordination
- **IV.** Psychosocial Characteristics:
  - **A.** Self-Concept
  - **B.** Motivation
  - **C.** Experience
  - **D.** Personality

Sensory Abilities

Safe and purposeful movement through the environment requires the traveler to take in, interpret, and react to information about the environment through which he or she is moving. Movement can take place without this environmental information, but the movement will neither be oriented nor necessarily safe. Many people have difficulty with independent travel because of deficiencies in their ability to receive or interpret environmental information.

Environmental information is gathered through the visual, auditory, vestibular, tactile, olfactory, proprioceptive, and gustatory senses. Vision is the most efficient of these and provides one with varied and rich information concerning the environment of travel, including traffic and traffic patterns, the path of travel, and obstacles and drop-offs within that path, as well as information that can be gained from signs (e.g., street and store names, the location of exits and rest rooms, transit information, the time to cross streets, and so forth), maps, and models. The auditory sense also provides long-range information concerning the environment, traffic patterns, and when it is safe to cross a street, in addition to information which may be gained from public address announcements (e.g., transit information) or through direct conversation. Other, more direct information may be gained from the vestibular proprioceptive–kinesthetic systems, tactile and olfactory senses as well.

The information gained from the senses must be processed before it is usable. Deficiencies in the information processing system may be caused by single or multiple impairments of the sense systems themselves or by problems in the perceptual mechanisms through which the person interprets the information picked up and delivered by the senses. Deficiencies in either system may pose barriers to travel, as can other conditions that affect one's ability to gain or process information.

Cognitive Abilities

The information gained must be turned into usable concepts (i.e., spatial and environmental) before it can be acted upon (Hill & Blasch, 1980). Mentally retarded individuals and individuals who have specific learning disabilities or cognitive impairments, especially if these are present from birth, are more likely to experience difficulty in developing adequate body, spatial and environmental concepts. These concepts are very important to orientation and subsequent environmental negotiation or wayfinding.

Purposeful negotiation of an environment requires the individual to establish and maintain orientation while traveling. To do this, the individual must understand the environment well enough to plan and execute routes, reverse routes, and use alternate routes when necessary. This requires an ability to store and recall information, solve problems, and make decisions, all of which may be difficult for persons with cognitive problems. Related to these skills is the ability to read maps or other representations of the environment as aids in planning a route or understanding an area. Problems with these skills may not pose insurmountable barriers to travel, but do pose limitations or a need for alternative solutions. Communication deficits often associated with cognitive problems (i.e., reading, aural comprehension, and oral–aural interaction) may limit the amount and type of information that may be available to the individual during the mobility process.

Deficiencies in the ability to solve problems that arise during travel may be due to the lack of appropriate concepts for doing so, failure to attend to relevant stimuli, problems with the process involved in reasoning and decision making, or the lack of efficient strategies for doing so (see Chapter 2). Some impairments, especially those that directly affect cognitive functioning, obviously affect a person's reasoning powers and therefore his or her problem-solving abilities. For others, difficulties with reasoning and problem-solving are related more to their lack of opportunity to be responsible for themselves, often resulting from a pattern of social interaction in which the person with the disability is never allowed to make decisions and suffer the consequences of wrong decisions. Without such experiences, a problem solving skill does not generally develop (Hughes et al., 1977).

Motor/Psychomotor Abilities

Purposeful negotiation of the environment requires more than the skills involved in orientation, it also depends upon the ability to move within and through the environment. One's ability to move may be affected by a number of factors including the actual ability to do so, posture, balance, gait, speed, endurance, strength, flexibility, agility, and motor control. Some individuals may be unable to move due to paralysis, while others may have difficulty in their ability to direct their movement based upon the sensory information they receive. In the former, the problem does not exist in the receptive mechanisms, but rather in the person's ability to produce accurate movements based upon the information received or because of neural disruption. This can cause difficulties in locomotion as well as in driving a vehicle (Bardoch, 1971). Others have problems negotiating various aspects of the physical environment (e.g., dealing with uneven terrain, stepping up curbs, traversing stairs without hand rails).

Some physical and neurological impairments involve the skeletal and neuromuscular components of the body that are responsible for a person's ability to stand upright and ambulate with an erect posture. Other impairments affect posture and gait indirectly through the difficulties a person has in perceiving correct posture and making changes in his own stance in relation to the vertical, or as a result of the reluctance of parents and teachers to expect and reinforce correct posture in children with disabilities.

Poor posture and gait can make movement through the environment inefficient, uncomfortable, or even impossible. Some posture and gait deficiencies make movement more precarious since they impair the reflexes through which the individual draws back from danger. Others make reactions slower and movements less precise (Aust, 1980). Reductions in strength, flexibility, and agility pose similar problems for the individual when dealing with terrain changes, steps, and curbs. Thus the individual's mobility may be limited by physical demands the environment places on the traveler (See Chapter 10). Similar restrictions may be imposed by reduced endurance and speed, especially as it affects the range of travel (see Chapters 5 and 15).

Psychosocial Characteristics

Psychosocial factors refer to the social and psychological variables that affect the way an individual relates to the social and physical environment in which he or she lives and travels (see Chapter 6). These variables affect one's expectations of self in terms of the types of behaviors that can or should be carried out, and the likelihood of successfully doing so. The latter is referred to as the sense of self-efficacy. "Efficacy expectations determine how much effort people will expend and how long they will persist in the face of obstacles and aversive experiences" (Bandura, 1977, p. 194). They are affected most of all by the cumulative effects of one's efforts and may be altered by one's experiences and interactions with others (Bandura, 1977). (For a complete treatment of psychosocial factors, see Chapter 6.)

Consideration of Other Factors

The degree to which any of the disabling conditions will affect one's performance is dependent upon a number of factors. The first is the history of the impairment or health problem experienced and the effect it has on personality, self-concept, and sensory, cognitive, and motor abilities. The second is the number of disabilities experienced and the interactive effect they have on performance. One need only examine the following list of potentially disabling conditions and their causes to appreciate the potential for different effects across individuals:

- **I.** Sensory Disabilities
  - **A.** Visual impairment

B. Hearing impairment

C. Vestibular and kinesthetic dysfunction

II. Circulatory Disorders

A. Arteriosclerosis

B. Heart disease

III. Orthopedic Disorders

A. Amputations

B. Arthritis

C. Muscular dystrophy

IV. Disorders of the Central Nervous System

A. Stroke
1. Spasticity
2. Rigidity
3. Hemiplegia

B. Neoplasm—tumors

C. Epilepsy

D. Cerebral palsy
1. Spasticity
2. Athetosis
3. Ataxia
4. Tremor and rigidity
5. Mixed types

E. Multiple sclerosis

F. Parkinson's disease

G. Spinal cord dysfunction
1. Paraplegia
2. Quadriplegia

H. Spina bifida

I. Traumatic brain injury (TBI)

V. Respiratory Disorders

A. Emphysema

B. Asthma and allergies

VI. Behavioral Disability

A. Attention Deficit Disorder (ADD)

B. Attention Deficit Hyperactivity Disorder (ADHD)

VII. Intellectual and Perceptual Disabilities

A. Specific learning disabilities (SLD)

B. Intellectual disabilities—mild (ID-Mi)

C. Intellectual disabilities—moderate (ID-Mo)

D. Intellectual disabilities—severe (ID-Severe)

E. Intellectual disabilities—profound (ID-Profound)

F. Emotional disability and mental illness

VIII. Geriatric Disorders (pathologies associated with aging)

IX. Endocrine Disorders

A. Obesity

B. Body disproportion

C. Diabetes

D. Body structural disorders
1. Gigantism
2. Dwarfism

X. Communicative Disorders

A. Articulation

B. Delayed speech development

C. Aphasia

The third consideration to keep in mind is that the disability associated with an impairment or illness varies in relation to type, location, extent, stability, and age of onset (LaGrow, 1992). And finally, it seems that disability has a variable effect on performance across individuals due to differences in self-concept, motivation, experience, and knowledge (Blasch & Welsh, 1980).

ENVIRONMENTAL DEMANDS OR CONSTRAINTS

Personal ability and the degree of environmental accessibility interact to produce functional mobility limitations. Constraints may arise from one's social environment, while demands are usually placed on the traveler by the physical environment. The social environment consists of those people whose actions affect the individual, including family members, rule and policy makers, environmental planners, service providers, the public in general, and others using the environment.

Social Environment

Family members and others in authority (e.g., teachers, principals, supervisors of day or residential facilities) may restrict an individual's opportunities for, and therefore experience with, travel in an attempt to protect that person from the dangerous and embarrassing aspects of travel. They may also do so because of a misconception, due to either ignorance or prejudice, of the individual's ability or potential for travel (see Chapter 6). Rule makers (e.g., principals, superintendents, law makers, people responsible for instruction) may wish to protect themselves or their employees (or constituents if in government) from potential environmental hazards, or they simply may not be concerned enough to fully consider the needs of anyone "outside of the norm." Environmental planners (e.g., architects, engineers, governmental planners, etc.) often fail to account for the needs of all users of the buildings, malls, streets, campuses, neighborhoods, and transit systems they design (see Chapter 10).

Service providers (e.g., information and transit personnel; clerks in stores, offices, and hotels; waiters and waitresses; sales personnel; and so on) may fail to provide the services that would enhance accessibility due to ignorance, embarrassment, or prejudice. The public in general may react curiously, insensitively, negatively, or in other ways that stigmatize the traveler and make it easier or more comfortable for them to simply stay at home. Other individuals in the general public (e.g., bike and skateboard riders, drivers, street merchants, and criminals) may restrict access to a given environment by their presence or their actions.

Physical Environment

The physical structure of the environment may place demands on people to perform at a level that is beyond their capacity. All people have limits in terms of the types of terrain they can traverse; however, some have real difficulties with ordinary environments that have been constructed with the able-bodied traveler in mind (Morgan, 1976). This may be true even after environmental modification. Those persons may only be able to travel safely and efficiently in low-demand environments (e.g., a single-story building with no stairs and easily opened doors) or those specifically designed to enhance accessibility (e.g., those with ramps and elevators provided for access, quality lighting and signage, accessible toilets and drinking fountains, removed or modified turnstiles and revolving doors) (see Chapter 10). Many factors must be considered when evaluating the potential effect of the environment on travel.

Environmental Factors

I. Social Factors
- **A.** Family responses
  - **1.** Overprotectiveness vs. support
  - **2.** Acceptance vs. rejection
  - **3.** Flexibility vs. inflexibility
- **B.** General public
  - **1.** Understanding vs. ignorance
  - **2.** Supportive assistance vs. prejudice

II. Physical Factors
- **A.** Buildings
  - **1.** Public
    - **a.** Entrances, doors, doorways, door handles
    - **b.** Stairs, ramps, and handrails
    - **c.** Hallways, corridors, and aisles
    - **d.** Floors and floor coverings
    - **e.** Toilet facilities

- f. Furniture
- g. Elevators and escalators
- h. Telephone locations
- i. Drinking fountains
- j. Suspended objects and projections
- k. Display islands
- l. Signage, e.g., raised numbers
- m. Concessions and vending machines
- n. Coat racks and cloakrooms
- o. Lighting

2. Commercial
    - a. Counters and aisles
    - b. Seating
    - c. Cafeteria lines—ordering and utensils
    - d. Box office
    - e. Turnstiles
3. Residential
    - a. Furnishings
    - b. Shower and tub
    - c. Kitchen counters, cupboards, appliances
    - d. Controls (light and heat)
    - e. Lighting

B. Residential neighborhoods
- a. Curbs, curb cuts, curb ramps, and gutters
- b. Crosswalks
- c. Traffic signals
- d. Signage
- e. Sidewalks, footpaths
- f. Driveways
- g. Manhole covers and gratings
- h. Mailboxes, fire hydrants, trash receptacles
- i. Overhanging branches, shrubbery, and fences
- j. Public telephones
- k. Drinking fountains

C. Business and shopping districts
- a. Parking, passenger loading zones
- b. Barricades
- c. Outdoor steps and stairs
- d. Projections, control boxes, and poles
- e. Parking meters
- f. Vending machines
- g. Furniture
- h. Landscaping, outdoor planters, and ornamental structures
- i. Sidewalks, footpaths

D. Metropolitan areas
- a. Street widths
- b. Crowd congestion
- c. Masking noises
- d. Safety islands
- e. Open excavation sites

E. Manufacturing/Industrial sites
- a. Entrances
- b. Gates
- c. Platforms, loading docks
- d. Industrial machines and equipment

F. Transportation systems
1. Bus, Trolley
    - a. Steps
    - b. Railings
    - c. Seating
    - d. Crowd congestion
    - e. Fare boxes and systems of payment
2. Subways, Elevated trains
    - a. Turnstiles

b. Platforms

3. Airplanes and trains

a. Terminals

b. Stations

c. Airports

4. Cars, taxis, and vans

G. Recreational facilities

1. Parks, monuments, historic sites, and trails

a. Width of walkways

b. Surface of walkways

c. Access to swimming facilities

d. Recreation equipment

e. Access to information and directions

2. Amusement parks

3. Athletic centers

III. Climatic Factors

A. Weather

1. Heat, cold

2. Rain, snow, hail

3. Humid, dry

4. Wind

B. Air quality

1. Pollution—pollen, car fumes

2. Altitude—high, low

The demands that environments (this includes work, education, and the health system) place on travel have a varying effect on individual performance. Some may be too complex or require too much memory, while others demand too much agility, speed, or endurance. Wide open spaces may prove to be troublesome for visually impaired individuals (Smith et al., 1992), while areas with tight passages may be impossible to traverse for persons in wheelchairs, and those without sidewalks restrict the elderly to their homes and yards (Long et al., 1990). The effect of the interaction between personal ability and environmental demands and constraints may be mediated through intervention.

INTERVENTION

Intervention may involve a number of strategies carried out on both a personal and societal level. These strategies include the modification of environments, advocating for the rights of the traveler, education of the public, and the provision of formalized and comprehensive mobility instruction to individuals with functional limitations. The first two aim to reduce the demands of the physical environment on the traveler. The third seeks to remove undue constraints imposed by the social environment, and the last is designed to enable the individual to circumvent those that remain.

I. Environmental Modification

A. Societal

B. Task and environmentally specific

II. Advocacy

A. Institutional or societal advocacy

B. Personal advocacy

III. Education and Instruction

A. Public education

B. Direct instruction

Environmental Modification

Environments may be physically modified to enhance their accessibility, reduce the demand they impose on performance levels, and make travel easier. Many of these modifications are relatively simple and inexpensive (e.g., physical barriers may be removed, ramps or handrails may be installed, lighting added, signage improved, route markers added, and memory cues provided). They may be done to improve the accessibility of environments in general. Federal law, the Americans with Disabilities Act (ADA), now requires state and local municipalities to meet standards of accessibility in all public places (see Chapter 10). As such, barriers to safe travel are being removed and accessibility to public places is being improved. Newly constructed environments are being built with these regulations in mind. Standards have been set for all public places. However, general modifications for accessibility (i.e., braille markings in elevators and curb cuts at intersections) are not yet in place in every environment, nor should they be expected for years to come. Furthermore, mandated modifications are not appropriate or sufficient for every need, since they are indeed general standards and cannot hope to account for the specific abilities or disabilities of every individual. Thus, some personal solutions may be required as well.

These solutions tend be both task and environment specific. Where possible, they may be made by the traveler, an instructor, or family member (e.g., those made around the home, school, or place of work). In other cases, appropriate authorities (e.g., transit or municipal) may have to be approached for action. In many instances, modifying the immediate environment may be the most effective intervention available.

Advocacy

Advocacy by and on behalf of persons with disabilities is a key to their successful integration in society. It was through large-scale advocacy that disabled persons' rights to equal opportunity, education, and access were recognized and protected by the law. Groups of and for people with disabilities continue to lobby to ensure gains made in the Architectural Barriers Act of 1968, the Rehabilitation Act of 1973 (with the 1992 amendments), and the ADA of 1990 (PL 101–336) are enforced and become reality. Institutional or societal advocacy is often required to get system-wide changes made. Yet, a more direct approach with local authorities is also required to meet individual needs.

In this case, specific barriers to an individual's independence and possible solutions for their travel may be addressed. The local transit authority, for example, may be approached directly to get a particular bus stop added or changed along a route to accommodate the needs of a given traveler by lowering demands for performance that may block his or her successful participation in everyday life. A street sign posing a hazard to an individual may be moved to ensure safety, or a business may be asked to comply with a local ordinance banning delivery vehicles from parking on the crosswalk. This may be done by the individual, a mobility instructor, a professional advocate, a consumer group, or through the organized efforts of associations.

Public Education

Educational programs may be provided for the public or to targeted groups (e.g., teachers, nurses, police, and architects) as another form of advocacy to reduce some of the social barriers or constraints that limit the individual's opportunity to travel. Programs may be designed to raise awareness of the abilities and needs of disabled travelers or provide specific instruction to those who are expected to meet those needs (i.e., transit personnel) (Uslan, 1990).

Individual Instruction

Direct instruction is required to teach the individual with functional mobility limitations the skills and strategies needed to cope with the demands of the environment, establish and maintain orientation, plan routes to reach destinations while circumventing obstacles, use public transit systems, and interact with the public and service providers during travel (Laus, 1977). Ideally, these services are individualized to meet the traveler's specific needs, provided on a one-to-one basis in the actual environments of travel and delivered by a qualified instructor (Welsh, 1972; Blasch & Welsh, 1980; Blasch, 1994; LaGrow et al., 1990).

Mobility instruction, as discussed in other chapters of this volume, encompasses many components; however, there is a primary focus on three general areas: devices, skills, and strategies. There are many mobility devices, such as wheelchairs, crutches, support canes, and walkers, as well as long canes, electronic travel aids (ETAs), and dog guides. These devices range from the very simple to the very sophisticated.

The second area involves the acquisition of skills. Basically a skill as such is proficiency or mastery in the performance of some task. The task may be using a compass, reading a map, taking a direction, or using a mobility aid. The skills that are taught in mobility instruction are predominantly cognitive and motor.

Finally, the area in which mobility instruction is exemplary in the fields of rehabilitation and special education is the use of strategies. Strategies are generally thought of as an ingenious plan, method, or effective way of getting a result. Many times individuals are forced to use their ingenuity to try some innovative or alternative behavior to circumvent some obstacle, or it may be the strategy of employing the use of a specific device such as a cane or walker. One specific example of an effective strategy is using assistance and taking charge of the situation. It is the strategies of how to ask for assistance, formulating the questions, repeating the answer, and possibly explaining to a pedestrian the best way to provide physical assistance. Once the strategies have been taught through a systematic curriculum of instruction, the individual then develops skill and proficiency in the application of these strategies. With the increase in skill level, there is also an increase in self-confidence and self-efficacy.

There are several key factors to the intervention component in mobility instruction that have proven extremely effective. One critical factor is providing individualized instruction. Teaching in independent travel requires individualized instruction. Because of the variety of components that are involved, it is unlikely that any two students will be able to proceed at the same rate. Attempting to teach two students at one time will result in danger for the students and inefficient instruction. Because part of the focus of mobility instruction must be on independence and individual problem solving, teaching with more than one person deprives one or the other of the students of the opportunity to learn to make decisions on their own and bear their consequences, which the student will have to do when traveling independently. Individualized instruction also enables the O&M specialist to structure the situation to reflect the level of complexity that is most needed by a particular student at that time in the learning process (Welsh, 1972).

Another critical instructional component is that instruction can be adequately provided only in natural environments similar to those in which the student will later travel. Although teaching in simulated and protected environments may be necessary for beginning instruction, it is not sufficient for the development of all needed skills. Natural or ecologically relevant environments are qualitatively different from the hallways of institutions such as schools and hospitals. In the students' routine environment there is a bombardment of stimuli and a variety of competing concerns such as existing dangers, the reactions of pedestrians, the possibility of getting lost, and the preoccupation with the actual business of the trip. The method that has proven to be the best way to prepare for such situations is instruction and practice in the real environment (Welsh, 1972). The importance of this concept for mobility instruction for multiply impaired individuals has been recently rediscovered and given great prominence (Gee, Harrell, & Rosenberg, 1987; Joffee & Rikhye, 1991; Bailey & Head, 1993).

Since mobility instruction has concentrated on teaching in the real environment, the mobility instructor has developed a unique knowledge and expertise in teaching environmental problem solving (see Chapter 6). Examples of specific environmental problem situations include what to do when confronted with a detour or barrier; if the elevator is not functioning; if veering occurs on a street crossing or in a parking lot; recovery from veering into a driveway or a street; and establishing one's location on a drop-off lesson, to mention a few. Aspects of this environmental problem-solving knowledge base are similar to those used by the person who participates in the sport of orienteering.

Traditionally, orienteering is a timed cross-country race in which the participants use a map and compass to plan the most efficient route between controls (checkpoints) on an unfamiliar course set in a large, wooded area. However, for the purposes of teaching environmental problem solving, courses can be set up anywhere—classrooms, playgrounds, and neighborhoods, and events can be held for a variety of purposes: to learn new settings, exercise, teach independent mobility (Blasch, 1981a, 1981b, 1984; Langbain, et al., 1981), promote inclusion (Blasch, 1994), and provide enjoyable activity. This activity, like O&M instruction and independent mobility, may be designed to improve the following skills: map-reading skills and orientation; landmark identification and use, distance estimation, use of compass directions for orientation, route following and planning, development of problem-solving and decision-making strategies, and practice in taking precautions against becoming lost or disoriented (Blasch, 1994).

Another important teaching component in mobility instruction is the need for lessons of graduated difficulty and responsibility. Various components have to be broken out of the total mobility task and presented sequentially. It is important to develop certain basic skills before the student can be expected to deal with other people in travel situations. For example, the student should be able to handle less congested areas of travel before proceeding to more complicated areas. A student should also develop confidence in her own travel abilities before she works on the skills of soliciting and using assistance. Although the particular sequence or approach may differ somewhat for individual students, and the approach used for persons with different disabilities may vary from that which has been most helpful for visually impaired persons, O&M specialists should be expert in planning sequenced lessons of graduated difficulty and responsibility. Such skill is necessary for work with persons with all types of mobility limitations, particularly as it relates to the development of the person's self-confidence in their travel abilities and the overcoming of any fears and anxieties that may exist.

Another common factor that has emerged in mobility instruction for people who are visually impaired is the synthesis of skills (self-efficacy and self-confidence). The synthesis of skills may be viewed as the whole of independent travel being greater than the sum of its parts (Chapter 11). No matter how expertly the student performs the various subskills in isolation, the various components frequently do not come together as smoothly as expected. Unless the student gets an opportunity to put it all together in practice situations with an O&M specialist available for feedback and assistance, it is likely that the student will not be able to learn to travel to full potential, at least not as soon as he or she might with such professional training.

Finally, one of the more important elements of mobility instruction is the designation of mobility instruction as the primary responsibility of one or more full-time staff members of an agency or program (Welsh, 1972). This is best done by the O&M specialist (Laus, 1974, 1977; Blasch, 1982; Williams et al., 1982; Brambila-Hickman & Denniston, 1984). Where mobility instruction of some sort is offered in programs for persons with limitations other than visual impairment, it is usually done by someone whose main responsibility lies elsewhere and who provides travel instruction only when time permits or when the need is so obvious and pressing that other duties must be put aside. Giving specific staff members responsibility for mobility instruction is an important step in the recognition and development of this service as an essential part of the program. The presence of an O&M specialist in a program also indicates that someone in the organization, who has a professional responsibility, will focus attention on this area and on the literature to learn how to improve the service. A designated person is able to devote full attention to this service without the distractions of other responsibilities.

Instructional Strategies

The strategies involved in the instruction of persons with functional mobility limitations are essentially the same as those used with persons who are visually impaired (Welsh, 1972; Blasch & Welsh, 1977; Blasch, 1981a). The program is individualized to account for the traveler's personal abilities and meet his or her specific needs (which may be even more varied than those presented by the visually impaired population, if this is possible) and is provided on a one-to-one basis.

Less emphasis, however, is placed on teaching the basics in the use of travel devices (if a travel device is necessary), since this is the responsibility of others (i.e., occupational and physical therapists) and is usually done before mobility in the outdoor or natural environment begins. On the other hand, more emphasis is placed on working and cooperating with other professionals. Less emphasis may be placed on sensory training and more on the development of routes and recovery techniques for those with cognitive impairments, and route planning to circumvent physical barriers for others. Similar attention is given to the use of public transportation and interaction with the public. These points are illustrated in some brief examples of providing mobility instruction to sighted individuals with disabilities. The following section discusses some of the routinely used techniques.

PROVIDING MOBILITY INSTRUCTION TO SIGHTED INDIVIDUALS WITH DISABILITIES

Intellectual Disabilities

Historically, travel training provided to students with intellectual disabilities was done in groups similar to field trips. In other cases, simulated environments of streets and storefronts were used. These methods tended to be very narrow in scope and were not very successful.

Many students with intellectual disabilities may have difficulties with reading (e.g., street signs or names of stores), memory, and verbal communication. Some techniques to circumvent this limitation is to use index cards (flash cards) with hand-drawn or photographed landmarks that can be laminated to protect against weather conditions. These cards can be used on a key ring or in a book form and sequenced for a specific route, or used to solicit assistance from the public. A productive mobility lesson is to have the student go into a store (prearranged with the store by the instructor) and ask for stationery or an advertisement with the store name and logo. Then the student can cut out the information and affix it to a flash card for future use as a visual reminder. Another helpful orientation tool is the use of an auditory cassette tape that gives a verbal step-by-step sequence of a route.

These activities also help to reinforce the use of appropriate landmarks (see Chapter 2). Often students with intellectual disabilities have not been taught to use primary landmarks, or they select inappropriate secondary landmarks such as a car or a barking dog. Instruction in the selection of stationary landmarks becomes an important aspect of the mobility lesson. One unique method involved a necklace made by the student with significant objects, like a charm bracelet. This allowed the student to focus on meaningful landmarks and the necklace served as a mnemonic to remember the route sequence. Often parents can be encouraged to have their sons give the directions when going to the store (e.g., turn right—or point—at Burger King). Although an individual may have an intellectual disability, this does not mean that he or she has trouble with orientation. It is not uncommon for students who cannot read to develop coping strategies when they are traveling on a new route in an unfamiliar area.

Map reading is another task that is often not taught because of preconceived expectations about individuals with intellectual disabilities. If the individual is unaware that maps are comprised of symbols representing the environment, start with pictures, photographs, or drawings of actual environments such as a classroom. Have the student point to the chair that she is sitting on in the picture. Then point to the window in the picture and have the student walk to the window. Gradually progress from the picture to symbolic representations on a map. If successful, progress to maps of the school, playground, home, neighborhood, and so on. Teaching the use of maps in this way is something that family members may also reinforce.

Another important aspect of the instruction is to teach an individual how to ask for information. This may begin with whom to ask. Generally, there is a great concern on the part of the parents and families of students with intellectual disabilities regarding the students' ability to make good judgments. There is a concern that the student may be vulnerable to abuse. Therefore, it is important to do role-playing and teach the student how to identify a "safe stranger." A safe stranger may be described as someone who is easily identified by a uniform or name tag (e.g., bank tellers, police, bus drivers). Mobility instruction provides opportunities for the student to role-play and demonstrate the ability to solve common travel problems, such as being approached by a stranger or getting lost. In the role-play, it is important to rehearse information-gathering questions and getting useful directions. In some cases the student may have a card with the address to show to the bus driver and a card of a different color with the return address to show to the bus driver when returning.

Crossing streets may be a challenge for some of these students. The most effective teaching strategy is one on one instruction and a lot of practice at street crossings in the student's community where they are likely to travel. The student may not be able to tell the instructor what type of street crossing they are making, but they must be able to demonstrate proficiency 100 percent of the time before the mobility instructor signs off on traveling alone.

One method used in the St. Paul, Minnesota, Public Schools is to videotape the student crossing streets and review the videotape in a classroom setting. Some students respond well when they observe their instructor making good or poor street crossings and are asked to evaluate. It is not uncommon for the student to be able to stand at a corner and accurately assess the street crossing and indicate when it is safe to cross. However, the student may never have been allowed to implement the decision, so they wait for a verbal cue from the mobility instructor or adult to verify their decision. Therefore, the mobility instructor may have to teach the student environmental decision-making and implementation. This may be accomplished by the behavioral procedure of fading. The mobility instructor may start with the student (who is extremely fearful) holding on to the instructor in the sighted guide technique, but with the student making the decision when to cross. The student continues to make the decision when to cross, but the progression of fading then has the mobility instructor stand next to the student, then directly behind, then 6 feet behind, and so on. This is an extremely important learning concept and may be the first time some individuals are allowed to make such decisions and act on them.

For those students who have trouble with problem solving, repetitive community-based travel experience seems to build a foundation upon which the student can draw information that they later are able to transfer to new and previously frustrating situations. The pivotal teaching tool on which students rely and base their problem-solving strategies is the "emergency information card." The emergency information card is a laminated card with emergency telephone numbers, names, addresses, a picture, and even pertinent medical information that the student keeps in their wallet. Reconstructing actual problems that the student has experienced while using the emergency information card in the community in a safe classroom setting provides opportunities for role playing solutions. Videotaping these role-playing situations becomes a useful tool for future students as well. Overall, the use of the emergency information card helps students develop a sense of self-assurance that enables them to learn how to solve problems. It is also valuable for the mobility instructor to have a copy of the same card. This is a safety precaution in case the student is lost and the mobility instructor has to ask people if they have seen the student. It is helpful to have a picture of the student.

Parents or caretakers may unintentionally foster dependence in the life of a person with an intellectual disability. Therefore, it is important to involve the parents or caretakers very early in the mobility program. Instructors may choose to invite parents and students to express their concerns and jointly strategize approaches to the mobility instructional sequence that will satisfy everyone. The instructor may also choose to invite parents or caretakers to observe lessons or help create the next lesson plan. Some of the parent's fears may be based on a limited knowledge of public transportation or their limited knowledge of problem-solving strategies. Other parental fears may be based on years of witnessing the student's high level of vulnerability. An effective teaching strategy is to teach the student the strategies for "what to do if . . . " For example, when the student is able to tell the instructor what they would do if a stranger approached, the support of the parents or caretakers is enlisted to role-play the "stranger approach." Some police community outreach programs may be willing to assist the mobility instructor in creating a "setup" where students are approached by a policeman out of uniform. The policeman offers them a ride or candy, or touches on whatever their particular area of vulnerability happens to be. The student's reaction to the undercover policeman is one measure of the student's ability to avoid dangerous situations.

Some students may exhibit inappropriate social behaviors. Some of these behaviors may keep store clerks or others from offering assistance or cause a bus driver to keep a student off a bus. Videotaping a student in a community setting and subsequently showing the videotape to the student may have a profound effect on his choice of community behaviors. Many of these same teaching procedures may be applicable to individuals with other disabilities.

Physical Impairments

The mobility instructor's objective is to give the student with orthopedic impairments as many opportunities to travel in as many community settings as possible.

There are resources available for the mobility instructor who is unfamiliar with assistive devices used by people with physical disabilities (see Chapter 15). It is sometimes helpful to borrow equipment and travel with a simulated functional mobility limitation for a period of time. Equipment technology is constantly changing, so it is important to attend local, regional, or national conferences to stay up to date. There is not enough written in current literature about community travel and assistive devices for physically disabled persons. However, one useful manual that details rules of the road for wheelchair users, including street crossings, is *A Wheelchair User's Manual for People with Spinal Cord Injury* (Blasch, Davies, & Shoup, 1981).

Many times a student is not given sufficient opportunities to practice street crossings. The ability to judge the distance of an oncoming car and the time it takes to cross the street safely is best done in the actual environment of travel. The effects of rain, snow, wind, and other weather conditions must be considered as well. It is also important for the wheelchair user to not only know how to ask for assistance, but also quickly explain to the pedestrian how to best manipulate the chair. Not unlike the Hine's Break and the sighted guide technique, this procedure to take charge to ensure that the assistance is appropriate is often needed at street crossings that are not accessible.

Two common problems facing a person with orthopedic impairments concern accessibility to various modes of transportation and accessibility to facilities. Lessons should be created that require the student to plan the route as completely as possible. This may include making arrangements for the student's choice of where to practice making a purchase; negotiating doors, elevators, ramps, people, obstructions, unexpected terrain changes; and handling a door-to-door paratransit system pick-up. In this process the student will invariably be confronted with the need to advocate for himself or herself. The mobility instructor can provide strategies for self-advocacy and environmental problem-solving by encouraging the student to be assertive in asking for assistance, getting help through difficult passageways, or by requesting that people move out of the way in crowded situations.

Specific Learning Disabilities

A learning disability is an invisible disability, yet it may produce as many limitations to independent mobility as any other disability. The most common problems experienced by people with specific learning disabilities (SLD) are the inability to read, reversal of letters and numbers, and an inability to follow directions that have been given verbally. However, it is also common for those individuals with SLD to have extreme difficulties with orientation. Getting up from one's desk and turning left rather than right is not uncommon. Remembering a sequence of directions may also be difficult. Asking students to describe the bus route from school to home or give directions to their grandmother's house that they travel every weekend may only produce a blank stare. These and other situations, such as an inability to dial their own telephone number, become very embarrassing for individuals with SLD.

A number of solutions to these problems have proven very successful. Teaching the use of sequential visual landmarks, such as turning toward the blue bulletin board, walking on the same side of the street as the sporting goods store, and crossing the street and going toward McDonalds are very helpful. It is also important to start with a specific route and establish a routine of using this route at a specific time or times each day. This may entail, for example, delivering the daily bulletins, using the same route every day and at the same time. Later, it is important to use the same route but at different times of the day. Methods to facilitate using this route would include drawing and using a map of the route and using written directions, depending on the reading capabilities of the individual, of the route. As the student becomes familiar and confident with the route, he or she should work with trying a detour ("Rather than going to the gym door and turning and walking down the 8th-grade hallway, today go to the trophy case and turn down the 7th-grade hallway") or an alternate route to the same destination. It is also very important to involve family members in the reinforcement of these orientation strategies. The individual must also be encouraged to use these strategies and implement them when traveling with friends or learning to go to a new destination.

Deafness or Hearing Impairments

For the mobility instructor who is teaching a student who is deaf or hard of hearing, it is important to learn sign language or enlist the services of a sign language interpreter. To be effective, it is important to break down the lessons into concrete parts and translate this information so it is understood. Similarly, it is important to have the mobility lessons in the natural environment. Present the lesson in its entirety first. Go through the entire route with the student without too much detail or explanation at first. Allow the student to visually absorb as much of the route as possible. Subsequent lessons will involve taking notes (by the student or the mobility instructor) of any unusual or permanent circumstances that the student has not noted previously (one-way streets, and so forth) and pointing these out.

Teaching the student how to solve travel problems includes social awareness as well as challenges with the environment. If the student seems to have problems with social graces (sitting too closely to other passengers on the bus, signing to a fellow students inside another passenger's "space," taking a seat on a bus that was designated for the elderly, and so forth), videotape the student in action and then view the tape and reenact these situations in a classroom or the student's home. Illustrate how the student intrudes upon another passenger and then strategize with the student on a more polite way to handle himself or herself in the community. This may be accomplished through role-playing. However, solving travel problems is much more effective if it is done on the spot, at the time of the problem, in the community. As with any type of mobility instruction, the instructor needs to develop a sense of when it is appropriate to intervene and when it is appropriate to allow the student to struggle a bit. However, some students may not know they have a problem. They may be unaware they are lost and continue traveling as if all is well. To allow a student to continue traveling in the wrong direction indefinitely will not necessarily serve a learning goal. It is better to allow the student to become slightly disoriented, but not too far from what is visually familiar. In later lessons when the student's visual scope of "what's familiar" broadens and he or she begins to connect whole blocks together in a cognitive map, the mobility instructor may find it of educational value to allow the student to travel in the wrong direction for a greater distance (see Chapter 6).

Making needs and wants known or asking directions involves preparing the student for an actual experience of being lost. Continually putting the student in a contrived situation will not make the experience meaningful. Wait for a "teachable moment" when students really need assistance, and then allow them to practice what they have learned and ask for help. For students who are deaf or hard of hearing, carrying a pad of paper and a pencil becomes as important as a wallet or billfold. For the student who is also intellectually disabled, the challenge may be how to clearly get a message across to a hearing person. Most likely, the initial experience will not be enough. But this experience can be role-played over and over again in the classroom or at home, and written phrases memorized for different situations. The other half of this challenge is the response the student receives from a clerk, security guard, or the general public. Persons offering assistance may give a verbal response instead of writing it down, or they may write their response down using words that are not understood. The student must be prepared to express what they need from the person as clearly as possible. When the student is unable to write in an emergency, body movements and gesturing may be useful. The mobility instructor can expect that this type of instruction may take several years or more to complete with weekly practice before the student is a safe and efficient independent traveler.

The person with a communication disorder has similar problems to the individual who is deaf or hard of hearing, and the solutions may be exactly the same. The main difference is that the individual can hear but is not able to speak. The problem solving and soliciting assistance strategies are much the same with the exception that this person may use an augmentative communication device or communication system with which the general public is probably not familiar. It is often valuable to role-play interactions with the public. The mobility instructor must work closely with the student's augmentative communication specialist or a speech and language pathologist to develop strategies for using the correct communication device or communication system in public.

Traumatic Brain Injury

Problems with short-term memory, maintaining orientation, map reading, and fear of independent travel are frequently outcomes of traumatic brain injury (TBI). The role of the mobility instructor is to assist the student with reentry into the community as an independent traveler after a probable long stint in a rehabilitation setting.

Teaching strategies generally focus on giving the person with TBI some tangible ways to maintain their orientation. Examples of this may be in the form of a mnemonic such as a charm bracelet or a written list of landmarks and turns. This strategy compensates for the three remaining problems that affect travel efficiency: short-term memory problems, map-reading problems, and fear of independent travel.

Instruction should begin with the student making a checklist of things to bring with him or her while traveling (i.e., wallet, identification, change for a phone call, flip chart or information book of the route, and so forth). Start with familiar locations and ask the student to select a route that he or she would like to master, such as the route to work or the grocery store. Develop a sequenced flip chart of written travel instructions or photographs of sequential landmarks to help stay oriented. If this route is a walking route, the student can hold the flip chart. If the student is a driver the circular file flip chart may be mounted on the dash board of the car.

The performance of students recovering from TBI may vary from day to day. Build in recovery strategies that students may use to help themselves if they become disoriented. Have students practice soliciting assistance, making a phone call on a pay phone, and providing the location where they became disoriented or their current location.

For students who want to advance their travel skills to unfamiliar indoor and outdoor areas, equip them with strategies that will help them stay oriented. Walk or drive through the new route once and teach them to use and carry a compass and tape recorder. Have the students describe the route they are taking on an audiotape. Subsequent lessons include observing students completing the route while they are listening to the tape, and eventually fading the student from using the tape if this is feasible. The range and level of travel complexity can best be mutually determined by the mobility instructor and the student, frequently discussing the student's readiness for more complex travel. If the student would like to work toward driving long distances to unfamiliar destinations, map-reading skills are helpful but not mandatory. Some of the pocket computers that sequentially list the routes, interstate services, and directions are very affordable. The traveler can also request that complex maps be simplified for easier reading or put on an audiotape. For people who cannot read a map because of difficulty using cardinal directions, mounting a compass on the car dashboard and adjusting their modified map so its directional arrow matches that of the car compass may prove helpful.

SUMMARY

This chapter illustrated some examples of teaching strategies and techniques for providing mobility instruction to sighted individuals with various disabling conditions. The intent is to provide the mobility instructor with a number of very applied examples, but not an exhaustive teaching curriculum for each disability. The examples and solutions cited for a specific disability are certainly not restricted to use with that particular disability, but may indeed be applied to any individual with a similar functional mobility problem.

As one would expect, less emphasis is placed on vision or the lack of it, with more attention placed on the consequences, causes, and treatment of other disabilities. The instructor must be familiar with the mobility strategies used for coping with various conditions. As a result, the instructor is more of an O&M specialist when it comes to dealing with disability groups, and is therefore more versatile. This is not so different from the demands currently placed on the O&M specialists who work with persons who are blind, who are increasingly teaching more individuals with multiple impairments and low vision, rather than totally blind travelers (Uslan, Hill, & Peck, 1989).

Currently, no single professional group has emerged to provide mobility instruction to those with functional mobility limitations. Where travel instruction of some sort is offered in programs for persons with limitations other than visual impairment, it is usually done by someone whose main responsibility lies elsewhere else and provides travel instruction only when time permits or when the need is so obvious and pressing that other duties must be put aside. Giving specific staff members responsibility for mobility instruction is an important step in the recognition and development of this service as an essential part of the program. The presence of mobility instructors in a program also indicates that someone in the organization has a professional responsibility for this area and is able to devote attention to this service without the distractions of other responsibilities (Blasch & Welsh, 1980).

O&M programs were originally designed to meet the needs of veterans who were adventitiously blinded during and immediately following World War II. Numerous modifications have been made since then to make O&M instruction more appropriate for persons of diverse ages, needs, and abilities (e.g., the very young, the very old, those with low vision, and the multiply impaired) (Uslan et al., 1989). It seems compelling that the profession of O&M continues to expand to include all persons with functional mobility limitations and emerges in the future as the profession responsible for providing services to learners with other mobility limitations.

Suggestions/Implications for O&M Specialists

1. Mobility services are available to other individuals with a variety of functional mobility limitations; however, these programs are generally limited in focus and thus fail to recognize the comprehensive nature of mobility as a skill area and the myriad of subtle factors involved in independent travel.
2. Independence in mobility involves a number of skills, including those required for ambulation or movement, environmental negotiation, and effective social interaction.
3. The potential for independent mobility is affected by the interaction between one's personal abilities, which is in turn affected by impairment, illness, age, and the environmental demands of travel. As the environmental demand increases, the potential for independence decreases. This interaction may be mediated or modified through an intervention. This intervention may be designed to reduce environmental demand or provide the traveler with the skills needed to deal with the environment, or both.
4. There are a number of factors that contribute to the degree to which any disabling condition will affect one's mobility.
5. The physical structure of the environment may place demands on people to perform at a level that is beyond their capacity. Accessibility reduces this environmental demand.
6. Interventions for independent mobility may involve a number of strategies carried out on both a personal and societal level.
7. Mobility instruction, as discussed in other chapters of this volume, encompasses many components; however, there is a primary focus on three general areas: devices, skills, and strategies.
8. There are several unique intervention components to mobility instruction, including individualized instruction; teaching in the natural environments; teaching environmental problem solving; lessons of graduated difficulty and responsibility; and the synthesis of mobility skills.
9. It is essential that one or more full-time staff members of an agency or program have primary responsibility for the mobility instruction.

ACTIVITIES FOR REVIEW

1. Develop a case for teaching mobility to disabled individuals other than the visually impaired. Has this been done before?
2. List the conditions that may affect mobility and produce a functional limitation in independent travel.
3. Describe the meaning of the formula: Mi = (Pa − Ed) + I and give a specific example.
4. Describe some of the social environmental constraints that restrict an individual's mobility.
5. Describe specific personal and societal interventions for independent mobility.
6. Describe a specific mobility device, skill, and strategy (not something for a visually impaired individual).
7. Describe orienteering and how it could be used to teach individuals with different functional mobility limitations.
8. Map-reading problems are common to individuals with some types of impairments. Define these impairments. How would you teach map reading differently?
9. Observe individuals with disabilities and evaluate their mobility skills. Are there any similarities with the mobility problems of individuals with a visual impairment?
10. Discuss if teaching O&M to individuals other than those with a visual impairment would detract from services for individuals who are blind and visually impaired?

PART FOUR

Progression of the Profession

CHAPTER 20

The Development of the Profession of Orientation and Mobility

William R. Wiener and Eileen Siffermann

Orientation and mobility (O&M) continues to grow and mature as a profession. A profession is generally considered to develop around a specific body of specialized knowledge and practice by persons educated in its application. Practitioners with common interests come together in professional associations to develop and share information, establish minimum qualifications, certify practitioners to possess certain competencies, and decide and enforce standards of professional conduct. This chapter is an effort to present a coherent picture of the O&M profession's emergence, status, and future directions.

EARLY DEVELOPMENTS

Gloucester Conference

In the early 1950s visitors to the Hines Veterans Administration Hospital studied the procedures initiated to rehabilitate veterans, but upon returning were unable to replicate the program with short-term training (Bledsoe, 1980). In 1953 the Reverend Thomas Carroll assembled a group of people in his home in Gloucester, Massachusetts, to discuss the dangers involved in allowing untrained persons to set themselves up as mobility experts (Koestler, 1976). It was felt that many in the work for those who were blind did not believe such formal instruction was necessary and were not yet ready to accept the standards some participants recommended.

National Conference on Orientation and Mobility

In June 1958 the U.S. Office of Vocational Rehabilitation identified the education of O&M specialists as its second highest priority in the area of preparing rehabilitation personnel (Voorhees, 1962). To implement this, the American Foundation for the Blind (AFB) funded a national conference that was held in 1959 to establish criteria for the basic selection of O&M personnel, develop a curriculum, and recommend the length of preparation and appropriate sponsorship.

This conference was a significant step in the establishment of O&M as a profession. A major decision was to establish the minimum preparation period for O&M specialists as 1 year of graduate study. This conference established the principle that O&M specialists should be sighted rather than blind. Although this point went against the thinking of many in the field, it was felt necessary to allow an instructor to move away and still provide for the client's safety. The conference further reinforced the need for extended preparation so instructors could habitually think about how to manage the problems of living without sight. The conference participants addressed the question of appropriate university settings and curriculum. Five recommended areas of study were techniques and practice of O&M, dynamics of human behavior as it relates to blindness, functions of the human body, study of the senses, and cultural and psychological implications of blindness.

The first grant to establish an O&M university program went to Boston College beginning in June 1960. The second O&M university program established in 1961 was at Western Michigan University (WMU), in Kalamazoo. The graduates of the new programs were in great demand. Stimulating this demand was the sponsoring of research and demonstration grants in O&M. These grants were intended to determine the value of skills in O&M preparation and the effectiveness of instructors educated in these techniques. Beginning in 1962, the Vocational Rehabilitation Administration (VRA) awarded 30 grants in 22 states that essentially paid the salaries of O&M specialists hired by participating schools and agencies.

Ad Hoc Committee Concerned with Mobility Instruction for the Blind

By 1966, recognition of the value of university-educated O&M specialists led to such a great demand that another conference, the Ad Hoc Committee Concerned with Mobility Instruction for the Blind, was held. Spurred on by the perceived need to come up with the greatest number of well-prepared O&M specialists in the shortest time, the committee reviewed the existing preparation programs and explored possibilities for increasing the number of O&M specialists. Because of this conference, the existing programs were encouraged to double their student enrollment, and the VRA was encouraged to continue its support for these programs and consider supporting new graduate and undergraduate programs. Several research studies were suggested to provide more empirical information about the need for O&M instruction and the actual knowledge and skills needed by O&M specialists. The necessity of studying the O&M needs of partially sighted persons received attention. As the demand for O&M specialists increased, so did preparation programs. The U.S. Office of Education sponsored O&M university programs that prepared graduates to instruct children with visual impairments. Meanwhile, the VRA began sponsoring new university O&M programs preparing instructors to service adults who were blind. The university O&M programs have become the primary means of articulating and delivering the body of knowledge that has become the core of the profession of O&M (see Table 20.1). A chronological listing of major events in development of O&M can be found in the appendix at the end of this chapter.

PROFESSIONAL ASSOCIATIONS

Another identified characteristic of a profession is the development of professional associations whose members come together to share information and act collectively to advance the profession's goals. The first association of those interested in O&M developed within the AAWB, American Association of Workers for the Blind (1895–1984) and AEVH, Association for the Education of the Visually Handicapped (1968–1984), formerly the AAIB, American Association of Instructors for the Blind (1871–1968). In 1984, AAWB and AEVH consolidated into AER, the Association for Education and Rehabilitation of the Blind and Visually Impaired.

At the 1964 AAWB convention, an informal meeting was held for all individuals interested in O&M. Persons attending discussed forming an association through which O&M specialists could exchange ideas, discuss common interests, receive current information, and provide for professional growth. At the request of the meeting participants, the AAWB Board of Directors approved a new interest group devoted to O&M.

Development of Mobility Interest Groups

The first meeting of the new interest group (Group IX) took place at the 1965 AAWB meeting, with much of the initial meeting devoted to the development of an organizational structure. In a parallel fashion, at the 1966 AAIB convention, following a general session on the development of the O&M preparation programs, a call was made for anyone interested in forming an O&M group. While the group was composed largely of persons who taught in schools, many issues and many members were the same as in AAWB. Interest Group IX, now AER Division Nine, gradually became the chief policy-generating body for O&M specialists. Organizations of O&M specialists also developed at the state and regional levels to exchange ideas and share information. Some of these developed within the chapter and regional structure of AER, while others developed independently.

DEVELOPMENT OF STANDARDS

One reason professionals come together in formal associations is to develop standards of education and preparation. The purpose is to ensure that those persons entering the area of service are of high caliber, by developing a method of identifying and recognizing those persons who have the necessary amount and type of preparation. O&M became involved in this process early in its history because of the widespread attention to accountability and certification issues that was occurring in other professions.

Commission on Standards and Accreditation of Services for the Blind

Influenced by a concern for accountability, AFB, in October 1961, began a study "to project the method, scope, and structure necessary to carry out an accreditation program in the field of work for the blind" (Commission on Standards and Accreditation of Services for the Blind, 1966), known as the COMSTAC report. The study recommended the formulation of standards for agency administration and service programs, and an organization to administer a nationwide system of voluntary accreditation based on them. From this the Commission on Standards and Accreditation of Services for the Blind (COMSTAC) was created. In 1961, COMSTAC initiated the process that led eventually to the development of standards and a process for certifying O&M specialists. As part of the process to establish accreditation of facilities and schools, COMSTAC appointed a Committee on Standards for Orientation and Mobility Services to conceptualize and express the role of these services, and the qualifications necessary to provide quality services. The committee later called for the establishment of an "appropriate body" to develop and implement standards for certification of O&M specialists. These standards would apply to those who were prepared in academic programs and those prepared in nonacademic settings while serving as O&M specialists at that time.

While COMSTAC was formulating its criteria and methods for evaluating and upgrading work for those who are blind, the O&M Interest Group within the AAWB was emerging and taking form. When the Interest Group met for the second time in 1966, the intent and standards of the COMSTAC group were known, and the challenge of establishing an appropriate body to develop and implement a certification process for O&M specialists was accepted by the group. At the 1966 AAWB convention the first certification committee was established.

Before the 1967 AAWB convention, the certification committee formulated standards based heavily on the standards recommended in the COMSTAC report. The educational qualifications called for graduation from an accredited graduate-level program that meets the standards outlined in the *COMSTAC Report* (1966), and membership in good standing in at least one professional organization. In addition, a time-limited grandfather clause was developed to allow for the certification of individuals who had been teaching as O&M specialists for a minimum of 5 years, and who met the physical and personal qualifications established. The initial certification standards established two levels of certification, provisional and permanent, which depended upon experience. A report of the certification committee was presented and accepted by the Interest Group at its 1967 meeting. The passed document also recommended that the National Accreditation Council (NAC), the accrediting body that resulted from COMSTAC, incorporate the use of certified instructors as an integral part of its requirement for O&M personnel in agencies and schools seeking accreditation. Interest Group IX then presented a resolution to the AAWB Board of Directors resolving that they approve the procedures and requirements for certification of O&M specialists by AAWB.

The passage of this resolution by the AAWB Board of Directors officially marked the beginning of certification in O&M. This certification would be granted by AAWB on the advice and recommendation of the Interest Group Certification Committee. AEVH was invited to appoint a member to the committee. In 1969 the first O&M specialists were certified by AAWB. The members of the Interest Group continued to evaluate the effect of the certification procedures and consider difficulties that arose with the intention of developing a fair and comprehensive set of standards.

By the time the AAWB O&M Interest Group convened in 1973, three new undergraduate preparation programs had developed. There was a need to change certification criteria to reflect undergraduate preparation. An Interest Group Certification Review Committee (CRC) was appointed to consider these changes and recommend specific curriculum standards. This committee realized that similar detailed standards were not available for graduate programs. At the 1975 meeting, this CRC proposed a temporary solution: grant certification to graduates of new preparation programs judged to be comparable to those whose graduates were currently being certified. Meanwhile, the CRC was directed to further develop university curriculum standards.

STANDARDIZATION OF PREPARATION AND CERTIFICATION

With this action, O&M as a profession moved toward the type of accountability and standardization needed to further the continuing expansion of the field. A standards proposal presented to the Interest Group at the 1977 AAWB convention was a comprehensive document that contained four distinct sections. The first section suggested standards for university programs, discussing the type and number of faculty members; addressed instructional requirements; considered questions of admission standards and evaluation procedures; and provided a detailed list of the curriculum content. The second section addressed the need for a formal process to review and approve university O&M preparation programs. The third section called for a revision in the certification standards. Instead of provisional and permanent certification, the proposal called for a change to baccalaureate and graduate certification, with both requiring periodic and ongoing continuing education and professional development. A final section of the CRC proposal suggested a special certification in the teaching of electronic travel aids. Although there was general support for these proposed changes, the Interest Group decided to take more time and solicit ideas from practitioners. At the 1979 AAWB convention, the Interest Group approved a modified proposal. It consisted of the standards from the previous proposal, along with new sections on competency based instruction and self-study guidelines.

The University Personnel Preparation Standards remained unchanged until after the consolidation of AAWB and AEVH. In 1986 an examination of the AER Division Nine Bylaws suggested structural changes were necessary to monitor and update the review process. The Division in 1988 approved updating the review process. In addition, the competency-based guidelines were updated. Finally, the Division voted to require a biennial program update for each of the previously approved university programs.

Functional Abilities Assessment of Certification Candidates

When formal O&M instruction began, sighted instructors were believed necessary to monitor the student and provide for safety from a distance. Initially the instructor works in close physical proximity to the student who is blind so that he or she can provide frequent instruction and easy feedback as required in the beginning stage of instruction. Later the instructor distances himself or herself to allow for more independence of the student. The instructor is required to evaluate the student's use of basic technique, subtle variations in techniques, changes in posture, gait, and other information communicated through body movements such as changes in level of comfort and anxiety, and student behaviors that correspond with environmental stimuli. To accomplish these goals, each instructor is required to monitor the student effectively from ever-increasing distances while still being able to quickly communicate potential danger if necessary.

The early certification of O&M specialists required that they be university educated; possess corrected vision of 20/20 acuity in each eye, with no field restrictions or evidence of a progressive visual loss; and be in good physical health. Over the years these visual criteria were gradually modified. In 1971 Interest Group IX changed the requirements to 20/40 acuity with a contiguous field of 120 degrees. This change was based on the vision requirements needed for a driver's license. It was believed that if individuals could drive a car with 20/40 vision, this should be suitable for observing students from a distance. In 1977 a Functional Abilities Checklist (FAC) was developed, which also included other functional characteristics deemed necessary to teach O&M. The visual component required evaluation of travelers and the environment under various illuminating conditions by the O&M specialist. The visual requirements included monitoring travelers from distances as great as 375 feet and assessing various travel situations that include scanning and perceiving an environmental configuration of no less than 300 degrees within 3 seconds, and tracking and describing traffic in a lighted intersection during average rush-hour traffic.

Development of the FAA

Following the development of the FAC, a debate developed regarding the appropriateness of requiring certain visual abilities of O&M specialists. In view of the continuing debate, Wiener, Bliven, Bush, Ligammari, & Newton (1992) conducted a study to determine the potential of individuals who were blind and partially sighted to monitor students from distances of up to 25 feet. The results indicated that there was a significant difference between the performance of the totally blind subjects and the sighted subjects. Blind subjects lagged behind their sighted counterparts by up to 4 seconds in their ability to recognize the occurrence of basic behaviors such as stopping, starting, turning, locating drop-offs and step-ups, detecting veering, and identifying contact with obstacles. In addition, significantly more errors were made in accuracy of identification of important travel behaviors. The authors cautioned, however, that blind subjects in the experiments were not prepared to function as mobility instructors and further study should be conducted to determine if such preparation could narrow the gap between sighted and blind subjects. As part of the same study, subjects who simulated acuities of 20/400 were also tested on their ability to monitor travelers. Comparison results between 20/400 and normal vision found no significant difference in monitoring performance between the two conditions. This suggested that a simulated acuity of 20/400 would be sufficient to monitor the variables presented in this study from distances of up to 25 feet.

Between 1988 and 1994, Division Nine labored to evaluate and revise its certification standards to parallel more closely the actual tasks required of O&M specialists. During this time Division Nine developed the Functional Abilities Assessment (FAA) to establish a more functional approach. Toward the completion of the FAA, the passage of the Americans with Disabilities Act (ADA) influenced the philosophy of Division Nine regarding the certification of O&M specialists with disabilities. In the past the certification standards required instructors to navigate stairs and monitor travelers from varying distances, without considering provisions for accommodations that would permit disabled individuals to serve as instructors. The standards, adopted by Division Nine at the 1994 AER conference, required shorter monitoring distances and recognized the need for alternative teaching strategies and accommodations for instructors who have disabilities.

The certification standards required that during the regular university clinical teaching experience, students must demonstrate their ability to monitor the travel behaviors of visually impaired persons for safety. In order to objectively measure monitoring performance with greater validity, a set of quantifiable competencies were established. In the context of successfully completing the requirements of the clinical teaching experience, students must demonstrate their ability to meet the minimum competencies for monitoring safe travel.

The distances required for monitoring were reduced to reflect the actual distances commonly used within the learning environment. A study by Chilens and LaGrow (1986) suggested that monitoring distances of 375 feet were not the norm. Through normative sampling, they found the range of monitoring distances to be from 1 foot to 50 feet, with the average monitoring distances ranging between 5 to 13 feet. These findings were verified through studies conducted by the Division Nine Functional Abilities Committee. In 1994 the new functional abilities assessment standards reflected these findings by establishing the monitoring distances between 6 and 20 feet.

The certification policy now requires that when an otherwise qualified person with a disability is unable to perform the monitoring tasks, the universities must explore the use of alternative strategies, accommodations, and auxiliary aids. Such determinations are to be made on a case-by-case basis and to be mutually agreed upon by the university and the disabled student. Alternative approaches can include adaptive techniques, use of adaptive equipment, and for some tasks, the use of assistants.

After Division Nine approval of the certification standards, the universities were unsure of how to efficiently implement the new standards. This created the need to bring the university personnel together to resolve the ambiguity. In March of 1995 the Division Nine Certification Standards Committee sponsored a conference on reasonable accommodation to explore alternative means by which students with disabilities could be taught to perform the essential job functions of O&M specialists (Wiener, Joffee, & LaGrow, 1995). Registrants included faculty members from each of the universities that prepare O&M specialists. The universities came together with disabled instructors to share ideas and field-test alternative approaches. At the conclusion of the conference it was agreed that a list of possible alternative approaches should be compiled and regularly updated. It was also decided that the standards for certification should be expanded to include all of the essential job functions required for safe and effective practice, and that those standards should also be used to evaluate university curricula. During the summer of 1995 the chairpersons of the Division Nine Certification Standards Committee, University Standards Committee, and Certification Committee came together to modify and expand the certification criteria as suggested and to put them into a format that would be useful to the universities, as well as licensure bodies. The standards document is known as the University Orientation and Mobility Competency Form (UOMC) (Joffee & Wiener, 1995). This document includes both academic and clinical competencies. Within the clinical criteria, the standards describe four monitoring distances that are based upon common practice: close (within arm's reach), intermediate (beyond arm's reach to 13 feet), distant (13 to 20 feet), and remote (beyond 20 feet). The competencies require O&M applicants, during university clinical experiences, to demonstrate proficiencies in monitoring that are specific to each of the distances. When a monitoring distance of more than 20 feet is selected, it is expected that the traveler has reached proficiency and does not require direct observation or intervention. At this distance the O&M specialist may use supplementary strategies for gaining information about student performance. For example, a candidate who is blind may choose to gather information about performance by consulting with an assistant or by asking the traveler questions after the completion of the lesson. At all distances the monitoring standards recognize alternative approaches that will allow disabled instructors to perform the essential job functions. These standards were passed by AER's Division Nine in March 1996.

Development of this policy evolved in a controversial environment. As early as 1981, the policy of requiring vision for admission to the Boston College Peripatology Program resulted in a review by the Office of Civil Rights (OCR). The Washington OCR directed the Boston OCR to examine the issue, "Is vision a necessary qualification to being a Peripathologist?" After a two-and-a-half–day review that included examination of records and meetings with the university administration, faculty members, and students, it was determined that the Boston College policy was not discriminatory. This decision was based upon the need to monitor the environment and the student consistently to ensure safety at an adequate distance without interfering in the interaction of the student with the public and the environment.

In 1983 litigation was initiated (*Shroeder v. AAWB*, and *Shroeder v. the New Mexico Board of Education*) to challenge the AAWB certification standards that required successful completion of a functional abilities test in order to gain certification. The plaintiff had graduated from the San Francisco State University Orientation and Mobility Personnel Preparation Program. The applicant was recommended for certification by his internship supervisors but was unable to demonstrate proficiency in all of the functional tasks required by the certification process in effect at that time. The Board of Directors of AAWB had voted to support the recommendation of Interest Group IX not to certify the applicant. The initiated lawsuit was based upon perceived violations of Section 504 of the Rehabilitation Act and various antitrust laws. The case against AAWB was later dismissed because the organization received no federal financial assistance, which is the requirement to be covered under Section 504. The case against the state of New Mexico continued forward because it had relied upon AAWB certification standards for issuing state certification. While it was hoped that the legal challenge would lead to a court decision that would establish firm legal direction, the litigation was instead dropped in 1987 by the plaintiff.

In another case, a student enrolled in the O&M curriculum at Texas Tech University in 1993 was found to have uncontrolled epileptic seizures that could result in an unreasonable risk of harm to the visually disabled students whom she would be teaching. After being counseled to withdraw over performance issues, she initiated litigation over the matter. In June 1995 (*McClure v. Texas Tech University*) a determination was made by the United States District Court for the Northern District of Texas that the plaintiff was not a qualified individual with a disability within the meaning of the applicable ADA law. It was further stated that "the only reasonable accommodation which would have addressed the safety issues under these circumstances would have required a substantial modification of the curriculum, the provision of assistance of a personal nature, or an undue financial hardship or administrative burden on the University." The court went on to say that neither the Rehabilitation Act nor the ADA requires an accommodation under these circumstances. The results of this decision are in agreement with *Southeastern Community College v. Davis* (1979) in which a deaf student within a nursing curriculum was found not to be a qualified individual with a disability within the meaning of the law. It therefore appears that a fundamental alteration of a university preparation program is not required to accommodate a student with a disability. Accommodations are appropriate only when they do not pose undue financial hardship or administrative burden on the university. It is with this understanding that Division Nine has pursued changes in its certification that provide for certification of persons with disabilities. Each applicant for certification must be able to demonstrate proficiency in essential job functions. The individual may use alternative procedures, auxiliary aids, or assistants, but those changes should not fundamentally alter the curriculum or cause undue hardship.

Controversy continues in regard to what is best (Blasch, 1996). The U.S. Department of Veterans Affairs (VA), in a request for opinion by their general counsel (October 1995), advised that "because of significant safety risks, the Rehabilitation Act of 1973 does not require the VA to hire O&M instructors who are totally blind . . . or to provide clinical training to totally blind students enrolled in affiliated colleges and universities." This advisory opinion, however, stated that the recommendation is based on practices, standards, technologies, and techniques currently utilized or available in the O&M field. The advisory opinion recognized that advocacy groups and professional organizations for people who are blind, such as AER, are studying possible reasonable accommodations that might be both effective and not overly burdensome. The advisory opinion concluded by saying that as such changes or improvements occur or become available, the VA will have to reexamine its programs to determine if reasonable accommodations might enable blind individuals to be hired as O&M professionals.

While the VA is opposed to the preparation and employment of O&M instructors who are visually impaired, the professional organization, AER, and Division Nine remain committed to certification of all individuals who can demonstrate that they can perform the essential functions of the job. The university programs are therefore admitting individuals with disabilities and exploring alternative means to achieve the desired performance outcomes. As this book went to press, individuals with disabilities were enrolled in university personnel preparation programs and several who had graduated have been certified by AER.

Evolution of Professional Certification

The O&M professional certification program was initiated in 1968 when AAWB Interest Group IX adopted procedures and requirements for certification of O&M specialists. In 1979 AAWB Interest Group IX voted to support two levels of certification: Initial Professional and Renewable Professional. The initial certification may be applied for immediately upon graduation from an approved university program. Applicants must submit a university transcript, endorsement of the O&M Code of Ethics, letters of reference, and a letter from the university indicating that the applicant has satisfactorily met the competencies listed in the UOMC form. The UOMC requires that the student meet both academic and clinical competencies (see Appendix B). Evaluation of the student's academic competencies is documented in the UOMC checklist by the university supervisor, and evaluation of the clinical competencies is documented by both a AER O&M-certified clinical field supervisor and the university. Upon expiration of certification, applicants are eligible to apply for renewable professional certification.

Renewable certification follows initial certification and requires renewal every 5 years. Applicants must submit a letter from their supervisor describing their professional performance and verifying the attainment of hours in the provision of O&M direct services, and present evidence of professional growth documented through activity points. The total professional activity points that are required vary by the amount of direct service hours performed over the 5-year period. Those who have taught fewer hours must engage in more professional activities. The professional activities approach is consistent with the standards set by most other professions, thus putting this requirement on par with the renewal activities of other professions such as social workers and occupational therapists. The O&M renewable professional certification becomes inactive when it has been expired for more than 5 years. To acquire certification again, an individual must reapply for Initial Professional Certification. Appendix B contains further information on initial and renewal Professional Certification Requirements.

In 1990 Division Nine recommended that individuals who possess a bachelor's or master's degree in a related field of study can become eligible for O&M certification by completing all O&M core curricula at an approved O&M university preparation program without graduating from that university. Individuals who possess a bachelor's or master's degree in a field not related to vision study can become eligible for O&M certification if they complete all the vision study courses in addition to the core curricula. Since the initiation of the O&M specialist certification in 1969, the progressive improvements within the certification program have demonstrated the growth of the profession itself. As of March 1997, 1,339 O&M specialists held AER O&M certification.

Canadian Certification

There have always been O&M specialists in Canada who graduated from preparation programs in the United States, but in addition there are instructors who received training through in-service preparation at the Canadian National Institute for the Blind (CNIB) and other facilities. Initially in-service training was necessary because resources did not exist within Canada to establish college-level preparation programs in O&M. In the early 1980s a movement developed to establish college preparation programs in Canada that would prepare O&M specialists. In 1985 a Task Force on Canadian O&M certification developed out of the need to establish standards for the certification of Canadian O&M instructors. Its focus was to provide national certification for all O&M training programs and instructors in Canada. The goal of the Task Force was to submit a proposal to Division Nine at the AER International Conference in 1986. Once accepted, the proposal would allow Canadian O&M instructors the opportunity to apply for AER certification. The issue of recognizing CNIB agency training as the equivalent of university personnel preparation was strongly rejected. The Division agreed, however, to the provision of accepting the CNIB applicants for initial certification under a "grandfather" provision for 2 years, which was later extended for 1 more year and extended again in 1995 for another year. Such certifications would be identified as a Canadian AER O&M certification and would be valid only in Canada. The other provision accepted by the Division was "to extend the opportunity to Canadian university-based training programs to seek recognition of their graduates, through the traditional process, with modifications aimed towards the Canadian experience" (Newcomer, 1986). The Division voted to permit Canadian university programs, for an interim 10-year period, to seek program recognition without being required to have a full-time faculty member in O&M. That provision has now expired, and Mohawk College has become the first Canadian personnel preparation program to meet the full AER university guidelines.

ETA Certification

In 1981 Interest Group IX took action on certification for teaching the use of Electronic Travel Aids (ETAs) by adopting a policy that contains ETA certification standards, ETA university curriculum guidelines, and the role of ETA manufacturers in the certification process. To receive ETA certification, an O&M specialist currently holding an O&M professional certification must satisfactorily complete an AER-sanctioned ETA course or workshop, and submit a competency-based checklist completed by the faculty representative or instructor of the ETA program. In 1992 an ad hoc committee began to consider revisions in the ETA certification program to keep pace with technological advancements.

Certification Appeals Process

In 1987 the AER International Board approved a policy by which individuals whose certification application had been denied by the certification committee may appeal that decision. The procedure calls for several levels of appeal. The first requires the certification committee to reconsider the application based on the appeal and additional documentation, and render a decision. Higher levels of appeal can be made to the Certification Review Committee of the Board of Directors of AER, and if necessary to the board itself.

REGULATING THE PROFESSION: A CODE OF ETHICS

Most discussions of the hallmarks of professions mention that activities which guarantee society members of a profession will use their specialized knowledge in a way that will benefit people who must avail themselves of members' services. As certification became more firmly established, O&M specialists realized it was insufficient to establish such a process without some mechanism to assure society that those who have entered the profession with the appropriate preparation also practice it in accord with acceptable and respected principles. In 1972 the O&M Interest Group appointed an ad hoc committee to investigate the feelings of the membership concerning the need for a code of ethics and to pull together some principles that might become a part of it.

Once established, a code can benefit several groups of people (Welsh & Wiener, 1977). Clients would benefit from the existence of an explicit statement of what was considered acceptable practice in O&M. Such a statement could encourage and reinforce the type of service that reflects the worth and dignity of clients and their right to confidentiality, safety, objectivity, participation in the decision making, and the highest quality services available. Administrators and employers would benefit from having a clear indication of what was considered acceptable practice in the profession against which they could evaluate the practice of their employees in O&M. The principles expressed in the code might also stimulate administrators to upgrade their O&M services when necessary.

The code of ethics was potentially beneficial for the O&M specialist. With a consensus statement of what was considered acceptable practice, the O&M specialist could operate in difficult situations with some assurance that their actions would be supported by their peers. Such assurance is particularly necessary today when malpractice is a concern in all professions. A code of ethics would provide a set of criteria against which disputed actions might be judged when claims of malpractice are brought against an O&M specialist. Such principles would protect O&M specialists from having their actions evaluated against criteria formulated by an opposing party in a court of law because of a particular claim. In addition, O&M specialists would have some support when they have to resist pressure from employers to participate in actions that are outside the scope of acceptable practice. This step in the profession's development would promote acceptance of O&M specialists among other disciplines, which in turn can lead to greater and more effective teamwork and collaboration.

With these goals in mind, the code of ethics committee surveyed O&M specialists for their ideas to ensure that whatever developed would represent the thinking of a wide range of members of the profession (Wiener et al., 1973). Those surveyed were asked whether a code of ethics was necessary and to react to a selection of principles culled from the codes of other professions that the committee thought might be applicable. Respondents were asked to suggest other principles that they thought should be considered and relate specific incidents they had experienced or knew about which they felt suggested ambiguous or unethical practice in need of clarification.

The responses suggested very strong support among O&M specialists for the idea of a code of ethics. The committee presented the drafted code at the Interest Group meeting during the 1973 AAWB convention. Various principles and sections were discussed and changes were made in the code, and it was officially adopted at the final meeting. However, the suggested procedures for enforcing the code of ethics and processing reports of unethical practice were not approved. These procedures were referred for further study and discussion. The application for certification was modified to include the new applicant's pledge of support for the code. An ethics committee was established as a standing committee within the Interest Group and assigned to continue to study the possibility of a formal review procedure, encourage an understanding of its principles, and continue to update the code when necessary. Appendix C contains the current Code of Ethics.

Code of Ethics Enforcement Process

A code of ethics is more useful if it has accompanying procedures that guide its application. In 1990 the AER International Board approved the Code of Ethics Enforcement Process. It is expected that the first action to be taken will be a communication between the complaining party and the accused. It is hoped that such a confrontation will result in resolution of the issue. In situations where resolution cannot be achieved, a formal process is available. The process involves a structure with a three-tier hierarchy consisting of (1) a Divisional Ethics Committee, (2) the Division Certification Committee, and (3) the AER Certification Review Committee. A final appeal is possible to the Board of Directors of AER.

RECRUITMENT INTO THE PROFESSION

During the 1979–1980 academic year, approximately 130 to 150 O&M specialists graduated from university programs (Wiener & Uslan, 1986; Uslan, Peck, & Kirchner, 1981). This number had dropped by 50 percent during the 1984–1985 academic year to a low of 74 graduates. Hatlen (1986) conducted a study that compared the number of advertised job openings in the blindness professions with the current university graduates who were available for employment. Advertised positions existed for 144 O&M specialists, while it was estimated that only 80 O&M specialists were available. The mismatch between supply and demand was dramatic.

Based on this precipitous change and a projected growth in the population of persons who are blind in the United States, Wiener and Uslan (1986) identified the potential personnel crisis in O&M. Particularly disturbing was the fact that during the mid-1980s several university programs were discontinued (Uslan, Hill, & Peck, 1989), and existing programs reportedly had trouble attracting applicants. Serious concerns were raised that the university system was unable to attract the students required to meet the nation's need for O&M specialists.

Initiatives to address the O&M personnel crisis were taken during the late 1980s. Under the leadership of the Affiliated Leadership League of and for the Blind (ALL) and AER, a cooperative program was launched to recruit prospective O&M specialists into university bachelor's and master's degree O&M programs.

Wiener and Joffee (1993) conducted a telephone survey of O&M programs in the United States and Canada to determine if recruitment efforts were having an impact. Their results suggest there was an increase in applications to and enrollment in university O&M programs. Fifteen university programs in the United States and one university and one agency training program in Canada were surveyed. It was found that university O&M programs in the United States and Canada were functioning at near full capacity and receiving applications from more students than could be accommodated. Since 1985 there has been a dramatic upswing in the number of individuals entering the field of O&M. Data indicates movement from a low of 74 graduates at the close of the 1984–1985 academic year to an enrollment of 186 in 1990, and there were many more qualified persons who applied to the programs than could be accommodated. It is thought that recruitment measures have had an impact on the enrollment in the university programs. The increase in enrollment may also be due to a general movement back toward service professions.

Many university programs began offering alternative preparation options that were successful in attracting students. Part-time, off-campus, and summer-only options were attracting nontraditional students, and second-career students, and were providing new opportunities for cooperative ventures between agencies, schools, and universities.

In 1989 AER and the National Council of State Agencies for the Blind (NCSAB) jointly surveyed service providers to determine the extent of the need for O&M specialists (Wiener, 1989). Surveys were sent to 450 agencies and schools and resulted in a 70 percent response rate. When asked to what degree the respondents had difficulty filling existing staff vacancies with certified O&M specialists during the past year, 16.5 percent responded with "absolutely impossible to fill," 33.3 percent responded with "great difficulty," 18.5 percent responded with "some difficulty," and 7.4 percent responded with "very easy to fill." When asked what educational qualifications are required for employment, 48.6 percent reported master's degrees, 56.8 percent reported bachelor's degrees, and 2.1 percent reported nonuniversity training.

When asked about the greatest unmet service need, the data indicated that multiply disabled individuals and elderly individuals topped the list with 34 percent and 23.4 percent, respectively. It was also found that 39.5 percent of the students receiving services were multiply disabled. Employers were asked: If compensation level or availability were not issues, what level of preparation would they prefer to see in their O&M staff? The results are given in Table 20.1.

Table 20.1 Desired Levels of Preparation

Master's degree	64.6 percent
Bachelor's degree	15.6 percent
Combination of the above—MA or BA with certification	12.8 percent
Associate's degree	1.6 percent
Nonuniversity training	8 percent

These results are consistent with the survey results by Welsh and Blasch (1974), indicating a preference among administrators to fill O&M positions with university-prepared O&M specialists.

While there is a shortage of O&M specialists, employers still insist on hiring O&M university graduates. University programs can flourish only in an environment which provides financial support for the operation of low-incidence programs that are not supportable from state funding. Each year the Office of Education in the U.S. government reviews grant proposals to support the preparation of O&M specialists. The total amount of money available has grown, but the amount of money available to individual universities continues to wane. The governmental policy has been one of limiting the number of students that can be served by any one university, and instead funding more universities with a lower level of support. While there has been an increase in the absolute level of funding, this increase has not kept pace with inflation. This approach has the effect of lowering the number of graduates accepted into the programs. Most recently the attempt at reducing the federal budget deficit has resulted in level funding for university preparation. Since the universities have the ability to attract sufficient numbers of students, and there continues to be difficulty in filling all the employment positions, it is hoped that increased funding to university personnel preparation programs will be implemented in the future.

Salary Levels for O&M Specialists

In the 1989 AER/NCSAB survey reported earlier (Wiener, 1989), an inquiry about current entry-level salary for new positions in O&M found that the mean salary for bachelor's degree O&M specialists was $19,977, and for master's degree O&M specialists was $22,446, with the highest salaries paid by public schools, followed by state agencies. It is significant to note that 46 percent of the employers who responded to this survey indicated that low salaries are a major factor that has interfered with recruitment efforts for employment. In a more recent salary survey (Wiener, Fauver, & Schwartz, 1995) it was found that in 1993 O&M specialists, within the first 3 years of employment, averaged a salary of $26,750. Although salaries are increasing, they are still significantly less than for comparable specialists such as physical therapists and occupational therapists.

ORIENTATION AND MOBILITY ASSISTANTS

Since the establishment of university personnel preparation in O&M, employers have favored hiring professionally prepared instructors (Welsh & Blasch, 1974; Wiener, 1989). However, there are too few O&M specialists to serve all of those who require consistent repetition to master critical skills (Wiener & Uslan, 1986). Various attempts have been made to train paraprofessionals, but none of these were widely replicated or adopted by the field (Wiener & Welsh, 1980).

In 1986 the Professional Issues Committee of Division Nine gathered information about the preparation and use of O&M assistants (OMAs). A questionnaire was developed and disseminated to over 1,000 members of Division Nine, which contained various questions about the concept of OMAs and the potential role or roles of OMAs in the delivery of O&M services. With a return rate of 40 percent it was found that 70 percent of the respondents supported the idea of OMAs and believed there was a role for such personnel (Wiener & Uslan, 1990). From the questionnaire the Professional Issues Committee developed a position paper (Wiener et al., 1990).

The Model

Early discussions centered on the creation of a viable training model. An in-service "trainer of trainers" model that included comprehensive standards, a strong evaluation component, and a certification program to ensure universal compliance was agreed upon. The trainer of trainers model included: (1) conducting a national workshop to prepare presenters from seven regions of the United States and Canada, (2) using the regional presenters in AER continuing education seminars to teach certified O&M specialists how to prepare and supervise OMAs using a competency-based program of approximately 200 hours of instruction and practice, and (3) establishing a certification program to provide consistent preparation and ensure adherence to AER standards. Violation of the standards by OMAs or their trainer-supervisors could result in disciplinary actions that would ultimately affect their certification. Beginning in the summer of 1991, OMA Seminars were conducted as part of the AER Continuing Education Program. Individuals wishing to become trainer-supervisors of OMAs learned how to train and supervise assistants at these seminars (Wiener & Hill, 1993).

Evaluation of the OMA Program

Between the years of 1990 and 1994, Division Nine prepared more than 130 trainer-supervisors of OMAs. In order to evaluate the effectiveness of the program, questionnaires were sent to all trainer-supervisors, and follow-up telephone calls were made to the 50 individuals who responded (Wiener, Lolli, & Huff, 1994). It was learned from the respondents that the trainer-supervisors had trained only 13 OMAs. The reasons for this low implementation rate were varied. Twenty-five percent reported that they did not have enough time to train the OMA within their regular work day. Thirty-nine percent reported that the role of the OMA was too restricted, 20 percent reported that the cost of in-service training the OMA was too high, and 54 percent reported that their facility did not have the funding necessary to hire an OMA.

Those who prepared OMAs found them to be a valuable asset. Two-thirds of those who had not established programs reported that they support the continuation of the OMA program, but would like to see changes to the program to broaden it and make it easier to access. Suggestions for change are divided among two categories. First, it was suggested that Division Nine expand the roles and responsibilities of the OMA; second, that the structure of the program be changed. It is expected that changes need to occur if the program is to become viable.

SPECIALTY AREAS WITHIN O&M

In the 1960s the success of independent travel experienced by the adult who was blind led to development of positions for university-prepared O&M specialists to work with school-age students. University programs expanded their targeted population to include course work, clinical teaching experience, internships, and student teaching with school-age students who were blind and visually impaired. To foster greater availability of qualified O&M specialists, universities began to offer dual program preparation that enhanced the abilities of itinerant teachers to provide O&M instruction. Later, as the need for early education was documented by the field of special education, emphasis was given to preparing O&M specialists for servicing preschool children with visual impairments. In addition, service providers often point out that people with multiple disabilities, and people who are elderly and blind, require unique expertise.

People with multiple disabilities require specialized O&M strategies such as infusion of instruction within the schedule rather than a pull-out model, shorter but more frequent instructional periods, and consultation with other staff and family on monitoring and reinforcing skills throughout daily travel opportunities. The development and use of adaptive mobility devices has had a positive impact on improved independent movement for persons with multiple disabilities, as well as preschoolers and elderly blind persons. Most university preparation programs include discussions on alternative programming for persons with multiple disabilities and, in addition, others provide opportunities for additional course work and clinical teaching experience.

In 1993, Western Michigan University launched the first federally-funded program specifically to prepare practitioners in O&M who will also receive extended preparation in gerontology. Students in such a sequence learn the skills to evaluate individuals and modify instruction to meet the needs of those who are elderly. Instructors learn how to functionally assess clients, teach modified mobility techniques, work with families and groups, and help elderly individuals access the existing network of aging services.

RESPONSIBILITY FOR PROFESSIONAL GROWTH

Continuing Education

Professionals are required to maintain knowledge of current practices and effective interventions, and continually add to their knowledge base. This can be accomplished through continued education in a number of ways. Professional conferences offer the opportunity to learn of innovative approaches in instruction and service delivery. Such opportunities are offered at the international, national, regional, state, and province levels. Many of these are sponsored by the blindness field and related fields, and are available to the individual O&M specialist. Efforts such as those of the International Mobility Conference (IMC) foster the goal by furthering the level of expertise for O&M specialists through an international exchange of ideas and information.

Upgrading the knowledge and skills of those who have already entered the profession is an ongoing effort. Renewed AER certification in O&M requires members to demonstrate that they have continued to study and learn about their area of expertise. This effort can often be facilitated through a formally structured mechanism of continuing education, with and without credit, that takes the form of seminars, telephone conferences, condensed university courses, workshops, correspondence courses, and participation in documented research.

There is urgent need for professionals to become active in the development and verification of knowledge related to their discipline. Like many professions, the knowledge and skills of O&M have grown largely from the practice experiences of the early practitioners. Although there is an ongoing effort to demonstrate and document the validity of this knowledge and move the profession ahead, more activity in this area is needed. O&M specialists must continue to gather and report information relating to practice through observation and research (see Chapter 24). All practitioners must be active in reading, responding to, and using new information. The profession's development will ultimately be measured by its contributions to a body of literature.

The O&M Archives

In an effort to gather, centralize, and maintain the documents that define and record the history of the profession, the O&M Archives was established at the Maryland School for the Blind in Baltimore. The room donated by the school includes displays and carefully cataloged papers and memorabilia. The Archives opened in June 1988 with the following goals: "to establish a setting where research into our profession's history is possible. Secondly, to create a visual and auditory display that gives visitors an appreciation of the exciting history of our profession—the humor, frustration, satisfaction, and rewards" (Sauerberger, 1988)."

FUTURE DIRECTIONS

Licensure and State Certification

Licensing is the granting by a state governmental agency to allow an individual sole authority to engage in practice in a specific arena. Permission is the basis of licensing, and such permission may be granted, denied, renewed, terminated, suspended, or revoked by the agency. In general, licensing boards control entrance into the occupation, and support and enforce the standards of practice among licensed practitioners. To further assure quality standards, credibility of the profession, public welfare, and gain entrance to third-party reimbursement, members of the O&M profession have explored establishing licensure. Since 1986 O&M specialists have been working toward licensure within some states. Obtaining licensure is not an easy political process. In most states the small numbers of O&M specialists make it difficult to obtain support. State licensure requires the development of a board to oversee the process. This board has to be financially self-supporting by the licensing fee (Hill, Hill, & Lebous, 1994). The limited numbers of O&M specialists in a state make financial self-sufficiency of a board unlikely. In an attempt to overcome this difficulty, some states have considered joining with boards of other professions or forming a board that combines various practitioners within the field of blindness.

Other alternatives to guarantee quality provision of O&M services have been examined. Included among them are state credentials and registries of qualified providers. In 1969 the California State Department of Education established a State Teaching Credential for O&M Instructors as a result of the efforts of the California Association of Orientation and Mobility Specialists (CAOMS). Consideration is being given to development of a state-by-state or province-by-province registry of O&M specialists that would support the standards achieved by the AER O&M certification program. In addition, AER has initiated plans to trademark the term "Certified Orientation and Mobility Specialist" (COMS). This would limit the use of the term to those who are certified by AER.

Third-Party Reimbursement

Some believe that having state licensure or a state credential in O&M would facilitate reimbursement for O&M services to individuals who are blind and visually impaired under private medical or governmental insurance plans. In the United States an effort is being made to have O&M included on the list of services for reimbursement on federal and state health insurance plans. However, O&M specialists need to be actively involved in the political process to change the law to allow reimbursement for services. In defining the O&M provider, a state-by-state effort needs to be made to support the standards now achieved by the AER O&M certification program.

Strengthening Certification

For the reasons stated above it is believed that universal licensure among the states and provinces may not occur in the near future. If the experience of other professions can serve as a guide, many years of hard work are needed to achieve such success. The field of occupational therapy, for example, has taken more than 20 years to achieve licensure in a majority of states. This was accomplished in part because of the large number of practitioners available in each state. The field of O&M, with only a fraction of the numbers, may find large-scale licensure a long-term goal. Licensure boards must be self-sustaining, and with limited numbers comes limited finances to support such an effort. Faced with this dilemma, the profession of O&M must find alternative ways of assuring that quality services are provided to consumers. At present, the strengthening of certification holds the greatest promise of ensuring quality. The future, therefore, should see a concerted effort to improve the certification process and gain further acceptance and credibility for the certification credential. Various other professional disciplines began their certification processes by utilizing their professional associations to be the certifying body. As the professions realized the conflict generated by having the professional association certify its own members, most associations established separate entities to certify their practitioners. Division Nine of AER is currently in a similar situation by virtue of having the professional association certify its own members. Future efforts will therefore have to focus upon establishing a certification program independent of AER. The Certification Review Committee of the Board of AER is currently exploring this option. Another method of strengthening certification is to develop a better means to ensure that practitioners possess the necessary knowledge and skills for effective practice. Currently, such assurance is limited to graduation from an approved university program and evaluation of the candidate's abilities by the university faculty and field supervisors. Other professions such as rehabilitation counseling, occupational therapy, and optometry insist upon an independent examination that evaluates the individual's knowledge base. Continued acceptance of the O&M certification credential will depend upon a similar approach. To further this goal, Division Nine has established an Ad Hoc National Certification Examination Committee and has charged it with the responsibility of developing a multiple-choice examination that will assess the certification applicant's academic knowledge and preparation for practice. Once established, passage of this test will be a necessary requirement before certification is granted.

International University Program Approval

The first steps have been taken to implement international program approval for university O&M preparation programs. At the 1992 AER conference, Division Nine declared that Massey University in Palmerston North, New Zealand, met all of the university guidelines. This permitted graduates of the program to apply for certification from AER. In 1996, AER granted permission for graduates of the Canadian Mohawk College O&M program who completed a baccalaureate degree to also apply for certification. Interest in further review of international programs has come from other countries. The question that remains is whether a universal set of guidelines should be administered, or if differential standards with different levels of certification should be established, based upon the country's comparable preparation level for other professionals. The potential exists for AER, through Division Nine, to have a greater impact upon O&M services worldwide.

Suggestions/Implications for O&M Specialists

1. In the early 1950s the services of orientors were recognized as having a positive impact on the independent travel of individuals who were blind and visually impaired. However, there were a limited number of persons prepared to provide mobility instruction. The model of the Hines Veterans Administration Hospital provided a structure to be replicated within the civilian population. A series of conferences led to the establishment of university preparation programs.
2. In the early 1960s professional associations of O&M specialists evolved so that practitioners could share information and advance the profession.
3. Influenced by the standards generated by the COMSTAC, the professional associations developed standards and a process for certification of O&M specialists.
4. Between the years 1975–1979, the professional association developed standards for personnel preparation and a process to review university O&M preparation programs. In 1988, an ongoing review of such programs was established.
5. Certification standards have become more functionally based, allowing for alternative approaches to perform the required competencies.
6. Certification evolved from a lifetime credential into a renewable process that requires continuing education to maintain knowledge and skills. An appeals process was established to contest decisions of the certification committee.
7. Specialty certifications were developed to assure quality instruction in the use of ETAs and for the training and supervision of orientation and mobility assistants.
8. Recognized professions function under a code of ethics that protects the interest of the student/client and the community. This code is enforced by the profession.
9. Limited organized efforts have been made to establish a recruitment effort on behalf of the profession. The university applications are sufficient to fill the available openings; however, within the service delivery systems, the supply of O&M specialists has not met the demand.
10. In an effort to meet the demand for more available O&M services and increase the amount of instruction provided to students, the profession implemented a program that established guidelines for the use of orientation and mobility assistants.
11. As the needs of persons who are blind changed, the demand for O&M services also changed. This reality impacted the personnel preparation programs and caused them to begin addressing the needs of various groups such as infants, toddlers, youth, multiply impaired individuals, people who are elderly, and those with low vision.
12. Professionals are responsible for maintaining current knowledge of best practice and advancing application of skills in the dynamic field of O&M while respecting its beginning and history.
13. O&M is a dynamic field that is developing within a changing environment. The directions influencing its future are licensure, third-party reimbursement, a stronger certification program which includes a national certification examination, and recognition of innovations in the area of university preparation.

ACTIVITIES FOR REVIEW

1. Recount the early events that led up to the development of the first university personnel preparation programs in O&M.
2. Explain the historical development of Division Nine of AER as the professional association for O&M specialists.
3. Discuss the development of standards in O&M in relation to standards setting at the time.
4. Outline the evolution of certification of O&M specialists from the initial standard of "perfect vision" to the current standard that emphasizes performance of essential functions of the job.
5. Explain the purpose of the Code of Ethics and who are its beneficiaries.
6. Identify and discuss the section of the Code of Ethics that deals with confidentiality.
7. Discuss the process and requirements of renewing certification in O&M.
8. How is the Code of Ethics enforced? What steps must be followed?
9. Explain the historical problems relating to recruitment into the profession and what steps have been taken to assure an adequate supply of practitioners.
10. Discuss the model that has been used to establish the orientation and mobility assistant program. What certifications accompany the model?
11. Discuss the development of specialty areas within O&M.
12. Discuss the possible future directions for the profession of O&M.

APPENDIX

Dates and Events which Influenced The Development of O&M

1860	Sir Francis Campbell experiments with long cane for "foot travel" at Perkins.
1872	*Blindness and the Blind—A Treatise on the Science of Typhology* by W. Hanks Levy.
1918–1925	Dog guides trained for blinded World War I veterans in France and Germany.
1929	Seeing Eye, Inc. founded in Nashville, Tennessee, and the first dog guide school in United States, incorporated.
1930	The first white cane ordinance passed sponsored by Peoria Illinois Lions Club.
1931	Lion's Club International voted to support the passage of white cane laws in every state.
1939–1945	World War II.
1944	*Facial Vision: The Perception of Obstacles by the Blind* by Supa, Cotzin, and Dallenback published.
1944	Hoover and others develop long-cane mobility techniques at Valley Forge Army Hospital. This was the real beginning of what has been called "foot travel." The term "orientation and mobility" was not common until the 1950s.
1945	The Surgeon General's office dispatched an orientor (C. Warren Bledsoe) from Valley Forge Army General Hospital at Phoenixville, Pennsylvania, to Dibble Army General Hospital at Menlo Park,

California, to teach the cane method.

1947 Opening of the Veterans Administration (VA) Hines Rehabilitation Center.

1947 First six O&M specialists selected at Hines VA Hospital—John Malamazian, Stanley Suterko, Alfred Dee Corbett, Edward Thuis, Lawrence Blaha, and Edward Mees.

1948 Russell C. Williams appointed as Chief of Hines Blind Unit.

1952 The film, *The Long Cane,* produced through the VA.

1953 Father Thomas J. Carroll of the Catholic Guild for the Blind in Boston mounts Gloucester Conference to define mobility instructor's role and training.

1954 Through the efforts of Mary E. Switzer, Director of the Office of Vocational Rehabilitation, the Vocational Rehabilitation Act supported demonstration grants in the area of preparation of O&M specialists.

1959 National Conference funded by AFB to establish criteria for the basic selection of mobility personnel, to develop a curriculum, and to recommend length of training and appropriate sponsorship.

1959 Ultrasonic Hand-Held Torch developed by Leslie Kay.

1960 *Instruction in Physical Orientation and Foot Travel, A Lesson Plan Outline,* published by The Industrial Home for the Blind, New York.

1960 Boston College starts first university program for O&M instructors. (Closed in May 1991.)

1961 Western Michigan University, Kalamazoo, second university training program established.

1961 Commission on Standards and Accreditation of Services for the Blind (COMSTAC).

1963 Standards for collapsible cane presented at Mobility Research Conference, MIT.

1964 *Mobility in Perspective* by Martha J. Ball published.

1964 First *Long Cane Newsletter* published, Vol. 1, No. 1, jointly by Boston College and Western Michigan University.

1964 *Specifications for the Long Cane* published by Veterans Administration.

1964 A petition approved by the AAWB Board of Directors for a new interest group devoted to O&M; Rod Kossick appointed as chairperson.

1964 Pathsounder was invented by Lindsay Russell while a consulting engineer with the Sensory Aids Evaluation and Development Center at MIT.

1965 First meeting of Interest Group IX (AAWB), Denver, Colorado.

1965–1966 Loyal E. (Gene) Apple serves as Chairperson of AAWB Interest Group IX.

1966 Ad Hoc Committee Concerned with Mobility Instruction for the Blind met in Washington, DC.

1966 At the AAWB Convention in Pittsburgh, Pennsylvania, Interest Group IX formed a committee to study the certification of O&M instructors.

1966 Mobility Group of AAIB established, Salt Lake City, Utah. Donald Blasch, first chairperson.

1966 California State University at Los Angeles training program in O&M was funded by VRA.

1966 Laser Cane was developed and manufactured by J. Malvern Benjamin and his colleagues at Bionic Instruments, Inc.

1966 Binaural Sensory Aid (forerunner to Sonicguide) developed by Leslie Kay at the University of Canterbury, New Zealand.

1966 First Interest Group newsletter published.

1966 California Association of O&M Specialists (CAOMS) established, designated as a "professional association" instead of a more general "mobility interest group." Active membership limited to O&M specialists; associate membership available.

1966 *COMSTAC Report* published.

1966 Florida State University established first undergraduate O&M training program.

1966 San Francisco State University established first graduate-level programs to prepare mobility instructors of children. Grant funded by U.S. Office of Education.

1966–1967 Fredick A. Silver serves as chairperson of AAWB Interest Group IX.

1967 Establishment of Midlands Mobility Center in England by Stanley Suterko.

1967–1968 John Malamazian serves as chairperson of AAWB Interest Group IX.

1967 After the AAWB Convention in Florida, Interest Group IX appointed an accreditation committee, later named Certification Standards Committee.

1968 AAIB became the Association for Education of the Visually Handicapped (AEVH).

1968 Gary Coker serves as chairperson of AEVH Mobility Interest Group.

1968–1969 Stanley Suterko serves as chairperson of AAWB Interest Group IX.

1968 Lawrence E. Blaha Award established in Division Nine of AAWB—Lawrence E. Blaha first recipient, Toronto, Canada.

1968 Interest Group IX adopted procedures and requirements for certification of O&M specialists; request sent to AAWB Board of Directors for approval.

1968 AAWB Board of Directors approved the certification procedures and requirements with the stipulation that the AAWB bylaws would need changing before certification can become a reality.

1968 *Demonstration of Home and Community Support Needed to Facilitate Mobility Instruction for Blind Youth* by Francis E. Lord and Lawrence E. Blaha published.

1969 Rotterdam Mobility Research Conference.

1969 California State Department of Education established a State Teaching Credential for Orientation and Mobility Instructors as a result of the efforts of the California Association of Orientation and Mobility Specialists. This is a definite step in the direction of

	high mobility standards in California public schools systems.
1969	AAWB appoints a committee representing various interests and geographical areas to implement the certification of O&M instructors.
1969	The AAWB Certification Committee met for the first time for the sole purpose of implementing the Certification Procedures as adopted by the membership at the 1968 convention, and approved by the AAWB Board of Directors.
1969	U.S. Office of Education funded two programs at the University of Pittsburgh and the University of Northern Colorado (dual certification).
1969	Model O&M Project for institutionalized mentally retarded blind—Boston College and Walter Fernald State School, Paul McDade.
1969	Model O&M Itinerant Project, Alameda County Public Schools, Haywood, California.
1969	First O&M certifications approved (56 for permanent certification and 40 for provisional certification), AAWB National Convention, Chicago, Illinois.
1969	Dr. Richard Hoover receives Blaha Award, Chicago.
1969–1971	Robert Mills serves as cochairperson of AEVH Mobility Group.
1969–1971	Robert H. Whitstock serves as chairperson of AAWB Interest Group IX.
1969	University of Pittsburgh O&M program begins. Funded by the U.S. Office of Education.
1970	Mobility conference held at Florida State University primarily for university personnel preparing O&M instructors at the university level. Universities represented: Boston College, California State College at Los Angeles, Florida State University, San Francisco State College, University of Pittsburgh, and Western Michigan University.
1970	*The First 15 Years at Hines* by John Malamazian published.
1970	New York State Association of Orientation and Mobility Specialists (NYSAOMS) established.
1970	San Francisco Low Vision Mobility Conference.
1971	*Distance Vision and Perceptual Training: A Concept for Use in the Mobility Training of Low Vision Clients,* by Loyal Apple and Marianne May published.
1971	*Low Vision Abstracts* begins publication.
1971	First Binaural Sensory Aids course taught in United States at Boston College and Western Michigan University.
1971	Vision requirements for O&M certification change from 20/20 and normal field to 20/40 acuity and field of 140 degrees.
1971	O&M certification "grandfather" clause expired.
1971	Undergraduate applicants for O&M certification defined.
1971	Interest Group IX to investigate the question of "Mobility Aides."
1971	First Regional Midwest O&M Non-Conference (NCOMA), Jacksonville, Illinois.

1971–1973	Robert Crouse serves as chairperson of AAWB Interest Group IX.
1971	G. William Debetaz received Blaha Award, Richmond, Virginia. First presentation of the Sir Francis Campbell cane.
1972	First Southeastern Orientation and Mobility Association (SOMA) Conference, Daytona Bleach, Florida.
1972	Pennsylvania Association of Orientation and Mobility Specialists (PAOMS) established.
1972	Stephen F. Austin University, Cleveland State University, and Talladega State College begin O&M programs (all undergraduate).
1973	*How Does A Blind Person Get Around?* published by AFB.
1973	O&M Paraprofessional Training Program funded by Virginia Commission for the Blind and RSA, directed by Robert Scheffe.
1973	O&M Code of Ethics adopted by AAWB Interest Group IX.
1973	Introduction of the Code of Ethics Enforcement Procedures, which was not accepted by Interest Group IX membership.
1973	Report of the Ad Hoc Committee on Mobility Aides presented to Interest Group IX.
1973	Stanley Suterko received Blaha Award, Cleveland, Ohio.
1973–1975	Bruce Blasch (elected), Frank Ryan (served) chairperson of AAWB Interest Group IX.
1974	Robert O. LaDuke serves as chairperson of AEVH Mobility Group.
1974	First comprehensive 6-week postgraduate courses in ETAs offered in United States at Western Michigan University.
1975	First questionnaire sent to Interest Group IX members on the role of paraprofessionals in the field of O&M.
1975	Low Vision Mobility Workshop at Western Michigan University.
1975	Hunter College, New York and University of Arkansas, Little Rock, begin O&M programs (terminated in 1982).
1975	AFB Conference on Travel in Adverse Weather, Minneapolis, Minnesota.
1975	Certification Committee of Interest Group IX includes representative from AEVH.
1975	Russell C. Williams received Blaha Award, Atlanta, Georgia.
1975–1977	William (Bill) Wiener chairperson of AAWB Interest Group IX.
1975	Establishment of the Interest Group IX Code of Ethics Committee.
1976–1978	David Loux serves as chairperson of AEVH Mobility Group.
1976	*Orientation and Mobility Techniques: A Guide for the Practitioner* by E. Hill and P. Ponder published by AFB.
1976	*Travel in Adverse Weather Conditions* by R. Welsh and W. Wiener published by AFB.
1977	Mowat Sensor developed by Geoff Mowat.
1977	A second O&M techniques book published, Center for Independent Living.

1977	Donald Blasch received Blaha Award, Portland, Oregon.
1977–1979	Robert Mills serves as chairperson of AAWB Interest Group IX.
1978–1980	Bob Bryant serves as chairperson of AEVH Mobility Group.
1978	Illinois O&M Association established.
1978	RSA funds university O&M programs for all disabilities ("Generic O&M") at University of Wisconsin, Madison (funding discontinued in 1983).
1979	First International Mobility Conference (IMC-1), Frankfurt, West Germany.
1979	ETA Certification for O&M specialist first considered.
1979	Vision requirements for O&M certification change from measured acuity/fields to functional vision requirements.
1979	Interest Group IX self-study and on-site review process of university O&M programs begins.
1979	Northern Illinois O&M program begins.
1979	Recognition of Talladego College O&M program by Interest Group IX (removed in 1990).
1979	Interest Group IX votes to support changes in certification requirements to provisional and professional; profession certification must be renewed every 5 years with documentation of professional activities.
1979	John D. Malamazian received Blaha Award, Oklahoma City, Oklahoma.
1979–1981	Kent Wardell serves as chairperson of AAWB Interest Group IX.
1979	Historian/Archivist, Berdell (Pete) Wurzburger, appointed by Interest Group IX chairperson.
1979	AAWB appoints a Board Committee to review certification documents presented for Board approval. Committee referred to as Certification Standards Committee, later named Certification Review Committee.
1979	Association of University Educators in O&M and Rehabilitation Training established.
1980–1982	Andrew S. Papineau serves as Beal Pickett cochairperson of AEVH Mobility Group.
1980	*Foundations of Orientation & Mobility* edited by R. Welsh and B. Blasch published by AFB.
1980	Recognition of University of Wisconsin O&M program by Interest Group IX. (removed in 1990).
1980	Recognition of Peabody College of Vanderbilt University O&M program by Interest Group IX (removed in 1995).
1981	Second International Mobility Conference (IMC-2), Paris, France.
1981	AFB (National O&M Consultant, Mark Uslan) takes over publication of *Long Cane News.*
1981	Formation of the Alliance, which served as a vehicle for the consolidation of AAWB and AEVH.
1981	Interest Group IX votes to support the requirements for ETA certification.
1981	John Eichorn received Blaha Award, Toronto.
1981–1982	James Liska serves as chairperson of AAWB Interest Group IX.

1982	Toni Heinze serves as chairperson of AEVH Mobility Group.
1982–1983	Gala Saber-Brooks serves as chairperson of AAWB Interest Group IX, Orlando.
1982	ETA Certification Standards approved by AAWB Board of Directors.
1982	Leadership Program (Doctoral Level) at Peabody starts.
1983	Lee Farmer receives Blaha Award, Phoenix, Arizona.
1983–1984	Stephen Sanford (AAWB) and Berdell Wurzburger (AEVH) cochairpersons of Division Nine.
1983	AFB funds National O&M Competency Study.
1983	Third International Mobility Conference (IMC-3), Vienna, Austria.
1983	Western Michigan University granted funds to look at professionals' attitudes toward the formation of a professional organization.
1983	Dominican College undergraduate O&M program begins (removed in 1988).
1983	Orientation and Mobility Association of Oregon (OMAO) established.
1983	Research and Demonstration Project (A. Bradfield)—Distance Vision Curriculum for O&M Instructors funded.
1983	NIHR Research and Demonstration Project, Pennsylvania College of Optometry/Peabody College—O&M for Low Vision Individuals funded.
1984	Geneseo (New York) O&M Program begins (lost funding in 1986).
1984	Peabody Preschool O&M Project (HCEEP Model Demonstration Project) is funded.
1984	AAWB and AEVH consolidate to become the Association for Education and Rehabilitation of the Blind and Visually Impaired (AER).
1984	Warren Bledsoe received Blaha Award, Nashville.
1984–1986	Patricia Coffey Bucci (elected, served 1984–1985); Jim Newcomer (served 1985–1986) chairperson of AER Division Nine.
1986	Recognition of Texas Tech University O&M program by Division Nine.
1986	Fourth International Mobility Conference (IMC-4), Jerusalem, Israel.
1986	*Electronic Travel Aids: New Directions for Research* published by National Research Council, Committee on Vision, Working Groups on Mobility Aids.
1986	Peggy Madera and Judy Davidhizer-Homes receive the First Citation for Excellence Award for outstanding O&M direct services presented by Division Nine, Chicago.
1986	Approved, revised Bylaws for Division Nine establishes seven Regional Directors and a Professional Issues Committee.
1986	Walter G. Olenek received Blaha Award, Chicago.
1986	"Provisional" O&M certification changed to "Initial Professional."
1986	Centralized processing through AER central office of O&M certification applications.

1986	Initiation of the "biannual review" of existing university preparation programs.
1986–1988	Jim Newcomer serves as chairperson of AER Division Nine.
1987	AFB sponsors The Visually Impaired Traveler in Mass Transit: Issues in O&M Conference, Washington, DC.
1987	Certification Appeals Process approved by the AER International Board.
1987	M. Kronick provides early discussion of alternative mobility devices (AMD) in *The "Wheel" Cane*, published in *Journal of Visual Impairment & Blindness.*
1988	The O&M Archives officially opened, Maryland School for the Blind, Baltimore, Maryland.
1988	"Mobility Assistant" Division Nine position paper supported by majority via the first mail ballot.
1988	Richard Welsh received Blaha Award, Montreal, Canada.
1988	Joan Levy received the Citation for Excellence Award, Montreal.
1988–1990	E. (Butch) Hill serves as chairperson of AER Division Nine.
1989	Fifth International Mobility Conference (IMC-5), Veldhoven, The Netherlands.
1989	*The Profession of Orientation and Mobility in the 1980s* by M. Uslan, E. Hill, and A. Peck, published by AFB.
1989	Sonic Pathfinder evolved out of the work of Tony Heyes at the Blind Mobility Research Unit at Nottingham University, England.
1990	Recognition of Northern Illinois University O&M program by Division Nine.
1990	*Preschool Orientation and Mobility Screening* by B. Dodson-Burk and E. Hill published by Division Nine.
1990	Hugo Vigorosa receives Blaha Award, Washington, DC.
1990	Judy Hayes receives the Citation for Excellence Award, Washington, DC.
1990	Approval of the revision of Division Nine Bylaws establishing the University Review, Research and Publication Review, International, Code of Ethics, Archives, and Continuing Education as standing committees. Election of officers will be by mail ballot.
1990	Position paper on "University Trained Mobility Specialists."
1990	Division Nine recommended that individuals who possess a bachelor's or master's degree in a related field of study can become eligible for AER O&M certification by completing all O&M core curricula at the same AER-approved O&M university preparation program. Requirements for individuals who possess a bachelor's or master's degree in a field not related to vision study were also approved. (Approved by the AER Board of Directors in 1992.)
1990–1992	Bruce Blasch serves as chairperson of AER Division Nine.
1990	Code of Ethics Enforcement Process approved by the AER International Board.

1990 *Access to Mass Transit,* edited by M. Uslan, A. Peck, W. Wiener, & A. Stern, published by AFB.

1991 Recognition of University of Texas at Austin O&M program by Division Nine.

1991 Regional Trainers Workshop of Orientation and Mobility Assistants at Western Michigan University.

1991 AER Board approved certification programs for Trainer/Supervisors of OMAs and Orientation and Mobility Assistants.

1991 Recognition of Massey University in New Zealand O&M program by Division Nine. First international O&M program recognized by AER.

1991 Sixth International Mobility Conference (IMC-6), Madrid, Spain

1992 Development of a computer model of cane techniques (RoboCane®) by Bruce B. Blasch and William De l'Aune.

1992 Recognition of Michigan State University O&M program by Division Nine.

1992 Recognition of Pennsylvania College of Optometry (PCO) O&M program by Division Nine.

1992 Division Nine recommends a revision to the professional activity requirement for AER certification renewal. This revision is comparable with other professional certification renewal activities.

1992 Butch Hill receives Blaha Award, Los Angeles, California.

1992 Darick Wright and Bonnie Dodson-Burk receive Citation of Excellence Award, Los Angeles.

1992 Establishment of the Newcomer-Hill Service Award. This award is to be presented at each international AER Conference by the Chair of Division Nine to recognize major contributions made to Division Nine during the previous 2 years. First recipient Susan S. Simmons, Los Angeles.

1992–1994 William Jacobson serves as chairperson of AER Division Nine.

1992 Recognition of University of Arizona O&M program by Division Nine.

1992 Central-Eastern O&M Association (COMA) first meeting.

1993 AER Board of Directors votes to remove the requirement of a physical examination or a completed physician's statement from O&M renewable professional certification.

1994 Seventh International Mobility Conference (IMC-7), Melbourne, Australia.

1994 Berdell H. "Pete" Wurzburger receives Blaha Award, Dallas, Texas.

1994 Colleen Calhoon and Carol Otten receive Citation for Excellence Award, Dallas.

1994 Sandy Kronick Distinguished Service Award received posthumously, Dallas.

1994 Dona Sauerburger receives the Newcomer-Hill Service Award, Dallas.

1994–1996 Dennis Lolli chairperson of AER Division Nine.

1996 Eighth International Mobility Conference (IMC-8), Trondheim, Norway.

1996 International Mobility Conference establishes the Suteiko-Cory Award.

1996 The Professional Standard for the Practice of O&M and the University Orientation and Mobility Competency Form approved by AER Division Nine.

1996 William Wiener receives Blaha Award, St. Louis, Missouri.

1996 Sharon O'Mara Maida receives Citation of Excellence Award, St. Louis.

1996 Kathleen Newman receives Sandy Kronick Distinguished Service Award, St. Louis.

1996 William Wiener and Elga Joffee receive Newcomer-Hill Service Award, St. Louis.

1996–1998 Eileen Siffermann serves as chairperson of AER Division Nine.

1996 Mohawk College, Ontario, Canada, recognized as an approved O&M program.

1996 Appointment of an ad hoc AER Division Nine committee to develop a national certification examination in O&M.

1997 Second edition of *Foundations of Orientation and Mobility,* edited by B. Blasch, W. Wiener, and R. Welsh, published by AFB Press.

1998 Ninth International Mobility Conference (IMC-9), Atlanta.

The authors wish to acknowledge the contribution of Everett Hill to the development of this chronology.

CHAPTER 21

Originators of Orientation and Mobility Training*

C. Warren Bledsoe

> Only the personal is great.
>
> —Disraeli

During the Christmas holidays of 1786 the children from Valentin Hauy's infant school for the blind in Paris were entertained for eight days at the palace of Versailles by King Louis XVI and Queen Marie Antoinette (Ross, 1951). They played with the royal children and gave demonstrations of what they had learned to astonished royal adults. This included complicated arithmetical calculations done in the head without benefit of tactile aids to thought or memory. The exactitude of results learned were vouched for by the pen and ink calculations of the Duc D'Angouleme, of whom we have the word of his learned uncle Louis XVIII that he was a sharp-witted youth before the Revolution drove him into exile and idleness (Daudet, 1913).

PROLOGUE

This is the first we know of one of the more spectacular skills which was to become the stock in trade of educators of the blind down through the 19th century, eventually termed "rapid arithmetic" in curricula of schools for the blind. Classical education of the blind in those decades included a number of highly developed special arts and techniques, such as touch reading and writing, tumbling, chair caning, and piano playing and tuning, but general competence in living without sight was left to the ingenuity of blind people themselves. This included those functions to which are directed the teaching skill which is termed "orientation and mobility" and was termed during its crude and early beginnings, simple "foot travel."

Formal orientation and mobility training of blind people was first attempted on an organized basis in the United States by the founders of the dog guide school known as Seeing Eye, Inc. (see Chapter 8). At that time the teaching of skills for living without sight had been in progress in this country for a century, guided originally by Dr. Samuel Gridley Howe, founder of the Perkins School for the Blind in 1832, whose broad-gauged genius permeated virtually every aspect of social progress from that year until his death in 1876. Howe's nearest approach to anything resembling

*A historical memoir of personal influences in the founding of orientation and mobility, in the writing of which the author has been greatly aided by reading *The Unseen Minority* by Frances A. Koestler. The historian who was there can have no better collaborator than the historian who was not.

The text of this chapter is reprinted from R. L. Welsh and B. B. Blasch, editors, *Foundations of Orientation and Mobility* (New York: American Foundation for the Blind, 1980), p. 581–624.

structured teaching of mobility was directed by one of his blind teachers during the 1860s. The teacher was Francis Campbell, who later was to emigrate to Britain and become the founder of the Royal Normal College and Academy of Music for the Blind in that kingdom, where he was naturalized and knighted in 1909 for his work as an educator of blind children and youth.

Commenting on what he termed "bodily training" at the Perkins School, Howe said it had been carried through with "more or less rigor" as he had been "seconded by assistants who had more or less faith in it" (Howe, 1872). Thus, with his habitual astuteness he stated a principle which subsequently governed everyone who has had success in the teaching of orientation and mobility in this century. Such teachers have found that people have abounded and still abound who are without such faith. Howe went on to reinforce his statement by mentioning Campbell's "system of physical training . . . carried to a high perfection." This was, he said, a form of training which could only be maintained persistently by those who possessed great natural pluck and personal magnetism. He mentioned rowing and swimming and floor scrubbing. But he said nothing which implied, even indirectly, that orientation and mobility were taught as part of a curriculum and stated with unaccustomed resignation that in the absence of such an individual as Campbell, the exercises he had mentioned "fall into comparative neglect." In this also he noted a principle all too familiar to experienced workers for the blind. To promote true self-management of blind people involves a never-ending effort. And this is not against inertia alone, for inertia in institutions can keep a thing going once it has gotten started whether it makes any sense or not. The effort combats something far more subtle and complex, a number of sensitivities which not only were to be revealed by the mobility teaching programs, but by resistance to those programs.

On this whole subject uninitiated members of society are often vocal in behalf of "a totally blind man I know who never had any lessons and does beautifully." And so indeed individuals have done down through the ages. The most noted of these was an Englishman named John Metcalf, who in the 18th century was a road builder and performed authenticated feats of getting about by himself on foot and on horseback, once guiding a sighted individual through a bog in dark of night. His doings were regarded by his contemporaries and by succeeding generations as little short of marvelous. To the present they are less so, for an old print shows he had a cane so long it was almost up to his hat. This instrument foreshadowed the principle on which one type of formal instruction was to be built when it finally arrived (Mannix, 1911/1976).

BENIGN SURREPTITIOUSNESS

That the long cane was not used earlier was perhaps due in part to what might be termed benign surreptitiousness, its rule being: In order to minimize the impact of blindness on others, do nothing that will make it clear to all that you are blind. This rule may also account for there having been no formal teaching. Those who claim that teachers of the blind have "always" taught orientation and mobility frequently end their protests by saying in effect that they thought at all costs it should be done unobtrusively, indeed in such a manner that the pupil hardly knew he was being taught. Few teachers now talk about such things, but Dr. Edward Allen, Director of the Perkins School (1907–1931), delivered a yearly lecture on what he termed "unconscious tuition" to the graduate students in the Harvard-Perkins course in special methods of teaching the blind.

One can hardly doubt that Campbell (who was extremely mobile himself with a moderately long cane) somehow taught his pupils mobility. His daughter-in-law, Mary Dranga Campbell, hearing an account of the orientation and mobility program of World War II, stated that it "resembled the work of my husband's father, Sir Francis Campbell." A journalist of the period, writing of Campbell's "faithful cane," said it "had brains, could almost talk, and ought to vote" (Willard, 1889).

That he was experimenting in the area of mobility during his Perkins days is revealed in an account of an inglorious mishap for which he was responsible. One of his detractors, Dennis Reardon, wrote of a rope procession which Campbell devised to enable students to go to the beach near the old Perkins School at South Boston. The rope was a long clothesline tied to a lot of broom handles some feet apart. One or two seeing leaders went first, 20 or more blind pupils holding onto handles and following.

The account goes on to say, "Well, one day the teacher who could see partially fell over a bank and brought all the others on top of him. Thereupon they all cast the whole contrivance into the water and left it there. The boys did it. It was he (Campbell) who put it in and we put it out" (Reardon, 1911).

Very much later at least one sophisticated orientation lesson was given by Campbell to a sighted individual. In the *Sunday School Chronicle* of July 8,1909, he is quoted as saying:

> The Duke of Westminster came to see the grounds [of the Royal Normal College] when I first planned them, and he told me that, instead of laying out a pleasure ground for my blind students, I had arranged so many death traps for them. But I blindfolded his lordship, and he found his way by signs all around the grounds and back to the house, and he left me a check for a thousand guineas as an expression of his delight at the provision which I had made for my students. ("An apostle," 1909.)

We may assume that Campbell carefully described the "signs" (present day mobility instructors would say landmarks) and that the Duke who was no ordinary duke, was a good listener. Certainly this was the best paid orientation and mobility lesson in history in the days when not only was a guinea five dollars and a quarter, but a dollar was a dollar.

EARLY TEACHERS

It may be assumed that other teachers, especially those who were blind, did something in the way of teaching their pupils "signs." Parents also were sometimes adroit in this regard. The noted Italian blind educator of the blind, Augusto Romagnoli, wrote of his father:

> He had no training, but at the same time he had not the prejudices of the professional teachers who often make mountains out of molehills. He loved me and made me share his own life. In the workshop I knew how to use the saw, the plane, and the compasses; anything that could not be touched he described to me in a few words. In the country, he taught me to walk beside him and to recognize by ear the proximity of a wall, a hedge, a tree or a ditch. He taught me to swim in the river when we bathed together. If there was a square to be crossed in a hurry, he made me cross it diagonally, explaining that the diagonal is the shortest way. (Romagnoli, 1931)

Definitely American teachers in the early 1900s cannot be said to have "made mountains out of molehills" where mobility was concerned. Indeed they did just the opposite. In 1910 Dr. Edward E. Allen, successor to Howe's successor at the Perkins School, made a survey visit to schools for the blind in Europe. Of German teachers of the blind he wrote:

> . . . the German's 'thoroughness or nothing' principle appeared to me to fill and run over. . . . The possession by the blind of the faculty for recognizing objects by the four senses, and the ability to locate themselves at any and at all times in space and to get about readily alone, is deemed by the Germans a too vitally important one to be left to haphazard. We leave our pupils to pick up this sort of thing, and they generally seem to do so. (Allen, 1969.)

Dr. Allen each year told his Harvard class that, "the care of the blind from the cradle to the grave," a concept he disapproved, was first said in

German. It is significant that in what is the first reference to formal teaching of orientation and mobility in the old Outlook for the Blind he was so politely skeptical of a pioneer program of that type. He seems to have transposed Howe's "comparative neglect" to "constructive neglect." For no mobility program was established at Perkins during the ensuing two decades of Allen's administration. And as Perkins went, so went most other schools for the blind in those days.

During the past 43 years, and particularly the last 25, which have been a time of intensive work to develop training programs in orientation and mobility, there has been recurrent speculation about why such action was not taken before.

In this speculation sometimes the obvious is overlooked. For example, the controlled environment of residential schools and other agencies for the blind gave their educators a false sense of achievement. The controlled environment often extended beyond the immediate property of the school or agency to neighborhoods beyond. Trolley cars stopped at spots convenient for the blind pupils. Housewives were careful to keep trash cans and tricycles off sidewalks in adjacent streets. Gradually the institution extended its domain to the community about it, shaping the neighbors' ways to its needs. True, a little beyond that everything was quite different, but very often even the pupil—indeed especially the pupil—was deceived until he went to college or sought a job in an unfamiliar environment. Another factor frequently overlooked is the simple truth that traffic hazards of the days before yesterday were in no way comparable to those of late 20th century America. Vehicles were noisier; sound patterns less sophisticated.

Not so obvious an impediment to the development of mobility training was shyness on the part of sighted individuals at invading the unique preserves of blind people over the barrier, "You'll never know what it is to be blind." This was abetted by doubt on the part of blind people that by looking there could be any important observation about what was truly efficient for a blind person. Yet the techniques which depend on the cane when they finally arrived undoubtedly came from visual perception by Dr. Richard E. Hoover. In the 1800s W. Hanks Levy, the noted blind British authority on blindness, seems to have evolved something close to the Hoover methods, yet missed what was to be the most important item of all, that the cane should always touch in front of the trailing foot, rather than the forward foot (Levy, 1872/1949). An observation after World War II of 337 veterans of blindness as well as war, revealed that only three had arrived at a realization that at least in dangerous places some such usage was prudent.

It would be false, however, to paint too bleak a picture of the blind of earlier decades. Very often indeed they got there on their own, sometimes with real skill, sometimes by the stumble and crash method, sometimes abetted by a little vision, frequently by the guidance of a sighted individual's elbow. Newell Perry, the noted California blind educator, managed to go all over the United States and Europe without regular guide or courier. Lord Kenswood, a visitor from Britain during the 1940s, mastered the use of public transportation in New York.

Late one night he alighted on an elevated platform at two in the morning and found himself totally alone.

> "Ah," he said to himself, "I am on a high place. I must be careful." I prodded with my cane and felt something soft and pliable. Then it spoke, saying, "I am blind drunk,' I said, 'I am blind, but I am not drunk. Let us help each other."

And they did.

Anecdotes such as that of Lord Kenswood on the elevated platform could be multiplied, for the good grace, capability, and humor of blind people of every age has been, and continues to be a far more reliable resource than is generally realized.

MRS. EUSTIS AND DR. HOOVER

Perhaps it is not too poetic or superstitious to say that the blind people of the United States were awaiting the arrival upon the scene of two people equal to their needs: Dorothy Harrison Eustis, the mother of the dog guide movement, and Dr. Richard E. Hoover, the father of orientation and mobility with the cane.

Quite different individuals, they never met, although Mrs. Eustis's years in work for the blind overlapped those of Dr. Hoover. She was born in 1886 and died in 1946 two years after Hoover began his training in cane technique at Valley Forge Army General Hospital. At that juncture it is unlikely that they would have communicated very effectively, for in the beginning the dog and cane people saw little need for one another, as is not the case today. One trait particularly may be noted in both, where blind people are concerned. This is irritation with workers for the blind who want to keep blind people in a prolonged state of gratitude for their rehabilitation. The work of both Mrs. Eustis and Dr. Hoover forever showed a keen desire to remove a lingering feeling of dependency after the cause of the dependency had become a thing of the past. Their greatest satisfaction was to encounter a blind individual using the methods they had devised. But it is unlikely that either was ever tempted to waylay a blind person and introduce him or herself as the inventor of the resource from which the blind person was benefiting. The inward sensitivity and respect for others which this betokens is as real as a cane or a dog. It was part of the "open sesame" which made it possible to develop acceptance of both dog and cane, and the professional descendants of Mrs. Eustis and Dr. Hoover have succeeded or failed in part because they have shared this sensitivity. But there was an equally important tangible factor in each case. The most important consideration with respect to any invention is that of work: work in the sense of performing, if it is a pump, pump, if it is a light, light, and work in the sense of serving the purpose for which it was designed, pump enough water for the family or town, put enough light in the lighthouse to warn a ship off the reef. Hoover had always thought a key factor in getting his technique accepted was 300 enormously durable, 6-oz (168 g) canes of thin-walled steel, which toward the end of the war was given an A-1 priority in a steel factory by request of the Surgeon General of the Army.

As well as being practical, Mrs. Eustis and Dr. Hoover were also daring. They took chances which other people cursed, sometimes under their breath, sometimes more loudly, but the curses neither dismayed them nor stopped them. A group of workers for the blind whom Mrs. Eustis had called together to advise her with regard to the inauguration of dog guide training began to argue among themselves vociferously, yet more vociferously, and yet more vociferously. From the edge of the group she and her associates simply detached themselves and went into the hall (it has been said on tiptoe—but that does not sound like Mrs. Eustis), where they agreed that whereas they would be accountable for the success or failure of the venture, they would do it their way. Whereupon they departed from the scene and for many years had little or no association with workers for the blind.

Late in Mrs. Eustis's life an episode which highlighted her point of view and independence occurred when she was offered one of the distinguished service awards in the field of work for the blind. She quite seriously proposed that it be given instead to the dog guides of Seeing Eye, and quite seriously was incensed when this proposal was coldly declined. Of an equally independent temperament, Dr. Hoover as a sergeant in the Medical Corps was asked if it would be beneath the dignity of his mobility instructors to clean the wards. He replied, "Aside from that, Colonel, they wouldn't have time to teach the blinded soldiers how to get around." The colonel accepted what he said and promoted him. When horseback riding was initiated in the War Blind Program another colonel opined that of course it would be necessary to keep the horses at a walk.

"No sir," said Sgt. Hoover, "we're going to start with men who have already ridden and canter the first day."

"But they're blind now," expostulated the Colonel. "You don't ride with your eyes," said Sgt. Hoover, "you ride with your legs."

"You don't have to tell me," said the Colonel heatedly, "I foxhunt."

And the blind men cantered the first day.

Mrs. Eustis was a woman with an electric nature at the interesting age of 43 when she established Seeing Eye, Inc. in 1929 . . . a divorcee who was in command of the respectful devotion of four adherents, each a strong character in his own right. It would be hard to say which of these was the key figure, but certainly her first blind pupil was indispensable. He was Morris Frank, a Hotspur of a young man. The second key figure was the man who was eventually called "Uncle Willie" by Seeing Eye graduates. Willie Ebeling was a retired business man and dog fancier who was a perfect dynamo for channeling the electric personalities with whom he was associated. His personal advice to other sighted workers for the blind frequently included, "Don't try to be a big shot, and don't crystallize resistance." The third of Mrs. Harrison's associates was a geneticist named Jack Humphrey, who had such a way with animals that he was said to have taught a camel to back up (supposedly impossible) and to have housebroken a horse (thought to have been unlikely).

Arriving on the scene a little later was William Debetaz, a young man from a French canton of Switzerland. A man of abounding energy and native intelligence, he was to become a past master at the art of teaching both dogs and people. Somewhat later arrivals (1934) were Mary Dranga Campbell and Elizabeth Hutchinson. Mrs. Campbell, a seasoned social worker and librarian, was a daughter-in-law of Sir Francis Campbell. Starting from this base, with a keen intellect she had developed a cold passion for excellence in work for the blind, had been almost everywhere and seen everything in the field. Her addition to the staff of Seeing Eye enabled Mrs. Eustis to maintain her own isolation from the field without losing sight of anything important it had to offer.

Miss Hutchinson had been trained as an occupational therapist. A woman of consummate good feeling, good manners, and common sense, she brought to a high state of effectiveness the social retraining of the clients in such matters as table etiquette, management of wardrobe, keeping track of possessions, those "weak" things of the world, which according to scripture "God has chosen to confound the mighty," and which can loom very large when blindness occurs (St. Paul, 1 Cor. 1.27).

Before she activated Seeing Eye, Mrs. Eustis had been the founder of Fortunate Fields (see Chapter 8 of this volume).

At this juncture it should be pointed out that as was the case with the training of children in orientation, German dog guide schools antedated the founding of Seeing Eye. Moreover, during the 1920s dog guides for the blind were an accepted resource for blind individuals in Germany. Over 4,000 were in use.

Dr. Gerhard Stalling, who had been a trainer of search dogs for the German Army during World War I, subsequently directed the opening of a school at Breslau where dogs were trained for the use of the blind. Breslau had long been a center of sophistication where blindness was concerned. In the early 1800s a school for the blind had been founded there by Johann G. Knie, a blind graduate of the University of Breslau, who was the first blind individual to be director of a residential school in Europe and a supreme realist about the senses through which blind children are educated. His school was described as a "melange of bells, rattles, drums, models of animals, machines, buildings," and he wrote a book entitled *A Guide to the Proper Management of Blind Children,* which was said to have been "gospel reading" in the world of the blind in the last century (Ross, 1951). This educational realism may well account for the fact that German educators got so much of a head start on the United States in mobility, at least where the dog guides were concerned. Over-preoccupation with the amenities of not "looking blind" can very seriously forestall special use of the fingers and also the nose.

"I smell many people," said a young deaf blind pupil walking into a crowded room. In the shocked hush of the group his wise teacher said with pioneering tact, "That's his way, folks. Be glad he can smell you."

VALLEY FORGE ARMY HOSPITAL

Social bolts of lightning are sometimes necessary in awakening tyros in work for the blind to the actualities of the situation. One in particular may be said to have set off the orientation and mobility program of Richard Hoover at Valley Forge Hospital.

Dr. James N. Greear, the eye chief at that hospital during World War II, was a past master at holding staff meetings. He had a special gift for putting everyone on one level.

Shortly after the Battle of the Bulge, newly blinded soldiers began to arrive in much greater numbers than they had previously. Seventeen came in one day, all of them much more recently wounded than any who had arrived previously. At the staff meeting that followed this development the staff maintained an exterior calm until close to the end of the meeting when the time came for the colonel to ask if anyone had any more questions, but not expecting any more.

"I have an observation to make," said Roberta Wilson, then a social worker at the hospital. "These patients who have just come in to the hospital are a shattered group. "

Discussion began all over again turning on the question of what the blinded soldiers needed most, but finally again led to a silence in the face of the large problem under consideration. This silence was broken by the matter-of-fact voice of Richard Hoover, who said, "I think the first thing they need is to know how to get around. We've been working on it, but not enough."

Then came the lightning.

"People say blind people in this country do a good job of getting around. I don't think they do a good job. I think they do a hell of a poor job."

To say that this was felt as an affront by the blind people in the room, both on their own behalf and for those who shared their handicap, would be a monstrous understatement. They ultimately forgave Hoover, became his believers, and one even became his pupil. But at the very time, as work for the blind had been shaped, and in view of what they had been led to believe about themselves, his words amounted to a crowning insult.

Fortunately they struck Col. Greear otherwise. Coming from an experienced teacher of the blind, they seemed to confirm what he had merely suspected, or at least hesitated to say, in his touchy role of ophthalmologist in charge of a program for the blind. He immediately reopened the question of training the soldiers in what was termed "foot travel," decided to strike while the iron was hot, and, with Hoover and several officers in his wake, set out impromptu for the office of the commanding officer of the hospital.

This was Col. Henry Beuuwkes, a fine old gentleman, who had eagles on his shoulders, and everything handsome in the way of accoutrements about him, for which the blinded soldiers had no respect whatsoever. Indeed he had been through several painful scenes when blinded soldiers had actually gotten into his office and pounded on his desk with their canes, demanding to know what was going to be done with and for them.

Relieved to have something practical offered that afternoon, he forthwith put all he had learned in the way of military administration into following out a prescription which Sgt. Hoover offered, and which the eye chief endorsed. This was not merely training in foot travel with the cane, but a large number of specially chosen, highly qualified instructors, a sufficient number to spend hours and hours teaching on an individual basis. To accomplish this, Col. Beuuwkes persuaded Major General Hayes to send Valley Forge Hospital panels of picked men, thirty at a time, from which the War Blind Service was allowed to choose "orientors." Regrettably the formula for this selection does not survive. However, it is reasonably certain that since Hoover had a hand in it, the words "common sense" found their way into whatever document was drawn up. Its product was a flow of excellent medical corpsmen whose very presence buoyed the atmosphere. This was the real beginning of what has been called "foot travel."

To avoid confusion, the term "orientation and mobility" will be used hereafter in this chapter, but this is a good place to say that the term was not common until the 1950s. Hoover and his associates adopted the term "foot travel" because it was believed that the term "orientation," which had previously been used, had gotten off to a sour start. "Foot travel" was chosen for its unpretentious, self-explanatory simplicity which it was hoped would be a point in its favor with the GIs. "Mobility" did not come into use until the initiation of a program at the Catholic Guild for the Blind after the war. It was at that agency the term "peripatology" was coined. The more sophisticated terms have accompanied the maturing of the art. The term "foot travel," however, was curiously appropriate to the almost Homeric atmosphere of Valley Forge.

The quality of the Valley Forge program was one of those paradoxes in human experience which those who shared in it find difficult to explain. Colonel Elliot Randolph, who succeeded Greear as eye chief, once shocked a roomful of Federal Security officials by saying that those who had worked on the war blind program at Valley Forge had had "fun." He himself was one of those lucky men to whom his work (ophthalmology) was "fun." This may well have been because he was always on the patient's side, not the kind ever to use his knife out of ambition or curiosity.

Despite many tragic factors which brought Valley Forge Hospital into existence, there is no doubt that it had about it an unaccountable "happy ship" quality. This has been described by Hoover himself in terms of the unusual talents of doctors and the community surrounding the hospital.

Other hospitals had somewhat similar resources, but did not have Hoover. He found a way not only to get the right men together to teach the soldiers, but knew how to handle both patients and corpsmen to get the best out of them. Also, by the time the selected panel of instructors came to the hospital, he had evolved both the idea of the light cane and the technique for making the most of it. This had come not only of observing with his eyes, but of blindfolding himself and experimenting, as have many of the gifted sighted pioneers, including Howe (Ross, 1951). It should be added that such pioneers are made of the stuff to ignore the protests of blind people who rush to tell them that they will never know what it is to be blind. But when results are good, the protesters forget they ever protested. Such was the case with respect to Hoover's system, but only after years of controversy.

RIVALRIES

Rivalries played their curious roles in the events which ultimately led to widespread acceptance of mobility training programs. The interested spectator from a good vantage point could not fail to observe what reminded him of a miniature war with a long series of skirmishes and battles. Animosities, affinities, egos, ids, and an occasional superego all played their parts. The intensity caused a good deal of comment among bystanders inexperienced in the ways of the human spirit consecrated to the improvement of life for blind people. To them it was unbelievable that there should be such heat for or against formal mobility training for the blind.

Part of the heat undoubtedly was generated by the fact that it was an impassioned time. The program began in a war and because of a war; a sort of holy war against Hitler, Mussolini, and the Japanese. This gave people who wore the uniform in those days a basic self-assurance for the time being with respect to their ways and doings. According to the law of the land, the war blinded until discharge belonged to the armed services.

Before they had lost their sight the word "belong" applied to them had carried no sinister connotation. But in the United States in this century as soon as you mention any blind person belonging to any agency whatsoever you are in trouble. Those who see blind people forever threatened by domination of the sighted are particularly sensitive on this point. At least one conversation between an ophthalmologist in uniform and the head of an agency for the blind got off to a bad start when the agency head told the ophthalmologist the blinded soldiers belonged to themselves. By World War II, work for the blind had reached such a point of strain on this subject that no one with any delicacy would use the term "belong," with regard to a client, in any sentence which could possibly be misconstrued. But with World War II, lo and behold! here were some blind people who actually did belong to the Army, the Navy, and the Marine Corps. And deep down in their hearts workers for the blind felt the glamorous war blinded should belong to them from the moment they were blinded. It should be taken into account that the people involved were in fact dedicated people, and that they were not contending for the riches of the world, but for the tough job of helping blind people learn to deal with their blindness. There were a number of armed camps which had been working and reworking uneasy truces with each other over the decades.

In one camp was the American Foundation for the Blind, commanded by its executive director, Dr. Robert Irwin, the champion of public school education for the blind. In the U.S. Office of Education was another camp commanded by Joseph Clunk, the architect of the national program of vocational placement of the blind, then in its infancy. In the education field Dr. Gabriel Farrell of the Perkins School had his camp, and Dr. Merle Frampton, principle of the New York Institute for the Blind, another. Farrell regarded Frampton as an archrival, Irwin regarded Frampton as an archenemy. A novice in work for the blind, though not at wheeling and dealing, Frampton was a long-term stormy petrel, an impassioned promoter of residential schools, sometimes called the Admiral Rickover of work for the blind.

This was not the end of the personality clashes among the influential. Irwin and Joseph Clunk turned deaf ears to each other. For two decades Irwin had been cultivating the Foundation's position of national leadership, and lately Clunk had been speaking for the blind of the nation from his ranking position in the federal government. Clunk had hopes that Congress would bestow the program for the rehabilitation of veterans on his office. This was a disturbing thought to Irwin.

There was, however, a rather loose-jointed confederation of opinion in the various camps which occupied the field, and there was one subject on which nearly everyone agreed. It was outrageous that the cream of challenges to their skill, the war blinded, should be where they could not be got at immediately and taken in hand by experienced practitioners.

Indignation over this was heightened by the fact that, as in other wars, the Surgeon General of the Army had made ophthalmologists responsible for the rehabilitation of the war blinded, and the field of work for the blind had been telling itself for two decades that ophthalmologists had made the war blind program of World War I a disaster. This had been said so often that even the people who did not believe it had given up putting in a word to the contrary, except to say the World War I program had forced the field to take a look at how it was organized nationally. This had produced a brief era of rare harmony during which the American Association of Workers for the Blind had joined forces with the American Association of Instructors of the Blind to found "a national clearing house for problems of the blind," and for this purpose established the American Foundation for the Blind.

When war clouds gathered in the early part of 1940, certainly it was time for another era of rare harmony, and at first it appeared one might ensue. With professional aplomb the American Association of Workers for the Blind had appointed Irwin chairman of a distinguished committee to advise the government about the "Care, Training and After Care of Persons Becoming Blind as a Result of the United States Defense Program and Possible Participation in the Present World War. "

RESPONSIBILITY

Frances Koestler, in *The Unseen Minority* (1976), describes how the committee went about its business sagaciously, issued a public warning against exploitation of the war blind, favoring the federal government's assumption of responsibility for the rehabilitation of the war blinded and, when Congress placed the responsibility with the Veterans Administration (VA), offered a clearcut plan for rehabilitation which theoretically could fit into the framework of Public Law 78–16, which authorized the VA to provide rehabilitation for disabled veterans.

But very shortly Irwin was writing,

> We have complications, growing out of the fact that the Veterans Administration, which is responsible for the rehabilitation of disabled veterans, has no jurisdiction over the men until they are discharged from the Army. Blinded men who may be kept in hospitals for months are under the Surgeon General of the Army or of the Navy. (Koestler, 1976.)

For the orientation and mobility program this was a godsend. Not a single leader in the field at that time would have backed Hoover's teaching the way Col. Greear did. The only one who came anywhere near having the connections and nerve to ask for so much manpower was Dr. Frampton. He had stolen a march on everyone and had himself put in charge of the Navy's program for rehabilitation of the handicapped at Philadelphia Naval Hospital. Yet visiting Valley Forge Hospital, he viewed the mobility training, and showed no sign of being impressed. In this he was no different from most other heads of agencies for the blind in the 1940s.

For a time one of the major points at issue between the Army and its critics, especially in the Office of Vocational Rehabilitation, was the emphasis put on orientation and mobility, and taught by sighted instructors!

It is strange to think in retrospect that many very fine leaders of the blind should have objected to the practice, still thinking as did Dr. Allen that the blind were best left to "pick up" mobility "on their own." (With perhaps a few pointers from some experienced blind person.) To be too hard on them for this would be equally benighted. Even the workers for the blind who had seen the war blinded of World War I had not seen what the staff at Valley Forge saw, soldiers flown back to the States within a few days of being abruptly and completely blinded. One of their few advantages was that they knew nothing about being blind and knew that they knew nothing, and were therefore amenable to early training as no large group of blind people had ever been before.

The numbers and situation of the war blinded not only produced the setting for simple experimentation and the organization of method. The needs of the men made them willing to submit to them.

It was strange and ironic that as it was being developed, a systematic approach to problems of blindness was criticized as the "Army way" of doing things, which of course meant ineptly. Indeed certain prominent state directors, some of whom were blind, "dug in" and were little fortresses against such practices until death or retirement parted them from the field. It should be said in fairness, however, that many of them had neither the experience nor the connections to obtain a clear idea of what was going on inside the service programs.

A good deal of confusion existed at the time, and continues in retrospect, over how the three army hospitals for the war blinded differed. Their differences were in theory quite clearcut, but practicalities blurred them. Valley Forge Army General Hospital at Phoenixville, Pennsylvania, and Dibble Army General Hospital at Menlo Park, California, were designated early in the war as centers for eye care, Valley Forge to serve eye casualties from the European Theater of Operations, Dibble those from the Pacific Theater. The need for giving them basic rehabilitation while in the hospital was almost immediately apparent, since many of them had disabilities which necessitated long-term hospitalization. Both programs grew by leaps and bounds through necessity, and many observers thought that no other installation for the blind was needed, although the committee Irwin had headed called for a rehabilitation center. Public Law 78–16 indicated that such a center should be operated by the VA.

The VA, however, was reluctant to involve itself. Its administrator, General Frank T. Hines, was against such a center on principle, based on his personal experience with the program for the war blinded of World War I. According to Dr. Irwin, it had been “a headache, and all the VA officials were a bit leery . . . ” (Koestler, 1976). General Hines and his assistants were even more leery of various agencies for the blind, which began to make plays for a contract to operate such a center, funded by the VA. This possibility was deeply disturbing to those who believed that the rehabilitation of the war blinded must be shouldered by the federal government. Such harmony as there had been on that subject was at an end. Opposing forces neutralized each other in conversations with VA officials, leaving them even more reluctant to run a rehabilitation center.

Meanwhile one agency was not in a position to wait on indecision and debate. This was the Army, which had a sizable number of eye casualties, some of whom had become the “war blinded” by late 1943, and were clamoring to be discharged from the service with or without rehabilitation.

AVON

The situation was taken in hand by Col. Derrick T. Vail, chief consultant in ophthalmology in the European Theater of Operations. He had exactly the temperament and capabilities the deadlock demanded. He was a very impatient man, very intelligent, had an impregnable reputation as a professor of ophthalmology at Northwestern University, and he stood in awe of no one. He came back from Europe to push for a center for the war blinded, and when he found the VA unwilling to budge, before anyone knew quite what was happening, he had persuaded the Surgeon General's office to assume responsibility for operating it. President Roosevelt signed an agreement authorizing the Army to operate a center. Other signatories were the Secretary of War, the Secretary of the Navy, the Chairman of the War Man Power Commission and the Administrator of Veterans Affairs.

Thus the program at Avon, Connecticut, came into existence. In time it was to receive almost as much criticism as had the War Blind Program of World War I. Its stated purpose was the social adjustment of the war blinded prior to discharge from the service. This was to include “mental adjustment as may be necessary to develop a proper attitude and a will to overcome the handicap” (Koestler, 1976). The staff at Avon took on this awesome charge with gusto, but there were certain immediate realities which hampered them from the start. The last program to be activated, it served trainees, many of whom had spent long months at one of the two general hospitals and often felt rightly or wrongly they had learned to manage their blindness. It was a moot question, moreover, from the beginning whether any lasting “adjustment” to blindness would take place before the men were out of uniform and while still at Avon.

Avon was like no setting most of the men had ever encountered before, or were ever likely to encounter again. A masterpiece of medieval academic architecture, idyllic, on a 2,000-acre estate, it would have offered the mystic or scholar an ideal retreat in which to while away eternity. But it was not ideal as a launching pad back to common daily living in the United States. Dr. Vail, while in England, had been exposed to the world-renowned, British war blinded institution, St. Dunstan's. He saw its American counterpart in Avon, but he was soon to discover the British model required very drastic modification to meet American concepts of rehabilitation. St. Dunstan's was monolithic, paternal, and there was not the slightest chance the American GIs would allow such an institution to be built around them.

It is a natural goal of virtually every severely handicapped American to mingle with the world. Certainly this was part of the philosophy of President Roosevelt, whose authorization of the Avon program limited the stay of the blinded service man to eighteen weeks. At the end of this time he would be discharged from the service. His further rehabilitation training and treatment would be provided by the VA, preferably in programs with the sighted. He could also if he chose elope from rehabilitative programs and institutions forever.

Avon's defenders, of whom there were a number, claimed that this was what they were promoting, but at least in one area their program took an unfortunate course toward that end. The training officer made the serious mistake of failing to recognize Hoover's work in orientation and mobility. Going even further, the Avon program espoused an old legend that a cane was unnecessary and insisted that trainees discard their canes on arrival at the installation.

In actual fact, to get about the premises of Avon without a cane was no great accomplishment. Its uneven floors and passageways offered many orientation cues, but more significantly it was a controlled environment, as much as any residential school for the blind. In lieu of cane training Avon invested heavy belief in the ability to detect obstacles through the sensation which has rather fancifully been called "facial vision," but which present-day mobility experts term "obstacle perception." This phenomenon has been demonstrated to be associated with hearing. Objects intercept sound waves and this absence of sound transfers itself to an illusion of cutaneous sensation.

More than the program at Valley Forge, the program at Avon was a program of entrepreneurs, who had somehow convinced themselves that teachers of the blind had been too steeped in tradition to exploit a God-given radar, available to blind people for the tuning in. This was in total disregard of common knowledge of the experienced—that "facial vision" only works for certain individuals, better on days when they are feeling well, that it is just not as reliable as touching an object with a cane and never, never warns of objects below the knees, or drop-offs such as curbs or the Grand Canyon.

With wasted fortitude, therefore, the Avon program undertook to persuade the blinded service men to dispense with their canes altogether, or if not that, to use them minimally away from Avon. Moreover, having considerable influence with the Surgeon General's office, for a time Avon personnel were able to convince the chief consulting ophthalmologist that this was correct policy and that it should prevail at Dibble Hospital. At Avon the policy gave way in the face of opposition from the blinded soldiers themselves. This came to a head when the uses of "facial vision" were exalted beyond measure in a 1945 *Saturday Evening Post* article,"They Learn to See at Avon Old Farms." Several hundred copies of the magazine lay unbought upon the counter of the Post Exchange at Avon, a grim admonition from the blinded soldiers. Those in charge of the program took the hint, and modified their position to the extent of having some token advanced cane training in downtown Hartford. This was hardly more than a gesture, but it accompanied an increased realization both at Valley Forge and the Surgeon General's office that Hoover's method was valid. As a result, in the summer of 1945 the Surgeon General's office dispatched an orientor from Valley Forge to Dibble to teach the cane method.

DIBBLE ARMY HOSPITAL

The Hoover method could hardly have been taken to a more unfriendly environment. Reliance on obstacle perception was virtually the religion of the staff, antedating the establishment of the Avon program. The anti-cane doctrine had been accepted as gospel by the eye chief, Colonel Norman Cutler, a brilliant ophthalmologist, whose responsibility for rehabilitation of the blind had been thrust upon him in the fortunes of war. He had quite naturally and sincerely begun by relying on the advice of his staff, confirmed by the sanction of the Surgeon General's office. However, following a visit to Valley Forge, he had begun to have doubts. After the *Saturday Evening Post* fiasco, he struck his colors and asked for a Valley Forge orientor to teach his staff the cane method.

When the Valley Forge orientor arrived at Dibble, the Colonel was much bedeviled by his blind staff members. Having heard it was correct practice to hire the visually handicapped, he had hired a number in quick succession, only to find that each thought he or she should be in charge of the program. All were unalterably opposed to the teaching of mobility as it was going forward at Valley Forge Hospital.

The Colonel also had on his hands a cadre of sighted instructors, not particularly well screened as they had been at Valley Forge. The blind staff had shown little inclination to share with them the facts of living as blind persons.

In conference with the Valley Forge instructor, they complained that one or more blind members of the staff had a habit of coming behind them, while they were in dealings with a blind soldier, and telling him he didn't have to do anything sighted people told him to do. This, they said, made teaching by facial vision uphill work. The Colonel himself had entered on his duties with a relatively fresh point of view toward the integrating of blind people into society. But he confessed to the Valley Forge instructor that he wondered if he should not persuade some of his wealthy friends to endow an institution like St. Dunstan's for their lifelong care.

By all this the blinded soldiers were relatively undamaged because of the mother wit God gave them. However, one of them had sat next to a congressman on a train and raised a curtain on the goings-on at Dibble as he had experienced them. The congressman had broken a story about this in the newspapers, and this was one of the factors which had led Dibble to seek help from Valley Forge.

For two months the Valley Forge mobility instructor gave lessons under the blindfold to the sighted corpsmen of Dibble. He also chose one soldier to teach. And one of the blind staff members did indeed shadow these lessons with some heart-to-heart talks, the nature of which could only be surmised. The blind soldier, a Kansan, did all that was expected of him, was competent with the cane, but kept his own counsel about his long-term intentions with regard to the mode of foot travel he would use. On this subject there were conflicting reports in after-years.

Simultaneously with the Kansan's training, the head mobility instructor at Dibble undertook to train a blinded soldier by the obstacle perception method for comparison with the cane method. This was a very impressive performance, which at least made the two instructors friendly journeymen in their trade. It is a curious fact, however, that several years after the war the Valley Forge instructor met the soldier (now a veteran) who had been trained by the Dibble method and discovered that the obstacle perception lessons had totally faded from his memory. This might seem to betoken the perfect job of rehabilitation which leaves no dependency whatsoever, had not the veteran in the intervening years adopted the use of a rather inadequate cane and technique for using it.

The war ended during the second month of the Valley Forge instructor's assignment to Dibble, and relatively little time remained for a program of training with the cane to develop momentum. George Gillispie, presently Chief of Service for the Blind in the central office of the VA, was a patient at Dibble at the time. He was given the task of showing the Valley Forge instructor what could be accomplished by the Dibble method. This he did extremely well. However, he now reports that he was given some lessons with the cane before leaving the hospital and that after leaving he paid for a course of lessons with the cane and has used one ever since.

The manner in which the Valley Forge method was received at Dibble Hospital was prophetic of the reception which was to greet subsequent efforts to offer it to the field, giving those who were interested in promoting it an inkling of what might be expected from the adult blind of the United States who had grown up in the school of hard knocks, won their way on their own and were proud of it. Both extremely hot and chillingly cold opposition came not merely from blind people who went without canes. One of the least sympathetic ridiculers of the Hoover method was the admirable, redoubtable cane user, Joseph Clunk. Wearing well-earned laurels for getting the federal program of vocational rehabilitation of the blind under way, he himself was a totally blind individual who could get anywhere he wanted to go, and he was absolutely dedicated to the cause of the blind. But he was very jealous of the prerogatives of blind individuals, and increasingly as the years went by could hardly bear to think of a sighted person having any say about the working of his program. His style early alienated him from doctors in charge of the war blinded, who kept him at arm's length. Offended at this, he regarded it as a real impertinence that foot travel was being taught to blinded soldiers by Hoover and his sighted helpers, including the author of this chapter.

Hitherto it has not seemed important in this narrative to say it was I who was the Valley Forge instructor at Dibble Hospital. However, the editors of this book have suggested that I must find some way of backing up my account of persons and scenes by identifying myself and the role I played in the evolving program of orientation and mobility. And I feel no compulsion in my retirement to withhold any of my experiences which may be of use to those who are now more active.

A CONGENITAL WORKER FOR THE BLIND

One of the most important of those experiences was being the son of my father, John Francis Bledsoe. He was just at the point of retirement when World War II came, having had a long career as an educator of the handicapped (1893–1941). As a young man, he had studied at the Harvard Graduate School of Education under Michael Anagnos, who had also taught principles of education of the handicapped to Anne Sullivan (Macy). With Anagnos my father read in the archives of the Perkins School, especially the theories of Samuel Gridley Howe. He was made superintendent of the Maryland School for the Blind in 1906 and immediately set about reorganizing it and rebuilding it according to Howe's "cottage family plan." The purpose of this was to make friends of teachers and pupils, give the pupils constant social acceptance and training and deinstitutionalize the school. For many years it was a model for educators updating their systems. In the war years he was perhaps the most venerable figure in the field of work for the blind, whose good will was sought by such diverse personages as Irwin, Farrell, and Frampton.

Thus I inherited some influence in work for the blind from my father. During World War II, I tried to put it to use, as had my father, for the good of the blind. And it is only fair I should give my version of what it did and how it worked.

A TRANSFER

The first evidence I had that I might have some force in the war blind program came in a letter, which I received in 1944 when I was a sergeant in the Air Force. It came from Major M. E. Randolph, Chief of the Ophthalmology Branch in the Office of the Surgeon General. It was a gracefully worded invitation to acquiesce in a transfer from the Air Force to the War Blind Program.

I had no doubt this letter was written more to my father's son than to me. Dr. Randolph had conversed with him and discovered, I think, that they had similar views on life and work.

Among other things Dr. Randolph was seeking the names of workers for the blind in the Army, in order to secure their transfers to his program. My father gave Dr. Randolph my address, but discouraged him from arranging the transfer in my case, because he felt his influence had unconsciously worked beyond its due to draw me into work for the blind. I was out and away, having just published a novel before going into the Air Corps, was working in a public relations office, was getting articles published in *Yank*, and my father was enjoying the fact that I was doing things on my own. He also was human enough to hope I could be kept out of the brewing squabbles over the war blinded, his experience with such contention having been the part of his work which he had enjoyed least. In actual fact I had grown more interested in work for the blind than either of us had expected, particularly in the squabbles and what caused them.

A TEACHER

When I graduated from Princeton in 1934, my father had rather cautiously and temporarily allowed me a teaching job at the Maryland School for the Blind. He was not averse to giving members of the family employment if he could get them at a good price. It was common practice in the past for schools for the blind. But he made it clear I must be out and away on my own in a reasonable time. In the meantime I had four very happy years coaching dramatics and teaching English as part of a superlative faculty.

One of my father's most fortunate professional accomplishments was the recruitment of Richard Hoover as mathematics teacher and athletic coach the school year of 1938–1939, during which I was away taking the Harvard course of special education of the blind. On my return Hoover and I got to know each other. It would be hard to overestimate the importance of the experience Hoover had with blindness in the setting of the school. He was with blind boys around the clock, living in the cottage with them, eating meals with them, teaching them and coaching term in athletics.

But at the school, as in every other school for the blind in the United States, we did not teach mobility, nor did it then appear necessary on a hundred acres of controlled environment in which the pupils spent as much as twelve years.

A lifetime in and around work for the blind was only half of my preparation for the war blind program. Equally important were two years of picaresque adventures in the Army after war broke out. As an enlisted man I found out at first hand something about soldiers, from whose lips I learned to appreciate the beauty and force of bad grammar, spoken by experts.

I at least learned enough about the Army to know what to do when I received Dr. Randolph's letter. I wrote to him immediately saying I was agreeable to the transfer. In about a month I received orders transferring me to Valley Forge Hospital.

On my train journey from Alabama to Pennsylvania I read in the newspapers that for the first time an enlisted man was being transferred from the higher priority Air Corps to the lower ranking Medical Corps. As the Air Corps had until then been the next thing to holy when demanding personnel, this gave me an inkling of the authority which had been generated in behalf of the war blinded. Afterwards I learned from Dr. Randolph that he had invoked Lt. General George H. Brett, commanding general of the Caribbean Air Force to get the transfer accomplished.

THE USE OF INFLUENCE

Here, if my self-revelation is to have any value at all, it is important that I give some personal experience and views with regard to the use of influence. Though I had not discussed my transfer at Craig Field, I had talked with some of my friends in work for the blind when on leave in Baltimore.

"Don't take it," said a surprising number of them, "unless they make you a ________." (Here various ranks above captain were mentioned.)

I was amazed at the naiveté of these suggestions both about the Army and influence where programs for blind people are concerned. You may be able to do that kind of bargaining where atomic physics is concerned. But any confidence man would have known this would be the sure way to lose the ears of perplexed officials who were seeking guidance in so delicate a side of the national catastrophe as blindness. It was also obvious in the situation described in Dr. Randolph's letter, as new and strange to me as to everyone else, the place to start was as near the bottom as possible and at the operating level.

It so happened that in the Valley Forge war blind program, when I was first assigned to it, rank was almost a disadvantage. The chief of the eye service, Lt. Col. James N. Greear, was far more eager to pick the brains of his noncommissioned specialists on blindness than his commissioned ophthalmologists. He listened to both Hoover and me, but better to Hoover, which I early detected, and from then on depended on Hoover to pass on my ideas to the Colonel or not, as he saw fit. He had arrived at Valley Forge before me, already absorbed a great deal of information about what had been done up until then, and had sized up the personalities involved shrewdly.

One of the first things Hoover and I had to get straight between us was what we thought of the budding fascination with obstacle perception. We gave it secondary rating. That was done together. I recall exactly when. In his open-minded way Hoover was giving it every opportunity in a long discussion we were having in a restaurant after all the patrons were gone. He said one of the authorities on obstacle perception would claim that an individual trained by the facial vision method could make his way through that room full of jumbled chairs without touching one: The chairs were hardly waist-high.

I said this went against everything I had ever seen, and he had ever seen.

He said, "You're right. We're going to have to use canes."

The next day he blindfolded himself and started working on his cane technique. I did not perceive what he did about its use until he went over it a number of times, as he was afterwards to do with hundreds of others, both sighted and blind. I did not see the advantage of the light cane until he explained it to me. Nor did I have anything to do with its manufacture, which, according to legend, he arranged by getting somebody to stop making part of a battleship for half an afternoon. However, when he had gotten the practicalities in hand, I learned to teach his technique, and taught it to the soldiers at Valley Forge. I also shared in teaching it to new instructors and gave several classes of them basic indoctrination in the ways of work for the blind before going out to Dibble Hospital.

ATTITUDES

One knotty question which we had to deal with early in our efforts was the extent to which you can train sighted people to be more graceful and considerate in their dealings with the blind. We found that you can, and there is very little doubt that our attention to this was one of the things which gave the Valley Forge program its happy ship quality. One of the tools we used in training the instructors was a short etiquette pamphlet, which spiced its message with a certain amount of surgical humor.

This was the forerunner of subsequent leaflets on guiding in which I had a hand at the VA and other agencies.

Colonel Greear was a staunch supporter of everything Hoover did, as was Col. Randolph later when he came to Valley Forge as chief of the eye service. Randolph's return to the role of physician and surgeon in the eye service there was a reward for yeoman service warding off ax grinders in the Surgeon General's office. It was not easy to tell them from the good citizens who could also be trying, at times, in their own way. Eventually the Surgeon General's office concluded that the best course was to pay formal attention to this latter category, who in many ways resembled the "hard core altruists" of the Harvard sociobiologist, Edward O. Wilson (Wilson, 1978).

Two such staunch souls were Dr. Irwin and Dr. Farrell. Irwin loathed all residential schools for the blind, based on a childhood aversion to the manure pile next to the athletic field at the Washington School for the Blind, where he had been a pupil. He had, nonetheless, managed to overcome this aversion to the extent of making friends with Farrell, who was a member of his board at the American Foundation for the Blind. Though director of the Perkins School, Farrell was far from a dyed-in-the-wool residential school man. Having been appointed to his job with no experience whatsoever in work for the blind (he had been a canon in the Episcopal Church, was a scholar, publicist, and organizer), he wore the scars of welcoming scorn from old timers in the field. But he wore them stoically, having managed to master his job, as he put it, by giving Perkins an organization, which it badly needed. By 1942 he was, on the whole, objective about subjects in work for the blind (with the exception of Dr. Frampton), and he had a sense of responsibility which went beyond his immediate domain, as is a tradition with directors of the Perkins School.

Correctly or incorrectly Irwin and Farrell regarded Avon as an extension of Frampton's power because its training officer, Capt. Blackburn, had once worked at Frampton's New York Institute.

Farrell had briefly aspired to be put in charge of the Army program as Frampton was of the Navy program, and when this did not materialize, he took up the role of éminence grise, joining forces with Irwin to influence the federal government at the highest possible levels. Before he had become director of the Perkins School, Farrell had been a clergyman too, and had the ear of Laura Delano, President Roosevelt's cousin, who was in the special confidence of the President, was in fact one of those in the room with him when he died. By managing this pipeline to the top prudently, Farrell gained entry to the programs for the war blinded.

At Valley Forge, Farrell was one of the first heads of a residential school to see an orientation and mobility lesson given, becoming thereby one of the first civilian workers for the blind to say kind words about it.

Undoubtedly it did not hurt the cause of the cane with Farrell that Avon had foolishly attempted to close its doors to him, and when he had to be admitted, kept what he dryly called a "bodyguard" with him when he went about. At Valley Forge he was much freer. I had gotten to know him quite well during the year I spent taking the Harvard course at Perkins, and he looked me up and aired his dissatisfactions with the war blinded program, telling me he was thinking very seriously of taking his views to the President through Miss Delano. I told him that I thought instead he should attempt to find out more about what the Army was trying to do, that I thought he could accomplish much more by making friends with the ophthalmologists and that Hoover's work was so valuable it should be a part of the Perkins program after the war. He nodded, but did not give himself away as to his intentions. I reported this conversation to Col. Greear, who took it with some irritation. I also told him I had heard there was a movement afoot to get the Surgeon General to appoint a citizens advisory committee on the war blinded and from my experience such a committee would be a good means of explaining the Army's good points to the field of work for the blind, which could not be ignored forever. He did not say "aye, yes, or nay." But not too long after that the committee was appointed and Farrell was made a member of it. It was almost a disaster.

CITIZENS ADVISORY COMMITTEE

The brainchild of Irwin, who chose its membership, included blue ribbon men and women. It was especially well laden with shining examples of successful blind people: Irwin himself, Philip Harrison, a World War I blinded veteran, who was head of the Pennsylvania program for the civilian blind, Peter Salmon, whose strong points were low vision and diplomacy, and at least one international status figure, Col. Edward Baker, in charge of Canada's blind program. The executives from agencies included at least two who had been hewers, haulers, fetchers, and carriers in their youth (Eber Palmer of the Batavia School for the Blind and Dr. Richard French of the California School). There was even that very necessary ingredient, the stormy petrel or radical, Father Thomas I. Carroll of the Catholic Guild for the Blind in Boston, pro tem chaplain at Avon.

The first meeting of the committee could hardly have had a more inauspicious beginning. Dr. Derrick Vail, who spoke for the Surgeon General, began by scolding the committee for interagency rivalries and lack of cooperation with the Army (Koestler, 1976). He was particularly irritated that Frampton had flatly refused to honor the Navy's commitment to make use of the program at Avon and made his refusal stick by invoking the influence of his friend Admiral Ross McIntyre, the President's physician. Dr. Vail was unaware that the members of the committee he was addressing, which included Irwin and Farrell, to a man or woman were hardly on bowing terms with Frampton. None had the slightest influence with him, nor cared to. Years later Vail told me ruefully he afterwards learned it was one of his brother ophthalmologists, Dr. Norbert Wiener, who had innocently encouraged the Navy's high-ranking officers to take their wayward course with respect to Avon. Nevertheless, Vail was right in thinking the committee had some negative views about the Army program, based not alone on vague rumors, but reports of a highly qualified emissary of Irwin's.

MISS GRUBER

Dr. Irwin never made the mistake of thinking he could get along without extensive vicarious use of eyesight, and for several months before the committee met he had had one of his representatives looking at the program of the war blinded. Early in 1945 he had appointed Kathern Gruber as director of the War Blind Service of the American Foundation for the Blind.

When he engaged her he wrote, "I am not quite sure what is needed. For quite a while your job is to find out what the government is not doing and why not. You can then accumulate the facts which we can lay before the proper government officials and get things going the right way" (Koestler, 1976).

Events were to show that Irwin's talents were at his best when he employed Kathern Gruber, but very soon he began to wonder if he had gotten more than he bargained for by saying to one of his assistants, "Miss Gruber would give the Foundation to those boys, and I love her for it, but you hold her down."

Moving into the war blinded scene, she was not merely an arresting and charming personality. She had brains and was a power in her own right by force of her overwhelming energy and absolute concentration on the good of the blinded service men. She was a seasoned professional in education of the blind, having been a resource teacher for blind pupils in the Minneapolis public schools, for whom she had managed to get summer jobs in the impossible job market of the depression.

Looking like a European queen in exile, she made her appearance at all the military hospitals where there were blinded military personnel. Elegant yet durable in war-worn conveyances and inns, she made friends wherever she went, but no one in those days ever called her by her first name. She was "Miss Gruber," so much a part of the war blinded years by that appellation that even those of us belonging to her own generation who have known her a long time have difficulty remembering to call her "Kay."

Helen Keller was at the time the Foundation's international representative, and she opened Miss Gruber's way into the military hospitals by paying visits to them first, explaining that Miss Gruber was to follow. Miss Gruber, when she arrived, had with her a notebook which sopped up information like a sponge. And if a blinded soldier, sailor, or marine had a need nobody knew how to deal with, she was sure to get wind of it, after which she would not rest, nor let others rest until a remedy had been found.

On her first visit to Valley Forge she saw the importance of the orientation and mobility program there, in the promotion of which she was to take a leading role. To start with, she described it to Irwin, persuaded him to keep an open mind on the subject, and finally give it active support. Also, she was highly effective in giving Irwin the information he needed to fence with the Surgeon General's representatives and make the citizens advisory committee effective, for despite its bad beginning the committee went into action successfully. This was due in large part to the discerning participation of Father Carroll, of whom she had made a friend, and whom she introduced to Irwin.

FATHER CARROLL

Much has been written about Father Carroll. Frances Koestler (1976) describes him at the time of World War II as a

> tall, Hollywood handsome young cleric endowed with a logical mind, a fighting spirit, and so deep a capacity for empathy with problems of blindness that the men in the rehabilitation centers fondly called him "Father Tom," while others, disregarding the fact that he was sighted, spoke of him as "the blind priest."

Father Carroll had entered work for the blind at the command of the Church. He often told of standing in a line of newly ordained priests and experiencing the quality of trauma he associated with loss of eyesight when he was assigned to the Catholic Guild for the Blind. A great parish priest was lost when he was assigned to the Guild. But the blind people of the United States acquired a priest who spent his life trying to serve them. Ecumenized long before the time of Pope John, Father Carroll was the deadly enemy of sanctimonious pity for blind people. He worked very hard at his job at the Guild, and he also burned the midnight oil studying blindness in all its phases. These lucubrations he was fond of calling "typhlology" after the definition in the *Oxford Dictionary*—"the science that deals with blindness." For years he wrote and rewrote his careful book, *Blindness: What It Is, What It Does, and What To Do About It* (Carroll, 1961).

An intense, not very pleased young man in the Avon days, his Irish sense of humor mellowed as the years went on, but he never lost his basic intensity, and in his later years kept a plain wooden coffin in his study, which his devoted secretary did her best to disguise as a couch. His spirit asserted itself in a tiny rugged cross which he left to be put in his hand when he was dead. On it was inscribed, "Everything must be built new." When Irwin had him appointed to the Surgeon General's advisory committee, he became the driving force that would not let the committee be blocked from effectiveness by courtesy and protocol. He had been at the grass roots as Avon's chaplain, and he was armed with facts. To some extent he had Vail's confidence, in part because he was clearly in favor of the Avon program, and indeed of continuing some form of federally controlled center for the war blinded after the war, a concept to which Vail was deeply committed. Father Carroll persuaded Irwin and Vail to arrange for three members of the committee to visit and inspect the Army installations for the war blinded, and also persuaded the committee to accept their invitations to go. The three were very well chosen: Peter J. Salmon, whose Industrial Home for the Blind was a model for agencies of its kind; Mrs. Lee Johnston, executive director of the Missouri Commission for the Blind, who had managed to make peace between social work and rehabilitation in her state; and Henry P. Johnson, executive director of the Florida Council for the Blind.

These solid citizens came back with a report which mollified Vail by its understanding of what the Army was trying to do. At the same time Peter Salmon, who was noted for being able to put plain facts in acceptable terms, pointed out that the Army program was alienating the war blinded from civilian organized work for the blind, on whom they might one day need to depend. He also admonished those who were in charge of the vocational training program at Avon for building "grandiose hopes."

Neither Father Carroll nor Vail wholly agreed with this latter criticism, but a new climate for exchange of opinions had been generated, and the committee was invited to make a second visit to the installations early in 1946. This they did, but to discover an entirely new set of problems, because with the war over, it was now in the wind that the Army was about to divest itself of all its programs for the war blinded. This was concomitant with a widespread determination to reform the VA and force the agency to face up to its responsibilities. Toward this end, President Truman had replaced General Hines with General Omar Bradley and appointed Maj. General Paul Hawley chief medical director. At the time, General Bradley had the type of charisma which is in eclipse in the world today. Just by going into the building and sitting down at his desk, he gave the country a feeling things were better at the VA. In the world of medicine General Hawley was also inspiriting. As an old army doctor he had accomplished the exceptional feat of giving civilian specialists in uniform a chance to work unhampered by military tradition, making of them an echelon of consultants in the European theater. In the VA one of his first measures was to negotiate the same arrangement between that agency and the same top-flight specialists as they went back into civilian life. Vail, Greear, and Randolph, all were to serve the VA in this capacity in the next several years, and it is a fact of history that without their support orientation and mobility would never have found a place to take root when the Army program was discontinued. And, without the cultivation afforded by the VA, it is almost certain it would have fallen into Howe's "comparative neglect."

In the face of these new developments, Irwin's advisory committee took the unusual, strategic step of disbanding, but not before volunteering itself intact to advise General Bradley. Against the advice of holdovers from the Hines administration, he accepted the offer. A VA Advisory Committee on the Blinded Veterans was appointed in March 1946. This gave Father Carroll as a member of the committee, and Miss Gruber at Chairman Irwin's elbow, the opportunity to use their brains, information, and zeal to sway the course of the VA program for the blind. They were not slow to go into action, which I observed at first hand, having been appointed special consultant to the VA Department of Medicine and Surgery a little earlier.

The previous summer Col. Vail had offered to have me commissioned in the Medical Corps as a reward for my labors. This I saw fit to decline. I had gotten to be a staff sergeant on my own in the Air Corps, and what I was doing in the Medical Corps I thought I could do as well or better in that grade. Col. Randolph did not dispute this, but kindly advanced my pay by giving me another stripe. Turning down the commission was to affect both my own fate and the fate of orientation and mobility. Enlisted men were mustered out of the service more rapidly than officers when the war ended. I was discharged from the Army in January of 1946, and thus the first person from Valley Forge or Avon to whom the new VA talked. It goes without saying that I did my duty by Hoover's "foot travel" program, and I can vouch for the fact that no one else from the Army program (except Hoover) would even have seen fit to mention it.

THE NEW VETERANS ADMINISTRATION

I found the iron hot. Dr. Donald Covalt was just then establishing a new medical rehabilitation program in the VA Department of Medicine and Surgery, with the full backing of General Hawley. I was assigned to look into the situation of 337 aging blind veterans of earlier wars, and see what should be done to bring service programs for them into line with up-to-date theory and practice. I spent six weeks traveling to nine centers, where I interviewed all 337 blinded veterans and made notes on their ways of getting about (Bledsoe, 1946). This left me more than ever convinced that it is a sad waste of good intentions and human power for the average blinded individual to work out his own methods of getting about without benefit of systematic instruction. Only three of the 337 men had worked out any approximation of Hoover's method of touching the cane to the ground in front of the trailing foot. All the old blind men seemed to be acting out a visual memory of how the cane was carried as a walking stick, exploring a little in front tentatively at dangerous points, but then bringing the cane back to the side. Suggestions that the cane should be wielded in an arc were greeted with objections about how this would "look." This is so natural a reaction that I decided it would take a lot of teaching, not only with the veterans of past wars, but of future wars to overcome it.

It was fortunate that it was Dr. Covalt to whom I reported this idea. No other official in Washington at the time who had authority in the rehabilitation of the blind would have thought they were important. Clunk at Federal Security had shown his utter scorn of what was going on at Valley Forge by destroying an entire consignment of 1,000 copies of the Valley Forge cartoon brochure. Covalt, however, as an expert in physical medicine, was extremely interested in body mechanics and how they needed retraining because of a disability. He was in natural agreement with what might be called Hoover's basic premise: that if common physical problems of self-management can be mastered by a newly handicapped person, most Americans have a basic philosophy to do what is known as "adjusting." He read my report promptly, and presented it favorably to General Hawley. Both of them approved my recommendations that the nine centers I had visited be revitalized by the introduction of orientation and mobility. For a start I had urged that each have a blind chief and one mobility instructor. I recruited chiefs for the homes which did not have them, and we arranged for them to go to Valley Forge Hospital for a two week indoctrination with the hope of recruiting instructors from among the corpsmen about to be discharged.

The Meeting

With the help of ophthalmologist friends from the Army, now civilian consultants to the VA Department of Medicine and Surgery, I was able to interest Covalt in establishing a new program at a hospital away from the other nine centers, unhampered by previous routines, which would serve newly blinded service men when the Army and Navy programs were closed out. This was the genesis of the program at Hines Hospital. Whether or not such a center should be operated was one of the major points at issue when Irwin's advisory committee met on May 25, 1946. Our accomplishments thus far gave Covalt and me seats at the meeting by request of Irwin, although the committee was actually the affair of the Vocational Rehabilitation Service of the VA.

Father Carroll took the initiative by asking 51 specific questions which he and Miss Gruber had developed with respect to the program for blinded veterans. The ensuing eight hours of discussion were a revelation with respect to the skill with which the old guard of the VA had learned to fence with critics. Some answers to questions were forthcoming, some promised another day, some made to appear irrelevant, some beyond the agency's mandate. All was said with bureaucratic ceremony and correctness. But nothing was said which gave Father Carroll, Miss Gruber, or me encouragement that the agency had any intention of coming to grips with one major responsibility: coordinating its entire program. And certainly there was a strong undercurrent of opposition not only to running a center in the Vocational Rehabilitation Service, but also in the Department of Medicine and Surgery. The VA officials were already mustering support for the idea of contracting for services with private agencies, including substitutes for blind rehabilitation centers, since, in fact, there were no centers in the present-day sense.

The Report

None of this was wholly unexpected by Father Carroll. Taking all the documents furnished by the VA, he composed a 21-page report which pushed hard for coordination of blinded veterans affairs, and for a basic rehabilitation center. But beyond that he set forth vigorously and succinctly what the agency had done and left undone; which it should not have. With the concurrence of the other members of the committee it was dispatched to General Bradley on Oct. 3, 1946. On Oct. 10th a polite acknowledgment was sent from General Bradley's office. Then further communication was not forthcoming for weeks.

In September, Irwin had employed me at the American Foundation for the Blind to edit the *Outlook for the Blind* and perform other functions. At the behest of Covalt he had allowed my other functions of assisting with plans to establish a VA hospital program for blinded veterans which he had decided to go ahead with. On visits to Washington I very soon concluded that the VA had buried the advisory committee's report. Then I heard from a knowledgeable source that the report was "dead." I also learned that those who had given the report this fate were opposing the idea of establishing a center according to Covalt's plan.

I asked Covalt if he minded if I took our copy of the report to General Hawley with a message that it was important. Almost as unorthodox as I, he gave his blessing.

GENERAL HAWLEY

It was a quarter of five in the afternoon, but I went immediately to one of the general's secretaries and had a parley with her explaining the circumstances. She took the document from me, went in to see the General and came back in a few minutes saying he would read the report that night and see me in the morning.

When I saw him that morning, he had indeed read the advisory committee's report, and it was quite clear to him what people inside the VA were up to. Also, he had made up his mind what to do about it, which was to go straight ahead with the plan to establish a blind program in a VA hospital, no matter what anyone thought about it. He spoke as though, naturally, I would help him, and naturally I did, though in the end it meant the finish of my career as an editor.

In 1969, I wrote an article for the *Blindness Annual,* which minutely dissected the happenings that culminated in the opening of the Hines Rehabilitation Center on July 4, 1947 (Bledsoe, 1969). Titled "From Valley Forge to Hines" with the subtitle "Truth Old Enough to Tell," it gives in detail the agonies through which we put ourselves in getting the program established. Reviewing this document after another decade, seeing in sharp focus forgotten scenes in which I participated, is a little like looking on a distant scene through a telescope. And as various contentions are seen in relation to each other, along with the thought, "How shocking!" comes also the thought, "How necessary!"

One of the reasons why the Hines Center emerged and has endured is because it was a polished bone of contention. It was justified and rejustified, and re-rejustified both in spoken and written words countless times. Every check and balance which General Hines had left as his legacy to the VA was used against it. I will not tell this tale again in this chapter, since it is available for those who care to study altruistic politics, and it had very little to do with orientation and mobility itself.

However, there was one practical question and one philosophical one which are significant in retrospect. Philosophically Irwin objected to all centers for the blind, because he was totally committed to the idea of integrating blind people with the sighted. Like Howe he was eternally mistrustful of any program which might evolve into a home or asylum, "charitable tyranny . . . the consequences a clannish spirit, a defiant disposition, restlessness and discontent" (Bledsoe, 1969). Irwin gave in to Miss Gruber and supported the center, also giving me a leave of absence to help set it up. But he never felt easy with it.

In the practical area, when I had my conversation with General Hawley, Father Carroll was still holding out for the center to be a continuation of Avon, and along with that he and I differed over the emphasis which Hoover and I put on orientation and mobility.

During the war Father Carroll had been steeped in Avon philosophy and was indeed one of its best influences. But no one at Avon had an attitude which was much more than patronizing toward the Hoover method. When eventually Father Carroll became a believer, he summed up his early doubts by saying the Valley Forge approach to rehabilitation had been to the psyche through the body, whereas it came natural to him to approach the body through the psyche. He always remained doubtful about one of the basic tenets of Hoover and Valley Forge, namely that the great majority of the war blinded had enough philosophy dormant in them to manage their souls if they were given the practical help they needed to function on a practical basis. At bottom it was not basic to Hoover's profession, either as an educator or later as a doctor, to pry into the soul. It was a requirement of Father Carroll's, to which he adhered in a decidedly unorthodox way, but to which he adhered. In any case, when he saw the effect of Hoover's work on the whole human being, he became a staunch supporter, though at times a wayward one. Once the Hines program was established, he became one of the indispensable influences which helped to keep it alive, and later to transplant its method outside the VA.

Not to go into the intricacies of the controversy over whether or not the VA should have a center, suffice it to say that it involved not only the VA Departments of Medicine and Surgery and the Vocational Rehabilitation Department, as main contenders, but all the outside ophthalmological consultants, the heads of several residential schools, including Frampton, the Administrator of Federal Security, the professor of ophthalmology at Johns Hopkins, who had his own plan for a civilian-veteran center, the Blinded Veterans Association, the Solicitor of the VA, the Bureau of the Budget, Father Carroll, who at one point denounced the VA to the press, and finally President Harry Truman, who transferred all responsibility for rehabilitation from the Army back to the VA on an ordinary business day (May 31, 1947).

General Bradley and General Hawley had only agreed to give the VA two years of service, and they were both due to retire Dec. 31, 1947. Hawley, having viewed the shilly-shallying over the blinded veterans program for two years, sent for me in early September and told me Bradley had asked him to straighten out the blind program. He said that if I would take on a specially created job as coordinator of blinded veterans affairs, which would cut across medical and vocational rehabilitation, he would use all the influence he had to see that I could act, that Bradley wanted the position in the Vocational Rehabilitation Department, but he would see to it that I had freedom to set up the center in medical at Hines Hospital. To get me started immediately he would give me a slot in the Department of Medicine and Surgery until the position was set up in Vocational Rehabilitation. I had very little faith in H. V. Stirling, the director of Vocational Rehabilitation who was "old VA," and I knew opposed to the establishment of the center, but I had great faith in Hawley and events proved I was justified. I agreed to his plan.

I was sworn in to the position in medical on Sept. 15, but my first weeks on the job established the fact that I would have no cooperation whatsoever from Vocational Rehabilitation. There was endless parleying between the personnel staffs of medical and vocational rehabilitation; efforts of the latter to eliminate my responsibility for establishment of the center from my job description; their suggestion that the original proposed grade and salary be cut in half; my acceptance of this while refusing to give up an iota of authority promised. To this there was no reply. Before I had agreed to take the position, Hawley had introduced me to Stirling, gone over the terms laid down by Bradley for my hiring, and he had concurred with everything the General had proposed, but now it was as though this had never been.

While these developments were occurring I did what I could to get the Hines center going, went out to Hines, started getting a building put in readiness, got equipment in process of procurement, seven positions set up and had suitable personnel available, but the fact that everyone knew I was in administrative limbo made them anxious, to say the least, about doing my bidding.

In December I set all these facts forth in a memorandum to General Hawley, expressing my anxiety over what would happen to the center when he and General Bradley were gone. I took the memorandum to the General and he read it at once.

After a pause to reflect, he said, "Well, I'm awfully sorry."

And I never heard anybody say these words as though he were more truly sorry.

Then he said, "I could go to Mr. Stirling and say, 'Jesus Christ!' and 'God damn it!' But it wouldn't do any good. Stay here in the Department of Medicine and Surgery and get the center going."

Which is what I did. In the end it was necessary for the General himself to stay on after January 1st as a special assistant to the new administrator.

Then he issued a classic memorandum on January 14, 1948:

> To: Deputy Chief Medical Director
> From: Special Assistant to the Administrator
> Subj: Reassignment of Mr. C. W. Bledsoe
>
> 1. The Administrator has directed me to straighten out the difficulties which have been threatening the agreement made by General Bradley with the representatives of welfare organizations for the blind.
> 2. This memorandum will, therefore, relieve Mr. C. W. Bledsoe from further duty in the Department of Medicine and Surgery and will assign him to my office.
> 3. You will continue to furnish Mr. Bledsoe with office space and clerical assistance.

General Hawley had seen the new administrator, Carl Gray, and made this highly unorthodox arrangement. Thus for a few months the blinded veterans had an unusually privileged chain of authority, and suspended upon it, the center was hoisted into position.

HINES VETERANS ADMINISTRATION HOSPITAL

General Hawley perceived very readily that the crucial factor in setting up the Hines center was the leadership of the chief, and was one of the few doctors in the VA who did not demur over the first principle which I laid down: that it must be a blind person and a veteran.

General Hawley said he would take care of money for supplies and equipment, but I must take care of personnel. However, he read, amended and approved the job description I wrote for the chief of the center, which I think in retrospect was the key to its success. It said:

> The Chief of Physical Medicine and Rehabilitation of the Blind at Hines Hospital will have charge of the key operation in the training program offered blinded veterans of the Veterans Administration. He is in immediate charge of a staff of seven of whom he is one, all of whom are assigned to Hines Hospital.
>
> The importance of his position and of the training operation is not to be measured by its size in relation to other programs in the Veterans Administration. It should be stressed that insofar as there is an operating unit for training blinded veterans inside the Veterans Administration, the unit at Hines will be that unit, and whoever is responsible for the training there will be responsible for the training of all blinded veterans who wish to receive training from the Department of Medicine and Surgery of the Veterans Administration. The Chief of Physical Medicine Rehabilitation for the Blinded at Hines will be responsible for the training of these men, for everything that happens to them from their arrival to their departure, for actually putting into effect all that we know, and all that is discovered with regard to this type of social adjustment.

No matter what is offered a blind person, from a martini to braille, it is likely to be compared with sight. It has to be good, and it runs a little better chance of acceptance if it is offered by a blind person. This is something which workers for the blind can very easily forget, and it is a fatal form of forgetting. It is an evil decade when sighted people forget to listen to the way blind people feel about what is done for them. Blind people are then likely to listen with only half a disbelieving ear to what sighted people tell them they see.

One of the subjects I had repeatedly discussed with the doctors in the VA was the importance of having a blind chief of the center. Physicians have a hard time with this thought because they are so habituated to the principle that the patient must not treat himself. However, one of the services which St. Dunstan's did the American war blinded was to get Vail used to the idea that the program should have a blind leader. Now, as we were setting up the Hines program, he had recently become chief consulting ophthalmologist to the VA, and he came to our assistance. During the long suspense over whether or not we were to have a center I had been able to canvass people still close to the blinded veterans about who would make a good chief, and, almost invariably, the name of Russell Williams was mentioned. The single most inspiring recollection I can call to mind from my working life is the thought that I implemented a recommendation from Hoover and others, sought Russell Williams out, and persuaded him to take the position as chief of the program at Hines if and when it was available.

Dr. Kelso Carroll was the manager of Hines Hospital in 1947 when we established the center. After the publication of "From Valley Forge to Hines" in 1969 he wrote me:

> Of course there will never be another blind center such as we had, and there will never be another Russ Williams. For my money Russ is one of the really true Americans—accomplished and dedicated to his work, family and country. Do you know the only information and direction I gave him when he first reported for duty? I told him how to get to the center, but probably insulted him by offering him a car to get there. Speaking thus of Russ is not to take anything away from you, Miss Gruber and others who did organize the center.

Carroll himself was the ideal doctor–administrator of a hospital, one of the best of the pre-war VA employees, who had served in the Army Medical Corps during World War II, and returned to the VA in the company of General Hawley. His temperament was in fine balance between the sanguine and the saturnine. His heart was not one "too soon made glad." But he knew what was good, and his retrospective praise of the center gave Williams and me better assurance than any other we ever received that the Hines program had done what it was intended to do. Since this is the case, despite Carroll's thought that there never will be another blind center like Hines, I think it is worth while recording the principles under which we activated the program.

THE WILLIAMS PRINCIPLES

The first principle was realism with respect to the fact of blindness. This was stated very clearly by Williams many years later when he was asked what he thought of the term "blind center."

> To this he replied,
>
> I'm not very fussy about whether you call it a rehabilitation center for the blind or a blind center: I don't mind either of these terms. I can't think what else you might call it and use the term blind, and I think the term blind should be used. To me blindness isn't an ugly word at all, and it seems to me that the people who think it is have very little faith in the ability of blind people to meet the conditions of life with all the resources at their disposal. I can't really involve myself very seriously in arguments over whether a center or a school can be blind in fact. This seems to me a classic time-waster around meetings and conventions. (Williams, 1965)

Along with realism a second principle which Williams and I held above every other consideration was the principle that a program for blind people depends on the steadiness of the personnel who make it up. Especially in a training period the vicarious use of the eyes of the sighted is crucial. Not only outstanding willingness, but outstanding dependability is required.

Williams and I made it clear from the beginning that we did not want an imposing center built for the program, that we wanted adequate, unpretentious quarters for it, but that we would settle for nothing but what we thought best in the way of personnel.

Concerning this we had some very "square" ideas, about which I will again let Williams speak for himself,

> The formula is rather simple: someone who really gets a sincere pleasure out of the growth of someone else and who just seems to have good standards—good level-headedness about him. There are certain guiding factors which are followed by people who have respect for other people. These are not the people who seem to live to depreciate other people, and seem to get a real satisfaction out of it . . . I don't think the center should be made up of people who are very far out in any direction. (Williams, 1965)

Speaking for myself in retrospect, I wanted everybody connected with the center to be a little better than I was–at everything except the kind of palace politics I had to learn to get the center approved. I wanted them all to be above that sort of thing, practicing the really high calling of teaching the blinded veterans how to get around. I was looking for the best type of supporters for a leader I regarded as indispensable. And in order to give double insurance to his leadership, remembering my experience at Dibble Hospital, I insisted that he be the only totally blind staff member to start with. This was my decision, based on my own worldly wisdom, for which I made it understood Russ Williams was not to be blamed, perhaps the only decision about which I did not even ask his opinion.

It was in implementing our ideas with respect to personnel that we made full use of the unusual authority which General Hawley had secured for us. For the time being we ran into very little opposition of any kind. Everyone seemed to be standing back and giving us room, our friends not to hamper us, our opponents hoping we would fall on our faces. In fact the opponents were making one more stand in the VA Solicitor's office, trying to block a technical bulletin announcing the opening of the center, but Williams and I decided to leave this to Hawley and Carroll, who at the last ditch went to Washington, defended the idea of the center roundly and got the technical bulletin released. In the long run the delay was to our advantage, since it gave us time to recruit and train personnel.

Recruiting

In view of the way the question of the center had been debated publicly and heatedly, recruitment possibilities were not promising at the beginning of 1947. The Valley Forge orientors had by then almost all been mustered out of the Army and had no difficulty finding jobs for themselves or getting admitted to college and universities under the G.I. Bill of Rights. During the war I had lost many of my personal contacts in work for the blind, and in any case most teachers of the blind adhered to the philosophy that what we were doing was unnecessary. However, I had one staunch friend at the Maryland School for the Blind, Stafford "Charlie" Chiles, a manual training teacher. Our first piece of recruitment luck was inducing him to take on the initiation of whatever manual training we were to have.

From then our recruitment was inside the VA with two exceptions. General Hawley had met Miss Gruber and decided forthwith to invite her to be a consultant to the program. Somewhat later Hoover was also appointed. From the time I left Valley Forge I had attempted to persuade the VA to associate Hoover with the orientation and mobility program. However, even before leaving Valley Forge, encouraged by Randolph, Hoover had decided to study medicine. Thereafter, although both the VA and I would have preferred to have him do the things I had been doing, he was no longer available and resisted all our enticements to draw him back. In the years since, blind people in the United States have had in him an ophthalmologist who can interpret their needs to his brother physicians with acumen, compassion, and firsthand knowledge. He has perhaps served as consultant on blindness to more agencies for the blind than any other ophthalmologist in the world. However, his first appointment was by no means a shoo-in. It fell to me to ask a distinguished doctor in the VA to appoint him, when he was a medical student, consultant to the Department of Medicine and Surgery. Fortunately, the doctor was E. H. Cushing, a man of vision, but I will never forget his face as he said, "A medical student!"

I said, "All I ask is that you interview him."

He did, sent for me, and simply nodded.

We also appointed Harry Spar, of the Industrial Home for the Blind in Brooklyn, as consultant on manual training, and he, Hoover, and Miss Gruber were the only representatives of work for the blind, looking over our shoulders, and at times taking an active part in the setting up of the center. Miss Gruber spent weeks at Hines assisting both in the selection process and training of the staff.

How we did this has been described twice elsewhere, both in "From Valley Forge to Hines" (Bledsoe, 1969) and from the instructor's point of view in "The First Fifteen Years at Hines" (Malamazian, 1970). It is worth reviewing, however, because it illustrates the effect of Williams' leadership qualities, which made the most of opportunities the rest of us put in his way.

At the time when I became associated with the VA, Dr. John Davis was fathering and bringing into the world the paramedical specialty of corrective therapy, a phase of physical medicine and rehabilitation nicknamed "the coach approach" and defined more formally as "exercise therapy." Davis was a psychologist who had been associated with Dr. Adolf Meyer, the psychobiologist, who when heading the psychiatric service at Johns Hopkins gave as much attention to training ward personnel as he did to his residents. Many of Davis' concepts were similar to those of Hoover, and he suggested that some of his corrective therapists could be retrained as orientation and mobility instructors. He further disclosed that the corrective therapists at Hines Hospital were a blue ribbon group, their nucleus having been formed by an elite unit trained in the Army medical corps by Dr. Allan Stinchfield. All were soldiers who had been wounded, reconditioned for combat and then selected to remain at the center, reconditioning other wounded soldiers. Obviously this gave promise of rather staunch and likable personality traits. The chief of the corrective therapy section at Hines, Carl Purcell, had been one of Stinchfield's unit. Williams was able to accomplish the very delicate bureaucratic maneuver of persuading him and his chief, Dr. Louis Newman, to allow us to interview the Hines corrective therapists and offer them the opportunity to be trained as orientation and mobility instructors. This was similar to our having a choice of the panels of specially selected men sent into Valley Forge Hospital, but even better since the corrective therapists had already proven themselves in many areas of importance to orientation and mobility. They had had education and experience in physical education, kinesiology, anatomy, psychology, remedial exercise, posture and gait training.

THE HINES PATTERN FOR INSTRUCTORS

Twelve men applied for the five orientation and mobility positions which had been established. All were interviewed by Williams, Miss Gruber, Stafford Chiles, and myself. Williams interviewed candidates by getting each to guide him on a long walk about the hospital. My interview consisted of giving each candidate a lesson in orientation and mobility blindfolded and then getting them to give the same lesson back to me while I wore the blindfold. Miss Gruber, always a superlative listener, then had a long talk with the candidate during which she extracted quantities of information both about him and the hospital. Stafford Chiles by contrast interviewed by talking man to man and, if the candidate was boastful, finding out what he was boastful about. After this we four spent hours discussing the candidates together, after which Williams meditated and made his decision. Some attention was paid to the papers of the candidates, but far more to our mere knowledge of humanity.

The names of the first six mobility specialists chosen suggest that the interviewers had something like divine guidance. They were John Malamazian, Stanley Suterko, Alfred Dee Corbett, Edward Thuis, Lawrence Blaha, and Edward Mees, each one almost apostolic in character, Malamazian as the St. Peter and Suterko as the St. Paul. All became past masters at the art of teaching orientation and mobility to blinded veterans and to other instructors. Malamazian became to Hines what Debetaz was to Seeing Eye, the preserver of its integrity year in and year out, eventually to be its first sighted chief without the slightest objection from anyone, including myself. Suterko was to become the missionary of the Hines methods to the outer world, first at other VA hospitals, then at Western Michigan University, and later outside the United States. Lawrence Blaha activated the training program for instructors at Los Angeles State. But before that, the six trained the first 80 blinded veterans to go through the Hines program, set in motion constant refinement of the Hoover method, and established an esprit de corps which was to make the staff perhaps the most stable unit in the entire VA and the most admired. In the 1950s more instructors were selected and trained to meet the needs of the Korean War blinded. The original six assisted Williams in recruiting and training this group, who for the next decade worked out methods which in the sixties were to become the substance of the master's degree university training programs, described in Chapter 20 of this volume.*

Williams had, and has, an extremely easygoing way of relating to people and the art of finding something in common with almost everyone he meets. Like Abraham Lincoln and King George V, he gives the deceptive impression that he is an ordinary man, whereas in fact he is most uncommon. Behind his unpretentious dignity is a very carefully thought out philosophy of rehabilitation, with principles and practices, which he hammered out on his own anvil and which he imparted to his staff day by day rather than in formal statements. The philosophy was never more active than when he chose personnel. He never made the mistake of employing an individual to serve the interests of anyone but the blinded veterans. He never made the mistake of employing an individual to rehabilitate him. The center was for the blinded veterans, not to rehabilitate its own personnel. But after hiring them Williams was constantly teaching his staff and learning from them. He had a real gift for choosing the creatively innovative and excluding the brilliant rebel program smasher. He had the great advantage of tapping the resources of corrective therapy at a stage which Alan Gregg described as "healthy adolescence" (Gregg, 1951). Working for Williams, boys became adults.

One of his happiest personnel choices was Donald Blasch, who went to Hines in 1951 as a counseling psychologist. Destined to his future position as chairman of the Department of Blind Rehabilitation at Western Michigan University, he very soon became Williams' philosophical sounding board, as well as a practical and profound psychotherapist for the blinded veterans in training. Blasch was very gifted in perceiving signs of mental health and strength which manifested themselves without the aid of therapy and not tampering with them.

RUSSELL WILLIAMS

Williams himself was a prime example of an individual whose handling of blindness a therapist would have been much put to it to improve. A technical sergeant in the artillery, he was blinded after the Normandy invasion, knew he was blind immediately, and was told in the hospital that he would be blind. He took it in such a way that the doctor who told him asked him to bolster the courage of a blind soldier in the next bed who the doctor did not feel was yet ready to be told he was blind. This Williams did.

The burden of another blinded veteran was put upon Williams within a few days of being told of his own prognosis. Whatever mystique is, he

*The names of these men, who deserve to be recorded, are Lee Farmer, Edward Polfus, Richard Russo, Richard Bugielski, Franklin Wood, James Lassen, James Enzinna, Cecil Miller, Raymond Brooks, Oscar Olivia, Norman Roche, Jack Henschen, Walter Olenek, Everett Bjork, Lloyd Widerberg, Berdel Wurzberger, Robert Cochman, Clovis Semmes, and Robert Smith.

has it, which Greear, Randolph, and particularly the ward officer, Dr. Linus Sheehan, readily perceived as he passed through Valley Forge and Avon.

He had been an Indiana schoolmaster and basketball coach before the war and they decided these were ideal qualifications to do the kind of counseling the other soldiers needed—a decision more pleasing to soldiers he served than to the personnel office, but the kind the eye chiefs had the authority to make if they chose, and they did so choose.

Though he had no degree in psychology or social work, and never would, he had observed everything the training programs had to offer at Valley Forge and Avon, where he was one of the soldiers who managed to acquit himself well without a cane. Back at Valley Forge, after conferring with Hoover, he took it up again and became a master at the art. In addition to learning the techniques of managing life without sight he had been observing the rehabilitation processes seething about him shrewdly, quietly, and compassionately. He had more than his share of people who saw possibilities in him and wanted to steer his career in one way or another. It was providential for the other blinded veterans that he chose the job at Valley Forge which took him back to the source of the war blind program and gave him an opportunity to see how it affected individuals and groups while no longer a part of it himself. In later years it was a recurrent phenomenon for trainees to want to emulate Williams' career. His reply to this was, "Not until you learn a good deal more about yourself, and all those people you want to help."

I believe it was at Valley Forge that he learned one of the most important lessons a blind leader of the blind can learn: to objectify beyond his own experience, not to think his way is the only way or that because he overcame a particular obstacle all blind people can, to determine in fact what it is reasonable to expect of all, or most, blind people.

By the time Williams came back to Valley Forge the staff there had more to offer in higher learning about blindness than any graduate school in the country. Not only was he associated with Hoover, but Martha Miller, a blind social worker, whom Irwin had been educating since her school days, became one of his colleagues, devoted to teaching him everything she knew. Paul Conlan, on leave from his position as head of the Michigan rehabilitation program, was his immediate supervisor. Louisa Walker, principal on leave from the South Carolina School for the Blind, and James Moxom, a blind graduate of the Maryland School for the Blind, both braille teachers, made friends with him, and were two more people who wanted to tell him what they knew, as was Ilah Oja, a typing teacher. These people organized themselves into a kind of morning seminar discussing with each other, case by case, what was emerging with respect to blindness in war. Miss Gruber was a frequent visitor, already sure in her own mind that Williams' fate was with the other blinded veterans. She formed a friendship with him that led to a remarkable correspondence which helped to build the Hines program.

Williams' philosophy of rehabilitation was best recorded in a series of statements he made for an interview on centers, which was published in the *Blindness Annual*, 1965 (Williams, 1965).

> There are some extremely difficult conditions imposed upon the staff of a center. It is a group of people interposed between two groups of doubters. On the one side of this staff is the client group who come in to this relationship without sufficient experience to realize that blindness can be lived out in quite a wholesome fashion.
>
> They are entering blindness for the most part, since we are talking about centers, after having seen. They have come from a seeing society and bring into blindness many of the attitudes which are generally found to exist among seeing people. So that's why I call them doubters, and they come to the center to have their doubts removed.

Williams' faith in his principles was put to the test many times, but never more than when the chief of physical medicine wanted to deny a blind epileptic patient the use of a wood lathe. Williams put his job on the line in this case because in his opinion the lathe was the only thing holding that particular veteran to his rehabilitation, and he said no one had the right to deprive him of the privilege of getting hurt.

Ever since Valley Forge we have been drawing to the attention of medical men the fact that it is as important to save a personality as to save a life, and this to me was very complete support of this idea.

ORIENTATION AND MOBILITY BOTTLED UP AT HINES

It will doubtless puzzle the present-day reader that the practices and principles developed in the Hines program should have remained almost exclusively resources of the veterans for a number of years. As an official responsible for the program, I have been reproached for this of late years almost as much as I was reproached for being one of the godfathers in the beginning.

Certainly VA officials had no desire to keep the art exclusively for their clients. Efforts were made in the 1950s to share the skills of Hines instructors with the field of work for the blind. But none of us realized then how time-consuming this would be. A few instructors whom Hoover trained in his spare time while he was at Johns Hopkins Medical School were a mere handful. Curious agencies sent representatives to Hines for periods of two weeks, but this did little more than confuse them about what was going on.

The Film

In 1952 the VA went to considerable trouble and expense to make a film, *The Long Cane,* depicting the Hines program (Veterans Administration, 1952). It was in one respect an enormous success, in another the next thing to a disaster. It was realistic. (Blinded veterans reenacted scenes from their lives in it.) It was so great an artistic success that it was shown at the Edinburgh Festival. It is one of the few training films of the 1950s which is still shown today. It proved a surefire mechanism to make converts of intelligent sighted public officials, including sighted workers for the blind. But the force of the message was so visual it was a dud as far as the blind population was concerned. This included important blind workers for the blind in positions of influence, whose minds were already made up that the Hines program was an impertinence because it was sprung from Valley Forge.

The makers of the film took too literally the "normality" of blind people and their "enjoyment" of movies. Quite a few years after the film had been made and shown I discovered that Hiram Chappell, one of the most knowing of Clunk's blind staff members, simply did not take in the basic action of Hoover's method, though he had sat through the film at least twice. A man of very fixed opinions, but also totally honest, he heard me say something one day which made him wonder if he had understood what the Valley Forge method was. When I demonstrated it to him by touch, he admitted he had never really understood it, and indicated he would have adopted it if he had been at the beginning of his career instead of at the end.

What we were up against with die-hard civilians, including those working in the rehabilitation field, became clear in 1953 when Father Carroll made an attempt to organize mobility instructors at what has always been referred to as "the Gloucester Conference." Though it was described in *Time* magazine, no formal report was ever published. An informal gathering which had great charm, it was actually sponsored by Father Carroll's family, who entertained 30 key people in work for the blind and kindred professions in summer cottages at Gloucester, Massachusetts. Father Carroll's purpose was to persuade the few mobility specialists then in existence to form a sort of association or union and thus persuade agencies for the blind to accept them as a legitimate part of rehabilitation services.

It was quite clear to the mobility specialists

after a few days that they could hardly hope for more than janitor or valet status from the agencies for the blind at the time. Russell Williams, Stanley Suterko, and I were all at the conference and saw this plainly. We decided that the only thing to do was let the Hines program prove itself under the protection of the VA without entangling alliances, at least for the time being. Elizabeth Hutchinson from Seeing Eye was also at the conference and she agreed with us. Father Carroll sent her and Williams out of the room three times to form a union. But they came back three times without a report.

Father Carroll was furious with all of us the night the conference broke up. But early the next morning, having been to mass, he told us goodbye with authentic forgiving grace. I thought then, and I think now, that we would have done harm had we followed the course he was promoting before expertise had been sufficiently perfected or demonstrated.

Punted Down the Field

Not until Joseph Clunk had been succeeded by another chief of services for the blind, and another, and another, did the hazards of bureaucracy produce a succès fou, which some might regard as an act of God. After the center at Hines had been set up, and at the end of the year I had agreed to give the project, I had resigned, intending fully to try my hand at novel-writing again. Almost immediately, however, I was asked to take consultant status in the VA, was called upon more and more when the Korean Conflict broke out, found myself interested as well as engaged, and finally was sworn in once again, this time as Chief of Services for the Blind in the Department of Medicine and Surgery. In that position I conducted a survey of the status of the war blinded in the postwar setting, a joint undertaking with Social Service. Within three months, 386 social workers visited 1,949 blinded veterans of World War II and Korea with service-connected disabilities, which was more than 98 percent of the entire group. I found things which needed to be done. Once again I was prodding people into action. My proddings wore out my welcome. Eventually a tight budget enabled officials to abolish my job with great regret and punt me down the field to the Office of Vocational Rehabilitation, a little uneasy about what I would do there.

This was in August 1958 and General Hawley wrote me a letter which said,

> the situation is very different from the days when General Bradley was administrator. He is a man completely immune to political pressures; and his only objective was to do well what was to be done. The only order he ever gave me was to make the best medical services possible. He never disapproved any recommendation I made to him and he gave me full authority to issue instructions in his name. This perfect atmosphere in which to do a creditable job disappeared on 30 November when he closed his desk and left the Veterans Administration. (Hawley, personal communication, 1958)

How right the general was we had already found when Dr. Carroll retired and Hines had a new manager, a congenital tamperer with everything God and man had ever created. On one of my visits to Hines before I left the agency I was startled to have him ask why I did not find a better job for Williams. This was about the time when the manager's own right-hand man said publicly that the blind center had brought Hines Hospital more authentic good will than all the rest of the hospital's programs put together.

It was plain to me as it was to others that the manager was dangerously ambitious to leave his mark by doing startling things, and along this line he would like to damp down the reputation of Williams and the center.

He was matched in central office by the coterie which was going about the business of ousting me by taking advantage of the shortage of funds to say that the blind program was in such good shape that my job was no longer necessary, especially in view of the small number of blinded veterans (a perennial bureaucratic bugbear to blind programs).

Some well-meaning friendly advisers in central office urged me to attempt to save my job by going to my congressman. This I declined to do, instead writing a letter to go up through the VA hierarchy to my superior and his and his, protesting against the abolition of the position, but stating that if it were retained I would under no circumstances occupy it. Imperviously the VA officials let my protest go through at all levels. I therefore continued my protest in a letter to President Eisenhower, asking for the privilege of an interview.

At this juncture apparently someone in the President's office called Sumner Whittier, newly appointed administrator of the VA, and suggested that he give personal attention to the blind program. He summoned me to an interview. In our conversation it was apparent that up to then he had been told very little about the story of the blinded veterans.

He said, however, that he had looked into the whole subject of my central office position and that "everything had been done wrong," that dealing with doctors was like beating on a soft pillow. Then he said he understood I was leaving the organization no matter what he did about the position, and I assured him this was the case. Then he asked me what I thought he should do. I had regained amateur status as a counselor of state.

Successors

I told him that in my opinion workers for the blind would never let him rest unless he retained the position and filled it, and if he appointed Williams to it the old guard in the VA would never dare touch him. Whittier had at least heard what a good job Williams was doing and protested that this would be a great sacrifice for the Hines program. I agreed, but told him there were 1,949 other blinded veterans with service-connected disabilities, that some of them were rising in the rehabilitation field and Williams could find a replacement for himself. I suggested Loyal E. Apple as an example.

This parting advice was my legacy to the old guard in the VA. Miss Gruber and Hoover backed it up vigorously, as did the Blinded Veterans Association, and Whittier actually followed it. Williams became as universal a favorite in central office as he had been at Hines, and from there was able to fend off the meddling of the Hines manager until he learned what not to tamper with. Apple was appointed to succeed Williams, and almost immediately there was a battle with the manager over whether the blinded veterans should be allowed to fill their own cigarette lighters. It ended in a compromise of sorts, however, which left the manager somewhat unnerved about the program, and thereafter he busied himself with other things and let his assistant deal with the blind center. Apple acquitted himself extremely well. He had been chosen for having some of the same characteristics as Williams, but distinct individuality, which subsequently found its way into the establishment of the center for blinded veterans at the Palo Alto Veterans Hospital. At that time John Malamazian became chief of the Hines center, a clear case of a man being chosen for his qualifications without regard to whether he was blind or sighted.

During the interregnum after Williams went to central office and before Apple was appointed, Donald Blasch came to the fore in the role of something more than a counseling psychologist. He was acting chief of the center for a number of months, and during that time acquitted himself with judgment as a stabilizing force which foreshadowed the major role he was to play in establishing the graduate program at Western Michigan University.

There is no doubt in my mind that the people in the VA who set up the chain reactions which moved several of us about on the chess board were trying to contain and restrain our creative spirits. That they should unwittingly have had an opposite effect accounts to some extent for what might be regarded as my superstition about the good auspices which governed the fate of orientation and mobility. It was extremely important that it be given time to mature unhampered by careless innovation for a decade, but equally important that it emerge to stand the test of general consumption at the end of that time. Events decided this in a way which strongly suggest the idea that, "There is a destiny which shapes our ends, rough-hew them as we will." This is sometimes a little hard to see in a time which glories in its rough hewing.

One of the unrecognized problems with American institutions is a national prejudice against anyone doing his job with easy comfortable grace as though he liked it, the assumption that without tension to the breaking point an individual is not earning his salt. We do not seem to want anyone to stay in any one spot long enough to get a firm grasp upon his situation. During my time in the VA there were four people in the hierarchy above me up to the president, making sixteen people with other things to do who could make or mar the program. Not one of the four in office knew what to do when we developed the crisis over my leaving. This is not so surprising when you consider they were short-termers with the entire medical and VA program to learn about during the short-term.

In the VA I began to learn how difficult it is to give even the most willing coprofessional in the helping professions a grasp of what work for the blind is all about. One unlucky administrator of the VA emerged from viewing a training film about Hines to say in the presence of reporters, "Well, I guess that will put the guide dog out of business."

After Seeing Eye had gotten the congressman from New Jersey to enlighten him, he was somewhat wiser, but not enough to refrain from boasting to a visiting blinded veteran that the VA was doing everything possible for the blinded veterans. This was at a time when the doctors were blocking the publication of the survey of blinded veterans which we had made, the familiar excuse being a shortage of funds, and the veteran, a sociologist from Harvard knowing this, drew it to the administrator's attention. The result was that the study was published, largely through force of the embarrassment, which has been the unfortunate motivation for a great many measures taken by the VA in behalf of blinded veterans. Most of the in-and-out administrators in my time were well-meaning men caught with want of knowledge about blindness, who never met their own specialists on the subject until they were in dire trouble.

MARY E. SWITZER

In the Office of Vocational Rehabilitation of the Department of Medicine and Surgery I found myself in an entirely different world from the VA. Mary Elizabeth Switzer was director of the agency, and a management improvement firm had just made a survey of her program which had summed up its report with "What Mary wants, Mary gets."

Fortunately what Mary wanted was "the good of the world," toward which she said she "connived," and she did night and day, seven days a week, with courage, stamina, salty common sense, lively, idealistic imagination, and, she said, "above all, hope."

Her excellent mind was in a head which seemed to have been sculpted for public appearances. Like the old Shakespearean actresses, she had large features. A fine fleece of silver white hair came to her beautifully modeled forehead in a widow's peak. She had a strong jaw and clear blue eyes. Her features which may have been formidable in earlier years had a weathered grace which both individuals and crowds found arresting and appealing. About the time I went to her organization, reporters had begun to write about her as a "grande dame." Certainly she had all the better elements that the term implies. Yet she was anything but a snob. "Great commoner" would have been a better description of her than "grande dame."

The first staff meeting at which I saw her preside was on the budget. Dwight Eisenhower was president and Maurice Stans was director of the Bureau of the Budget.

Miss Switzer sat for a long time listening to

the croaking of her misanthropes. One of her legs was crossed over the other, and she was swinging her foot as though she were kicking Plato's "large and sleepy horse, the State."

When the lugubrious finally stopped talking she spoke, saying, "Well, if I were in Mr. Stans' position, I might do as he does. Everyone knows there is a double standard. One for the military and one for the rest of us. But I've decided not to get emotional about it, because when we get into Congress, we've got the votes."

The votes she did indeed have. As time went on her prestige at hearings in Congress was unique. Her skill at extracting money from the legislators for her thousands of research and demonstration grants for the good of the physically handicapped was proverbial.

Presiding over the grants, she wore grandma half-moon glasses and knitted, but could keep track of the cash approved from grant to grant better than those with pencils in hand. It almost goes without saying that, after her early years understudying and supporting individuals who were at the top, when she first emerged as head of an agency, there was some unrest among the males about her, who at first mistook her style for weakness and fretted themselves unduly over her knitting at meetings. They would have estimated her more wisely, as they afterwards learned to do, if they had spent a little less of their lives reading about statistics and a little more about Elizabeth I of England, the Empress Maria Theresa of Austria, and Catherine the Great of Russia. Like the strong queens in history, Mary Switzer was feminine in her speech, in her surroundings, in personal dealings. And gradually she got people to see there was nothing wrong with her ways, no deficiency in logic, nor on occasion unalterable resolution.

Like the above-mentioned women heads of state, she had long-term trusted supporters, including the secretaries of Health, Education, and Welfare, as they came and went.

"She always weeps when they go," said Joseph Hunt, her right-hand man, "but ends up by practically marrying the next one."

Her devil's advocate was Samuel Marta, an old Bureau of the Budget man, whom she dispatched to the VA to see what we were up to when we did the social work follow-up study of blinded veterans. The chasm between the VA and HEW was so great I cared very little about his criticism, which we had not invited, and which had to do with our not attempting to pry into the personal incomes of the veterans with service-connected disabilities. Apart from this I had an impression he acquired a reluctant admiration for the work we had done. I believe it was on the strength of this with strong backing from Miss Gruber and Father Carroll that Miss Switzer welcomed me into her agency.

I had had two encounters with her before that. One was over the abortive attempt made by Dr. Alan Woods, the professor of ophthalmology at Johns Hopkins, to establish a joint civilian—veteran center for the newly blinded. The other was over the spending of $25,000 left in the care of an ophthalmologist to be spent for the benefit of the blind. Mary Switzer and I had tried to get him to set up revolving loan funds to make it possible for truculent promising young blind people to buy and pay for psychiatry without benefit of agency supervision. But the ophthalmologist was all surgeon, said there were no good psychiatrists in his city, and gave the money to the agencies.

When I went to HEW, Mary Switzer had just persuaded Louis Rives to take the job of Acting Chief of Services for the Blind, and I was put on his staff. I had met him only once before, at an American Association of Workers for the Blind convention. He had made a statement at one session concerning the VA, some detail of which I disagreed with, but I was sufficiently impressed by him not to take the floor and correct him on the spot. After the meeting we had had a brief pleasant exchange, and I thought he gave hope of better things with respect to orientation and mobility in HEW. But, this was dashed when I heard he was not interested in being Chief of Services for the Blind permanently, and was only acting at the convenience of Miss Switzer. But there is an old rule of institutions that there is nothing so permanent as the temporary, and he remained a reluctant, but superlative head of the unit for almost ten years. During that time rehabilitation of the blind had a kind of golden age. Ten million dollars was spent on 183 research and demonstration projects of wide diversity.

LOUIS RIVES

Rives was, and is, an accomplished negotiator with the better traits of a southern gentleman and a Yankee horse trader. He has a not-unbecoming cloak of cynicism, which he can wear against the chill of the world, but I very shortly discovered he was a warm-hearted, spacious man, with a magnificent brain. And I never had a difference with him over what was worth a good laugh, or what a good laugh is worth. I suppose it is necessary to mention that he is blind, but in no one that I ever knew did it seem more incidental. A graduate of the William and Mary Law School, he had worked in the Office of General Council of Health, Education, and Welfare and then had done a great service for the Office of Vocational Rehabilitation in designing the state–federal agreements to implement the Vocational Rehabilitation Act of 1954.

Rives had a real gift for using whatever personnel he had under him. His indoctrination in rehabilitation had been through a course in vocational placement given by Clunk, where he had heard little good of the VA program, but he listened to what I had to say about orientation and mobility, and I presume also to Hiram Chappell, with whom I became great friends, having lunch with him every day, and thereby disabusing him of the misconceptions he had gotten from seeing *The Long Cane.* I do not know whether Rives would recall that I pressed the subject of orientation and mobility too enthusiastically, but in any case it was clear in time he was making ready to invest.

During the weeks of my getting acquainted with Rives and Hiram Chappell, I saw little of Miss Switzer, but it was her habit to find some means of getting personally acquainted with every member of her staff and communicating with them directly at will. One day she asked for a copy of my novel, which I furnished her.

It so happened that one of the most sympathetic characters in the book is a spinster librarian with a great sense of civic responsibility, a heart of gold, and a caustic tongue. It was almost a portrait before I met her of Miss Switzer's lifelong friend, unofficial consultant and sounding board, Isabella Diamond, who was Treasury librarian for twenty-five years. My book has brought me many more friends than work for the blind has, and such was the case with Miss Diamond and Miss Switzer, whom it gave the feeling that I understood their mission and purpose in life. Miss Switzer then began to consult me directly on many subjects, including orientation and mobility.

At this juncture Rives revealed how broad-gauged he was. He told me frankly he saw this situation developing, and though it sometimes bypassed him, he knew I would keep him informed and communicate with Miss Switzer for the good of the blind. This I can honestly say that I did. Rives himself had an excellent relationship with her. His predecessors had foolishly tried to exclude her from decision making with regard to services for the blind. He made use of her brain and powers of persuasion to the full. When Miss Diamond retired as Treasury librarian he brought her also into the fold by making her editor of the newly established *Blindness Annual* of the American Association of Workers for the Blind, which was to become the organ through which orientation and mobility got a hearing nationally. Miss Diamond's focus on blindness was an extremely important pipeline into Miss Switzer's consciousness. They were on a par intellectually. Miss Switzer had a Radcliffe-trained brain, and Miss Diamond had gone to Bryn Mawr. They had a house together and forever pooled their wits against ignorance, superstition, and every other kind of skulking evil which might impede the flourishing of the human race. Rives and I saw to it that rehabilitation of the blind had a regular place on the agenda, and orientation and mobility came into its own as will be seen by the following letter of June 30, 1960, written to Sumner G.

Whittier, Administrator, Veterans Administration, with its "great commoner" postscript.

Dear Mr. Whittier:

For several years we have watched with interest the development of the Veterans Administration program of physical re-training of newly blinded veterans at the Veterans Administration Hospital at Hines, Illinois. Our advisors agree that in improving methods and techniques in this important aspect of a blind person's life, the system established by Mr. Russell Williams and his group of orientation therapists at Hines Hospital, has no counterpart elsewhere.

At the same time, the Office of Vocational Rehabilitation has become increasingly aware of the need for basic training of blind people in general competence, especially in the management and handling of themselves as blind persons. With this in mind we have made a training grant to Boston College to enable that institution to train mobility instructors of the blind, not only in motor skills, but in some depth concerning the psychological implications of what they are doing and the nature of social responsibility entailed in rehabilitation.

I have long had a very real concern that our two agencies use the resources available to blind people in a cooperative way. I see clearly a need for exchange, both of ideas and people, and I would like to make this possible. It is very clear that on a country-wide basis there will have to be more courses and different kinds of courses in mobility, not only for blind people but for their instructors. Though the authorities on the subject so far have tended to avoid refresher courses for instructors, we see this as one of the primary needs of the present. This possibility and others I would like to have freely and cooperatively discussed between our two agencies.

In my opinion this would best be accomplished if we could arrange for responsible group action by members of our staffs most familiar with these matters, both in theory and in detail. It seems it would also be wise to draw into in these counsels persons from Boston College and other training institutions as they entered the field.

I understand a real respect exists between your Chief of Blind Rehabilitation, Mr. Russell Williams, and our Chief of Services to the Blind, Mr. Louis H. Rives, Jr., each of whom is blind and each of whom contributes a different type of experience to rehabilitation.

Without our mutual action I am afraid a skill which is really useful will not reach the great majority of blind people for many years to come. This is something so important to the future of blind people that I think you and I should get together personally and see to it that the machinery is set up and the policies are carried out which will make sure that something good and lasting is accomplished.

Sincerely yours,
Mary E. Switzer
Director

Hon. Sumner G. Whittier
Administrator
Veterans Administration
Washington 25, D.C.
cc: Mr. Hunt
Mr. Garrett

P.S. A fascinating effort but we need to bring the boys together.*

Orientation and Mobility Grants

The grant to Boston College which Mary Switzer mentioned in her letter to Sumner Whittier inaugurated the use of Vocational Rehabilitation during the decade of the sixties to fund a massive constellation of orientation and mobility grants which were vehicles for much of the progress described by Wiener and Sifferman in Chapter 20. In *Blindness* (1971) under the title "Orientation and Mobility Fans Out" the remarkable breakthrough which occurred has been delineated succinctly with impressive statistical detail. In this national and then international movement Donald Blasch proved to be an indispensable

*Written by hand by MES on original

pivot figure in conjunction with Dean George Mallinson at Western Michigan University. Blasch now knows more orientation and mobility instructors and more about them than anyone in the world who is not one. Unfortunately in work for the blind it is simply not true that no one is indispensable. Many good services come to a halt when people die, and would never have existed without them in the first place. In my opinion Blasch is one of the elements without which orientation and mobility would not have spread as it has.

Wiener and Sifferman (chapter 20) show that the spur which was to set so many people in motion was a conference held in June 1960 at the American Foundation for the Blind. Out of the conference came support of the graduate courses at Boston College, Western Michigan University, and California State of Los Angeles. Out of the graduate courses came the instructors who put into operation demonstrations of orientation and mobility teaching in 30 communities in 22 states. Paid for by the Vocational Rehabilitation Administration, it was these demonstrations which finally convinced agencies for the blind that mobility instruction was a basic and legitimate part of rehabilitation service for the blind.

An important lesson in public administration would be lost if it were not recorded that at the time Miss Switzer made these grants they were regarded by respected experts on blindness as a most dubious investment. Indeed it was still a rather unpopular dubious investment, and it would have helped to solidify her popularity with some heads of state agencies for the blind if she had turned her back on orientation and mobility altogether. It was only through the skillful diplomacy of Louis Rives and H. A. Wood that the idea of endorsing orientation and mobility was given approval by the National Council of State Agencies for the Blind as "something Mary and Lou want."

Miss Switzer was a firm believer in putting money into her causes and talking about them in language that could be understood. She was tireless both in making speeches to skeptical audiences and keeping guardianship of her budget at every stage. She never lost sight of the fact that most audiences, including congressional committees, needed to learn the ABCs of rehabilitation over and over and that you cannot run services for the severely handicapped without cash.

"You can't get people behind causes," she often admonished her staff, "by talking to yourselves."

After she had acquired a certain number of honorary degrees (she had twenty-two), she declined to accept any more unless she were invited to accept with a speech about rehabilitation. The speeches were simple, to the point and practical, drawing attention to such facts as the income taxes paid by rehabilitants after receiving rehabilitation services.

"Nothing turns Mary on like a budget," said her successor John Twiname.

"She's tough. That means we respect her over here," said James Hyde, a blinded veteran who had risen high in the councils of the Bureau of the Budget.

The remarkable thing about such a statement from a budget man was that Mary Switzer often frightened her own staff by the originality and scope of her programs, such as dance therapy for the deaf at Gallaudet, appreciation of art for the blind, and when she first began to support it, orientation and mobility undoubtedly seemed rash to some of her veteran staff. Fears of her in fiscal matters were generated in part because she was the first big spender in the federally financed rehabilitation program, following frugal beginnings in the 1920s, the Depression, and World War II. Roosevelt himself had been remarkably skeptical about money spent on rehabilitation. To one of the rehabilitation experts of his time is attributed the dictum, "Nothing large, expensive, or technical."

Accounting

This was not Mary Switzer's policy by any means. To some people she seemed extravagant in administering public funds. In my opinion she was generous, but prudent, and I paid close attention over the course of more than ten years to money she spent on research and training programs for the blind. In fact, this became one of my particular functions in Services for the Blind along with being the guardian of orientation and mobility and optical aids projects. Beginning in 1965 Miss Switzer made me coauthor of a yearly account of where and how vocational rehabilitation money was spent on programs for the blind. This was published each year in *Blindness Annual.* Services for the Blind was the only unit in Vocational Rehabilitation which published such reports, separated from material on other categories of the disabled, and in a publication which reached a large number of workers in the specialty reported.

From these reports it is a matter of public (and easily available) record that from 1960 until 1970 Mary Switzer's administration paid $3,200,000 as matching funds to universities for salaries of faculty and fellowships for students learning to teach orientation and mobility in the master's degree programs. This was at Boston College, Western Michigan University, and California State.

In the same ten years the Vocational Rehabilitation Administration paid $1,113,298 to thirty communities as seed money to pay the salaries of instructors in demonstration programs. It fell to me to draft the guidelines of these projects and follow their progress.

During the demonstration period approximately 1,500 blind individuals, including blind children, were given an average of 30 lessons each in orientation and mobility, making the cost per lesson about $25 at the demonstration stage. Extravagant this may appear to some people, but, if you believe, as I do, that orientation and mobility is one of the secrets of preserving the personality of the individual who loses his sight, the cost is on a par with psychotherapy, and not excessive. An overwhelming demand for mobility instructors which followed the demonstration projects seemed to confirm this emphatically.

The very first day at Valley Forge, talking with the first World War II blinded veteran to whom I was assigned, to get things straight in my own mind, I asked him if he minded the fact that I had not been in combat, and was not blind.

He said, "No. I'm glad you haven't been in combat, haven't been hurt, and if you're going to teach me, I'm glad you can see."

There was nothing whatsoever I had to add to that man's philosophy or management of his emotions, or his grace under pressure.

But other instructors and I did teach him orientation and mobility. He was grateful, and I think it kept him from becoming a handicapped person.

Defenders

Nevertheless, all such experience notwithstanding, hardly had the training grants at universities been approved before their opponents began to suggest that if they were a success, federal aid should be phased out. And when they were a success this thought was spoken more loudly. To this kind of talk, when everyone had had their say, Mary Switzer paid no attention, perceiving that in the face of the obstacles to be overcome only an unremitting attack over a long period of time would answer. In continuing to support the graduate programs both she and blind people were fortunate in the lieutenants she had who were immediately responsible for her programs for the blind. Louis Rives, her assistant, Joseph Hunt and Cecile Hillyer, in charge of training grants, whether or not they were believers in Miss Switzer's ideas, carried them through with vigor and efficiency as though they were. Both Hunt and Rives, who were superb public officials, became staunch defenders not only of orientation and mobility, but of the standards of the graduate schools.

But it was Mary Switzer who was its champion defender, both with words and money.

Once when she was lunching with a group of educated bureaucrats, none but she was able to translate the second motto on the back of the American dollar bill.

She freely rendered into English: "Annuit coeptis novus ordo seclorum," as: "A new order of the ages favors our undertakings."

No one ever spent the federal dollar toward such a hope more devotedly than she. Her support of orientation and mobility continued to the very end of her life, both with power and discernment. Indeed it seemed to have become a prime example for her of what she wanted to give handicapped people, as can be seen from the following memorandum which she wrote to her successor John Twiname on February 1, 1971, a few months before she died.

> I have been thinking almost constantly about our conversation the other day concerning the cuts in the training programs and what it will mean for our handicapped people and those we have the responsibility for training to serve them.
>
> As I told you, I feel the most telling evidence of the effectiveness of the vocational rehabilitation training programs is the record of where the students go after they are trained. One of the most graphic studies is in the field of mobility instruction for the blind and visually handicapped. The attached copy of an article, which appeared in the January 1971 issue of *Long Cane News*, contains just the type of data that should be available for every single specialty. The sooner it is available the more effective can be the case for not cutting away this important program at a time when we are trying to bring more effective and efficient services to everyone.
>
> You will note from this article that there is practically no slippage at all in the graduates of mobility programs away from work with blind and seriously visually handicapped people. You will note also that the distribution of these instructors is about what you would expect and what you would think would be right. The largest percentage are in public schools, state agencies serving the blind, and private agencies serving the blind—these would be, of course, lighthouse, rehabilitation centers (many of which are under private auspices), etc. Residential schools have another 18 percent which is excellent and probably should be higher. I would suggest that you ask people in other fields to get you similar documentation. Naturally, I will be glad to help in any way possible.

No one knew better than Mary Switzer that the acceptance of the programs she offered to blind people came very largely from interpretation of them by Rives. His ability to make use of even the most unorthodox methods in gaining his ends made collaboration with him exhilarating in the extreme. A case in point was a device we used to promote the orientation and mobility program after he had sold the idea to the higher echelons in the National Council of State Agencies for the Blind and we wanted to reach the House of Commons, so to speak, as well, many of them blind, who had heard unsettling rumors about feats of foot travel they might be called upon to perform.

The Skit

In discussing how we might reach them, I pointed out to Rives that I thought the film *The Long Cane* had produced some opposite results from those intended, because its message was so visually conveyed. In presenting our case to workers in the field through the American Association of Workers for the Blind, we should do it entirely orally and tactilely. A presentation was to be made at the association's 1960 convention. I wrote a humorous skit entitled "Propaganda for Living" in the manner of an Alfred Hitchcock movie, based on the realization that the audience would be overwhelmingly seasoned workers for the blind, half of them blind, and unsentimental about blindness. The skit was recorded on a disc, to be followed by a question and answer session in which Hoover, Father Carroll, and Rives participated. We then arranged for Hoover and half a dozen mobility instructors to give individual demonstrations to the blind members of the audience. The audience reacted from the start as we had hoped. Doubtless they were the only audience to be found anywhere who would have laughed heartily when a blind man who refused to use a cane landed under a train. The punch line came after sound effects of a train whistle, a train chugging into the station, and then silence, broken by the words, "Inasmuch as it has pleased God to take unto himself our beloved brother, at least he went his own way." The record did what *The Long Cane* had not because it was in a medium which depended on vision not at all. As soon as the meeting broke up, flocks of blind people came forward for demonstrations which continued through the day.

It should be said, however, that *The Long Cane* continued to be an enormous success in letting sighted people know what orientation and mobility is all about. With the sighted, "Propaganda for Living" was often found to produce an adverse reaction, even among audiences presumably sophisticated with respect to rehabilitation. The record cost seven dollars, the film thirty-two thousand. It would be hard to say which did most to promote orientation and mobility. In my opinion the record marked an important turning point in the acceptance of orientation and mobility. But Miss Switzer and Miss Diamond, who liked the movie very much, and undoubtedly espoused mobility in part because of it, could not bear the record, even though they granted it had the desired effect on the audience for which it had been written. Laughter at blindness as a rule is best left to blind people themselves. But seven years after the Gloucester Conference, with no appreciable progress in the outer world, and an excellent program bottled up at Hines, it seemed time for a desperate ill to be overthrown by a desperate remedy.

The lengths to which those with an antipathy toward the orientation and mobility program would go in opposition were demonstrated the night before the session at which "Propaganda for Living" was played. A hardened scoffer at the emphasis put on orientation and mobility training, much given to convention antics and buffoonery, undertook to keep Rives at a very lengthy symposium, in fact kept him talking until five in the morning, hoping he would beg off from presiding the next day and giving his very necessary blessing. But Rives proved as staunch as Socrates, at dawn took a dip in the ocean instead of going to bed, and managed the morning session with panache. Hoover was his guide swimming, one of the countless times he has stood by the cause of orientation at every level, from sitting among the elders of the land to giving a lesson to one of his patients who needs it then and there, the only ophthalmologist in the country capable of doing this, and probably the only one willing. He also understands resistance to his methods as well as anyone alive today.

It will never be safe to assume that controversy over the very fundamentals of work for the blind will be over. To be outdone with this circumstance, to say that people "ought not to be that way" is one of the common reactions of "rookies" and "tyros" in the field.

EPILOGUE

To understand why people have been, are, and are likely to be with respect to problems of blindness is one of the many reasons to study the history of human experience with regard to this particular phenomenon. It is also basic to resolutions of current controversies. There are certain very important lessons workers for the blind have at hand for the learning from the long internecine war waged over orientation and mobility. It is the second war of its kind the field has experienced in this century, the first having been over punctography, the great contention between the promoters of braille and the promoters of New York Point, termed "The War of the Dots" by Robert Irwin in his memoirs (Irwin, 1955).

The first lesson from both wars is that people who deal with human problems should not expect to have calm sailing. In retrospect, it is rather surprising that anyone should have expected tranquil waters for such an innovation as the long cane, used not to whack passing tree stumps, but to locate curbs off which the bearer was expected to step onto a street he was then expected to cross. On this subject I would like to acknowledge a statement I made for Hoover to publish in the *Blindness Annual* of 1968.

> It is hard to please me, I confess, with anything written about methods of teaching blind people mobility. What might be termed an executive or "administrative" view of this part of work for the blind frequently finds its way into print full of statements that tell nothing at all. Almost never is there a real impression of pupil and teacher working their way, minute by minute, quarter hour by quarter hour, foot by foot, rod by rod, fighting a hard battle which is part of the so-called adjustment to blindness, by which is meant also getting on top of rage, jealousy and frustration which are brought forth and dealt with by pupil and teacher. I object to bland language and pretense that it is no trick to master the art of seeming a gracious being under these circumstances, much less actually becoming one. Too often language used to describe all that goes into the struggle of blind people to be mobile is far too tender. Blindness is not a tender thing, nor are most of the means to surmount it. They are for the brave and the faithful, who are rather difficult to describe in official or scientific language. (Hoover, 1968)

Many years later Dr. Hoover gave a retrospective prescription for dealing with these complex difficulties at one of the many meetings which were held in the U.S. Department of Health, Education, and Welfare for the perpetuation of his work. This unpublished document of six pages reveals as well as any other what is required in theory, strategy, and tactics for surmounting these difficulties.

> It is only when the trainee feels secure and comfortable in the instructor–trainee relationship that he will do his best and the instructor be the most helpful to him.
>
> The most ideal combination for this type of therapy is when there is a collaboration between the instructor and trainee, each learning from the other. Many times he cannot be patterned after a preconceived plan but must always be modified and adapted to the particular needs of a particular life situation. . . .
>
> You might say that we must give the trainee a series of opportunities to gratify certain basic needs which are present in varying degrees in all types of inability or struggles.
>
> If one were to outline the basic needs I think you could do it in five attempts.
>
> The best method of alleviating tension is known to be bodily activity. Next to this is the need to talk. I include those both in the same category because they both afford an opportunity for an individual to discharge pent-up feelings and can provide a companion upon whom the individual depends for understanding and guidance.
>
> There is nothing unimportant, so particular attention must be paid to everything that is done and everything that is heard. It is impossible to set down any general rules but one might say, (a) listen patiently, (b) do not interrupt, (c) think along with the patient, (d) show a real interest and personal warmth to what is going on, and (e) avoid criticism and argumentation.
>
> The second basic need is the need to be told what to do. If one suffers from an inability, a discomfort, and is in emotional distress, he needs definite support and guidance. He would like to depend on someone who is certain of himself and knows just what to do to alleviate our misery and suffering and at the same time provide him with methods of carrying on by himself. The value of routines and schedules of exercise, rest, and recreation may be attributed in part to this basic human need. Sometimes we want to be freed from having to think for ourselves.
>
> The third need is the need to be accepted.

One who has just recently been maimed or handicapped is tense, worried and uncomfortable, and anxious.

We should evaluate the trainee thoroughly, then discuss why it is thought certain methods should be learned or taught. Do not allow ourselves to portray we feel he is foolish, stupid, or unscientific with his questions or his attempts to use his own methods. He may be testing our interest in him as a person as well as seeking further reassurance. Make the patient feel that he is a collaborator. Tell him how he is doing. Use his own words as much as possible in order to tell him what it is he needs and what it is he is accomplishing. He will be impressed by our sincere interest and feel that we consider him worthwhile and intelligent. Do not make the mistake of trying to minimize his difficulties. He knows he has difficulties, and we cannot change this by minimizing them.

We must not be afraid to speak the truth, if it seems indicated. Probably the individual will be complimented by our personal interest in his illness, in his troubles and feel encouraged to do his best and to tackle other problems.

The fourth basic need is the need to be oneself. Encourage him to do what he really wants to do. Also guide him into doing some of the things that we know will be necessary for him. He will gradually learn to think of himself and for himself, and with it will come a sense of freedom of action and a feeling of well being.

The fifth and final basic need is that of the need for the trainee to finally emancipate himself from the influence of the instructor, because he must at some time leave the controlled protective environment and finally face even more stark reality. Lessons and routine should be reduced and finally discontinued. Be sure he is not exchanging one set of problems for another which will limit his activities and keep him a semi-invalid continuing to rely on someone to tell him what to do and to be with him. One might emphatically state that the patient is not a good traveler until he is completely capable and comfortable in doing this on his own, feeling free to act like any other healthy emotionally secure individual, in keeping with his personal needs and social interest. (Hoover, personal communication, 1976)

Suggestions/Implications for O&M Specialists

1. In the history of formal education programs for people who are blind or severely visually impaired, formal instruction in O&M is relatively recent. O&M specialists need to realize that they are members of a new profession that has not yet been fully integrated and accepted in the blindness field.
2. While many individuals who are blind developed over the centuries their own idiosyncratic methods of independent travel, the significance of the developments at Valley Forge Hospital and at the Hines Veterans Administration Hospital following World War II was the development of a standardized system of travel instruction that could help each person develop his or her own level of independent travel.
3. The tradition of O&M specialists learning the techniques they will teach by working under blindfold themselves goes back to Richard Hoover's work at Valley Forge. It is also in the tradition of Samuel Gridley Howe and other sighted persons who have successfully pioneered advances in the fields of education and rehabilitation of the people who are blind. O&M specialists need to appreciate the background and importance of this aspect of their education, even though it adds to the cost of training.
4. At the time of World War II, existing civilian organizations serving people who were blind felt that the development of rehabilitation programs for blinded military personnel should have been their prerogative. The successful growth of the innovative approach to O&M resulted from the status of the new program within the Office of the Surgeon General and later the Veterans Administration, where it was sheltered from the politics of work for the blind until it was able to clearly demonstrate its success.
5. Much of what was accomplished to develop O&M as a professional discipline required the knowledgeable interest and support of key decision-makers such as General Paul Hawley, Mary Switzer, Louis Rives, and others. In practically every case, these individuals had to be personally convinced by those knowledgeable about O&M in regard to what it was, how it operated, and why it was important. O&M specialists need to realize this part of their mission and responsibility has not changed and continues to this day. A quote attributed to Miss Switzer by the author is, "You can't get people behind causes by talking to yourselves."
6. In this chapter's Epilogue, Hoover's analysis of the human dynamics that occur between instructor and student in the O&M training situation is quoted. Hoover's philosophy, which emphasized the importance of the role of the student as a full collaborator in the training, genuinely accepted and respected by the instructor, has formed the basis of the interpersonal relationship which has been central to the success of O&M instruction since its inception.

ACTIVITIES FOR REVIEW

1. This chapter identified several attitudes that contributed to the slow growth of formal training in O&M. Discuss what the following three attitudes have in common and whether there are any current manifestations of them in the field of work for those who are blind. The attitudes are as follows:
   - Campbell's successors at Perkins did not have sufficient faith in his system of "bodily training;"
   - "A totally blind man I know never had any lessons and does beautifully;"
   - In order to minimize the impact of blindness on others, do nothing that will make it clear to all that you are blind.
2. Discuss how the environments of residential schools did not encourage the development of formal instruction in O&M.
3. Identify three personality characteristics shared by Dorothy Harrison Eustis and Richard Hoover that contributed to their success as developers of mobility systems for people who are blind.
4. Identify the sources of rivalries that existed between the civilians who were responsible for work for persons who were blind during World War II, and those who were assigned to carry out the military's responsibility for rehabilitating blinded military personnel. How did these rivalries affect the subsequent acceptance of the long-cane techniques in the civilian population?
5. Each of the three rehabilitation centers for blinded military personnel established during World War II initially approached travel instruction differently. Describe the different approaches to instruction that were initially characteristic of the Valley Forge Hospital program, the Dibble Hospital program, and the Avon Old Farms program.
6. Discuss the findings and the importance of Bledsoe's study of 337 aging veterans who were blind from previous wars in Veterans Administration centers around the country in 1946.
7. Analyze the meaning of Father Carroll's comment that his early doubts about the Valley Forge program were a result of the fact that the Valley Forge approach to rehabilitation had been to the psyche through the body, whereas it came natural to him to approach the body through the psyche.
8. Identify and discuss three philosophical principles that Russell Williams brought to his position as the first chief of the blind rehabilitation center at the Hines VA Hospital.
9. Analyze Mary Switzer's 1971 memo to John Twiname in light of the current emphasis on the importance of outcome measurements.
10. Discuss the role of the skit titled "Propaganda for Living" in the efforts to gain acceptance for formalized instruction in O&M.
11. Analyze the need for O&M instruction being offered as one-on-one instruction in light of Hoover's formula for the relationship that should exist between the O&M specialist and the trainee.

CHAPTER 22

The Development of the Profession of Orientation and Mobility Around the World

Nurit Neustadt-Noy and Steven J. LaGrow

A cane, stick, staff, or bamboo pole has been used by persons who are blind for travel purposes throughout history. References to blind persons using such devices can be found in writings of the ancient Hebrews, Greeks, and Chinese. The systematic use of a cane as a travel aid was first described in England over 120 years ago (Levy, 1872). Yet the long cane was not adopted for widespread use until it was introduced in the United States at the end of World War II as part of a comprehensive system of instruction and travel known as orientation and mobility (O&M) (Bledsoe, 1969).

This chapter tracks the dissemination of O&M as an instructional system around the world. Although some of this movement has been documented in the literature, most has not. As a result, a great deal of the information presented in this chapter was gathered informally from colleagues who come together every two and one half years to participate in the International Mobility Conferences (IMC), and through responses to mail surveys. As a result, there are gaps in the information provided and unevenness in the presentation across the various countries and regions of the world, and perhaps some errors. In spite of these deficiencies, this overview is an initial step in the process of documenting this phenomenon. Those responsible for the introduction of O&M in each country and region have not been named because identifying everyone proved impossible. However, an appendix specifies the contributions of a number of people who have participated in this process.

This chapter (1) identifies the events or organizations responsible for stimulating the development of O&M in each country or region, (2) describes the instructional programs available for training O&M instructors, (3) develops a chronology of dissemination of the profession around the world, and (4) recognizes the various cultural, political, and economic factors affecting this process. Where possible, the material gives the reader a feeling for the differences among countries and regions of the world in terms of the ratio of instructors to population, the service models used, the educational requirements for entry into the profession, and the development of professional organizations and grouping where they have occurred. These objectives should be used as a rough guide when reading this chapter.

Thanks to all the individuals who collaborated by providing useful and valuable information. Their special efforts enabled the writing of this chapter. Special thanks to Tom Blair, whose private archives and his love of and ability to document historic events served as the basis for the survey used in producing this chapter.

THE UNITED KINGDOM AND NORTHERN AND WESTERN EUROPE

Formal O&M techniques were accepted in England following a series of studies conducted between 1964 and 1966 to determine their efficacy. In the first of these, the current practices used for teaching mobility skills in both Great Britain and the United States were compared. The system in use at Hines Veteran Administration (VA) Hospital was viewed favorably (Fraser of Lonsdale, 1965). A recommendation was made to have a blind individual from England sent to Hines and Western Michigan University for training with the express purpose of subjecting him to the "American training methods" for further evaluation of these procedures (Blasch, 1971). This was done in 1965 under the sponsorship of St. Dunstan's, one of Great Britain's largest organizations for the blind. Later that same year, two instructors were brought from the United States to England to instruct a few "select St. Dunstaners." The parties involved were sufficiently impressed with the results of this training to seek funding from the Viscount Nuffield Foundation to establish Midlands Mobility Center (MMC) as a nonresidential O&M training program. Instructors from the United States were brought to England to establish the curriculum and train a limited number of mobility instructors for the center (Figure 22.1).

In 1965, a similar study of existing service options was conducted under the joint auspices of the American Foundation for the Blind (AFB), the American Foundation for Overseas Blind (AFOB), and the Royal National Institute for the Blind (RNIB). This led to the establishment of a short-term course run at the RNIB's Assessment Center at Torquay in 1967 to train four instructors for that organization (Blasch, 1971). In a parallel project, another mobility specialist from the United States spent 6 months the following year establishing O&M courses at the Royal School for the Blind and St. Vincent's School for Blind and Partially Sighted Children. By the end of 1969, the MMC had an established program with four full-time instructors, and RNIB, St. Dunstan's, and the Birmingham Royal Institute for the Blind had joined to establish the National Mobility Center (NMC) to train mobility instructors for the United Kingdom. Over 400 instructors were trained there in the first 20 years of its operation, many of whom were from European (e.g., Germany, Denmark, Holland, and Belgium) and Commonwealth Nations (e.g., Australia, New Zealand, South Africa, and India).

Sweden

Although widespread acceptance of O&M in Europe did not occur until the British conducted their experiments with O&M, Sweden established its O&M training as early as 1952, after the first instructor was trained at Hines VA Hospital in the United States. Presently all O&M instructors in Sweden are trained at the Stockholm Institute of Education Department of Special Education. In a country with a population of 8.8 million, approximately 75 O&M instructors are practicing today.

The Netherlands

The Netherlands also started O&M for the first time in 1952 on a small scale. This was done at the Royal Institute for the Blind in Hulzon-Bussuem. The Dutch followed closely the studies done by the British, drawing similar conclusions about the suitability and desirability of O&M instruction. Following these studies, they brought an American O&M instructor to Holland for 6 months, with the help of the RNIB and St. Dunstan's, for the purpose of setting up a training program. However, organized training of O&M instructors didn't start until 1990. Since then, 12 instructors and 60 teachers and therapists have graduated from this program. The Dutch are now in the process of forming a professional association of O&M instructors. Among all O&M training centers in Europe, the Dutch are the only ones to use a street-crossing technique recommended by Levi (1872) in which the traveler raises the cane to

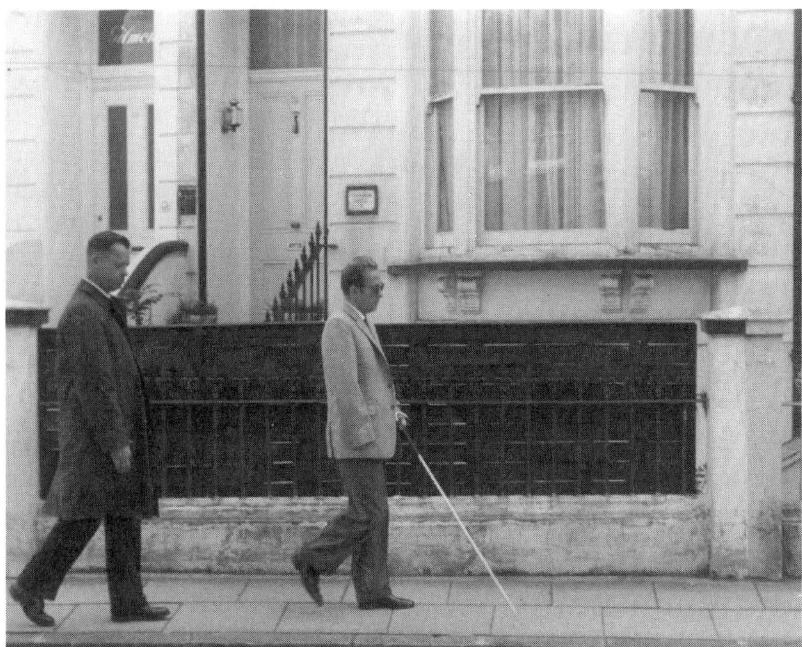

Figure 22.1. An instructor (Stanley Suterko) and a mobility student from St. Dunston's, September 1965.

shoulder height and holds it out parallel to the ground while crossing.

Denmark

Denmark commenced its own O&M training courses in 1970 soon after the first Danish instructor was trained in Birmingham, England. Over 141 instructors have since graduated from the Danish training center, with 65 instructors practicing in the country. Throughout the years they have provided training to more than a dozen instructors from Norway, Iceland, Ireland, Greece, Greenland, Turkey, and Finland.

Finland

The Finns, who were among the first foreigners to be trained by the Danish, went on to introduce O&M into the curriculum for persons who are blind in their country in 1972. Shortly thereafter, they started their first O&M course. In 1984, the Finnish Central Federation of the Visually Handicapped (FCFVH) established a 1-year course for the training of O&M specialists (Ojamo, Ruponen, Paiula, & Hirn, 1990).

Norway

In Norway O&M was started at the Huseby School for the Blind in 1964 by a physical education teacher who was trained in Sweden and at Western Michigan University. Soon after another instructor was trained at NMC in Birmingham, and in 1968 an O&M program started at the Tambartun School for the Blind, in the north. Both schools turned into resource centers in early 1990. The first Scandinavian course for O&M was conducted at Huseby in 1971 with 12 participants representing Denmark, Finland, Sweden, and Norway. In 1985 the first university training program was established in Oslo and 12 instructors were trained. Funding difficulties caused the termination of the young program, which reopened in 1995; 12 O&M students were admitted. About

50 O&M instructors are currently members of the National Norwegian Association of O&M instructors.

France

In 1968–1969, the AFOB conducted two workshops in Paris. Representatives of fourteen nations from four continents participated in these workshops (Blasch, 1971). The French Mobility Center at Marly Le Roi was founded in 1980 training 6–8 French instructors each year. In 1992, this center changed its name to the Association pour les Personnes Aveugles ou Malvoyants (Association of the Blind and Visually Impaired) (APAM). Approximately 100 instructors have been trained to date by the center, of which 15 were for the French regions of Switzerland, 1 was from Zaire and 3 from Spain.

Portugal

Among others, the first four instructors from Portugal were trained at the early Paris courses. They went on to teach mobility to persons who are blind and later to train trainers.

Germany

Formal O&M instruction began in the former West Germany in 1974 after the first two instructors from Germany completed their training at the NMC in Britain. They introduced O&M to children at the School for the Blind in Marburg. They began to train other instructors in these techniques at the Mobility Center in Marburg in the 1970s. In 1979, the Institute for Rehabilitation and Integration of the Sight Impaired (IRIS) was founded in Hamburg and since then provides training for mobility instructors and rehabilitation teachers generally throughout Europe, but especially for Germany and others from the German-speaking regions of Austria and Switzerland.

Spain

ONCE (Organización Nacional de Ciegos Españoles), the National Organization of the Blind in Spain, has run numerous courses, training over 100 instructors since the early 1980s. Spanish, American, and European instructors have provided training in the practical skills of mobility while professors from various Spanish universities have provided the theoretical course work. A number of other Spanish instructors have qualified at the NMC in Britain and the IRIS in Germany as well.

Italy

Two IRIS-trained instructors ran national O&M courses in Italy in 1989 and 1990. The first course was organized by the Italian Union of the Blind and funded by the Ministry of Labor; it was run in Milan. Seven instructors from all regions of Italy participated. The second course was held in Rome, where four more instructors were trained. As of 1991, there were 13 O&M instructors trained in Italy, and 12 more were trained until 1996 (Von Prondzinski, 1991).

Belgium

In the early 1980s a few people from the Flemish part of Belgium attended a short O&M course in the Netherlands. In 1988, two professionals already working for a number of years—one from the Flemish part and one from the French-speaking part of Belgium—were trained in Birmingham, England and Boston. Nevertheless, although Brussels has become the capital of the European Common Market (ECM), where funds are distributed to support many social projects in Europe, Belgium's visually impaired people were left out of the sponsorship. No professional preparation programs have yet developed there. As a result, no training programs are a part of the schools for persons who are blind, nor for visually impaired adults and elderly persons of Belgium.

Greece

Greece has become the latest of the European countries to offer O&M services in a formalized manner. Although O&M was first introduced at the KEAT School for the Blind in Athens in the mid-1980s, it was not until 1994 that the first six Greek university graduates were sponsored by the ECM to be trained in Denmark to form a new cadre of instructors in that country. Their practice module of the course was held in Athens so that they could experience the Greek environment. They were dually qualified in O&M and activities of daily living (ADL) and are employed by the Panhellenic Association of the Blind (Poulea, 1994). In 1995, the newly trained instructors trained four instructors in the Island of Rhodes.

Differences in O&M

The acceptance of O&M across Europe has been uneven, possibly reflecting historical differences in the development of services to people who are visually impaired in general. Numerous examples of this uneven development can be cited. Dog guides, for example, have been in use in Germany since 1916, more than 60 years before O&M was first offered in Marburg and nearly 70 years before dog guides were to become available in Spain (Alcala, 1991). The white cane was introduced in Great Britain in the 1920s, more than 40 years before formal O&M training was adopted in Great Britain and elsewhere. Yet the white cane generally did not come into use in the rest of Europe until it was introduced as a component of O&M training. O&M was introduced in Sweden in 1952, 40 years before it was introduced in Greece. Electronic travel aids (ETAs) were first introduced in Birmingham, England in the 1950s, almost 30 years before they began to appear throughout Europe (one of the first courses for instructors in the use of the Sonicguide® in Europe was run in Denmark in 1977).

The O&M programs established in Great Britain and Western and Northern Europe also reflect these differences in the development of services to persons who are visually impaired, as well as the myriad of differences in the cultures and economies represented in this region. The programs range in length from 12 weeks to 18 months, with the number of hours of training under the blindfold or other simulation ranging from a low of 80 to a high of 350 hours (Neustadt, 1990). The prerequisites for entry into the courses vary greatly. In Portugal, for example, all O&M instructors are qualified teachers; in England they are required to first have a qualification in social work; in Finland they must hold a university degree (but in an unspecified area); other countries require completion of high school only. A number of programs are run by agencies, while others are at the postgraduate level. Graduates of these programs may receive only organizational acknowledgment of their skills, a diploma or certificate from the organization, a university degree, or a graduate degree. There is no generally recognized certification body for the whole of Europe. All the programs are generally small, accommodating 6 to 15 students per session. Some have been in operation for more than a quarter of a century while others are virtually brand new. As a result, the number of O&M instructors available in each country varies greatly as well. For example, there are nearly 500 qualified instructors in Great Britain (population 54 million), over 100 in Spain (population 38 million), 240 in Germany (population 79 million), about 65 in Denmark (population 5 million), 30 in Finland (population 5 million) and 12 in Greece (population 10 million).

O&M instructors may have a choice of private contract work or agency employment as is done in Denmark and Germany; work for any number of agencies as is the case in Great Britain; or have only one national agency to work for, as is the case in Spain, Greece, and Finland. As different as the training programs are, the qualifications held, and the places in which they may be employed, O&M instructors in Europe appear to be remarkably similar to one another and not all that different from the Americans who influenced them. In one study that sought to compare European (i.e., the sample included British, as well as Western and Northern Europeans) and American

O&M instructors, no differences were found in terms of age, sex, and presence of visual impairment, years of experience in the field, the types of agencies they work for, and the distribution of the age of clients served (Cory et al., 1991). The only apparent differences found were in their level of education (i.e., university level education of the American respondents versus nonuniversity certificates of the Europeans), and the degree of vision of the clients they served (i.e., 29 percent of the clients served by the Americans were considered to be totally blind, as opposed to 49 percent for the Europeans).

The travel environments and the transportation systems vary across countries and may vary greatly from those in the United States. Von Prondzinski (1991) provides a succinct, but colorful, description of urban areas in Italy:

> The cities are beautiful and old, the streets are narrow and full of life and the traffic seems chaotic. The city street maps often have more resemblance to a maze than a chessboard, and it seems as though the town planners of the time didn't like the idea of using a rectangle as the basis for constructing a building or a district. In some cities, it is impossible to find a single building which is rectangular in form, surrounded by four footpaths. (Von Prondzinski, 1991, p. 183)

The Europeans started the first truly international forum for O&M by establishing the biannual International Mobility Conference (IMC). The first of these was held in Germany in 1979. Subsequent meetings have taken place in France, Austria, Israel, the Netherlands, Spain, Australia, and Norway; the United States will host the IMC for the first time in Atlanta in 1998.

EASTERN EUROPE AND THE FORMER SOVIET UNION

Most rehabilitation services in Eastern Europe and the former Soviet Union revolve around factory operations and union membership. These services are centrally run, economically independent programs. Chances for employment, pay, and benefits are relatively good under this system. Emphasis is placed on work with the belief that rehabilitation is most successful if it is linked directly and immediately to vocational training and placement (Spungin, 1990). Less emphasis is placed on independence, which is seen as a Western concept and viewed suspiciously by the various governments making up the Eastern Bloc (Wiener, 1991).

The spread of O&M as a system and a profession to Eastern Europe was therefore affected by this political view as well. As a result, no significant developments in this area occurred until the loosening of controls in the late 1970s.

Poland

O&M was not introduced in Poland, for example, until loosening of controls occurred, even though the importance of independent travel had been recognized back in the 1920s and was included in the first curriculum for teachers of blind and visually impaired students (Kuczynska-Kwapisz, Kwapisz, & Adamowicz-Hummel, 1991). The first mobility specialists in Poland were trained in 1979 at a 6-week workshop conducted at the Laski Institute for the Blind by two O&M specialists from the United States (Figure 22.2). A number of short workshops conducted by the Polish Association of the Blind, together with the Center for Continuous Education of Teachers, and based on the curriculum introduced at the Laski workshop, followed (Kuczynska-Kwapisz et al., 1991).

In 1983, a 75-hour course in O&M was added to the curriculum for teachers of persons who are visually impaired at the Maria Grzegorzewska College of Special Education. Poland's first full program for the preparation of O&M specialists began in 1989 under the coordination of a graduate of the Laski Workshop at the same college. These courses are intended for specialists who plan to teach O&M full time. They require a master's degree, current employment working with visually impaired persons, and 2 years of experi-

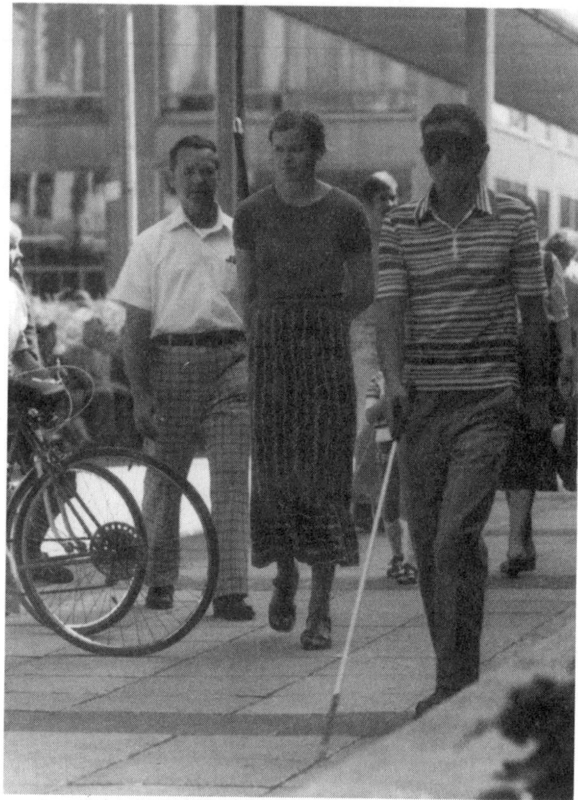

Figure 22.2. A mobility student and a blindfolded student receive training by a mobility specialist (Stanley Suterko) in Poland.

ence for entry. There are 12 students in each class (Kuczynska-Kwapisz et al., 1991).

In 1994, O&M curriculum was introduced at the graduate level, and soon after in 1995 an extended 4-year partnership project with U.S.-based AWARE (Association for World Action in Rehabilitation and Education) was sponsored by the Soros Foundation. The program is open to Polish and Eastern European participants.

Czechoslovakia

In Czechoslovakia experience began with the long cane in 1976. At the time the Czechs had no literature or previous studies to rely upon. They worked with sighted persons under occlusion to develop techniques for the Czechs' use. When they finally gained access to literature from the West, they found their methods to be remarkably similar to those used in the United States and the rest of Europe, with variations noted in rhythm and grip only (Wiener, 1991).

O&M training was provided to both children and adults in Czechoslovakia following the 1976 experiments, until it was banned in 1981 as an "imperialistic method" (Wiener, 1991). Other, more socialistic methods were then developed by the Federation of Invalids, which were ideologically correct but never actually used. Some schools continued to allow mobility specialists to run courses in O&M, but only after hours and without pay. This situation continued until 1989, when more professional practices were again allowed (Wiener, 1991).

Hungary

In 1978, the first Hungarian instructor was trained in East Germany in a course for Eastern European countries. Soon after completing the course, four colleagues from the School for the Blind were trained. In 1980, these four conducted a course in basic techniques for eight volunteers from the Association of the Blind. In the same year, the first organized rehabilitation center offering O&M, ADL, and other adjustment skills was established. This rehabilitation center has also become the training center for instructors and has trained seven instructors to replace those who have since departed. Since 1992, the Budapest Teacher's College incorporated O&M in its curriculum for all special education students (Pronay, 1995).

Romania

The school for the blind in Cluj, Romania, was the first in that country to include O&M in its curriuculum in 1994, following the return of one of its teachers from a training course in Birmingham, England. The practical aspects of life, such as independent mobility and independent skills of daily living, are regarded in Romania as unimportant. Heavy emphasis is placed on academic achievements; thus very little time is left for students to practice or enjoy independent mobility until they graduate from high school. In fact, instruction in O&M is only permitted after normal school hours.

Estonia

Although the long cane was not formally taught in Estonia until recently, persons who were blind learned to value the use of it by themselves (Kalso & Koiv, 1995). The formal education of teachers and instructors in the Russian and Baltic states was done by correspondence through the Department of Education at the University of St. Petersburg. From 1993 to 1995 a group of nine instructors from various cities in Estonia have received instruction in O&M at Tartu from Finnish instructors. This course was held in short modules and emphasized basic cane skills.

Lithuania

The education of persons who are blind in Lithuania started at the beginning of this century, but the interest in independent mobility skills increased only in the 1980s after a few articles were translated from foreign language journals into Lithuanian. The first organized O&M course took place in 1991 and lasted 6 weeks. Twelve Lithuanian O&M instructors were trained by Polish instructors. In 1996, another course was offered, and 13 instructors were trained. As these instructors are all teachers of the visually impaired, O&M became an additional qualification.

Adult O&M services are provided by the Lithuanian Training Center for the Blind in Vilnius. Since 1991, White Cane Day has been celebrated in the country to increase the awareness of and interest in independent mobility skills of persons who are blind.

Future Trends

The advances in the development of O&M in this part of the world in the 1980s may very well be reversed by the collapse of the Soviet Union that occurred in the 1990s, and the economic chaos which has followed. This probably will hold true for all services to persons who are blind in these countries, and especially to those in the republics that make up the former Soviet Union, which enjoyed distinctly economic advantages from a centrally run system (Spungin, 1990).

THE SOUTH PACIFIC AND ASIA

The development of O&M as a profession in the South Pacific and Asia has been uneven, with the more Westernized and more economically developed countries adopting the profession earlier and more completely. Not surprisingly, Australia and New Zealand were among the first nations in this region to adopt O&M as an integral part of their services to persons who are blind and visually impaired. These two areas are essentially Western nations in culture, language, and economy. The man-made environment (e.g., cities, blocks, streets, intersections) is more similar to that found in the United States than even in Britain and Europe.

Australia and New Zealand

Australia

Interest in O&M was generated in Australia and New Zealand following presentations at the First Rehabilitation Conference in Melbourne, Victoria, Australia, in 1963. A number of short courses were run at the Royal Victorian Institute for the Blind following this conference. During the late 1960s other agencies for persons who are blind in Australia and New Zealand began to investigate the need for the provision of O&M services through a series of reciprocal visits with agencies in Britain and the United States (Blasch, 1971). The first O&M instructor in Australia to complete a full O&M training program did so at the National Mobility Center in Birmingham, England, in 1970 (Stroud, 1993).

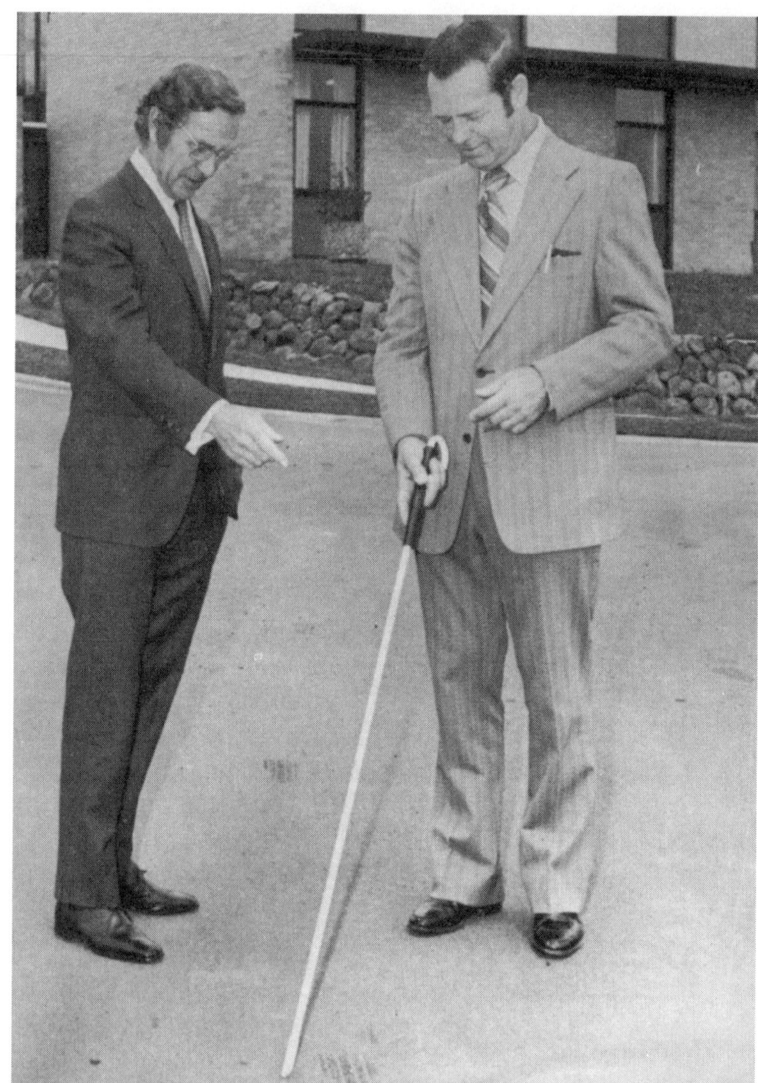

Figure 22.3. Stanley Suterko, right, discussing long-cane technique with J. K. Holdsworth, director of the National Guide Dog and Mobility Training Center, Kew, Victoria, Australia.
Source: *Guide Dog Magazine, 8,* 1973.

In 1971, the Australian National Council for the Blind, in conjunction with the Australian Council on Rehabilitation for the Disabled, obtained funding for a 2-year period through the Federal Department of Social Security to run a series of instructors' courses in which a total of 21 instructors were trained (Pressey, 1986). This original course was run by two instructors from the United States, with the assistance of lecturers from Melbourne and Monash Universities. The course was modeled on the one run at Western Michigan University, with modifications where appropriate (Pressey, 1986). The Royal Guide Dogs for the Blind Associations of Australia took up the training of O&M specialists, following the completion of the original grant, on a fee-paying basis to organizations wishing to have staff trained (Figure 22.3). This program continues today in conjunction with LaTrobe University in Melbourne. Other programs are offered by Victoria and Renwick Colleges in New South Wales, as well. The latter are primarily affiliated with teacher-training courses, with their graduates working in the schools and at the School for the Deaf and Blind.

The majority of O&M instructors in Australia work for the Royal Guide Dogs Associations as part of their overall mobility services. Many are dually qualified as either Guide Dog instructors or ADL instructors and may provide services from a center or in the client's place of residence. Most of these instructors belong to and are certified by the Orientation and Mobility Instructors Association of Australasia (OMIAA), which was founded in 1971 following the completion of the first training program. The OMIAA has established its own certification requirements and adopted the Code of Ethics of Division Nine of the (U.S.) Association for the Education and Rehabilitation of the Blind and Visually Impaired (AER). Currently, the OMIAA has approximately 100 members in Australia and New Zealand (Stroud, 1993).

New Zealand

O&M techniques were adopted in New Zealand in the early 1970s as well. However, New Zealand did not start its own training program until the late 1980s. Prior to that, instructors were either sent to Australia or Britain for training or imported from Australia, Britain, Canada, various European countries (e.g., Sweden and Germany), or the United States. In 1988, the Royal New Zealand Foundation for the Blind (RNZFB) provided a grant to Massey University to establish an O&M training program. This program was established as an endorsement to its existing postgraduate Diploma in Rehabilitation, and is recognized by both the AER and OMIAA Accreditation Committees. New Zealanders are active in the OMIAA and have been from its beginning. All O&M instructors in New Zealand (approximately 25 at this time) are employed by the RNZFB and either work out of one its four regional offices or 13 service centers, or from Homai College, the school for persons who are blind in Auckland. The majority of services are provided on an itinerant basis, with most instructors providing both O&M and ADL services.

Pacific Islands

A number of instructors from the Pacific Islands have attended short courses in the region and are providing O&M services in their home countries. Yet there have been no O&M training programs established in the islands to date.

Japan

The differential growth of O&M as a profession across the emerging economies of Asia reflect the difference in economic development in those countries. Japan, one of the most developed economies in the world, is the only country in Asia to have adopted O&M on a large scale basis, with more than 500 instructors trained in the area of O&M to date. The development of the profession of O&M in Japan roughly paralleled that in Australia. The first rehabilitation program in Japan to include an O&M component was established at the Nippon Lighthouse for the Blind in Tokyo in 1965 with the help of the American Foundation of Overseas Blind (AFOB). In 1970, 1972, 1973, and 1974, short courses of 4 months in duration were conducted by the Nippon Lighthouse in conjunction with the AFOB and run by O&M instructors from the United States to provide staff from various agencies and schools from around the country with training in O&M techniques. In 1975, staff from the Nippon Lighthouse began to run their own courses.

At the same time the National Rehabilitation Center for the Disabled in Tokyo also began to train O&M instructors. Its program was 1 year in length and included training in ADL as well.

In 1991 the Ministry of Social Welfare started a training course for rehabilitation workers. This program provides a dual qualification in O&M and ADL. The course is 1 year in duration and requires an undergraduate degree for entry.

Hong Kong

O&M is also offered as part of the curriculum at the Ebenezer School and Home for the Blind in

Hong Kong and by the Hong Kong Society for the Blind in their adult rehabilitation program. O&M training was first offered in Hong Kong in 1975 through a workshop sponsored by the AFOB. Six instructors were trained in that original course. Since that time, instructors have been sent overseas for training or have received in-service training from the Society for the Blind. Fifteen instructors have been trained since 1979; eight of those were trained at the NMC in Britain, three in the Philippines, one in Australia, and three by in-service. Of those, only eight remain in the field. Turnover of staff is an obvious problem in Hong Kong. This is partly due to the lack of status associated with the position, the frustrations associated with teaching O&M in Hong Kong, and the ready availability of other higher status and higher paying positions in the colony.

The density of population and congestion in the streets makes mobility very difficult in Hong Kong, as does the belief that contact with the cane of a person who is blind will bring three years of bad luck, among other superstitions and prejudices related to blindness in Chinese culture. The same conditions have affected the development of services in Singapore and Taiwan, two other countries in the region with rapidly expanding economies.

Taiwan

Although O&M has been included in the curriculum in the School for the Blind in Taiwan since 1966, they have had difficulty keeping trained staff. The first full-time training course for O&M instructors was established in 1991 at Normal University with the cooperation of Western Michigan University.

Singapore

Singapore is one of the more prosperous nations in the region, yet services for persons who are blind are not well developed. Short courses have been run in Singapore under the auspices of the Singapore Association of the Blind since 1984, with the last run in 1994.

At the present there are only two O&M instructors practicing, due to the same frustrations and high rate of turnover of trained staff seen in Hong Kong and Taiwan.

Other Asian Countries

The other, less prosperous nations of the region have worked cooperatively with international nongovernmental agencies to develop services and train local staff. Most of those persons work in community-based rehabilitation (CBR) programs.

> They have been trained in short, intensive courses which are practical in orientation and geared to meet the needs and conditions of a particular local community. The goal of the training is to equip the field worker with the skills needed to help blind persons lead more productive lives within their families and communities. Therefore, emphasis is placed on skills that improve the functioning of a person in his everyday life. This includes orientation and mobility, activities of daily living, basic education, gardening skills, arts and crafts, and when appropriate, work skills. Since the educational backgrounds of the field workers vary considerably, training is more "hands on" and practical than theoretical. (Horton, 1986, p. 255)

The first of these short courses was offered in Malaysia in 1967 under the sponsorship of the AFOB. Participants were from Malaysia, South Korea, India, Singapore, Hong Kong, Japan, Thailand, and the Philippines (Figure 22.4). A separate initiative was conducted in South Vietnam (Kossick, 1970) at the same time under the sponsorship of the World Rehabilitation Fund. The latter was conducted to train instructors to meet the needs of the victims of the war in that country (Figures 22.5 and 22.6).

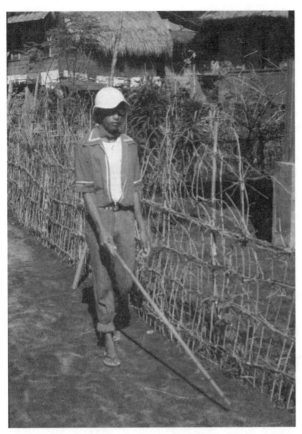

Figure 22.4. A man who is blind who underwent a rehabilitation course in the Philippines.

Source: Helen Keller International. Reprinted with permission.

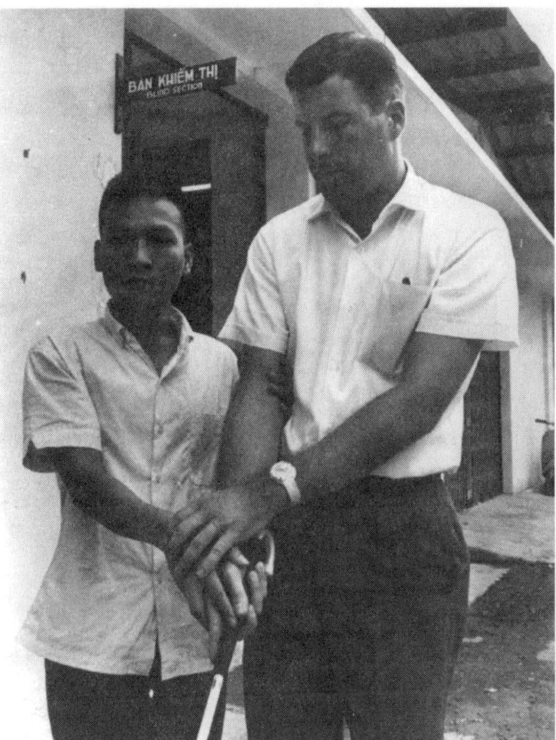

Figure 22.5. An instructor (Rodney Kossick) teaching a blinded Vietnamese ranger to use proper cane technique.

Indonesia

The first training program for O&M instructors in Indonesia was run in 1978 under the sponsorship of Helen Keller International (HKI), in collaboration with the Indonesian Department of Education and Culture and funding from United States Aid for International Development (USAID). This course was recognized by the Indonesian Government in 1981. A permanent training program was established at IKIP Teachers Training College in Bandung. Since its establishment in 1981, more than 130 instructors have gone through the course.

Thailand and the Philippines

The first short course run in Thailand in 1984 was sponsored by Thailand's Ministry of Education and conducted with the help of Christoffel Blinden Mission (CBM). A follow-up was run in 1985 to further develop the skill of the participants. A similar course was run by the CBM in the Philippines in 1988, in partnership with the Rehabilitation Foundation and Social Welfare and the Ministry of Education, for 15 participants. The course was run at the Asian Institute of Tourism, a part of the University of the Philippines. A second course was run in 1989 for 14 participants in Quezon City. Other courses were run on the island of Mindanao for school teachers and field workers from the Department of Social Welfare. Course work currently is offered in O&M from the Philippine Normal University for credit toward a graduate degree in O&M and other formal qualifications in special education.

People's Republic of China

O&M was introduced to the People's Republic of China rather late in comparison to other coun-

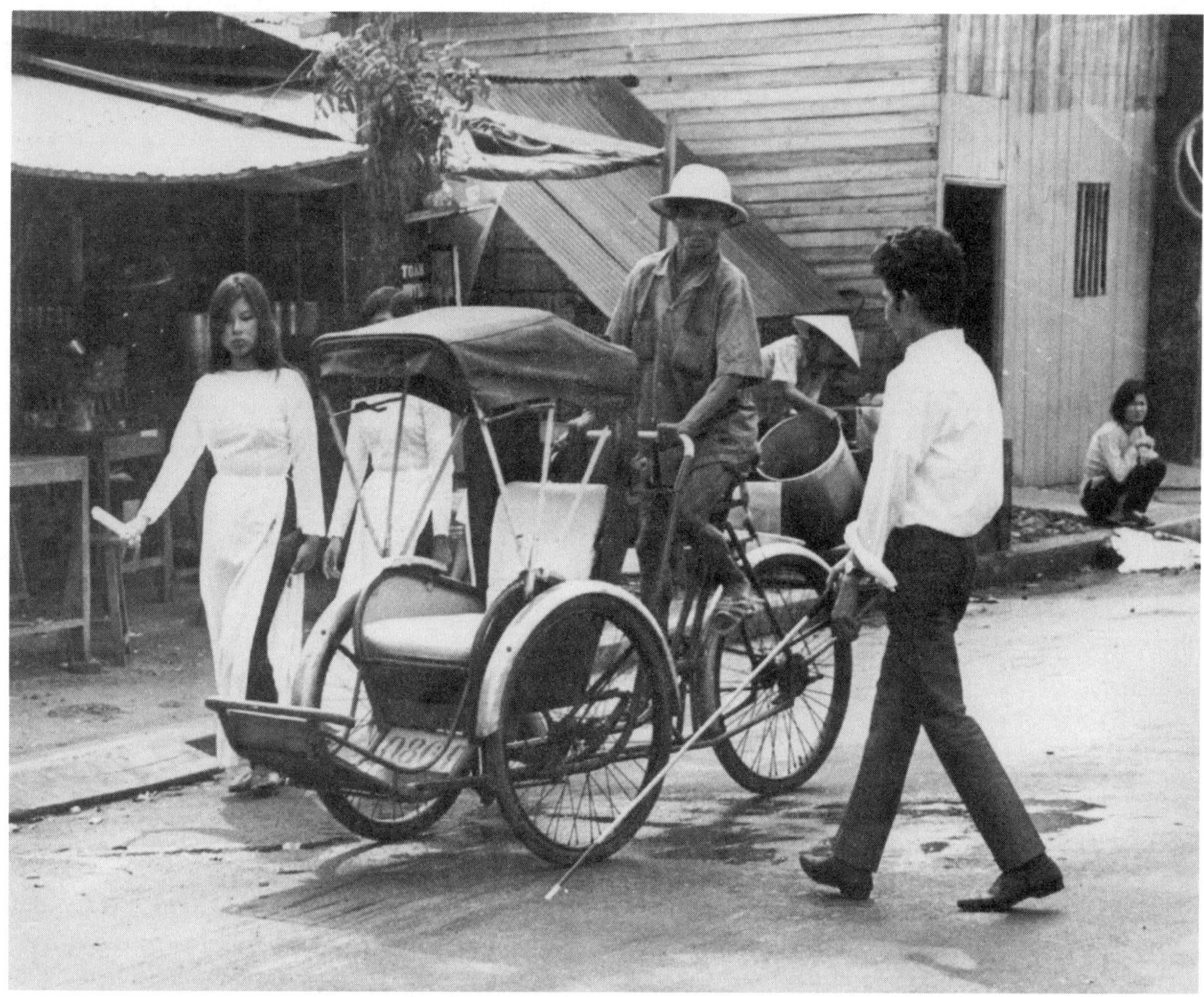

Figure 22.6. A blinded veteran crossing the street for morning tea.

tries in the region. This was primarily due to China's closed-door policy and Mao's Cultural Revolution (Miaode & Hong, 1994). The first training program in O&M in China was sponsored by the CBM with the Amity Foundation and the Golden Key Center, and approved by the Ministry of Education. This course was run at the School for the Blind in Beijing in June 1989 for 11 individuals. The theory of basic, practical, and rural training was conducted at and near the Beijing School for the Blind by specialists from the CBM, with the advanced practical training taught in Beijing and its suburbs (Blair, 1990). This first short course was to be the customary 3 months in duration, but was terminated earlier due to the unrest following the Tiananmen Square incident. A second course was run in 1990 at Nanjing Special Education College, 500 miles south of Beijing, located in a semirural area 14 miles from the city. Fifteen teachers from different parts of China participated in the course. Hundreds of O&M instructors have since been trained by participants of these initial courses (Blair, 1990).

O&M is now a mandated part of the curriculum in the Schools for the Blind in China, with more than 50 percent of those pupils having received O&M services in the 5 years following its introduction to China. Despite these apparent gains, the overwhelming majority of the seven-million-plus visually impaired people in China will probably never receive these services. The majority of people in China live in rural towns where less than 4 percent of the population of blind children attend schools (Miaode & Hong, 1994). Adults have virtually no access to O&M. Little time is available for receiving the training, as they must work to eat, have no expectation of such services, and live in environments that simply are not conducive to independent travel (Miaode & Hong, 1994).

INDIA, BANGLADESH, PAKISTAN, AND SRI LANKA

India

Services for persons who are blind and visually impaired in India are well established.

> They include special and residential schools, vocational training centers, agricultural training centers, Braille presses, Braille libraries, talking book production centers, rehabilitation centers for newly blind persons, mobility training programs, placement programs, a research training center, teacher training and staff training programs, nurseries for preschool blind children, homes for ageing blind persons, and even a small unit for deaf–blind persons. In addition, a number of special aids and equipment for blind persons, including Braille wristwatches, are now being manufactured in India. However, services are unevenly distributed and are inadequate to meet the needs of the nation. (Ahuja, 1990, p. 272)

The number of visually impaired persons in India ranges from 4 to 9 million, depending on the definition used (Singh, 1990). The smaller figure includes only those who can count fingers from 3 feet or less, the larger figure includes those who meet the legal definition of blindness (Singh, 1990). Only about 10 percent of all children who are blind (as defined by finger counting) receive any form of education, and less than 1 percent of all blind adults receive rehabilitation services (Ahuja, 1990). Both economic conditions and cultural and religious beliefs contribute to a general complacency and apathy toward blindness, by both those who are blind and those who are not (Ahuja, 1990). These conditions have hindered a further expansion of services.

Although there are a relatively large number of agencies for persons who are blind in India (over 200 schools for the blind and 100 institutions and agencies), there is a huge population to serve, which constitutes more than 1/10 of all the blind people in the world, most of whom (i.e., more than 80 percent) live in rural towns and villages (Ahuja, 1990; Singh, 1990). A number of community-based rehabilitation initiatives have been launched since the 1970s to provide services in the rural sector (Singh, 1990). Many of these programs have included O&M services.

The first O&M training program was established at Dehra Dun in North India under the auspices of India's Social Welfare Department, with the help of an O&M instructor from the United States. This program was later transferred to New Delhi and the Blind Relief Association. In 1975, the CBM sponsored a training program to train 25 instructors for South India. The National Association of the Blind sponsored a series of introductory courses in O&M for 20 teachers from different parts of the country in Bombay in 1977. This course was run with both financial and instructional assistance from Australia. In 1981, the National Association for the Blind conducted another training course in Bombay. In that same year, the YMCA College of Physical Education in Madras in South India established an O&M training program with the help of the CBM.

Bangladesh

Similar economic conditions and cultural and religious beliefs exist in Bangladesh and Pakistan. As a result, the vast majority (i.e., over 90 percent) of people who are blind in these countries have no access to O&M services. The services that are available have been provided by local instructors trained in local programs or in other Asian countries in CBM-sponsored programs. The first local O&M training program in Bangladesh was run in 1977 under the joint sponsorship of the Department of Social Welfare and the Swedish Federation of the Visually Handicapped. This course was designed for special education teachers from the schools for the blind and resource rooms around the country. O&M has officially been included in the school curriculum for blind children since 1985, but only partially provided due to the lack of availability of qualified instructors. The Bangladesh Dristihin Foundation and University of Dhaka started training programs in 1990 and 1993, respectively, to address this problem.

Pakistan and Sri Lanka

In Pakistan, CBM and the Pakistan Association for the Blind ran a number of short courses to train O&M instructors between 1985 and 1988. Most of this work centered on the needs of those at the Peshawar refugee camps. However, the mismatch between need and resources is so great in Pakistan and the likelihood of being able to train and employ the thousands of O&M specialists required is so low that recent efforts have concentrated on the dissemination of practical advice and hints for safe adaptations through radio services. Ten O&M instructors are active in Sri Lanka. The first one was trained in 1984 in India. Physical fitness is part of O&M training there.

THE MIDDLE EAST AND AFRICA

As in the South Pacific and Asia, the development of the profession of O&M in the Middle East and Africa has been uneven. The more Westernized countries of Israel and South Africa adopted it early, while most countries in the region offer little in the way of O&M services.

Israel

The exception in the Middle East is Israel, which offered its first short course for O&M instructors in 1965 with the help of the HKI. Persons already working as home teachers for blind persons were trained to provide O&M instruction as well. Thus, instructors were dually qualified from the very beginning. A series of short courses were offered for home teachers until 1977, when the first university-affiliated course was offered jointly by the Ministry of Labor and Social Affairs, Haifa University, and Migdal Or (the American–Israeli Lighthouse). This course was approximately 1 calendar year in duration. At the end, 24 students graduated with dual competency in O&M and ADL, or O&M and preschool education (Siegel, 1986). Since then, similar courses have been offered about every other year, with 4 to 12 graduates per class. There are currently over 60 O&M instructors practicing in Israel, most of whom are active members in the Israel Association of Education and Rehabilitation Association (IAER). There are another group of 40 instructors working in Gaza and the West Bank under the Palestinian authority. They were trained in three groups of 12, 14, and 18. The first two groups were trained in the early 1980s under the sponsorship of the CBM, with the help of instructors from the American–Israeli Lighthouse (Zaga, 1986). The third group was trained in 1993 under the auspices of the West Bank Civil Administration, with the help of both Israeli and Palestinian O&M specialists. The courses were 6 to 12 weeks in duration, with continuing education workshops and update seminars through the years. Most Palestinian instructors are dually qualified, like their Israeli counterparts.

Other Middle Eastern Countries

Instructors in this part of the world encounter a great mix of cultures, beliefs, traditions, and environments in which to work. For example, in Israel, there are Jewish people who have come from all parts of the world and Arabs from Moslem,

Christian, and Druse backgrounds. There are humanists and fundamentalists of all faiths. Each group has its own attitudes toward blindness. The range of attitudes displayed covers the spectrum of possibility, as do the range of environments in which people must travel. This area has modern cities with planned neighborhoods, traffic and traffic jams, the narrow lanes of the Old City, rural villages, and refugee camps, all of which require different skills for their safe and efficient negotiation, as do the more subtle barriers erected by society (e.g., social stigma regarding blindness) (Siegel, 1986; Zaga, 1986).

Other societies in the Middle East are more homogeneous and less influenced by Western trends. Although there are some O&M services available throughout the region (e.g., Amman, Jordan; Cairo, Egypt; Lebanon; the United Arab Emirates; and Yemen) where a handful of O&M instructors are available to deal with vast numbers of people who are blind, there has been no acceptance of the profession or the need for it. The physical layout of the environment, economic realities, and cultural values of the region are not conducive to its growth.

Africa

A similar pattern has emerged in Africa, with South Africa being the only country to adopt O&M on a large scale. O&M was first introduced in South Africa in 1969 as a supplement to Dog Guide training. It soon became considered a complementary, rather than supplementary, skill. By 1974, the South African Guide Dog Association had established an O&M training program with courses offered annually. From 1986, they have included ADL skills as well. These courses are of 9 month's duration, followed by a 3-month internship at the employing agency. More than 100 instructors have been trained by this school since its inception. Shorter courses (e.g., of 4.5 months' duration) were offered in 1978, 1983, and 1987 to train O&M instructors to work exclusively with those who live in rural areas. It is estimated that this population makes up between 60 to 70 percent of all visually impaired persons in South Africa (Higgerty & Rhodes, 1991). Although the size of the villages they live in vary, the lack of a systematic and structured man-made environment with paved streets and footpaths is the common denominator of these rural environments. The Bundubasher slip-on tip was developed and special cane techniques have been devised to aid travel in these areas (Higgerty & Rhodes, 1991). The newly formed state of Botswana started offering some O&M training at the schools for the blind after the College of Special Education in Sweden assisted in 1995 by training local school teachers in basic techniques.

As in the Middle East, a number of economic, cultural, linguistic, political, and geographic barriers exist in Africa that impede the spread of O&M to the rest of the continent (Chigadula, 1991; Daka, l991; Sehlz, 1986). The environment is simply not conducive to independent travel. In most cases, travelers who are blind are not protected by white cane or traffic laws. There are few sidewalks or raised footpaths for the use of pedestrians. Those that are available are not reserved for pedestrians alone, but are shared with shops and traffic of all sorts (Chigadula, 1991). Furthermore, few African countries have the resources to meet even the most basic needs of the vast majority of blind people.

For most countries, subsistence issues are more pressing than the acquisition of independent living skills (Sehlz, 1986). Where services are available they are generally limited in scope and range. In Ethiopia, for example, there are only two local O&M instructors for the estimated half a million people who are blind, and there are no sources of canes within the country—all are sent from outside as donations (Maru, 1990). In Eritrea, the neighboring country, there is no formal training in O&M. In Malawi, the only O&M services available are those provided by specialist teachers of visually impaired children (Chigadula, 1991). Lesotho offers O&M services from the Resource Center School for the Blind in the capital Maseru. The four O&M instructors working there were trained as teachers for the blind at College Montfort in Malawi in 1970, 1975, and 1992.

Zambia cannot afford to produce the standard typhlo cane. They therefore must rely on the use of bamboo or rattan canes and foreign aid and expertise.

Instructors have been trained in Ghana for the various countries of the West African subregion through the combined efforts of the Ghana Society for the Blind and the CBM. Two courses were run in 1988 for this purpose. However, they were only 2 and 4 weeks in duration. The CBM was also heavily involved in basic training of O&M instructors in Kenya in 1978, 1980, and 1985. In the beginning, training programs were geared for school teachers and O&M instructors. Between 1985 and 1994, more than 44 O&M instructors were trained by the Kenya Institute of Special Education (KISE) (Mwangi, 1994). Their training was modified to meet the unique problems of mobility in Kenya, such as the irregular surfaces of the roads which makes cane use very difficult, the paucity of landmarks, and the adverse weather conditions that characterize the country (Saya, 1993).

When the Norwegians made arrangements to host IMC-8, they decided to sponsor a group of educators in the field of blindness from Uganda to attend the conference. This cooperation led to the development of the O&M curriculum and training of instructors in Uganda.

THE AMERICAS

Canada

As stated earlier, the profession of O&M began in North America in the United States following World War II (see Bledsoe, Chapter 21 of this volume). It was adopted in Canada soon after and is offered as one of the seven core services provided by the Canadian National Institute for the Blind (CNIB), a nonprofit rehabilitation agency founded in 1918 (Magarrell, 1990). CNIB is the agency primarily responsible for the delivery of services in all territories and provinces of Canada, with the exception of the province of Quebec. In Quebec, services are provided by the province as a right of citizenship. Quebec funds three agencies: the Centre Louis-Hébert and the Institut Nazareth et Louis-Braille are for its French-speaking citizens, and the Montreal Association for the Blind is for those who speak English.

The CNIB has traditionally trained its own O&M instructors, although Mohawk College has been running an O&M course since the early 1990s. Quebec has sent its instructors to various universities in the United States or to CNIB for training. A university training program was begun in the early 1980s at Université de Sherbrooke.

Latin and South America

O&M services in Latin and South America are not nearly as well established as they are in North America. O&M was first introduced in South America in Brazil in the 1960s. At that time an instructor from the United States ran a short course for 15 instructors. Only one of those first participants went on to teach O&M, and he is still practicing today. Over the years he has trained a number of other instructors. Currently there are approximately 30 instructors in Brazil.

The CBM, HKI, and ONCE have cooperated with various local organizations over the years to train instructors in Bolivia, Colombia, Chile, Costa Rica, Ecuador, Paraguay, and Peru. These countries have had difficulty retaining O&M instructors due to the low pay and status typically afforded to teachers and others in similar professions. Most services available in this region are provided to children attending either schools for the blind or integrated public schools. In Argentina, O&M services are provided from high school onward. This tradition is being challenged by local O&M instructors, who have taken the position that O&M should start as early as possible. In 1995, the International Council for the Education of the Visually Impaired (ICEVI) invested in organized courses to train eight O&M instructors from

Nicaragua; Honduras; Guatemala; Panama; and Mexico, where O&M instruction in the schools has been provided for some time (Piccione, 1995).

SUMMARY

The profession of O&M has spread throughout the entire world in the past 40 years, albeit unevenly. The skills and techniques making up the system of instruction and travel that constitute the body of knowledge known as O&M were initially developed in the United States and adopted in the United Kingdom, Western and Northern Europe, Canada, and the rest of the Americas. These practices soon spread to Australia, New Zealand, Japan, and South Africa, where they were adopted on a large scale. The way O&M is practiced in these places is remarkably similar, despite differences in political and educational systems, language, population density, and man-made environments. In fact, the techniques used and the professional values that underlie the training of instructors and the provision of services to visually impaired persons are more similar than different. This is quite unique, considering the fact that the built environments are so different, as are the educational, social, and cultural institutions. Yet the similarity in values and standard of living seem to overcome the obvious differences between these countries. However, as one would expect, more variance occurs in the less economically developed, non-Western countries, where both the standard of living and the values of the cultures are more markedly different.

In the old Eastern Bloc, for example, the values and practices of the profession have been viewed as being blatantly Western and unacceptable. In the Middle East, Asia, and the Pacific Islands, they are often seen as being at odds with the values and beliefs of the culture and therefore as somewhat irrelevant or impractical. In other places, the values are acceptable, but the practices are not relevant to the economic or social circumstances in which they must be delivered. As a result, the systems of delivery have been adapted to meet the needs, beliefs, and resources available for the provision of services to people who are blind and visually impaired. In many parts of Asia and the Far East, for example, O&M is provided by a generalist who provides all the forms of support needed, including vocational, recreational, and educational rehabilitation. The specialization common to the practice of O&M in most Western countries is not practical in rural Asia, nor is the goal of independence necessarily valued as the outcome of O&M training. In many parts of the world this goal is seen as being immature and at odds with the communal values of interdependence and cooperation.

In other parts of the world, the issues of subsistence take priority over those of independence. In parts of Africa, for example, the cost of a long cane is prohibitive, let alone the expenses involved in providing the training to go with the cane. This has also been seen to be the case in Bangladesh, Pakistan, and rural China.

Despite all of the differences and difficulties in the world, the profession has spread and continues to develop. Today, there is no continent where O&M is not taught. Surely this trend will continue, but with it will come greater variations in the techniques we know as O&M and the style in which these services are provided. The differences in the backgrounds and approaches of those teaching O&M may also grow, as will their training and professional values. Yet one hopes these differences will reflect the needs of the persons receiving these services and prove that the profession is growing as it evolves to meet the myriad needs of the people of the world.

Suggestions/Implications for O&M Specialists

1. The fact that O&M has been accepted on every continent on Earth suggests that it has a robustness in relevance and efficacy that transcends cultural, economic, political, and environmental differences. Parallels in its emergence across nations and continents can be drawn, with its evolution moving from a system of instruction designed for adults who are adventitiously blind to one that also has relevance for all sectors of the blind and visually impaired population, including very young, very old, and multiply impaired persons.
2. The British accepted O&M after a period of assessment and evaluation in their own country. This was essentially the first time these techniques were systematically investigated in a place where the environment varied in many significant ways from the place where these systems were devised. The widespread and rapid acceptance of O&M in the United Kingdom confirmed the adaptability of the strategies across environments.
3. The British, through the National Mobility Center, were instrumental in disseminating O&M techniques throughout Europe and the Commonwealth. The Swedes and Danes had a similar effect in Northern Europe, as did the Germans in Western Europe. During the 1960s and 1970s there was a concerted effort to establish O&M throughout much of what was thought of as the Western or developed world.
4. The similarities among British, European, and American O&M instructors in terms of the clientele they served, the agencies they worked for, and the ways they provided services were significant. Similarities among instructors and their places of employment became less apparent as the profession spread to Asia and the so-called developing world.
5. The more economically developed and Westernized countries of Asia, Africa, and the Middle East adopted the profession of O&M earlier and more completely than their neighbors. Yet the sharing of cultural values appeared to be more of a determinant of this trend rather than simple economics.
6. A minimum level of prosperity is necessary before O&M emerges as a priority. In many parts of the world issues of subsistence must take priority over independence.
7. The values inherent in the "culture of rehabilitation" in general and those relating specifically to O&M may at times be at odds with cultural variables. In some cultures, the emphasis placed on independence in O&M is at odds with the interdependent and collective nature of the society. In others, the emphasis on specialization and professionalism, which often marks the profession, may be seen as either irrelevant or impractical.
8. The disparity in the way the profession of O&M has emerged between North and South America may be reflective of both cultural and economic differences in this region.

ACTIVITIES FOR REVIEW

1. Trace the development of O&M from the United States to Britain and Northern and Western Europe. Identify the agencies and training organizations responsible for the spread of this profession and the lines along which it seemed to spread.
2. Describe the barriers to the spread of O&M to Eastern Europe before the collapse of the Soviet Union. Were these primarily cultural, political, or economic?
3. Describe the spread of O&M in Asia and the South Pacific. Identify the cultural and economic variables that affected its dissemination in this region.
4. Describe "community-based rehabilitation" as it emerged in Southeast Asia and its influence on the spreading of O&M in Asia, India, and Africa.
5. Trace the development of O&M in Asia, India, and Africa, and identify the agencies and training organizations responsible.
6. Describe the unique manner in which the profession of O&M emerged in South Africa, and identify any other region in the world that could follow a similar pattern.
7. Describe the spread of the profession of O&M in the Americas. Compare the differences in the development of this profession in North and South America. Identify the cultural and economic factors that may have influenced these developments.
8. Identify the agencies and training organizations most responsible for the development of O&M in Canada, the United States, and South and Central America, respectively.
9. What would you predict to be the future of O&M as a profession in the various regions of the world in the 21st century? Which factors do you forsee as being most likely to affect the profession in the future?

APPENDIX

Early Participants in the Dissemination of O&M

Many individuals and agencies have participated in the process that resulted in the dissemination of O&M throughout the world. Some of those have been identified below.

Alfred Leonard directed the initial studies on O&M for the Medical Research Council of England.

Walter Thorton was the blind traveler sponsored by St. Dunstan's to receive O&M training at Western Michigan University and the Blind Rehabilitation Center at Hines Veterans Administration Medical Center.

Dr. Leonard and Mr. Thorton went together to set up Midlands Mobility Center (MMC) in the United Kingdom.

Stanley Suterko (during 1966–1967) and Robert Crouse (during 1967–1969) trained the first British O&M instructors at MMC.

William Goodman conducted the AFOB/RNIB study in the United Kingdom.

Lee Farmer trained the first instructors for the RNIB at the Torquay Assessment Center.

Robert LaDuke trained O&M instructors at the Royal School for the Blind and St. Vincent's School for the Blind and Partially Sighted in the United Kingdom.

Mary Cane was the first director of National Mobility Center (NMC) in the United Kingdom (for 1969–1973).

Jeane Kenmore headed O&M courses from the AFOB's Paris office.

Armando Ramalho, Moura e Casto, Luis de Barros, and Julia Pavia were the first Portuguese O&M instructors trained in Paris.

Liche was the first West German O&M instructor trained at the NMC. Beatrice and Jochen Fischer founded the first West German Mobility Center to train O&M instructors. Pam and Dennis Cory founded the IRIS in Hamburg.

Anta Ryman was the first Swedish O&M instructor who was trained in the United States.

W. J. J. Kooyman was the first O&M instructor in the Netherlands.

Ritva Kuuskooki was the first Finnish instructor who trained in Denmark in 1971–1972.

Maria Grzegorzewska was an early educator whose teaching and writing formed the cornerstone of education and rehabilitation for people who were visually impaired in Poland.

Stanley Suterko and Daniel Nelson provided the training for the course at the Laski Institute in Poland.

Jadwiga Kuczynska-Kwapisz is a Laski graduate who coordinated the first professional preparation course in O&M at the Maria Grzegorzewska College of Special Education.

Pavel Wiener developed cane techniques through experimentation and was one of the first O&M instructors in Czechoslovakia.

Jack Wilkingson was the first Australian trained in O&M techniques.

Tom Beaton completed the O&M course at the NMC in Britain in 1970. He was the first professional O&M instructor in Australia and one of the founders of OMIAA.

Rod Kossick and James Liska were the O&M instructors from the United States who ran the first training program in Australia.

Rod Kossick and Genevieve Caulfield ran the O&M training course in South Vietnam.

W. Ban and Brian Peel were early O&M instructors in New Zealand and among the founders of the OMIAA.

Steven LaGrow set up the first O&M training program at Massey University in New Zealand.

Zimmerman of the AFOB helped the Nippon Lighthouse establish the first independent living training center in Japan.

Bob Jaekle, Loyal Apple, and Bill Walkowiak ran the early workshops for the Nippon Lighthouse.

Mr. Osuki and Ms. Tsujiuchi were the first Japanese O&M instructors. They went on to be the chief instructors in the ensuing workshops run by the Nippon Lighthouse.

Jim Leja from Western Michigan University helped Normal University in Taipei establish an O&M training course; Bob Jaekle ran the course for the AFOB in Malaysia.

Kirk Horton ran O&M courses in Asia for the CBM, HKI, and Perkins-Hilton Foundation.

Dr. Claude Chambet founded the O&M training center at Mary Le Roi near Paris.

Tom Blair ran the first short course for the Singapore Association for the Blind, the first short course for HKI in Indonesia, the first course for the CBM in China, and the short courses in both Thailand and the Philippines for the CBM; in all cases he was assisted by local staff.

Irham Hosni and Yan Sujano were graduates of the first short course in Indonesia.

Hans Murrl and Heinz Degenhardt were the first trainers of O&M in courses for Eastern European countries.

The AFOB was the international extension of the American Foundation for the Blind; later it was changed to Helen Keller International.

ONCE is the Association of the Blind in Spain, which assists Latin American countries in developing rehabilitation and O&M services.

IMC is the International Mobility Conference meeting for O&M instructors, which is held every two-and-a-half years.

Division Nine is the O&M division and the largest division at AER.

CHAPTER 23

The Administration of Orientation and Mobility Programs for Children and Adults

Robert J. Crouse and Michael J. Bina

The responsibilities for both the orientation and mobility (O&M) specialist and the administrator in delivering and administering O&M services within education and rehabilitation settings are challenging. Although O&M instructors are responsible for direct one-to-one delivery of these services, education and rehabilitation administrators are responsible for the management of the O&M program and supervision of the direct service provider. This chapter attempts to assist both the O&M specialist and the administrator in accomplishing their individual and shared responsibilities in ensuring that the best possible services are delivered with the necessary frequency to benefit the most students in light of various constraints and realities. Accomplishing this charge and meeting this responsibility is enhanced when the O&M specialists and administrators work cooperatively, are resourceful, plan carefully, remain flexible, and have an ongoing commitment to professional standards and respect for the student.

The material is divided into four subsections. First, federal and state laws and regulations that mandate individualized services for children and adults with disabilities are reviewed. Second, suggested solutions to overcome various challenges in administering O&M programs are presented. Third, standards of high-quality programs are discussed. And fourth, issues and responsibilities related to personnel recruitment, mobility assistants, continuing education, ethics, liability, and insurance are addressed.

FEDERAL AND STATE LAWS

In the 1970s landmark federal laws were passed that resulted in sweeping changes in the ways that education and rehabilitation services were to be provided. With the passage of the Rehabilitation Act in 1973 and the Education for all Handicapped Children Act in 1974, agency and school personnel were required to implement major changes in procedures and programming. These laws have been amended numerous times, but their intent has stayed the same in that the provisions in these laws provide for services to which disabled children are entitled and for which adults may apply.

The Rehabilitation Act, as amended, and the Individuals with Disabilities Education Act (IDEA), while focusing on services to two different age groups, share many commonalities. Foremost among these is the guarantee of legal due process procedures to protect individual rights such as confidentiality, notice, consent, and appeal. The laws require comprehensive assessments to determine individual needs and development of Individualized Education Programs (IEPs) or Individualized Written Rehabilitation Plans (IWRPs), and that special education services be provided at no cost to parents or students. While most rehabilitation services are for adults with an employment goal, in some cases rehabilitation clients may be expected to pay for some expenses, such as college tuition.

The Rehabilitation Act Amendments of 1992 place greater emphasis on providing services to individuals with the most severe disabilities as a first priority and the achievement of the individual's employment objective as the primary goal. A person with a severe disability is defined as:

1. an individual whose disability is permanent, chronic, or cyclical in nature;
2. an individual who has a severe physical or mental impairment that seriously limits two or more life functions (mobility, communication, self-care, self-direction, interpersonal skills, work tolerance, or work skills) in terms of employment outcome; and
3. an individual whose program can be expected to require vocational rehabilitation services over an extended period of time.

The regulations of the Act require that an IWRP be developed for all eligible applicants. The IWRP must clearly indicate that the employment objective is consistent with the individual's capability and include statements of goals and intermediate rehabilitation objectives. The IWRP must also spell out specific services that are to be provided along with specific goals, objectives, and time frames in which these services are to be achieved. O&M services are provided for in several sections of the Act, including Title I and Title VII, Chapter 2 ("Independent Living Services for Older Individuals Who Are Blind").

The Rehabilitation Act is a state and federal partnership that requires a monetary sharing of federal dollars and state-matching funds (78 percent federal contribution with a state match of 22 percent). The Rehabilitation Act also requires each state to develop an approved State Plan that addresses the intent, purpose, and regulations contained in the Act and indicates how services are to be provided.

The Individuals with Disabilities Education Act mandates that a comprehensive assessment be done by a multidisciplinary team as the foundation for the development of an IEP. The IEP specifies the required special education and related services, along with targeted goals, objectives, and timelines to meet the student's identified needs. Related services are defined as those provisions that are necessary for individuals with disabilities to benefit from special education. Examples of related services are occupational therapy, physical therapy, and special transportation. O&M is recently listed in IDEA-related services. O&M services are now specified in law and can also be specified on an IEP as a required related service. Therefore, in common—but not universal—practice, O&M is written into IEPs even though it was not formerly listed as a primary or related service. A few states have specified O&M as a related service in their respective state special education laws, and some require certification of personnel in this specialty.

In 1994 the Council of Schools for the Blind (COSB) and the Association for Education and Rehabilitation of the Blind and Visually Impaired (AER) proposed changes in federal law and regulations whereby O&M training would be specified as a related service (Association for Education and Rehabilitation of the Blind and Visually Impaired, 1994). The rationale for O&M being included as a related service is that with its inclusion, parents and service providers—and particularly special education administrators—unfamiliar with the unique needs imposed by blindness will be reminded about the potential benefits of O&M service. It is currently being proposed as a related service in the reauthorization of IDEA.

SERVICE DELIVERY OPTIONS

Federal law requires special education services to be provided in the least restrictive environment (LRE). The rationale for the LRE legal concept is the preference that placements be in settings as near as possible to the student's or client's home, and with nondisabled individuals to the maximum extent possible. The concept of LRE implies that there be a series of options from which to choose a placement where the student's needs can be met to the greatest extent without unnecessary restriction. The regulations that implement the federal laws provide for "a continuum of alternative placements." For school-age children, these placements include special schools that have residential and day components, and local education agency placements which have various options including regular education classroom, pull-out services, resource and self-contained rooms, and itinerant services. O&M services can be provided in any of these placements.

Since the late 1980s strong emphasis has been placed on full inclusion of students in regular education classrooms (The Association for Persons with Severe Handicaps, 1994; Hehir, 1994; Joint Organizational Effort, 1994). Full inclusion is not a federal or state law, but a strong philosophical model that advocates for elimination of all special placements where students are pulled out of regular classrooms. If full inclusion were to be implemented on a wide-scale basis, the continuum of alternative placements would be eliminated, leaving only the regular education classroom. This would have a tremendously adverse effect on the provision of O&M to school-age children.

How can O&M services be delivered within the regular classroom when a majority, if not all, mobility lessons require the student to be taught in environments away from the class, for example, indoor settings, residential neighborhoods, and business areas? Is it necessary for students to be taught in these areas in order for them to learn and apply the O&M skills? Recognition that O&M is a legitimate reason to pull a student out of a regular classroom is gaining wider acceptance by professionals (Hatlen & Curry, 1988), state departments of education (C. Allman, personal communication, 1994), and federal· officials (Hehir, 1994).

O&M services are provided in a wide variety of administrative structures and program settings. In most cases employers directly contract and employ mobility staff on the agency's or school's payroll with full benefits. In some cases, mobility staff are hired on a subcontract basis, part time or full time. In the past 20 years there has been a significant growth in service provided by private contractor mobility specialists working for schools and agencies. The principle employers of O&M specialists are:

- *Private, not-for-profit agencies.* The agencies provide center-based and community-based (itinerant) mobility services to a wide age range of clients, from preschoolers to elders.
- *State rehabilitation agencies.* These state-supported services can be either rehabilitation center-based or community-based services, and serve adults and some high-school-age students.
- *Statewide schools for children who are blind.* These state-operated or private schools provide regular school curricula in addition to blindness-specific instruction on a day, residential, or outreach basis. In many schools for the blind the number of students with multiple disabilities has increased significantly. This increase has necessitated careful program planning to meet the complex needs of students.
- *Local education agencies.* These are local, county, and regionalized school districts supported by local taxes and state funds. They have the responsibility of providing regular and special education services to all children, including the approximately

10 percent of the population who have physical, cognitive, emotional, or sensory disabling conditions that interfere with achievement in school.

Within the above education or rehabilitation settings, instruction can be provided through either a center-based or itinerant service delivery model. The model of service delivery used depends on whether the caseload is "clustered" in a small geographic area or "decentralized," that is, sparsely spread over a wide geographic region. In cases where the caseload is clustered or centralized, instructors are able to provide services out of one school or agency. In cases where the caseload is decentralized and spread geographically, these instructors must utilize an itinerant model.

There is no one perfect service delivery model. Each has unique advantages and disadvantages. The trend in recent years has been toward itinerant or community-based models for both children and adults.

Irrespective of the service model in which mobility services are provided, good planning is essential. Effective program planning addresses these issues: (1) the population served, (2) the framework and constraints of the agency, school, or organization in which it must operate, (3) the goals and objectives of the mobility program, (4) the size and geographical area to be served, and (5) the ages, developmental levels, and needs of the clients and students.

The well-designed mobility program will take into account all of these variables in developing a written plan of service. The following sections discuss planning issues relevant to the various types of service models.

Center-Based Service Delivery

O&M services provided in center-based adult rehabilitation programs and in statewide schools for blind children have a distinct advantage over services provided on an itinerant basis. Having students clustered in one location eases scheduling difficulties, provides ready access to clients and O&M training areas at or near the agency or school, allows more time for direct student and client instructional time, alleviates the lost time spent in driving great distances, and enhances the acquisition of O&M skills by being able to schedule students and clients on a more frequent basis than is possible in itinerant situations.

Another major advantage for O&M specialists who work in a rehabilitation center or school for blind children is the support, encouragement, and guidance that is available from other professionals who are trained and experienced in blindness-specific areas. In contrast, professionals who provide services on an itinerant basis often feel isolated because of an inability to discuss issues, validate strategies, and share concerns with other professionals.

Residential rehabilitation centers and schools for children who are blind that serve large geographic areas typically are not able to provide this training in the client's home community. In some cases the agency or school instructors are able to refer the client to a local O&M specialist, or are able to do home visits so that transfer of learned skills to the client's home community can be implemented at the conclusion of the student's training program.

Itinerant or Community-Based Programs

While itinerant or community-based programs have the advantage of providing services in the students' home neighborhoods, these services present the greatest challenge in both instructional and program planning. The biggest challenge in providing services on an itinerant basis is the necessity of having to drive long distances between various schools or clients' homes.

Within the itinerant service delivery option, the O&M specialist must be adept at managing time, traveling distances, and scheduling students for instruction. The advantage of providing instruction in a person's home area, particularly for adults, is that instruction is provided in the areas in which they later will be traveling. This ideal learning opportunity reduces the need for transfer of learning. Lessons can be designed to specific destinations along actual routes that the individual will use on a daily basis after training is complete.

A major disadvantage of providing services on an itinerant basis is that the O&M specialist must constantly be planning lessons in different settings for each and every student. This presents a major challenge to consistently plan well-organized and time-efficient lessons.

Another problem faced by the itinerant O&M specialist is the size of the caseload and the size of the area to be served. The larger that each of these variables is, the less frequently students or clients can be seen. From a learning standpoint, two or three lessons per week is preferred over one lesson per week. There are advantages in serving fewer students and having them complete the O&M program than to stretch out instruction over an extended period of time. In actual practice this is not always possible, given the preference and prohibition against placing students or clients on waiting lists. As a result, more individuals receive instruction, but often in greatly diminished frequencies.

Itinerant O&M specialists in heavily populated school districts have the advantage of serving a majority of their caseload in a relatively small geographic region. On the other hand, O&M instructors employed in rural areas or sparsely populated districts are typically required to travel extensively to work with students who are spread out geographically.

ADMINISTRATIVE CHALLENGES

When the primary purpose of O&M instruction is closely analyzed, the uniqueness of this service provision becomes readily apparent. First, blindness or impaired vision may seriously impact and often restricts an individual's ability, confidence, and motivation to travel independently. Second, traveling without sight through various environments does involve risks and dangers of a magnitude unlike other subjects or skill areas. Third, unlike most instructional subjects in which students can be grouped in large numbers, most O&M services must be provided on an individualized, one-to-one basis. This uniqueness and concern for safety is often criticized on the basis of comparing the cost-effectiveness of delivery of O&M services on a one-to-one basis to the expenditures of an elementary teacher who has a class of 20–30 students in one class. Fourth, because blindness is a low-incidence disabling condition, students are typically spread out and not geographically concentrated. Also, because of the low incidence of blindness, the general population are unfamiliar with blindness and do not have "common knowledge" of the mobility needs of people who are blind and visually impaired.

Administrators need to be aware of the visibility factor in terms of public relations when they have O&M instructors working in the community. The public becomes very aware of instructors working with students in neighborhoods and business areas. This may provide extremely valuable public relations within the community and give the public a better understanding of the direct service provided by the organization. Some agencies and schools provide instructors with jackets, shirts, or other such items to identify the agency.

O&M specialists, along with special education and rehabilitation administrators, face various constraints and challenges as a result of the uniqueness associated with providing this service. Foremost among these challenges is the establishment of selection criteria and attempting to respond to the great demand for these services, personnel availability, limited resources, the limited number and geographic spread of the university training programs, time constraints, the threat of student injury and potential liability, the trend toward generic services, accountability and outcome measures, and finally, the increasing complexity of the needs of a changing population. While many of these constraints present formidable obstacles, it is important for the O&M specialist and the administrator to work together to plan; problem solve; explore alternative strategies; and exercise flexibility, creativity, and patience in implementing programs.

Selection Criteria

Many schools and agencies have established selection criteria and priorities for students or clients referred for O&M services. The types of selection criteria include, but may not be limited to, the following items: (1) the need to get to and from a job, training program, or school, or within a training facility or school; (2) the need to get to and from the agency using public buses or paratransit; (3) the most pressing need to the student, to establish an independent living status; and (4) the question of whether the student is a danger to himself or herself or others in the environment.

The mobility specialist may or may not have much input concerning these selection criteria for new students. It is advisable that mobility specialists be involved in the establishment of selection polices and their advice be solicited when making these decisions.

Personnel Availability

Due to recent innovative recruitment and program modifications by university training programs, the critical shortage of O&M specialists has been significantly reduced (see Chapter 20). Among these innovative efforts are summer university classes for professionals currently employed in education or rehabilitation services who wish to be certified in O&M; they complete their programs in three or four summer sessions. Also, an off-campus program delivered to rural areas where staff of agencies cannot attend the university has been implemented. Some employers, in order to recruit and employ mobility personnel, have paid the expenses or sponsored students enrolled in the university programs with the provision they return to the organization upon graduation and work for a predetermined period of time.

Recent initiatives in Congress to balance the federal budget threaten future funds available for university personnel preparation programs. Such action would negate the gains that have been made in recent years toward meeting the demand for O&M personnel across the country.

Administrators must be aggressive in their recruitment efforts to attract mobility personnel to their organization, including consideration of paying expenses for travel to the agency or school for an interview and observation of the program. Those administrators who are not proactive in their recruitment efforts will have prolonged vacancies in their mobility positions.

Limited Resources and Third-Party Reimbursement

Third-party reimbursement includes payment for special education or rehabilitation services by a private insurance carrier or public program such as Medicare. Many rehabilitation centers have worked with clients who were injured on the job and are covered by worker's compensation laws. A limited number of private insurance carriers also cover rehabilitation costs due to non-work related accidents or illnesses—they usually require a negotiated program length and specific cost estimates.

There is currently movement among rehabilitation providers, beginning with those agencies with low vision clinics, to obtain reimbursement under the Medicare program (Massof et al., 1995). Medicare has Part A, which is in-hospital coverage, and Part B, which is reimbursement of medical care provided by the physician and other related professionals. A few agencies have been able to bill for parts of low vision services when such services are provided by ophthalmologists or optometrists; it is a complicated reimbursement program that follows a medical model format. More recently, low vision clinics based on the medical model have begun billing for activities of daily living (ADL) services (similar to reimbursement of services for occupational therapy) and O&M services similar to reimbursement for physical therapy. Many restrictions, rules, and regulations apply to these services and how and where they can be delivered.

Third-party billing requires a complex coding and reimbursement system in which the doctor and clinic must be registered as a provider with the insurance company handling the Medicare program for that state.

Time Constraints

Time is clearly a valuable commodity in education and rehabilitation settings. O&M instructors and administrators are regularly faced with time constraints that impact and restrict student scheduling and assigning personnel to students.

Typically, in an educational setting, students who are blind or visually impaired have classes that are required of all students (e.g., mathematics, reading, science, etc.); in addition, they have classes that are blindness-related (e.g., braille, adapted physical education, resource period, etc.). Matching mutual time availability for students and specialized personnel is a most difficult challenge. This is compounded in cases where O&M instructors provide itinerant services split between two or more school buildings in one district or between separate school districts with multiple sites.

Time additionally becomes a critical variable given that the typical school period is 50 minutes. This does not leave much instructional time whenever training is scheduled off the school grounds and requires travel to and from residential or business areas. The challenge is further complicated given the expansion of services to new populations. Whereas instructors in the early 1970s focused primarily on higher functioning middle- and high-school-age students; today O&M personnel have responsibility for an expanded caseload of students from preschool to adults who range from above to significantly below grade- and age-functioning levels. This often translates into decreased instructional time and increased travel time between schools, given that special education programs for students of different ages are seldom in the same school building. The same difficulty exists within rehabilitation settings due to increased caseloads caused by expansion of services, such as those for elderly blind students. As in educational settings, it is a challenge in rehabilitation agencies to include all the critical-need areas, such as adjustment and vocational counseling and daily living skills training, which compete with mobility for a slot in the schedule.

Typically in most schools and agencies the number of students waiting to receive services is greater than the capacity of the service faculty. As a result, either some students or clients are delayed in receiving the services or are provided services on a more limited basis than normal. Often students can be scheduled only two or three periods per week, given scheduling difficulties and the availability of instructors. Ideally, as in any area of instruction, concentrated O&M instruction on a daily basis is more desirable than training on a less concentrated and frequent basis. Achievement of skills is enhanced when students have regular and frequent opportunities to apply and practice what they have previously learned. This is especially critical for young children or developmentally delayed students, who have difficulty generalizing skills from one situation to another.

In many adult rehabilitation settings it is possible to provide more frequent instruction. The student may have a one-hour mobility lesson in the morning and a one-hour lesson in the afternoon. In some phases of the program it is possible to concentrate instruction in two consecutive one-hour periods of instruction. In educational settings, such scheduling opportunities, while possible, are much more challenging, given the many required subjects and scheduling conflicts. However, in some educational settings, after-school lessons or summer school programs allow more frequent and regularly scheduled O&M instruction.

It is not uncommon for O&M specialists to be challenged and questioned regarding the necessity to work with only one student at a time. These challenges center on the fact that other skill and subject areas, such as reading and physical education, are traditionally taught in instructional settings where the teacher has responsibility for more than one student per period. In these situations, however, the students are not involved in complicated learning activities or the dynamically changing environments that students and instructors face in typical O&M scenarios, such as traffic situations. In typical O&M training settings in which there are ever-present dangers, it is imperative to provide one-to-one supervision and instruction specifically tailored to meet the unique needs of an individual, rather than the general needs of a group of individuals. Although questioning the necessity for one-on-one instruction has diminished in the last 20 years, O&M instructors are still questioned by administrators who are not familiar with the travel needs of people who are blind. Typically, once the rationale for one-to-one instruction is explained, the administrator realizes individualized instruction is in the best interests of students, clients, and the school or the agency.

Paperwork Demands

Another major factor related to time constraints are paperwork requirements. Increased paperwork in the past two decades is a result of many factors. These are heightened accountability, the need for documented paper trails as a legal protection, and demand that services be goal directed and outcome based. Administrators should allow sufficient time in the mobility instructor's schedule for assessment, report writing, development of objectives, planning, and documentation of student progress. Personal computers have been effectively used to improve time efficiency in the development of individualized programs and meet the demands for documentation. In such programs, comprehensive listings of goals and objectives have been identified and are "deposited" in a "bank" from which instructors can later "withdraw" specifics to particular students' needs. Use of these computerized goals and objectives can also be used to record student progress, and have the potential to be used as a database for future program evaluation and research.

Student Injury and Liability Threats

O&M training involves balancing carefully calculated risks with exercised precautions, as students are expected to negotiate challenging environments. The possibility of student injury during O&M instruction, or after completion of training, and the subsequent potential for agency, administrator, or O&M specialist liability presents an ever-present administrative concern. Later in this chapter these critical administrative concerns will be discussed in more detail in the section on legal liability.

Generic Service Trend

Blindness-specific programs in both rehabilitation and education settings are being threatened by the trend toward generic services. Generic services that are designed to meet broad, general needs typically are less expensive than blindness-specific services, but do not provide the specific skill instruction necessary for effective functioning. Given the present—and likely future—economic climate, the trend away from specialists to generalists is expected to increase as a cost-saving strategy.

The generic approach to service provision ignores the inherent unique qualitative difference of various disabling conditions. Since the impact and needs imposed by blindness, deafness, and physical impairments are qualitatively and uniquely different, it is unlikely that generic services will be successful in responding to these needs. The service responses must be as diverse as the disabling conditions themselves.

Both the rehabilitation and education fields are similarly affected by the trend of generic services. Within rehabilitation the trend toward umbrella-type state agencies and away from separate services or commissions for the blind is an ever-increasing reality (Johnson, 1993). This concept has become a new model for delivery of services in which all individuals with widely varying disabilities and needs are served by staff generalists, as opposed to specialists. Within education, the trend toward full inclusion threatens specialized services. Proponents of full inclusion advocate for elimination of all special class placements, leaving all services to be provided only in the regular classroom (Joint Organizational Effort, 1993). Grimmelsman (personal communication, 1994) provided an example of the dangerous trend toward generic services within one state where job coaches were required to teach their clients who were blind how to travel to and from their places of employment.

Accountability and Staff Support

Administrators must balance the demand for accountability with the need to provide support of staff. They must ensure good bottom-line management and produce high-impact results while simultaneously supporting personnel who are directly responsible for client and student achievement. The administrator must strive for outcomes and results while being responsive to staff needs by providing budgetary and interpersonal support as necessary.

One of the primary responsibilities that an administrator has is providing feedback and evaluation of the O&M instructor's performance. Most agencies and schools have developed formalized evaluation systems that are used on an annual basis. In many cases these evaluation systems are not tied into direct instructional effectiveness, but rather focus on general professional and employment factors such as responsibility, interpersonal relations, attendance, and other factors. Many agencies and schools have implemented developmental supervision models where the administrator utilizes coaching-type skills to assist the teacher to improve direct instructional skills. The supervisor observes the lessons on a regularly scheduled basis throughout the year and meets with the teacher to provide feedback, reinforce desired instructional behaviors, and discuss possible alternative strategies. These developmental supervision models emphasize professional growth on an ongoing basis rather than as an end-of-the-school-year activity. With this ongoing feedback the O&M specialist has the opportunity to try new strategies and methodologies within a supportive environment.

In many cases, such as in public school programs, the administrator may not have formal training or experience in blindness. However, these individuals are expected to provide guidance, support, accountability, and supervision of highly specialized O&M instructors. The O&M specialist in such cases can assist and has a responsibility to provide opportunities for the supervisor to learn about the needs of individuals who are blind and, in particular, O&M services. This can be accomplished by providing reading material, setting up opportunities for direct observation of instruction, and providing a supervisor with the names and telephone numbers of experienced administrative peers in neighboring school districts or agencies. As supervisors gain more knowledge about blindness and O&M, they will be in a better position to understand and respond to the uniqueness of this service.

Expansion of O&M Services to Populations with Complex and Unique Needs

In the past 20 years there has been a steady increase in the expansion of services to individuals who are elderly, preschool children, and children and adults with multiple disabilities. This positive expansion of service has created a challenge particularly for staff who have not previously received specialized training in their preparation programs to meet the needs of preschoolers, elderly, or multiply disabled children and adults.

This expansion of services and the need to provide staff with the skills to respond to and meet the needs of these populations has created a great demand for comprehensive staff development opportunities. Administrators and O&M specialists should take advantage of university course work, staff development programs, and continuing education programs within their district, school, agency, or professional organization.

Continuing Education

Special attention must be given to ensuring that staff remain current with new trends, advances, and methodology in blindness and related fields. This is a shared responsibility between O&M specialists and their supervisors. Research in the blindness field indicated that "rust-out" was more of a phenomenon than "burnout" among professional staff in public and residential schools for children who are blind (Bina, 1982). It is important that O&M personnel, like all staff, attend workshops, seminars, and professional conferences. Maintaining O&M certification requires the participation in specified professional activities.

STANDARDS OF HIGH-QUALITY O&M PROGRAMS

The development of high-quality O&M programs is dependent upon specific components. Specific standards for O&M programs have been a part of the standards developed by the field and implemented by the National Accreditation Council for Agencies Serving the Blind and Visually Handicapped (NAC) since its origin. The following outline highlights the basic ingredients that are critical in ensuring the provision of quality services to students and clients.

1. *Personnel:*
   - **a.** Staff are graduates of approved university programs and achieve and maintain AER certification.
   - **b.** A supervisory evaluation and feedback system is implemented.
   - **c.** Opportunities for continuing education are provided.
2. *Program Components:*
   - **a.** Mobility program goals are tied into agency or school mission.
   - **b.** Program is well-organized, goal directed, and outcome oriented.
   - **c.** Adequate program support and resources are provided.
   - **d.** The program is student or client centered and responsive to the needs of consumers and families.
   - **e.** The program allows individualized program design and reinforcement.
   - **f.** The program is interdisciplinary in its approach and features communication systems, collaborative efforts, and has internal and external program evaluation measures to gain feedback from consumers, employers, family members, and other professionals.
3. *Administrative Accountability and Support:*
   - **a.** Mobility services are an integral part of the agency or school mission.
   - **b.** Clear written policies and procedures are established.
   - **c.** Fiscal support is provided to meet program needs.

Individual Program Planning

It is widely accepted that learning is enhanced when instruction is presented in a logical, sequential, and motivating manner. It is also widely accepted that instructors cannot approach the learning process with one prescription for all students and clients. Different approaches may be necessary for different individuals who have varying needs and learning styles. The skills for safe, efficient, and independent O&M are commonly listed in unit outlines based on travel environments (indoor, residential, business) or are established in a developmental sequence from simple to complex skills (basic skills, advanced cane travel, public transportation skills).

In the past most O&M programs, particularly at adult rehabilitation centers, used sequential unit outlines and standardized written lessons that all participants were expected to complete before moving on to the next series of lessons. The ultimate objective was to have all students complete all of the standardized lessons in a sequential manner. Today most programs do not follow such a regimented instructional model, because it is not always appropriate for their students or the setting in which they are providing services.

Nevertheless, it is extremely important that today's O&M specialists utilize sound unit- and lesson-planning methods in designing instructional plans for their students or clients. The O&M specialist must balance the need to learn specific skills in a sequential manner with the need to focus on the immediate needs of the student to catch a bus, walk safely to the mailbox, etc.

Good lesson plans delineate the instructional objective, which may be a concept, a technique, or skill to be learned, and the setting in which the lesson will be performed. Plans include how the lesson will be presented and how the student's performance will be evaluated (see Chapter 12 of this volume). It is critical that instructors and their supervisors recognize the importance of committing adequate time in evaluation of student or client needs and goals in developing written lesson plans.

Legal Liability

We live in a society where people file lawsuits against one another for seemingly inconsequential reasons. In spite of the fact that ever-increasing numbers of people who are blind are traveling safely and independently throughout their communities, the general public finds such accomplishments astonishingly remarkable. Certainly there are dangers involved and risks associated with independent travel in the environment without vision or with severely limited vision. The questions therefore arise, "What happens if a student is injured during the course of mobility training or after the program was completed?" "Can the O&M specialist be held liable?"

The best protection against liability is to apply precautions that minimize the chance of student injury. To be negligent, the O&M specialist must be proven negligent. Negligence is conduct that falls below a prescribed standard established for the protection of others. The professional standard is what a reasonable and prudent O&M specialist, acting in good faith, would or should have done in a particular situation. This standard would be presented by a professional panel of peers who would testify on what they personally felt was reasonable and prudent conduct. They would rely on established criteria and guidelines in the AER O&M Code of Ethics (see Appendix C), specified in accreditation standards, certification requirements, agency or school policy, lesson plans, and in the professional literature. A jury then would consider if the acts of the O&M specialist were reasonable, prudent, and acceptable professional behavior compared to the established standard.

For negligence to be proven, four conditions must be met: (1) the O&M specialist must have owed the student the duty of supervision and appropriately valid instruction; (2) there was a failure on the part of the O&M specialist to discharge that duty either by doing or not doing something; (3) actual injury must have occurred; and (4) a foreseeable, close, causal connection between the failure and the injury must be shown.

If any of these four conditions can be proven not to apply, an O&M specialist is most likely not to be found negligent. The first condition, in almost all cases, applies. The O&M specialist clearly owes the student a duty, especially if the individual is still in training, and in many cases this duty extends even after the student has "graduated" from training, particularly if the O&M specialist incorrectly or inadequately instructed a student. The panel of peers would establish if there was failure on part of the O&M specialist to discharge his or her duty in accordance with acceptable standards by either omitting a critical element in the instructional process or committing an act which contributed to the third condition, that is, the student injury.

O&M specialists must use good judgment and precaution in designing instructional plans that foresee potential dangers to their students, and then take steps to avoid them. Instructors must insure that their students fully understand and can safely use skills before they are advanced to new or more complex travel environments. Instructors, as a precaution, should avoid progressing students too quickly through the designed training program when there are indications or evidence they do not fully grasp the concepts or cannot apply the required skill in all situations. It is critical that the lessons provided and the acquisition of skills are carefully documented in the student's case file. For example, if they have learned to use stoplights at busy intersections safely, the case file should document how many times they did so under the supervision of the O&M specialist. An added precaution against liability and a good practice is to divulge to students, clients, and families the risks involved in O&M training. (Concerns related to risk, the potential for student injury, liability issues, and safeguards are discussed in detail in "The Legal Implications of Solo Experiences in Orientation and Mobility Training" [Bina, 1976]).

Banja (1994) presents a thorough discussion on the ethical and professional issues regarding instructors informing their students as to the potential risks and dangers involved in independent travel. Banja contends that other than the Mobility Coverage Profile and Safety Index (MCPSI) (RoboCane®) developed by B. Blasch and W. De l'Aune in 1992, mobility professionals do not have scientific methods of risk assessment by which to properly inform mobility students of the frequency or risks involved in independent travel. However, the issue of risk determination brings into focus ethical issues that mobility instructors need to attend to before, during, and at the conclusion of their program of instruction with each student.

Three items must be discussed with each student. They are as follows:

1. Since mobility is a physical skill learned in a variety of environments, there is risk of injury. The one-to-one O&M specialist-to-student ratio is designed, as much as is humanly possible, to lessen the chance of injury during the learning process.
2. The design of the plan of instruction will attempt to meet the student's objectives in acquiring O&M skills; for example, does he or she wish to travel in quiet, relatively residential neighborhoods only, or wish to travel independently in more complex environs, crossing busy streets and using public transportation? The O&M specialist needs to inform the student that risk taking increases as the complexity of the environment increases.
3. Finally, at the end of the course of instruction, the O&M specialist should discuss with the student his or her weaknesses and strengths in relation to what the plan of instruction included and the student's goals in independent travel. These points need to be documented in the final report in the student's case file or record. If a student has limitations, these must be stated and discussed in detail. The mobility specialist cannot guarantee the traveler will be accident free in independent travel any more than a driver's license insures that an operator of a motor vehicle will be accident-free.

Having the student of legal age sign an informed consent statement in which he or she acknowledges the potential and possible danger in traveling without sight in various environments is a recommended precaution and safeguard. However, these informed consent statements do not absolve the O&M specialist or an agency from liability in cases where there is negligence. Such disclosure serves as documentation which is evidence that the O&M specialist and the agency or school informed the student or their family of potential dangers and associated risks.

Liability Insurance

Another protection against legal liability is liability insurance provided by the employer or obtained by the employee through a private company.

Many states, schools, or agencies, according to common law of governmental immunity or nonliability principal, cannot be sued. Likewise, many nonprofit agencies, based on the English precedent of charitable immunity, also cannot be sued. However, even though the state or school or agency cannot be sued, the immunity often enjoyed by them does not extend to the O&M specialist. Although many states are waiving their sovereign immunity and removing charitable immunity, thus allowing these entities to be sued, this offers no additional protection for the employee. The injured party may still seek damages from the O&M specialist in addition to the legal action taken against the governmental agency. In some states where sovereign immunity has been retained, these states are permitted to carry liability insurance for their employees. Some states have adopted a "save harmless" concept, where the state gives the school district permission to "save" from "harm" a teacher from the possible financial burden of a court settlement when actions were done in good faith within the scope of employment. Within this category are many states who are self-insuring and would provide legal protection or pay legal fees and damages out of their own pockets. These states have sufficient assets to assume the burden of payment without purchasing liability insurance from an outside source. It is important that instructors employed under such circumstances have appropriate liability assurances that the employer will cover costs of both legal defense and any subsequent damages if the employee acted in good faith within the scope of his employment.

O&M instructors should request specific written information from potential or current employers regarding the exact status and extent of their legal liability protection. Even though an employer may provide either liability insurance coverage or "hold harmless" protection guarantees for their employees, instructors should also investigate taking out personal liability insurance as a supplement to existing coverage. Many professional organizations and teacher's unions offer professional liability coverage for reasonable premiums. Additionally, O&M specialists are encouraged to check with their homeowner's insurance company, which likely covers only personal and typically not professional liability protection. Generally, this type of liability protection has a business pursuit exclusion clause and does not cover a homeowner in the scope or performance of his or her employment. Often homeowner coverage can be extended to cover an individual in the scope of their employment by paying an additional premium. Also, if instructors are considering professional liability insurance, they should research what is considered adequate coverage for their particular employment situation to assure adequate coverage. O&M specialists who contract their services to schools and agencies typically by definition are not considered employees, and therefore are not entitled to benefits and protection typically afforded employees. Therefore many freelance contract instructors must obtain their own insurance coverage; however, during negotiation of the contract, it would not be considered unreasonable for the O&M specialist to inquire regarding the employer's willingness either to pay all or part of the premium or extend existing liability coverage afforded to regular agency or school employees.

A final concern is automobile insurance. O&M specialists need to understand the legal limits of insurance as it pertains to using their own vehicles to carry out their job. It is nearly impossible for an employer to purchase insurance coverage on property it does not own. In other words, an agency or school cannot purchase insurance coverage on an instructor's vehicle, because they do not own this equipment. In case of an accident, the O&M specialist's automobile insurance policy must cover all passengers transported on company business. Instructors need to examine the extent of liability, personal injury, and property damage their policy covers if their car is used for business purposes.

Some employers are able to provide a commercial auto rider provision, but such coverage only adds on to the O&M specialist's personal insurance. Such plans rarely supplant the need for O&M specialists to provide their own automobile insurance.

MOBILITY AS A CAREER

The field of O&M has grown tremendously in the last 25 years. Personnel employed in O&M range from those working as mobility assistants to O&M specialists with baccalaureate and graduate degrees. Others have become supervisors of mobility services in educational programs or rehabilitation services. Many people started out in direct services, and with experience and further education or training became administrators of agencies, college or university faculty, or researchers. Since mobility is a key factor in independence for children and adults, many opportunities exist in the fields of education, rehabilitation, and the fast-growing field of gerontology. Some professionals have taken expertise learned in O&M for visually impaired individuals and provide O&M instruction to sighted individuals with other disabilities (see Chapter 19).

Furthermore, many professionals have combined the discipline of mobility with other service areas, such as rehabilitation teaching, subject matter teaching, or gerontology. Personnel with dual preparation and certification have become extremely valuable assets to programs serving specialty populations or rural areas.

SUMMARY

The delivery of high-quality O&M services is the responsibility of O&M specialists and program administrators in agencies or schools. Mobility services are provided by a wide variety of organizations, both public and private, and delivered in center-based or community-based settings.

Mobility service providers today face many challenges, including a diverse population, time constraints in which to provide instruction, and ever-increasing caseloads. Other challenges include trends in the fields of education and rehabilitation away from highly specialized services, such as movement from O&M to generic delivery systems. Liability issues and adequate protection against potential lawsuits must be addressed in setting up mobility programs.

The development of quality O&M services within any organizational structure or physical environment is accomplished by (1) employing well-qualified O&M staff, (2) providing effective communication and supervisory systems, (3) creating a mobility program that reflects the mission of the organization, (4) being student oriented, and (5) providing adequate fiscal support.

Suggestions/Implications for O&M Specialists

1. Effective O&M services occur when administrators and O&M specialists work cooperatively, exercise good program planning, retain flexibility in scheduling, secure adequate resources, and are committed to professional standards for the program.
2. The Amendments to the Rehabilitation Act of 1992 changed the focus on clients to be served by placing a priority of service on individuals defined as having severe disabilities.
3. The Individuals with Disabilities Act (IDEA) does not mandate O&M services as a required service, but allows for O&M to be included in the Individualized Education Program (IEP) as a related service.
4. Caseload size and frequency of instruction are considerations that O&M specialists must address when planning and managing an itinerant program model.
5. The importance of good lesson planning and time management is paramount when implementing an effective O&M program.
6. Despite the trend toward generic services in adult rehabilitation and the push for inclusion in education, a strong case can be made for specialized O&M services, particularly when safety issues are a concern.
7. The recipe for developing quality O&M programs includes a mixture of hiring qualified personnel and a clearly defined and related mission for O&M services to the overall program, along with good financial support, a focus on students, and clearly written policies and procedures.
8. O&M specialists must understand the conditions that prove or disprove negligence in regard to questions of liability. They must also practice caution and exhibit good judgment in assessing student progress.
9. O&M specialists need to verify liability and automobile insurance coverages when planning a program, in order to determine the need for supplementary coverage.

ACTIVITIES FOR REVIEW

1. Describe what is meant by the term "severe disability" with regard to the Amendment to the Rehabilitation Act of 1992.
2. List the required components of all IWRPs.
3. Explain how O&M services are made a part of the IEP under the federally mandated IDEA.
4. Compare the advantages and disadvantages of center-based vs. itinerant instructional models.
5. Compare and prioritize selection criteria to be used in selecting students for O&M services. Discuss differences in selection criteria for adult rehabilitation programs and school programs.
6. Discuss the justification you would give an administrator who asks you why you can't work with more than one person at a time.
7. Discuss the importance of documentation of student progress in regard to potential liability issues.
8. Describe the major components that

should be included in developing instructional plans.

9. Devise solutions to solve problems for overcoming the time constraints of both center-based and itinerant O&M services.

10. Discuss the safety and limitation issues that should be reviewed with students or clients at the conclusion of their instructional program. How should this be documented in the case file?

CHAPTER 24

Research and the Mobility Specialist

William R. De l'Aune

Would it not be far better to let things go on as they are and hope that somehow something will emerge, while we create a valuable impression that we are really trying to solve the problems of blind mobility and in the process satisfy all sorts of personal needs? Put in this underhand way I do not suppose anybody would answer the question in the affirmative. And yet, broadly speaking we are apparently and quite cheerfully prepared to let things go on as they are, using as excuses that we do not really know what blind mobility is all about, that it is some mysterious craft at best, and that almost anything is worth trying regardless of rationale, cost, raising of false hopes, and the rest. All this would just about be all right if there were unlimited resources in manpower and finance, if there were not urgent problems crying out to be solved to make life just a little bit more tolerable for all or some of our users rather than provide a haven for just one or two.

—J. Alfred Leonard (1973)

The topics covered in this chapter are concerned primarily with the way research fits into the field of orientation and mobility (O&M) and the role that the practitioner plays in this grand scheme. They will focus on issues concerning the many possible designs of research projects rather than on the analysis of the data. Readings and lectures on details of research design and methodology are available and should be consulted to expand coverage of these topics. Some knowledge of statistical procedures is necessary for data analysis, and such information is obtainable through books, mathematically oriented friends, computer programs, and inexpensive statistical calculators. As a result, this once-insuperable hurdle to the "numerically challenged" is no longer as formidable.

Research can be thought of as a rather ritualized way of organizing and understanding the superficially chaotic world around us. The information gained through this process can and should be shared with others who might benefit from it. Because mobility specialists have access to observations in a greater variety of situations than could ever be hoped for in the laboratory, it is not unreasonable to expect them to share in the task of expanding the state of knowledge about their work. The practitioner can make such a contribution by going through the effort of structuring situations so that events are more reliably observed, making the commitment to process the resulting observations and then accurately and honestly relaying the results to fellow professionals. This effort will not only help colleagues, but will sharpen the practitioner's skills in assessing the validity of conclusions reached from other research.

DIFFERENT RESEARCH APPROACHES

"You get what you pay for," is a common expression. In research the entity purchased is knowledge. Payment is extracted through the effort and skill of the investigator in the currency of the control that researcher is able or willing to exert on subjects and their environments. In the course of this chapter we will discuss descriptive, exploratory, and experimental designs. Although the more elegant (and more controlled) research designs are "better" in the sense that they provide information with greater confidence, they may be too constrained and not prove to be practical in the everyday world of the mobility specialist. This is because the designs may demand too narrow a focus, result in ethical dilemmas, or create irreconcilable problems of control. An investigator should evaluate a number of different research approaches before any study is undertaken. The investigator must make the decision of which one to use based on the merit of the design for the specific situation and not on the basis of what method is "best" in a more abstract sense. Although it might be assumed that a super sleek, handmade sports car is "better" than the sort of car most of us are likely to drive, how adequately would it serve us in our daily automotive needs? How long, for example, would this extraordinary means of transportation remain locked in your garage waiting for the perfect, long, sunny day?

Descriptive or Naturalistic Observation

In the naturalistic approach, the researcher observes things in a natural setting in as unobtrusive a manner as possible and records and interprets his or her observations. This can be done as casually as a mobility specialist recording the progress of a client or group of clients, or in as rigidly structured a manner as the actuarial tables generated by insurance companies based on huge data sets. The effort expended by the investigator to systematically integrate and honestly report on relevant features of a large number of observations, and the skills with which these efforts are invested, determine the quality of the descriptive information.

One of the cardinal principles of the naturalistic approach is that the information gained must remain *descriptive.* Because the researcher has chosen to remain detached from the situation being observed, there are simply too many variables out of experimental control to justify any claims of causality. An instructor may note, for example, that all of her clients seem to have trouble learning to cross a certain intersection, and may suggest or hypothesize reasons for the difficulty. These hypotheses can be the subject of another more in-depth study, but when using the descriptive observational approach, one can only make concrete statements that describe the observations made concerning the difficulties one's clients are having with this task, and the relevant phenomena associated with these observations.

Exploratory, Correlational, or Psychometric Analysis

In the exploratory, correlational, or psychometric analysis, the naturalistic techniques of observation are processed at a more formal level. Once again, while not extensively intervening in the situation, the researcher might want to test the hypothesis that the difficulty in learning to cross an intersection is related to the density of traffic at the time of the lesson. The records of clients' progress could be studied to ascertain whether intersections with less traffic tend to give clients less difficulty. The mobility specialist-researcher might even want to inject more effort and skill into the enterprise by taking a random sample of his or her clients and observing their difficulty (as measured by some wonderfully quantifiable factors, such as the time it took them to learn independent crossing at a specific intersection successfully) and the density of traffic flow at the time of training (perhaps measured in cars per minute). From data obtained from this imaginary

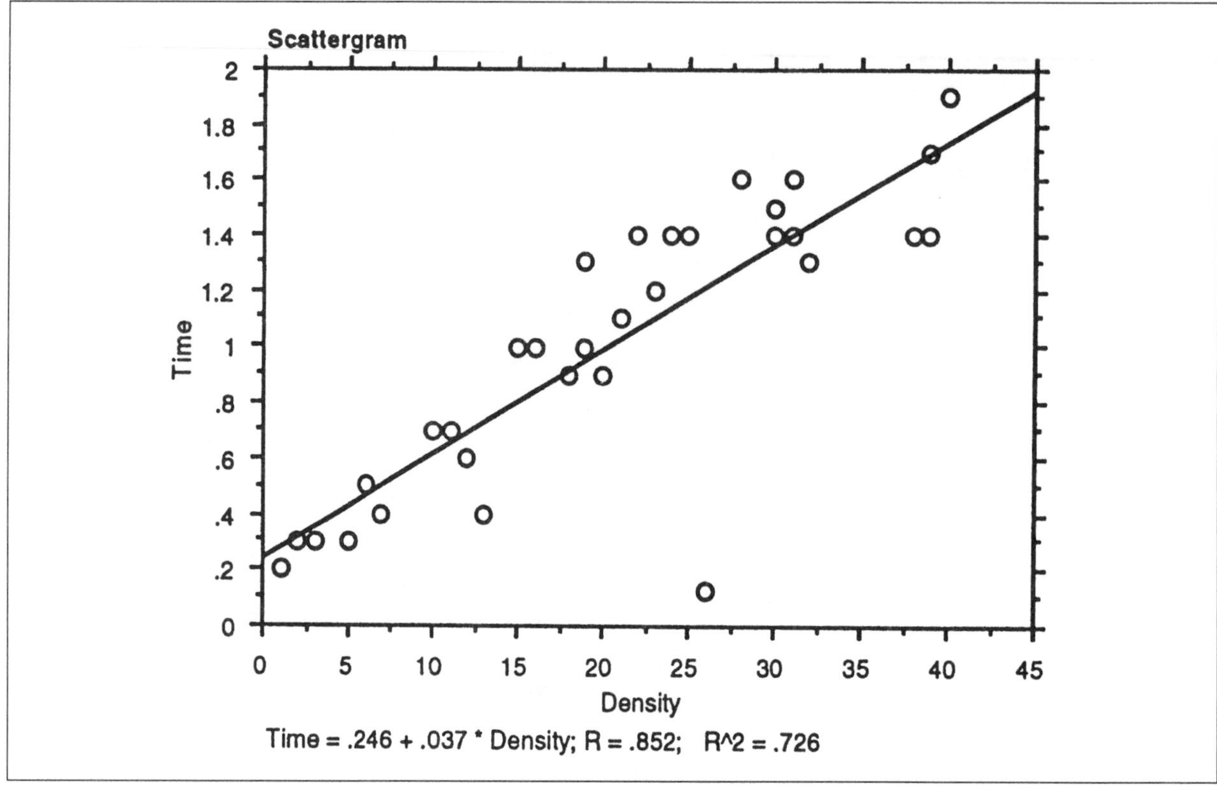

Figure 24.1. Graph showing an imaginary relationship between learning time and traffic density.

project, a graph such as the one shown in Figure 24.1 might be generated.

Analysis of this imaginary data with an inexpensive statistical calculator or a basic statistics program on a personal computer results in a correlation of 0.852 between learning time and traffic density. Most computer programs will give the equation of the line that best fits the data. (Using the equation shown at the bottom of the figure, one can predict the training time by multiplying the traffic density by 0.037 and adding 0.246 to that product.) Squaring the computed correlation of 0.852 indicates that 73 percent of the total variation in learning time can be explained by this best-fitting line, a highly significant amount.

Although enthusiastic about the findings, our budding researcher will be careful to report the correlation between traffic density and learning time as simply a *relationship*. The informed researcher is aware that a statement indicating that the increase in learning time was *caused* by the increase in traffic density is unwarranted. Once again, too little control was exerted on all of the extraneous influences to justify such a statement.

The real cause of the observed relationship may have been the complicated signal systems that go hand in hand with busy intersections. It may have been the low blood-sugar levels of the clients at the 5 P.M. exposure to the more dense rush-hour traffic. It could have been due to countless other things that were simply linked to the density of traffic variable. Although none of these possible contributing factors make the statement that there is a relationship between learning time and traffic density any less valid, they do make the causal statement false. Even if none of these contributing factors existed, because they cannot be ruled out logically, the causal statement cannot logically be made.

The Experimental Design

The basic rule of the experimental method is to keep all factors, except two, constant and then observe the effects of varying the one (the independent variable) on the behavior of the other (the dependent variable). If the introduction of the independent variable is associated with a statistically significant change in the dependent variable and if the assumption that all factors except the two variables in question have been held constant (or neutralized by random sampling techniques) is valid, then the hypothesis of change in the dependent variable being caused by the change in the independent variable is supported. The support of this causal hypothesis can be strengthened by replication of the findings, using similar protocols and different groups of subjects. This approach provides the most powerful design available to a researcher.

If the intrepid researcher-mobility specialist now wishes to go all the way and test the hypothesis that traffic density does increase learning time by the experimental approach, he or she would find himself or herself very busy. First, potentially confounding factors such as temperature, level of pollution, level of noise, and lighting would have to be controlled. There are a number of ways that this could be accomplished. An indoor intersection could be created in a tightly controlled laboratory setting so that all of these confounding variables would be held constant. An outdoor intersection could be carefully scheduled and controlled so that the confounding variables varied, but within in an acceptably narrow range. The levels of the confounding variables could be left to chance, carefully recorded, and statistically equalized (covaried) in the statistical analysis. Once these issues were settled, our researcher would then set up a formal hypothesis such as, "A heavy traffic rate, as defined by a flow of 20 or more cars a minute, will result in an increase in learning time to successfully cross the intersection without sight when compared to a light traffic rate, as defined by fewer than 20 cars a minute." After securing a random sample of subjects to neutralize potential confounding factors in the population such as level of anxiety, hearing problems, intelligence, or motor disabilities, the researcher would record the time required for instruction when traffic rates (which were under his or her control, of course) were more than or equal to 20 cars per minute or less than 20 cars per minute. If the results of the test statistic allowed the rejection of the null hypothesis (the statistically tested statement that there would be no differences between the two conditions of traffic density, as opposed to the difference predicted by the research hypothesis), the researcher could then discuss his or her experimental results that *support* the notion of causal link between traffic density and learning time.

Single-Subject and Small-Sample Designs

Single-subject experimental designs have proved particularly attractive to service providers in conducting clinical research. While this design can be used to evaluate interventions with small groups of subjects, it is particularly appealing to the clinician because it allows evaluation of interventions with a *single* client. Single-subject experiments compare baseline (generally notated as "A") and treatment or intervention phases (generally notated as "B") in terms of observed behaviors of the subject. Normally the subject is observed and behavioral data are recorded (e.g., number of collisions with obstacles during a one-hour mobility lesson) until a relatively stable baseline is observed. Using the same example of clients who have difficulties crossing a particular intersection, the researcher introduces the intervention (perhaps the use of an electronic travel aid), and data is recorded in the same manner. Typically, the comparison is replicated over time: the intervention is withdrawn, baseline measurements are repeated, and the intervention is reintroduced. This is called a withdrawal or reversal design and can be schematically represented as an A–B–A–B protocol.

The comparison can also be made across different *behaviors* (e.g., number of obstacle collisions and stumbles counted), *subjects* (two or more subjects would go through the process), or *environments* (same protocol in different places). The effectiveness of the treatment is determined by visual inspection of the charted data. The interpretation of the data resulting from this research design can be ambiguous, as opposed to the clear-cut acceptance or rejection of a null hypothesis resulting from the statistical tests possible in designs using groups of subjects. On the other hand, single-subject designs fit well with clinical practice and give service providers a framework that can assist them in evaluating interventions with an effort not significantly greater than that expended in the careful recording of clinical observations. Much more information relevant to single-subject research designs and their assets and limitations can be found in Kazdin (1978) and Yin (1989).

EXAMPLES OF MOBILITY RESEARCH

The three basic types of behavioral research (descriptive, exploratory, and experimental) are not so nicely separated. The research literature is replete with examples of studies straddling these arbitrary divisions. Rather than thinking of categories of research, it may be more productive to think of research approaches as lying on a continuum in which the amount of certainty attributable to the results is proportional to the amount of experimental control exerted by the researcher.

This question of control is central to our discussion of research and its place in O&M. Although good research and experimental design are worthwhile goals, a lot of research questions present both practical and ethical problems in exerting this control. Examples of how several projects have dealt with this consideration may illustrate the variety of solutions possible. It should be noted that these examples do not represent any attempt at fairness in sampling of the research. They were chosen to illustrate the main points of the chapter. The author's research and that of his friends feature prominently simply because it is more comfortable to point out limitations of designs one has helped to implement than to critique the work of others.

Descriptive Designs

Foundations of Mobility Research: Theory and Speculation

Psathas' (1976) article "Mobility, Orientation, and Navigation: Conceptual and Theoretical Considerations," is an attempt to establish a theoretical framework that is laid almost independently of systematic real-world observations. Much loved by the classic Greeks, this approach exhibits a concern with semantic clarity and the minute details of task description that helps researchers to formulate their thoughts in a much more precise manner than otherwise possible. Although it is easy to dismiss this sort of effort as mere "armchair speculation," it must be remembered that mobility represents a young area of study that is extremely ill-defined. It is in just this type of situation that rumination over concepts and theories becomes very important.

Nowhere is this better illustrated than in the evaluations of many of the electronic mobility devices. The question asked seems relatively straightforward: "How well does this device assist an individual with a visual impairment to meet her mobility needs?" The process of answering of such a question is anything but straightforward. Even after the characteristics of the particular visually impaired person in question are resolved (they are, after all, members of an incredibly heterogeneous population with varying degrees of visual loss and travel needs), a way of defining and quantifying mobility needs and performance must be devised for testable data to be generated. How can the complex man–machine performance be evaluated if the performance itself is tenuously defined?

Is mobility performance the speed at which the individual moves from point A to point B; the amount of coverage his cane, dog guide, or electronic travel aid (ETA) provides; the directness of his route; the security he feels in his movement; the safety with which he travels; the independence of his travel; or is it rather a composite of a lot of separate things, each weighted differently for each person, based on individual needs? If it is the latter, then professionals have to sit back and piece the bits of this puzzle together so that the framework of a testable theory of mobility will have a firm foundation upon which to build. The significance of the "armchair" contributions brought by Psathas and other mobility theorists to this cause will be judged by the magnitude of the response it precipitates from researchers and practitioners in the field, and how well it lends itself to and stands up under empirical testing.

Data-Based Theory Building

Research undertaken by Weisgerber and Hall (1975) under contract from the Veterans Administration serves as an example of a more observational approach to this same problem of clarification and definition. A compendium was developed by filtering the opinions and observations of researchers and practitioners in the field of O&M into logical subdivisions of the overall "mobility task." The authors divided the environmental sensing needs of people who are blind into four major sections, each of which is further divided into topical areas. The topical areas were each given a working definition, a rationale, examples of effective and ineffective behaviors, and a listing of those requisite behaviors that are thought to be components of that particular topical area. These behaviors are observable, and as such, lend themselves to the quantification researchers lust after.

Although significantly less lively reading than a mystery novel, the mobility specialist who plunges into this work is afforded a glimpse of his or her profession from a fresh perspective. At worst, the nitpicking nature of a system such as this provides a forum through which debate can take place on the appropriateness of the inclusion of various tasks. The compendium might also provide material for the preparation of skill area "checklists" to be used in measuring the progress of clients. The most exciting potential contribution that can come from an endeavor of this sort provides an objective, quantifiable basis for understanding and responding to the mobility needs of persons who are blind.

Knowledge-Based Theory Building

A more empirically based level of speculation is represented by some research recently completed at the Atlanta Rehabilitation Research and Development (R&D) Center, the O&M Task Safety Project. In this project, a conference of experts in the field of O&M convened in Atlanta. From this meeting a complex matrix of O&M tasks, environments, skills, and functional prerequisites (sensory, motor, and cognitive) was generated. The matrix was incorporated into a knowledge-based, computer-driven expert system, which was designed to determine if an individual with specific training and specified sensory, motor, and cognitive functions can accomplish specific O&M tasks in specified environments with an acceptable level of safety. Once this system was developed, it was used as a tool to achieve consensus with a second panel of experts. Areas of disagreement were targeted for expansion and refinement of the knowledge base. The primary product was not the computer-driven expert system, but the knowledge base for O&M task safety, generated by the best professional judgment of the field.

Model-Based Theory Building

A more tightly focused method in this vein from the Atlanta Rehabilitation R&D Center is the long-cane coverage modeling program, RoboCane®) (Blasch & De l'Aune, 1992). In this effort, a much simpler physical concept, the motion of the cane through space and the effect of this motion in clearing the path for the traveler, is modeled and an overhead point of view of the traveler is graphically depicted on a personal computer. This program allows the mobility specialist to input physical variables that describe an individual's cane technique (i.e., hand height, sweep width, cane length), and then view a graphic display showing the resultant coverage. Based on these data, the computer is able to calculate the percentage of coverage provided by the cane, the ratio of the coverage provided by the cane to the total area needing coverage (e.g., the width of the body for above-ground objects, or the soles of the feet for drop-offs). This model has been validated through a comparison of the results of the video analysis of actual cane users with the output of the RoboCane®) program. The power of such a modeling program lies in the ability of the mobility specialist to change characteristics and immediately view the consequences. What would result if the client shortened her stride length? What if the client used a different length cane? What if the client centered his hand better? All of these questions can be answered quickly and simply by the software. Such a model is limited to this simple mechanical analysis of the cane. It does not take into account all of the variables discussed by the mobility experts in the O&M Task Safety Project, but we can be much more confident of its conclusions because it examines a simpler, more mechanistic subset of the complex behavior we call mobility. It should be noted that the percentage coverage value computed by this model could be used as a dependent variable in future studies using descriptive, exploratory, or experimental designs.

The Survey: A Detailed Example of a Common Method

A major type of descriptive research in mobility is represented by the survey. Smith, De l'Aune, and Geruschat (1992) were interested in mobility problems related to vision loss. This survey study was based on Smith's dissertation that illustrated both the numerous assets and problems associated with this design. As such we will examine the methods used in the study rather than the study's results.

What better source of information on her topic than a survey of the individuals with vision loss and their mobility instructors? Smith used two national surveys (one open-ended and one forced-choice), which were administered separately to mobility practitioners and their clients. Persons with low vision were instructed to answer the surveys with only themselves and their own specific mobility problems in mind. Mobility practitioners were asked to answer the same questions, about the client filling out the survey, as well as about the low vision population in general.

The open-ended survey was relatively easy to construct. The respondent was asked one question about what were considered to be the top five, ranked in order, mobility problems experienced by them (the client), their client's problem (the mobility professional), and then problems for the low vision population in general (the mobility professional). The closed-ended survey was constructed from a literature review of low vision mobility problems and through opinions of an expert panel of reviewers consisting of both mobility professionals and consumers. This survey addressed 12 separate areas representing potential mobility problems. Each area was divided into four questions representing different specific problems in these domains. For each potential mobility problem the respondent was asked to rate the level of difficulty on a scale of 0 to 3 with 0 indicating "no problem" and 3 indicating "big problem." The expert panel reviewed the instrument for content and clarity and the revised form was subjected to pilot testing by a small sample of mobility professionals and consumers. The survey was then administered by phone with the open-ended questions asked first in order not to bias the subject's response.

The minimum sample size was determined by the accuracy required to differentiate between the intervals in the forced-choice survey instrument. With four possible response numbers (0–3) there were three intervals between the choices (approximately 33 percent of the response range), requiring an accuracy of at least 15 percent to interpret the data. Using data from a previous pilot survey, a conservative estimate of 67 percent was derived for the population rate of stated difficulty with mobility tasks. Employing this estimated rate of difficulty in a formula for estimating sample size error (Kalton, 1983), the appropriate sample size was determined to be a minimum of 78 subjects or 39 mobility practitioner–client pairs.

To obtain this sample, a national list of mobility practitioners was acquired from the Association for Education and Rehabilitation of the Blind and Visually Impaired (AER). Mobility practitioners were contacted via a cover letter briefly describing the study. Assurances of confidentiality and anonymity were provided. Participants were required to provide their own responses, contact their most current client with low vision, and work back in their client roster until a willing eligible client participant was found. Once this was accomplished, the surveys were administered by phone.

Reliability can be expressed as the accuracy of an instrument. A reliable instrument is free from error and provides repeatable consistent results. To assess *inter-rater reliability,* 20 percent of the phone surveys were scored by two different recorders with a kappa statistic used to assess agreement. Inter-rater reliability of placement of open-ended responses into selected categories was also performed. To assess *test–retest reliability,* 20 percent of the surveys were retested at approximately a 3- to 5-day interval. *Internal consistency* of the survey was assessed through the use of Cronbach's alpha.

Validity can be expressed as the usefulness of an instrument. A valid instrument fulfills the purposes that prompted the examiner to administer it. Because no standardized published instrument existed for measuring the mobility problems of persons with low vision, *criterion validity* (comparing results from this instrument with a "gold standard" instrument) could not be established. *Content validity* of the survey was addressed by the original literature review and expert review of the instrument.

The analysis of the data was relatively simple in the case of the closed-ended questions. Numerical responses to four questions in each area were added together to obtain an estimate of the degree to which the respondents thought each of the 12 potential problem areas was actually a problem. These scores were compared with each other to determine what was the greatest problem. Scores from clients were compared with those obtained from their instructors to determine differences in perceptions of problems between the two groups. Client characteristics (i.e., degree of remaining vision, age, sex) were used to group the clients and examine if different client types perceived mobility problems in different ways.

The open-ended responses, so easily written, were more difficult to analyze. The entire set of open-ended responses was first examined to determine a set of categories within which the answers could fit. The responses were then put into these categories and frequency tabulations were generated. Although this was difficult, it was manageable because of the limited size of the sample. With a large survey, analysis of open-ended questions is extraordinarily labor-intensive. Readers should remember this before they go through all the pain and effort of designing and undertaking a survey project, only to end up with data that cannot be analyzed in their lifetime.

Exploratory Designs

Multivariate Data Analysis

In 1977, De l'Aune and Needham illustrated one of the products of a multivariate analysis approach used by the research program of the Eastern Blind Rehabilitation Center of the Veterans Administration. The computer coding of a large array of patient characteristics (the basic data profile consists of 113 demographic, physical, and psychological variables for each veteran) made it possible to "observe" the characteristics of a large number of clients who are blind. Among other things, it was possible to compute mean values for different variables on the center's clients. Histograms were plotted to illustrate characteristics, such as age distribution of the client population. The computer could also easily compare the depression scores from the Minnesota Multiphasic Personality Inventory (MMPI) of different categories of blinded veterans (e.g., nondiabetic blinded veterans versus diabetic blinded veterans). Correlations could be generated between age and MMPI depression scores. Indeed, it was possible to compute correlations between every variable and every other variable

(6,328 distinct correlations). At the 0.05 level of significance, this number of correlations would be expected to randomly provide the investigators with 316 statistically significant relationships and a lot of publications!

It should be obvious that such a system is vulnerable to abuse. It should be equally obvious that exploratory data analysis has value. Especially in the absence of significant prior research addressing this scope of client characteristics, such a data set and statistical analysis techniques have tremendous power to define relationships and major factors involved with rehabilitation and all of its component parts. When performance on a device was added to the variable list and analyzed for relationships with the items on the client data profile, the researchers were able to make some sense out of the clinical observation, "Some people just seem to do better than others." The initial correlative studies can be used to identify major predictive factors and direct the investigators into studies of a more specific nature. They also provide preliminary data that are valuable in the design of screening, pretraining, and lesson plans for the devices or skills.

Three-Factor Measurement

A similar, although much more narrowly focused, technique was employed in the assessment of mobility performance by a group at the University of Nottingham (Armstrong & Heyes, 1975). By concerning themselves with and monitoring three factors assumed to be linked to the elusive concept called "mobility skill," the researchers were able to construct performance profiles of individuals who were blind and using dog guides, long canes, ultrasonic spectacles, and the Swedish laser cane. The first factor, safety, was measured by recording the frequency of unintentional physical contact with various parts of the environment and the frequency of unintentional departures from the sidewalk, both mid block and at the end of the block (Armstrong & Heyes, 1975). The second factor, efficiency, was measured by both the walking speed and the smoothness or continuousness of the walking. Smoothness was defined as the ratio between the length of time taken by the person to cover a specific distance and the proportion of that time during which he was actually physically moving forward (Armstrong & Heyes, 1975). The final factor, psychological stress, was measured by monitoring the average stride length of the subject. All of these data were gathered while the subject traveled on a standard outdoor route.

It should be noted that even with all of the computer coding mentioned in the previous study and the sophisticated videotaping used by this group, these studies are still dealing with observational and correlational techniques.

Heightened Controls

Researchers at the Department of Electrical Engineering, University of Canterbury, Christchurch, New Zealand (Kay, 1976), went even further and controlled such variables as lighting and temperature as their subjects were electronically tracked in a 60 × 40 foot (18 × 12 m) enclosure. As the subject moved, signals were generated by a computer under the command of the experimenters. These were presented to the subject as indications of imaginary objects in the laboratory. Through their investigations of the optimum signals for effective perception of the imaginary objects, the researchers planned to design mobility devices employing these signals. In this case the investigators were not only observing the behavior of their subjects while they travel in a highly controlled, standardized environment, but they were also presenting controlled stimuli to them. The resulting data were therefore capable of being much cleaner than those obtained in any of the methods previously cited.

The tight focus, the very aspect of this work that makes it so methodologically attractive, also makes it essential that all of the other "human factor" variables that are not considered explicitly in the design are canceled out by random sampling techniques. As a chain's strength is defined by the strength of its weakest link, so is the strength of a research project defined by its weakest aspect. Because of the difficulties encountered in samples from the extremely heterogeneous visually impaired population, this factor usually provides the truest test of a study's worth. The sophistication lavished on the instrumentation could be lost if poor sampling techniques are used in subject selection.

One must also keep in mind that the results from laboratory settings such as this one are not automatically applicable to the universe outside. If a display proves to be significantly more effective in this setting, we cannot assume that these results will generalize into the highly variable environment of the real world. However, this approach does provide us with the *best estimate* we can obtain.

Heightened Control in a More Natural Setting

A study by Guth and LaDuke (1995) provides an example of a tight case study research design executed and reported in a terse, economical manner. Four pedestrians who were blind served as subjects in three 15-trial sessions. The subjects' tendency to veer was examined on videotapes made while participants walked across an asphalt tennis court. The information obtained from such a project can be regarded as very high in quality due to the design, sampling, and analysis.

It is still difficult to be able to generalize the results from data obtained from such a small sample observed on a smooth, obstacle-free surface. Also, one could argue that such a narrow focus contributes little to filling in the large gaps of knowledge in the mobility field. However, it is difficult to dispute the argument that if complex mobility problems were broken down into such manageable chunks, they could eventually be solved.

Experimental Design

Single-Subject Design

LaGrow and Murray (1992) provided an excellent and practical example of how a single-subject research design can be used to measure the effectiveness of a low vision rehabilitation intervention. A simple reversal design (baseline–intervention–baseline–intervention) was discussed by the authors and is illustrated in Figure 24.2. This A–B–A–B protocol is considered appropriate for the assessment of the efficacy of an intervention in which learning is not the primary concern (e.g., light, contrast, complexity, and image size). For example, if image size is the intervention (independent variable), time needed to complete a standardized reading task (the dependent variable) with 8-point print (baseline), time needed with 16-point print (intervention), time needed with 8-point print, and time needed with 16-point print can be recorded. From the resulting graph, the effectiveness of doubling the size of the image can be visually evaluated. The authors pointed out that this simple design is most appropriate when only one level of the intervention is used. However, things are seldom this simple. They noted Faye (1976) recommends that when prescribing an optical device, a *range* of magnifications should be evaluated.

For this type of problem the authors used a variation of the reversal design, the alternating treatment design. This more elaborate single-subject design not only indicates if the intervention is effective, but which of the tested levels of the intervention has the greatest effect on the dependent variable. The authors wanted to determine which of two levels of magnification was most effective in allowing a client to read maps and graphs, as measured by the time required to identify certain characteristics of the maps and graphs. The authors employed a design represented as A–B–B′–A–B′–B′C–B. "A" stands for the baseline phase (no magnification). "B" stands for the phase in which two levels of magnification were presented. During this B phase the level of magnification to be used in the intervention was *selected.* "B′" stands for the intervention phase in which the selected magnification is *used.* The next A represents a return to the baseline level of magnification followed by B′, a return to the intervention phase. The authors then increased the complexity of the design by looking at another

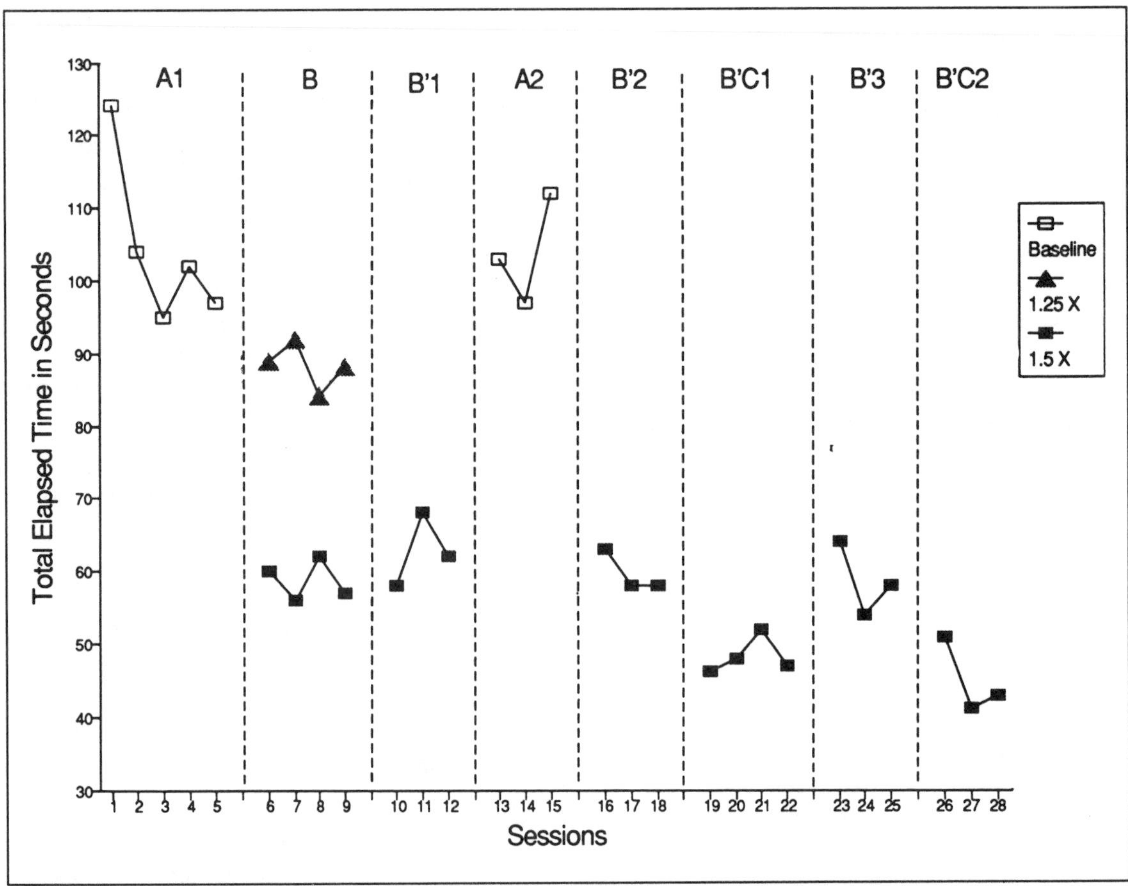

Figure 24.2. The total elapsed time taken to identify specified countries when a map reproduced (A) without increasing the size or contrast, (B) increasing the map 1.25 times and 1.5 times the original size, and (B′C) enlarging the map with added contrast is read.

Source: From S. LaGrow & S. Murray, 1992. Use of the alternating treatment design to evaluate intervention in low vision rehabilitation. *Journal of Visual Impairment & Blindness, 86*(10), 435–439.

intervention. "B′C" represents an additive phase in which the contrast level of the materials was enhanced. The final return to B′ was used to evaluate if any change in the dependent variable seen in the additive phase was due to the use of higher contrast.

LaGrow and Murray's study has elegance and simplicity, and shows the clinical relevance of single-subject techniques. Their report (1992) is well worth reading to obtain the level of detail required for an appreciation of this particular design and to gain some insights as to how it might be applied to a mobility practice.

Control Group Design

Up to this point no examples of studies in the mobility field utilizing a classic, grouped experimental design have been cited. This is not because of a lack of such studies, but because of the lack of any "major" clinical research being carried out in this manner. The focus of such studies is by definition very narrow. This incremental approach to increasing knowledge keeps the research clean, but tends to make the results less interesting to practitioners. The necessity of withholding a potentially beneficial treatment to the control group also poses ethical problems of severity in direct relationship to the degree of expected benefit.

De l'Aune, Scheel, and Needham (1974) used such a design. They exposed an experimental group to an acoustic training experience for approximately 300 seconds. Next, their performance in detecting lateral openings in a corridor was compared to the performance of a control group not exposed to the training. The statistical analysis of the results indicated that the performance of the experimental group was significantly higher than that of the control group.

This design provided very high-quality information about the efficacy of this particular training technique for the analysis of lateral openings in the hallway used in the experiment, but no information was provided as to the generalizability or durability of the training effect. It could be concluded that the increase in performance was brought about by the exposure to the stimuli used in the training session.

APPROACH TO RESEARCH

This chapter has introduced a wide range of research being done in the O&M field. All of the different designs have their advantages and disadvantages. They all have problems that compromise the reliability of the information they provide. All practitioners will have the same sorts of problems, and like the researchers cited, practitioners must not be deterred from undertaking projects of interest. The remainder of this chapter addresses problems with sampling not previously discussed, recommends a pragmatic approach to research design, and finally offers suggestions for doing research in the area of follow-up.

Sampling

Sample Size

One of the more pervasive trouble spots is the sampling of subjects from the client population. How many subjects should one have? The statistical power of an experiment is usually computed to determine how large a sample to use or how effective a given sample size will be. In other words, the statistical power tells us how sensitive a design will be in testing the null hypothesis. More subjects will result in increased sensitivity. The traditional feeling (especially in areas of research where there is a difficulty in obtaining subjects) is that "the bigger the sample, the better the study." However, this can be abused—a study using a large sample can be so sensitive to group differences that differences between groups can be determined to be statistically significant while remaining clinically irrelevant. For example, the author could design a study testing a drug to lower body temperature with thousands of subjects in the experimental and control groups. This would result in a sensitivity that might measure temperature differences between the drug users (experimental group) and the placebo users (control group) to a small fraction of a degree. Although a reduction in temperature of a few hundredths of a degree might be found to be statistically significant in such a study, the clinical significance of this small a change would be minimal. Power analysis allows one to determine how large a sample is needed to be sensitive to *the smallest change the researcher considers to be relevant.* Wiener (1971) provides more information on this subject, but it would probably be better for readers to speak with a statistician in determining power.

Sampling Problems

Visually impaired subjects bring to our research projects a multitude of variables that are not under our control. In theory, the best method of working around this is through the use of *random sampling* techniques in the hope that the differences between clients will cancel themselves out. This, however, requires fairly large samples drawn from even larger populations, a luxury not available to many researchers in this field.

In a given geographic area, the visually impaired population is not always numerous enough to provide a good subject pool from which to draw a random sample. In addition, some of the potential subjects may not be willing to participate in research projects, giving the investigator the additional concern of having his or her few subjects come from a nonrandom sample. This particular problem is especially apparent in some technical device evaluations, where one suspects only the very device-oriented segment of the target population participated. This self-selection factor has a major impact on the generalizability of the research results from studies of this type.

Even if good sampling opportunities present themselves, researchers run into confounds caused by major differences in the functional visual attributes of the sample. If the population is compartmentalized into subgroups based on visual abilities and stratify the sample, the limited population size is taxed further. If standardization on vision is imposed by blindfolding all of the visually impaired subjects, the sample is homogenized, but overlooks the effects of useful residual vision on the task in question.

There are many other sampling problems intrinsic to this population. Differences between individuals experiencing vision loss adventitiously or congenitally should be considered in any project. The problem of varying levels of novelty in the sightless experience due to duration of loss is another matter of concern. The age of the subjects is a major factor. Differences in the experiences of visually impaired persons who grow old versus elderly persons who become visually impaired have only recently been noted.

Of course, one can solve most of the sampling problems by using sighted subjects in the studies made artificially "blind" by the use of blindfolds or low vision simulators. One would then be confronted with all sorts of additional questions, such as abnormally high anxiety levels induced by the blindfolds, prior experience advantages of the "real" blind people, ad infinitum. The generalizability of data generated from such a study becomes a matter of great concern.

If all of these basic problems are added to the difficulty of designing or finding tests appropriate to the dimensions about which assessment is desired in the first place, this seems to be a hopeless situation. It seems patently impossible to eliminate all of the problems. There is no solution, but there is a strategy.

Compromise

The strategy for dealing with the problems listed above is not very satisfying, but it is the same as used by researchers in other, more traditional, scientific fields: a compromise! The researchers must try to do the best they can with the situation they have. The ideal of an experimental design should be approached as closely as possible, but valid investigations should not be deferred simply because the ultimate in scientific rigor is unobtainable.

When the work of other researchers in the field is read, this must be kept in mind. It is permissible to utter a sad, "tsk, tsk," when a methodological "error" is spotted, especially if the reader can visualize a way in which the source of the flaw could be minimized without adding additional problems. This should be brought to the author's attention, but in the meantime the study should still be read and the information valued in relationship to the rigor of the work. *All studies are flawed.* A responsible investigator will call these flaws to the attention of his or her audience and explain the reasons for their presence and the consequences they may have on the results.

This all boils down to a reassertion of the validity of the variety of ways in which research, the contribution of knowledge to the field, is possible. The practical applications of this pragmatic research philosophy may be made more apparent if we examine possible solutions to a common research question that readers may wish to address.

Follow-Up

If one can assume that some sort of follow-up is desired to assess the effectiveness of one's services, what would be the best way to accomplish this? The answer, as might be expected, is a resounding, "It depends!"

The "best" way would probably be to observe the client in his or her home environment at various times after the delivery of the services in question and directly ascertain the effectiveness of the services. The "ideal" would include preintervention observations against which the postintervention observations could be compared. To this, a control group for whom no services had been provided should be added. For example, a group of randomly sampled clients may have been observed experiencing independent travel an average of 15 minutes a day before mobility training. After training, this group may have averaged 4 hours a day of independent travel, contrasting sharply with the 15 minutes a day average maintained by the control group. This data would indicate a spectacularly effective mobility training program.

Not only would this experimental design pose ethical problems because of the unannounced observation and the arbitrary withholding of services for the control group, but it would be incredibly costly and difficult to do. A lot of time and effort could be saved by simply visiting the client after the delivery of services and asking her how much he or she traveled now as opposed to the amount of traveling done immediately before training.

This method gives the same general information as in the previous example, but forces one to assume that the client had an accurate knowledge of this information and was providing undistorted answers. The practitioner could never be certain if the client was trying to please the agency by reporting an excessive improvement or attempting to purposely minimize the benefit of the training for personal reasons. The interviewer could make note of corroborative evidence, such as the condition of the client's cane (especially tip wear) or the comments and observations of the family, in an attempt to make the data more valid. Better yet, the O&M instructor could visit in person and observe the client in an appropriate travel situation.

If a personal visit is not possible because of time or the distance involved, a phone follow-up could be a viable alternative. All of the problems involving validity present in the preceding method would remain. It would be possible, however, to speak to the client's family after the formal part of the interview and attempt to verify the statements.

Another even less expensive alternative is that of a mail follow-up. In addition to the normal problem of questionnaire reliability, the researcher faces—with persons who are visually impaired—varying degrees of difficulty in their independently answering the questionnaires. If sighted assistance is required, then possible social pressures may act to influence the responses. One also now has a problem of a significant number of individuals who may choose not to respond at all. This may bias the sample and give data on only a selected number of the clients.

Three ways have been examined to attack this rather simple problem. Each method has inherent levels of confidence in the information gathered. Each method is different in terms of cost, both in terms of time and money; none are "ideal." One thing remains certain, even the method that gives the least amount of information will provide more than what would be obtained if no type of follow-up were attempted. The method used should be the best for the given situation, considering the resources available.

SUMMARY

The purpose of this chapter was to encourage practitioners to become personally involved with research. It is acknowledged that the bulk of the material presented, however, has covered little but the difficulties encountered in doing this. It has shown that the research of the "professional researchers" in mobility is far from being without fault or beyond criticism. And now, to pile insult onto injury, the practitioner is encouraged to enter this arena of ambiguity.

The reason is thus: The opening quote by Alfred Leonard. The O&M field cannot afford to turn its back on the gaps in the present knowledge of mobility. Information is needed and practitioners have the best access to it. As professionals, there is a mandate to share this information and assist in building the body of knowledge of the profession.

Research should be well-thought out and carefully executed, but not considered immune to criticism. Because all of the systems have flaws, valid comments on these flaws are desirable. Clear statements from the researcher on the limitations of the study are the most desirable of all, but constructive criticism from others should always be welcomed. Readers should not be afraid of reviews before doing a project. A research proposal should be reviewed by an institutional Human Investigations Committee, where it will be evaluated with a sensitivity for subject protection and ethical issues. A research and development committee should also review proposals for methodological adequacy. In addition, peers should review a proposal to determine its practical significance.

After the project results are reported, criticism should still be welcome. Methodologic criticism, if valid, can be used to improve future research efforts. The results may not mean what the researcher had originally thought they meant, because of a design flaw or the volatile and variable nature of some of the situations and most of the subjects studied, but the results will have meaning. This meaning may be crucial to the work of another researcher.

In a similar vein, comments endorsing the nature of a design, but denouncing the trivial nature of the results should bother the researcher only a little. Trivial findings are not as nice as big Nobel Prize-level findings, but there simply are not enough of those kinds of findings to go around. The determination of the importance of a research result is usually through hindsight in a historical perspective, so the researcher may even have the last laugh, albeit posthumously. The normal function of "trivial" findings is to serve as a piece of a jigsaw puzzle involving a "major" problem.

The one criticism a researcher should never have to endure is an accusation of dishonesty. Results should be respected, even if they are not as impressive as one had hoped, or if they failed to match original expectations. Research increases knowledge in an incremental fashion, and every bit of information helps the process along. Misinformation or data presented in a manner intended to mislead the reader or misrepresent the results are never justified.

This chapter was not intended as a work to refer to in designing a research project. There are other books available (e.g., Rowntree, 1981) and other individuals to consult who can serve much more adequately in this mission than a short piece such as this. Practitioners need to read and talk a lot about research design and statistical methods before becoming *seriously* involved with research. Ask colleagues and favorite teachers for their recommendations.

This chapter was intended as an encouraging agent, a sort of cheerleader for research. If one still feels shaky about the project lying dormant in one's head, talk it over with a professor or an experienced researcher. You will find that very few of us have unlisted phone numbers.

Suggestions/Implications for O&M Specialists

1. In using a descriptive or naturalistic approach, the researcher observes things in a natural setting in as unobtrusive a manner as possible and records and interprets his or her observations. The information gained from this type of approach must remain descriptive because of the large number of variables beyond experimental control.
2. In an exploratory, correlational, or psychometric approach, the observations are processed at a more formal level. The data are described statistically and relationships and associations are examined. As with the descriptive approaches, too little experimental control is exerted on the variables observed to express more than statements of association.
3. In an experimental approach, all factors except two are kept constant. The researcher observes the effects of varying one (the independent variable) on the behavior of the other (the dependent variable). A change in the dependent variable associated with change in the independent variable *supports* a causal relationship. It is rare that sufficient control is present over "all other factors" to justify a definitive statement of causality.
4. Single-subject designs are attractive to service providers because they are based on interventions with a single client. They represent a framework that, although not terribly more complex than that found in the careful recording of typical clinical observations, allows the evaluation of interventions and the progress of clients.
5. Reliability can be expressed as the accuracy of an instrument. Interobserver (rater) reliability, test-retest reliability, and internal consistency are all types of reliability assessments.
6. Validity can be expressed as the usefulness of an instrument. Content validity and criterion validity are types of validity.
7. Forced-choice items in a survey instrument are more difficult to prepare, but are easier to analyze. Open-ended items are easier to prepare but more difficult to analyze and interpret.
8. The number of subjects in a study (the sample size) is determined by the degree of sensitivity to association or difference required by the research question. To be relevant, a study's statistically significant resolution should be similar to resolution required by clinical significance.
9. Research studies, particularly in clinical rehabilitation, are complex and almost inevitably flawed. These flaws result in limitations in the studies, but do not invalidate the information gained.
10. Because of their access to clinical information and insights, it is mandated that practitioners share this information with their profession by conducting or becoming involved with research.
11. Research results may be flawed or disappointing, but they should never be dishonest. Misinformation or data presented in a manner intended to mislead the reader or misrepresent the results are never justified.

ACTIVITIES FOR REVIEW

1. Review a mobility research paper and identify the research questions, the type of approach used to answer the question, the independent and dependent variables, the method of analysis, the results, and the conclusions. Are the conclusions appropriate in light of the data? Justify your last response.
2. In the previously reviewed mobility research paper, describe another (hopefully simpler) way to answer the research questions. What are the problems and advantages to your approach? Do you think your approach is better than the one used in the paper?
3. Certain mobility situations may activate dimensions of trait anxiety identified by Endler (1983). Describe a study that could test this supposition.
4. Describe a mobility problem and an intervention. How could the intervention be evaluated using a single-subject design?
5. A researcher has come up with a mobility technique to speed up travel. In an experiment with a large number of subjects (and a large amount of money), she has found that the time to travel a route has decreased at a statistically significant level with the new technique. The average time to complete the route with the standard technique was 4 minutes. The average time to complete the route with the new technique was 3 minutes and 57 seconds. Are you impressed with this statistically significant gain? Why not? What would you think a clinically relevant decrease in time for traveling the route would be?
6. One type of validity not discussed in this chapter is construct validity. Find a source that describes construct validity and summarize it in your own words.
7. A common method for describing the central point of a list of values that measures an attribute of a group (e.g., age) of subjects is the mean or average value of that attribute for the group. A common method for describing the variation of those values is the range. Another method for describing the variation is the standard deviation. Find a source that describes how the standard deviation is computed and summarize this computation in your own words.
8. Discuss the sources of information used for questions 6 and 7 with your peers. Which are the simplest and most easily understood sources? Remember the sources you feel comfortable with for future reference.
9. Should you report the results of an experiment that you have conducted that leads to a conclusion that you do not personally believe? Why?
10. Despite the fact that the sources you've found that take you beyond this chapter are difficult to read, the author of this chapter feels very strongly that you, as a practicing mobility instructor, should be actively involved with both critically reviewing the research of others and doing your own research in mobility. Why should you go through the trouble?

EPILOGUE

The Future

During the time between the publication of the first edition of this text and the current edition, the profession of orientation and mobility (O&M) has grown and matured. For the first edition, it was not possible to turn to O&M specialists to author all of the chapters. The editors had to seek several authors outside of O&M who could apply the principles of their disciplines to address the needs of O&M. With the maturing of the discipline, the editors of the current edition in almost every case were able to identify at least one O&M specialist to prepare each of the chapters. Further evidence of the maturing of the profession can be found by examining the citations at the end of this volume. A quick glance through these references will show the reader that a large proportion of research has been conducted directly by O&M specialists. One of the key ingredients in the maturing of a profession is the development of its knowledge base. O&M has taken the responsibility of extending its knowledge base by examining its assumptions and experimentally validating its conceptual foundations, as well as its procedural strategies. The next steps for the discipline are to evaluate its effectiveness, extend its horizons to serve individuals with other disabilities, adapt instruction to the changing populations and the changing environment, make use of appropriate emerging technology, and keep its service delivery models consistent with best practices.

EVALUATION OF EFFECTIVENESS

The profession of O&M is developing at a time when everyone is required to prove the worth of the services that are provided. Throughout the human service fields there is a cry to establish outcome measurements that demonstrate the effectiveness of services. Providing O&M in such an environment requires practitioners to evaluate instruction and document its effect on the children and adults who are served. It is no longer enough to simply say that practitioners do "good work" or that they "touch lives." O&M specialists must make a concerted effort to measure performance outcomes. This provides a challenge to develop a common vocabulary and establish tools to document the changes in performance that occur as a result of instruction. Currently the U.S. Department of Veterans Affairs and the National Accreditation Council for Agencies Serving the Blind and Visually Handicapped are working together to establish measurement instruments that can be used by agencies to evaluate their effectiveness. In a similar way some private agencies are being encouraged by the United Way to evaluate the outcomes of their services. As part of this movement, the professionals in the area of O&M must agree on measures that will document service effectiveness and contribute to this process. In the years ahead, continued emphasis will be placed on standards and indicators to evaluate services.

SERVICES FOR INDIVIDUALS WITH OTHER FUNCTIONAL MOBILITY LOSSES

The process of O&M instruction has led to an awareness that many individuals with disabilities other than visual impairments are subject to O&M limitations and may benefit from formal mobility instruction. In the years to come, instructors will be called upon to address the needs of these persons who have functional limitations in travel. The dimensions of travel problems have been the basis for an emerging noncategorical model of mobility (see Chapter 16 of this volume). Preparing O&M specialists to provide instruction to individuals with various disabilities other than blindness is a necessary step for the future. This will entail developing a comprehensive university preparation curriculum that encompasses all disabilities, expanding certification, and networking with new service providers. The first step toward this expansion has been achieved through the awarding of a grant to address these tasks. Western Michigan University (WMU), working in association with organizations and people in the disability movement (the Association for Education and Rehabilitation of the Blind and Visually Impaired, the Association for Retarded Citizens, the Eastern Paralyzed Veterans Association, the United Cerebral Palsy Association, the Association for the Help of Retarded Children, the Research and Training Center on Traumatic Brain Injury, the U.S. Department of Veterans Affairs, the State University of New York, consumers of services, and various service providers), has been awarded a grant from Project ACTION of the National Easter Seals Society to determine practice competencies, establish a curriculum, develop a national certification examination, and plan a certification process for practitioners. The present plan is to establish a process that will include development of new university programs to prepare practitioners at undergraduate and graduate institutions, as well as to expand the current university programs in blindness to incorporate the additional competencies that will prepare instructors to teach independent travel to individuals with various disabilities. Activities are also under way to secure funding to offer continuing education for currently practicing O&M specialists so that they will be able to increase their knowledge base to serve this expanded population.

CHANGING POPULATIONS

Services to adults and children who are visually impaired have changed as a result of changing needs of the client population. In addition to meeting the travel needs of people with no functional vision, O&M specialists have taken on the additional responsibility of helping people with low vision use their vision effectively while traveling. They have embraced low vision teaching strategies, which include teaching the use of unaided vision to identify the critical features of the environment, and teaching the use of optical devices to reach out and examine the details in the environment. O&M specialists are also finding that they are working with more individuals who are elderly or have multiple impairments. This has necessitated instructors to become more comfortable with new devices such as the adaptive mobility devices (AMDs) and other adaptive equipment such as walkers, orthopedic canes, wheelchairs, and other assistive devices. Instruction itself has changed and increased its emphasis on meeting immediate needs of the student in addition to the more traditional approach of teaching toward generalization to new environments. In work with multiply impaired children, assessment has focused upon transdisciplinary evaluation, which reduces the number of new practitioners introduced to the child and establishes less complicated communication with parents. Instruction has also expanded to include more emphasis on work with infants and toddlers. Early work starts with involvement of the parents and often proceeds to instruction with AMDs or special canes for children. Based on the changing populations, personnel preparation programs will need to assess practice needs continually, and modify their programs accordingly.

Statistics show that 12 percent of the population is elderly, and this is expected to grow to 18 percent in the years to come. It is also known that more than 70 percent of people who are blind are 65 years old or older. As Crews and Clark in Chapter 14 of this volume indicated, almost 2.7 million people over 65 years of age have severe visual impairment; by the year 2030, as baby boomers enter the ranks of the elderly, the numbers will increase to 6 million. The rate of severe visual impairment is proportionally greater in the upper age categories (Nelson & Dimitrova, 1993). Individuals between the ages of 65 and 74 experience severe visual impairment at the rate of 47 per 1,000; between the ages of 75 and 84 the rate changes to 99 per 1,000. For those over the age of 85, the prevalence rate is 250 per 1,000. With this growing number of visually impaired elderly will come a need for O&M specialists to provide service. The techniques and strategies that young people use to travel may not be the same as those needed by elderly people. An understanding of older individuals, their capabilities, and their limitations will help instructors provide better training. Increased emphasis on aging will need to take place in the university personnel preparation programs as more and more elderly people experience visual impairment.

Many elderly individuals who are blind do not have an employment goal but are in need of O&M services to permit them to achieve independent functioning. Although the Rehabilitation Act of 1973 (as amended) provides rehabilitation services to assist these individuals to become independent homemakers, the emphasis of this act is to return working-age individuals to gainful competitive employment in integrated settings. Older individuals will therefore need a source of rehabilitation funding that is not tied to employment. Title VII, Chapter 2 of the Rehabilitation Act is designed to meet this need and will take on more and more importance in serving these individuals. Funding for this program, however, has been less than $10 million for the entire nation. With such a low level of funding, few practitioners can be hired to meet the needs of older persons. Higher appropriations will be needed so that O&M services can be provided. A second approach is to tap into the expanding field of health care to pay for O&M services. However, O&M has not been on the list of services that are reimbursable for Medicare, Medicaid, or other forms of third-party reimbursements. Opportunities for reimbursement may appear, however, as managed care continues to develop and integrated health care systems take on more responsibility for functional impairments, rather than just clinical health care. In the future, a funding source will be needed so that O&M can become a routine part of services for older individuals with vision loss.

THE CHANGING ENVIRONMENT

The Americans with Disabilities Act, through its accessibility guidelines [*Americans with Disabilities Act Accessibility Guidelines* (ADAAG)], and the Uniform Federal Accessibility Standards from the Architectural Barriers Act have designated scoping requirements that serve to make the environment more accessible. The guidelines provide specifications for such features as protruding objects, head room, signage, landmarks, stairs, and elevators. In addition, guidelines have been suggested to serve as a warning of impending danger in such places as corners, where there are wheelchair cuts, and along the edges of platforms in rapid-rail environments. Although statistics show that visually impaired travelers find it difficult to detect perpendicular streets at sloping corners (Bentzen & Barlow, 1995) and at times miss platform drop-offs (Uslan, Peck, Wiener, & Stern, 1990), usage of tactile warnings in these locations has not yet been universally accepted. An expansion of such warning indicators throughout the environment will be necessary so that visually impaired travelers can more consistently detect streets and hazards.

Semi-actuated and fully actuated traffic signals are presenting difficulties for many travelers who are blind. Traffic-actuated controllers, unlike pretimed controllers that have fixed cycle times, change according to variations in the volume, location, and speed of traffic. Such actuated controllers are most often found at intersections where traffic volume is irregular, or where it is necessary to maximize traffic volume on a main street that contains a large flow of traffic. These controllers now account for approximately 50 percent of the traffic signals in the United States, and their numbers will continue to increase. If only one car is present at an intersection, these signals do not allow sufficient time for a pedestrian to cross the street. They sense the presence of the car and allow just enough time for the car to go through the intersection before changing back, and do not consider the time requirements for a pedestrian to complete a crossing. This becomes a problem for blind travelers, who depend upon the start-up surge of a car to signal when it is time to cross. Although there is often a pedestrian control button to regulate the flow of traffic, the totally blind traveler may not know of its existence or may have trouble finding it. A solution to this problem will have to be found that will allow both efficient control of the traffic and safe methods for blind people to cross the street. In the future it will be important for O&M specialists to form a working coalition with traffic engineers to examine traffic control issues and thus prevent future problems from arising.

External bus announcements represent an opportunity for visually impaired travelers to increase the information available for them at bus stops. While sighted people are able to identify an approaching bus through visible signage, people with visual impairments are often unable to easily identify the correct bus and must solicit assistance of a sighted passerby, or board the bus to ask the driver the route number of the bus. The *Americans with Disabilities Act Accessibility Guidelines* (*ADAAG*) outlines standards for presenting information that is usable by persons with visual disabilities. Standard 1192.35 (Public Information System) indicates that buses should be equipped with a public address system to announce stops and provide other passenger information within the vehicle. Similar information would be most useful if it could also be made available to pedestrians waiting at a bus stop through external speakers employed outside of the bus. Although *ADAAG* stops short of requiring announcements to be employed externally to assist individuals identify buses while waiting at stops, research is under way to study its feasibility and effectiveness (Wiener, Ponchillia, Joffee, & Kuskin, 1997). It is therefore hoped that external announcements or a comparable system will be required in the future.

EMERGING TECHNOLOGY

Current electronic travel aids (ETAs) have focused upon either indicating a clear path in front of the individual as he or she walks or expanding the individual's ability to sense the presence or absence of objects farther ahead or to the sides. In the near future a generation of devices may be available that will provide detailed information about the individual's position in the environment. Electronic orientation aids (EOAs) like Strider in the United States and MoBIC in Europe are anticipated to provide detailed information regarding location and will be able to identify when an individual has deviated from a planned route. The system functions by triangulating on 3 of 24 global positioning satellites and uses this information to pinpoint the location of the traveler. When this is combined with a map of the area and appropriate software to translate this information from a longitude and latitude into a verbal description of the environment, the individual is able to gain needed information about surroundings and location.

The transition from traditional analog tactile maps to digital maps and global positioning systems (GPS) provides new potential to enhance orientation. The new generation of electronic orientation aids promises potential for independent route planning and orientation within the environment. At the same time however, the new technology will challenge practitioners to discover the best ways of teaching the use of these devices. Research will need to be conducted to determine how best to interface the systems with the user who is blind.

In a similar way, new types of signage may bring forth additional information for orientation. As described in Chapter 9 of this volume, infrared and frequency modulation signage are being used to provide detailed information that is helpful in wayfinding. Such "signs" are being used to assist individuals in public buildings and in rapid-rail environments. Use of this technology may expand in the future to include applications that will further enhance travel. Use of such information as a part of traffic control, for example, could provide information about the intersection and the timing of the light.

Audible pedestrian traffic lights have been in use for decades, but most recently they have been gaining in popularity. Such pedestrian signals have been used at difficult-to-interpret intersections and proven to be helpful. Standardization of these systems, however, will be necessary if they are to be universally understood by travelers who are blind.

New electronic visual aids are beginning to appear which may help individuals with specific visual impairments. The Low Vision Enhancement System (LVES) and the Magnicam V-Max are devices that utilize a video image and autofocusing to improve contrast, image quality, and other visual characteristics. Additional study of these devices and their possible use for mobility are needed in the future.

Technology is also being used to provide objective analysis of devices and mobility techniques. Biomechanical motion analysis incorporating videography is a method of recording and displaying information about movement that allows quantitative measures to be directly obtained from digitized video images. These measures allow researchers to measure instantaneous velocity, acceleration, and linear and angular displacement. Thus, videography bridges the gap between the mathematics and observation in the comparison, description, and evaluation of motion. The use of movement analysis in rehabilitation is best known for analyzing the gait of amputees to monitor the rate and effectiveness of therapy. This technology is particularly applicable to the movement involved with blind or low-vision mobility. This technology allows for the development and validation of a new generation of software for the O&M specialist. An example of such software is RoboCane®), which allows both researchers and clinicians to evaluate cane coverage afforded to visually impaired travelers by either their existing or modified cane techniques for specific travel hazards (Blasch & De l'Aune, 1992). By demanding an objective set of parameters describing the traveler and cane technique, it promotes documentation of travel characteristics that serve as "snapshots" in the rehabilitation process, or as part of O&M instruction. Future directions for this type of software include computer modeling of some specific low-vision conditions, ETAs, and modeling of an individual's home environment.

SERVICE DELIVERY AND PERSONNEL PREPARATION

The Individuals with Disabilities Education Act (IDEA) guarantees that all children who have disabilities will receive a free, appropriate public education. Periodically parts C through G of this act are reauthorized. Within these discretionary sections is reference to "related services" that are necessary for children with disabilities to benefit from special education. These related services consist of a nonexhaustive list of examples of critical services such as occupational therapy, speech pathology and audiology, and counseling services. Clearly absent from this list is the provision of O&M for children who are blind. Without being specified in the list of examples, O&M is less likely to become a part of services that are provided for blind and visually impaired children. It has been the goal of the O&M profession to further ensure the provision of independent travel instruction for students who require the service. To reach this goal, practitioners across the nation have contacted their legislative representations asking for O&M to be included in the list of examples of related services when IDEA is reauthorized. A change in the statute has occurred and that O&M will be considered for each child who requires such service.

Empowerment and consumer choice have become the defining elements in both rehabilitation and education. Through the years as the Rehabilitation Act of 1973 has been reauthorized, various changes have taken place to increase consumer control. Beginning in 1973, a pilot initiative for the first Client Assistant Program (CAP) was established to provide clients with the ability to challenge the decisions made regarding their rehabilitation programs. The provision was later made permanent in 1984. In a similar fashion, the Individual Written Rehabilitation Plan (IWRP), which originated in 1973, has gradually been modified to ensure more client involvement in the development of the plan. The 1992 amendments to the Rehabilitation Act established a pilot project to evaluate greater consumer choice in the selection of service providers. The 1997 regulations for the Rehabilitation Act reaffirm the desire to provide consumers with control of their programs. In the arena of education, the Individual Education Program (IEP) and its accompanying due process rights have given parents the ability to exercise control of goals and objectives. Braille bills in various states have further attempted to provide parental control over the reading media taught to children.

As the Rehabilitation Act and IDEA are reauthorized, consumer control will once again be in the forefront of the minds of the legislators. The trend toward empowerment and choice will lead to new attempts at providing consumers with the tools that will give them more say in the development and implementation of their programs. In the area of O&M this trend will certainly affect the instructional process. Consumers and their families will continue to have active involvement in the development of programing. It is even possible that someday a voucher system may be used for adults to select their own service providers. In any event all attempts should be made to provide consumers with the specific instruction that they desire and the information that they need to make informed choices. In order to take advantage of freedom of choice, consumers will need access to reports of outcome measures so that they can properly choose instruction or agencies.

Since the 1992 reauthorization of the Rehabilitation Act of 1973, funding for university personnel preparation programs has remained static. Each year the same amount of $39.6 million has been authorized to support preparation of rehabilitation personnel. Because of this level funding, university programs in the rehabilitation sector have been forced to do more with less. The amounts of grant awards have not kept pace with rising tuition and inflation. Students who receive tuition assistance and stipends often must also work long hours so that they can support themselves. University programs that prepare personnel for working with children in low-incidence categories have also been faced with uncertainties. The U.S. Office of Special Education Programs has advocated for regionalization of the university programs. It is not known if the current level of support for low incidence personnel preparation programs will continue under this new arrangement. If we are to meet the needs of both children and adults, the personnel preparation programs must be maintained and must receive increasing levels of funding so that appropriately prepared professionals can be graduated.

CONCLUSION

The field of O&M has made great strides in extending its knowledge base and modifying its practices to adapt to the changing milieu. The chapters in this textbook are evidence of this expansion and growth. They share the current state of the art, which has occurred as a result of the research of O&M specialists and from the application of research from other disciplines. The profession will grow and prosper as long as it continues to expand its knowledge base and is responsive to the needs of the people it serves.

References
Appendixes
Glossary
Resources
Index

REFERENCES

Ad Hoc Committee on Mobility Instruction for the Blind. (1966). *Report of the National Conference Vocational Rehabilitation Administration.*

Adelson, E., & Fraiberg, S. (1974). Gross motor development in infants blind from birth. *Child Development, 45,* 114–126.

Ai, E., & Luckie, A. (1994). In T. Cohen, M. A. Sande, & P. A. Volberding (Eds.), *The AIDS knowledge base* (2nd ed., Section 5.28, pp. 3–4). Boston: Little, Brown.

Aiello, J., & Steinfeld, E. (1980). *Accessible buildings for people with severe visual impairment* (Report No. HUD-PDR-404). Washington, DC: U.S. Department of Housing and Urban Development, Office of Policy Research.

Ajuha, S. C. (1990). Rehabilitation of visually handicapped Indians: The problem and the numbers. *Journal of Visual Impairment & Blindness, 84*(6), 270–273.

Alcal, A. T. (1991, September 9–12). *O.N.C.E. Guide-Dog Foundation: First center for dog training in Spain.* Paper presented at the Sixth International Mobility Conference, Madrid, Spain.

Allen, E. (1969). Impressions of institutions for the blind in Germany and Austria. *Blindness Annual,* 1969, 220–224. (Originally published in *The New Outlook for the Blind,* February 1910 and Spring 1910.)

Allen, K. E., & Marotz, L. (1994). *Developmental profiles: Pre-birth through eight.* Albany, NY: Delmar.

Alloy, L. B., & Seligman, M. E. P. (1979). On the cognitive component of learned helplessness and depression. *Psychology of Learning and Motivation, 13,* 219–276.

Allport, G. W. (1961). Pattern and growth in personality. New York: Holt, Rinehart & Winston.

Alvarez Reyes, D. (1993). Deaf-blind Education: "Access to Context." *Journal of the International Association for the Education of deaf-blind People, 12,* 5–9.

American Automobile Association. (1957). *How to drive* (p. 58). Washington, DC: Author.

American Council of the Blind. (1991). Resolution 91-25: Development of appropriate sound emitting equipment for electrically powered vehicles. Tampa, FL: Author.

American Foundation for the Blind. (1960). Mobility and orientation—A symposium. *New Outlook for the Blind, 54*(3), 77–94.

American National Standards Institute. (1980). *American national standard for buildings and facilities: Providing accessibility to and usability for physically handicapped people* (A117.1). New York: Author.

American National Standards Institute (ANSI). (1989a). *American national standard specifications for audiometers.* ANSI S3.6-1969, revision 1989. New York: Author.

American National Standards Institute (ANSI). (1989b). *Specifications for hearing aid characteristics.* ANSI S3.22-1987. New York: Author.

American Speech-Language-Hearing Association. (1997). *Guidelines for audiologic screening.* Rockville, MD: Author.

Americans with disabilities act accessibility guidelines for buildings and facilities. (1991). Washington, DC: U.S. Architectural and Transportation Barriers Compliance Board.

An apostle to the blind. (1909, July 8). *Sunday School Chronicle.* (Sir Francis J. Campbell Papers, Library of Congress, Box 34.)

Anderson, J. R. (1995). *Learning and memory: An integrated approach.* New York: Wiley.

Anderson, J. R., & Bower, G. (1983). *Human associative memory.* Washington, DC: Winston.

Anderson, J. R. (1985). *Cognitive psychology and its implications* (2nd ed.). San Francisco: W. H. Freeman.

Andrews, S. K. (1985). The use of capsule papers in producing tactual maps. *Journal of Visual Impairment & Blindness, 79*(9), 396–399.

Angwin, J. P. B. (1968a). Maps for mobility—1. *New Beacon, 52,* 115–119.

Angwin, J. P. B. (1968b). Maps for mobility—2. *New Beacon, 52,* 143–145.

Anthony, T. L., Fazzi, D. L., Lampert, J. S., & Pogrund, R. L. (1992). Movement focus: Orientation and mobility for young blind and visually impaired children. In R. L. Pogrund, D. L. Fazzi, & J. S. Lampert (Eds.), *Early focus: Working with blind and visually impaired children and their families* (pp. 80–111). New York: American Foundation for the Blind.

Apple, L. E. (1962). Factors in mobility rehabilitation which experience has proven useful. *Proceedings of the Mobility Research Conference.* New York: American Foundation for the Blind.

Apple, L. E. (1971). *Report on low vision and mobility.* American Association of Workers for the Blind Annual Conference, Richmond, VA.

Apple, L. E., & Blasch, B. B. (1976). Workshop on low vision mobility. *Bulletin of Prosthetics Research,* 10–26, 46–138. Department of Medicine and Surgery. Washington, DC: Veterans Administration.

Apple, L. E., & May, M. (1970). *Distance vision and perceptual training: A concept for use in mobility training of low vision clients.* New York: American Foundation for the Blind.

Apple, M., Apple, L. E., & Blasch, D. (1980). Low vision. In R. Welsh & B. Blasch (Eds.), *Foundations of orientation and mobility* (pp. 187–223). New York: American Foundation for the Blind.

Appleyard, K. (1976). *Planning a pluralistic city.* Cambridge, MA: MIT Press.

Architectural and Transportation Barriers Compliance Board. (1991). *Americans with disabilities accessibility guidelines.* Washington, DC: U.S. Department of Transportation.

Arias, C., Curet, C. A., Moyano, H. F., Joekes, S., & Blanch, N. (1993). Echolocation: A study of auditory functioning in blind and sighted subjects. *Journal of Visual Impairment & Blindness, 87*(3), 73–77.

Armitage S. E., Baldwin, B. A., & Vince, M. (1980). The fetal sound environment of sheep. *Science, 208,* 1173–1174.

Armstrong, J. D. (Ed.). (1973). *The design and production of maps for the visually handicapped.* Mobility Monograph No. 1. Nottingham, England.

Armstrong, J. D., & Heyes, A. (1975). The work of the Blind Mobility Research Unit. In K. Kwatny & R. Zuckerman (Eds.), *Proceedings of Conference: Devices and systems for the disabled.* Philadelphia: Temple University.

Arthur, P., & Passini, R. (1992). *Wayfinding: People, signs and architecture.* New York: McGraw-Hill.

Ashmead, D., Davis, D., & Northington, A. (1995). Contribution of listener's approaching motion to auditory distance perception. *Journal of Experimental Psychology: Human Perception and Performance, 21,* 239–256.

Ashmead, D., Hill, E., & Talor, C. (1989). Obstacle perception by congenitally blind children. *Perception and Psychophysics, 46*(5), 425–433.

Aslin, R. N., & Smith, L. (1988). Perceptual development. *Annual Review of Psychology, 39,* 435–473.

Aslin, R. N., Pisoni, D. B., & Jusczyk, P. W. (1983). Auditory development and speech perception in infancy. In P. H. Mussen (Series Ed.) & M. M. Haith & J. J. Campos (Vol. Eds.), *Handbook of child psychology* (4th ed.). *Vol. II: Infants and developmental psychology.* New York: Wiley.

Association for Education and Rehabilitation of the Blind and Visually Impaired. (1994). *Association for Education and Rehabilitation of the Blind and Visually Impaired Conference Resolutions.* Dallas: Author.

Association for Persons with Severe Handicaps. (1993). A resolution on inclusive education. In J. M. Kauffman & D. P. Hallahan (Eds.), *The illusion of full inclusion: A comprehensive critique of a current special education bandwagon* (pp. 314–316). Austin, TX: PRO-ED.

Atkinson, R. C., and Shiffrin, R. M. (1968). Human memory: A proposed system and its component processes. In K. Spence & J. Spence (Eds.), *The psychology of learning and motivation* (Vol. 2). New York: Academic Press.

Ault, C. (1976). The low vision person—"A marginal man." *Bulletin of Prosthetics Research,* 88–122. Workshop on low vision mobility. Department of Medicine and Surgery. Washington, DC: Veterans Administration.

Aust, A. M. D. (1980). Kinesiology. In R. L. Welsh & B. B. Blasch (Eds.), *Foundations of orientation and mobility* (pp. 37–71). New York: American Foundation for the Blind.

Austin, T., & Sleight, R. (1952). Accuracy of tactual discrimination of letters, numerals, and geometric forms. *Journal of Experimental Psychology, 43,* 239–249.

Ausubel, D. P. (1960). The use of advanced organizers in the learning and retention of meaningful verbal material. *Journal of Educational Psychology, 51,* 267–272.

Ausubel, D. P. (1963). *The psychology of meaningful verbal learning.* New York: Grune & Stratton.

Ausubel, D. P., & Yousser, M. (1963). Role of discriminability in meaningful parallel learning. *Journal of Educational Psychology, 54,* 331–336.

Ausubel, D. P., Novak, J. D., & Hanesian, H. (1978). *Educational psychology: A cognitive view* (2nd ed). New York: Holt, Rinehart & Winston.

Axelson, P. W., Thomas, P. H., Chesney, D. A., Coveny, J. L., & Eve-Anchassi, D. (1994). Trail guides with universal access information. *RESNA '94* (pp. 306–308), June 17–22. Rehabilitation Engineering Society of North America. Nashville, TN.

Azar, G., & Lawton, A. (1964). Gait and stepping as factors in the frequent falls in elderly women. *Gerontologist, 4,* 83–84.

Baca, L. M., & Cervantes, H. T. (1989). Bilingualism and bilingual education. In L. M. Baca & H. T. Cervantes (Eds.), *The bilingual education interface* (2nd ed., pp. 23–24). Columbus, OH: Merrill.

Bailey, B. R., & Head, D. (1993). Orientation and mobility services to children and youth with multiple disabilities. *RE:view, 25*(2), 57–UN64.

Baird, A. A., & Goldie, D. (1979). Activities and experiences develop spatial and sensory understanding. *Teaching Exceptional Children, 11,* 116–119.

Baird, A. S. (1977). Electronic aids: Can they help blind children? *Journal of Visual Impairment & Blindness, 71*(3), 97–101.

Baker, L. D. (1973). Blindness and social behavior: A need for research. *New Outlook for the Blind, 67*(7), 315–318.

Baldwin, J. D., and Baldwin, J. E. (1986). *Behavior principles in everyday life.* Englewood Cliffs, NJ: Prentice Hall.

Baldwin, V. (1993). "Population/Demographics: Presentation." In J. W. Reiman and P. A. Johson (Eds.), Proceedings from the National Symposium on Children and Youth Who Are Deaf-Blind (pp. 53–66). Monmouth, Oregon: Teaching Research Publications.

Ball, M. (1964). Mobility in perspective. In *Blindness annual.* Washington, DC: American Association of Workers for the Blind.

Bandura, A. (1977). Self-efficacy: Toward a unifying theory of behavioral change. *Psychological Review, 84,* 191–215.

Bandura, A. (1986). *Social foundations of thought and action: A social cognitive theory.* Englewood Cliffs, NJ: Prentice Hall.

Bandura, A. & Adams, N. E. (1977). Analysis of self-efficacy theory of behavioral change. *Cognitive Therapy and Research, 1,* 287–308.

Bandura, A., & Walters, R. H. (1963). *Social learning and personality development.* New York: Holt.

Bandura, A., Reese, L., & Adams, N. E. (1982). Microanalysis of action and fear arousal as a function of differential levels of perceived self-efficacy. *Journal of Personality and Social Psychology, 43,* 5–21.

Banja, J. D. (1994). The determination of risks in orientation and mobility services: Ethical and professional issues. *Journal of Visual Impairment & Blindness, 88,* 401–409.

Barac-Cikoja, D., & Turvey, M. (1991). Perceiving aperture size by striking. *Journal of Experimental Psychology: Human Perception and Performance, 17,* 330–346.

Barber, P. A., Turnbull, A. P., Behr, S. K., & Kerns, G. M. (1988). A family systems perspective on early childhood special education. In S. L. Odom & M. B. Karnes (Eds.), *Early intervention for infants and children with handicaps: An empirical base* (pp. 179–198). Baltimore: Brooks.

Bardach, Joan L. L. (1970). Psychological factors in the handicapped driver. *Psychological Aspects of Disability, 17*(1), 10–13.

Barker, R. G., Wright, B. A., Meyerson, L., & Gonick, M. R. (1953). *Adjustment to physical handicap and illness: A survey of the social psychology of physique and disability.* New York: Social Science Research Council.

Barker, L. M. (1994). *Learning and behavior: A psychological perspective.* New York: Macmillan.

Barker, P., Barrick, J., & Wilson, R. (1995). *Building sight: A handbook of building and interior design solutions to include the needs of visually impaired people.* London: Royal National Institute for the Blind.

Barlow, J., & Bentzen, B. L. (1995). *Cues blind travelers use to detect streets.* Technical Report. Cambridge, MA: U.S. Department of Transportation, Federal Transit Administration, Volpe National Transportation Systems Center.

Barraga, N. C. (1964). *Increased visual behavior in low vision children.* New York: American Foundation for the Blind.

Barraga, N. C. (1986). Sensory perceptual development. In G. T. Scholl (Ed.), *Foundations of education for blind and visually handicapped children and youth* (pp. 83–98). New York: American Foundation for the Blind.

Barraga, N. C., & Morris, J. E. (1980). *Program to develop efficiency in visual functioning: Sourcebook on low vision.* Louisville, KY: American Printing House for the Blind.

Barth, J. L. (1982). The development and evaluation of a tactile graphics kit. *Journal of Visual Impairment & Blindness, 76*(6), 269–273.

Barth, J. L., & Foulke, E. (1979). Preview: A neglected variable in orientation and mobility. *Journal of Visual Impairment & Blindness, 73*(2), 41–48.

Bassett, I., & Eastmond, J. (1964). Echolocation: Measurement of pitch versus distance for sounds reflected from a flat surface. *Journal of the Acoustical Society of America, 36,* 911–917.

Battelle Memorial Institute, Human Affairs Research Center & Ilium Associates, Inc. (1976). *Transit user information aids: An evaluation of consumer attitudes.* Washington, DC: U.S. Department of Transportation, Urban Mass Transit Administration.

Baumgart, D., Johnson, J., & Helmstetter, E. (1990). *Augmentative and alternative communication systems for persons with moderate and severe disabilities.* Baltimore, MD: Paul H. Brookes.

Beattie, P. (1995). Testimony at Washington Metropolitan Area Transit Authority hearing on platform edge detection, Washington, DC, March 3, 1995.

Bekesy, G. von. (1928). Zur Theorie des Horens. Die Schwingungsform der Basilarmembran. *Physik Zeitschrift, 29,* 793–810.

Beliveau-Tobey, M., & De l'Aune, W. (1991). *Identification of roles and functions of orientation and mobility specialists.* Jackson, MS: Mississippi State Rehabilitation Research and Training Center on Blindness and Low Vision.

Beliveau-Tobey, M., & Smith, A. (Eds.). (1980). *The interdisciplinary approach to low vision rehabilitation.* Stillwater: Oklahoma State University, National Clearinghouse on Rehabilitation Information.

Benjamin, J. (1968). A review of the Veterans Administration blind guidance device project. *Bulletin of Prosthetics Research, 10*(9), 64.

Bennett, J. D. (1991). The fallacy of timing methods. *Re:view, 23,* 75–83.

Bentzen, B. L. (1972). Production and testing of an orientation and travel map for visually handicapped persons. *New Outlook for the Blind, 66*(8), 249–255.

Bentzen, B. L. (1973). Transfer of learning from school setting to life style in a habilitation program for multiply handicapped blind persons. *New Outlook for the Blind, 67*(7), 297–300.

Bentzen, B. L. (1977). Orientation maps for visually impaired persons. *Journal of Visual Impairment & Blindness, 71*(5), 193–196.

Bentzen, B. L. (1980). Orientation aids. In R. Welsh & B. Blasch (Eds.), *Foundations of orientation and mobility* (pp. 291–355). New York: American Foundation for the Blind.

Bentzen, B. L. (1983). Tactile specifications of route configurations. In J. Wiedel (Ed.), *Proceedings: First International Symposium on Maps and Graphics for the Visually Handicapped.* Washington, DC.

Bentzen, B. L. (1984). Accessibility: Guidelines for blindness professionals. *Yearbook of the Association for Education and Rehabilitation of the Blind and Visually Impaired* (pp. 2–12).

Bentzen, B. L. (1989a). Considerations in the design of tactile maps for use by visually impaired travelers on rail rapid transit. *Enhancing the use of rail rapid transit by visually impaired travelers* (Report No. UMTA-MA-06-0141–88–7) (Vol. 7). Washington, DC: U.S. Department of Transportation.

Bentzen, B. L. (1989b). Specifications for letters and numerals for touch reading. *Enhancing the use of rail rapid transit by visually impaired travelers.* (Report No. UMTA-MA-06-0141-88-9). Washington, DC: U.S. Department of Transportation, Urban Mass Transportation Administration.

Bentzen, B. L. (1991). Spatial updating in the blind: Effects of training with air sonar versus sounding objects. (Doctoral dissertation, Boston College, 1991). *Dissertation Abstracts International—*B *52/11,* p. 611.

Bentzen, B. L. (1994). Detectable warnings in transit facilities: Safety and negotiability. Washington, DC: Federal Transit Administration and Project ACTION of the National Easter Seal Society.

Bentzen, B. L. (1996). Transit vehicle signage for persons who are blind or visually impaired. *Journal of Visual Impairment & Blindness, 90,* 352–356.

Bentzen, B. L., & Barlow, J. (1995). Impact of curb ramps on safety of persons who are blind. *Journal of Visual Impairment & Blindness, 89,* 319–328.

Bentzen, B. L., & Easton, R. D. (1995). *Specifications for transit vehicle next stop messages.* Newton, MA: Carroll Center for the Blind.

Bentzen, B. L., & Mitchell, P. A. (1993). *Audible signage as a wayfinding aid: Comparison of "Verbal Landmarks" versus "Talking Signs."* Unpublished manuscript.

Bentzen, B. L., & Mitchell, P. A. (1995). Audible signage as a wayfinding aid: Comparison of Verbal Landmark® versus Talking Signs®. *Journal of Visual Impairment & Blindness, 89,* 494–505.

Bentzen, B. L., & Peck, A. (1979). Factors affecting traceability of lines for tactile graphics. *Journal of Visual Impairment & Blindness, 71,* 264–269.

Bentzen, B. L., Crandall, W. F., & Myers, L. (in press). Use of remote infrared signage in a complex transit station by persons having cognitive disabilities. *Journal of Visual Impairment & Blindness.*

Bentzen, B. L., Jackson, R. M., & Peck, A. F. (1981a). *Techniques for improving communication with visually impaired users of rail rapid transit systems* (Report No. UMTA-MA-003608103). Washington, DC: U.S. Department of Transportation, Urban Mass Transportation Administration.

Bentzen, B. L., Jackson, R. M., & Peck, A. F. (1981b). *Selection of tokens and orientation of farecards by visually impaired users of rail rapid transit* (Report No. UMTA-MA-11-0036-4). Washington, DC: U.S.

Department of Transportation, Urban Mass Transportation Administration.

Bentzen, B. L., Nolin, T. L., & Easton, R. D. (1994a). *Detectable warning surfaces: Color, contrast and reflectance* (Report No. VNTSC-DTRS-57-93-P-80546). Cambridge, MA: U.S. Department of Transportation, Federal Transit Administration, Volpe National Transportation Systems Center.

Bentzen, B. L., Crandall, W. F., Chigier, B., Warden, G. F., & Carosella, L. (1995a, February 1–2). Comprehensive wayfinding system for transportation services: Talking Signs® and Speak2Directions. *Proceedings: Orientation and Navigation Systems for Blind Persons.* University of Hertfordshire, Hatfield, England.

Bentzen, B. L. Nolin, T. L. Easton, R. D. Desmarais, L., & Mitchell, P. A. (1993). *Detectable warning surfaces: Detectability by individuals with visual impairments* (VNTSC-DTRS57-92-P-81354 and VNTSC-DTRS57-91-C-0006). Final report. U. S. Department of Transportation, Federal Transit Administration, Volpe National Transportation Systems Center, and Project ACTION, National Easter Seal Society.

Bentzen, B. L., Nolin, T. L., Easton, R. D., Desmarais, L., & Mitchell, P. A. (1994b). *Detectable warnings: Safety and negotiability on slopes for persons who are physically impaired.* Federal Transit Administration and Project ACTION of the National Easter Seal Society.

Bentzen, B. L., Nolin, T. L., Easton, R. D., & Mitchell, P. A. (1995c). *Signage specifications for transit vehicles: Human factors research.* Berlin, MA: Accessible Design for the Blind.

Berg, R., Jose, R., & Carter, K. (1983). Distance training techniques. In R. Jose (Ed.), *Understanding low vision* (pp. 277–316). New York: American Foundation for the Blind.

Bergman, M. (1957). Binaural hearing. *Archives of Otolaryngology, 66,* 572–578.

Berlá, E. P. (1972). Behavioral strategies and problems in scanning and interpreting tactual displays. *New Outlook for the Blind, 66*(8), 277–286.

Berlá, E. P. (1973). Strategies in scanning a tactual pseudomap. *Education of the Visually Handicapped, 5,* 8–19.

Berlá, E. P., & Butterfield, L. H. (1977). Tactile political maps: Two experimental designs. *Journal of Visual Impairment & Blindness, 71*(6), 262–264.

Berlá, E. P., & Murr, M. J. (1975). The effects of noise on the location of point symbols and tracing a line on a tactile pseudomap. *Journal of Special Education, 9,* 183–190.

Bigelow, A. (1991). Spatial mapping of familiar locations in blind children. *Journal of Visual Impairment & Blindness, 85*(3), 113–117.

Bigelow, A. (1992). Locomotion and search behavior in blind infants. *Infant Behavior and Development, 15,* 179–189.

Bina, M. J. (1982). Morale of teachers of the visually handicapped: Implications for administrators. *Journal of Visual Impairment & Blindness, 76*(3), 121–128.

Bina, M. J. (1976). The legal implication of solo experiences in orientation and mobility training. *New Outlook for the Blind, 69*(6), 225–231.

Blair, T. (1990). *History of O&M in China and the Far East.* Unpublished manuscript.

Blank, R. (1957). Psychoanalysis and blindness. *Psychoanalytic Quarterly, 26,* 1–24.

Blasch, B. B. (1975). The use of the long cane by clients with visual acuity of 10/200 as an aid or an identification device. *Low Vision Abstracts, 2*(2), 8.

Blasch, B. B. (1978). Blindisms: Treatment by punishment and reward in laboratory and natural settings. *Journal of Visual Impairment & Blindness, 72*(6), 215–230.

Blasch, B. B. (1981a). *Foundations for mobility instruction: A mobility model. In Proceedings of the Second International Mobility Conference.* Paris: IMC2.

Blasch, B. B. (1981b). *Independent mobility training to increase the activities of independent living for disabled individuals* (Project No. #19132). Madison: Wisconsin Division of Vocational Rehabilitation.

Blasch, B. B. (1982). *Mobility training for use of existing public transportation services.* Final Report (Grant Proposal No. 19935 (ICI)). Madison: Wisconsin Council of Developmental Disabilities.

Blasch, B. B. (1984). *Orienteering for persons with developmental disabilities* (Project No. ADD #07DD0273/13). Madison, WI: Department of Health and Human Services, Office of Human Development Services.

Blasch, B. (1994). *Spatial orientation and wayfinding in elderly persons.* Final report.

Blasch, B. B. (1994a). *The effects of inclusion on cognitive performance and affective behavior through an orienteering program.* Unpublished doctoral dissertation, Athens: University of Georgia.

Blasch, B. B. (1994b, February). *The mobility therapist and the non-exclusive mobility model.* Paper presented at the Seventh International Mobility Conference, Melbourne, Australia.

Blasch, B. B. (1994c). The non-exclusive model of mobility and the mobility therapist. *Visions in Mobility: Proceedings of the Seventh International Mobility Conference.* Melbourne, Australia: Royal Guide Dogs Associations of Australia.

Blasch, B. B. (1996). Focus on the needs of clients, not instructors. *Journal of Visual Impairment & Blindness, 90*(1), 5–7.

Blasch, B. B., & Brouwer, O. (1983). Innovative uses and content of maps for persons with visual impairment. In J. Wiedel (Ed.), *Proceedings of the First International Symposium on Maps and Graphics for the Visually Handicapped.* Washington, DC.

Blasch, B. B., & De l'Aune, W. R. (1992). A computer profile of mobility coverage and a safety index. *Journal of Visual Impairment & Blindness, 86*(6), 249–254.

Blasch, B. B., & Long, R. (1994). Environmental information needs for wayfinding by special populations. Veterans Administration Merit Review Final Report: Department of Veterans Affairs, Rehabilitation R&D Services.

Blasch, B. B., & Stuckey, K. A. (1995). Accessibility and mobility of persons who are visually impaired: A historical analysis. *Journal of Visual Impairment & Blindness, 89,* 417–422.

Blasch, B. B., & Welsh, R. (1977). Orientation and mobility training for persons from all handicapped groups. In *Proceedings of the Biennial Convention,* American Association of Workers for the Blind, Portland, OR.

Blasch, B. B., & Welsh, R. L. (1980). Training for persons with functional mobility limitations. In R. L. Welsh & B. B. Blasch (Eds.), *Foundations of orientation and mobility* (pp. 461–476). New York: American Foundation for the Blind.

Blasch, B., Davies, M., & Shoup, E. (1981). *A wheelchair user's manual for people with spinal cord injury.* Madison: University of Wisconsin.

Blasch, B. B., De l'Aune, W., & Blasch, E. (1996). New concepts and cane techniques based on research from RoboCane®. *Proceedings from the International Mobility Conference 8.* Trondheim, Norway.

Blasch, B. B., Kynast, L., & Manuel, S. (1995). *Pilot Study of the Walkmate.* Unpublished manuscript.

Blasch, B., LaGrow, S., & De l'Aune, W. (1996). Three aspects of coverage provided by the long cane: Obstacle, surface and foot placement preview. *Journal of Visual Impairment & Blindness, 90,* 295–301.

Blasch B. B., Long, R. G., & Griffin-Shirley N. (1989). Results of a national survey of electronic travel aid use. *Journal of Visual Impairment & Blindness, 83,* 449–453.

Blasch, B. B., Welsh, R. L., & Davidson, T. (1973). Auditory maps: An orientation aid for visually handicapped persons. *New Outlook for the Blind, 67*(4), 145–158.

Blasch, D. (1971). Orientation and mobility fans out. *Blindness 1970–71 AAWB Annual* (pp. 9–18). Washington, DC: Association of Workers for the Blind.

Blasch, D., & Apple, L. (1976). Severe visual impairments: Part I. In K. Wardell (Ed.), *Selected articles from the long cane news* (pp. 26–28). Los Angeles: California State University at Los Angeles, Department of Special Education.

Bledsoe, C. W. (1945). They learn to see at Avon Old Farms. *Saturday Evening Post.*

Bledsoe, C. W. (1946). *Survey of World War I blinded veterans in hospitals and homes.* Unpublished report.

Bledsoe, C. W. (1965). The "blind center": Ideal or spectre. *Blindness,* 28–31.

Bledsoe, C. W. (1980). Originators of orientation and mobility training. In R. L. Welsh and B. B. Blasch (Eds.), *Foundations of orientation and mobility,* (pp. 581–624). New York: American Foundation for the Blind.

Bledsoe, W. (1969). From Valley Forge to Hines: Truth old enough to tell. *American Association of Workers for the Blind Blindness Annual,* 97–142.

Blind Childrens Center. (1986). *Move with me: A parents' guide to movement development for visually impaired babies.* Los Angeles: Author.

Boehm, R. (1986). The use of echolocation as a mobility aid for blind persons. *Journal of Visual Impairment & Blindness, 80*(9), 953–954.

Book, A., & Garling, T. (1981). Maintenance of orientation during locomotion in unfamiliar environments. *Journal of Experimental Psychology: Human Perception and Performance, 7,* 995–1006.

Bosbach, S. R. (1988). Precane mobility devices. *Journal of Visual Impairment & Blindness, 82*(8), 338–339.

Brabyn, J., & Brown, B. (1990, March). *Low vision mobility: Problem analysis using photographic methods.* Paper presented at the meeting of the International Conference on Low Vision, Melbourne, Australia.

Brabyn, J., & Foulke, E. (1987). Transcripts from an observational study of experienced blind pedestrians. Unpublished raw data.

Brabyn, J., & Foulke, E. (1988). Orientation and mobility research. In *1988 Report of progress: Rehabilitation Engineering Center of the Smith-Kettlewell Eye Research Institute* (pp. 21–23 and Appendix pp. 1–5). San Francisco: The Smith-Kettlewell Eye Research Institute.

Brady, F. (1988). *A singular view: The art of seeing with one eye* (4th ed.). Annapolis, MD: Author.

Brambila-Hickman, B., & Denniston, K. (1984). *Mobility training curriculum for developmentally disabled adults.* Dearborn Heights, MI: Wayne County Associations for the Retarded.

Branch, L. G., Horowitz, A., Carr, C. (1989). The implications for everyday life of incident self-reported visual decline among people over age 65 living in the community. *Gerontologist, 29,* 359–365.

Bransford, J. D., & Stein, B. F. (1984). *The ideal problem solver.* San Francisco: Freeman.

Bransford, J. D. (1979). *Human cognition: Learning, understanding, and remembering.* Belmont, CA: Wadsworth.

Bransford, J. D., Sherwood, R. D., Vye, N. J., & Rieser, J. (1986a). Teaching thinking and problem solving: Research foundations. *American Psychologist, 41,* 1078–1087.

Brazelton, T. (1977). Effects of maternal expectation on early infant behavior. In S. Cohen & T. Comiskey (Eds.), *Child development: Contemporary perspectives.* Itasca, IL: Peacock Press.

Brennan, V., Peck, F., & Lolli, D., (1992). *Suggestions for modifying the home and school environment.* Watertown, MA: Perkins School for the Blind.

Briskey, R. J. (1972). Binaural hearing aids and new innovations. In J. Katz (Ed.), *Handbook of clinical audiology* (pp. 572–578, 590–601). Baltimore: Williams & Wilkins.

Brody, S. J. (1986). Preface. In S. J. Brody & G. E. Ruff (Eds.), *Aging and rehabilitation: Advances in the state of the art.* New York: Springer.

Brody, S. J., & Ruff, G. E. (Eds.) (1986). *Aging and rehabilitation: Advances in the state of the art.* New York: Springer.

Brothers, R. J., & Huff, R. A. (1972). *Manual of suggested activities for the development of sound localization skills.* Louisville, KY: American Printing House for the Blind.

Brown, C., & Bour, B. (1986). Movement analysis and curriculum for visually impaired preschoolers. In *A resource manual for the development and evaluation of special programs for exceptional students: Vol. V–K.* Tallahassee: Florida Bureau of Education for Exceptional Students, Department of Education.

Bryant, N. W., & Jansen, W. A. (1980). In R. L. Welsh & B. B. Blasch (Eds.), *Foundations of orientation and mobility* (pp. 452–459). New York: American Foundation for the Blind.

Bugliarello, G., Alexandre, A., Barnes, J., & Wakstein, C. (1976). *The impact of noise pollution–A socio-technological introduction* (pp. 81–92). New York: Pergamon.

Burch-Sims, G. P., & Ochs, M. T. (1992). The anatomical and physiologic bases of otoacoustic emissions. *Hearing Journal, 45*(11), 9–10.

Bürklen, K. (1932). *Touch reading of the blind* (F. K. Merry, Trans.). New York: American Foundation for the Blind.

Burklen, K. (1924). *Blinden-psychologie.* Leipzig: Verlag von Johann Ambrosius Barth.

Burlingham, D. (1965). Some problems of ego development in blind children. *Psychoanalytic Study of the Child, 19,* 95–112.

Burton, G. (1993). Non-neural extensions of haptic sensitivity. *Ecological Psychology, 5,* 105–124.

Burton, G. (1994). Crossing without vision of path gaps. *Journal of Motor Behavior, 26,* 147–161.

Bushnell, E., & Boudreau, J. (1993). Motor development and the mind: The potential role of motor abilities as a determinant of aspects of perceptual development. *Child Development, 64*(4), 1005–1021.

Butler, D. L., Acquino, A. L., Hissong, A. A., & Scott, P. A. (1993). Wayfinding by newcomers in a complex building. *Human Factors, 35,* 159–173.

Byrne, R. W., & Slater, E. (1983). Distances and directions in the cognitive maps of the blind. *Canadian Journal of Psychology, 37,* 293–299.

Campos, J., Hiatt, S., Ramsay, D., Henderson, C., & Svejda, M. (1978). The emergence of fear on the visual cliff. In M. Lewis & L. Rosenblum (Eds.), *The development of affect.* New York: Plenum.

Carhart, R. (1958). The usefulness of the binaural hearing aid. *Journal of Speech and Hearing Disorders, 23,* 42–51.

Carkhuff, R. (1972). New direction in training for the helping professions: Toward a technology for human and community resource development. *Counseling Psychologist, 3*(3), 12–30.

Carroll, T. J. (1961). *Blindness: What it is, what it does, and how to live with it.* Boston: Little, Brown.

Casals, B. C., & Valiña, M. C. (1991). The acquisition of spatial awareness from verbal descriptions in blind and sighted people. *Proceedings: Sixth International Mobility Conference* (Book 1, pp. 35–46). Madrid, Spain.

Casey, S. M. (1978). Cognitive mapping by the blind. *Journal of Visual Impairment & Blindness, 72*(7), 297–301.

Cattell, R. B. (1965). *The scientific analysis of personality.* Baltimore: Penguin.

Centers for Disease Control. (1994). *HIV/AIDS Surveillance Report, 6*(1). Atlanta: Author.

Chalkley, T. (1982). *Your eyes.* Springfield, IL: Charles C Thomas.

Chang, T. M. (1986). Semantic memory: Facts and models. *Psychological Bulletin, 99,* 199–220.

Chen, D., & Smith, J. (1992). Developing orientation and mobility skills in students who are multihandicapped and visually impaired. *Re:view, 24*(3), 133–139.

Chen, S. (1990). How Japan accomodates its bus travelers. In M. M. Uslan, A. F. Peck, W. R. Wiener & A. Stern (Eds.), *Access to mass transit for blind and visually impaired travelers* (pp. 97–99). New York: American Foundation for the Blind.

Chew, S. (1986). The use of traffic sounds by blind pedestrians. *Dissertation Abstracts International, 47,* 08B. (University Microfilms No. AAG8627007.)

Chigadula, R. T. (1991, September 9–12). *Orientation and mobility training requisites of the blind and low vision people.* Paper presented at the Sixth International Mobility Conference, Madrid, Spain.

Chilens, D., & LaGrow, S. (1986). *Use of normative sampling to set standards for observational distances required.* Unpublished master's thesis, Western Michigan University, Kalamazoo.

Cholden, L. S. (1958). *A psychiatrist works with blindness.* New York: American Foundation for the Blind.

Clark, J. G. (1981). Uses and abuses of hearing loss classification. *Asha, 23,* 493–500.

Clarke, K. (1988). Barriers or enablers? Mobility devices for visually impaired multihandicapped infants and preschoolers. *Education of the Visually Handicapped, 20,* 115–132.

Clarke, K. (1992). A comparision of the effects of mobility training with a long cane and a precane device on the travel performance of preschool children with severe visual disabilities. *Dissertation Abstracts International,* 53 (5-A), pp. 1476–1477-A. (University Microfilms No. 92–27, 252.)

Clarke, K. L., Sainato, D. M. & Ward, M. E. (1994). Travel performance of preschoolers: The effects of mobility training with a long cane versus a precane. *Journal of Visual Impairment & Blindness, 88,* 19–30.

Clifton R. K. (1985). The precedence effect: Its implications for developmental questions. In S. E. Trehub, B. S. Schneider (Eds.), *Auditory development in infancy* (pp. 85–99). New York: Plenum.

Clifton, R. K., Morrongiello, B. A., Kulig, J. W., David J. M. (1981). Newborns' orientation toward sound: possible implications for cortical development. *Child Development,* 52, 833–838.

Coker, G. (1979). A comparison of self-concepts and academic achievement of visually handicapped children enrolled in a regular school and in a residential school. *Education of the Visually Handicapped, 11,* 67–76.

Coleman, C. L., & Weinstock, R. F. (1984). Physically handicapped blind people: Adaptive mobility techniques. *Journal of Visual Impairment & Blindness, 78*(3), 113–117.

Colenbrander, A. (1977). Dimensions of visual performance. *Opthalmology Transactions, American Academy of Opthalmology and Otolaryngology, 83,* 332–337.

Commission on Standards and Accreditation of Services for the Blind. (1966). *The COMSTAC report.* New York: Author.

Connell, B. R. (1987). Environmental and behavioral contributions to falls in the elderly. In D. Lawrence, R. Habe, A. Hacker, & D. Sherrod (Eds.), *People's needs/planet management, paths to co-existence* (Proceedings of the 18th Annual Environmental and Design Research Association Conference). Washington, DC: Environmental Design Research Association.

Coon, N. (1959). *A brief history of dog guides for the blind.* Morristown, NJ: The Seeing Eye.

Corn, A. (1983). Visual function: A theoretical model for individuals with low vision. *Journal of Visual Impairment & Blindness, 77*(8), 373–377.

Corn, A. L. (1986). Low vision and visual efficiency. In G. T. Scholl (Ed.), *Foundations of education for blind and visually handicapped children and youth* (pp. 99–117). New York: American Foundation for the Blind.

Corn, A. L., & Koenig, A. J. (1996). *Foundations of low vision: Clinical and functional perspectives.* New York: AFB Press.

Corn, A. L., & Sacks, S. Z. (1994). The impact of nondriving on adults with visual impairments. *Journal of Visual Impairment & Blindness, 88*(1), 53–68.

Corn, A., Ferrell, K., Spungin, S., & Zimmerman, G. (1996). *What we know about teacher preparation programs in blindness and visual impairments.* Paper prepared for the NASDE Policy Forum, Training Educators to Work with Students Who Are Blind or Visually Impaired. Washington, DC.

Cory, D., Neustadt-Noy, N., Geruschat, D., Smith, A., Beliveau-Tobey, B., & De l'Aune, W. (1992). *Characteristics of orientation and mobility instructors in Europe and the USA: A comparison study.* Paper presented at the International Mobility Conference, Madrid, Spain.

Cotzin, M., & Dallenbach, K. (1950). Facial vision: The role of pitch and loudness in the perception of obstacles by the blind. *American Journal of Psychology, 63,* 485–515.

Cowen, E., Underberg, R., Verillo, R., & Benham, F. (1961). *Adjustment to visual disability in adolescence.* New York: American Foundation for the Blind.

Craik, F. I. M. (1979). Human memory. *Annual Review of Psychology, 30,* 63–102.

Crandall, W. F., Bentzen, B. L., & Myers, L. (1995a). *Remote infrared signage for people who are blind or print disabled: A surface transit accessibility study.* Final report. Washington, DC: U.S. Department of Transportation, Federal Transit Administration and Project ACTION of the National Easter Seal Society.

Crandall, W. F., Bentzen, B. L., Myers, L., & Mitchell, P. A. (1995b). *Transit accessibility improvement through Talking Signs® remote infrared signage: Administration and evaluation.* Final report. Washington, DC: U.S. Department of Transportation, Federal Transit Administration and Project ACTION of the National Easter Seal Society.

Cratty, B. J. (1965). *Perceptual thresholds of nonvisual locomotion (Part 1).* Los Angeles: University of California.

Cratty, B. J., & Sams, T. A. (1968). *The body-image of blind children.* New York: American Foundation for the Blind.

Cratty, B. J., & Williams, H. (1966). *Perceptual thresholds of nonvisual locomotion (Part 2).* Los Angeles: University of California.

Crews, J. E. (1994). The demographic, social and conceptual contexts of aging and vision loss. *Journal of the American Optometric Association, 65,* 63–68.

Croce, R. V., & Jacobson, W. H. (1986). The application of two-point touch cane technique to theories of motor control and learning: Implications for orientation and mobility training. *Journal of Visual Impairment & Blindness, 80*(6), 790–793.

Curry, S. A. & Hatlen, P. H. (1988). Meeting the unique educational needs of visually impaired pupils through appropriate placements. *Journal of Visual Impairment & Blindness, 82,* 417–424.

Daka, C. P. (1991, September 9–12). *Orientation and mobility: A Zambian perspective.* Paper presented at the Sixth International Mobility Conference, Madrid, Spain.

Darwin, C. (1873). Origin of certain instincts. *Nature, 7,* 417–418.

Daudet, E., & Stawell, Mrs. R. (Trans.). (1913). *Madame royale* (pp. 235–236). New York: George H. Doran.

Dauterman, W. L. (1972). *Manual for the Stanford Multi-Modality Imagery Test.* New York: American Foundation for the Blind.

Davey, G. C. L. (1992). Classical conditioning and the acquisition of human fears and phobias: A review and synthesis of the literature. *Advances in Behavior Research and Therapy, 14,* 29–66.

Davidson, T. (1973). A survey of developments in a new field: Orientation and mobility for the low vision person, Part III. *Low Vision Abstracts, 1*(5), 1–7.

de Beni, R., & Cornoldi, C. (1988). Imagery limitations in totally congenitally blind subjects. *Journal of Experimental Psychology: Learning, Memory, & Cognition, 14,* 650–655.

DeCasper, A. J, & Fifer, W. P. (1980). Of human bonding: Newborns prefer their mothers' voices. *Science, 208,* 1174–1176.

de Haas, C., & Weisgerber, R. A. (1978). Environmental sensing selection evaluation and training system (ESSETS): Environmental sensing selection and matching. Palo Alto, CA: American Institutes for Research.

De l'Aune, W. R. (1980). Research and the mobility specialist. In R. L. Welsh & B. B. Blasch (Eds.), *Foundations of orientation and mobility* (pp. 653–662). New York: American Foundation for the Blind.

De l'Aune, W., & Needham, W. (1977). In M. Cannon (Ed.), *Proceedings* of *the Fifth New England Bioengineering Conference* (pp. 111–115). Personality Determiners of Successful Prosthetic and Sensory Aid Use. New York: Pergamon.

De l'Aune, W., Scheel, P., & Needham, W. (1974). Methodology for training indoor acoustic environmental analysis in blinded veterans. *Journal of the International Research Communications System, 2,* 1212.

De l'Aune, W., Lewis, C., Dolan, M., Grimmelsman, T., & Needham, W. (1976, April). *Two sensory aids having profound effects on the blind.* Paper presented at the IEE International Conference on Acoustics.

De l'Aune, W., Lewis, C., Needham, W., & Nelson, J. (1977). Speech compression: Personality correlates of successful use. *Journal of Visual Impairment & Blindness, 71*(2), 66–70.

DeLoache, J. S. (1991). Symbolic functioning in very young children: Understanding of pictures and models. *Child Development, 62,* 736–752.

DeLoache, J. S., & Marzolf, D. P. (1992). When is a picture not worth a thousand words: Young children's understanding of pictures and models. *Cognitive Development, 7,* 317–329.

Department of Transport. (1991). *Disability Unit Circular 1/91: The use of dropped kerbs and tactile surfaces at pedestrian crossing points.* London: Author.

De Witt, J. (1988, July). *BIOVISION—20/20 by 2020: A systematic concept for developing an artificial visual prosthesis.* Paper presented at the Douglas C. Macfarland Seminar at the Biannual Meeting of the Association for Education and Rehabilitation of the Blind and Visually Impaired, Montreal, Quebec, Canada.

Diamond, M. D., Weiss, A. J., & Grynbaum, B. (1968). The unmotivated patient. *Archives of Physical Medicine and Rehabilitation, 49,* 281–284.

Diderot, D. (1916). Letter on the blind in early philosophical works (M. Jourdian, Trans.) (pp. 68–141). Chicago and London: Open Court Publishing.

Dodds, A. G. (1989). Motivation reconsidered: The importance of self-efficacy in rehabilitation. *British Journal of Visual Impairment, 7,* 11–15.

Dodds, A. G., Howarth, C. T., & Carter, D. C. (1982). The mental maps of the blind: The role of previous experience. *Journal of Visual Impairment & Blindness, 76,* 5–12.

Dodds, A. G., Ferguson, E., Ng, L., Flannigan, H., Hawes, G., & Yates, L. (1994). The concept of adjustment: A structural model. *Journal of Visual Impairment & Blindness, 88,* 487–497.

Dodson-Burk, B., & Hill, E. W. (1989a). *An orientation and mobility primer for families and young chil-*

dren. New York: American Foundation for the Blind.

Dodson-Burk, B., & Hill, E. W. (1989b). *Preschool orientation and mobility screening.* Alexandria, VA: Division IX of the Association for Education and Rehabilitation of the Blind and Visually Impaired.

Dolanski, V. (1931). Do the blind sense obstacles? *And There Was Light, 1,* 8–12.

Downs, R. M., & Liben, L. S. (1990). Getting a bearing on maps: The role of projective spatial concepts in map understanding by children. *Children's Environments Quarterly, 7,* 15–25.

Dressler, F. B. (1893). On the pressure sense of the drum of the ear and facial vision. *American Journal of Psychology, 5,* 344–350.

Dunst, C. J., & Trivette, C. M. (1988). Toward experimental evaluation of the Family, Infant and Preschool Program. In H. Weiss & F. Jacobs (Eds.), *Evaluating family programs.* New York: Adline.

Dunst, C. J., Trivette, C. M., & Deal, A. (1988). *Enabling and empowering families: Principles and guidelines for practice.* Cambridge, MA: Brookline Books.

Durrant, J. D., & Lovrinic, J. H. (1995). *Bases of hearing science.* Baltimore: Williams & Wilkins.

Dyer, D., & Smith, A. (1972, Fall). The effects of vision utilization on distance vision efficiency. *Low Vision Abstracts, 2*(3), 13.

Dykes, J. (1992). Opinions of orientation and mobility instructors about using the long cane with preschool-age children. *RE:view, 24,* 85–92.

Eames, E. & Eames, T. (1994). *A guide to guide dog schools* (2nd ed.). New York: Baruch College Guide Dog Book Fund.

Easterbrook, J. A. (1959). The effect of emotion on the utilization and the organization of behavior. *Psychological Review, 66,* 183–201.

Easton, R. D., & Bentzen, B. L. (1980). Perception of tactile route configurations by blind and sighted observers. *Journal of Visual Impairment & Blindness, 74*(7), 254–257, 261–265.

Easton, R. D., & Bentzen, B. L. (1987). Memory for verbally presented routes: A comparison of strategies used by blind and sighted people. *Journal of Visual Impairment & Blindness, 81*(3), 100–105.

Edman, P. K. (1992). *Tactile graphics.* New York: American Foundation for the Blind.

Ehresman, P. (1995). Free-standing canes. *RE:view, 27*(1), 15–23.

Eichorn, J. R., & McDade, P. R. (1969). *Teaching orientation and mobility to the mentally retarded blind.* Chestnut Hill, MA: Boston College Peripatology Program.

Ekehammer, B. (1975). Interactionism in personality from a historical perspective. *Psychological Bulletin, 81,* 1026–48.

Elias, H. (1974). A tactile guidestrip for blind pedestrians. *New Outlook for the Blind, 68*(7), 322–323.

Emerson, D. L. (1981). Facing loss of vision: The response of adults to visual impairment. *Journal of Visual Impairment & Blindness, 75*(2), 41–45.

Endler, N. S. (1980). Person-situation interaction and anxiety. In K. L. Kutash & L. B. Schlesinger (Eds.), *Handbook of stress and anxiety* (pp. 249–266). San Francisco: Jossey-Bass.

Endler, N. S. (1983). Interactionism: A personality model, but not yet a theory. In M. M. Page (Ed.), *Personality: Current theory and research* (pp. 155–200). Lincoln: University of Nebraska Press.

Epstein, R. A., & Meyer, R. G. (1970, January). *Output measurements for the Laser Cane.* Cincinnati, OH: Laser Laboratory, Children's Hospital Research Foundation, Medical Center, University of Cincinnati.

Erin, J. N., & Corn, A. L. (1994). A survey of children's first understanding of being visually impaired. *Journal of Visual Impairment & Blindness, 80,* 132–139.

Evans, B. W., Fellows, J., Zorn, M., & Doty, K. (1980). Cognitive mapping and architecture. *Journal of Applied Psychology, 65,* 474–478.

Farina, A., Holland, C. H., & Ring, K. (1966). Role of stigma and set in interpersonal interaction. *Journal of Abnormal Psychology, 71,* 421–428.

Farmer, L. W. (1975). Travel in adverse weather using electronic mobility guidance devices. *New Outlook for the Blind, 69*(10), 433–439, 451.

Farmer, L. W. (1980). Mobility devices. In R. L. Welsh & B. B. Blasch (Eds.), *Foundations of orientation and mobility* (pp. 357–412). New York: American Foundation for the Blind.

Faye, E. E. (Ed.). (1984). *Clinical low vision.* Boston: Little, Brown.

Feather, N. T. (1966). Effects of prior success and failure on expectations of success and subsequent performance. *Journal of Personality and Social Psychology, 3,* 287–298.

Feddersen, W. E., Sandel, T. T., Teas, D. C., & Jeffress, L. A. (1957). Localization of high frequency tones. *Journal of the Acoustical Society of America, 29,* 988–991.

Felson, D., Anderson, J., Hannan, M., Milton, R., Wilson, P., & Kiel, D. (1989). Impaired vision and hip fracture: The Framingham study. *Journal of the American Geriatric Society, 37,* 495–500.

Felton, B., & Kahana, E. (1974). Adjustment and situationally bound locus of control among institutionalized aged. *Journal of Gerontology, 29,* 295–301.

Fernald, A. (1992). Human maternal vocalisations to infants as biologically relevant signals: An evolutionary perspective. In J. H. Barkow, L. Cosmides, & J. Tooby (Eds.), *The Adapted mind: Evolutionary psychology and the generation of culture* (pp. 392–428). New York: Oxford University Press.

Ferrell, K. A. (1979). Orientation and mobility for preschool children: What we have and what we need. *Journal of Visual Impairment & Blindness, 73*(4), 147–150.

Ferrell, K. A. (1985). *Reach out and teach: Meeting the training needs of parents of visually and multiply handicapped young children.* New York: American Foundation for the Blind.

Ferrell, K. A., & Suvak, P. A. (1996). *Educational outcomes for Colorado students with visual impairments: Final report.* (Available from Division of Special Education, University of Northern Colorado, Greeley, CO 80639.)

Fifer, W. P., Moon, C. (1988). *Auditory experience in the fetus.* West Caldwell, NJ: Telford Press.

Finestone, S., Lukoff, I., & Whiteman, M. (1960). *The demand for dog guides.* New York: Research Center, New York School of Social Work, Columbia University.

Finley, F., Cody, K., & Finizie, R. (1969). Locomotion patterns in elderly women. *Archives in Physical Medicine and Rehabilitation, 50,* 140–146.

First European Symposium on Tactual Town Maps for the Blind. (1984). General Report. Brussels, Belgium.

Fisk, S. (1986). Constant contact technique with a modified tip: A new alternative for long-cane mobility. *Journal of Visual Impairment & Blindness, 80*(10), 999–1000.

Fluharty, W., McHugh, J., McHugh, M., Willits, P., & Wood, J. (1976). Anxiety in the teacher–student relationship as applicable to orientation and mobility instruction. *New Outlook for the Blind, 70*(4), 153–156.

Fordyce, W. (1971). Behavioral methods in rehabilitation. In W. Neff (Ed.), *Rehabilitation psychology.* Washington, DC: American Psychological Association.

Foulke, E. (1964). Transfer of a complex perceptual skill. *Perceptual and Motor Skills, 18,* 733–740.

Foulke, E. (1971). The perceptual basis for mobility. *American Foundation for the Blind Research Bulletin, 23,* 1–8.

Foulke, E. (1983). Spatial ability and the limitations of perceptual systems. In H. Pick and L. Acredolo (Eds.), *Spatial orientation: Theory, research, and application.* New York: Plenum.

Foulke, E. (1985). The cognitive foundations of mobility. In D. Warren & E. Strelow (Eds.), *Electronic spatial sensing for the blind: Contributions from perception, rehabilitation, and computer vision.* Boston: Martinus Nijhoff.

Foy, C. J., Kirchner, D., & Waple, L. (1991). The Connecticut precane. *Journal of Visual Impairment & Blindness, 85*(2) 85–86.

Foy, C. J., Von Scheden, M. & Waiculonis, J. (1992). The Connecticut pre-cane: Case study and curriculum. *Journal of Visual Impairment & Blindness, 86*(4), 178–181.

Fraiberg, S. (1968). Parallel and divergent patterns in blind and sighted infants. *Psychoanalytic Study of the Child, 23,* 264–300.

Fraiberg, S. (1977). *Insights from the blind.* New York: Basic Books.

Franck, L. (1990). Effect of a cane with microprism reflecting tape on the nighttime visibility of blind rural travelers. *Journal of Visual Impairment & Blindness, 84*(1), 8–10.

Franks, F., & Kephart-Cozen, C. (1982). *Introduction to map study I: Representing a known environment symbolically on simple maps.* Louisville, KY: American Printing House for the Blind.

Fraser of Lonsdale. (1965). *Chairman's notes: Long cane technique.* Review, St. Dunstan's, October. No. 558, Vol. 50, pp. 3–4.

Freeman, R. D., Goetz, E., Richards, D. P., & Groenveld, M. (1991). Defiers of negative prediction: A 14-year follow-up study of legally blind children. *Journal of Visual Impairment & Blindness, 85*(9), 365–370.

Freidson, E. (1965). Disability as social deviance. In M. Sussman (Ed.), *Sociology and rehabilitation.* Washington, DC: American Sociological Association.

Freud, S. (1961). Two encyclopedia articles. In J. Strachy (Ed. and Trans.), *The standard edition of the complete psychological works of Sigmund Freud* (Vol. 18). London: Hogarth. (Original work published in 1923.)

Frostig, M., & Horne, D. (1964). *The Frostig program for the development of visual perception: Teacher's guide.* Chicago, IL: Follett.

Fulton, J. P., & Katz, S. (1986). Characteristics of the disabled elderly and implication for rehabilitation. In S. J. Brody & G. E. Ruff (Eds.), *Aging and rehabilitation: Advances in the state of the art* (pp. 36–46). New York: Springer.

Gallon, C., Oxley, P., & Simms, B. (1991). *Tactile footway surfaces for the blind.* London: Transport and Road Research Laboratory, Department of Transport.

Gardner, H. (1985). *The mind's new eye: A history of the cognitive revolution.* New York: Basic Books.

Garling, T., Lindberg, E., & Mantyla, T. (1983). Orientation in buildings: Effects of familiarity, visual access, and orientation aids. *Journal of Applied Psychology, 68,* 177–186.

Garvey, P. (1994). *Changeable message sign visibility* (DTFH61-91-C-00042). Draft interim report. Washington, DC: Department of Transportation, Federal Highway Administration.

Gaunet, F., & Thinus-Blanc, C. (1995). Exploratory patterns and reactions to spatial change: The role of early visual experience. In B. G. Bardy, R. J. Bootsma, & Y. Guiard (Eds.), *Studies in perception and action III.* Mahwah, NJ: Lawrence Erlbaum.

Gaver, W. W. (1993). How do we hear in the world: Explorations in ecological acoustics. *Ecological Psychology, 5,* 285–314.

Gee, K., Harrell, R., & Rosenberg, R. (1987). Teaching orientation and mobility skills within and across natural opportunities for travel: A model designed for learners with multiple severe disabilities. In L. Goetz, D. Guess, & K. Stremel-Campbell (Eds.), *Innovative program design for individuals with dual sensory impairments* (pp. 127–157). Baltimore, MD: Paul H. Brooks.

Gelfand, S. A. (1990). *Hearing: An introduction to psychological and physiological acoustics.* New York: Marcel Dekker.

Genensky, S. M., Barry, S. N., Bikson, T. H., & Bikson, T. K. (Eds.). (1979). *Visual environmental adaptation problems of the partially sighted: Final report.* Santa Monica, CA: Center for the Partially Sighted.

Gentner, D. (1989). The mechanisms of analogical reasoning. In S. Vosniadou & A. Ortony (Eds.), *Similarity and analogical reasoning.* Cambridge, England: Cambridge University Press.

Georgia Institute of Technology. (1985). *Signage for low vision and blind persons: A multidisciplinary assessment of the state of the art* (Contract No. 300-83-0280). Draft final report. Washington, DC: Architectural and Transportation Barriers Compliance Board.

Gerber, S. (1974). *Introductory learning science.* Philadelphia: W. B. Saunders.

Gerson, L. W., Jarjoura, D., & McCord, G. (1989). Risk of imbalance in elderly people with impaired hearing or vision. *Age and Ageing, 18,* 31–34.

Geruschat, D. R. (1985). *Illumination and low vision mobility: Final report.* Washington, DC: National Institute of Handicapped Research. (Grant No. 1231413680A1.)

Geruschat, D. R., & De l'Aune, W. (1989). Reliability and validity of O&M instructor observations. *Journal of Visual Impairment & Blindness, 83*(9), 457–460.

Geruschat, D. R., Neustadt-Noy, N., & Cory, D. (1994). *Roles and functions of mobility instructors who attended IMC5 and IMC6.* Paper presented at the International Mobility Conference, Melbourne, Australia.

Gibson, E. J. (1969). *Principles of perceptual learning and development.* New York: Appleton-Century-Crofts.

Gibson, J. J. (1958). Visually controlled locomotion and visual orientation in animals. *British Journal of Psychology, 49,* 182–194.

Gibson, J. J. (1962). Observations on active touch. *Psychological Review, 69,* 477–491.

Gibson, J. J. (1966). *The senses considered as perceptual systems.* Boston: Houghton Mifflin.

Gibson, J. J. (1979). *The ecological approach to visual perception.* Boston: Houghton Mifflin.

Gill, J. M. (1973a). *Design, production and evaluation of tactual maps for the blind.* Unpublished doctoral thesis, University of Warwick, Coventry, England.

Gill, J. M. (1973b). Method for the production of tactual maps and diagrams. *American Foundation for the Blind Research Bulletin, 26,* 203–204.

Gill, J. M. (1996). *Smart cards: Interfaces for people with disabilities.* London: Royal National Institute for the Blind.

Gill, J. M. (Ed.) (1994). *Smart cards and disability: Proceedings of the COST 219 Seminar.* Helsinki, Finland.

Gill, J. M., & James, G. A. (1973). A study on the discrimination of tactual point symbols. *American Foundation for the Blind Research Bulletin, 26,* 19–34.

Gillman, A. E., Simmel, A., & Simon, E. P. (1986). Visual handicaps in the aged: Self-reported visual disability and quality of life of residents of public housing for the elderly. *Journal of Visual Impairment & Blindness, 80*(2), 588–590.

Gipsman, S. (1981). Effect of visual condition on use of proprioceptive cues in performing a balance task. *Journal of Visual Impairment & Blindness, 75*(2), 50–54.

Goetz, L., Guess, D., & Stremel-Campbell, K. (Eds.). (1987). *Innovative program design for individuals with dual sensory impairments* (pp. 127–157). Baltimore, MD: Paul H. Brooks.

Goetzinger, C. P. (1978). Word discrimination testing. In J. Katz (Ed.), *Handbook of clinical audiology* (2nd ed.). Baltimore: Williams & Wilkins.

Goffman, E. (1963). *Stigma: Notes on the management of a spoiled identity.* Englewood Cliffs, NJ: Prentice Hall.

Golledge, R. G. (1991). Tactual strip maps as navigational aids. *Journal of Visual Impairment & Blindness, 85*(7), 296–301.

Golledge, R. G., Costanzo, C. M., & Marston, J. R. (1995). *The mass transit needs of a non-driving disabled population.* Final report. Santa Barbara: University of California Achievement Field Station PATH.

Golledge, R. G., Doherty, V., & Bell, S. (1995). Acquiring spatial knowledge: Survey versus route-based knowledge in unfamiliar environments. *Annals of the Association of American Geographers, 85,* 134–158.

Golledge, R. G., Loomis, J. M., Klatzky, R. L. (1994). *Auditory maps as alternative to tactile maps for wayfinding.* Paper presented at the Fourth International Symposium on Maps and Graphics for the Visually Impaired, São Paulo, Brazil.

Gómez, J. P. (1991). Urban elements which limit the mobility of the visually impaired and suggestions for their elimination. *Proceedings of the Sixth International Mobility Conference,* Madrid, Spain.

Goodman, A. (1965). Reference zero level for pure tone audiometry. *Asha, 7,* 262–263.

Graham, M. D. (1968). *Multiply impaired blind children: A national problem.* New York: American Foundation for the Blind.

Grantham, D. W. (1995). Spatial hearing and related phenomena. In E. Carterette & M. Friedman (Series Eds.) & B. Moore (Vol. Ed.), *Handbook of perception and cognition: Hearing* (2nd ed., pp. 297–345). New York: Academic Press.

Green, D., & Swets, J. (1966). *Signal detection theory and psychophysics.* New York: Wiley.

Greenough, W., Black, J., & Wallace, C. (1987). Experience and brain development. *Child Development, 58,* 539–559.

Gregg, A. (1951). *Corrective therapy, the adolescent profession.* Unpublished lecture.

Griffin, D. R. (1958). *Listening in the dark.* New Haven, CT: Yale University Press.

Griffin, H. (1981). Motor development in congenitally blind children. *Education of the Visually Handicapped, 12,* 106–111.

Guth, D. A. (1992). Space saving statistics: An introduction to constant error, variable error, and absolute error. *Peabody Journal of Education, 67*(2), 110–120.

Guth, D., & LaDuke, R. (1994). The veering tendency of blind pedestrians: An analysis of the problem and literature review. *Journal of Visual Impairment & Blindness, 88,* 391–400.

Guth, D., & LaDuke, R. (1995). Veering by blind pedestrians: Individual differences and their implications for instruction. *Journal of Visual Impairment & Blindness, 89*(1), 28–37.

Guth, D. A., Hill, E. W., & Rieser, J. J. (1989). Tests of blind pedestrians' use of traffic sounds for street-crossing alignment. *Journal of Visual Impairment & Blindness, 83*(9), 461–468.

Guth, D., Rieser, J., & Yen, L. (1995, July). *Toward understanding long canes as perceptual tools: Tapping, stirring, and scraping to identify stuff by sound and touch.* Paper presented at the Eighth International Conference on Perception and Action, Marseille, France.

Hahn, W. L. (1908). Some habits and sensory adaptations of cave-inhabiting bats. *Biology Bulletin, 15,* 135–193.

Hall, C. S. (1954). *A primer of Freudian psychology.* New York: World.

Hall, G., Rabelle, A., & Zabihaylo, C. (1994). *Audible traffic signals: A new definition.* Montreal: Institut Nazareth et Louis-Braille & Montreal Association for the Blind.

Hamilton, W. (1980). *Electric automobiles: Energy, environmental, and economic prospects for the future.* New York: McGraw-Hill.

Haneline, R. L. (1992). [ETAs and dog guides.] Unpublished raw data.

Hapeman, J. (1993). *The effects of blended curbs on the ability of nonvisual travelers to detect intersections.* Unpublished Master's project, Department of Blind Rehabilitation, Western Michigan University, Kalamazoo.

Hapeman, L. B. (1967). Developmental concepts of blind children between the ages of 3 and 6 as they relate to orientation and mobility. *International Journal for the Education of the Blind, 17,* 41–48.

Harford, E., & Barry, J. (1965). A rehabilitative approach to the problem of unilateral hearing impairment: The contralateral routing of signals (CROS). *Journal of Speech and Hearing Disorders, 30,* 121–128.

Haring, N. G., & Schiefelbusch, R. L. (1967). *Method in special education.* New York: McGraw-Hill.

Harley, R. K. (1963). Verbalisms among blind children. *American Foundation for the Blind, Research Services No. 10.* New York: American Foundation for the Blind.

Harley, R. K., Merbler, J. B., & Wood, T. A. (1975). The development of a scale in orientation and mobility for multiply impaired blind children. *Education of the Visually Handicapped, 8,* 1–5.

Harley, R. K., Wood, T. A., & Merbler, K. B. (1980). An orientation and mobility program for multiply impaired blind children. *Exceptional Children, 46*(5), 326–331.

Harley, R. K., Long, R. G., Merbler, J. B., & Wood, T. A. (1987). Orientation and mobility for the blind multihandicapped young child. *Journal of Visual Impairment & Blindness, 81*(8), 377–381.

Harrell, L., & Akeson, N. (1987). Preschool vision stimulation: *It's more than a flashlight!* New York: American Foundation for the Blind.

Harris, J. (1948). Discrimination of pitch: Suggestions toward method and procedure. *American Journal of Psychology, 61,* 309–322.

Hart, V., & Ferrell, K. A. (1985). Parent/Educator cooperative efforts in education of the visually handicapped. In G. T. Scholl (Ed.), *Quality services for blind and visually handicapped learners: Statements of position.* Reston, VA: Division of the Visually Handicapped, Council for Exceptional Children.

Hartridge, H. (1920). The avoidance of objects by bats in their flight. *Journal of Physiology, 54,* 54–57.

Hatlen, P. H. (1986). *A report on the mismatch between the supply of and demand for instructors in the field of visual impairment.* Unpublished manuscript.

Hauger, J. S., Safewright, M. P., Rigby, J. C., & McAuley, W. J. (1994). *Detectable warnings project: Report of field tests and observations.* Final report. Washington, DC: U.S. Architectural and Transportation Barriers Compliance Board.

Havens, L. L. (1967). Dependence: Definitions and strategies. *Rehabilitation Record, 8*(2), 23–28.

Havlik, R. J. (1986, September 19). Aging in the eighties, impaired senses for sound and light in persons age 65 and over: Preliminary data from the supplement on aging to the National Health Interview Survey: United States, January–June, 1984. *Advance Data,* No. 125.

Hayes, J. R. (1988). *The complete problem solver* (2nd ed.). Hillsdale, NJ: Lawrence Erlbaum.

Head, D. (1979). A comparison of self-concept scores for visually impaired adolescents in several class settings. *Education of the Visually Handicapped, 10,* 51–55.

Hecox, K. (1975). Electrophysiological correlates of human auditory development. In L. B. Cohen & P. Salapatek, (Eds.), *Infant perception: From sensation to cognition* (Vol. 2, pp. 151–191). New York: Academic Press.

Hehir, T. (1994). OSEP [Office of Special Education Programs] director interview. *The Association for Education and Rehabilitation of the Blind and Visually Impaired Report, 11,* 1, 3–6.

Heller, M. A., & Schiff (1991). *The psychology of touch.* Hillsdale, NJ: Lawrence Erlbaum.

Heller, T. (1904). *Studien zur blinden Psychologie.* Leipzig: Wilhelm Englemann.

Herman, J., Chatman, S. P., & Roth, S. F. (1983). Cognitive mapping in blind people: Acquisition of spatial relationships in a large scale environment. *Journal of Visual Impairment & Blindness, 77,* 161–166.

Herman, J., Herman, T. G., & Chatman, S. P. (1983). Constructing cognitive maps from partial information: A demonstration study with congenitally blind subjects. *Journal of Visual Impairment & Blindness, 77,* 195–198.

Herman, R. (1982). A therapeutic approach based on theories of motor control. *International Rehabilitation Medicine, 4,* 185–189.

Herms, B., Elias, H., & Robbins, D. (1974). *Guidestrips for visually handicapped pedestrians.* Paper presented at Third National Seminar on the Planning, Design, and Implementation of Bicycle and Pedestrian Facilities, San Diego, CA.

Heyes, A. (1993). *Sonic Pathfinder training manual,* Kew, Australia: Royal Guide Dogs Association of Australia.

Higgerty, M., & Rhodes, M. (1991, September 9–12). *Rural travel in South Africa.* Paper presented at the Sixth International Mobility Conference, Madrid, Spain.

Higgins, S. (1985). Movement as an emergent form: Its structural limits. *Human Movement Science, 4,* 119–148.

Hill, E. W. (1971). Hill Performance Test on Selected Positional Concepts. Chicago: Stoelting.

Hill, E. W. (1971). Mobility and concept development for low vision children. *Low Vision Abstracts, 1*(2), 5.

Hill, E. W. (1981). *The Hill performance test of selected positional concepts.* Chicago: Stoelting.

Hill, E. W. (1986). Orientation and mobility. In G. T. Scholl (Ed.), *Foundations of education for blind and visually handicapped children and youth* (pp. 315–340). New York: American Foundation for the Blind.

Hill, E. W., & Blasch, B. B. (1980). Concept development. In R. L. Welsh & B. B. Blasch (Eds.), *Foundations of orientation and mobility* (pp. 265–290). New York: American Foundation for the Blind.

Hill, E. W., & Ponder, P. (1976). *Orientation and mobility techniques: A guide for the practitioner.* New York: American Foundation for the Blind.

Hill, E. W., Dodson-Burk, B., & Smith, B. A. (1989). Orientation and mobility for infants who are visually impaired. *RE:view, 21*(2), 57–60.

Hill, E. W., Rosen, S., Correa, V., & Langley, M. (1984). Preschool orientation and mobility: An expanded definition. *Education of the Visually Handicapped, 16,* 58–72.

Hill, E. W., Rieser, J. J., Hill M.-M., Hill, M., Halpin, J., and Halpin, R. (1993). How persons with visual impairments explore novel spaces: Strategies for good and poor performers. *Journal of Visual Impairment & Blindness, 93*(8), 295–301.

Hill, J. W. (1973). Limited field of view in reading lettershapes with the fingers. In F. Geldard (Ed.), *Cutaneous communication systems and devices.* Austin, TX: Psychonomic Society.

Hill, K., & Horton, M. (1985, April). *Validation of a classroom curriculum teaching elementary school students test-taking skills that optimize test performance.* Paper presented at the annual meeting of the American Educational Research Association, Chicago.

Hill, M. (1994). The introduction and possible development of Greater Manchester's smart card system for public transport. In J. M. Gill (Ed.), *Smart cards and disability: Proceedings on the COST 219 Seminar.* Helsinki, Finland.

Hill, M. M., Hill, E. W., & LeBous, C. (1994). Toward the establishment of state licensure for orientation and mobility specialists. *Journal of Visual Impairment & Blindness, 88*(3), 201–205.

Hill, M. M., Dodson-Burk, B., Hill, W. W., & Fox, J. (1995). An infant Sonicguide intervention program for a child with visual disability. *Journal of Visual Impairment & Blindness, 88,* 329–336.

Hines, S. S. (1990). The impact of fear on blind and visually impaired travelers in rapid rail systems. In M. M. Uslan, A. F. Peck, W. R. Wiener & A. Stern (Eds.), *Access to mass transit for blind and visually impaired travelers.* New York: American Foundation for the Blind.

Hirsh, I. J. (1950a). Binaural hearing aids: A review of some experiments. *Journal of Speech and Hearing Disorders, 15,* 114–123.

Hirsh, I. J. (1950b). The relation between localization and intelligibility. *Journal of the Acoustical Society of America, 22,* 196–199.

Hnath-Chisolm, T. (1994). Cochlear implants and tactile aids. In J. Katz (Ed.), *Handbook of clinical audiology* (4th ed.). Baltimore: Williams & Wilkins.

Hollins, M. (1985). Styles of mental imagery in blind adults. *Neuropsychologia, 23,* 56–566.

Hoover, R. E. (1946). Foot travel at Valley Forge. *Outlook for the Blind and Teachers Forum, 40*(9), 246–251.

Hoover, R. E. (1950). The cane as a travel aid. In P. Zahl (Ed.), *Blindness* (pp. 353–365). Princeton, NJ: Princeton University Press.

Hoover, R. E. (1968). The Valley Forge Story. *Blindness,* 55–78.

Horak, F., Shupert, C., & Mirka, A. (1989). Components of postural dyscontrol in the elderly: A review. *Neurobiology of Aging, 10*(6), 727–738.

Horowitz, A. (1995). Aging, vision loss, and depression. *Aging and Vision News, 7*(1), 1, 6–7.

Horton, K. (1986). Delivery of orientation and mobility services through community based rehabilitation programs in Asia. In N. Neustadt, S. Merin, & Y. Schiff (Eds.), *Orientation and mobility of the visually impaired.* Jerusalem: Heiliger.

Hoshmand, L. (1975). "Blindisms:" Some observations and propositions. *Education of the Visually Handicapped, 7*(2), 56–60.

Howard, I. P., & Templeton, W. B. (1966). *Human spatial orientation.* New York: Wiley.

Howe, G. (1872). *Forty-first annual report of the trustees of the Perkins Institution and Massachusetts School for the Blind.* Boston: Perkins Institution and Massachusetts School for the Blind.

Hoyt, L., & Hudson, J. W. (1981). Dog guide dialogs. *Journal of Visual Impairment & Blindness, 75,* 62.

Huebner, K. M., Prickett, J. G., Welch, R., & Joffee, E. (Eds.). (1995). *Hand in hand: Essentials of communication and orientation and mobility for your students who are deaf–blind.* New York: AFB Press.

Hughes, M. C., Smith, R. B., & Benitz, F. (1977). Travel training for exceptional children. *Teaching Exceptional Children, 1*(4), 90–91.

Hughes, R. (1967). Orientation and mobility for the partially sighted. *International Journal for the Education of the Blind,* 119–120.

Humphrey, E., & Warner, L. (1934). *Working dogs.* Baltimore: Johns Hopkins Press.

Humphries, T., Snider, L., & McDougall, B. (1993). Clinical evaluation of the effectiveness of sensory integrative and perceptual motor therapy in improving sensory integrative function in children with learning disabilities. *Journal of Occupational Therapy Research, 13*(3), 163–182.

Huss, C. P. (1984). A multidisciplinary approach to driving for the visually handicapped. *Rehabilitative Optometry, 2,* 10–11.

Huss, C. P. (1988). Model approach—low vision driver's training and assessment. *Journal of Vision Rehabilitation, 2*(2), 31–44.

Hyman, M. (1972). Social psychological determinants of patient's performance in stroke rehabilitation. *Archives of Physical Medicine and Rehabilitation, 53,* 217–226.

Illinois Office of Education. (1973). *A curriculum guide for the development of body and sensory awareness for the visually impaired.* Springfield, IL: Illinois Office of Education.

Institute of Transportation Engineers. (1989). *A toolbox for alleviating traffic congestion.* Washington, DC: Author.

Institute of Transportation Engineers. (1995). *Improving traffic signal operations: A primer.* Washington, DC: Author.

International Standards Organization (ISO). (1985). *ISO Normal equal loudness contours for pure tones under free-field listening conditions.* ISO/R225-1985. Geneva: International Standards Organization.

Irwin, R. (1955). *As I saw it.* New York American Foundation for the Blind, 1955.

Jackson, D. M. (1977, March). *Electronic travel aids in the urban environment.* Paper presented at the Conference on Orientation and Mobility in Urban Environment, sponsored by American Foundation for the Blind, New York.

Jacobson, W. (1979). Complementary travel aids for the blind persons: The Sonicguide used with a dog guide. *Journal of Visual Impairment & Blindness, 73*(1), 10–12.

Jacobson, W. H. (1993). *The art and science of teaching orientation and mobility to persons with visual impairments.* New York: AFB Press.

James, G. A. (1972). Problems in the standardization of design and symbolization in tactile route maps for the blind. *New Beacon, 56,* 87–91.

James, G. A. (1975). Kit for making raised maps. *New Beacon, 59,* 85–90.

James, G. A., & Gill, J. M. (1974). Mobility maps for the visually handicapped: A study of learning and retention of raised symbols. *American Foundation for the Blind Research Bulletin, 27,* 87–98.

James, G. A., & Swain, R. (1975). Learning bus routes using a tactual map. *New Outlook for the Blind, 69*(5), 212–217.

James, W. (1890). *Principles of psychology* (Vol. 2). New York: Holt.

Jan, J., Freeman, R., & Scott, E. (1977). *Visual impairment in children and adolescents.* New York: Grune & Stratton.

Jan, J., Sykanda, A., & Groenveld, M. (1990). Habilitation and rehabilitation of visually impaired and blind children. *Pediatrician, 17,* 202–207.

Jan, J., Robinson, G., Scott, E., & Kinnis, C. (1975). Hypotonia in the blind child. *Developmental Medicine and Child Neurology 17,* 35–40.

Jannson, G. (1990). Non-visual guidance of walking. In R. Warren & A. Wertheim (Eds.), *Perception and control of egomotion* (pp. 507–521). Hillsdale, NJ: Lawrence Erlbaum.

Jansson, G. (1991). The control of locomotion when vision is reduced or missing. In A. E. Patla (Ed.), *Adaptability of human gait.* North Holland: Elsevier.

Javal, E. (1905). *On becoming blind.* New York and London: Macmillan.

Jervis, F. (1959). A comparison of self-concepts of blind and sighted children. In *Guidance programs for blind children.* Watertown, MS: Perkins School for the Blind.

Joffee, E., & Rikhye, C. H. (1991). Orientation and mobility for students with severe visual and multiple impairments: A new perspective. *Journal of Visual Impairment & Blindness, 85*(5), 211–216.

Joffee, E. (1988). A home-based orientation and mobility program for infants and toddlers. *Journal of Visual Impairment & Blindness, 82*(7), 282–285.

Joffee, E. (1995). The ADA: How blindness organizations are responding. *Journal of Visual Impairment Blindness News Service.* Vol. 89(2), pp. 22–23.

Joffee, E. (n.d.). *We can do it together: Mobility for students with multiple handicaps* [Videotape]. New York: American Foundation for the Blind Shoe String Video.

Joffee, E., & Wiener, W. (1995). Strengthening certification standards. *AER, Division Nine—Orientation and Mobility Newsletter,* Fall 1995, 4–5.

Johnson, G. (1994). Administration, advocacy, and evolution. *Journal of Visual Impairment & Blindness, 88,* 484–485.

Joint Organizational Effort. (1993). Full inclusion of students who are blind and visually impaired: A position statement. In J. M. Kauffman & D. P. Hallahan (Eds.), *The illusion of full inclusion: A comprehensive critique of a current special education bandwagon* (pp. 307–309). Austin, TX: PRO-ED.

Jose, R. T. (Ed.). (1983). *Understanding low vision.* New York: American Foundation for the Blind.

Jose, R. T., & Springer, D. (1975). Optical aids: An interdisciplinary perscription. *New Outlook for the Blind, 67*(1), 12–18.

Juurmaa, J. (1965). An analysis of the components of orientation mobility and mental manipulation of spatial relationships. *Report of the Institute of Occupational Health,* August, No. 28.

Juurmaa, J. (1973). Transposition in mental spatial manipulation: A theoretical analysis. *American Foundation for the Blind Research Bulletin, 26,* 87–134.

Kalloniatis, M., & Johnston, A. (1994). Visual environmental adaptation problems of partially sighted children. *Journal of Visual Impairment & Blindness, 88,* 234–243.

Kalso, A., & Koiv, A. (1995). *On history: Teaching orientation and mobility for blind in Estonia.* Unpublished manuscript.

Kalton, G. (1983). *Introduction to survey sampling.* Beverly Hills, CA: Sage.

Kantner, R., Clark, D., Allen, L., & Chase, M. (1976). Effects of vestibular stimulation on nystagmus response and motor performance in the developmentally delayed infant. *Physical Therapy, 42,* 399–413.

Karnes, T., Schiedeck, J., & Postello, T. (1994). *Hazards of protruding objects.* Unpublished manuscript.

Kates, L., & Schein, J. (1980). *A complete guide to communication with deaf-blind persons.* Silver Spring, MD: National Association of the Deaf.

Kay, L. (1974). A sonar aid to enhance spatial perception of the blind: Engineering design and evaluation. *Radio and Electronic Engineer, 44*(11), 605–627.

Kay, L. (1976). *Sensory Perception Laboratory Newsletter.* Christchurch, New Zealand: Department of Electrical Engineering, University of Canterbury.

Kay, L. (1980). The Sonicguide, long cane, and dog guide: Their compatibility. *Journal of Visual Impairment & Blindness, 75*(7), 277–280.

Kazdin, A. E. (1978). Methodological and interpretive problems of single-case experimental designs. *Journal of Consulting and Clinical Psychology, 46*(4), 1978, 629–642.

Keane, G. (1965). Auditory rehabilitation for hearing-impaired blind persons. *Asha Monograph, 12,* 31–51.

Kellog, W. N. (1962). Sonar systems of the blind. *Science, 137* (3528), 399–404.

Kemp, B., Brummel-Smith, K., & Ramsdell, J. W. (Eds.) (1990). *Geriatric rehabilitation.* Boston: Little, Brown.

Kemp, B. (1990). The psychosocial context of geriatric rehabilitation. In B. Kemp, K. Brummel-Smith, & J. W. Ramsdell (Eds.), *Geriatric rehabilitation* (pp. 41–57). Boston: Little, Brown.

Kennedy, J. M. (1995, May). *Raised line drawings.* Paper presented at the National Orientation and Mobility/Rehabilitation Teaching Conference, Lake Joseph, Ontario.

Kennedy, J. (1993). *Drawing and the blind: Pictures to touch.* New Haven, CT: Yale University Press.

Kephart, J. G., Kephart, C. P., & Schwarz, G. C. (1974). A journey into the world of the blind child. *Exceptional Children, 40,* 421–427.

Kermoian, R., & Campos, J. (1988). Locomotor experience: A facilitator of spatial cognitive development. *Child Development, 59,* 908–917.

Kerr, N. (1983). The role of vision in "visual imagery" experiments: Evidence from the congenitally blind. *Journal of Experimental Psychology: General, 112,* 265–277.

Kidwell, A. M., & Greer, P. S. (1973). *Sites, perception and the nonvisual experience: Designing and manufacturing mobility maps.* New York: American Foundation for the Blind.

Kiester, E. (1990). *AIDS and vision loss.* New York: American Foundation for the Blind.

Killion, M. (1978). Revised estimate of minimal audible pressure: Where is the missing dB. *Journal of Acoustical Society of America,* 63, 1501–1505.

Killion, M. C., Staab, W. J., & Preves, D. A. (1990). Classifying automatic signal processors. *Hearing Instruments, 41,* 24, 26.

Kirchner, C. (1990). Trends in the prevalence rates and numbers of blind and visually impaired schoolchildren. *Journal of Visual Impairment & Blindness, 84*(9), 478–479.

Kirchner, C., & Lowman, C. (1988). Sources of variation in the estimated prevalence of visual loss. In C. Kirchner (Ed.), *Data on blindness and visual impairment in the U.S.* (pp. 3–10). New York: American Foundation for the Blind.

Kirchner, C., & Peterson, R. (1980). Blind and visually impaired nursing home residents: Some social characteristics and services received. *Journal of Visual Impairment & Blindness, 74*(10), 401–403.

Kirchner, C., & Peterson, R. (1980). Multiple impairments among noninstitutionalized blind and visually impaired persons. *Journal of Visual Impairment & Blindness, 74*(1), 42–44.

Kirkwood, D. H. (1990). 1990 U.S. hearing aid sales summary. *Hearing Journal, 43*(12), 7–13.

Kitano, H. (1973). Highlights of institute on language and culture: Asian component. In L. A. Bransford, L. M. Baca, & K. Lane (Eds.), *Cultural diversity and the exceptional child* (pp. 14–15). Reston, VA: Council for Exceptional Children.

Klatzky, R. L., & Lederman, S. J. (1987). The intelligent hand. In G. Bower (Ed.), *The psychology of learning and motivation: Vol. 21,* (pp. 121–151). San Diego, CA: Academic Press.

Klatzky, R. L., Golledge, R. G., Loomis, J. M., Cicinelli, J. G., & Pellegrino, J. W. (1995). Performance of blind and sighted persons on spatial tasks. *Journal of Visual Impairment & Blindness, 89,* 70–82.

Klatzky, R. L., Loomis, J. M., Golledge, R. G., Cicinelli, J. G., Doherty, S., & Pelligrino, J. W. (1990). Acquisition of route and survey knowledge in the absence of vision. *Journal of Motor Behavior, 22,* 19–43.

Klausner, S. Z. (1969). *Disabled families: A study of a link between the social contributions of the disabled and the retardation of their rehabilitation in the family context.* Philadelphia: Center for Research on the Acts of Man.

Kleck, R., Ono, H., & Hastorf, A. (1966). The effects of physical deviance upon face to face interaction. *Human Relations, 19,* 425–436.

Knight, J. (1972). Mannerisms in the congenitally blind child. *New Outlook for the Blind, 66*(9), 297–302.

Koenig, W. (1950). Subjective effects in binaural hearing. *Journal of the Acoustical Society of America, 22,* 61–62.

Koestler, F. A. (1976). *The unseen minority.* New York: The David McKay.

Kohler, I. (1964). Orientation by oral clues. *American Foundation for the Blind Research Bulletin, 4.*

Kossick, R. (1970). Activating a program for the blind in South Vietnam. *American Association of Workers for the Blind Blindness Annual,* 25–54.

Kottke, F. H., Halpern, D., Easton, J. K. M., Ozel, A. T., & Burrill, C. A. (1978). Training and coordination. *Archives of Physical Medicine and Rehabilitation, 59,* 567–572.

Kozel, B. (1995). Diabetes and orientation and mobility training: An added challenge. *Journal of Visual Impairment & Blindness, 89,* 337–342.

Krahe, B. (1992). *Personality and social psychology: Towards a synthesis.* London: Sage.

Kronick, M. K. (1987). Children and canes: An adaptive approach. *Journal of Visual Impairment & Blindness, 81*(2), 61–62.

Kuczynska-Kwapisz, J., Kwapisz, J., & Adamowicz-Hummel, A. (1991, September 9–12). *Orientation and mobility services in Poland.* Paper presented at the Sixth International Mobility Conference, Madrid, Spain.

Kuhl, P. (1987). Perception of speech and sound in early infancy. In P. Salapatek, L. B. Cohen (Eds.), *Handbook of infant perception,* Vol. 2. New York: Holt.

Kuhl, P. (1991). Human adults and human infants show a "perceptual magnet effect" for the prototypes of speech categories, monkeys do not. *Perception and Psychophysics, 5*(2), 93–107.

LaDuke, R. O., & Welsh, R. L. (1980). Educational aspects. In R. L. Welsh & B. B. Blasch (Eds.), *Foundations of orientation and mobility* (pp. 527–548). New York: American Foundation for the Blind.

LaForge, R. G., Spector, W. D., & Sternberg, J. (1992). The relationship of vision and hearing impairment to one-year mortality and functional decline. *Journal of Aging and Health, 4*(1), 126–148.

LaGrow, S. J. (1986). Assessing optimal illumination for visual response accuracy in visually impaired adults. *Journal of Visual Impairment & Blindness, 80*(8): 888–895.

LaGrow, S. J. (1992). *The rehabilitation of visually impaired people.* Auckland, New Zealand: Royal New Zealand Foundation for the Blind.

LaGrow, S. J., & Blasch, B. B. (1992). Orientation and mobility services for older persons. In A. L. Orr (Ed.), *Vision and aging: Crossroads for service delivery* (pp. 255–287). New York: American Foundation for the Blind.

LaGrow, S., & Mulder, L. (1989). Structured solicitation: A standardized method for gaining travel information. *Journal of Visual Impairment & Blindness, 83*(9), 469–471.

LaGrow, S., & Murray, S. (1992). Use of the alternating treatment design to evaluate intervention in low vision rehabilitation. *Journal of Visual Impairment & Blindness, 86*(10), 435–439.

LaGrow, S. J., & Weessies, M. J. (1994). *Orientation and mobility: Techniques for independence.* Palmerston North, New Zealand: Dunmore Press.

LaGrow, S., Blasch, B., & De l'Aune, W. (1997). The efficiency of the touch technique for surface and foot-placement preview. *Journal of Visual Impairment & Blindness,* 91, 47–52.

LaGrow, S. J., Kjeldstad, A. & Lewandowski, E. (1988). The effects of cane-tip design on three aspects of nonvisual travel. *Journal of Visual Impairment & Blindness, 82*(1), 13–16.

LaGrow, S. J., Wiener, W. R., LaDuke, R. O. (1990). Independent travel for developmentally disabled persons: A comprehensive model of instruction. *Research in Developmental Disabilities, 11,* 289–301.

Lambert, L. M. & Lederman, S. J. (1989). An evaluation of the legibility and meaningfulness of potential map symbols. *Journal of Visual Impairment & Blindness, 83*(8), 397–403.

Landau, B., Spelke, E., & Gleitman, H. (1984). Spatial knowledge in a young blind child. *Cognition, 16,* 225–260.

Langbain, E., Blasch, B., & Chalmers, B. (1981). An orienteering program for blind and visually impaired persons. *Journal of Visual Impairment and Blindness, 75,* 273–276.

Langley, M. (1980). *The teachable moment and the handicapped infant.* Reston, VA: ERIC Clearinghouse on Handicapped and Gifted Children, Council for Exceptional Children. (ERIC Document Reproduction Service No. E0191254.)

Lappin, J. S., & Foulke, E. (1973). Expanding the tactual field of view. *Perception and Psychophysics, 14,* 237–241.

Large, T. (1982). The effects of attitudes upon the blind: A reexamination. *Journal of Rehabilitation, 6,* 33–35.

Laus, M. D. (1977). *Travel instructions for the handicapped.* Springfield, IL: Charles C Thomas.

Laus, M. D. (1974). Orientation and mobility instruction for the sighted trainable mentally retarded. *Education and Training of the Mentally Retarded, 9*(2), 20–73.

Leary, B., & von Schneden, M. (1982). *"Simon Says" is not the only game.* New York: American Foundation for the Blind.

Lederman, S. J., & Klatzky, R. L. (1987). Hand movements: A window into haptic object recognition. *Cognitive Psychology, 19,* 342–368.

Lee, D. (1980). The optic flow field: The foundation of vision. *Philosophical transactions of the Royal Society of London, Series B, 290,* 169–179.

Lee, D., Young, D., & McLaughlin, C. (1984). A roadside simulation of road crossing for children. *Ergonomics, 27,* 1271–1281.

Lehtinen-Railo, S., & Juurmaa, J. (1994). Effect of visual experience on locational judgments after perspective changes in small scale space. *Scandinavian Journal of Psychology, 35,* 175–183.

Leonard, J. A. (1966). *Aids to navigation: A discussion of the problem of maps for the blind traveler.* Paper presented at St. Dunstan's International Conference on Sensory Devices for the Blind, London.

Leonard, J. A. (1969). Static and mobile balancing performance of blind adolescent grammar school children. *New Outlook for the Blind, 63*(3), 65–72.

Leonard, J. A. (1973). The evaluation of blind mobility. *American Foundation for the Blind Research Bulletin, 26,* 73–76.

Levack, N. (1991). *Low vision: A resource guide with adaptations for students with visual impairment.* Austin: Texas School for the Blind and Visually Impaired.

Levi, J. M., & Schiff, W. (1966). Study of texture discrimination. *Development of raised line drawings as supplementary tools in the education of the blind* (Final report, September, Project No. RD-1571-S) (Appendix B). Washington, DC: Department of Health, Education and Welfare, Vocational Rehabilitation Administration.

Levy, W. H. (1872). *Blindness and the blind.* London: Chapman and Hall.

Levy, W. H. (1949, April). Blindness and the blind, *New Outlook for the Blind,* 106–110. (Originally published in 1872).

Lewin, K. (1936). *Principles of topological psychology.* New York: McGraw-Hill.

Lewis, B. (1978). Sensory deprivation in young children. *Child: Care, Health, & Development, 4,* 229–238.

Liben, L. S., & Downs, R. M. (1993). Understanding person–space map relations: Cartographic and developmental perspectives. *Developmental Psychology, 29,* 739–752.

Liddicoat, C. M., Meyers, L. S., & Lozano, E. (1982). A comparison of two sets of nonbraille elevator symbols. *Journal of Visual Impairment & Blindness, 76,* 194–196.

Linder, T. W. (1990). *Transdisciplinary play-based assessment: A functional approach to working with young children.* Baltimore, MD: Paul H. Brookes.

Linder, T. W. (1993). *Transdisciplinary play-based intervention: Guidelines for developing a meaningful curriculum for young children.* Baltimore, MD: Paul H. Brookes.

Locke, E. A., & Latham, G. P. (1985). The application of goal-setting to sports. *Journal of Sports Psychology, 7,* 205–222.

Locke, E. A., Shaw, K. N. Saari, L. M., & Latham, G. P. (1981). Goal setting and task performance: 1969–1980. *Psychological Bulletin, 90,* 125–152.

Long, R. G. (1985). The relationship of visual behavior to mobility performance and beliefs in persons with low vision. *Dissertation Abstracts International, 47,* 501A.

Long, R. G. (1992). *Housing accessibility for individuals with visual impairment or blindness.* Raleigh, NC: Center for Housing Design.

Long, R. G., Boyette, L. W., & Griffin-Shirley, N. (1996). Older individuals and community travel: The effect of vision impairment. *Journal of Visual Impairment & Blindness, 90,* 314–324.

Long, R. G., McNeal, L., & Griffin-Shirley, N. (1990). *The effect of visual loss on mobility of elderly persons* (Research Grant No. 133 GH 70038). Final Report. National Institute on Disability and Rehabilitation.

Long, R. G., Reiser, J. J., & Hill, E. W. (1990). Mobility in individuals with moderate visual impairments. *Journal of Visual Impairment & Blindness, 84*(3): 111–118.

Loomis, J., & Lederman, S. (1986). Tactual perception. In K. Boff, L. Kaufman, & J. Thomas (Eds.), *Handbook of perception and human performance. Vol. 2: Cognitive processes and performance.* New York: Wiley.

Loomis, J. M., Klatzky, R. L., Golledge, R. G., Cicinelli, J. G., Pellegrino, J. W., & Fry, P. A. (1993). Nonvisual navigation by blind and sighted: Assessment of path integration ability. *Journal of Experimental Psychology: General, 122,* 73–91.

Lord, F. E. (1969). Development of scales for the measurement of orientation and mobility skills of young blind children. *Exceptional Children, 36*(2), 77–81.

Lord, S., Clark, R., & Webster, I. (1991). Visual acuity and contrast sensitivity in relation to falls in an elderly population. *Age and Ageing, 20,* 175–181.

Lowenfeld, B. (1964). *Our blind children, growing and learning with them* (2nd ed.). Springfield, IL: Charles C Thomas.

Lukoff, I. (1972). Attitudes toward the blind. In *Attitudes toward blind persons.* New York: American Foundation for the Blind.

Luxton, K., Banai, M., & Kuperman, R. (1994). The usefulness of tactual maps of the New York City subway system. *Journal of Visual Impairment & Blindness, 88,* 75–84.

Lydon, W. T., & McGraw, M. L. (1973). *Concept development for visually handicapped children: A resource guide for teachers and other professionals working in educational settings.* New York: American Foundation for the Blind.

Lyon, J. (1985). *Playing God in the nursery.* New York: W. W. Norton.

MacDonald, A. P., & Hall, J. (1971). Internal-external locus of control and perception of disability. *Journal of Counseling and Clinical Psychology, 36,* 338–343.

MacDonald, J. D., & Gillette, Y. (1984). *Turn-taking with communication: ECO treatment module.* Columbus: Ohio State University.

MacLean, W., & Baumeister, A. (1982). Effects of vestibular stimulation on motor development and stereotyped behavior of developmentally delayed children. *Journal of Abnormal Child Psychology. 10*(2), 229–245.

Macmillan, N. A., & Creelman, C. D. (1991). *Signal detection: A user's guide.* Cambridge: Cambridge University Press.

MacWilliam, L. J. (1980). A curriculum for teaching clients to use landmarks while traveling. *Journal of Visual Impairment & Blindness, 75*(7), 269–272.

Magarrell, G. (1990). Services for visually impaired adults in Canada. *Journal of Visual Impairment & Blindness, 84,* 283–285.

Mager, R. F. (1967). *Preparing instructional objectives.* Belmont, CA: Fearon.

Malamazian, J. D. (1970). The first 15 years at Hines. In *Blindness annual* (pp. 59–75). Washington, DC: American Association of Workers for the Blind.

Manchester, D., Woollacott, M., Zederbauer-Hylton, N., & Marin, O. (1969). Visual, vestibular and somatosensory contributions to balance control in the older adult. *Journal of Gerontology, 4,* M118–127.

Mancil, G. L., & Owsley, C. (1988). 'Vision through my aging eyes' revisited. *Journal of the American Optometric Association, 59,* 288–294.

Mandler, G., & Sarason, S. (1952). A study of anxiety and learning. *Journal of Abnormal and Social Psychology, 47,* 166–173.

Mannix, J. B. (1976). John Metcalf: Blind Jack of Knaresborough. *Blindness* 94–103. (Originally published in 1911.)

Manton, K. G., Corder, L. S., & Stallard, E. (1993). Estimates of change in chronic disability and institutional incidence and prevalence rates in the U.S. elderly population from the 1982, 1984, and 1989 National Long Term Care Study. *Journal of Gerontology: Social Sciences, 48*(4), S153–S166.

Markus, H. (1977). Self-schemas and processing information about the self. *Journal of Personality and Social Psychology, 35,* 63–78.

Markus, H., & Nurius, P. (1986). Possible selves. *American Psychologist, 41,* 954–969.

Marmor, G. (1977). Age at onset of blindness in visual imagery development. Perceptual and Motor Skills, 45, 1031–1034.

Marron, J., & Bailey, I. (1982). Visual factors and orientation-mobility performance. *American Journal of Optometry and Physiological Optics, 59*(5), 413–426.

Martin, F. (1994). *Introduction to audiology.* Englewood Cliffs, NJ: Prentice Hall.

Martinuik, R. G. (1979). Motor skill performance and learning: Considerations for rehabilitation. *Physiotherapy* (Canada), *31*(4), 187–202.

Maru, A. A. & Cook, H. J. (1990). Education of blind persons in Ethiopia. *Journal of Visual Impairment & Blindness, 84*(6), 265–267.

Massachusetts Institute of Technology (MIT). (1965, October 31). *Final report to Vocational Rehabilitation Administration, Department of Health, Education, and Welfare, Washington, D.C. From Sensory Aids Evaluation and Development Center,* Cambridge, MA: Author.

Massof, R. W., Dagnelia, G., Deremeik, J. T., DeRose, J. L., Alighai, S. S., & Glasner, N. M. 1995. Low vision rehabilitation in the U.S. health care system. *Journal of Vision Rehabilitation, 9*(3), 3–23.

Mattingly, W. (1976). A study to evaluate the effectiveness of an intervention of utilization of residual vision on the independent mobility of persons with low vision. *Low Vision Abstracts, 2,* 3.

Maxim, H. (1912). The sixth sense of the bat. *Scientific American* (Suppl.), 148–150.

McClenaghan, B. A. (1983). Motor rehabilitation, application of instructional theory. *Physical Educator, 40,* 2–7.

McClure, R. (1995, June). Texas Tech University, In the United States District Court for the Nothern District of Texas Lubbock Division, Civil Action No. 5: 94-CV-185-C, p. 8.

McCrae, R. R., & Costa, P. T. (1987). Validation of the five-factor model of personality across instruments and observers. *Journal of Personality and Social Psychology, 52,* 81–90.

McDonald, P., vanEmmerik, R., & Newell, K. (1989). The effects of practice on limb kinematics in a throwing task. *Journal of Motor Behavior, 21,* 245–264.

McFarlin, D. B., & Blascovich, J. (1981). Effects of self-esteem and performance feedback on future affective preferences and cognitive expectations. *Journal of Personality and Social Psychology, 40,* 521–531.

McGean, T. K. (1991). *Innovative solutions for disabled transit accessibility* (Report No. UMTA-OH-06-0056-91-8). Washington, DC: U.S. Department of Transportation, Urban Mass Transportation Administration.

McPhee, W., & Magleby, F. L. (1960). Success and failure in vocational rehabilitation. *Personnel and Guidance Journal, 38,* 497–499.

Mehr, E. B., & Freid, A. N. (1975). *Low vision care.* Chicago: The Professional Press.

Meighan, T. (1971). *An investigation of the self-concept of blind and visually handicapped adolescents.* New York: American Foundation for the Blind.

Memorandum of Communication. (1995, October 23). Department of Veterans Affairs, Request for Opinion—O&M Training by Blind Instructors, p. 12.

Mettler, R. (1987). Blindness and managing the unseen environment. *Journal of Visual Impairment & Blindness, 81,* 476–481.

Mettler, R. (1994). A cognitive basis for teaching cane travel. *Journal of Visual Impairment & Blindness, 88*(4), 338–348.

Mettler, R. (1995). *Cognitive learning theory and cane travel instruction: A new paradigm.* Lincoln: State of Nebraska, Department of Public Institutions.

Meyerson, L. (1963). Somatopsychology of physical disability. In W. Cruickshank (Ed.), *Psychology of exceptional children and youth.* Englewood Cliffs, NJ: Prentice Hall.

Miaode, Z. & Hong, L. (1994, January). *Introduction, current situation and strategies of orientation and mobility skills on China's mainland.* Paper presented at the Seventh International Mobility Conference, Melbourne, Australia, pp. 112–125.

Millar, S. (1981). Crossmodal and intersensory perception and the blind. In R. D. Walk & H. L. Pick (Eds.), *Intersensory sensory integration.* New York: Plenum.

Millar, S. (1994). *Understanding and representing space: Theory and evidence from studies with blind and sighted children.* Oxford: Clarendon Press.

Miller, G. A., Galanter, E. H., & Pribram, K. H. (1960). *Plans and the structure of behavior.* New York: Holt, Rinehart & Winston.

Miller, J. (1967). Vision: A component of locomotion. *Physiotherapy, 53,* 326–332.

Miller, P. H. (1983). *Theories of developmental psychology.* San Francisco: W. H. Freeman.

Mills, A. W. (1958). *Journal of the Acoustical Society of America, 30,* 237–246.

Mills, A. W. (1960). Lateralization of high-frequency tones. *Journal of the Acoustical Society of America, 32,* 132–134.

Mims, F. M., III. (1972, June). Eyeglass mounted mobility aid. *Journal of the American Optometric Association,* 673–676.

Minuchin, S. (1974). *Families and family therapy.* Cambridge, MA: Harvard University Press.

Mitchell, M. (1988). *Pathfinder tactile tile demonstration test project.* Miami: Metro-Dade Transit Agency.

Monbeck, M. (1973). *The Meaning of blindness.* Bloomington: Indiana University Press.

Monighan-Nourot, P., Scales, B., VanHoorn, J., & Almay, M. (1987). *Looking at children's play: A bridge between theory and practice.* New York: Teachers College Press.

Montgomery, P. (1981). Assessment and treatment of the child with mental retardation. *Physical Therapy, 6,* 1265–1271.

Moore, J. E. (1984). Impact of family attitudes toward blindness/visual impairment on the rehabilitation process. *Journal of Visual Impairment & Blindness, 78*(3), 100–106.

Moore, S. (1984). The need for programs and services for visually handicapped infants. *Education of the Visually Handicapped, 16,* 48–57.

Morgan, M. (1976). Beyond disability: A broader definition of architectural barriers. *American Institute of Architects Journal,65*(5), 50–53.

Morris, J. E., & Nolan, C. Y. (1963). Minimum sizes for areal type tactual symbols. *International Journal for the Education of the Blind, 13*; 48–51.

Morrongiello, B. A. (1988). Infants' localization of sound along two spatial dimensions: Horizontal and vertical axes. *Infant Behavioral Development 11,* 127–143.

Morrongiello, B. A. & Clifton, R. K. (1984). Effects of sound frequency on behavioral and cardiac orienting in newborn and five-month-old infants. *Journal of Experimental Child Psychology 38,* 429–446.

Morrongiello, B. A. & Gotowiec, A. (1990). Recent advances in the behavioral study of infant audition: The development of sound localization skills. *Journal of Speech, Language, Pathology, and Audiology, 14,* 51–63.

Morrongiello, B. A. & Rocaa, P. T. (1987). Infants' localization of sounds in the vertical plane: Estimates of minimum audible angle. *Journal of Experimental Child Psychology, 43,* 181–193.

Mouchet, E. (1938). Un Nuevo Capitaula de Psicofisiologia: el Tacto a Distanci o Sentibo de les Obstaclos en los Ciegos. *An. Inst. Piscol., 2,* 419–441.

Mueller, H. G., Grimes, A. M., & Erdman, S. A. (1983). Subjective ratings of directional amplification. *Hearing instruments, 34,* 14–16.

Muir, D. W. (1985). The development of infants' auditory spatial sensitivity. In S. E. Trehub & B. S. Schneider (Eds.), *Auditory development in infancy* (pp. 51–83). New York: Plenum.

Muller, M., & Wehner, R. (1988). Path integration in desert ants, Cataglyphis fortis. *Proceedings of the National Academy of Sciences, 85,* 5287–5290.

Murakami, T., & Shimizu, O. (1990). Platform accidents in Japan. In M. M. Uslan, A. F. Peck, W. R. Wiener, & A. Stern (Eds.), *Access to mass transit for blind and visually impaired travelers* (pp. 112–115). New York: American Foundation for the Blind.

Murakami, T., Aoki, S., Taniai, S., & Muranaka, Y. (1982). Braille blocks on roads to assist the blind in orientation and mobility. *Bulletin of the Tokyo Metropolitan Rehabilitation Center for the Physically and Mentally Handicapped,* 11–24.

Murakami, T., Ohkura, M., Tauchi, M., Shimizu, O., & Ikegami, A. (1991, December 3–4). An experimental study on discriminability and detectability of tactile tiles. *Proceedings of the 17th Sensory Substitution Symposium,* Tokyo.

Murray, M., Kory, R., & Clarkson, B. (1969). Walking patterns in healthy old men. *Journal of Gerontology, 24,* 169–178.

Musselwhite, C. R. (1986). *Adaptive play for special needs children.* San Diego, CA: College-Hill Press.

Mwangi, A. (1994). *The blind in Kenya.* Unpublished manuscript.

Myers, S. O., & Jones, C. G. E. F. (1958). Obstacle experiments: Second report. *Teacher of the Blind, 46,* 47–62.

National Mapping Council of Australia. (1985). *A national specification for tactual and low vision town maps.* Canberra: National Mapping Council of Australia.

National Research Council. (1986). Electronic travel aids: New directions for research. Washington, DC: National Academy Press.

Neff, W. (1979). *Success of a rehabilitation program: A follow-up study of the vocational adjustment center* (Monograph 3). Chicago: Jewish Vocational Center.

Neisser, U. (1976). *Cognition and reality.* San Francisco: W. H. Freeman.

Nelson, K. A. (1987). Statistical brief # 35: Visual impairment among elderly Americans: Statistics in transition. *Journal of Visual Impairment & Blindness, 81,* 331–334.

Nelson, K. A., & Dimitrova, G. (1993). Statistical Brief # 36: Severe visual impairment in the United States and in each state, 1990. *Journal of Visual Impairment & Blindness, 86*(3), 80–85.

Nelson, R. (1987). *Transportation noise reference book.* Boston: Butterworths.

Neustadt, N. (1990). *A survey of European O&M training programs.* Paper presented at the Third European Seminar, Helsinki, Finland.

Neve, J. Jorritsma, F. & Kinds, G. F. (1994). The Visual Advice Center Eindhoven: An experiment in Dutch low vision care. In A. C. Kooijman, P. L. Looijestijn, J. A. Welling, & G. J. Wildt (Eds.), *Low vision research and new developments in rehabilitation.*

New York City Board of Education. (1986). *AIDS: A special report on Acquired Immunodeficiency Syndrome* (p. 3). New York: NYC Board of Education.

Newby, H. A., & Popelka, G. R. (1992). Audiology (6th ed.). Englewood Cliffs, NJ: Prentice Hall.

Newcomer, J. (1986, Winter). Canadian certification details. *Division Nine Newsletter,* p. 4.

Noble, W. G. (1975). Auditory localization and its impairment. *Maico Audiological Library Series, 14*(Report One).

Nolan, C. Y. (1971). Relative legibility of raised and incised tactual figures. *Education of the Visually Handicapped, 3,* 33–36.

Nolan, C. Y., & Morris, J. E. (1971). *Improvement of tactual symbols for blind children* (Final report, Project No. 5-0421; Grant No. OEG-32-27-0000-1012). Louisville, KY: American Printing House for the Blind.

Norton, F. T. (1960). Training normal hearing to greater usefulness: A progress report. *New Outlook for the Blind, 54*(6), 199–205.

Nurion Industries. (1992). *Polaron: Opening new words for the blind.* Frazer, PA: Author.

O'Donnell, B. A. (1988). Stress and the mobility training process: A literature review. *Journal of Visual Impairment & Blindness, 82*(4), 143–147.

O'Donnell, L., & Smith, A. (1994). Visual cues for enhancing depth perception. *Journal of Visual Impairment & Blindness, 88,* 258–266.

O'Mara, B. (1989). *Pathways to independence: Orientation and mobility skills for your infant and toddler.* New York: The Lighthouse.

O'Neil, M. J. (1992). Effects of familiarity and plan complexity on wayfinding in simulated buildings. *Journal of Environmental Psychology, 12,* 319–327.

Ochaíta, E., & Huertas, J. A. (1993). Spatial representation by persons who are blind: A study of the effects of learning and development. *Journal of Visual Impairment & Blindness, 87*(2), 37–41.

Ojamo, M., Ruponen, T., Paija, L., & Hirn, H. (1990). The rehabilitation of visually impaired persons in Finland. *Journal of Visual Impairment & Blindness, 84*(6), 294–295.

Olshansky, S., & Beach, D. (1975, August). Special report. *Rehabilitation Literature.*

Olson, D. R., & Pau, A. S. (1966). Emotionally loaded words and the acquisition of a sight vocabulary. *Journal of Educational Psychology, 57,* 174–178.

Owen, S. (1985). Maintaining posture and avoiding tripping. *Clinics in Geriatric Medicine, 1,* 581–599.

Owsley, C., Sekuler, R., & Siemsen, D. (1983). Contrast sensitivity through adulthood. *Vision Research, 23,* 689–699.

Palazesi, M. A. (1986). The need for motor development programs for visually impaired preschoolers. *Journal of Visual Impairment & Blindness, 80*(2), 573–576.

Papousek, H. (1961). Conditioned head rotation reflexes in infants in the first month of life. *Acta Paediatrica* (Stockholm), *50,* 565–576.

Parkes, D. (1994). *Multi-media audio-tactile maps and plans: A sound-space for blind users.* Paper presented at the Fourth International Symposium on Maps and Graphics for the Visually Impaired, São Paulo, Brazil.

Parkes, D. (1995). Access to complex environments for blind people: Multi-media maps, plans, and virtual travel. Proceedings, Seventeenth International

Cartographic Conference, Barcelona, Madrid: Spain. Book 2, 2449–2460.

Parkes, D., & Dear, R. (1991). Making and using high resolution audio-tactile orientation and mobility plans and maps with the NOMAD system. *Proceedings, Sixth International Mobility Conference* (Book 1, pp. 329–336). Madrid, Spain.

Parsons, S. (1986). Function of play in low vision children: Part 2. Emerging patterns of behavior. *Journal of Visual Impairment & Blindness, 80*(6), 777–784.

Passini, R., Dupré, A., & Langlois, C. (1986). Spatial mobility of the visually handicapped active person: A descriptive study. *Journal of Visual Impairment & Blindness, 80*(8), 904–907.

Peck, A. F., & Bentzen, B. L. (1987). *Tactile warnings to promote safety in the vicinity of transit platform edges* (Report No. UMTA-MA-06-0120-87-1). Washington, DC: U.S. Department of Transportation, Urban Mass Transportation Administration.

Peck, A. F., & Uslan, M. (1990). The use of audible traffic signals in the U.S. *Journal of Visual Impairment & Blindness, 84,* 547–551.

Peck, A. F., Tauchi, M., Shimizu, O., Murakami, T., & Okhura, M. (1991). *Tactile tiles for Australia: A performance evaluation of selected tactile tiles under consideration for use by the visually impaired in Australia.* Unpublished manuscript, Association for the Blind, Brighton Beach, Victoria, Australia.

Peck, J. E. (1994). Development of hearing. Part I: Phylogeny. *Journal of American Academy of Audiology, 5,* 291–299.

Peck, J. E. (1995). Development of hearing. Part III: Postnatal development. *Journal of American Academy of Audiology, 6,* 113–123.

Pelli, D. G. (1986). The visual requirements of mobility. *Proceedings of the International Symposium on Low Vision, Centre for Sight Enhancement, University of Waterloo, Ontario, Canada.* Toronto: Springer.

Peponis, J., Zimring, C., & Choi, Y. K. (1990). Finding the building in wayfinding. *Environment and Behavior, 22,* 555–590.

Periera, L. (1990). Spatial concepts and balance performance: Motor learning in blind and visually impaired children. *Journal of Visual Impairment & Blindness, 84*(3), 109–111.

Perrott, D. R., & Elfner, L. F. (1968). Monaural localization. *Journal of Auditory Research, 8,* 185–193.

Peter Muller-Munk Associates. (1986). *Information system for low vision persons* (ED Contract No. 300-85-0186). Washington, DC: U.S. Architectural and Transportation Barriers Compliance Board.

Pfaffenberger, C. J., Scott, J. P., Fuller, J. L., Ginsburg, B. E., & Biefelt, S. W. (1976). *Guide dogs for the blind: Their selection, development, and training.* Amsterdam: Elsevier.

Phares, J. E. (1976). *Locus of control in personality.* Morristown, NJ: General Learning Press.

Piccione, L. (1995). Latin American region. *The Educator, 8*(1).

Pick, H. L., Jr. (1980a). Perception, locomotion and orientation. In R. L. Welsh & B. B. Blasch (Eds.), *Foundations of orientation and mobility* (pp. 73–88). New York: American Foundation for the Blind.

Pick, H. L., Jr. (1980b). Tactual and haptic perception. In R. L. Welsh & B. B. Blasch (Eds.), *Foundations of orientation and mobility* (pp. 89–114). New York: American Foundation for the Blind.

Pinedo, A. H. (1995). In *Models of paratransit eligibility.* Washington, DC: Project ACTION, National Easter Seal Society.

Pogrund, R. L., & Rosen, S. J. (1989). The preschool blind child *can* be a cane user. *Journal of Visual Impairments & Blindness, 83*(9), 431–439.

Pogrund, R. L., Fazzi, D. L., & Schreier, E. M. (1993). Development of a preschool "Kiddy Cane." *Journal of Visual Impairment & Blindness, 87*(2), 52–54.

Pogrund, R. L., Healy, G., Jones, K., Levack, N., Martin-Curry, S., Martinex, C., Marz, J., Roberson-Smith, B., & Vrba, A. (1993). *Teaching age-appropriate purposeful skills: An orientation and mobility curriculum for students with visual impairments.* Austin: Texas School for the Blind and Visually Impaired.

Pollack, M. C. (1975). Special applications of amplification. In M. C. Pollack (Ed.), *Amplification for the hearing impaired* (pp. 243–256). New York: Grune & Stratton.

Ponchillia, P. E., & Kaarlela, R. (1986). Post-rehabilitation use of adaptive skills. *Journal of Visual Impairment & Blindness, 80*(4), 665–669.

Ponchillia, S. V. (1993). Complications of diabetes and their implications for service providers. *Journal of Visual Impairment & Blindness, 87*(9), 354–358.

Pope, A. M., & Tarlov, A. R. (1991). *Disability in America: Toward a national agenda for prevention.* Washington, DC: National Academy Press.

Potter, L. E. (1995). Small-scale versus large-scale spatial reasoning: Educational implications for children who are visually impaired. *Journal of Visual Impairment & Blindness, 89,* 142–152.

Poulea, K. (1994, January). *Independent living of the visually impaired in Greece: Past and present.* Paper presented at the Seventh International Mobility Conference, pp. 103–106. Melbourne, Australia.

Preiser, W. F. E. (1985). A combined tactile/electronic guidance system for visually impaired persons in indoor and outdoor spaces. *Proceedings of the International Conference on Building Use and Safety*

Technology. Washington, DC: National Institute of Building Sciences.

Pressey, N. (1986). Position paper on orientation and mobility instructor training programs within Australia. *Orientation and Mobility Instructors Association of Australasia Journal of Orientation and Mobility, 11*(2), 10.

Pressley, M., & Levin, J. R. (Eds.). (1983). *Cognitive strategy research: Educational applications.* New York: Springer.

Pressley, M., Goodchild, F., Fleet, J., Zajchowski, R., & Evans, E. D. (1989). The challenges of classroom strategy instruction. *Elementary School Journal, 89,* 301–342.

Pronay, B. (1995, May). Paper presented at European Seminar, Prague.

Psathas, G. (1976). Mobility, orientation and navigation: Conceptual and theoretical considerations. *New Outlook for the Blind, 9,* 385–391.

Putnam, P. B. (1979). *Love in the lead.* New York: E.P. Dutton.

Pyfer, J. (1988). Teachers, don't let your students grow up to be clumsy adults. *Journal of Physical Education, Recreation, and Dance, 59,* 38–42.

Pyykko, I., Jantti, P., & Aalto, H. (1990). Postural control in elderly subjects. *Age and Ageing, 19,* 215–221.

Rand Corporation. (1975). *Information transfer problems of the partially sighted: Recent results and project summary* (RK-1770). Washington, DC: U.S. Department of Health, Education and Welfare.

Rasch, P., & Burke, R. (1965). *Kinesiology and applied anatomy* (2nd ed.). Philadelphia: Lea and Febiger.

Reardon, D. (1911). [Statement in Campbell Papers at the Perkins School Library]. Unpublished manuscript.

Reeve, J. (1992). *Understanding motivation and emotion.* New York: Harcourt Brace Jovanovich.

Rice, C. E. (1967). Human echo perception. *Science, 155,* 656–664.

Rice, C. E., & Feinstein, S. H. (1965). Echo detection ability of the blind: Size and distance factors. *Journal of Experimental Psychology, 70,* 246–251.

Richterman, H. (1966). Mobility instruction for the partially seeing. *New Outlook for the Blind, 60*(8), 236–238.

Rider, E., & Rieser, J. (1988). Pointing at objects in other rooms: Young children's sensitivity to perspective structure after walking with and without vision. *Child Development, 59,* 480–494.

Rieser, J. J. (1991). Development of perceptual-motor control while walking without vision: The calibration of perception and action. In H. Bloch & B. Berenthal (Eds.), *Sensory motor organization and development in infancy and early childhood.* The Netherlands: Kluwer.

Rieser, J., & Frymire, M. (1995, November). *Locomotion without vision is coupled with knowledge of real and imagined surroundings.* Paper presented at the 36th Annual Meeting of the Psychonomic Society, Los Angeles.

Rieser, J., & Garing, A. (1994). Spatial orientation. *Encyclopedia of human behavior, Vol. 4* (pp. 287–295). New York: Academic Press.

Rieser, J., Garing, A., & Young, M. (1994). Imagery, action, and young children's spatial orientation: It's not being there that counts, it's what one has in mind. *Child Development, 65,* 1262–1278.

Rieser, J. J., Guth, D. A., & Hill, E. W. (1982). Mental processes mediating independent travel: Implications for orientation and mobility. *Journal of Visual Impairment & Blindness, 76*(6), 213–218.

Rieser, J. J., Guth, D. A., & Hill, E. W. (1986). Sensitivity to perspective structure while walking without vision. *Perception, 15,* 173–188.

Rieser, J., Halpin, J., & Hill, E. (1993).Unpublished study, Vanderbilt University, Nashville, TN.

Rieser, J. J., Hill, E. W., Taylor, C. R., Bradfield, A., & Rosen, S. (1992). Visual experience, visual field size, and the development of nonvisual sensitivity to the spatial structure of outdoor neighborhoods explored by walking. *Journal of Experimental Psychology: General, 121,* 210–221.

Rieser, J. J., Hill, E. W., Rosen, S., Long, R. G., Taylor, C., & Zimmerman, G. (1985). *The locomotion and mobility of low vision persons. Final report.* Washington, DC: National Institute of Handicapped Research. (Grant No. 1231413680A1).

Rieser, J. J., Lockman, J. J., & Pick, H. L. Jr. (1980). The role of visual experience in knowledge of spatial layout. *Perception and Psychophysics, 28,* 185–190.

Rieser, J., Pick, H. L. Jr., Ashmead, D., & Garing, A. (1995). Calibration of human locomotion and models of perceptual-motor organization. *Journal of Experimental Psychology: Human Perception and Performance, 21,* 480–497.

Rintelmann, W., Harford, E., & Burchfield, S. (1970). CROS for blind persons with unilateral hearing loss. *Archives of Otolaryngology, 91,* 284–288.

Rochester-Genesee Regional Transportation Authority. (1995). *Automated on-board next stop route announcement system using GPS technology.* Final report. Washington, DC: U.S. Department of Transportation Federal Transit Administration and Project ACTION of the National Easter Seal Society.

Rogers, C. (1951). *Client-centered therapy.* Boston: Houghton Mifflin.

Romagnoli, A. (1931). The training of teachers of the blind. In H. Lende, E. McKay, and S. C. Swift (Eds.), *Proceedings of the World Conference on Work for the Blind.* New York: American Foundation for the Blind.

Romains, J. (1924). *Eyeless sight* (G. K. Ogden, Trans.). New York and London: Putnam.

Rosen, S. (1986). Assessment of selected spatial gait patterns of congenitally blind children (Doctoral dissertation, Vanderbilt University, 1986). *Dissertation Abstracts International, 47,* 3000A.

Rosen, S. (1989). [Gait, balance, and veering tendency in congenitally blind children and youth]. Unpublished raw data.

Rosen, S. & Pogrund, R. (1994). [Comparative study of blind six- to eight-year olds: Cane and non-cane users]. Unpublished raw data.

Rosenbaum, D. (1991). *Human motor control.* San Diego, CA: Academic Press.

Rosenbloom, A. A. (1992). Physiological and functional aspects of aging, vision, and visual impairment. In A. L. Orr (Ed.), *Vision and aging: Crossroads for service delivery* (pp. 47–68). New York: American Foundation for the Blind.

Ross, A. O. (1992). *The sense of self: Research and theory.* New York: Springer.

Ross, I. (1951). *Journey into darkness, The story of the education of the blind* (p. 103). New York: Appleton-Century-Crofts.

Rossano, M. J., & Warren, D. H. (1989). The importance of alignment in blind subjects' use of tactile maps. *Perception, 18,* 805–816.

Rothkope, E. Z. (1965). Some theoretical and experimental approaches to problems in written instruction. In J. D. Krumboltz (Ed.), *Learning and the educational process.* Chicago: Rand McNally.

Rotter, J. B. (1966). Generalized expectancies for internal vs. external control of reinforcement. *Psychological Monographs, 80,* 1–28.

Rouse, D., & Worchel, D. (1955). Veering tendency in the blind. *New Outlook for the Blind, 49,* 115–119.

Rowntree, D. (1981). *Statistics without tears.* New York: Charles Scribner's Sons.

Rubel, E. W. (1985). Auditory system development. In G. Gottlieb & N. A. Krasnegor (Eds.), *Measurement of audition and vision in the first year of postnatal life: A methodological overview* (pp. 53–90). Norwood, NJ: Ablex.

Russell, L. (1966). Travel Pathsounder and evaluation. In R. Dufton (Ed.), *Proceedings on the Conference on the Evaluation of Sensory Devices for the Blind* (pp. 293–297). London: St. Dunstan's.

Rutherford, W. (1886). A new theory of hearing. *Journal of Anatomy and Physiology, 21,* 166–168.

SafeTech International, Inc. (1993). *WalkMate™: The new generation electronic travel aid.* Palisades Park, NJ: Author.

Sailor, W., Wilcox, B., & Brown L. (Eds.). (1980). Methods of instruction for severely handicapped students. Baltimore: Paul H. Brooks.

Sanders, D. (1971). *Aural rehabilitation.* Englewood Cliffs, NJ: Prentice Hall.

Sauerberger, D. (1988, May). O&M archives opening soon. *Division Nine Newsletter,* p. 11.

Sauerburger, D. (1989). To cross or not to cross: Objective timing methods of assessing street crossings without traffic controls. *RE:view, 21,* 153–161.

Sauerburger, D. (1993). *Independence without sight or sound: Suggestions for practitioners working with deaf-blind adults.* New York: American Foundation for the Blind.

Saya, F. (1993). Mobility training in Kenya. *British Journal of Visual Impairment, 6,* 83.

Sayers, B. M., & Cherry, E. C. (1957). Mechanism of binaural fusion in the hearing of speech. *Journal of the Acoustical Society of America, 29,* 973–987.

Schenkman, B. (1986). Identification of ground materials with the aid of tapping sounds and vibrations of long canes for the blind. *Ergonomics, 29,* 985–988.

Schenkman, B., & Jansson, G. (1986). The detection and localization of objects by the blind with the aid of long-cane tapping sounds. *Human Factors, 28*(5), 607–618.

Schiff, W., & Foulke, E. (Eds.). (1982). *Tactual perception: A sourcebook.* New York: Cambridge University Press.

Schiff, W., & Isikow, H. (1966). Stimulus redundancy in the tactile perception of histograms. *Development of raised line drawings as supplementary tools in the education of the blind* (Final report, September, Project No. RD-1571-S) (Appendix C). Washington, DC: Department of Health, Education and Welfare, Vocational Rehabilitation Administration.

Schmidt, R. A. (1991). *Motor learning and performance: From principles to practice.* Champaign, IL: Human Kinetics.

Schneekloth, L. (1989). Play environments for visually impaired children. *Journal of Visual Impairment & Blindness, 83*(4), 196–211.

Scholl, G. T. (Ed.). (1986). *Foundations of education for blind and visually handicapped children and youth.* New York: American Foundation for the Blind.

Schone, H. (1984). *Spatial orientation: The spatial control of behavior in animals and men.* Princeton, NJ: Princeton University Press.

Schulman-Galambos, C., & Galambos R.(1979). Brainstem evoked response audiometry in newborn hearing screening. *Archives of Otolaryngology, 105,* 86–90.

Schulz, P. J. (1977). Reactions to the loss of sight. In T. J. Pearlman, G. Adams, & S. H. Sloan (Eds.), *Psychiatric problems in ophthalmology.* Springfield, IL: Charles C Thomas.

Scott, J. (1962). Critical periods in behavioral development. *Science, 138,* 949–958.

Sehlz, A. (1986). Programs for the visually impaired in developing countries. In N. Neustadt, S. Merin, & Y. Schiff (Eds.), *Orientation and mobility of the visually impaired.* Jerusalem: Heiliger.

Sekuler, R., & Blake, R. (1994). *Perception* (3rd ed.). New York: McGraw-Hill.

Sekuler, R., & Hutman, L. (1980). Spatial vision and aging. I: Contrast sensitivity. *Journal of Gerontology, 35,* 692–699.

Seligman, M. E. P. (1975). *Helplessness: On depression, development and death.* San Francisco: W. H. Freedman.

Seybold, D. (1993). Investigating stress associated with mobility training through consumer discussion groups. *Journal of Visual Impairment & Blindness, 87,* 111–112.

Shearer, D. E., & Shearer, M. S. (1976). The Portage Project: A model for early childhood intervention. In T. D. Tjossem (Ed.), *Intervention strategies for high risk infants and young children* (pp. 335–350). Baltimore, MD: University Park Press.

Sherwood, D. (1988). Effect of bandwidth feedback knowledge of results on movement consistency. *Perceptual and Motor Skills, 66,* 535–542.

Shibata, H. (1976). Visual training and mobility training for the person with low vision. *Low Vision Abstracts, 2,* 3.

Shimizu, O., Murakami, T., Ohkura, M., Tanaka, I., & Tauchi, M. (1991). Braille tiles as a guiding system in Japan for blind travelers. *Proceedings of the Sixth International Mobility Conference,* Madrid, Spain.

Shingledecker, C. (1983). Measuring the mental effort of blind mobility. *Journal of Visual Impairment & Blindness, 77*(7), 334–339.

Siegel, I., & Murphy, T. (1970). *Postural determinants in the blind (the influence of posture on mobility and orientation).* Chicago: Visually Handicapped Institute.

Siegel, S. A. (1986). Orientation and mobility instructors: The Israeli model. In N. Neustadt, S. Merin, & Y. Schiff (Eds.), *Orientation and mobility of the visually impaired.* Jerusalem: Heiliger.

Simon, E. P. (1984). A report on electronic travel aid users: Three to five years later. *Journal of Visual Impairment & Blindness, 78*(10), 478–480.

Singh, T. B. (1990). Services for the visually impaired in India. *Journal of Visual Impairment & Blindness, 84*(6), 286–293.

Siqueland, E. R., & Lipsitt, L. P. (1966). Conditioned head turning in human newborns. *Journal of Experimental Child Psychology, 3,* 356–376.

Skellenger, A. C., & Hill, E. W. (1991). Current practices and considerations regarding long cane instruction with preschool children. *Journal of Visual Impairments & Blindness, 85*(3), 101–104.

Skinner, B. F. (1953). *Science and human behavior.* New York: Macmillan.

Skinner, B. F. (1974). *About behaviorism.* New York: Knopf.

Slavin, R. E. (1991). *Educational psychology: Theory into practice* (3rd ed.). Boston: Allyn & Bacon.

Sliney, D. H., & Freasier, B. C. (1969, August). *Evaluation of a Laser Cane.* (Radiation Protection Special Study No. 42-089-69170, p. 17), U.S. Army Environmental Hygiene Agency.

Smedslund, J. (1978). Bandura's theory of self-efficacy: A set of common sense theorems. *Scandinavian Journal of Psychology, 19,* 1–14.

Smith, A. J. (1976, Spring). Orientation and mobility and low vision training without aids: Trends and needs. *Low Vision Abstracts, II*(3).

Smith, A. J. (1987). Low vision orientation and mobility: Strategies for assessing and enhancing visual efficiency in the environment. In C. Tee, W. Ng, G. Omar, & L. Fee (Eds.), *First Asia-Pacific seminar on low vision: Proceedings of the seminar* (pp. 77–91). Kuala Lumpur, Malaysia: Malaysians Association for the Blind.

Smith, A. J. (1990). Mobility problems related to vision loss: Perceptions of mobility practitioners and persons with low vision. *Dissertation Abstracts International, 51*(5). (University Microfilms No. 9026646.)

Smith, A. J., & Cote, K. S. (1982). *Look at me.* Philadelphia: Pennsylvania College of Optometry.

Smith, A. J., & Geruschat, D. R. (1983). *Developmental assessment of standard training protocols for the use of fresnel prisms for persons with peripheral field defects: Effects of independent travel and psycho-social adjustment. Final report.* The Low Vision Research and Training Center, Pennsylvania College of Optometry. Washington, DC: National Institute for Handicapped Research. (Grant # 12314136801A.)

Smith, A. J., & O'Donnell, L. M. (1991). *Beyond arm's reach: Enhancing distance vision.* Philadelphia: Pennsylvania College of Optometry.

Smith, A. J., De l'Aune, W., & Geruschat, D. R. (1992). Low vision mobility problems: Perceptions of O&M specialists and persons with low vision. *Journal of Visual Impairment & Blindness, 86*(1), 58–62.

Smith, M., Chetnik, M., & Adelson, E. (1969). Differential assessments of "blindisms." *American Journal of Orthopsychiatry, 39,* 807–817.

Snell, M. (Ed.). (1983). Systemic instruction of the moderately and severely handicapped. Columbus, OH: Merrill.

Society of Automotive Engineers of Japan. (1977). *Research and development of electric vehicles in Japan.* Agency of Industrial Science & Technology, Ministry of International Trade and Industry.

Sokolov, V. E., & Kulikov, V. F. (1987). The structure and function of the vibrissal appparatus in some rodents. *Mammalia, 51,* 125–138.

Sonksen, P. M., Levitt, S., & Kitzinger, M. (1981, June). *Motor development in the visually disabled child.* Paper presented at the International Symposium on Visually Handicapped Infants and Young Children, Tel Aviv.

Southeastern Community College v. Davis, 442 U.S. 397 No. 78–711 (1979).

Speaks, C. E. (1992). *Introduction to sound: Acoustics for the hearing and speech sciences.* San Diego, CA: Singular Publishing Group.

Speigler, M. D. (1983). *Contemporary behavioral therapy.* Palo Alto, CA: Mayfield.

Sperling, D. (1995). *Future drive.* Washington, D.C.: Island Press.

Spielberger, C. D. (1972). Anxiety as an emotional state. In C. D. Spielberger (Ed.), *Anxiety: Current trends in theory and research* (Vol. I). New York: Academic Press.

Spungin, S. J. (1990). The Eastern Bloc and the Soviet Union in transition: What of services to blind persons? *Journal of Visual Impairment & Blindness, 84*(6), 260–261.

Staab, W. J. (1978). *Hearing aid handbook* (pp. 16–23). Phoenix: Author.

Staab, W. J. & Lybarger, S. F. (1994). Characteristics and use of hearing aids. In J. Katz (Ed.), *Handbook of clinical audiology* (4th ed., p. 662). Baltimore: Williams & Wilkins.

State of Florida. (1983). *A resource manual for the development and evaluation of special programs for exceptional students: Vol. V–E: Project IVEY: Increasing visual efficiency.* Tallahassee: Author.

State of New York. (1986). *Diabetes and your eyes.* Albany: Department of Health.

Stremel, K., Perreault, S., Welch, T. R. (1995). Strategies for classroom and community. In K. M. Huebner, J. G. Prickett, T. R. Welch, & E. Joffee (Eds.), *Hand in hand: Essentials of communication and orientation and mobility for your students who are deaf-blind* (pp. 411–444). New York: AFB Press.

Stephens, B., & Grube, C. (1982). Development of Piagetian reasoning in congenitally blind children. *Journal of Visual Impairment & Blindness, 76*(4), 133–143.

Stephens, R., & Longley, A. (1995). An orientation and navigation system for blind and partially sighted people. *Proceedings of the European Conference on the Advancement of Rehabilitation Technology,* Lisbon, Portugal.

Stevens, A. (1993). A comparative study of the ability of totally blind adults to align and cross the street at an offset intersection using an alternating versus non-alternating audible traffic signal. Unpublished master's thesis, Université de Sherbrooke, Sherbrooke, Québec, Canada.

Stevens, J. (1991). Thermal sensibility. In M. A. Heller & W. Schiff (Eds.), *The psychology of touch* (pp. 61–90). Hillsdale, NJ: Lawrence Erlbaum.

Stevens, S. S., & Newman, E. B. (1936). The localization of actual sources of sound. *American Journal of Psychology, 48,* 297–306.

Stone, R. (1990, August 20). An artificial eye may be within sight. *The Washington Post,* p. A03.

Stonequist, E. (1937). *The marginal man.* New York: Scribners.

Stotland, E., & Canon, L. K. (1972). *Social psychology: A cognitive approach.* Philadelphia: W. B. Saunders.

Stover, D. (1995). Radar on chip. *Popular Science, 246*(3), 107–116.

Straw, L. B., Harley, R. K., & Zimmerman, G. J. (1991). A program in orientation and mobility for visually impaired persons over age 60. *Journal of Visual Impairment & Blindness, 85*(3), 108–113.

Strelow, E. R. (1983). Use of binaural sensory aid by young children. *Journal of Visual Impairment & Blindness, 77*(9), 429–438.

Strelow, E. R. (1985). What is needed for a theory of mobility? Direct perception and cognitive maps—Lessons from the blind. *Psychological Review, 92,* 226–248.

Strelow, E. R., & Brabyn, J. A. (1982). Locomotion of the blind controlled by natural sound cues. *Perception, 11,* 635–640.

Stroud, P. (1993). History of the Orientation and Mobility Instructors Association of Australasia. *Orientation and Mobility Instructors Association of Australasia Journal of Orientation and Mobility, 11*(2), 3.

Sullivan, R. F. (1988). Transcranial ITE CROS. *Hearing Instruments, 39,* 11–12, 54.

Supa, M., Cotzin, M., & Dallenbach, K. M. (1944). "Facial vision:" The perception of obstacles by the blind. *American Journal of Psychology, 57,* 133–183.

Suterko, S. (1967, December). Long cane training: Its advantages and problems. *Proceedings of the Conference for Mobility Trainers and Technologists* (pp. 13–18). Cambridge: Massachusetts Institute of Technology.

Suterko, S. (1973). Life adjustment. In B. Lowenfeld (Ed.), *The visually handicapped child in school* (pp. 279–317). New York: John Day.

Sutherland, D., Olshen, R., Cooper, L., & Woo, S. (1980). The development of mature gait. *Journal of Bone and Joint Surgery, 62A*(3), 336–353.

Tait, P. E. (1972). The implications of play as it relates to the emotional development of the blind child. *Education of the Visually Handicapped, 4*(2), 52–54.

Talor, C. (1993). *Sensitivity to changes in perspective as a function of onset of blindness, point of observation, and number of targets.* Doctoral dissertation, Vanderbilt University, Nashville, TN.

Taraya, E. (1995). *Executive summary: Guidestrips for visually disabled/blind pedestrians.* City and County of San Francisco: Department of Public Works, Office of the Disability Access Coordinator.

Taylor, M., & Lederman, S. (1975). Tactile roughness of grooved surfaces: A model and the effect of friction. *Perception and Psychophysics, 17,* 23–26.

Tellevik, J. M. (1992). Influence of spatial exploration patterns on cognitive mapping by blindfolded sighted persons. *Journal of Visual Impairment & Blindness, 86*(5), 221–224.

Templer, J. A. (1992). *The staircase: Studies of hazards, falls, and safer design.* Cambridge, MA: MIT Press.

Templer, J. A., & Wineman, J. D. (1980). *The feasibility of accomodating elderly and handicapped pedestrians on over-and-undercrossing structures* (FHWA-RD-79-146). Washington, DC: Federal Highway Administration, U.S. Government Printing Office.

Templer, J. A., Wineman, J. D., & Zimring, C. M. (1982). *Design guidelines to make crossing structures accessible to the physically handicapped.* Final Report #DTF-H61-80-C-00131). Washington, DC: Federal Highway Administration, Office of Research and Development, Environmental Division.

Tennyson, R. D., & Park, O. (1980). The teaching of concepts: A review of instructional design literature. *Review of Educational Research, 50,* 55–70.

The Seeing Eye Inc. (1984). [The Mowat Sensor Project.] Unpublished raw data.

The Seeing Eye Inc. (1992). [Survey of mobility instructors.] Unpublished manuscript.

Thompson, D. (1993). *The promotion of gross and fine motor development for infants and toddlers: Developmentally appropriate activities for parents and teachers.* Reston, VA: ERIC Clearinghouse on Handicapped and Gifted Children, Council for Exceptional Children. (ERIC Document Reproduction Service No. ED361104.)

Thyer, B. A., & Stocks, J. T. (1986). Exposure therapy in the treatment of a phobic blind person. *Journal of Visual Impairment & Blindness, 80,* 1001–1003.

Tielsch, J. M., Sommer, A., Witt, K., & Royall, R. M. (1990, February). Blindness and visual impairment in an American urban population: The Baltimore Eye Study. *Archives of Ophthalmology, 108,* 286–290.

Tijerina, L., Jackson, J. L., & Tornow, C. E. (1994). *The impact of transit station platform edge warning surfaces on persons with visual impairments and persons with mobility impairments* (Battelle Contract No. FE-6591/BK). Columbus, OH: Washington Metropolitan Area Transit Authority.

Tolman, E. C. (1932). *Purposive behavior in animals and man.* New York: Century.

Toole, T., McColskey, D., & Rider, R. (1984). Retention of movement cues by visually impaired persons. *Journal of Visual Impairment & Blindness, 78*(10), 487–490.

Toronto Transit Commission. (1990, September). *Tactile edge warning systems evaluation.* Toronto, Canada: Author.

Transport and Road Research Laboratory. (1983). *Textured pavements to help blind pedestrians.* London: Department of the Environment, Department of Transport.

Trehub, S. E., Schneider, B. A., Morrongiello, B. A., & Thorpe, L. A. (1988). Auditory sensitivity in school-age children. *Journal of Experimental Child Psychology, 46,* 273–285.

Trehub, S. E., Schneider, B. A., Morrongiello, B. A., & Thorpe, L. A. (1989). Development changes in high-frequency sensitivity. *Audiology, 28,* 241–249.

Truschel, L. (1906). Der sechste Sinn der Blinden. *S.f. Exp. Padagogik, 3,* 109–142; *4,* 129–155; *5,* 66–77.

Tulving, E. (1983). *Elements of episodic memory.* Oxford: Clarendon Press.

Tulving, E. (1985). How many memory systems are there? *American Psychologist, 40,* 385–398.

Turnbull, G. I. (1982). Some learning theory implications in neurological physiotherapy. *Physiotherapy, 68*(2), 38–41.

Tuttle, D. W. (1984). *Self-esteem and adjusting with blindness.* Springfield, IL: Charles C Thomas.

Tuttle, D. W. (1986). Family members responding to a visual impairment. *Education of the Visually Handicapped, 18*(3), 107–116.

Tuttle, D. W. (1987). The role of the special education teacher-counselor in meeting students' self-esteem needs. *Journal of Visual Impairment & Blindness, 81,* 156–161.

Tyler, R. S., & Schum, D. J. (Eds.). (1995). *Assistive devices for persons with hearing impairment.* Boston: Allyn & Bacon.

Ungar, S., Blades, M., & Spencer, C. (1995). Visually impaired children's strategies for memorising a map. *British Journal of Visual Impairment, 13,* 27–32.

Ungar, S., Blades, M., & Spencer, C. (1996). The ability of visually impaired children to locate themsleves on a tactile map. *Journal of Visual Impairment & Blindness, 90,* 526–535.

Ungar, S., Blades, M., Spencer, C., & Morsley, K. (1994). Can visually impaired children use tactile maps to estimate directions? *Journal of Visual Impairment & Blindness, 88,* 221–233.

Ungar, S., Blades, M,, & Spencer, C. & Morsley, K. (in press). Teaching visually impaired children to make distance judgments from a tacile map. *Journal of Visual Impairment & Blindness.*

Uslan, M. M. (1990). In-service training for bus drivers. In M. M. Uslan, A. F. Peck, W. R. Wiener, & A. Stern (Eds.), *Access to mass transit for blind and visually impaired travelers* (pp. 91–93). New York: American Foundation for the Blind.

Uslan, M. M., Hill, E., & Peck, A. (1989). *The profession of orientation and mobility in the 1980s: The AFB competency study.* New York: American Foundation for the Blind.

Uslan, M. M., Peck, A., & Kirchner, C. (1981). Demand for orientation and mobility specialists in 1980. *Journal of Visual Impairment & Blindness, 75*(1), 8–12.

Uslan, M. M., Wiener, W. R., & Newcomer, J. (1990). The rapid rail training seminar. In M. M. Uslan, A. F. Peck, W. R. Wiener, & A. Stern (Eds.), *Access to mass transit for blind and visually impaired travelers* (pp. 45–52). New York: American Foundation for the Blind.

Uslan, M. M., Peck, A. F., Wiener, W. R., & Stern, A. (Eds.). (1990). *Access to mass transit.* New York: American Foundation for the Blind.

U.S. Select Committee on Aging (1991). *Aging America: Trends and projections, 1991 Edition.* Washington, DC: Author.

Vallerand, R. J., Deci, E. L., & Ryan, R. M. (1985) Intrinsic motivation in sport. In K. B. Pandolf (Ed.), *Exercises and sports sciences review* (Vol. 15, pp. 389–425). New York: Macmillan.

Vanderheiden, G. (1995). *Talking fingertip: Access to touchscreen kiosks and ATMs for blindness and low vision.* Madison: University of Wisconsin Trance Center.

Van Sohn, A. (1985). *Diabetes, vision impairment, and blindness.* New York: American Foundation for the Blind.

Vaughn, D. G., Asbury, T., & Riordan-Eva, P. (1995). *General ophthalmology* (14th ed.). Norwalk, CT: Appleton & Lange.

Veterans Administration. (1952). *The Long Cane* [Film].

Villey, P. (1930). *The world of the blind: A psychological study* (pp. 101–131). London: Duckworth.

von Bekesy, G. (1967). *Sensory inhibition.* Princeton, NJ: Princeton University Press.

von Hofsten, C. (1985). Perception and action. In M. Freese & J. Sabini (Eds.), *Goal directed behavior: The concept of action in psychology* (pp. 80–109). Hillsdale, NJ: Lawrence Erlbaum.

Von Prondzinski, S. (1991, September 9–12). *Italy starts orientation and mobility activities.* Paper presented at the Sixth International Mobility Conference, Madrid, Spain.

Voorhees, A. (1962). Professional trends in mobility training. *New Outlook for the Blind,. 56*(1), 3–9.

Wainapel, S. F. (1989). Attitudes of visually impaired persons toward cane use. *Journal of Visual Impairment & Blindness, 83,* 446–448.

Waiss, B., & Cohen, J. M. (1992). The functional implications of glare and its remediation for persons with low vision. *Journal of Visual Impairment & Blindness, 86*(1), 28.

Walker, D., Grimwade, J., & Wood, C. (1971). Intrauterine noice: A component of the fetal environment. *American Journal of Obstetrics and Gynecology, 109,* 91–95.

Walker, J. E., & Shea, T. M. (1980). *Behavior modification: A practical approach for educators* (2nd ed.). St. Louis: Mosby.

Wardell, K. T. (1980). Environmental modifications. In R. L. Welsh & B. B. Blasch (Eds.), *Foundations of orientation and mobility* (pp. 477–525). New York: American Foundation for the Blind.

Wardlow, D. (1974). A nine months drop out study, Hot Springs Rehabilitation Service. In B. Cobb (Ed.), *Special problems in rehabilitation.* Springfield, IL: Charles C Thomas.

Warren, D. (1984). *Blindness and early childhood development* (2nd ed.). New York: American Foundation for the Blind.

Warren, D. (1994). *Blindness and children: An individual differences approach.* New York: Cambridge University Press.

Watson, D., & Watson, M. (1993). *A model service delivery system for persons who are deaf-blind.* University of Arkansas Rehabilitation Research and Training Center for Persons Who Are Deaf or Hard of Hearing, Little Rock: University of Arkansas.

Weinberg, R., Bruya, L., Longino, J. & Jackson, A. (1988). Effect of goal proximity and specificity on endurance performance of primary grade children. *Journal of Sport and Exercise Psychology, 10,* 81–91.

Weisgerber, R., & Hall, A. (1975). *Environmental sensing skills and behaviors* (VA Contract No. V101 (134) P-163). Palo Alto, CA: American Institutes for Research.

Weisman, J. (1981). Evaluating architectural legibility: Wayfinding in the built environment. *Environment and Behavior, 13,* 189–204.

Welsh, R. L. (1972). Cognitive and psychosocial aspects of mobility training. In *Blindness Annual,* 1972, 99–

109. Washington, DC: American Association of Workers for the Blind.

Welsh, R. L. (1980). Topic 3. Visually impaired older persons. In R. Welsh & B. Blasch (Eds.), *Foundations of orientation and mobility* (pp. 420–428). New York: American Foundation for the Blind.

Welsh, R. L., & Blasch, B. B. (1974). Manpower needs in orientation and mobility. *New Outlook for the Blind, 68*(10), 433–443.

Welsh, R. L., & Blasch, B. B. (1980). Training for persons with functional mobility limitations. In R. L. Welch & B. B. Blasch (Eds.), *Foundations of orientation and mobility* (pp. 461–476). New York: American Foundation for the Blind.

Welsh, R. L., & Wiener, W. R. (1977). The code of ethics for orientation and mobility specialist: A progress report. *Journal of Visual Impairment & Blindness, 71*(5), 222–224.

Werker, J. F., & Tees, R. C. (1992). The organization and reorganization of human speech perception. *Annual Review of Neuroscience, 15,* 377–402.

Werner, L. A., & Gillenwater, J. M. (1990). Pure-tone sensitivity of 2- to 5-week old infants. *Infant Behavior and Development, 13,* 355–375.

Wernick, J. (1985). Use of hearing aids. In J. Katz (Ed.), *Handbook of clinical audiology* (3rd ed., pp. 911–935). Baltimore: Williams & Wilkins.

Wever, E. G. (1949). *Theory of hearing.* New York: Wiley.

Whetnall, E. (1964). Binaural hearing. *Journal of Laryngology and Otology, 78,* 1079–1089.

Whiteman, M., & Lukoff, I. (1965). Attitudes toward blindness and other physical handicaps. *Journal of Social Psychology, 66,* 134–145.

Whitener, B. (1981). *The electric car book.* Louisville, KY: Love Street Books.

Wiedel, J. W., & Groves, P. A. (1969a). Designing and reproducing tactual maps for the visually handicapped. *New Outlook for the Blind, 63,* 196–201.

Wiedel, J. W., & Groves, P. A. (1969b). *Tactual mapping: Design, reproduction, reading and interpretation* (Final report, University of Maryland, Project No. DR-2557DS). Washington, DC: Department of Health, Education and Welfare, Vocational Rehabilitation Administration.

Wiener, F. M. (1947). On the diffraction of a progressive sound wave by the human head. *Journal of the Acoustical Society of America, 19,* 143–146.

Wiener, H. (1974). An attributional interpretation of expectancy-value theory. In B. Wiener (Ed.), *Cognitive views of human motivation* (pp. 51–69). New York: Academic Press.

Wiener, P. (1991, September 9–12). *Mobility training in Czechoslovakia before 1989 and today.* Paper presented at the Sixth International Mobility Conference, Madrid, Spain.

Wiener, W. R. (1989). [Personnel shortages in orientation and mobility. AER & NCSAB Joint Survey]. Unpublished data.

Wiener, W. R. (1992). Orientation and mobility. In Wiener, W. R. *Accommodation and accessibility: Implementing the ADA on a local level.* New York: American Foundation for the Blind.

Wiener, W. R. (1993). An innovative model for training orientation and mobility assistants. *Journal of Visual Impairment & Blindness, 87*(5), 134–137.

Wiener, W. R., & Carlson-Smith, C. (1996). The auditory skills necessary for echolocation: A new explanation. *Journal of Visual Impairment & Blindness, 90* (1), 21–35.

Wiener, W. R., & Goldstein, B. (1977). A spectral analysis of traffic sounds in residential, small business, and downtown areas. Unpublished manuscript.

Wiener, W. R., & Joffee, E. (1993). The O&M personnel shortage and university training programs. *RE:view, 25*(2), 67–73.

Wiener, W. R., & Uslan, M. (1986). The crisis in O&M in manpower. *Long Cane News, 5*(1), 1–4.

Wiener, W. R., & Uslan, M. (1990). Mobility assistants: A perspective on new service providers. *RE:view, 22*(2), 56–68.

Wiener, W. R., & Vopata, A. (1980). Suggested curriculum for distance vision training with optical aids. *Journal of Visual Impairment & Blindness, 74,* 49–56.

Wiener, W. R., & Welsh, R. L. (1980). The profession of orientation and mobility. In R. L. Welsh & B. B. Blasch (Eds.), *Foundations of orientation and mobility* (pp. 625–651). New York: American Foundation for the Blind.

Wiener, W., Fauver, R., & Schwartz, M. (1995). Survey of salaries of professionals in the field of blindness. *RE:view, 26*(4), 149–157.

Wiener, W. R., Joffee, E., & LaGrow, S. (1995, Spring). Conference on reasonable accommodations. *Division IX Newsletter,* pp. 3–8.

Wiener, W. R., Lolli, D., & Huff, R. (1994). Evaluation of the OMA program. Presentation at the 1994 AER International Conference.

Wiener, W. R., Bliven, H. S., Bush, D. Ligammari, K., & Newton, C. (1992). The need for vision in teaching orientation and mobility. *Journal of Visual Impairment & Blindness, 86*(1), 54–57.

Wiener, W. R., Deaver, K., DiCorpo, D., Hayes, J., Hill, E., Manzer, D., Newcomer, J., Pogrund, R., Rosen, S., & Uslan, M. (1990). The orientation and mobility assistant. *RE:view, 22*(2), 69–78.

Wiener, W. R., Hill, E., Barlow, J., Deniston, T., Fall, L., Fergusen, C., Gerlech, K., Griffin-Shirley, N., Hill, M. M., Joffee, E., Kossick, R., Leja, J., Lolli, D., Scheffle, R., Uslan, M. & Richardson, J. (1991). *Curriculum guidelines for training orientation and mobil-*

ity assistants [training manual]. Alexandria, VA: Association for Education and Rehabilitation of the Blind and Visually Impaired.

Wiener, W. R., Lawson, G., Naghshineh, K., Brown, J., Bischoff A., & Toth, A. (submitted 1997). The use of traffic sounds to make street crossings. Manuscript in preparation.

Wiener, W. R., Ponchilla, S., Joffee, E., & Kuskin, (1997). External bus speaker and their effectiveness with visually impaired persons. Manuscript in preparation.

Wiener, W. R., Welsh, R., Hill, E., LaDuke, R., Mills, R., & Mundy, G. (1973). The development of a code of ethics for orientation and mobility specialists. *Blindness,* 6–16.

Willard, F. (1889). *Glimpses of 50 years.* Boston: Women's Temperance Publication Association.

Williams, B., Hoff, H., Millaway, S., & Cassidy, M. (1982). *Project OMNI—Orientation & Mobility for Needed Independence: A pre-requisite orientation & mobility skills development curriculum.* Norristown, PA: Montgomery County Intermediate Unit No. 23.

Williams, R. (1965). How a center can be run for the rehabilitation of blind people. In *Blindness annual* (pp. 32–48). Washington, DC: American Association of Workers for the Blind.

Williams, T. F. (1984). *Rehabilitation in the aging.* New York: Raven.

Willoughby, D., & Duffy, S. (1989). *Handbook for itinerant and resource teachers of blind and visually impaired students.* Baltimore, MD: National Federation of the Blind.

Wilson, E. O. (1979, Nov.–Dec.). Altruism. *Harvard Magazine, 80,* 23–28.

Winer, B. J. (1971). *Statistical Principles in Experimental Design* (2nd ed.). New York: McGraw-Hill.

Winter, D., Patia, A., Frank, J., & Walt, S. (1990). Biomechanical walking pattern changes in the fit and healthy elderly. *Physical Therapy, 70*(6), 340–347.

Wittrock, M. C. (1986). Students' thought processes. In M. C. Wittrock (Ed.), *Handbook of research on teaching* (3rd ed.). New York: Macmillan.

Wolk, S., & Kurtz, J. (1975). Positive adjustment and involvement during aging and expectancy for internal control. *Journal of Consulting and Clinical Psychology, 43,* 173–178.

Wolpe, J., & Lazarus, A. A. (1966). *Behavior therapy techniques: A guide to the treatment of neuroses.* New York: Pergamon.

Wolpe, J., Salter, A., & Reyna, L.. (1964). *The conditioning therapies.* New York: Holt, Rinehart & Winston.

Woollacott, M., Debu, B., & Mowatt, M. (1987). Neuromuscular control of posture in the infant and child: Is vision dominant? *Journal of Motor Behavior, 19*(2), 167–186.

Worchel, P. (1951). Space perception and orientation in the blind. *Psychological Monographs: General and Applied, 65,* 1–27 (Whole No. 332).

Worchel, P., & Ammons, C. (1953). The course of learning in the perception of obstacles. *American Journal of Psychology.*

Worchel, P., & Dallenbach, K. (1947). Facial vision: Perception of obstacles by the deaf-blind. *American Journal of Psychology, 60,* 502–553.

Worchel, P., & Mauney, J. (1950). The effect of practice on the perception of obstacles by the blind. *Journal of Experimental Psychology, 41,* 170–176.

Wright, J. C., & Mischel, W. (1987). A conditional approach to dispositional constructs: The local predictability of social behavior. [Special issue.] *Journal of Personality and Social Psychology, 53,* 1159–1177.

Wright, B. (1960). *Physical disability—a psychological approach.* New York: Harper and Row.

Wright, H. N., & Carhart, R. (1960). The efficiency of binaural listening among the hearing-impaired. *Archives of Otolaryngology, 72,* 789–797.

Yin, R. K. (1989). *Case study research: Design and methods.* London: Sage.

Yngström, A. (1991). The tactile map—The surrounding world in miniature. *Proceedings: 6th International Mobility Conference* (Book 1, pp. 223–238). Madrid, Spain.

Yost, W. A. (1994). *Fundamentals of hearing* (p. 78). New York: Academic Press.

Zaga, M. (1986). Development of orientation and mobility program in a developing country. In N. Neustadt, S. Merin, & Y. Schiff (Eds.), *Orientation and mobility of the visually impaired.* Jerusalem: Heiliger.

Zelazo, P. (1984). "Learning to walk:" Recognition of high order influence. In L. Lipsitt & C. Rovee-Collier (Eds.), *Advances in infancy research* (Vol. 3). Norwood, NJ: Ablex.

Zemlin, W. R. (1988). *Speech and hearing science: Anatomy and physiology* (2nd ed.). Englewood Cliffs, NJ: Prentice Hall.

Zimmerman, G. J. (1990). Effects of microcomputer and tactile aid simulations on the spatial ability of blind individuals. *Journal of Visual Impairment & Blindness, 84,* 541–546.

Zweibelson, I., & Barg, C. F. (1967). Concept development of blind children. *The New Outlook for the Blind, 61*(7) xxx–xxx.

University Orientation and Mobility Competency Form

Academic Competencies

All referenced distances are approximate (estimated rather than actual measurements).

Applicant is rated "yes" or "no" for each competency.

A# **MEDICAL ASPECTS OF BLINDNESS AND VISUAL IMPAIRMENT**

A-1 The candidate has demonstrated knowledge and understanding of the visual system and how it works.

A-2 The candidate has demonstrated knowledge and understanding of the etiology of visual impairments and the effects of these impairments on visual functioning.

A-3 The candidate has demonstrated knowledge and understanding of the roles and functions of low vision clinics.

A-4 The candidate has demonstrated knowledge about the resources for low vision devices and care.

A-5 The candidate has demonstrated a basic knowledge and understanding of hearing impairments and the impact of hearing impairments on auditory functioning and communication.

A-6 The candidate has demonstrated basic knowledge and understanding of the following health conditions and disabilities: alcoholism and substance abuse, AIDS, deafness, stroke or cerebral vascular accidents, traumatic brain injury, mental retardation, cerebral palsy, amputations, epilepsy, diabetes mellitus, spinal cord injury, pulmonary dysfunction, multiple sclerosis, cardiovascular disease, rheumatic disease, and mental illness.

A-7 The candidate has demonstrated a knowledge of the roles of the professionals involved in the health care and rehabilitation of persons with the conditions in A-2, A-5, and A-6, above.

B# **SENSORY MOTOR FUNCTIONING**

B-1 The candidate has demonstrated knowledge and understanding of the basic development, anatomy, physiology, perceptual processes, and training of each sensory system (visual, auditory, vestibular, kinesthetic, touch, olfactory, proprioceptive) and the interrelationships of these systems.

B-2 The candidate has demonstrated knowledge and understanding of the common pathologies associated with each sensory system and the implications for orientation and mobility.

B-3 The candidate has demonstrated knowledge and understanding of perception as it pertains to cognition, sensation, attention, memory, cognitive mapping, orientation, and the utilization of information conveyed through sensory stimulation.

B-4 The candidate has demonstrated knowledge and understanding of the manner in which sensory information affects safety and access in travel environments.

B-5 The candidate has demonstrated knowledge and understanding of sound measurement, classifying and quantifying hearing loss, the special auditory needs of persons with visual impairments, the use of hearing aids by persons with visual impairments, auditory training programs, and the uses of audiometric data for traffic interpretation.

B-6 The candidate has demonstrated knowledge and understanding of the rudimentary practices used for screening of hearing function, including the use of hearing questionnaires and localization tests.

(*continued on next page*)

Appendix A. University Orientation and Mobility Competency Form

University Orientation and Mobility Competency Form (*continued*)

B-7 The candidate has demonstrated knowledge and understanding of the mechanics of human locomotion and the psychomotor factors influencing mobility such as sensory awareness, integration of reflexes, muscle tone, and coordination, as well as problems with balance, posture, gait, endurance, strength, flexibility, agility, and coordination.

B-8 The candidate has demonstrated knowledge and understanding of the principles of nonvisual locomotion including movement theories, theories of spatial orientation, veering and its remediation.

C# **PSYCHO-SOCIAL ASPECTS OF BLINDNESS AND VISUAL IMPAIRMENTS**

C-1 The candidate has demonstrated a basic beginning knowledge and understanding of the different counseling theories such as psychodynamic, person-centered, gestalt, cognitive, rational emotive, behavioral, and reality therapy.

C-2 The candidate has demonstrated knowledge and understanding of the psycho-social consequences of congenital and adventitious blindness.

C-3 The candidate has demonstrated knowledge and understanding of the adjustment process that may accompany visual impairment and concomitant disabilities.

C-4 The candidate has demonstrated knowledge and understanding about the impact of vision loss on the family and the strategies available to include family members, caregivers, and support systems as encouragers of independence.

C-5 The candidate has demonstrated knowledge and understanding of the impact that motivation, fear, anxiety, self-concept, self-efficacy, and social interactions have on the educational and rehabilitative processes.

C-6 The candidate has demonstrated knowledge and understanding of the importance of establishing appropriate interaction skills and rapport with students and their families or significant others.

C-7 The candidate has demonstrated knowledge and understanding of the importance of counseling students about setting mobility goals, choosing a mobility system, and other topics related to the use of mobility skills for daily living.

C-8 The candidate has demonstrated knowledge of the resources that are available to assist students to deal with psycho-social problems that affect O&M learning or performance.

C-9 The candidate has demonstrated knowledge and understanding of the impact on learners of socio-cultural factors, including social class identification, ethnic/racial background, and cultural group attitudes toward blindness.

C-10 The candidate has demonstrated knowledge and understanding of society's attitudes toward blindness and visual impairments and the methods for affecting attitude change that can be utilized by both the instructor and the student.

C-11 The candidate has demonstrated knowledge and understanding of the importance of discussing and analyzing the feelings and reactions they may have in response to working with persons with visual impairments and persons with multiple disabilities.

C-12 The candidate has demonstrated knowledge and understanding of the available coping strategies and community resources that may be used by the student and the instructor for resolving issues related to physical losses, trauma, and death.

(*continued on next page*)

University Orientation and Mobility Competency Form (*continued*)

D#	**HUMAN GROWTH AND DEVELOPMENT OVER THE LIFESPAN**
D-1	The candidate has demonstrated knowledge and understanding of the principles of child development.
D-2	The candidate has demonstrated knowledge and understanding of the typical and atypical sensorimotor development patterns of children and youth who are blind or visually impaired.
D-3	The candidate has demonstrated knowledge and understanding of the effects of visual impairments on affective, psychomotor, and cognitive development and processes.
D-4	The candidate has demonstrated knowledge and understanding of how the developmental patterns of children with visual impairments affect the acquisition and performance of O&M skills and techniques.
D-5	The candidate has demonstrated knowledge and understanding of the aging process.
D-6	The candidate has demonstrated knowledge and understanding of how the aging process affects the acquisition and performance of O&M skills and techniques.
D-7	The candidate has demonstrated knowledge and understanding of the manner in which students' attitudes toward O&M instruction may change over the lifespan.
D-8	The candidate has demonstrated knowledge and understanding of the strategies and methods that are used to teach O&M to students of all ages.
D-9	The candidate has demonstrated knowledge and understanding of effective ways to convey information about the implications of the developmental patterns associated with blindness and visual impairments over the lifespan to students and their families, other professionals, and individuals in the community.
E#	**CONCEPT DEVELOPMENT**
E-1	The candidate has demonstrated knowledge and understanding of the role that body image, spatial, temporal, positional, directional, and environmental concepts play in moving purposefully in the environment.
E-2	The candidate has demonstrated knowledge and understanding of the effects of visual impairment and blindness on concept development and the manner in which persons who are blind or visually impaired acquire and utilize conceptual information.
E-3	The candidate has demonstrated knowledge and understanding of the manner in which individuals who are blind or visually impaired acquire and use body image, spatial, temporal, positional, directional, and environmental concepts.
E-4	The candidate has demonstrated knowledge and understanding of the published lists of concepts that are related to O&M.
E-5	The candidate has demonstrated knowledge and understanding of the manner in which concept development is incorporated in conducting O&M assessments, designing and implementing O&M programs, and evaluating students' progress.
E-6	The candidate has demonstrated knowledge and understanding of the manner in which mental retardation and other concomitant disabilities affect the acquisition and utilization of concepts by students who are blind or visually impaired.
E-7	The candidate has demonstrated knowledge and understanding of the methods and strategies used to adapt concept development instruction for students with mental retardation and other concomitant disabilities.

(*continued on next page*)

University Orientation and Mobility Competency Form (*continued*)

E-8 The candidate has demonstrated knowledge and understanding of the value of communicating information about the relationship between concept development, visual impairment, and O&M to students' families and significant others, and to other professionals involved in the students' special education or rehabilitation program.

F# MULTIPLE DISABILITIES

F-1 The candidate has demonstrated knowledge and understanding of the effects of additional impairments, including sensory, sensorimotor and physical impairments, mobility impairments not related to blindness, mental retardation, learning disabilities, diabetes, organic brain damage, and challenging behaviors on the orientation process and on mobility.

F-2 The candidate has demonstrated knowledge and understanding about the effects of deaf-blindness on communication, orientation, and mobility.

F-3 The candidate has demonstrated knowledge and understanding of the environmental demands that affect the mobility of visually impaired students with physical and sensorimotor impairments as well as the factors to consider when evaluating these students' travel environments.

F-4 The candidate has demonstrated knowledge and understanding of the unique assessment and instructional needs of learners with multiple impairments, and learners who are deaf-blind.

F-5 The candidate has demonstrated knowledge and understanding of the multidisciplinary, interdisciplinary, and transdisciplinary approach to instruction for students with multiple impairments and students who are deaf-blind.

F-6 The candidate has demonstrated knowledge and understanding of the instructional strategies and methods used, including the use of specialized communication systems, modes, devices and adapted mobility systems and devices, for teaching students with multiple impairments and students who are deaf-blind.

G# SYSTEMS OF ORIENTATION AND MOBILITY

G-1 The candidate has demonstrated knowledge and understanding of the use of the long cane as a mobility system.

G-2 The candidate has demonstrated knowledge and understanding of the different types of long canes, adapted canes, and adaptive mobility devices, and their strengths and limitations as travel tools considering individual travel needs and travel environments.

G-3 The candidate has demonstrated knowledge and understanding of the techniques used to prescribe canes, adapted canes, and adaptive mobility devices.

G-4 The candidate has demonstrated knowledge and understanding of the construction, assembly, and maintenance of the long cane and adaptive mobility devices, knows the nomenclature of the cane and its parts, is aware of resources for procuring long canes and other devices, and has demonstrated proficiency in maintaining and repairing canes and adaptive mobility devices.

G-5 The candidate has demonstrated knowledge and understanding of the dog guide as a mobility system, the methods and strategies for providing orientation assistance to a dog guide user, and knows the process for making referrals to dog guide training centers.

G-6 The candidate has demonstrated knowledge and understanding of electronic travel aids (ETAs) and their use and application as a supplementary mobility system, knows how ETAs are classified, and is knowledgeable about the basic principles of operating commercially available ETAs.

G-7 The candidate has demonstrated knowledge and understanding of optical and non-optical devices and their use and application as a supplementary mobility system; knows and understands how optical and non-optical devices are classified, their basic principles of operation, and the various ways persons with visual impairments can use these devices in travel environments.

(*continued on next page*)

University Orientation and Mobility Competency Form (*continued*)

G-8 The candidate has acquired knowledge and understanding about the use of ambulatory aids such as support canes, walkers, crutches, and wheelchairs and the manner in which these devices are used by persons who are blind or visually impaired.

G-9 The candidate has demonstrated knowledge and understanding of the relative advantages and disadvantages of the mobility systems, including the long cane, optical and non-optical devices, ETAs, and the human guide for a range of persons with blindness and visual impairments, and can communicate this information effectively to students and their families.

H# ORIENTATION AND MOBILITY SKILLS AND TECHNIQUES

H-1 The candidate has demonstrated knowledge and understanding of the human guide techniques and their applications including: position and grip, transferring sides, narrow passageways, accepting or refusing assistance, doorways, stairways, and seating.

H-2 The candidate has demonstrated knowledge and understanding of basic skills and their applications including: upper hand and forearm, lower hand and forearm, and trailing techniques, squaring-off, taking direction, and locating dropped objects.

H-3 The candidate has demonstrated knowledge and understanding of the cane techniques and their applications in indoor and outdoor environments including: diagonal cane and touch technique, touch technique modifications, including three point touch, touch and slide, touch and drag, constant contact technique, and the use of the cane for shore lining.

H-4 The candidate has demonstrated knowledge and understanding of the techniques for using adaptive mobility devices for children and adults in indoor and outdoor environments.

H-5 The candidate has demonstrated knowledge and understanding of the methods used to handle the long cane including: cane grip, placement, and manipulation; utilizing the cane to contact and examine objects, and handling the cane when switching from one side of a human guide to another.

H-6 The student has demonstrated knowledge and understanding of techniques used for familiarization to indoor and outdoor environments including: the use of landmarks, clues and cues, search patterns, and numbering systems.

H-7 The candidate has demonstrated knowledge and understanding of the techniques used for soliciting assistance and declining assistance, when necessary.

H-8 The candidate has demonstrated knowledge and understanding of orientation and travel skills including: route planning, direction taking, distance measurements and estimations, utilization of compass directions, recovery techniques, analysis and identification of intersections and traffic patterns, use of traffic control devices, techniques for crossing streets, techniques for travel in indoor environments, outdoor residential, small business and business districts, mall travel, and travel in rural areas.

H-9 The candidate has demonstrated knowledge and understanding of the O&M skills and techniques used for travel on public and private transportation.

H-10 The candidate has demonstrated knowledge and understanding of the O&M skills and techniques used to negotiate public conveyor systems including elevators, escalators, people movers, and revolving doors.

H-11 The candidate has demonstrated knowledge and understanding of modifications to O&M skills and techniques that are appropriate for students with unique individual needs.

(*continued on next page*)

University Orientation and Mobility Competency Form (*continued*)

I#	INSTRUCTIONAL METHODS, STRATEGIES AND ASSESSMENT
I-1	The candidate has demonstrated knowledge and understanding of the basic principles of learning theory, including: classical conditioning, operant conditioning, cognitive theory, memory and information processing, guided and discovery learning, and the manner in which these theories relate to O&M instruction.
I-2	The candidate has demonstrated knowledge and understanding of the media and materials that are used to support O&M instruction, (e.g., visual, tactile, and auditory maps and models, graphic aids, and tape recorded information), proficiency in designing and producing instructional materials, and knowledge of the resources for obtaining commercially available media and materials.
I-3	The candidate has demonstrated knowledge and understanding of the observational techniques that are appropriate for O&M instruction.
I-4	The candidate has demonstrated knowledge and understanding of the strategies and methods used to select, design, and implement non-clinical procedures for assessment and instruction in the use of sensory information in travel environments.
I-5	The candidate has demonstrated knowledge and understanding of the strategies and methods used to design and implement instructional programs using the optical and non-optical devices recommended by eye care professionals for use in travel environments.
I-6	The candidate has demonstrated knowledge and understanding of the strategies and methods used to assess environments for accessibility and safety.
I-7	The candidate has demonstrated the knowledge and understanding of the strategies and methods used to analyze and select environments for introducing, developing, and reinforcing O&M skills and techniques.
I-8	The candidate has demonstrated knowledge and understanding of the strategies and methods for selecting an appropriate position (i.e., in front of, behind, or to the side of the student) for effective instruction and student safety as the student advances through the O&M program.
I-9	The candidate has demonstrated knowledge and understanding of the importance of selecting and maintaining appropriate distances between the instructor and the student as the student progresses from early learning situations when skills are introduced to advanced learning when skills are applied to environments of various types and complexities.
I-10	The candidate has demonstrated knowledge and understanding of the commonly used distances between the instructor and the student: *close* (arm's length), *intermediate* (from approximately beyond arm's length to 13′), *distant* (approximately 13′ to 20′), and *remote* (beyond 20′).
I-11	The candidate has demonstrated knowledge and understanding of the considerations involved in selecting monitoring distances (close, intermediate, distant, and remote) to promote skill development, safety, and independence.
I-12	The candidate has demonstrated knowledge and understanding of the use of "drop-off" lessons for the assessment of O&M skills, and knows the strategies and methods for selecting, designing, and implementing "drop-off" lessons.
I-13	The candidate has demonstrated the knowledge and understanding of the strategies and methods used to develop and conduct "solo" (independent) lessons and independent travel experiences.

(*continued on next page*)

University Orientation and Mobility Competency Form (*continued*)

I-14 The candidate has demonstrated knowledge and understanding of the strategies and methods used to communicate with students about instructional travel experiences during which the distance between the instructor and the student is remote.

I-15 The candidate has demonstrated knowledge and understanding of the role of the rehabilitation counselor, rehabilitation teacher, special education teacher, adapted physical education teacher, occupational therapist, physical therapist, social worker, and other related professionals who may be involved in interdisciplinary, multidisciplinary, or transdisciplinary instruction.

I-16 The candidate has demonstrated knowledge and understanding of standardized and non-standardized O&M assessment instruments, and knows how to conduct assessments using these instruments.

I-17 The candidate has demonstrated knowledge and understanding of the appropriate procedures used to assess O&M skills and foundation areas such as motor, cognitive, and sensory skills.

I-18 The candidate has demonstrated knowledge and understanding of the strategies and methods used to analyze, interpret, and utilize O&M assessment information for selecting, designing, and implementing O&M programs consistent with individual needs.

I-19 The candidate has demonstrated knowledge and understanding of the strategies and methods for using assessment information to maintain ongoing evaluation of student progress and implement program modifications and remediation appropriately.

I-20 The candidate has demonstrated the knowledge and understanding to analyze and interpret assessment reports from related professional fields, and has demonstrated the ability to utilize information in these reports in conjunction with O&M assessments.

I-21 The candidate has demonstrated knowledge and understanding of the strategies and methods used to conduct O&M assessments and instruction in itinerant, school, and center based settings.

I-22 The candidate has demonstrated knowledge and understanding of the strategies and methods used to conduct assessments, and to select, design, and implement O&M instruction that accommodates cultural and lifestyle differences.

I-23 The candidate has demonstrated knowledge and understanding of the strategies and methods used to evaluate the effects of health conditions, physical, and sensory impairments on the orientation process and on mobility.

I-24 The candidate has demonstrated knowledge and understanding of the strategies and methods used to assess sensory motor functioning.

I-25 The candidate has demonstrated knowledge and understanding of the strategies and methods used to assess psycho-social needs related to O&M instruction.

I-26 The candidate has demonstrated knowledge and understanding of the strategies and methods used to assess human growth and development over the lifespan for planning and implementing O&M instruction.

I-27 The candidate has demonstrated knowledge and understanding of the strategies and methods used to assess concept development, and to select, design, and implement instruction for concept development that is consistent with students' O&M needs.

I-28 The candidate has demonstrated knowledge and understanding of the specific strategies and methods used to assess the O&M skills of students who are deaf-blind, and to select, design, and implement O&M instruction that meets the needs of students who are deaf-blind.

(*continued on next page*)

University Orientation and Mobility Competency Form (*continued*)

J#	**HISTORY AND PHILOSOPHY OF O&M**
J-1	The candidate has demonstrated knowledge and understanding of the major historical events leading to the establishment of university personnel preparation programs in O&M.
J-2	The candidate has demonstrated knowledge and understanding about the history and philosophy of educational and rehabilitation practices as they relate to O&M instruction.
J-3	The candidate has demonstrated knowledge about the development and nature of O&M programs and services in countries around the world.
J-4	The candidate has demonstrated knowledge and understanding of the Code of Ethics for O&M specialists.
J-5	The candidate has demonstrated knowledge and understanding of the accrediting processes for educational and rehabilitation facilities.
J-6	The candidate has demonstrated knowledge and understanding about the certification standards for O&M specialists, O&M trainer-supervisors and O&M assistants.
J-7	The candidate has demonstrated knowledge and understanding of the history of the profession of O&M as well as ongoing and new developments in the following areas: long cane and adaptive mobility devices, dog guide programs, low vision services, ETAs, university personnel preparation programs, recruitment, and personnel development.
J-8	The candidate has demonstrated knowledge and understanding of the strategies and methods that are used to empower students and their families to be informed and effective consumers of special educational and rehabilitation services in O&M.
J-9	The candidate has demonstrated knowledge and understanding of the strategies and methods use to advocate with consumers for quality programs and services for persons who are blind or visually impaired.
K#	**PROFESSIONAL INFORMATION**
K-1	The candidate has demonstrated knowledge and understanding about the sources of current literature pertinent to the profession of O&M.
K-2	The candidate has demonstrated knowledge and understanding about the professional organizations relevant to the practice of O&M, and knows about the services they provide.
K-3	The candidate has demonstrated knowledge about how to maintain professional competence and stay abreast of new information and evolving trends pertinent to the profession of O&M.
K-4	The candidate has demonstrated knowledge and understanding of the basic research approaches used to study O&M including descriptive, exploratory, experimental, and single subject design.
K-5	The candidate has demonstrated knowledge and understanding of the considerations involved in evaluating new ideas, instructional techniques, and research findings in the field of visual impairment and blindness including: sampling problems, ethical issues, and design compromises related to research and demonstration projects conducted with small samples.
K-6	The candidate has demonstrated knowledge and understanding of how to evaluate the strengths and limitations of research reports pertinent to the practice of O&M.
K-7	The candidate has demonstrated knowledge and understanding of national and local environmental accessibility standards.

(*continued on next page*)

University Orientation and Mobility Competency Form (*continued*)

L# **DEVELOPMENT, ADMINISTRATION, AND SUPERVISION OF O&M PROGRAMS**

L-1 The candidate has demonstrated knowledge and understanding of the O&M service delivery models including: the residential rehabilitation center, the nonresidential rehabilitation center, and itinerant rehabilitation services; residential and special school programs, community based itinerant and resource room school programs.

L-2 The candidate has demonstrated knowledge and understanding of the kinds of practice models available for O&M specialists including: staff positions in educational, rehabilitation, and health care settings, private contracting of direct care O&M services, and independent consulting.

L-3 The candidate has demonstrated knowledge and understanding of the major federal and state/provincial legislation and policy affecting the preparation of personnel in O&M and the provision of O&M services for persons with visual impairments.

L-4 The candidate has demonstrated knowledge and understanding of local, state/provincial, and national resources that support the effective provision of O&M programs and services.

L-5 The candidate has demonstrated knowledge and understanding of the role of the O&M specialist, the O&M assistant, and other personnel involved in interdisciplinary, multidisciplinary, and transdisciplinary approaches to providing service to persons with visual impairments.

L-6 The candidate has demonstrated knowledge and understanding of the methods used to develop and organize O&M programs.

L-7 The candidate has demonstrated knowledge and understanding of the issues involved with student safety and instructor liability.

L-8 The candidate has demonstrated knowledge of the sources of products used in the delivery of O&M services.

L-9 The candidate has demonstrated knowledge and understanding of the indicators of quality O&M instruction including: individualized clinical assessment, program development, and planning; and service delivery that is responsive to individual needs, age appropriate, respects multicultural differences, and provides appropriate follow-up.

L-10 The candidate has demonstrated knowledge and understanding about designing O&M instructional goals, objectives, and implementing instructional programs that are compatible with service delivery systems and available resources by considering: planning that is responsive to students' training needs and the availability of personnel, equipment, and materials; providing written schedules that reflect the O&M instructor's activities, and submitting written reports consistent with the administrative requirements of the service delivery system.

L-11 The candidate has demonstrated knowledge and understanding of the systems used for appropriate record keeping in the provision of O&M programs and services.

L-12 The candidate has demonstrated knowledge and understanding of the roles, training levels, and procedures appropriate for O&M assistants, ancillary personnel, and volunteers with respect to the provision of O&M services.

L-13 The candidate has demonstrated knowledge and understanding of appropriate communication about students' O&M program, including goals and progress, to family members and significant others, and knows how to carry out this communication in the context of client confidentiality.

L-14 The candidate has demonstrated knowledge and understanding about how to plan and conduct in-service presentations and workshops about O&M skills, and knows how to conduct these workshops and presentations.

(*continued on next page*)

University Orientation and Mobility Competency Form (*continued*)

L-15 The candidate has demonstrated knowledge and understanding about how to plan and present effective public education programs related to topics in O&M.

Clinical Practice Competencies

All referenced distances are approximate (estimated rather than actual measurements).

Demonstration of competence during supervised clinical hours (examines application of assessment, instruction, and monitoring). *Applicant is rated "yes" or "no" for each competency.*

CL-1 The candidate has demonstrated proficiency in establishing rapport and interacting with students.

CL-2 The candidate has demonstrated proficiency in seeking and accessing records and resources within a facility.

CL-3 The candidate has demonstrated proficiency in evaluating students utilizing appropriate assessment tools, methods, and settings for developing instructional programs.

CL-4 The candidate, in various environments, has demonstrated the ability to evaluate the manner in which a student with low vision uses visual information for travel with residual vision and nonoptical devices. The candidate will also demonstrate these abilities with optical devices after consultation with a low vision eye care specialist.

CL-5 The candidate has demonstrated proficiency in designing and implementing activities, with and without nonoptical devices, to maximize the use of functional vision in travel environments. The candidate will also demonstrate these abilities with optical devices after consultation with a low vision eye care specialist.

CL-6 The candidate has demonstrated proficiency in evaluating functional hearing.

CL-7 The candidate has demonstrated proficiency in designing and implementing activities, with and without hearing aids, to maximize the use of functional hearing.

CL-8 The candidate has demonstrated proficiency in teaching the application of techniques used to maximize use of auditory information.

CL-9 The candidate has demonstrated proficiency in writing behaviorally stated goals and objectives based on evaluation findings that are realistic and appropriately sequenced.

CL-10 The candidate has demonstrated skills in planning, conducting, and evaluating lessons according to the individual's learning style, stage of development, age, or other unique personal attributes that affect learning.

CL-11 The candidate has demonstrated proficiency in planning and delivering lessons that have a stated goal, appropriate site or setting, clear instructions, and stated desired behavior or action.

CL-12 The candidate has demonstrated the ability to obtain, construct, and utilize instructional materials that are appropriate for the student's level of functioning and the particular lesson.

CL-13 The candidate has demonstrated proficiency in designing instructional programs based on knowledge of the various means and levels of communication, and how the communication affects lesson planning and implementation as well as the student's response to instruction.

CL-14 The candidate has demonstrated proficiency in observation skills, the ability to interpret and analyze observations, and the flexibility to change lessons and program sequence based upon observations.

(*continued on next page*)

University Orientation and Mobility Competency Form (*continued*)

CL-15 The candidate has demonstrated proficiency in writing anecdotal notes that are concise and contain pertinent information.

CL-16 The candidate has demonstrated proficiency in providing timely, accurate, and effective feedback to a student regarding progress within a lesson and within a program.

CL-17 The candidate has demonstrated proficiency in consulting with the client, family, and other appropriate personnel regarding the student's O&M program, while respecting agreed upon parameters of confidentiality.

CL-18 The candidate has demonstrated proficiency in modifying or adapting instruction in situations or environments that may affect an O&M lesson, such as adverse weather, fatigue, emotional upset, unexpected noise, construction, etc.

CL-19 The candidate has demonstrated proficiency in acknowledging and effectively dealing with a student's needs, fears, dependency, unrealistic goals, personality, socioeconomic level, living arrangement, or the effects of degenerative or sudden onset of disease.

CL-20 The candidate has demonstrated proficiency in establishing and maintaining an appropriate position and physical distance between the instructor and the student for effective instruction, while maintaining a level of awareness for student safety considering the instructional circumstances, lesson site, and student skills.

CL-21 The candidate has demonstrated discretion in the timing of interventions with students indicating appropriate understanding of the student's need for support and opportunities to achieve independence throughout the instructional process.

CL-22 The candidate has demonstrated proficiency in teaching students to use their remaining senses in establishing their position, location, and direction in relationship to the travel environment.

CL-23 The candidate has demonstrated proficiency in teaching body awareness, body image, body parts, and body movement.

CL-24 The candidate has demonstrated proficiency in teaching environmental concepts.

CL-25 The candidate has demonstrated proficiency in teaching laterality, directionality, positional/relational, spatial, measurement and temporal concepts.

CL-26 The candidate has demonstrated proficiency in selecting, designing, and implementing nonclinical procedures for instruction in the use of residual vision, as well as other remaining senses, with consultation as appropriate.

CL-27 The candidate has demonstrated proficiency in distinguishing between a clue and a landmark and in teaching a student to use them appropriately.

CL-28 The candidate has demonstrated proficiency in providing appropriate clues during instruction, and requesting appropriate responses from the student.

CL-29 The candidate has demonstrated proficiency in teaching kinesthetic, visual, and auditory distance awareness.

CL-30 The candidate has demonstrated proficiency in teaching compass directions, and the application of compass directions to labeling corners at intersections.

CL-31 The candidate has demonstrated proficiency in teaching the use of indoor and outdoor numbering systems.

CL-32 The candidate has demonstrated proficiency in teaching the following in appropriate travel environments: human guide technique, protective techniques, direction taking, retrieving dropped objects, trailing, execution of turns, self-familiarization.

(*continued on next page*)

University Orientation and Mobility Competency Form (*continued*)

CL-33 The candidate has demonstrated proficiency in teaching cane techniques in appropriate travel environments, such as: diagonal cane technique, touch, touch and slide, touch and drag, three point touch, and continuous contact technique, techniques for ascending and descending stairs, storage of the cane, cane techniques for object negotiation, entry and exit through doors, and manipulation of the cane when traveling with a human guide.

CL-34 The candidate has demonstrated proficiency in teaching sidewalk travel.

CL-35 The candidate has demonstrated proficiency in teaching students to identify the location of intersecting sidewalks.

CL-36 The candidate has demonstrated proficiency in teaching corner detection and negotiation.

CL-37 The candidate, when monitoring at close (arm's length) distances, has demonstrated the ability to determine that a student has arrived at a drop off in indoor environments.

CL-38 The candidate has demonstrated the ability to effectively monitor the student as the student approaches a stair drop-off, to identify the position of the cane tip in relation to the stairs as the student descends, and to make contact with the student, as appropriate, while the student negotiates the stairs.

CL-39 The candidate, when monitoring at close (arm's length) and intermediate distances (from approximately beyond arm's length to 13′), has demonstrated the ability to identify adequate and inadequate cane techniques.

CL-40 The candidate, when monitoring at close (arm's length) and intermediate distances (from approximately beyond arm's length to 13′), has demonstrated the ability to determine that a student reacts appropriately to obstacles.

CL-41 The candidate, when monitoring from close (arm's length), intermediate (from approximately beyond arm's length to 13′) and distant positions (approximately 13′ to 20′), has demonstrated the ability to determine effectively, in any manner, the position, movement, and safety of the student at all times.

CL-42 The candidate, when monitoring from close (arm's length), intermediate (from approximately beyond arm's length to 13′), and distant positions (approximately 13′ to 20′), has demonstrated the ability to communicate effectively to the traveler, in any manner, that the traveler must come to an immediate stop.

CL-43 The candidate, when monitoring from a close distance (arm's length), has demonstrated the ability to determine, within 2 seconds of its occurrence, that the student has stopped or has failed to stop at street corners.

CL-44 The candidate has demonstrated proficiency in teaching alignment using environmental sounds and lines of reference.

CL-45 The candidate has demonstrated proficiency in teaching street crossings.

CL-46 The candidate, at stop sign and traffic light controlled intersections, has demonstrated the ability to accurately assess that the student has chosen the correct moment to cross the street.

CL-47 The candidate has demonstrated the ability to determine the correctness of alignment of a student at stop sign and traffic light controlled intersections.

CL-48 The candidate, when monitoring from an intermediate distance, at stop sign or traffic light controlled intersections, has demonstrated the ability to identify vehicles turning in front of the student from the parallel and onto the perpendicular street.

(*continued on next page*)

University Orientation and Mobility Competency Form (*continued*)

CL-49 The candidate, when monitoring from an intermediate distance, has demonstrated the ability to determine if the student has veered unsafely during a crossing (beyond the crosswalk lines or the distance equivalent).

CL-50 The candidate has demonstrated proficiency in teaching travel skills to students in complex environments such as areas with random hazards and drop-offs, areas not previously traveled, and areas with congested pedestrian travel.

CL-51 The candidate has demonstrated proficiency in teaching cane techniques in environments with escalators, revolving doors, turnstiles, and elevators.

CL-52 The candidate has demonstrated proficiency in teaching use of traffic controls.

CL-53 The candidate has demonstrated proficiency in teaching students to negotiate service stations, parking lots, and railroad tracks.

CL-54 The candidate has demonstrated proficiency in teaching use of public transportation.

CL-55 The candidate has demonstrated proficiency in teaching appropriate skills and procedures for independent travel in the following areas: indoor, residential, business, rural, and special areas (e.g., malls, campuses).

CL-56 The candidate has demonstrated proficiency for communicating with students about travel experiences for which the distance between the instructor and the student is remote (beyond 20′) and for which immediate physical or verbal communication may not take place.

CL-57 The candidate has demonstrated the ability to effectively determine the appropriateness of the student's interaction with the public and to evaluate these interactions with the student.

CL-58 The candidate has demonstrated proficiency in teaching modifications for adverse weather conditions and seasonal travel.

CL-59 The candidate has demonstrated proficiency in assisting students to choose the most appropriate mobility system (cane, dog, ETA) to meet the student's needs at a particular time.

CL-60 The candidate has demonstrated proficiency in planning, implementing, and/or adapting lessons that incorporate the use of a dog guide or ETAs.

CL-61 The candidate has demonstrated proficiency for developing efficient and effective scheduling for O&M programs.

CL-62 The candidate has demonstrated proficiency in writing evaluation reports that describe specific tasks, conditions, and responses, and that contain recommendations based on the interpretation of these evaluations.

CL-63 The candidate has demonstrated proficiency in writing concise progress reports containing pertinent information.

CL-64 The candidate has demonstrated proficiency in maintaining ongoing records and files.

CL-65 The candidate has demonstrated proficiency in meeting with appropriate personnel to ensure accurate follow-through with established skills, techniques, and program sequence.

CL-66 The candidate has demonstrated respect for student confidentiality.

CL-67 The candidate has demonstrated proficiency in locating professional information and resources.

CL-68 The candidate has demonstrated proficiency in developing and maintaining professional relationships.

CL-69 The candidate has demonstrated proficiency in providing in-service education and continuing education to assist related professionals to function as effective interdisciplinary, multidisciplinary and transdisciplinary team members.

CL-70 The candidate has demonstrated conduct consistent with the Orientation and Mobility Code of Ethics.

APPENDIX B

Initial and Renewable Professional Certification Requirements for Orientation and Mobility

AER Initial Professional Certification in Orientation and Mobility may be applied for if the applicant has completed required course work from one of the approved university/college programs (Table 1) in orientation and mobility. This certification does not require any previous O&M experience and is not renewable. This certification is granted for a period of five (5) years.

Applicants must submit one copy of their transcript reflecting completion for credit of the required core curricula from their O&M preparation program. The transcript must show the date when either a bachelor's or master's degree was awarded. Two letters of reference are required. One should be from the AER-approved O&M program faculty, or the director of the program where the applicant attended, documenting successful completion of the program and the fulfillment of the competency requirements. The second letter of reference should be from the clinical experience/internship supervisor. If the applicant already has 1 year of full-time teaching experience in O&M, a detailed letter from the employer/supervisor may be substituted for the internship reference letter. As with other professions, applicants are asked to sign and date the Statement of Endorsement of the Orientation and Mobility Code of Ethics. The completed application form is to be submitted with the application fee to AER.

AER Renewable Professional Certification in Orientation and Mobility follows Initial Certification and requires renewal every five (5) years.

Applicants must submit a photocopy of their most current certification. All applicants must have previously held Initial or Renewable Certification in Orientation and Mobility which can be verified by the AER central office. A letter from the applicant's supervisor is required which describes the applicant's professional performance and verifying the attainment of direct service hours. The completed Professional Activity Requirement Verification Form, along with supporting documentation, is to be submitted with the application form and fee to AER.

The calculation of required professional activity points is dependent on the range of direct service hours as verified by the applicant's supervisor(s). If over 5 years, the applicant has over 6,000 hours of direct service, the required number of professional activity points is 100. If the range is 2,500 to 6,000 of direct service hours, the required number of professional activity points is 200. If the range is 500 to 2,499 of direct service hours, the required number of professional activity points is 400. If the range is 0 to 499 of direct service hours, the required number of professional activity points is 600.

The areas of professional activities are continuing education, college credit, professional conference, professional presentation, professional service, mentorship/supervision, peer ob-

Table 1 AER Approved Programs in Orientation & Mobility

AER Approved University Program	Years (60–96)
Boston College (G)	60–91
Western Michigan University (G)	61–96
Florida State University (U & G)	66–96
San Francisco State University (G)	66–96
California State University, Los Angeles (G)	67–96
University of Pittsburgh (G)	69–96
University of Northern Colorado (G)	69–96
Talladega College (U)	72–83
Stephen F. Austin State University (U)	72–96
Cleveland State University (U)	72–86
University of Arkansas (G)	75–96
Hunter College (G)	75–81
University of Wisconsin (G)	78–81
Peabody College/Vanderbilt (G)	80–95
Dominican College (U)	83–87
SUNY Geneseo (G)	84–86
Michigan State University (G)	84–96
Texas Tech University (G)	85–96
Northern Illinois University (G)	90–96
Massey University (New Zealand) (G)	91–96
University of Texas at Austin (G)	91–96
University of Arizona (G)	92–96
Pennsylvania College of Optometry (G)	92–96
University of Massachusetts at Boston (G)	94–96
Mohawk College (Canada) (U)	96

servation, publication in a newsletter, curriculum development, educational project, publication of an article or book chapter, and publication of a book. Points must be acquired from at least three (3) different areas. Point values vary per activity. Any professional activity performed outside the direct service hours can be considered within these professional activities. Special educational projects need to be preapproved by AER Division Nine Certification Committee.

An individual holding either AER Initial or Renewable Professional Orientation and Mobility Certification is referred to as a Certified Orientation and Mobility Specialist (COMS).

APPENDIX C

Code of Ethics for Orientation and Mobility Specialists

Preamble

Orientation and mobility specialists (peripatologists) recognize the significant role that independent movement plays in the overall growth and functioning of the individual and are dedicated to helping each individual attain the level of independence necessary to reach his or her full potential. Orientation and mobility specialists gather, develop, and utilize specialized knowledge in accomplishing this with all professions, the possession of specialist knowledge obligates the practitioner to protect the rights of the individuals who must avail themselves of the particular service. To assure the public of our awareness of this obligation, we commit ourselves to this Code of Ethics.

In order to fulfill this obligation, orientation and mobility specialists pledge themselves to standards of acceptable behavior in relation to the following five commitments: Commitment to the Student; Commitment to the Community; Commitment to the Profession; Commitment to Colleagues and Other Professionals; and Commitment to Professional Employment Practices.

It is the responsibility of each orientation and mobility specialist to adhere to the principles in the Code and encourage colleagues to do the same.

1. Commitment to the Student

1.1 The orientation and mobility specialist will value the worth and dignity of each individual.

1.2 It is the responsibility of the orientation and mobility specialist to strive at all times to maintain the highest standards of instruction.

1.3 The orientation and mobility specialist will take all reasonable precautions to insure the safety of the student and to protect the student from conditions which interfere with learning.

1.4 The orientation and mobility specialist will respect the confidentially of all information pertaining to the student. He or she will not divulge confidential information about any student to any individual not authorized by the student to receive such information unless required by law or unless withholding such information would endanger the safety of the student or the public.

1.5 Before beginning instruction with the student, the orientation and mobility specialist will make every attempt to obtain and evaluate information about the student which is relevant to the orientation and mobility instruction.

1.6 The orientation and mobility specialist will respect the rights of the student and/or parent/guardian to participate in decisions regarding the instructional program.

1.7 Decisions regarding continuing or discontinuing instruction will be made with the student and will be based upon evaluation of the student's needs, abilities, and skills.

The decisions will be made in the student's best interest independent of personal or agency convenience.

1.8 The orientation and mobility specialist will provide sufficient information regarding the various types of orientation and mobility guidance devices and will explore with the student which device will best meet specific needs.

1.9 The orientation and mobility specialist will seek the support and involvement of the family and/or guardian in promoting the student's instructional goals and in advancing his or her continued success. This will include sharing information with the family that will facilitate the student's welfare and independence, but not communicating information which violates the principles of confidentiality.

1.10 The orientation and mobility specialist will ask the consent of the student and/or guardian before inviting others to observe a lesson or before arranging to have the student photographed or tape-recorded.

1.11 The orientation and mobility specialist will make all reports objective and will present only data relevant to the purposes of the evaluation and instruction. When appropriate, the orientation and mobility specialist will share this information with the student.

1.12 The orientation and mobility specialist will endeavor to provide individuals involved with the student with sufficient knowledge, instruction and experiences relative to orientation and mobility so as to facilitate the goals of the student.

1.13 The orientation and mobility specialist will not dispense or supply orientation and mobility equipment unless it is in the best interest of the student.

1.14 The orientation and mobility specialist will not allow consideration of personal comfort or convenience to interfere with the design and implementation of necessary travel lessons.

1.15 The orientation and mobility specialist will be responsible for services to students who are referred and will provide adequate ongoing supervision when any portion of the service is assigned to interns or student teachers who are enrolled in orientation and mobility university programs, with the understanding that each individual will function under strict supervision.

1.16 The orientation and mobility specialist will make every attempt to see that follow-up service is provided at the completion of instruction.

2. Commitment to the Community

2.1 The student will not be refused service by the orientation and mobility specialist because of age, sex, race, religion, national origin or sexual orientation.

2.2 The student shall not be excluded from service because of the severity of his or her disabilities unless it is clearly evident that he or she cannot benefit from the service. The orientation and mobility specialist will attempt to influence decision making which establishes the rights of individuals to receive service.

2.3 The orientation and mobility specialist will contribute to community education by defining the role of orientation and mobility in the community, by describing the nature and delivery of service, and by indicating how the community can be involved in the education and rehabilitation process.

2.4 The orientation and mobility specialist will not engage in any public education activity that results in the exploitation of his or her students. Exaggeration, sensationalism, superficiality and other misleading activities are to be avoided.

3. Commitment to the Profession

3.1 The orientation and mobility specialist will seek full responsibility for the exercise of professional judgment related to orientation and mobility.

3.2 To the best of his or her ability, the orientation and mobility specialist will accept the responsibility, throughout the career duration, to master and contribute to the growing body of specialized knowledge, concepts and skills which characterize orientation and mobility as a profession.

3.3 The orientation and mobility specialist will interpret and use the writing and research of others with integrity. In writing, making presentations, or conducting research, the orientation and mobility specialist will be familiar with and give recognition to previous work on the topic.

3.4 The orientation and mobility specialist will conduct investigations in a manner which takes into consideration the welfare of the subject, and report research in a way as to lessen the possibility that the findings will be misleading.

3.5 The orientation and mobility specialist will strive to improve the quality of provided service and promote conditions which attract suitable persons to careers in orientation and mobility.

3.6 The orientation and mobility specialist will, whenever possible, support and participate in local, state, and national professional organizations.

3.7 The orientation and mobility specialist will accept no gratuities or gifts of significance over and above the predetermined salary, fee, and/or expenses for professional service.

3.8 The orientation and mobility specialist will not engage in commercial activities which result in a conflict of interest between these activities and professional objectives with the student.

3.9 The orientation and mobility specialist involved in development or promotion of orientation and mobility devices, books or other products, will present such products in a professional and factual way.

3.10 The orientation and mobility specialist will report suspected and/or known incompetence, or illegal or unethical behavior in the practice of the profession.

3.11 The orientation and mobility specialist will strive to provide fair treatment to all members of the profession and support them when unjustly accused or mistreated.

3.12 Each member of the profession has a personal and professional responsibility for supporting the orientation and mobility code of ethics and maintaining effectiveness.

4. Commitment to Colleagues and Other Professionals

4.1 The orientation and mobility specialist will engage in professional relationships on a mature level and will not become involved in personal disparagement.

4.2 The orientation and mobility specialist will communicate fully and openly with colleagues in the sharing of specialized knowledge, concepts, and skills.

4.3 The orientation and mobility specialist will not offer professional services to a person receiving orientation and mobility instruction from another orientation and mobility specialist, except by agreement with the other specialist or after the other specialist has ended instruction with the student.

4.4 When transferring a student, the orientation and mobility specialist will not commit a receiving specialist to a prescribed course of action.

4.5 The orientation and mobility specialist will seek harmonious relations with members of other professions. This will include the discussion and free exchange of ideas regarding the overall welfare of the student and discussion with other professionals regarding the benefits to be obtained from orientation and mobility services.

4.6 The orientation and mobility specialist will not assume responsibilities which are better provided by other professionals who are available to the student.

4.7 The orientation and mobility specialist will seek to facilitate and enhance a team effort with other professionals. In such situations where team decisions are made, the orientation and mobility specialist will contribute information from his or her own particular perspective and will abide by the team decision unless the team decision requires that he or she act in violation of the code of ethics.

5. Commitment to Professional Employment Practices

5.1 The orientation and mobility specialist will apply for, accept, or offer a position on the basis of professional qualification and will act with integrity in these situations.

5.2 The orientation and mobility specialist will give prompt notification of any change of availability to the agency or school where he has applied.

5.3 The orientation and mobility specialist seeking to hire other specialists will give prompt notification of change in the availability or nature of a position.

5.4 The orientation and mobility specialist will respond factually when requested to write a letter of recommendation for a colleague seeking a professional position.

5.5 The orientation and mobility specialist will provide applicants seeking information about a position with an honest description of the assignment, conditions of work, and related matters.

5.6 The orientation and mobility specialist will abide by the terms of a contract or agreement, whether verbal or written, unless the terms have been falsely represented or substantially changed by the other party.

5.7 The orientation and mobility specialist will not accept positions where proven principles of orientation and mobility practice are compromised or abandoned, unless the position is accepted with the intention of amending or modifying the questionable practices and providing that they do not participate in the behavior which violates the code of ethics.

5.8 The orientation and mobility specialist will adhere to the policies and regulations of the employer except where he or she is required to violate ethical principles indicated in this code. To avoid possible conflicts, the orientation and mobility specialist will acquaint the employer with the contents of this code.

5.9 The orientation and mobility specialist may provide additional professional service through private contracts, as long as these services remain of the highest quality and do not interfere with the specialist's regular job duties.

5.10 The orientation and mobility specialist will not accept remuneration for professional instruction from a student who is entitled to such instruction through an agency or school, unless the student, when fully informed of the services available, decided to contract privately with the specialist.

5.11 The orientation and mobility specialist will establish a fee for private contracting in cooperation with the contracting agency or school that is consistent with the reasonable and customary rate of that particular geographic region.

5.12 When providing additional service through private contracts, the orientation and mobility specialist will observe the agency or school's policies and procedures concerning outside employment including the use of facilities.

Adopted by Interest Group IX of the American Association of Workers for the Blind, July 1973, and by its successor, the Association for Education and Rehabilitation of the Blind and Visually Impaired.
Revised by AER Division Nine, July 1990.
Approved by AER International Board, April 1991.

GLOSSARY

AAIB (American Association of Instructors for the Blind, 1871–1968) An association of professionals who work with children who are blind; the predecessor of AEVH.

AAWB (American Association of Workers for the Blind, 1895–1984) An association of professionals who work with adults who are blind.

Achromatopsia A congenital defect in or absence of cones, resulting in the inability to see color and reduced clear central vision.

Acquired brain injury Injury to the brain that occurs after the first few years of life.

Acquired immunodeficiency syndrome *See* AIDS

Activities In classical conditioning, one type of secondary reinforcer that includes shopping, listening to music, and playing games.

ADAAG (Americans with Disabilities Act Accessibility Guidelines) Regulations implementing Title III of the Americans with Disabilities Act that make public accommodations accessible to and usable by persons with disabilities.

Advance organizer Developed by Ausubel, an initial statement or visual presentation about the subject to be learned that provides a structure for the new information and relates it to information the individual already possesses.

Adventitious Occurring or appearing later in life.

AER (Association for Education and Rehabilitation of the Blind and Visually Impaired) An association, established in 1984, of professionals who work with children and adults who are blind or visually impaired.

AEVH (Association for the Education of the Visually Handicapped, 1968–1984) An association of professionals who work with children who are blind or visually impaired.

Afference Feedback from the body about its movements. *See also* Efference

AIDS (acquired immunodeficiency syndrome) A viral disease transmitted by the human immunodeficiency virus (HIV). It is transmitted only through specific, at-risk behaviors and cannot be contracted by casual contact. *See also* HIV

AIDS-related dementia A mental disorder associated with AIDS that is caused by a direct invasion of the brain structures by HIV. Symptoms can include depression, loss of affect and appetite, problems with sleep, confusion, and forgetfulness. The first signs of dementia include difficulty concentrating, impaired recent memory, and slowness of thought. *See also* AIDS; HIV

Air conduction threshold Intensity level at which signals presented through earphones or sound field are detected 50 percent of the time.

Albinism The congenital absence of pigment in the iris and choroid that causes light sensitivity and reduced acuity.

Ambulatory aids Appliances that provide physical support for moving through the environment, including such devices as wheelchairs, walkers, crutches, and support canes.

American Manual Alphabet A one-handed system of fingerspelling commonly used in the United States.

American Sign Language (ASL) A language used by people who are deaf, the concepts and vocabulary of which are comprised of signs produced with movements of the arms and hands, facial expression, and body language, and that has its own morphology, semantics, and syntax.

Amplification The process of increasing the magnitude of a signal through power, current, or voltage.

Amputation The surgical removal of a limb (or portion of a limb).

Amsler grid A graphlike card used to determine central field losses, as in macular degeneration.

Angina pectoris A heart condition characterized by decreased circulation of blood to the heart muscle.

Aniridia A congenital malformation (usually incomplete) of the iris, accompanied by nystagmus, photophobia, reduced visual acuity, and often glaucoma.

Annunciator A technology that presents over a loudspeaker information that is being displayed electronically in print.

ANSI (American National Standards Institute) The creator of ANSI A117.1, an industry standard based on a consensus process, that provides specifications for making the built environment accessible to and usable by persons with disabilities.

Anxiety A diffuse reaction to a vague or not clearly perceived threat.

Aphakia The absence of the lens, usually resulting from the removal of a cataract.

ARC (AIDS-related complex) A diagnosis made if a person tests positive for the HIV virus and has a set of specific symptoms, including loss of appetite and skin rashes. Usually thought of as a less severe and intermediate form of AIDS, it can nonetheless be severe, disabling, and sometimes fatal. *See also* AIDS

Astigmatism A refractive error caused by spherocylindrical curvature of the cornea or lens; corrected with a cylindrical lens.

Audible signage A system that makes information in print signage available through spoken messages; may be either announced on a loudspeaker or heard privately using a hand-held receiver.

Audible traffic signal A signal that indicates the onset of a pedestrian walk cycle using tones, clicks, musical phrases, or speech. These are integrated into pedestrian signals and may also function as an auditory beacon.

Audiogram A standard graph used to record hearing thresholds for sounds at different frequencies.

Audiometer An instrument used to measure a person's hearing for a variety of signals, such as pure tones and speech.

Auditory maps Verbal descriptions and directions that are recorded on a cassette or disk and played on a tape or disk recorder.

Auditory nerve The group of nerve fibers that carry impulses relating to both hearing and equilibrium from the inner ear to the brain.

Backward chaining In behavioral learning theory, teaching the last substep or link in the chain of substeps first, and then the next-to-last substep or link, and so on. The other substeps are linked to the chain in this manner until the entire task is learned.

Base of support An area located within the outer circumference of all points of contact of the body with the ground or other supporting surface.

Behavioral learning theory A set of principles that attempts to explain learning in terms of observable changes in the behavior of a person. *See also* Classical conditioning; Operant conditioning.

Behavior theory A set of principles that contends that behavior is primarily determined by external environmental influences, particularly by the consequences of one's actions as one interacts with the environment.

Behind-the-ear (BTE) hearing aid A personal amplification device that is contoured to fit behind the ear.

Binocular vision Vision that uses both eyes to form a fused image in the brain and results in three-dimensional vision. *See also* legal blindness

Blindness The inability to see; the absence or severe reduction of vision.

Body concept Knowledge of the parts of the body, their function, and their spatial relationship to other body parts.

Bond guide The emotional connection that must exist between a blind handler and his or her dog guide if the dog is to perform properly.

Bone conduction threshold Intensity level at which signals presented through a bone conduction vibrator are detected 50 percent of the time.

Body planes Theoretical division of the body into halves (left/right, top/bottom, front/back).

Braille A system of raised dots that enables functionally blind persons to read and write by touch.

Brainstem auditory evoked response (BAER) tests A procedure used to record electrical activity evoked from the auditory portion of the eighth nerve and brainstem by presenting stimuli through earphones or a bone conduction vibrator.

Brittle diabetes A type of diabetes, usually characterized by little or no natural production of insulin by the body, in which small amounts of carbohydrates or protein can cause great increases in blood glucose. Poor control of this type of diabetes usually results in extreme daily swings in blood sugar.

Bus lift A platform that raises or lowers to lift people who use wheelchairs or who are otherwise unable to climb steps into and off of buses.

Cartographic orientation A systematic spatial arrangement of places in an environment in a recognizable pattern resembling geometric figures, such as a street grid pattern with rectangular blocks.

Cataract A clouding of the lens, which may be congenital, traumatic, secondary to another visual impairment, or age related.

Central auditory system The auditory neural pathways, nuclei, and centers in the brain beyond the synapse of the eighth nerve fibers in the cochlear nuclei of the brainstem.

Center of gravity Point within the body (or body segment) which, if supported, would then support the rest of the body (or segment) without toppling.

Central nervous system (CNS) Portion of the nervous system consisting of the brain and spinal cord.

Cerebral palsy A neurological condition affecting body movement and coordination. Caused by injury to the motor centers of the brain prenatally, at birth, or during the first few years of life

Certification A voluntary process that culminates in the granting of a certificate which indicates that an individual is recognized as meeting all the criteria necessary for practice within a profession.

Certified Orientation and Mobility Specialist (COMS) The title given by the AER to individuals who meet all certification standards to teach orientation and mobility.

Chronic health impairments Medical conditions that affect internal organs and systems, such as heart conditions, respiratory conditions, or circulatory conditions.

Clamps (tie-downs) Special clamps or straps on buses that attach to wheelchair frames to prevent rolling as the bus moves

Classical conditioning A category of behavioral learning theory that can be used to change behavior by pairing a neutral stimulus that typically would not elicit a response with an unconditioned stimulus that naturally elicits a response. *See also* Behavioral learning theory

Clearance The amount of room a dog guide allows for its master, including overhead.

Clearance error A dog guide's mistake that results in the person who is blind or visually impaired bumping something or someone.

Closure In cognitive learning theory, the principle that people organize their perceptions so that they are as simple and logical as possible. People fill in the gaps in perceptions as necessary to make sense of the total presentation.

CMS (changeable message sign): An electronic sign that uses flip-dot, LED, or LCD technology.

Cochlea The auditory portion of the inner ear, located in the petrous portion of the temporal bone.

Cochlear implant Wire electrodes placed in a nonfunctional cochlea and attached to an induction coil buried surgically under the skin behind the ear. When activated by sound, the electrodes stimulate a healthy auditory nerve.

Code of ethics A standard intended to assure that those who have entered a profession have the appropriate preparation and that they practice in accordance with acceptable and respected principles.

Cognition A general concept embracing all the various modes of knowing, perceiving, remembering, imagining, conceiving, judging, and reasoning.

Cognitive learning theory A set of principles that attempts to explain learning in terms of the mental processes that a person uses to more fully understand some concept or strategy.

Cognitive map Knowledge of a specific spatial layout, which includes object-to-object relationships.

Coloboma A congenital cleft in some portion of the eye, caused by the improper fusion of tissue during gestation; may affect the optic nerve, ciliary body, choroid, iris, lens, or eyelid.

Color vision The perception of color as a result of the stimulation of specialized cone receptors in the retina.

Commands Directions given to dog guides.

Commodities In classical conditioning, one type of secondary reinforcer that includes such items as toys, books, clothes, and jewelry.

Compression An increase in the density of particles in a medium leading to an instantaneous increase in sound pressure.

COMSTAC (Commission on Standards and Accreditation) A commission, created in 1961, to study the development of standards in providing services for people who are blind or visually impaired.

Concept A mental representation, image, or idea of concrete objects, as well as of intangible ideas, such as feelings.

Conceptual knowledge Information about general patterns, such as the layout and traffic patterns of typical intersections. Also called Semantic knowledge.

Conditional dispositional construct A concept which suggests that certain traits or dispositions affect behavior only under certain conditions or in certain situations.

Conditioned response A learned response to a stimulus.

Conductive loss Hearing loss resulting from a lesion or disease in the outer ear, the middle ear, or both.

Confrontation visual field testing A method for making a functional assessment of peripheral vision.

Congenital Present at birth.

Congestive heart disease A medical condition characterized by a weakening of the heart muscle that impairs the heart's ability to pump blood.

Constant contact technique A standard touch technique in which the cane tip remains in contact with the ground at all times.

Continuous reinforcement In behavioral learning theory, a reinforcement after every successful behavior.

Contrast sensitivity The ability to detect differences in grayness and background.

Coordination Harmonizing of activity by the nervous system in order to organize movement.

Correction In dog guide handling, a reprimand. May be verbal, such as "No!" or a "leash correction," which is a sharp, quick pull-release on the leash connected to the dog's collar.

Crawl To move forward on one's belly.

Creep To move forward on one's hands and knees.

Criterion-referenced test An assessment of an individual's development of certain skills in terms of absolute levels of mastery, in which the items are objective and arranged in a hierarchical order of sequential skills.

Critical periods Developmental periods during which specific skills are learned most easily.

CROS (contralateral routing of signals) hearing aid An amplifying system in which a microphone picks up sound on the side of an impaired ear and sends it electrically to a normal or near normal ear.

Crutch Ambulatory aid, made of either wood or aluminum, consisting of a vertical post handgrip and either an underarm supported (underarm crutch) or forearm support (Lofstrand/Canadian/Forearm crutch).

Deaf-blindness Concomitant hearing and visual impairments, the combination of which may present unique communication, learning, developmental, orientation and mobility, and social needs.

Deafness A loss of hearing that is so severe that it is nonfunctional for the ordinary activities of daily living.

Decibel (dB) A unit for expressing the relative intensity or loudness of sounds.

Decondition The process of eliminating or greatly reducing a conditioned response that may be detrimental to learning a desired outcome.

Dependency A class of behaviors capable of eliciting positive attending and ministering responses from others.

Depth perception The overlapping of two slightly dissimilar images from the two eyes to give three-dimensional vision.

Desensitization A multistage process that begins by extinguishing conditioned fear responses to stimuli far removed from the target situation. The target behavior is systematically approached in small steps, with time allowed for the conditioned fear response to extinguish at each step.

Detectable warning A walking surface that has been demonstrated to be reliably detectable under foot and with a long cane; functions as a stop sign for persons with visual impairments.

Detection error A mistake in judging the presence or absence of an important environmental feature or event.

Developmental arrest Cessation of the developmental process in a specific area, such as walking.

Diabetes mellitus A disease characterized by inability to fully utilize glucose as a source of energy.

Diabetic retinopathy Disease of the retina associated with long-standing diabetes; it takes the form of degeneration of the retinal blood vessels, which show fluid leakage in early stages, and hemorrhages, leading to possible blindness, in late stages.

Diagonal cane technique A cane technique used in familiar indoor areas, in which the cane is held in one hand and is positioned diagonally across and in front of the body.

Diffraction The bending or scattering of sound waves around an object.

Directionality The ability to move the body when given various positional terms, such as right, left, forward, and over.

Discount transit fare Reduced rates for bus, subway, or other transportation offered by some districts to people who are older or impaired.

Discovery learning A teaching strategy in which the material to be learned is discovered by the learner. The task given is a problem to be solved.

Disposition theory A system of concepts which holds that the consistency in an individual's actions can be explained by the presence of relatively stable personal factors or traits.

Division Nine The division of AER that serves the professional community of orientation and mobility specialists.

Dog guide By agreement between the Seeing Eye, Leader Dogs for the Blind, and Guide Dogs for the Blind, *dog guide* is the generic term for dogs that are trained to guide blind people. The terms *guide dog, leader dog,* and *seeing eye dog* properly refer only to dogs trained at those respective schools.

Doppler effect The increase in frequency of a sound because of the compression of sound waves and the shortening of wavelength as distance decreases between a sound source and an object.

Dorsal kyphosis Excessive forward bending of the upper spine.

Drop-off lesson A means of evaluating and teaching orientation skills in which the instructor purposefully does not identify the place where the lesson is to begin, gives the student a specific site to be located, and asks the student to interpret the environment independently and to use all problem-solving skills required to travel to the specified location.

Dynamic balance Balance required during such movements as walking or running.

Dynamic visual acuity The ability to discriminate and identify objects when the person is stationary and targets are moving and when both the person and the targets are moving.

Dynamic visual field The potential functional field range when a person moves through the environment.

Eccentric viewing Intentionally looking to one side of an object that provides the best visual acuity.

Echolocation (obstacle perception) The use of reflected sound (including ambient sound) to detect the presence of objects, such as walls, buildings, doors, and openings.

Efference Motor control commands to the muscles. *See also* Afference

Egocentric The orientation individual is at the center, so that the environment is related to a person's own body using such terms as right, left, in front of, and behind.

Electronic orientation aid (EOA) A device used for orientation and navigation that may be external to the user or carried with the traveler.

Electronic travel aid (ETA) A mobility device (head borne, caneborne, chest worn, or handheld) that extends the range of sensory awareness of the traveler with a visual impairment beyond the fingertip, cane, or dog guide. ETAs emit ultrasound vibrations or laser beams that probe the environment and provide tactile or auditory signals or both.

Emergency information card (EOC) A laminated information card with emergency telephone numbers, names, addresses, a picture and, if necessary, medical information.

Emphysema A lung disease that can result in shortness of breath.

Environmental concepts The knowledge of environmental features, such as the size, shape, color, and texture of telephone poles, parking meters, and sidewalks and of the spatial regularities of features in built environments.

Environmental flow The lawful changes in traveler's distances and directions to things in the surroundings that change during locomotion.

Environmental negotiation *See* Wayfinding

Environmental regularity The use of the predictability of built environments as an aid in establishing and maintaining orientation and in making educated guesses about the location of objects or environmental features relative to one another. For example, parking meters are next to streets; restrooms and water fountains in buildings typically are near one another; elevator doors are in consistent locations in a building across floors.

Episodic knowledge Information about particular places and events—of particular "episodes" of experience.

Eustachian tube The tube connecting the middle ear and the nose-throat area, which equalizes pressure on both sides of the tympanic membrane.

Eversion Outward rotation of the ankles that places the body's weight on the instep.

Expectancy motivation The combined influence of perceived self-efficacy and anticipated outcomes on behavior.

External locus of control A person's tendency to consider reinforcements or punishments received as resulting from outside forces such as luck, chance, or fate over which the individual has no control.

Extinction In behavioral learning theory, the concept that when a reinforcer is no longer present, many behaviors that have been reinforced will be weakened and ultimately disappear or become extinct.

Familiar environment Any indoor or outdoor physical setting in which the student has traveled previously.

Familiar intensity Knowledge of the loudness of a particular sound source and how that sound varies with one's distance from the sound source.

Familiarization The organized process of learning the arrangement of a room, building, or other area by using systematic strategies to locate landmarks and relate their location to other locations or features in the environment. Perimeter, gridline, and reference point familiarization strategies are used most commonly by individuals who are visually impaired. Also called Self-familiarization.

Family systems theory A set of principles used in counseling originally proposed by Minuchin that states that families act as systems independent of the individual actions of its members.

Fear A flight or avoidance reaction that an individual has to a specific threat or danger.

Feedback In classical conditioning, one type of secondary reinforcer that gives an individual information about his or her own behavior.

Feedback loop Interplay of sensory inputs and motor outputs to coordinate movement.

Figure-ground In psychology, the attempt to discriminate among the figures in complex figural presentations; to separate the figure from the background.

Fixed interval In behavioral learning theory, a schedule of reinforcement in which the behavior is reinforced on a set time schedule so long as the behavior that is to be strengthened is being performed correctly when the time for the reward occurs.

Fixed ratio In behavioral learning theory, a schedule of reinforcement in which the reinforcer is administered after a fixed number of successful behaviors.

Foot-placement preview A situation that occurs when the cane tip strikes the surface where the foot will be placed.

Forearm trough A curved, metal tray that can be attached to crutches to enable one to support weight on the forearm instead of on the hand.

Four-H program (4-H) An educational and social program for children, originally to teach agricultural and homemaking skills to farm children. Many dog guides begin their training in the homes of children who are raising the dogs as 4-H projects.

Frequency In acoustics, the number of vibrations, repetitions of compressions, and rarefactions of a sound wave that occur at the same rate over a period, generally one second, and psychologically perceived as pitch.

Fresnel prisms A series of plastic prisms applied to regular eyeglass lenses that are used to correct eye deviations or to displace peripheral information onto areas of the retina.

Frontal plane Theoretical division of the body into front and back halves.

Functional mobility limitation The interaction between one's personal abilities, and the environmental demands of travel. As the environmental demand increases, the potential for functional mobility limitations also increases. This interaction may be mediated or modified through an intervention to reduce environmental demand, to provide the traveler with the skills needed to deal with the environment, or to both.

Gait A person's pattern of walking.

Geographic information system (GIS) An electronic database consisting of an atlas of geographic information, such as streets and landmarks.

Gestalt A term derived from German that means configuration or organization. In cognitive learning theory, it defines the world into meaningful wholes rather than isolated stimuli. In other words, the whole is greater than the sum of its parts.

Glare An annoying sensation produced by too much light in the visual field that can cause both discomfort and a reduction in visual acuity.

Glaucoma A condition characterized by an increase in intraocular pressure, visually associated with a buildup of aqueous fluid, that may cause damage to the the optic nerve and eventual visual field defects if left untreated.

Global positioning system (GPS) An electronic position-sensing technology based on orbiting satellites which communicate with portable transmitters and receivers that, in interaction with a geographic information system, can inform users of their exact location and relationship to landmarks or coordinates.

Glucose A simple sugar, present in blood and other tissues, which serves as the major source of immediate fuel for the cells in the body.

Gross motor milestones Gross motor skills such as sitting, crawling, and walking that generally appear at specific points in the course of motor development.

Guided learning A more regimented and passive teaching strategy in which the same type of solutions are needed to solve similar problems.

Handling The skill of working with an individual dog guide in such a way that it gives the best possible result, maximizing the individual dog's strengths while minimizing its weaknesses.

Haptic perception The ability to identify objects by size, shape, and feel.

Hearing impairment A departure from normal hearing sensitivity.

Heel strike The contact of the heel with the ground as the foot steps down.

Hemianopsia Blindness in one half of the field of vision in one or both eyes.

Hemiplegia Paralysis on one side (either left or right) of the body.

High guard The position in which the arms are held with hands between shoulder and head height to facilitate balance when standing and walking.

HIV (human immunodeficiency virus) A virus that selectively attacks and destroys cells of the body's immune system, leaving the infected person without the body's defenses against infections. *See also* AIDS

Hyperopia (farsightedness) A refractive error caused by an eyeball that is too short; corrected with a convex (plus) lens.

Hypoglycemia Low blood glucose level; insulin "reaction," insulin shock; may occur with or without observable clinical symptoms.

Hypotonia Low muscle tone.

Immittance tests Tympanometry and acoustic reflex tests that require no behavioral response from the subject.

Independent movement The act of moving through the environment in a safe and efficient manner.

Individualized Education Program (IEP) A written plan of instruction by an educational team for a child who receives special education services that includes the student's present levels of educational performance, annual goals, short-term objectives, specific services needed, duration of services, evaluation, and related information. Under the Individuals with Disabilities Education Act (IDEA), each student receiving special services must have such a plan.

Individualized Written Rehabilitation Plan (IWRP) A plan developed to meet the specialized rehabilitation needs of an individual (21 years of age or older).

Individualized Transition Plan (ITP) A written plan developed by an educational team to establish specific transition goals and to identify instructional objectives that support a student's postschool goals, primarily community living and integrated employment. A requirement of the Individuals with Disabilities Education Act (IDEA).

Information point Two or more features of a travel environment that by themselves do not convey specific information about one's location in space, but when juxtaposed permit traveler's to locate themselves relative to their surroundings For example, the fire hydrant next to the newspaper box specifies a particular location on a block that has several fire hydrants and newspaper boxes.

Infrasonic Sounds below the normal hearing range for frequency (below 20 Hz).

Inner ear The innermost portion of the ear, which is embedded in the petrous portion of the temporal bone and contains the cochlea, which houses the sensory receptors for hearing, and the utricle, saccule, and semicircular canals, which house the receptors for balance.

Insulin The hormone secreted by the cells of the pancreas. Required by most tissues in order to utilize glucose for energy.

Intelligent disobedience A dog guide's actions when it disobeys its handler's command because obedience would put handler and dog at risk. Especially refers to traffic work.

Intensity The amplitude of particle vibration that is psychologically perceived as loudness.

Interdisciplinary team model A team approach in which professionals from different disciplines undertake independent assessments of a student but carry out program development as a collective effort.

Intermittent claudication A medical condition characterized by an inability of the circulatory system to pump sufficient blood (into the legs, for example) to the muscles during exercise.

Internal locus of control A person's tendency to consider reinforcements or punishments received as resulting from his or her own efforts.

In-the-canal (ITC) hearing aid A personal amplification system that is located mostly or entirely within the external ear canal.

In-the-ear (ITE) hearing aid A personal amplification system that fits into the ear canal and the concha.

Juno walk (harness) A term used by many dog guide schools to refer to a walk with an instructor simulating a dog's work while holding and pulling a harness or a harness handle. Used to teach basic techniques and to assess a student's or applicant's needs and abilities before accepting an applicant into a dog guide program or matching the applicant with a dog.

Keratoconus A hereditary degenerative disease that is manifest in adolescence or later, in which the cornea thins and becomes cone shaped and vision is reduced.

Ketoacidosis (ketosis) An acute metabolic state that can occur in diabetes when blood levels of insulin are inadequate. Toxic acids accumulate in the blood, ketones appear in the urine, and dehydration occurs. If untreated, it can result in coma and death.

Ketone A toxic product produced in the liver from fats if glucose cannot enter the cells; occurs when insulin levels are inadequate.

Kinesiology The study of movement.

Kinesthesia The awareness of movement that results from the interaction of tactile, proprioceptive, and vestibular inputs.

Kinetic labyrinth The portion of the vestibular system that registers the direction of head movement.

Landmark, primary An environmental feature that is detectable to visually impaired travelers, that is always present, and that is not likely to be missed as one travels a route.

Landmark, secondary Any environmental that is intermittent or that may not be encountered by travelers as they travel a route. Examples are a fan in a water fountain or an object on the sidewalk opposite to the traveler.

Laterality The complete motor awareness of both sides of the body; the recognition of right and left (i.e., from an egocentric perspective).

Layout The distances and directions that relate objects to each other in one's environment.

Learned helplessness A psychological state that results when an individual perceives that events in his or her environment are uncontrollable.

Legal blindness Term used to define conditions that make individuals eligible for government and agency benefits and services. An individual who is legally blind has a visual acuity of 20/200 or less in the better eye with the best correction or a visual field of no more than 20 degrees.

Lens The part of the eye that changes shape to adjust the focus of images from various distances into a sharp image on the retina.

Levels of processing theory The concept that the more thoroughly one can process information, the more likely it is that one can move the information from short-term to long-term memory.

Licensure The granting of permission by a state governmental agency to allow an individual sole authority to engage in practice in a specific arena.

Localization The ability to orient oneself to the environment through the use of the sense of hearing; the determination of the direction of a sound source.

Localization error A mistake in judging the or direction to an environmental feature or event.

Locomotor skills Abilities, such as creeping, crawling, and walking, that are used to move in the environment.

Locus of control A characteristic way in which a person views the source of the events or outcomes she experiences.

Long arch The arch of the foot formed by the ligaments that run from the heel to the base of the toes.

Long-range goals The measure of performance to be obtained by the end of the educational or rehabilitation program.

Low guard The position in which the arms are held with hands at the sides and close to the hips, in order to facilitate balance when standing and walking.

Low vision A visual impairment even with best correction, but with the potential for use of available vision, with or without optical or nonoptical compensatory visual strategies, devices, and environmental modifications.

Lumbar lordosis The posterior curvature of the lower spine resulting in a swayed back.

Macular degeneration A progressive loss of central vision caused by a degeneration of the retinal cones.

Magnifiers Devices that increase the size of an image through the use of lenses or lens systems.

Map Two-dimensional visual, tactile, or tactile-visual representation of spatial layout having information perceptible to vision, touch, or both.

Medium guard The position in which the arms are held with hands between waist and shoulder height in order to facilitate balance when standing and walking.

Middle ear The portion of the ear extending inward from the tympanic membrane (the eardrum); an air-filled cavity containing three ossicles, their attachments, and the eustachian tube.

Mixed hearing loss A hearing impairment that results from both a conductive and a sensorineural problem in the same auditory system.

Mobility The act or ability to move from one's present position to one's desired position in another part of the environment safely, gracefully, and comfortably. *See also* Orientation

Mobility coverage The scope or range of environmental preview information provided to the traveler about the path of travel.

Mobility systems Canes, electronic devices, and dog guides that serve as extensions of a person's senses to help the individual determine obstacles and changes in the terrain of the path of travel.

Mobility techniques A set of specific skills and strategies, developed for persons who are visually impaired or deaf-blind or who have additional impairments, that help individuals remain safe while traveling.

Model Three-dimensional representation of an object or spatial layout.

Motivation A factor or group of factors which is thought to influence behavior.

Motor output The movement of one or more body parts

Multidisciplinary team model A team approach in which several professionals from different disciplines work independently to conduct assessments of a student, write and implement separate program plans, and evaluate the student's progress with the parameters of their own disciplines.

Muscle tone The underlying neurological activity in the muscles that provides motor readiness for movement.

Myopia (nearsightedness) A refractive error resulting from an eyeball that is too long; corrected with a concave (minus) lens.

NAC (National Accreditation Council) for Agencies Serving the Blind and Visually Handicapped The accrediting body for agencies serving people who are blind and visually impaired.

Negative punishment In behavioral learning theory, the removal of a valued or prized stimulus to weaken the occurrence of a particular behavior.

Negative reinforcement In behavior learning theory, the strengthening of a behavior by the removal of an aversive stimulus.

Nephropathy Degeneration of the small blood vessels in the kidney that seriously compromises kidney function.

Neurological impairment A medical condition that affects the brain, spinal cord, or peripheral nerves.

Neuropathy A loss of the myelin coating from peripheral nerves that results in reduced functioning. Symptoms vary depending upon which nerves are involved, but can include numbness or pain in the extremities, impotence, or poor bladder control.

New psychological situation A situation in which the location of positive goals and the path by which they can be reached are not clearly perceived by an individual.

Night blindness A condition in which visual acuity is diminished at night and in dim light.

Numbering systems A systematic use of numbers to identify buildings or rooms within a building.

Nystagmus An involuntary oscillation of the eyes, usually rhythmical and in one direction; may be side to side or up and down.

Object concept The knowledge that objects have mass and occupy space; the knowledge of classes of objects and of their physical and functional properties.

Object preview The detection of objects in one's path of travel.

Object-to-object spatial relationships The spatial relationship between objects or places that do not change with self-movement.

Occupational therapist A trained professional who specializes in infant gross motor development and in the development and functioning of fine motor skills.

Operant conditioning A category of behavioral learning theory that involves the use of pleasant and unpleasant consequences to change behavior. It is based on the premise that if an act is followed by a satisfying change in the environment, the likelihood that the act will be repeated in similar situations is reinforced or increased. *See also* Behavioral learning theory

Ophthalmologist A physician who specializes in the medical and surgical care of the eyes and is qualified to prescribe ocular medications and to perform surgery on the eyes. May also perform refractive and low vision work, including eye care examinations and other vision services.

Opportunistic infections Infections that are potentially life threatening to a persons with compromised immune systems.

Optic atrophy The degeneration or malfunction of the optic nerve, characterized by a pale optic disk.

Optometrist A health care provider who specializes in refractive errors, prescribes eyeglasses or contact lenses, and diagnoses and manages conditions of the eye as regulated by state laws. May also perform low vision examinations.

Orientation The knowledge of one's distance and direction relative to things observed or remembered in the surroundings and keeping track of these spatial relationships as they change during locomotion. *See also* Mobility; Orientation.

Orientation and mobility (O&M) The field dealing with systematic techniques by which blind and visually impaired persons orient themselves to their environments and move about independently. *See also* Mobility; Orientation

Orientation and mobility (O&M) assistants Paraprofessionals who are trained and certified to practice specified skills under the direction of orientation and mobility specialists.

Orientation and mobility (O&M) specialist A professional who specializes in teaching travel skills to visually impaired persons, including the use of canes, dog guides, or sophisticated electronic traveling aids, as well as the sighted guide technique.

Orienteering An activity in which the participants use a map and possibly a compass to plan and execute the most efficient route between controls (checkpoints) on an unfamiliar course.

Orthopedic impairment A medical condition that affects the bones, muscles, and joints

Osteoarthritis A medical condition characterized by pain in and damage to joints.

Otoacoustic emissions (OAEs) tests A procedure for measuring sounds in the external ear canal that are generated by movement of the outer hair cells in the cochlea and transmitted through the middle ear.

Outcome expectations A person's assessment of the likelihood that a particular behavior will produce a particular outcome.

Outcomes Observable, measurable goals.

Outer ear Outermost portion of the ear containing the pinna and the ear canal and separated from the middle ear by the tympanic membrane.

Out-toeing The outward turning of the feet away from the direction of travel when walking.

Overlearning In behavioral learning theory, for example a raising of the criteria needed to learn a skill. Instead of expecting a skill to be learned if an individual does it correctly five times, the instructor expects learning to be achieved if the individual does it correctly ten times.

Paratransit services Door-to-door transportation services available in some cities to the elderly or people with impairments.

Passing Behavior by a person designed to conceal a salient aspect of that individual's identity.

Path integration The tracking of self-to-object spatial relationships over the space and time of one's movements

Pedal guards Small rims on the edges of wheelchair pedals that protect the toes from contact with objects.

Perception In psychology, the way in which a person interprets and organizes stimuli. The ability to obtain information about the characteristics, identity, and location of objects and events by looking, listening, touching, and using other forms of active, direct observation.

Perceptual-motor coordination To harmonize the forces and directions of one's actions with the perceived sizes, distances, and directions of the things in one's surroundings.

Performance criteria The standard used to determine if a short-term goal has been accomplished.

Perimeter, gridline, reference point Strategies for systematic exploration of a space in order to acquire spatial information.

Peripheral auditory system The outer ear, middle ear, inner ear, and the auditory or cochlear portion of the cranial nerve (CN VIII).

Peripheral nervous system (PNS) The portion of the nervous system consisting of the nerves that leave the spinal cord and travel to the distant parts of the body.

Peripheral vision The perception of objects, motion, or color outside the direct line of vision or by other than the central retina.

Pes planus Flat feet.

Pfui Correction word used by some dog guide schools.

Phase The position of a particle within its vibratory cycle or the position of pressure change that occurs within a complete cycle of a sound wave.

Physical therapist A professional who specializes in the development and functioning of gross motor skills.

Polarcentric orientation The use of compass directions, such as north, southeast, and west, that are based on the location of the North Pole.

Polio Viral condition affecting the spinal cord that results in partial or full paralysis of affected body parts.

Procedural knowledge Information about the correct way in which to accomplish things and where to do them.

Positive punishment In behavioral learning theory, the use of an aversive stimulus to weaken behavior.

Positive reinforcement In behavioral learning theory, the use of the environment as a stimulus to strengthen a behavior.

Postural sway The movement of the body when standing (or upper body when sitting) in a "figure-8" pattern at the head in order to compensate for ongoing subtle changes in the alignment of body parts over the body's center of gravity.

Posture The vertical alignment of body parts over the body's center of gravity.

Preferred visual field The location (in space) at which an individual seems to notice the most objects in the environment.

Primary reinforcers In classical conditioning, the use of innately pleasurable stimuli, such as food and water, to reinforce a behavior.

Procedural memory The ability to recall how to do something, particularly a physical task.

Profession A field of practice developed around a specific body of specialized knowledge and practiced by persons educated in its application.

Proprioception The sense, or perception, of the relative positions and movements of parts of the body, independent of vision. *See also* Kinesthesia

Prosthesis An artificial substitute for a diseased or missing body part.

Psychoanalytic theory A system of concepts first advanced by Sigmund Freud which holds that behavior is largely determined by unconscious forces that trace their source to early developmental experiences.

Punisher In behavioral learning theory, a consequence that reduces a specific behavior.

Rarefaction An area of reduced density and pressure in a sound carrying medium.

Reactions The mature movement patterns that develop in infancy and support coordinated movement throughout life.

Reciprocal arm swing The normal forward and backward movement of the arms (concurrent with the movement of the opposite leg) when walking.

Reciprocal determininsm *See* Social cognitive theory

Reflection A sound energy bouncing off a baffle, thereby changing its direction and perhaps its phase.

Reflexes The primitive movement patterns present in infants that support early movement.

Reflexive actions Action responses to certain specific sets of external conditions. They are designed to occur automatically whenever a person encounters a particular set of circumstances.

Refraction A change in the direction of sound wave propagation because of a change in speed while passing from one medium through another.

Refractive errors Conditions such as myopia, hyperopia, and astigmatism caused by corneal irregularities, in which parallel rays of light are not brought to a focus on the retina because of a defect in the shape of the eyeball or the refractive media of the eye.

Reinforcer In behavioral learning theory, any consequence that strengthens or increases the frequency of a behavior.

Replacement (student) A student returning for a second or subsequent dog guide.

Retinal detachment The separation of the retina from the underlying choroid, nearly always caused by a retinal tear. It usually requires surgical intervention to prevent loss of vision.

Retinitis pigmentosa A group of progressive, often hereditary, retinal degenerative diseases that are characterized by decreasing peripheral vision; some progress to tunnel vision, whereas others result in total blindness if the macula also becomes involved.

Retinopathy of prematurity A series of retinal changes, from mild to total retinal detachment, seen primarily in premature infants. Believed to be connected to the immature blood vessels in the eye and their reaction to oxygen, but may be primarily the result of prematurity with very low birthweight. Functional vision can range from near normal to total blindness.

Retrocochlear hearing loss A hearing impairment resulting from a pathology beyond the cochlea.

Rheumatoid arthritis A medical condition characterized by pain and damage of joints.

RoboCane A computer software program that models an individual's gait, cane position, and movement. The program provides a three-dimensional analysis of the obstacle preview of the cane coverage.

Rote travel Travel characterized by movement from one landmark to another along a known path with little knowledge of the spatial relationships of the landmarks to one another and little flexibility in the route traveled from one location to another.

Safe stranger A person, such as police, bus drivers, bank tellers, who is easily identified by a uniform or name tag as belonging to a non-threatening group.

Safety or efficiency trade-off A decision in which safety is compromised to enhance efficiency or in which efficiency is compromised to enhance safety.

Sagittal plane The theoretical division of the body into left and right halves.

Scale A term that expresses the relationship between the size of an area mapped and the size of the map.

Scanning The systematic use of head and eye movement to search for targets.

Schemes In cognitive learning theory, a network of connected facts and concepts.

Scoliosis Sideways curvature of the spine.

Scotoma A gap or blindspot in the visual field that may be caused by damage to the retina or visual pathways. Each eye contains one normal blind spot, corresponding to the location of the optic nerve head, which contains no photoreceptors.

Secondary reinforcers In classical conditioning, a reinforcers so closely associated with primary reinforcers that an individual will be motivated to act based on receiving the secondary reinforcer itself.

Self-concept The collection of thoughts and feelings one has about oneself.

Self-efficacy A person's judgments of his or her capability to organize and execute courses of action required to attain designated types of performances.

Self-esteem The affective dimensions of one's self-concept.

Self-initiated movement Movement initiated in the absence of encouragement or other intervention from another person.

Self-to-object spatial relationships The spatial relationships between a traveler and objects in the surroundings that change predictably with self-movement.

Semantic memory A person's ability to mentally organize concepts and facts into networks of connected ideas or relationships called schemes. Each person stores these schemes in different ways.

Sensation In psychology, the way in which information is actually received by the sensory apparatus.

Sensorineural hearing loss A hearing impairment resulting from a dysfunction somewhere within the inner ear or beyond.

Sensory input Sensory information received from the environment.

Sensory-motor phase Piaget's first stage of intelligence, in which knowledge is tied to the content of specific sensory input or motor actions.

Sensory receptors Receptors located in the skin, muscles, and joints that receive sensory information, which is then sent to the brain through the peripheral nerves and spinal cord.

Shaping behaviors In behavioral learning theory, the molding of a behavior so that it gradually comes to approximate the desired end state.

Short-term objectives Specified measurable outcomes along the way to achieving a long-range goal.

Signal-detection theory The principles by which to understand and characterize errors made during detection judgments.

Signal-processing hearing aid An amplification system that produces output different from its input.

Skill A proficiency or mastery in the performance of some task, as, for example, reading a map using a mobility aid or using the long cane.

Snellen chart A chart used for testing central visual acuity, usually at distances of 20 feet, that consists of lines of letters, numbers, or symbols in graded sizes down to specific measurements. Each size is labeled with the distance at which it can be read by the normal eye.

Social cognitive theory Concepts advanced by Bandura contending that a personality develops through a process of reciprocal determinism, which refers to the continuous interaction of personal and environmental factors and the person's own behavior.

Social reinforcers In classical conditioning, one type of secondary reinforcer that includes praise, approval of others, and personal attention.

Sound A series of disturbances in the density of particles in an elastic medium.

Sound field A space where sound waves are present.

Sound level meter An instrument used to measure sound pressure levels.

Spatial concept The understanding of the spatial location of two or more objects relative to one another, using, for example, such prepositions as over, under, and behind; right and left; North, South, East, and West.

Spatial orientation The process of establishing and maintaining one's position in space relative to objects that cannot be perceived directly, and the process of learning the spatial relationships among objects in a place.

Spatial updating The process of keeping track of the effect of self-movement on spatial relationships to objects that cannot be perceived directly.

Speech recognition threshold The lowest level at which 50 percent of two-syllable words can be recognized; the lowest level at which one can just start to understand speech.

Spina bifida A medical condition leading to partial or full paralysis of the lower body caused by incomplete formation of the spine.

Spotting A procedure by which one monitors the movement of another, in readiness to assist if balance is lost.

State anxiety A transitory experience of unpleasant, consciously perceived feelings of tension and apprehension.

Static balance The ability to maintain a static posture such as sitting or standing.

Static utricle The portion of the vestibular system that signals the position of the head in space, responding to sudden tilting movements of the head as well as to linear acceleration and deceleration.

Static visual acuity The ability to discriminate and identify a variety of stationary targets when the viewer is stationary.

Static visual field The ability to describe the outermost objects seen in the stationary field of vision; the outer boundaries of the visual field.

Stereotypes Repetitive movement patterns.

Stigma A label or behavior that indicates some deviation from a norm or standard.

Strategy An ingenious plan or method or effective way of producing a result.

Stride length The distance between successive steps of the same foot.

Stride width The distance between the feet in a plane perpendicular to the line of travel.

Subway gap The narrow space between a subway car and the platform.

Support cane An ambulatory aid, made of wood or aluminum, that consists of a single vertical post with a handgrip at hip height. The cane may have a single point of contact on the ground or may have a base consisting of three or four small legs.

Suprathreshold speech recognition test A procedure for assessing the functional ability to hear and understand speech.

Surface preview The detection of changes in the surface to be traveled, most notably those associated with changes in the plane itself, such as stairs or curbs, and texture (e.g., rough or smooth).

Systematic desensitization A therapeutic use of conditioning principles to help a person learn to cope with extreme anxiety or fear.

Tactile map A map on which information is perceptible to touch.

Tangent screen A technique for plotting visual field within 30 degrees of fixation.

Task analysis In behavioral learning theory, the careful breakdown of the desired terminal behavior into sufficiently small subtasks so that each increment in performance toward the final goal is readily achievable.

Telemicroscope A lens system in which an adaptation called a reading cap is used on a telescope to provide additional plus lens power to an existing system, transforming the telescope into a viewing device for intermediate distances.

Telescope A lens system that makes small objects appear closer and larger.

Tendons The fibrous bands that attach to the bones on each side of a joint.

Third-party reimbursement Payment for services from recognized payers such as Medicare, Medicaid, HMOs, and private insurance companies

Token reinforcers In classical conditioning, one type of secondary reinforcer that might include money, grades, or passes to go out at night or on weekends.

Topocentric orientation The individual's ability to relate his or her position and the position of other aspects of the environment to an identifiable landmark.

Touch technique (two-point touch technique) A specific cane technique used by travelers with visual impairments in outdoor and unfamiliar indoor areas. The cane is swung from side by side, low to the ground, touching down at each end of the arc.

Tracing Visually following single or multiple stationary lines in the environment, such as hedge lines, roof lines, or baseboards.

Tracking Visually following a moving object.

Trait anxiety A stable disposition to experience anxiety frequently and intensely in response to a wide range of situations.

Transdisciplinary team model A team approach in which professionals from different disciplines cooperate and collaborate during initial assessment and planning phases of designing a student's educational program and offer ongoing support and input.

Transfer Moving from one support surface (e.g. a wheelchair) to another (e.g., a car seat).

Transverse arch The arch of the foot formed by the ligaments running from the instep to the outside edge of the foot.

Transverse plane The theoretical division of the body into top and bottom halves.

Ultrasonic Sounds above the normal hearing range for frequency (above 20,000 Hz).

Unconditioned response A reflexive action that results from a biological predisposition, such as salivation caused by the smell of food.

Unfamiliar environment Any indoor or outdoor physical setting to which the student has never been exposed.

Unit One way of referring to a dog guide team.

Universal design Architectural design having the goal that all elements should be accessible to (or adaptable for the use of) all persons, including those with impairments.

Universal precautions Steps that human service providers take to prevent the spread of infection.

University personnel preparation standards Standards that are used by AER to approve programs that prepare orientation and mobility (O&M) specialists.

Variable interval ratio In behavioral learning theory, a schedule of reinforcement in which the reinforcement is not always available and the person being reinforced has no idea when such reinforcement will occur; the reinforcement averages out to a certain time for each correct behavior.

Variable ratio In behavioral learning theory, a schedule of reinforcement in which the number of behaviors required for reinforcement is unpredictable, although it is certain that the behavior will eventually be reinforced and that rate of reinforcement will average out to a certain number for a specific number of correct behaviors.

Verbal aid Spoken or written descriptions of spatial layouts and routes of travel.

Vestibular system The portion of the inner ear that provides feedback about the rotary acceleration, linear acceleration, and tilt of the head

Visual acuity The sharpness of vision with respect to the ability to distinguish detail, often measured as the eye's ability to distinguish the details and shapes of objects at a designated distance; involves central (macular) vision.

Visual field The area that can be seen when looking straight ahead, measured in degrees from the fixation point. Also called Field of vision.

Visual contrast The difference in the amount of light reflected from one region of space to the next.

Walker An ambulatory aid, generally made of aluminum, that consists of four tall legs and a horizontal frame, often U-shaped, at the top.

Wayfinding The act of moving through the environment with purpose (e.g., to reach a destination).

RESOURCES

This resource guide is intended as a starting point for orientation and mobility professionals who are seeking information for themselves and their clients on pertinent government agencies, national organizations that provide information, consumer education materials, services, and referrals to services for blind and visually impaired individuals. Professional organizations of interest to orientation and mobility specialists are also included here. The American Foundation for the Blind (AFB) acts as a national clearinghouse for information about blindness and visual impairment, operates a toll-free national hotline, and is a source of additional information. The National Technology Center at AFB ([212] 502-7642) is a repository of information about assistive technology.

An essential part of working with blind or visually impaired individuals is providing information about a wide variety of products and services they may require. An extensive listing of sources of products and services may be found in the *Directory of Services for Blind and Visually Impaired Persons in the United States and Canada,* published by AFB Press. The *Directory* also has a listing of university programs in various states offering training in the area of orientation and mobility. Some classic reference works in the field of orientation and mobility that readers may wish to consult include *Foundations of Orientation and Mobility,* edited by Richard L. Welsh and Bruce B. Blasch, *Orientation and Mobility Techniques: A Guide for Practitioners,* by Everett W. Hill and Purvis Ponder, and *The Art and Science of Teaching Orientation and Mobility to Persons with Visual Impairments,* by William H. Jacobson, which are available from AFB Press, and *Orientation and Mobility: Techniques for Independence,* by S.J. LaGrow and M. Weessies, available from Division Nine of the Association for Education and Rehabilitation of the Blind and Visually Impaired (see the listing that follows). Readers should note that the organizations and sources of products and services listed have been included here for resource purposes only, and inclusion does not constitute an endorsement of any kind.

American Council of the Blind
1155 15th Street, N.W., Suite 720
Washington, DC 20005
(202) 467-5081 or (800) 424-8666
FAX: (202) 467-5085
E-mail: ncrabb@access.digex.net
URL: http://www.access.digex.net
Promotes effective participation of blind people in all aspects of society. Provides information and referral, legal assistance, scholarships, advocacy, consultation, and program development assistance. Interest groups include the Deaf-Blind Committee and the Council of Citizens with Low Vision International. Publishes *The Braille Forum.*

American Foundation for the Blind
11 Penn Plaza, Suite 300
New York, NY 10001
(212) 502-7600 or (800) 232-5463
TTY/TDD: (212) 502-7662
FAX: (212) 502-7777
E-mail: newyork@afb.org
URL: http://www.afb.org
Provides services to and acts as an information clearinghouse for people who are blind or visually impaired and their families, professionals, organizations, schools, and corporations. Stimulates research and mounts program initiatives to improve services to visually impaired persons; advocates for services and legislation; maintains the M. C. Migel Library and Information Center and the Helen Keller Archives; provides information and referral services; operates the National Technology Center and the Career and Technology Information Bank; produces videos and publishes books, pamphlets, the *Directory of Services for Blind and Visually Impaired Persons in the United States and Canada,* and the *Journal of Visual Impairment & Blindness.* Maintains the following offices throughout the country in addition to the headquarters' office:

AFB Midwest
401 N. Michigan Avenue, Suite 308
Chicago, IL 60611
(312) 245-9961
FAX: (312) 245-9965
E-mail: chicago@afb.org

AFB Southeast
National Initiative on Literacy
100 Peachtree Street, Suite 620
Atlanta, GA 30303
(404) 525-2303
FAX: (404) 659-6957
E-mail: atlanta@afb.org
E-mail: blmit@afb.org

AFB Southwest
260 Treadway Plaza
Exchange Park
Dallas, TX 75235
(214) 352-7222
FAX: (214) 352-3214
E-mail: afbdallas@afb.org

AFB West
111 Pine Street, Suite 725
San Francisco, CA 94111
(415) 392-4845
FAX: (415) 392-0383
E-mail: sanfran@afb.org

Governmental Relations Group
820 First Street, N.E., Suite 400
Washington, DC 20002
(202) 408-0200
FAX: (202) 289-7880
E-mail: afbgov@afb.org

American Printing House for the Blind
1839 Frankfort Avenue
Louisville, KY 40206-0085
(502) 895-2405 or (800) 223-1839
FAX: (502) 899-2274
E-mail: info@aph.org
URL: http://www.aph.org
Administers an annual appropriation from Congress to provide textbooks and educational aids for legally blind students. Also produces materials in braille and large print and on audiocassette; manufactures computer-access equipment, software, and special education devices for visually impaired persons; and maintains an educational research and development program and a reference-catalog service.

Association for Education and Rehabilitation of the Blind and Visually Impaired
4600 Duke Street, Suite 430
Alexandria, VA 22304
(703) 823-9690
FAX: (703) 823-9695
E-mail: aernet@laser.net
Promotes all phases of education and work for people of all ages who are blind and visually impaired, strives to expand their opportunities to take a contributory place in society, and disseminates information. Certifies rehabilitation teachers, orientation and mobility specialists, and classroom teachers. Subgroups include Division Nine, Orientation and Mobility. Publishes *RE:view, AER Report, Job Exchange Monthly,* and *RT News,* a quarterly newsletter.

Blinded Veterans Association
477 H Street, N.W.
Washington, DC 20001-2694
(202) 371-8880 or (800) 669-7079
FAX: (202) 371-8258
Encourages and assists all blind veterans to take advantage of rehabilitation and vocational training benefits, job placement assistance, and other aid from federal, state, and local resources by means of a field service program. Promotes extension of sound legislation and rehabilitation through liaison with other agencies. Through 48 regional groups and field service offices, operates a volunteer service program for blinded veterans in their communities and provides information and referral services.

Canadian National Institute for the Blind
1929 Bayview Avenue
Toronto, ON M4G 3E8, Canada
(416) 480-7580
FAX: (416) 480-7677
E-mail: natgovernment@east.cnib.ca
URL: http://www.cnib.ca
Provides services to people who are blind or visually impaired through a network of divisional offices throughout Canada.

Council for Exceptional Children
Division of the Visually Impaired
1920 Association Drive
Reston, VA 22091-1589
(703) 620-3660 or (800) 328-0272
TTY/TDD: (703) 620-3660
FAX: (703) 264-9494
Acts as a professional organization for individuals serving children with disabilities and children who are gifted. Is the largest such international organization, with 17 specialized divisions. Primary activities include advocating for appropriate government policies; setting professional standards; providing continuing professional development; and helping professionals obtain conditions and resources necessary for effective professional practice. Publishes numerous related materials, journals, and newsletters.

Council of U.S. Guide Dog Schools
c/o Guiding Eyes for the Blind
611 Granite Springs Road
Yorktown Heights, NY 10598
(914) 245-4024
Provides consultation on dog guide schools.

Helen Keller International
90 Washington Street, 15th Floor
New York, NY 10006
(212) 943-0890
Provides consultation and assistance to developing nations to help them establish programs to prevent blindness and to educate and rehabilitate blind children and adults.

Helen Keller National Center for Deaf-Blind Youths and Adults
111 Middle Neck Road
Sands Point, NY 11050
(516) 944-8900 (voice/TDD)
FAX: (516) 944-7302
Provides technical assistance to facilitate the transition of deaf-blind youths from educational services to community-based adult services.

National Accreditation Council for Agencies Serving the Blind and Visually Handicapped
260 Northland Boulevard, Suite 236
Cincinnati, OH 45246
(212) 683-5068 (Will change after 10/1/97)
FAX: (212) 683-4475
Provides a national process for the development and updating of standards for agencies, schools, and programs serving people with visual impairments. Also develops and implements an accreditation program based on those standards.

National Association for Parents of the Visually Impaired
P.O. Box 317
Watertown, MA 02272-0317
(800) 562-6265
FAX: (617) 972-7444
Provides support to parents and families of children and youths who have visual impairments. Operates a national clearinghouse for information, education, and referral. Publishes a newsletter *Awareness.*

National Federation of the Blind

1800 Johnson Street
Baltimore, MD 21230
(410) 659-9314
FAX: (410) 685-5683
URL: http://www.nfb.org
Strives to improve social and economic conditions of blind persons, evaluates and assists in establishing programs, and provides public education and scholarships. Interest groups include the Committee on the Concerns of the Deaf-Blind. Publishes *The Braille Monitor* and *Future Reflections.*

National Rehabilitation Association
633 Washington Street
Alexandria, VA 22314
(703) 836-0850
TTY/TDD: (703) 836-0849
FAX: (703) 836-0848
Serves as a membership organization for professionals in the field of rehabilitation and as an advocate for the rights of persons with disabilities. Publishes the *Journal of Rehabilitation* and *Contemporary Rehab.*

Royal National Institute for the Blind
Technical Development Department
224 Great Portland Street
London W1N 6AA
England
44-21-643-9912
Conducts research, publishes directories of international research in blindness, and supplies equipment for persons with visual impairments to an international market.

U.S. Department of Education
330 C Street, S.W.
Washington, DC 20202
(202) 205-9316
Administers a wide variety of programs and procedures relating to people who are blind or visually impaired. The Office of Special Education and Rehabilitative Services (OSERS), (202) 205-5465, oversees federal personnel preparation programs and special education policies. The Office of Special Education Programs, (202) 205-5507, administers the Individuals with Disabilities Education Act and related programs for the education of children with disabilities. The Rehabilitation Services Administration (RSA), (202) 205-5482, administers grants and oversees programs related to the vocational rehabilitation of blind and visually impaired persons.

U.S. Department of Veterans Affairs
Blind Rehabilitation Service
810 Vermont Avenue, N.W.
Washington, DC 20420
(202) 535-7637
Provides a wide variety of services, including orientation and mobility instruction, to blinded U.S. military veterans.

INDEX